Community Child Health and Paediatrics

Edited by

David Harvey FRCP, DCH
Senior Lecturer in Paediatrics and Chairman, Department of Paediatrics and Neonatal Medicine, Royal Postgraduate Medical School, Hammersmith Hospital, London

Marion Miles FRCP, DCH
Consultant Community Paediatrician and Honorary Senior Lecturer, St Mary's Hospital and Medical School, London

and

Diane Smyth MD, FRCP, DCH
Consultant Community Paediatrician and Honorary Senior Lecturer, St Mary's Hospital and Medical School, London

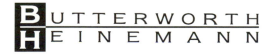

BUTTERWORTH
HEINEMANN

Butterworth-Heinemann Ltd
Linacre House, Jordan Hill, Oxford OX2 8DP

℟ A member of the Reed Elsevier plc group

OXFORD LONDON BOSTON
MUNICH NEW DELHI SINGAPORE SYDNEY
TOKYO TORONTO WELLINGTON

First published 1995

© Butterworth-Heinemann Ltd 1995

British Library Cataloguing in Publication Data
Community Child Health and Paediatrics
  I. Harvey, David
  618.92

ISBN 0 7506 1323 8

Library of Congress Cataloguing in Publication Data
Community child health and paediatrics/edited by David Harvey,
  Marion Miles, and Diane Smyth.
  p.   cm.
  Includes bibliographical references and index.
  ISBN 0 7506 1323 8
  1. Community health services for children.   2. Paediatrics.
  I. Harvey, David (David Robert)   II. Miles, Marion.   III. Smyth,
  Diane.
  [DNLM: 1. Child Health Services.   2. Paediatrics.   WA 320 C7346]
  RJ101.C644   94–11861
  362.1'9892–dc20   CIP

Typeset by TecSet Ltd, Wallington, Surrey
Printed and bound in Great Britain by Butler & Tanner, Frome, Somerset

Contents

Preface

It has been exciting to witness the growth and recognition of community child health over the last twenty years. As is conventional, the preface is the last section of the book to be written. It so happens this comes just after the death of Professor Donald Court who did so much to develop the speciality of community child health. We record his death with sadness. It makes us again reflect on the changes that have taken place in community child health and paediatrics since the middle 1970s when the *Court Report* was published. The committee for that report recognized the critical importance of prevention in child health, including the necessity for making this an integral part of primary health care. They also recognized the need for a speciality of paediatricians trained in developmental, educational and social paediatrics working mainly but not exclusively in the community. Although the report was in part criticized at the time, many of its proposals have since been implemented. There is increasing recognition that consultants in general paediatrics should often be responsible for children in both the hospital and community settings.

The gestation of this book has been longer than we had hoped. This has produced complications because there have been profound changes in the practice of community child health over the last few years and they are still rapidly occurring. As editors we have been very concerned this might make some terminology in the book seem out of date, but we believe the principles of care remain the same. In the local organization of care in the UK, we knew at the outset of planning this book that *area health authorities* had disappeared, but *district health authorities* have since gone the same way. Now hospitals and surrounding localities are often governed by *Trusts* and it sometimes seems that, rather than improving services by healthy friendly rivalry, they are often determined to regard other Trusts with suspicion and even hostility. Co-operation and communication between Trusts and units is also made more difficult by the frequency with which some health workers change their names from the descriptive titles with which we were more familiar.

We are grateful indeed to the contributors of this book who have responded with kindness and patience to all our queries and questions and the inevitable delays that have occurred. We are also grateful to our secretaries who have so willingly supported our efforts.

We hope this book will be a basic text for those working in community child health and general paediatrics and also prove valuable to those studying for examinations at all stages. In the past the speciality of paediatrics has often seemed too concerned with illness and hospital-based care. It is now well accepted that much of this care has moved out into the community.

Contributors

Adjaye, Nellie   MSc, MB, BS, FRCP
Consultant Community Paediatrician, Honorary
Medical Advisor, Sickle Cell Society [UK], Preston Hall
Hospital, Maidstone, Kent

Atkins, Carol   Bsc[Hons], SRD
Paediatric and Renal Dietician, St Mary's Hospital,
Paddington, London

Ayton, Margaret   MA, RGN, RHU
Assistant to the Chief Nursing Officer, Newcastle
Health Authority, Newcastle-Upon-Tyne

Bagnall, Pippa   BA, RGN
Previously Professional Head of School Nursing,
Riverside, now Director of The Queen's Nursing
Institute, London

Barnes, Pamela   Cert Ed[SKTC Dip] BAC
Chairman, Hospital Play Staff Examination Board,
formerly District Play Co-ordinator, South Manchester
Health Authority, Manchester, Lecturer in Early
Childhood Education, City College, Manchester

Bellman, Martin   MD, FRCP, DCH
Consultant Paediatrician, Camden and Islington
Community Services NHS Trust, Honorary Clinical
Senior Lecturer, University College London

Borzyskowski, Matgorzata   MB, BS, FRCP
Consultant Neurodevelopmental Paediatrician,
Newcomen Centre, Guy's Hospital, London

**Brock, Sue   DSA Cert Child Care, AIMSW,
CCETSW Award Practice Teaching, Dip NLP**
Psychotherapist in Clinical Training, Metandia Trust,
Trainee Practitioner NLP

Brook, Charles   MD, FRCP
Professor of Paediatric Endocrinology, The Middlesex
Hospital, London

Bryan, Elizabeth   MD, FRCP, DCH
Honorary Consultant Paediatrician, Director of the
Multiple Births Foundation, Queen Charlottes &
Chelsea Hospital, London

Bungay, Christine   SRP, MCSP
Superintendent Physiotherapist, Child Development
Centre, St George's Hospital, London

Chan, Michael   MBE, MD, FRCP
Senior Lecturer and Honorary. Consultant
Paediatrician, Department of Tropical Paediatric &
International Child Health, Liverpool School of
Tropical Medicine, Liverpool

Charlton, Anne   PhD, MEd, BA
Director of the Cancer Research Campaign Education
& Child Studies Research Group, Department of
Public Health & Epidemiology, University of
Manchester, Manchester

Clark, Brenda   BSc(Hons), SRD
Chief Dietician, Royal Hospital for Sick Children,
Glasgow

Cooklin, Alan   MB, ChB, FRCPsych
Consultant in Family Psychiatry, Marlborough Family
Service, Founding Director, Institute of Family
Therapy, London

Cooper Robinson, Jean   OBE, PhD, FCST
Formerly Principal of the National Hospitals College
of Speech Sciences, London

Cordeiro, Mario   MD
Consultant Community Paediatrician, Clinical
Lecturer in Child Health, Member of National Child
and Adolescent Health Committee, Lisbon, Portugal

Cullen, Deborah   BA
Secretary to the Legal Group of British Agencies for
Adoption and Fostering, London

Curtis, Hazel   MD, MRCP
Consultant Community Paediatrician, Department of Paediatrics, Torbay Hospital, Torbay

Daniels, Harry   PhD, BSc
Institute of Education, London

Davies, Bethan   MEd, MRCS, LRCP
Formerly Consultant Audiological Physician, Audiology Department, Charing Cross Hospital, London

Davies, Murray   MBA, DipASS, CQSW
Regional Director NSPCC Cymru/Wales and Midlands, Cardiff and West Bromwich

Davies, Pamela   MD, FRCP, DCH
Formerly Reader in Paediatrics, Institute of Child Health and Consultant Paediatrician, Hammersmith Hospital, London

Dawson, Neil   BSc[Hons], PGCE
Teacher and Family Therapist, Marlborough Family Service, London

de Sousa, Carlos   MD, BSc, MRCP
Consultant and Senior Lecturer, Regional Paediatric Neurology Centre, St George's Hospital, London

Dodge, John   MD, FRCP, DCH
Professor of Child Health, The Nuffield Department of Child Health, The Queen's University of Belfast, Institute of Clinical Sciences, Belfast, N Ireland

Drake, Chris   LBISt, Dip OTC
Principal Orthotist, Queen Mary's University Hospital, London

Dreifuss, Fritz   MB, FRCP, FRACP
Professor of Neurology, Department of Neurology, School of Medicine, University of Virginia Health Sciences Centre, Charlottesville, Virginia, USA

Edwards, Bridget   FRCP
Consultant Paediatrician Parkside NHS Trust and Central Middlesex Hospital NHS Trust, London

Elkan, Judith   BA, MACP
Principal Child Psychotherapist, Department of Child and Adolescent Psychiatry, St Mary's Hospital, London

Elston, John   BSc, FRCS
Consultant Ophthalmic Surgeon, Oxford Eye Hospital, Oxford

Emond, Alan   MA, MB, BChir, MD, MRCP
Consultant Community Paediatrician, Institute of Child Health, Royal Hospital for Sick Children, Bristol

Fletcher, Patrick   MSc
Educational Psychologist, Royal Borough of Kensington and Chelsea, London

Garralda, M. Elena   MD, MPhil[Psych], FRCPsych. DPM
Professor of Child and Adolescent Psychiatry, St Mary's Hospital and Medical School, University of London, Central Middlesex Hospital, London

Gillon, Raanan   BA, MB, BS, FRCP, Hon RCM
Director, Imperial College Health Service, Imperial College of Science, Technology and Medicine, London

Goodyear, Helen   MB, ChB, MRCP
Lecturer, Honorary Senior Registrar, The Hospital for Sick Children, Great Ormond Street, London

Golding, Jean
Professor of Paediatric and Perinatal Epidemiology, Institute of Child Health, University of Bristol, Bristol

Green, Stuart   MA, FRCP
Paediatric Neurologist, Senior Lecturer in Paediatrics and Child Health, Institute of Child Health, Birmingham

Harper, John   MD, MRCP
Consultant Paediatric Dermatologist, The Hospital for Sick Children, Great Ormond Street, London

Harvey, David   FRCP, DCH
Senior Lecturer in Paediatrics and Chairman, Department of Paediatrics and Neonatal Medicine, Royal Postgraduate Medical School, Hammersmith Hospital, London

Heckmatt, John
Consultant Paediatrician (Community), Bushey Health Centre, Watford

Hobbs, Chris   BS, MRCP, DobstRCOG
Consultant Community Paediatrician, St James' University Hospital, Leeds

Hogan, James   BDS, MSc, DPD
Specialist in Dental Public Health, Paddington Community Hospital, London

Hunt, David   FRCS
Consultant Orthopaedic Surgeon, St Mary's Hospital, London

Jenkins, Sue   MRCP, DCH, FRCP
Consultant Community Paediatrician, City and East London Family and Community Health Services, Department of Community Child Health, St Leonard's Hospital, and Queen Elizabeth Hospital for Sick Children, London

Kingsley, Mary   MA[Lond], BSc[Lond], Dip VH, Cert Ed. Teaching H.I. Children,
Head of Service for Children with a Visual Disability, Barnet Local Educational Authority

Kurtz, Zarrina   MSc, FFPHM
Consultant in Public Health Medicine, South Thames
Regional Health Authority and Honorary Senior
Lecturer, St. George's Hospital Medical School,
London

Kverndal (née Keating), Diana   MCSP
Formerly Superintendent Physiotherapist, Child
Development Centre, St Mary's Hospital, London

Lansdown, Richard   PhD, FBPsS, CPsychol
Consultant Psychologist, Department of Psychological
Medicine, Great Ormond Street Hospital for Children
NHS Trust, London, and Honorary Senior Lecturer,
Institute of Child Health, London

Lenton, Simon   DRCOG, FRCP
Community Paediatrician, Bath

Lessing, Daniela   MSc, MB, ChB, MRCP, DCH
Consultant Community Paediatrician, The Slough
Child Development Centre, Slough

Lethem, Jane   MPsychol, BA, AFBPS
Head Clinical Psychologist, Department of Child
Psychiatry, St Mary's Hospital, London

**Levinge, Alison   RMth, LESM(MT), currently re-
searching for a PhD**
Music Therapist, Stapleton, Bristol

Logan, Stuart   MB, ChB, MSc, MRCP
Community Paediatric Teaching Unit, Department of
Paediatric Epidemiology, Institute of Child Health,
University of London, London

Macfarlane, Aidan   FRCP
Consultant in Public Health Medicine, Oxfordshire
District Health Authority, Oxford

McKinlay, Ian   FRCP
Senior Lecturer in Community Child Health,
Department of Developmental Medicine, Salford
Health Authority, Royal Manchester Children's
Hospital, Manchester

Manzur, Adnan
Clinical Fellow, Division of Neurology, British
Columbia Children's Hospital, Vancouver, Canada

Marlow, Neil   DM, MA, MB, BS, FRCP
Consultant Senior Lecturer in Child Health [Neonatal
Medicine], St Michael's Hospital, Bristol

Mayall, Berry   PhD
Assistant Director, Social Science Research Unit,
Institute of Education, University of London, London

Miles, Marion   FRCP, DCH
Consultant Community Paediatrician and Honorary
Senior Lecturer, St Mary's Hospital and Medical
School, London

Mitchell, John   FRCP
Formerly Fellow in Health and Clinical Management,
Kings Fund College, King Edward's Hospital Fund for
London, London

Mok, Jacqueline   MD, FRCP[Ed], DCH
Consultant Paediatrician and Part-time Senior Lecturer
and Department of Community Child Health,
Edinburgh, and The Regional Infectious Disease Unit,
City Hospital, Edinburgh

Moodley, Molly
Inspector for Special Education, of the former Inner
London Education Authority, London

Nicoll, Angus   MSc, MRCP
Consultant, Public Health Laboratory Service,
Communicable Disease Surveillance Centre, London

Oates, Kim   MD, FRCP, FRACP, DCH
Douglas Burrows Professor of Paediatric and Child
Health, The University of Sydney, and Chairman,
Division of Medicine, The Children's Hospital,
Camperdown, Australia

Papadatos, Costas   MD
Professor of Pediatics [Emeritus], University of Athens,
Greece

Papadatou, Danai   PhD
Associate Professor of Psychology, School of Nursing,
University of Athens, Greece

Peers, Judith   EDT, EDH, FEATC
Head Dental Therapist, Community Unit, Wembley
Hospital, Middx

Polnay, Leon   FRCP, DCH
Reader in Child Health, Nottingham Community
Health, Nottingham

Pryce-Jones, Elizabeth MB, ChB, DCH
Formerly Principal Physician [Child Health] Merton,
Merton and Sutton District Health Authority and,
Honorary Secretary 'The Medical Officers of Schools
Association' London

Renton, Mirjana
Senior Child Psychotherapist Department of Child and
Adolescent Psychiatry, St Mary's Hospital, London

Richards, Anthony   MB, BS, FRCS
Consultant ENT Surgeon, Charing Cross Hospital,
London

Richardson, Heather   FRCP [Ed], DCH
Consultant Paediatrician, Clinical Director of
Community Child Health Services, Community and
Priority Services Unit, Thanet and Canterbury Health
Care Trust, Canterbury

Riley, Judith   DPhil, MA, MSc, Cert Ed.
Deputy Director and Fellow in Management
Education, King's Fund College, King Edward's
Hospital Fund for London, London

Roberts, Susan   Dip CST, MCST
Chief Speech Therapist, Child Development Centre,
Royal Liverpool Children's Trust, Liverpool

Rosenbloom, Lewis   MB, FRCP, DCH
Consultant Paediatric Neurologist, Royal Liverpool
Children's Trust, Liverpool

Ross, Euan   MD, FRCP, MFPHM, DCH
Professor and Head of Department, Department of
Community Paediatrics, King's College School of
Medicine & Dentistry, King's College London, London

Russell, Philippa   LLD Hon
Director, Council for Disabled Children, London

Schwartz, Ruby   MB, BS, D.Obst, RCOG, FRCP
Consultant Paediatrician, Central Middlesex Hospital,
London

Sheppard, Sarah MSc
Formerly Principal Audiological Scientist, Children's
Hearing Assessment Centre, General Hospital,
Nottingham, now Research Fellow, Department of
Experimental Psychology, University of Sussex,
Brighton

Sibert, Jo   MD, FRCP, DCH
Professor of Community Child Health, Llandough
Special Children's Centre, Penarth, South Glamorgan

Smyth, Diane   MD, FRCP, DCH
Consultant Community Paediatrician and Honorary
Senior Lecturer, St Mary's Hospital and Medical
School, London

Sonksen, Patricia   MD, D.Obst, RCOG, MRCP
Senior Lecturer in Developmental Paediatrics, The
Institute of Child Health and Honorary Consultant
Paediatrician, Great Ormond Street Hospital for
Children NHS Trust, London

Spoudeas, Helen   MB, BS, MRCP
Senior Registrar/Honorary Lecturer in Paediatric
Endocrinology, The Middlesex Hospital, London

Stanley, Fiona   MD, MSc, FFPHM
Director, Western Australian Research Institute of
Child Health, Perth, and Professor, Department of
Paediatrics, The University of Western Australia,
Nedlands, Australia

Stewart-Brown, Sarah   PhD, MFPHM, MRCP
Consultant in Public Health Medicine, Department of
Public Health Medicine, Worcester and District Health
Authority, Worcester

Taylor, Brent   PhD, MB, ChB, FRCP, FRACP
Professor of Community Child Health, The Royal Free
Hospital, London

Taylor, David   MD, MSc, FRCP, FRCPsych
Formerly Professor of Child and Adolescent
Psychiatry, University of Manchester, Manchester

Thomas, Andrew   DPhil, BA, CPsychol, AFBPsS, FSS
Qualitative Research Unit, Social and Community
Planning Research, London

Thomas, Lennox   MA CQSW
Formerly Senior Probation Officer, Associate Member
of The British Association of Psychotherapists,
London, Visiting Teacher to the Tavistock Clinic,
London, Senior Lecturer Department Psychiatry
University College, London, Clinical Director
NAFSIYAT, The Intercultural Therapy Centre, London

Thompson, Elizabeth   MD, FRACP
Formerly Consultant Clinical Geneticist, The Kennedy-
Galton Centre, Clinical Research Centre, Northwick
Park Hospital, London

Thornhill, Diana   BA, DBO[T]
Head Orthoptist, Orthoptic Department, Western
Ophthalmic Hospital, London

Touwen, Bert
Professor of Neurology, Department of Developmental
Neurology, University Hospital, Groningen, The
Netherlands

Wadland, Bryan   BA, DSA
Formerly Divisional Education Social Work Manager,
Inner London Education Authority, London

Waine, Colin OBE, FRCGP, FRC Path
Immediate Past Chairman, The Royal College of
General Practitioners, London, Director of Primary
Care, Sunderland Health Commission, Sunderland

Warren, Inga   DipCOT
Head Occupational Therapist, Children's Services,
St Mary's Hospital and Medical School, London

Watson, Joyce   MD, MFCM, MRCGP, DA, DPH
Deceased. Formerly Vice President & Medical Advisor,
The Society for the Prevention of Solvent Abuse, St
Mary's Chambers, Stone

Wharton, Brian   MBA, MD, DSc, FRCP, DCH
Director-General, British Nutrition Foundation,
London, formerly Rank Professor, Department of
Human Nutrition, University of Glasgow, Royal
Hospital for Sick Children, Glasgow

Whiting, Mark   MSc, BNur, RGN, RSCN, NDN, RHV
Paediatric Home Care, St Mary's Hospital and Medical
School, London

Zeitlin, Harry   MD, FRCP, FRCPsych
Professor, Academic Department of Psychiatry,
University College, London

Chapter 1

Introduction

Marion Miles and Diane Smyth

Community-based health services for children began in the UK over 200 years ago. Since then many factors have contributed to their development including the changing attitudes and expectations of society. Our current child protection system provides a good example and demonstrates the development of a caring service in response to public rejection of a previously accepted practice, namely child cruelty. Other examples include sophisticated support services for children with disabilities who would previously have been hidden away but are now openly integrated into the community. Major events such as war have also shaped the services by drawing attention to the ill health of children and the need to support single parent families. More recently the establishment of the National Health Service has facilitated the development of paediatrics as a speciality.

Initially the emphasis of the community child health service was on prevention and the identification of physical ill health by regular inspection and review, thus filling any gaps left by family practitioner and hospital services.

Now, with increasing rapidity, roles are changing. The artificial barriers between the work of family doctors and community and hospital-based paediatricians are being eroded. The role of parents and carers as effective health protectors and providers has been recognized, releasing community health professionals from a supervisory role and allowing them to be selectively more supportive.

Although there is now more agreement at national level about the desirable content of surveillance and health promotion programmes for children and young people, the fragmentation of the health service into Trusts and units could result in greater variability at local level. It will become even more important for community child health services to retain a traditional public health approach since community paediatricians will need to promote health care programmes based on local population needs. The statutory requirements of social and educational services and recent legislation continue to require close inter-agency working. There are fundamental changes taking place within these agencies as well as the National Health Service, so that maintaining valuable working relationships is essential but provides further challenges to all child health practitioners.

This book will be of particular use to all child health professionals especially those working or planning to work outside hospital against a changing and some-times turbulent background. We have drawn no clear dividing line between general paediatric topics and those encountered in the practice of community child health, but items which relate to the care of acutely ill children are omitted since they are fully addressed in other textbooks.

The book starts by setting epidemiological parameters and then describes growth and development and the services designed to promote them optimally. Specific problems that are separately addressed include child protection and child care law, neurological, language and learning disorders and problems associated with sensory loss. Relevant orthopaedic conditions and physical illnesses are discussed, together with challenging issues such as behaviour problems and bereavement.

Since it was not the intention to describe UK services in isolation, an important section on community services in developing countries is included. Finally, the professionals involved in delivery of the service and, most importantly, parents who are the major health carers of children are considered together with the support services available to them.

What this book provides therefore, is a snapshot of community child health care as it is delivered at the present time. Services are changing but the development of a combined child health service continues.

Chapter 2

Epidemiology

Zarrina Kurtz and Fiona Stanley

The uses of epidemiology in community paediatrics

Epidemiology is the study of the distribution and determinants of disease frequency in human populations. It is based on the tenet that disease is not distributed randomly, and that what determines the patterns of frequency tells us about the disease process. Epidemiology forms the scientific basis of public health medicine. It is recognized that there are important areas of interface between the work of community paediatricians and consultants in public health medicine. A joint working party with representatives from the Faculty of Public Health Medicine and the British Paediatric Association[1] listed these areas as:

1 Monitoring screening programmes
2 Organizational aspects of immunization programmes
3 Liaison with other organizations
4 Organization and management of health education and health promotion programmes
5 Health advocacy
6 Community approaches to prevention
7 Training of other health professionals
8 Planning and developing children's services
9 Information and evaluation.

In many instances community paediatricians undertake a significant proportion of public health work for children, and epidemiology is a crucial component of the specialist skills required for this and other aspects of their work. Its uses include providing a community diagnosis, completing the clinical picture, describing natural history, identifying causes and risks, identifying syndromes, providing normal values, and planning and evaluating health services.[2]

1 Providing a community diagnosis of child health problems and risks

Using epidemiological methods, a description of characteristics of the population provides a health profile. This will include how many children there are overall and the proportions in different age groups; whether to expect the numbers to increase or not depending upon the birth rate, survival and migration in recent years; the number of children living in families in underprivileged circumstances and therefore having particular risks to health and difficulties in receiving health services; whether there are localities with clusters of poor quality or overcrowded housing, and whether indicators of health such as immunization uptake are different in children living in or attending clinics in such localities. A health profile can be used to determine the content of a community child health service and where to concentrate the delivery. Trends over time will help in planning and may give an indication of the effects of health service or other interventions.

In making a community child health profile, routinely published statistics such as the distribution of infant deaths by birthweight of babies born in each Regional Health Authority (RHA) in England and Wales are available.[3] Conceptions, teenage conceptions and their outcome rates are also available for the mother's usual RHA of residence.[4] Where 15% or more of the total live births are to mothers born outside the UK, District Health Authority (DHA) birth rates are also published.[4] This information may suggest not only the need for additional neonatal and community services in a particular Regional or District Health Authority but also give clues as to why the population in some localities is at higher risk. Local and further detailed studies may then be carried out in order to target preventive programmes appropriately. An example is a recent analysis showing higher perinatal mortality rates in immigrant mothers compared with those born in the UK with variation between

DHAs and between different ethnic groups.[5] These findings may indicate ways in which health services in different districts deal more or less effectively with babies and mothers at risk and may also give clues to the aetiology of perinatal risk and suggest strategies for prevention.

Routinely available data on immunization uptake have shown for many years that average national uptake figures conceal large regional variations and even larger variations between districts. Inner city DHAs can be identified as having the lowest uptake (Table 2.1). These findings have led to community paediatricians in DHAs with poor uptake making special provision such as walk-in immunization clinics offering specialist advice and immunization by health visitors in the home.[6,7] The impact of such activities can be evaluated by continuing to monitor these rates.

Sometimes in order to make a community diagnosis, a special survey will be carried out. A recent survey identified a much higher prevalence of dental disease in children of Vietnamese immigrants than others living in Lambeth, Lewisham and Southwark, associated with the length of time spent in this country, and indicating a need for a special preventive programme for this ethnic group.[8]

The community paediatrician will want to up-date the community diagnosis at regular intervals through surveillance. National surveillance of important preventable conditions such as congenital rubella syndrome can identify the success or otherwise of rubella immunization programmes.[9] Another example is the monitoring system set up in 1964 following recognition of the risk to babies whose mothers had

taken thalidomide during pregnancy, for reporting congenital malformations detected within 7 days of birth. Now clusters in time or place of cases of malformations can be identified, raising suspicion and leading to action much more rapidly than had been possible before.[10]

2   Completing the clinical picture

The hospital paediatrician's view of child health problems and disease conditions is likely to be limited both with regard to the types of problem that exist and to the range of manifestations of any one condition. In addition, individual paediatricians are likely to have different experiences due not only to real differences in morbidity at different times and in different localities but also to different thresholds for referral to their care.[11] The community paediatrician may have a similarly limited perspective of different conditions considered in a clinical context. However, since there is a responsibility to consider the overall health problems of a child population, broader information is needed.

The epidemiological approach in identifying all cases in the community irrespective of severity or stage of illness enables a representative picture of a condition to be built up, which is the basis for determining an unbiased prognosis. For example, the proportion of children with febrile convulsions who later develop afebrile seizures was found to range from 2.6% to 76.9% in 19 studies based on clinic attenders. However, seven population-based studies indicated a

Table 2.1 Immunization 1987/88: Two year uptake rate of children born in 1985

	Whooping cough (%)	Polio (%)	Measles (%)
England	73	87	76
Regional health authority range	64 Mersey	83 Mersey and SE Thames	70 NE and SE Thames
	80 Wessex	94 Wessex	85 South Western
Thames regions	70–76	83–91	70–77
Inner London district health authorities			
Brent	59	67	56
Paddington	55	62	54
Riverside	58	68	57
Hampstead	65	60	24
Bloomsbury	34	51	51
Islington	67	79	65
City and Hackney	60	69	58
Newham	58	69	50
Tower Hamlets	63	73	68
West Lambeth	51	66	45
Camberwell	58	67	48
Lewisham and N. Southwark	61	74	64
Richmond, Roehampton and Twickenham	65	76	66
Wandsworth	63	74	62

Source: Kurtz, Z. From Vaccination and immunization summary information from forms KC50, KC50A and KC51, Department of Health, England SM12B, 1989 (unpublished).

consistently lower proportion, between 1.5% and 4.6%.[12] Children admitted to hospital with febrile convulsions are more likely to have had prolonged seizures, however, if follow-up includes those managed at home by the general practitioner, the outlook is much more encouraging.[13]

A number of sources of information may be needed to obtain a comprehensive and accurate picture of a disease or condition. For conditions such as cerebral palsy, epilepsy, child abuse, drug abuse in adolescence, and learning difficulties, some, but not all of the affected children may be known differentially to the health authority, education authority, social services department, police department, local pharmacies, and voluntary organizations. For other conditions, such as speech and language problems, it is extremely difficult to obtain a true and comprehensive idea of morbidity because the sources of data available do not reflect the real extent of the problems, as they are based solely on referrals which, in turn, may be dependent on the availability of specialist resources.

3 Describing the natural history of disease

Many paediatricians may see only the tip of the iceberg of disease as it is usual for presentation to occur at severe or late stages. Population-based surveys can quantify the extent of mild and more serious manifestations of a condition, and the likely outcome by a certain age or after a defined length of disease history. Follow-up of a representative sample of cases can describe the full natural history and the risk of developing complications for an individual. For example, a survey of secondary school children would reveal about two per thousand with insulin-dependent diabetes by the age of 16 years.[14] If the survey included immunological analyses, pancreatic islet cell antibodies would be found in a higher proportion indicating children at risk of developing diabetes, particularly among the siblings of those with clinically manifest disease.[15] Complications such as retinopathy would be found in some of those with diabetes if the survey included young adults, and in a greater proportion if a wider age range was sampled.

A recent analysis of the heights of children followed up at the ages of 7, 11, 16 and 23 years shows that less than one-third of both boys and girls who are very short (below the 5th centile) at age 7 years become short adults (Table 2.2).[16] It also found that of the 120 girls who were short at 7 years but above the 10th centile at 23 years, 89 (74%) were already above the 10th centile when measured at 16 years. In the boys, catch-up growth tended to occur a few years later. This type of information is essential in giving clinical advice to children presenting with short stature and to their parents.

4 Identifying causes and risk factors

Many regard this as the main contribution of epidemiology to the study of disease. Concepts of causation are described fully and clearly by Rothman (see Further reading). Exposure to a causal factor results consistently in higher risk of disease and where it is possible to prevent exposure or at least to prevent the initiation of pathology, primary prevention of the disease process can be attempted, as in immunization against measles. It is increasingly recognized that many diseases are the result of a number of factors each of which increases the risk either additively or exponentially. In conditions such as juvenile onset diabetes,[17] hypertension,[18] obesity,[19] only some of the risk factors may be known and the way in which they interact not properly understood. In these conditions we usually rely, at present, on early detection of the disease process with the offer of treatment to prevent symptoms from developing. This is called secondary prevention and is the basis of selective screening, as for neural tube defects in pregnancy.

Failure of take-up of preventive services can be an important risk factor. This is exemplified in an outbreak of 30 cases of measles, with one death, in a primary school in Somerset, which had a high overall immunization uptake rate of 91%. Among the role of cases, 87% had not been immunized.[20] Although the role of important factors associated with many conditions are known, for example the role of maternal smoking in low birthweight and of parental smoking

Table 2.2 Outcome of cases with height deficiency at 7 years[16]

| | Age 7 | At 5th and 10th centile at later ages | | |
		Age 11	Age 16	Age 23
Boys				
<5th centile	174 (100)	87 (50.0)	86 (49.6)	55 (31.6)
From <5 to <10th	- -	42 (24.1)	31 (17.8)	25 (14.3)
Girls				
<5th centile	211 (100)	129 (61.1)	75 (35.5)	60 (28.4)
From <5 to <10th	- -	31 (15.0)	47 (22.2)	31 (14.6)

in respiratory disease in children, preventive activities which largely rely on health education have had limited success. In the prevention of childhood injuries, health education to modify parents' behaviour is again a key strategy, but has proved disappointing. However, markedly lower rates of injury have followed legislation on the requirement to wear seat belts, to make children's night clothes from flameproof material stating clearly on the garment when this is not the case, and to dispense aspirin in child-resistant containers.[21]

5   Identification of syndromes

The way in which patterns of disease cluster can lead to differentiation of single disease conditions into different groups. Mental retardation (children with IQs below 70) clusters differently with parents' social class depending on whether it is mild or severe.[22] Children with IQ below 50 appear to show no social-class bias but, in mild mental retardation, there is a strong social-class bias. A study conducted in Aberdeen found mild mental retardation unassociated with evidence of brain damage to be 28 times commoner in children of unskilled or semi-skilled fathers than in non-manual groups from the same population.[23] Overcrowding, large families, and low educational standards in parents have all been found to be associated. These findings, together with those from studies in twins and adopted children, strongly suggest that most mild mental retardation arises from a combination of genetic and adverse environmental factors. In only a minority of cases, especially in middle-class children with a clear history of cerebral damage, can single-factor aetiology, such as birth trauma or infection be identified. Improved preventive and management strategies can now be specifically tailored towards these separate syndromes.[22]

6   Providing normal values

A major part of medical practice depends upon recognizing signs of disease, and this depends to a large extent upon distinguishing what is abnormal from what is normal. This knowledge is gained from data collected from a number of people so that a full range of the characteristic of interest can be defined, as well as the usual experience described according to the mean or average, the median and the mode (see glossary). The information must be collected from a large enough number of people so that all possible values of the characteristic are included in the range, and the people should be representative of the population from which they come. Only then can the characteristics of an individual be assessed usefully against the group experience.

Every day in clinical practice with children we measure height and weight and assess whether an individual child's growth gives cause for concern by comparing his or her measurements against charts derived from measuring many children's heights and weights and giving the range and average values to be expected for a particular chronological age. Recently, in the UK, it has been recognized that individual children's growth is being compared with standards that were derived at a time when socioeconomic circumstances were different, affecting the overall pattern of growth in the child population, and also derived from a population of different ethnic composition.[24] This has led to the collection of new epidemiological information in order to develop up-to-date standards for comparison and standards that are specific for different ethnic populations. In order to identify important deviations at an earlier stage, intrauterine growth charts have been developed in the same way.

In assessing normality, what occurs often is usually considered normal and what occurs infrequently abnormal. This is a statistical definition based on the frequency of a characteristic in a defined population, but it may be misleading in medical terms. People with very high or very low values of a characteristic may or may not be 'diseased'; for example they are with regard to high blood pressure but they are not with low blood pressure or high IQ, both conditions usually considered to be desirable. When certain numerical values have been shown to be regularly associated with symptomatic disease or predictive of underlying pathology or of future symptoms, they can then define health problems. In the range of values of a characteristic, it will often be necessary to decide upon a cut-off point above or below which it is decided that disease is present, or that treatment will be effective; for example, at what height level, age, and growth rate should treatment for short stature be started? In other conditions, such as inborn errors of metabolism, a different type of biological observation indicates abnormality, depending upon its presence or absence, without a range of values giving rise to varying likelihood of disease. A description of how clinical phenomena are measured, expressed, and distributed among unselected people can be found in Fletcher, Fletcher and Wagner (see Further reading). Ways in which data can be summarized and techniques for analysis are also described.

7   Planning and evaluating health services

In planning health services, the needs of the population must be described. For this, measures of health and disease are collected and routinely up-dated, as accurately and with as complete coverage as possible. Data such as the local birth rate and the rate of low birthweight births, that are essential in making the community diagnosis, are the foundation for planning. It may be important to distinguish health problems that can be influenced by health service intervention

– needs for services – from needs defined according to morbidity and mortality rates. Special studies may be required to identify groups who are at particular risk such as homeless families living in temporary accommodation.

Data about the current use of services give some measure of need, but more of demand and availability. These include, for example, admission rates to neonatal intensive care and special care baby facilities, and the length of stay. But it is also necessary to find out whether there are adequate resources for the number of babies who need them, including enough of the right kind of equipment and sufficiently skilled staff. Are the procedures carried out in neonatal intensive care known to be effective, and how many babies survive and with what degree of impairment? This evaluation needs epidemiologically-based methods and the findings must inform further planning.

The structure, process and outcome of services all need to be assessed for evaluation.[25] Epidemiological methods are critical in deciding whether components of the service are effective and in monitoring its overall efficiency in achieving its aims. This will include assessment of unmet need, over-costly or wasteful service use, and unwanted side-effects. Changes in indicators of health can be monitored over time, before and after introduction of services, and in different districts which have different patterns of service. Methods used in evaluating community development projects have been described.[26] Case-control studies and randomized controlled trials are also used to test carefully-defined hypotheses. While randomized controlled trials are the most important method of evaluation, they are not always possible or necessary and can be long and expensive. Although problems with random allocation and non-response seriously biased the results, the study designed to examine the effect of extra health visitor intervention on unexpected deaths in infants in Sheffield is a good example of a randomized controlled trial.[27] More recent examples include investigation of the effect of a home visit accompanied by the giving of specific advice compared with a national television campaign and a local health education programme, in improving safety in the home,[28] and a randomized controlled trial of surgery for glue ear.[29]

Epidemiological methods

Epidemiology is about counting and measuring, but what is most important is the relationship of what is counted or measured to the population at risk. The measures used are measures of frequency – incidence and prevalence. *Incidence* is the rate of occurrence of new cases that arise within a defined population within a defined time period. New cases can be diseases such as measles, events such as admission to hospital, birth or death, or occurrence of a risk factor such as low birthweight. The following are measures of incidence:

- Measles notifications which in 1988 in England and Wales were 170.66 per 100 000 population. The highest rates were in children aged 11 months with a rate of 2229.86 per 100 000.
- There were 4.3 stillbirths per 1000 total births in the UK in 1992.
- Admissions in 1985 for children aged under 14 years to paediatric departments (excluding special care baby units) in the Oxford Region were 221.2 per 1000 children.

Incidence is of particular interest in searching for the causes of disease because comparing rates will give clues as to what may be giving rise to higher or lower figures. Incidence rates are used for monitoring health and for evaluating the effects of health care programmes. To establish the incidence of a particular condition, a follow-up or cohort study is needed.

Incidence is also the basic expression of the risk of developing a disease, being admitted to hospital, being born with low birthweight, etc. The differing risk in people exposed to a particular factor compared with those not exposed is called the relative risk. The proportion of the risk that is due to exposure to the particular risk factor is called the attributable risk.

Prevalence is the amount of a disease or condition that exists in a defined population at a particular time – the point prevalence. Period prevalence describes the proportion of a population affected by disease over a defined period and includes all cases present at the beginning of the period plus the new cases that arise during that period, using as denominator an average figure for the number in the population at risk over the time period.

Prevalence is particularly useful in describing the load of chronic illness. A distinction must be made between prevalence and cumulative incidence. For example, 4.1 per thousand is commonly quoted as the prevalence of epilepsy in children aged 11 years in the UK.[30] However, epilepsy is an episodic condition and some 11-year-old children with a history of seizures will no longer be having fits nor taking anticonvulsant medication. The cumulative incidence in a cohort of children was found to be 5.3 per 1000 up to the 12th birthday, but the prevalence of epilepsy (that is active epilepsy) was 4.3 per 1000 at the age of 11 years in the same sample of children.[31]

The prevalence of a condition depends upon the incidence and upon the recovery or death rate. A large proportion of children in a community such as a school may develop conditions such as mild coughs and colds but, because they recover within a day or two, only a small proportion of the school is ill at any one time. Even though the annual incidence of juvenile-onset diabetes is of the order of between 4.4 and

11.6 per 100 000,[32] because it is a life-long condition, the prevalence in children by school-leaving age is of the order of two per 1000.[14] Prevalence may be determined from cross-sectional studies and surveys.

The usefulness of measures of frequency depends crucially upon the way in which cases (the numerator) and the population at risk (the denominator) are defined. Again, prevalence rates for epilepsy in children vary widely in different studies, and some of the variation will be because what constitutes a case of epilepsy is defined differently in different studies.[33]

The way in which a disease is defined may change over time: some of the increasing proportion of postneonatal mortality from 'sudden death, cause unknown' is attributed to transferred causes of death likely to have been previously classified as respiratory conditions; so that comparison of the same condition when the same disease label is used may not be accurate.[34] Care must also be taken when comparing conditions as they occur in different places and in different groups of people, since the same labels may not be used for the same conditions. An important example is behaviour disorder within the school population. This is characterized as a medical condition differently by teachers, doctors and families, and by those from different ethnic backgrounds. It must be said that there is considerable confusion even within medical and scientific circles as to how best to classify these disorders. Accuracy is also important when defining exposure to a risk factor such as lead in the environment, or radiation.

Definition of the denominator is equally important. The population at risk indicates those who are susceptible to the disease under consideration. For example, although it may be helpful to examine the incidence of mumps in relation to the total child population when assessing the uptake of MMR (measles, mumps, rubella) immunization, if the rate of mumps orchitis were being examined, it would not be meaningful to include girls in the denominator. The term person-years may be used to give an accurate denominator for exposure rates in a population group where some people may move out of it during the study period and a different number may move in. A denominator may for example be limited to a defined age or occupational group.

Epidemiological studies

Epidemiological studies may be divided broadly into two types – descriptive and analytic. Descriptive studies may also be called observational studies. Observations are made about disease occurrence in the population of interest and the frequency of disease related to particular characteristics of the population. Three kinds of characteristics are examined: time, person and place. Characteristics of time may be linear, comparing time past with later time, or recurrent, such

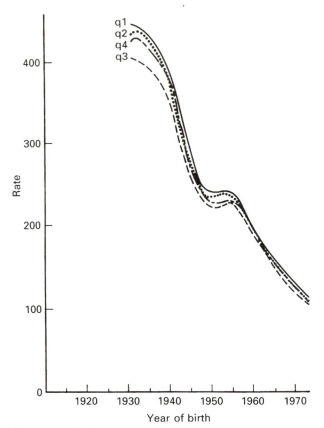

Figure 2.1 Stillbirth rates, by quarter (q) of the year, England and Wales. Rates per 10^4 live births. Curves based on 7-year moving average of rates for the years 1928–78.[35]

as the association with the time of day or season. For example, analysis of seasonal variation in stillbirth rates (Figure 2.1) and of deaths under the age of one year was used to examine seasonal changes in rates over time and whether there was correlation between seasonal rates and temperature.[35] Characteristics of place may be related to geographical position such as north or south, to ecological features such as mountain or seaside, to urban or rural features, or to administrative boundaries between countries or regions. Startling geographical differences have been described in the incidence of neural tube defects within a few hundred miles, between West Glamorgan and districts in London.[36] There are many characteristics of people that may be examined but the most useful include age, sex, race or ethnic group, position in the family, number of siblings, socioeconomic group, and occupation. Figure 2.2 shows childhood mortality by age, sex and social class for all causes of death and for motor vehicle traffic accidents.[37]

Examples of descriptive studies include observation of the fall in notifications for whooping cough over the years during which nutrition and living conditions improved, with a further dramatic fall on the introduction of immunization in 1957 and the rise following the widely publicized controversy in 1976 suggested that

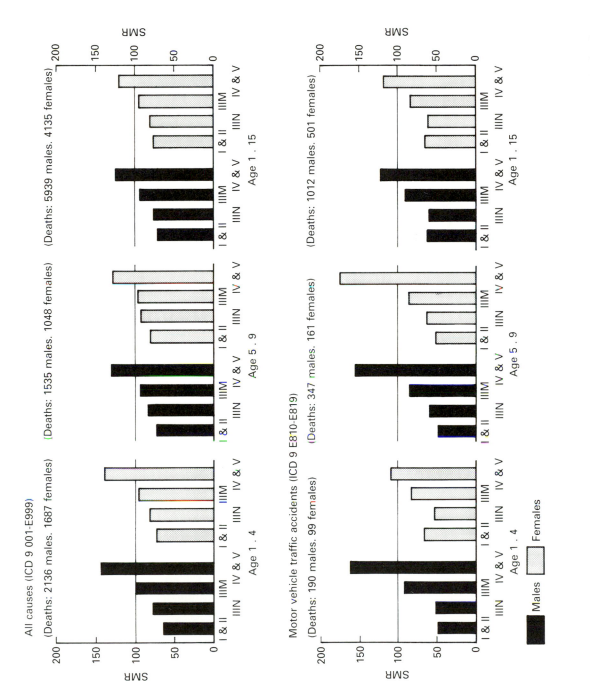
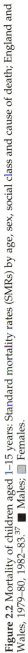

Figure 2.2 Mortality of children aged 1–15 years: Standard mortality rates (SMRs) by age, sex, social class and cause of death; England and Wales, 1979–80, 1982–83.[37] ■ Males; ▨ Females.

pertussis vaccine caused brain damage (Figure 2.3).[38] A recent example of a descriptive prevalence study is of dental disease among Vietnamese immigrants in East London. The mean number of decayed, missing or filled teeth in 5 year-olds in three boroughs was found to be 8.3 in Vietnamese children, none of whom were caries free, compared with a mean of 2.07 in other children, 50% of whom were caries free. The extent of the role in dental disease of other factors such as social class and length of time lived in this country was also examined.[8]

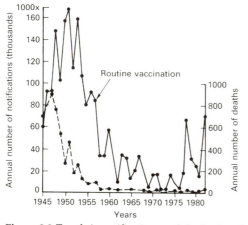

Figure 2.3 Trends in notifications and deaths for whooping cough in England and Wales.[38] - - - - Notifications; —— Deaths.

Descriptive studies may include follow-up of a population some of whom are exposed to certain risk factors, to ascertain the frequency of disease outcome in those exposed compared with those who are not. These follow-up studies are also called cohort studies and they may be carried out even in retrospect – the exposure experience of a population can be related to the frequency of disease when that outcome has already occurred. The follow-up of women during pregnancy which described the reduced birthweight in babies of smokers is an example of such a descriptive cohort study.[39]

Descriptive studies may suggest hypotheses about the cause or course of disease. Analytic studies are set up in order to test a hypothesis. Analytic studies may be case-control or intervention studies. Cohort follow-ups may also be designed so that analyses can be carried out to test a hypothesis.

In a case-control study, people with the condition to be studied are selected as the cases. The hypothesis as to whether their condition is caused by a particular risk factor is tested by comparing them with control subjects, selected in all other ways to be as like the cases as possible. The degree of exposure to the risk factor is measured in both groups and the rates compared.

Case-control studies can be done rapidly and may be used for rare disease conditions but if the results are to be useful, it is important that the cases are represen-

tative of all people with the condition to avoid selection bias. For example, general recommendations should not be made about the relation of mother's smoking to low birthweight babies if the mothers studied smoked only one brand of cigarette or lived on a single housing estate. Great care must be taken, for this reason, to define the cases accurately, for example, the exact level of birthweight that is meant by low birthweight. Either at the stage of design or analysis, the variables that are known or suspected to be associated with the outcome of interest must be taken into account. For instance, with low birthweight as outcome, key variables would include mother's height, ethnic group, socioeconomic group and parity. Controls need to be matched with cases, on an individual basis for possible confounding factors (see glossary), or by ensuring that the grouped characteristics of the controls are similar to those of the cases. Statistical methods are also available to allow for potential confounding factors in subsequent analysis. Difficulties with case-control studies include lack of knowledge at the time of the study of all the factors that may affect the condition under study. If the cases and controls are different with respect to this unknown factor as well as to the exposure that is specifically being investigated, the relative effects of the two risk factors cannot be estimated. Other difficulties can arise if memory or recording of the risk factor is different in cases and controls (recall bias). It is known that people with a disease are more likely than those without it to recall events that are possibly linked to its onset. Being aware of and attempting to control for selection and recall bias is important. In spite of these inherent problems to case-control studies, they are an extremely useful epidemiological tool. A case-control study was used to examine the risks of pertussis vaccine by comparing the immunization experience of children admitted with acute neurological disorders, with controls.[40]

Cohort studies are necessary to calculate risks of disease. The exposures and the outcomes to be measured must be carefully defined at the outset. Levels of exposure that relate to particular types of outcome can be estimated and the effect of other risk factors taken into account, without depending on recall. Problems can arise, mainly due to cost and to losses from the original sample, if follow-up is needed over long periods before the outcome of interest occurs, and if a large population is needed to obtain a sufficient number of outcomes to allow the statistical significance of association with the risk factors to be calculated. In the UK three cohort studies have been carried out, each based upon all births in one week in 1946, 1958 and 1970 respectively.[41–43] Important aspects of children's health have been followed into adult life and the natural history of conditions such as asthma and vision defects have been charted.[44,45] Recently follow-up of babies born to mothers with cytomegalovirus (CMV) infection have shown the risk of serious defects arising by the age of 5 years to be 10%; this brings into question whether screening of all mothers would be a wasteful use of resources.[46]

Intervention studies are carried out to test the effect of the addition or removal of a treatment or risk factor on the risk of disease. The effect of adding fluoride to the water supply on prevalence of dental caries in children was tested by comparing two similar populations. In one district fluoride was added in 1956 while the other was left with unfluoridated water (Table 2.3).[47]

Table 2.3 The effect of fluoridation on dental caries, Watford and Sutton study

Proportion of children caries-free before and after fluoridation		
	Watford (fluoridated in 1956)	Sutton (non-fluoridated)
Children aged 3–7 years.	Deciduous teeth	
1956	19% (631)	25% (449)
1965	50% (677)	38% (665)
Children aged 8–10 years.	Permanent teeth	
1956	14% (560)	14% (474)
1967	42% (345)	23% (254)

From: *Reports on Public Health and Medical Subjects*[(47)]

Other epidemiological studies are concerned with developing methodologies for service evaluation or for research into health problems; for example, the development of a scoring system to identify babies at risk of sudden infant death syndrome.[48]

> An epidemiologic study is properly viewed as an exercise in measurement, with accuracy as the goal. Design strategies are intended to reduce the sources of error, both systematic and random. Reduction of random error improves the precision of the measurement, whereas reduction of systematic error improves the validity of the measurement. (Rothman, see Further reading)

All epidemiological findings are based upon associations between an effect, that is a disease or impairment with a cause or a risk factor, that is an environmental or personal characteristic. If an association is found, it is more likely to be causal if the association is strong. There is a high relative risk if it can be replicated in different populations in different situations, if the cause precedes the effect, if lower levels of the causal exposure are associated with lower levels of the effect

(the dose/response relationship), if removal of the cause is associated with removal of the effect, and if there is a biologically plausible mechanism whereby the cause can produce the effect in question, particularly if it can be demonstrated experimentally.

More than a brief outline of epidemiological methods is beyond the scope of this chapter. It is important that the community paediatrician should have sufficient understanding of the essential principles behind epidemiological methodology to read the medical literature critically and to evaluate study design and results in areas of particular interest. The paediatrician should also be able to use appropriate epidemiological investigations to evaluate child health problems. Before designing and carrying out an epidemiological study, further reading of texts given in the list at the end of this chapter is recommended, as well as obtaining advice from members of a local department of epidemiology.

Sources of data

Routinely collected data

A large variety of data related to health and disease are collected and published regularly on a national basis; in many cases figures are also given for each region and district. Most of these statistics are produced by the Office of Population Censuses and Surveys (OPCS) and published by Her Majesty's Stationery Office (HMSO). A considerable volume of data is collected that is not published but is often available on request to OPCS.

The national census is undertaken every 10 years, most recently in 1991, and provides baseline data about the population. Estimates of population are made at intervals between census years. Information is available on the total population for area of residence, type of housing, size of household, occupation, date of birth, and sex. In 1991 information on self-reported ethnic group was collected for the first time.

Mortality data, derived from death certificates, offer information based on all but about a hundred deaths a year. They are the most reliable indicator of health status particularly for changes over time, since cause of death has been recorded in the UK for 150 years. Care must be taken in interpreting mortality data because of errors and inconsistencies in the completion of death certificates and the way in which the information is coded. For example, systematic under-reporting of suicide is known to have occurred while it was illegal to commit suicide and still continues because of the stigma attached to this cause of death. For the same reasons there has been under-reporting of HIV infection and AIDS. Cause of death is coded according to an agreed classification system, the International Classification of Disease (ICD), which is periodically up-dated and expanded to incorporate new knowledge. The system is now undergoing a tenth revision. Changes in the incidence of sudden infant death syndrome are partly attributable to changes in the way deaths from unknown cause have been classified and coded.

Care must also be taken when comparing mortality experience between different populations. Overall or crude mortality rates may be misleading if the composition of the populations is different with respect to factors that have powerful effects on the death rate. The most important of these is age. Age-specific rates will clarify the situation. Standardization is a technique used to estimate a summary figure for comparative mortality that also takes into account relevant differing population structure.

Since 1975, records of deaths occurring in infants aged under one year have been routinely linked to their birth records and this has allowed monitoring of infant death rates by birthweight and other variables such as mother's country of birth (Table 2.4).[5]

Routinely collected data describe morbidity less satisfactorily because they are collected only as a result of contact with health services. Information is limited to hospital inpatients and attendance at general practice and to certain special categories of condition such as abortions, congenital malformations, communicable diseases and cancer. Statistics are regularly published on a 10% sample of all patients discharged from hospital, as part of the hospital inpatient enquiry (HIPE). The hospital activity analysis (HAA) relates to all patients discharged, collected by each DHA and available to individual hospital departments. Data are gathered on patient characteristics and variables such as diagnosis, length of stay and type of referral but are not collected for outpatients, nor is it possible to identify re-admissions or the outcome of treatment.

Information about patient use of general practice services is collected on a continuing basis from a number of sentinel practices throughout the country, chosen to include practices of different types (single-handed/health centre, urban/rural, etc). Three larger scale national morbidity surveys giving more detail about patients and conditions seen in general practice have been carried out, the most recent in 1981–1982.[49] From these, it is possible to say that 98.5% of children aged 0–4 years consult their general practitioner every year and that the highest proportion do so because of upper respiratory tract problems. Consultation rates in the youngest children are higher than for any other age group, whereas in children aged 5–14 years the rate of 66.9% is lower than other age groups.

Information about self-reported illness and use of health services is published annually in the General Household Survey, along with a range of information on health, housing, employment, education, transport, social services and social support, obtained from a sample of households.

Certain disease conditions have special data collection and reporting systems. The longest running of these concerns communicable disease surveillance by the Public Health Laboratory Service, and information is collated, analysed and published by the Communicable Disease Surveillance Centre in the form of weekly reports and regular reviews. Rapid identification of outbreaks is made possible through this national reporting system, as well as analysis and specialist interpretation of longer-term trends, for example of the spread of HIV infection or the incidence of congenital rubella syndrome.

Special analyses are carried out which may be useful in monitoring or studying aspects of health. Linking of records from different sources is a well-established example. Linkage between morbidity records and census characteristics for patients in a sample of 25 practices in England and Wales gives important details

Table 2.4 Birthweight specific perinatal mortality rates* by country of birth of mother (1982–85, England and Wales)[5] (Number of deaths in parentheses)

Mother's country of birth	Birthweight (g)					
	All weights	<2500 g	2500–2999 g	3000–3499 g	3500–3999 g	4000 g+
United Kingdom	10 (22 503)	94 (14 107)	7 (2899)	3 (2418)	2 (1203)	3 (550)
Irish Republic	10 (279)	98 (166)	8 (36)	3 (32)	2 (20)	2 (6)
India	12 (576)	68 (353)	6 (89)	4 (67)	3 (23)	7 (11)
Bangladesh	14 (225)	81 (132)	8 (38)	5 (31)	4 (10)	12 (6)
East Africa	13 (351)	66 (241)	5 (51)	3 (27)	2 (8)	11 (8)
West Africa	13 (149)	102 (95)	9 (20)	4 (18)	2 (5)	3 (3)
Caribbean Commonwealth	13 (288)	84 (178)	5 (27)	4 (33)	2 (10)	10 (13)
Pakistan	19 (1022)	115 (600)	11 (156)	5 (110)	6 (63)	12 (35)

*Rounded to nearest integer.

EPIDEMIOLOGY 13

about differential use of primary care by socioeconomic groups.[50] A special study linking details from prescriptions dispensed, patient characteristics such as age and sex and records of hospital admissions, obstetric deliveries, and deaths has shown how hypotheses about the adverse effects of drugs especially on the fetus could be generated and tested by these means.[51] A particular type of linkage provides the information that is available from the cancer registry. This includes demonstrating increased survival of children with lymphatic leukaemia over the past 25 years (Figure 2.4).[52]

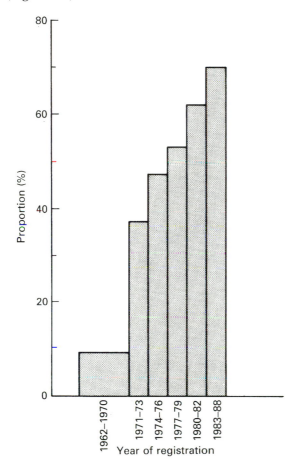

Figure 2.4 Five-year survival of children under 15 years of age with acute lymphocytic leukaemia by year of registration.[52]

Regularly updated statistics are published, not directly on health topics, but covering many aspects of interest such as distribution of income from the Family Expenditure Survey,[53] and employment status and ethnic composition of the population from the Labour Force Survey.[54] Disadvantages of routinely collected statistics are that there may be a lengthy interval between collection of the data and publication, and that they may not be generally applicable so that details appropriate to a particular subject being investigated have not been collected.

Specially collected data

Useful sources include a number of national surveys carried out by the OPCS on aspects of children's health, such as diets of British schoolchildren[55] based on the National Food Survey, surveys of smoking[56] and of alcohol[57] use in children, and the national disability survey.[58] The Health Education Authority also publishes its own survey results, for example, about schoolgirl mothers,[59] and has been responsible for health related behaviour surveys of school pupils aged between 11 and 16 covering the past 10 years.[60]

In 1986 the British Paediatric Surveillance Unit (BPSU) was established, providing a unique system for the study of rare conditions in children. Annual reports have documented, among other information, that after public warnings in 1986 about the use of aspirin for children and in spite of improved reporting, the annual totals of cases of Reye's syndrome fell to 27 in 1988/9 compared with a peak of 90 in 1983/4 and were the lowest since reporting began in 1981.[61]

Data for the management of local services are usually collected in the form of registers, such as local authority disability registers, which were set up originally to administer the provision of statutory welfare benefits and continuing care. They are notoriously difficult to maintain; for example, the health service input related to children with cerebral palsy may come from several different clinicians working in hospital, a special centre, the community services or primary care. Registers have limitations depending upon what they are used for, and in particular, mild and very severe cases may not be included if they do not merit services. Only a handful, such as the North East Thames Region cerebral palsy register,[62] set up as a research project, have complete case finding and standard case ascertainment and can therefore be used to obtain accurate prevalence information and for planning and evaluating services. There can be serious difficulties when considerations of confidentiality influence what information is recorded, for example on the child protection register.

Opportunities for local surveillance are limited, largely because accurate data collection is difficult. A much discussed example is the lack of figures in many DHAs for injuries in children in order to identify particularly dangerous situations. A special reporting system covering all Inner London Education Authority (ILEA) schools[63] was developed to describe all accidents occurring in a particular environment related to defined populations. This has been used to study the number and type of accidents occurring in school playgrounds, upon which recommendations for safety standards have been made. A collaborative project with the local police has been reported from Newcastle where the postcoded address of local children injured in road traffic accidents is recorded at the time of routine coding for the Central Police Computer.

Information on home address was not available from routine police data. Information from the six month pilot phase of the project showed, among other things, that the highest rates of injury at all ages occurred in areas of social deprivation.[64]

Many district health authorities now have computerized recording of health service activity in pre-school children, such as immunization, health problems, and the number of children with hearing defects. A national module for this has been developed which ensures standard and compatible recording of data across districts. However some districts use individually different systems which do not allow easy comparison. A national school health module has also been developed but is not yet widely in use. These computerized information systems offer the potential basis for monitoring child health and for research.[65]

A most valuable overview of research and local child health projects in England and Wales was published in 1984 and has since been updated every couple of years.[66] This reports findings on levels and types of health problems, resources, and service use that may be used as the basis for estimates in other localities, as well as suggesting approaches to service delivery and suitable methodologies for evaluative and other research.

Patterns of childhood mortality, morbidity and handicap

Children's health problems have changed considerably even since the current framework for a community paediatric service was outlined by the Court Committee in 1976.[67] There have been striking changes in incidence, notably of infectious diseases.[68] Children with many conditions now survive longer, so that more children who would previously have died in infancy are living with chronic illnesses such as cystic fibrosis, at least into early adulthood. Advances in knowledge have led to the recognition of earlier and milder stages of certain disorders such as phenylketonuria and hypothyroidism for which treatment is available and known to influence the likelihood of developing complications. In addition there are now available effective strategies for managing the more severe stages of an increasing number of conditions, such as congenital heart disease, renal abnormalities and Duchenne muscular dystrophy, which previously would have been left untreated.

Mortality at all ages and from all causes has declined. The principal causes of death in children over the age of one year now are injuries and accidents, congenital anomalies, malignancy, and respiratory disease.[34] These conditions also cause considerable morbidity. Improved medical care means that many children now survive after a diagnosis of cancer, with chronic respiratory disease, and congenital anomalies, and following very severe accidents. Survival, however, is often accompanied by disability and handicap. Levels of self-reported long-standing illness have risen in 5–15 year olds, as for all other ages, since the early 1970s.[69] However, children over the age of 5 years are usually considered to be the healthiest age group in the population because they have lower mortality rates,[70] lower hospital admission rates,[71] and lower consultation rates in general practice[49] than other age groups. These and other routinely published national and local statistics offer a largely incomplete picture of health status and of health problems in children and adolescents.[72,73] This is mainly because the data are based upon the use of services. Information is particularly patchy for certain groups such as deprived families and those who live in the inner city because of their patterns of use of services.[74]

Mortality

The highest proportion of all deaths in children aged from 0 to 14 years occurs during the first year of life: 73.1% of all deaths. Infant mortality in England and Wales was 7.4 per thousand live births in 1991, the lowest rate recorded to date. There has been steady improvement in mortality in the first year of life over the past few decades and this has largely been due to improvements in perinatal and neonatal rates while postneonatal rates have remained steady (Figure 2.5).[3] The main causes of death in the perinatal period are low birthweight and congenital malformations. Postneonatal deaths are dominated by cot deaths, complications in low-birthweight neonatal survivors and congenital malformations. Infections as a cause of death have fallen but are still important in poorer families. Thus postneonatal mortality has become less useful as a social indicator.

Congenital malformations have increased as a proportion of all infant deaths: 26% of 6000 deaths in 1985. However, as a proportion of all stillbirths, congenital malformations have fallen from 18% in 1975 to 9% in 1985. Most of our advances have been in identifying the affected fetus in utero which means that prevention depends on the parents' painful choice as to whether to terminate the pregnancy. Careful ascertainment of neural tube defects by prenatal detection and of birth outcome has shown a fall in birth prevalence. This fall is partly accounted for by selective termination and partly by a spontaneous reduction the cause of which is unknown. It has been estimated that the annual incidence at birth of anencephaly and spina bifida fell by 80% between the average annual incidence for the years 1964–72 (3.15 per thousand) and the incidence in 1985 (0.62 per thousand).[75] About one third of this reduction can be attributed confidently to prenatal detection and selective termination of pregnancy.

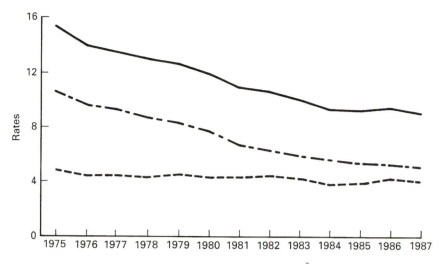

Figure 2.5 Infant mortality rates, 1975–87: England and Wales.[3] — Infant deaths; – – – Neonatal deaths; - - - - Postneonatal deaths

Because reporting of termination for malformed babies can be incomplete, and probably more so than for notification of births with neural tube defects, the impact of screening is likely to be greater than these figures suggest.[75]

Injuries remain the commonest single cause of death after the first year of life, accounting for 30% of deaths. Accidents were responsible in 1988 for 49% of deaths from all causes in children aged 5–19 years, and 57% in 15–19 year olds.[76] In this latter age group, motor vehicle accidents caused 57% of the deaths from accidents and 32% of all deaths. Fatalities represent only a very small fraction of the overall toll of childhood accidents (Table 2.5).

Table 2.5 Child casualties by age and severity (all reported casualties – Great Britain 1988)

	Severity			
Age of child	Fatal	Serious	Slight	Total
0–4	105	1234	5992	7331
5–7	85	1719	6685	8489
8–11	120	2539	10276	12935
12–15	152	3417	13597	17166
All children	462	8909	36550	45921

Morbidity

Infectious disease and respiratory conditions

It is estimated that infectious diseases still cause about 10% of deaths in children aged 0–15 years. It is well known that there is considerable under-reporting of infectious illnesses and that there are difficulties in assessing their true impact upon children's health.[68]

Beside the major improvements in incidence and rates of cure, new infections have emerged, such as those due to the human immunodeficiency virus (HIV), and others have increased in incidence, for example food poisoning and salmonellosis usually associated with inadequate cooking of poultry or cross-contamination in kitchens. There are also newly susceptible children such as those who are immuno-compromised due to HIV infection or drug treatment for leukaemia. There can be a false sense of complacency in the UK about continuing dangers from diseases that have become less common, which include the major preventable infections of childhood. National immunization cover against measles is now 92%[75] exceeding for the first time the WHO target of 90% by 1990[79] – necessary to eliminate the disease, but the rate varies between 65% and 99% in individual districts and a new national target of 95% by 1995 has now been set. Measles can still be a most unpleasant illness with the risk of serious complications in many children.

Respiratory disease remains a major problem in children, accounting for 5–10% of deaths, 20% of hospital admissions and a third of illness episodes in general practice. Asthma is probably the most important disabling condition in school-age children and responsible for much school absence.[80] Comparatively higher rates of infectious illness,[68] accidents,[81] and lower respiratory tract infections[38] are found among children in the inner city than those living elsewhere.

Disability and handicap

Estimates of the number of children with disabilities vary between 2% and 20%, depending upon the ways in which disability is defined and the ages included.

The Warnock committee[82] reported that 2% of children had a continuing need for special provision because of severe difficulties with learning. These include children with severe problems related to vision, hearing, speech, physical and neurological function associated with conditions such as cerebral palsy and epilepsy, and psychological problems. Disabilities likely to have a significant effect on the ability to carry out normal everyday activities were found in 3.8% of 5–9 year olds and 3.5% of 10–15 year olds in the recent OPCS national survey of disability in Great Britain.[58] Nearly two thirds of these children had more than one disability. The most common disability was behaviour disorder, found in 2.1% of children overall. If certain chronic illnesses associated with high levels of functional impairment such as cerebral palsy, cystic fibrosis, spina bifida, and leukaemia are included, the estimated prevalence is of the order of 5%, according to a review of recent American surveys.[83] Prevalence figures of 20% include children with milder functional impairments such as uncomplicated asthma, correctable visual or hearing impairments, and moderate emotional disturbance.[82]

Prevalence estimates in the UK are based mainly upon local studies of individual conditions such as asthma[38] and epilepsy,[84] from time-limited registers such as the South East Thames cerebral palsy register, or from the national birth cohort studies, for example for diabetes.[14] While some careful local studies exist, the way in which cases are defined as well as the choice of characteristics of the population studied means that findings may not be generally applicable. The cohort studies are now becoming largely out-of-date. The first collection of statistics for a complete year since the 1981 Education Act came into force in April 1983 on the number of pupils with statements of special educational needs shows the percentage in all pupils in maintained schools varying between education authorities, from 0.2 in Wigan to 2.3 in inner London and 2.6 in Buckinghamshire. Statemented and special school pupils as a percentage of all pupils ranged from 1.1 in Barnsley to 3.1 in inner London and 3.2 in Bedfordshire.[85] The variation is now well recognized to be due more to local constraints on the number of pupils who can be statemented than to the true prevalence of pupils with severe learning disabilities.

Psychological problems

Children with chronic illness and disability, particularly those with intellectual and educational retardation, have been shown repeatedly to have higher rates of accompanying psychological problems.[86] Sixty-five per cent of all children with disability in the OPCS national survey had behavioural disability, while the overall rate of disability due to behaviour in children living in private households was 2.1%.[58] Psychological disorders have become more important in all children,

and there are increases in the rates of depression, suicide and attempted suicide[87] and of a number of other conditions such as eating disorders, including both obesity[88] and anorexia.[89] The overall prevalence rate of psychiatric disorder in middle childhood is twice the rate in urban (25%) as in rural areas (12%).[90] These are largely non-specific emotional disorders characterized by fearfulness, phobias, anxiety and depression, and conduct disorders.[91] Childhood psychological problems are associated with parental mental disorder, marital disharmony, overcrowding, reduced neighbourhood support and social cohesiveness, and high levels of life stress and life events. In children aged 4 and 5 years, entering Inner London Education Authority (ILEA) schools in 1986, behavioural problems were recorded on average in 48 per thousand children.[92] However, definition of the defects identified at the school entry medical examination is not standardized and there are no measures of severity. There were large variations in the rate of behavioural disorders and of all health problems (from 43% to 66%) in different DHAs. Information is not collected which would allow further exploration of the reasons for these differences.

Health behaviour

Patterns of physical activity among British schoolchildren have recently revealed that many children seldom undertake the amount of physical activity believed to benefit the cardiopulmonary system, although boys are more active than girls.[93]

Smoking and the use and abuse of alcohol, solvents, and other drugs are now an established part of the lives of many children. These behaviours potentially have serious health consequences in children and young people and may lead to the establishment of patterns that endanger health throughout life. There was some improvement in the proportion of children who smoke in the 1980s, but the rates are still worrying and the proportion is declining less in girls than boys. In 1988, 8% of children aged 11–15 years in England and Wales admitted to smoking regularly (at least one cigarette a week) and a further 5% admitted to occasional smoking. The prevalence of smoking increases rapidly with age, with 17% of boys aged 15–16 smoking regularly and 22% of girls.[94]

The proportion of young people who drink alcohol has increased over the last 30 years; they are starting earlier and drinking more.[95] Alcohol is a contributing factor in 45% of fatal road accidents involving young people.[96] Between 0.5% and 1% of secondary school children now abuse solvents which cause about 100 deaths a year.[97]

Almost one child in ten in England and Wales was born to a teenage mother in 1988[98] and fertility in this age group is at its highest level since 1975. Teenage pregnancy is associated with a variety of physical problems for the mother, low birthweight of the child, and high rates of fetal, perinatal and maternal mortality.[99] Many of these ill effects are related to low socio-economic status, unemployment, poor housing and social environment, low educational achievements, lack of support and stable relationships, inexperience, isolation, depression and poor levels of attendance at antenatal and other clinics.[99] A pregnant teenager is a relatively rare occurrence for an individual school which may find it more difficult to cater for all the physical, medical, social, residential and educational needs of the expectant mother and baby.[100] Local education authorities vary in their policies for the education of pregnant girls, and many of those below the statutory leaving age receive no more education once they have become pregnant.[101] Teenage parenthood is a characteristic associated with child abuse,[102] and in children of teenage mothers a disproportionate number of accidents and hospital admissions and a higher incidence of sudden infant death syndrome have been reported.[99]

Child neglect and abuse are now more widely recognized. Although population data upon which to assess trends are not reliable, National Society for the Prevention of Cruelty to Children (NSPCC) registers indicate a substantial rise in the number of cases (34% in 1986) and continuing links between child abuse and stress, unemployment, and low income in the family.[103] In 1989, 3.5 per 1000 children under 18 years old were on child protection registers in England, with a range of 8.2 per 1000 in inner London to 1.8 per 1000 in East Anglia. A recent survey has provided evidence that at least 10% of men and women have been sexually abused before the age of 16.[104] There is better understanding now of the immediate and permanent harm that may result from sexual abuse and of ways in which children at risk may be identified.

Racial harrassment was first recognized officially as an issue for schools in a Home Office report published in 1981.[105] In 1987 the Commission for Racial Equality published the results of a study which showed that racial harrassment is a widespread problem in education and that many local education authorities and institutions have yet to address it effectively.[106] Just as more subtle expressions of harrassment are difficult to define, so is the range of effects that it may have on children's health, well-being, and equality of opportunities.

Dental health

Children's dental health has improved greatly over recent years.[107] Fifty-four per cent of 5 year olds are now free from caries[108] but about 20% of children have 80% of their teeth decayed, missing or filled. Children in social classes IV and V are those with most disease and are least likely to have had dental care. Children in some ethnic minority groups either have more disease or else have similar disease rates but obtain less treatment.[109]

Deprivation and health

Multiple deprivation is associated with well documented risks to health.[110] Adult mortality rates for a number of important and preventable diseases are much higher in inner London than outer London, and are also high in other conurbations in England.[111] Ill health in parents is known to be associated with increased risks of a number of health problems in their children, including accidents[112] and behaviour disorders.[113]

Growth is perhaps the most important single measure of the health of children. There is a positive national trend towards taller children, but from 1979 to 1986 this has ceased. The Department of Health has documented the consistent finding from a number of representative national studies that short stature is associated with lower social class,[114] and shorter height in inner city children has been shown in Liverpool.[115] Inner city children and children from ethnic minority groups are shorter on average than a representative national population sample, with the exception of Afro-Caribbean boys and girls.[116]

There is accumulating evidence of the contribution to ill health of specific factors such as poor housing,[117] and homelessness.[118] Children of unemployed fathers and of those in unskilled occupations, and of single and poor parents also have higher risks to health.[21,119] Uptake of preventive services is lower in deprived communities as shown by immunization rates by the age of 2 years in the 14 inner London health districts in 1987/88. These averaged 55% for pertussis and 58% for measles, in comparison with a national range among health districts from 51% (W Lambeth) to 94% (W Surrey and NE Hants) for pertussis, and from 24% (Hampstead) to 96% (Wycombe) for measles (see Table 2.1).

Children from ethnic minority backgrounds tend to live in more deprived conditions[116] and also to have specific health problems such as sickle cell disease, rickets and tuberculosis.[120] Among both professionals and families from ethnic minority groups, there tends to be poor understanding of how to provide and to make effective use of appropriate services. This is due largely to different cultural expectations and to difficulties with language.[121]

Summary: opportunities and advocacy

Epidemiological methods provide an essential tool for the critical evaluation of the work of community paediatricians. It is now also of prime importance to apply these techniques to the systematic study of patients' needs for and satisfaction with services.

Clear opportunities for investigation in these areas are now presented because of the high profile given in the 1990 NHS and Community Care Act to a consumer-led service and to the need for audit of medical work. It is recognized that research is needed in many aspects of the discipline of community paediatrics. Specific projects that have been identified as priorities include outcomes and effectiveness of child health surveillance programmes, intervention studies with disadvantaged populations, and the ways in which parents use services.[122] Children's rights are under widespread discussion at this time fuelled by the need to implement the United Nations Convention on the Rights of the Child which was ratified by the UK in December 1991. The community paediatrician is in a position of special responsibility to act as advocate for children's well-being. Although there are many instances where the paediatrician must make decisions in the best interests of the individual child, making similar decisions in relation to groups of vulnerable children or children as a group within the population is less familiar territory. Epidemiological information provides the crucial evidence for children's needs and for improvements in health that would justify the use of resources in particular ways. Case histories cannot carry sufficient weight. Building on studies such as those carried out by Margaret Stacey[81] and Vera Carstairs,[74] with sound background knowledge of local children's health problems and of local service organization, the community paediatrician can use simple epidemiological data and research methodology to gather evidence by which to encourage particular directions of development of services for children.

Glossary

Bias or systematic error: occurs when observations consistently do not record truly what is being measured.

selection: this occurs when observations are made on a group of people that have been selected so that the proportions do not reflect the situation in the total population. A type of selection bias (response bias) occurs when a sufficiently large number of a study sample refuse to take part or cannot be included, so that information is gathered from a group that is unrepresentative with respect to relevant characteristics.

information: occurs when observations are consistently incorrect due to techniques employed in obtaining them. There are two main sources:

measurement: where the methods of measurement are consistently dissimilar among groups under observation.

observer: where the observer records or recalls information consistently differently among groups, not accurately influenced by true differences.

confounding: occurs when two factors are interrelated and it is incorrectly concluded that one of the factors is the causal agent.

Disability: any restriction or lack of ability (due to an impairment) in performing an activity in a manner or range considered normal for a human being.[124]

Handicap: a disadvantage for a given individual, resulting from a disability or impairment, that limits or prevents the fulfilment of a role that is normal for that individual.[124]

Impairment: any loss or abnormality of physiological or anatomical structure.[124]

Incidence: the rate of occurrence of new cases in a defined population within a specified time period.

Mean or average: the sum of the observations divided by the total number of observations.

Median: the point where the number of observations above equals the number below.

Mode: the most frequently occurring value.

Morbidity: the experience, usually in a population or group, of ill health or disease, or both.

Percentile, decile, quartile, etc: the proportion of all observations falling between specified values.

Precision: is lack of random error.

Predictive value: the probability of disease, given the results of a screening or diagnostic test. Positive predictive value is the probability of disease in a person with a positive (abnormal) test result. Negative predictive value is the probability of not having the disease when the test result is negative (normal). Predictive value is an answer to the question: if a patient's test result is positive (negative) what are the chances that the patient does (does not) have the disease?

Prevalence: the number of cases present within a defined population at one point in time (point prevalence), or within a defined period of time (period prevalence).

Prevention:[123]

primary: affects the agent of disease, vector or host so that the disease process cannot be initiated.

secondary: stops progression of the disease following detection of previously unrecognized disease.

tertiary: alleviation or prevention of disability or handicap following impairment by disease.

Random error: is the effect that chance or unpredictable factors can have on observations. It can be minimized in principle by making the observations on as near to the total population as possible, or in practice, by careful selection of the study sample.

Range: from lowest to highest value in a distribution.

Repeatability: is the extent of agreement between repeated measurements. Repeatable measurements may be valid or systematically invalid.

Risk:

absolute: the incidence of disease.

attributable: the incidence of disease in those exposed to a risk factor less the incidence in those not exposed.

relative: the incidence of disease in those exposed to a risk factor divided by the incidence in those not exposed.

Sensitivity: the proportion of people who genuinely have a condition who, on screening, test positive for the condition. A sensitive test will rarely miss people who have the condition.

Specificity: the proportion of people who do not have a condition who, on screening for that condition, test negative. A specific test will rarely misclassify people without a condition as having the condition.

Standard deviation: the absolute value of the average difference of individual values from the mean.

Standardization: is a technique employed so that two rates can be compared between populations that are different with respect to another factor known to influence the rates under consideration. An example of this is the standardized mortality ratio (SMR).

Validity: is lack of systematic error. It is the extent to which a method provides the assessment of that which it purports to measure. Two general kinds of validity may be distinguished:

internal validity is the degree to which the results of an observation are correct for the patients being studied; it applies to the particular conditions of the particular group of subjects being observed, and is threatened by bias and random variation.

external validity is the degree to which the results of an observation are generalizable or hold true in other settings, and is threatened by sampling bias

References

1 Faculty of Public Health Medicine and the British Paediatric Association. *Together for Tomorrow's Children*. Report of a Joint Working Party. London: BPA, 1990.

2 Morris, J.N. *Uses of Epidemiology*, 3rd edn. London: Churchill Livingstone, 1975.

3 Office of Population Censuses and Surveys. *Mortality Statistics for England and Wales 1991*. Perinatal and infant: social and biological factors. Series DH3 no 25. London: HMSO, 1993.

4 Office of Population Censuses and Surveys. *Birth Statistics 1989*: series FM1 nos 18 and 19: England and Wales. London: HMSO, 1991.

5 Balarajan, R., Botting, B. Perinatal mortality in England and Wales: variations by mother's country of birth (1982–85). *Health Trends* 1989; **21**: 79–84.

6 Hall, R., Williams, A.L.J. Special advisory service for immunisation. *Arch Dis Child* 1988; **63**: 1498–1500.

7 Jefferson, N., Sleight, G., Macfarlane, A. Immunisation by a nurse without a doctor present. *Br Med J* 1987; **294**: 423–4.

8 Todd, R., Gelbier, S. Dental caries prevalence in Vietnamese children and teenagers in three London boroughs. *Br Dent J* 1990; **168**: 24–26.

9 Tobin, J.O'H., Sheppard, S., Smithells, R.W., Milton, A., Noah, N., Reid, D. Rubella in the United Kingdom 1970-1983. *Reviews of Infectious Diseases*. 7, suppl. 1;

March–April 1985. Chicago: University of Chicago, 1985.

10 Office of Population Censuses and Surveys. *Congenital Malformation Statistics for England and Wales 1988*. Series MB 3 no. 4. London: HMSO, 1990.

11 Anderson, H.R. Increase in hospital admissions for childhood asthma: trends in referral, severity, and readmissions from 1970 to 1985 in a health region of the United Kingdom. *Thorax* 1989; **44**: 614–19.

12 Ellenburg, J.H., Nelson, K.B. Sample selection and the national history of disease. Studies of febrile seizures. *J Am Med Assoc* 1980; **243**: 1337–40.

13 Ross, E.M., Peckham, C.S. Seizure disorder in the National Child Development Study. In: Rose F.C., ed. *Research Progress in Epilepsy*. London: Pitman, 1983: 46–59.

14 Kurtz, Z., Peckham, C.S., Ades, A.E. Changing prevalence of juvenile-onset diabetes mellitus. *Lancet* 1988; ii, 88–90.

15 Bottazzo, G.F., Pujol-Borrell, R., Gale, E. Auto-immunity and diabetes: progress, consolidation and controversy. In: Alberti, K.G.M.M., Krall, C.P., eds. *The Diabetes Annual* 2. Amsterdam: Elsevier Science Publishers BV, 1986: 13–29.

16 Greco, L., Power, C., Peckham, C.S. Adult height and weight of children 'short normal' and underweight children. (Forthcoming).

17 Diabetes Epidemiology Research International. Preventing insulin dependent diabetes mellitus: the environmental challenge. *Br Med J* 1987; **295**: 479–81.

18 de Swiet, M., Fayers, P.M., Shinebourne, E.A. Blood pressure in four and five-year old children: the effects of environment and other factors in its measurement – the Brompton study. *J Hypertens* 1984; **2**: 501–505.

19 Peckham, C., Stark, O., Moynihan, C. Obesity in school children: is there a case for screening? *Public Health* 1985; **99**: 3–9.

20 O'Brien, J., Hill, A. Outbreak of measles in a primary school. *Communicable Disease Report 88/89*. London: CDSC, 1988.

21 Golding, J. Child health and the environment. In: Alberman, E.D., Peckham, C.S., eds. Childhood epidemiology. *Br Med Bull* 1986; **42**: 204–211.

22 Graham, P.J. Behavioural and intellectual development. In: Alberman, E.D., Peckham, C.S., eds. Childhood epidemiology. *Br Med Bull*. 1986; **42**: 155–162.

23 Richardson, S.A. Family characteristics associated with mild mental retardation. In: Begab, M.J., Hayward, H.C., Garber, H.L., eds. *Psychosocial Influences in Retarded Performance*. Baltimore: University Park Press, 1981.

24 Chinn, S., Price, C.E., Rona, R.J. Need for new reference curves for height. *Arch Dis Child* 1989; **64**: 1545–1553.

25 Colver, A. Measuring child health. British Paediatric Association Community Paediatric Group Newsletter, Spring 1989: 1–2.

26 Stewart-Brown, S. Evaluation of community development projects. BPA Community Paediatric Group Newsletter, Spring 1989: 3–5.

27 Carpenter, R.G., Emery, J.L. Final results of study of infants at risk of sudden death. *Nature* 1977; **263**: 724–725.

28 Colver, A.F., Hutchinson, P.J., Judson, E.C. Promoting children's home safety. *Br Med J* 1982; **285:** 1177–80.

29 Black, N.A., Sanderson, C.F.B., Freeland, A.P., Vessey, M.P. A randomised controlled trial of surgery for glue ear. *Br Med J* 1990; **300:** 1551–56.

30 Ross, E.M., Peckham, C.S., West, P.B., Butler, N.R. Epilepsy in childhood: findings from the National Child Development Study. *Br Med J* 1980; **1:** 207–210.

31 Kurtz, Z., Tookey, P., Ross, E. The incidence and prevalence of epilepsy in children and young people in the United Kingdom. (Submitted for publication.)

32 Baum, J.D., Metcalfe, M.A., Gale, E.A.M., Jarrett, R.J. National survey of childhood onset diabetes 1988. *Arch Dis Child,* 1989; **64:** 1221.

33 Kurtz, Z., Tookey, P., Ross, E. The epidemiology of epilepsy in childhood. In: Ross, E., Chadwick, D., Crawford, R., eds. *Epilepsy in Young People.* Chichester: John Wiley, 1987: 13–21.

34 Pharoah, P.O.D. Perspectives and patterns. In: Alberman, E.D., Peckham, C.S., eds. Childhood epidemiology. *Br Med Bull* 1986; **42:** 119–126.

35 Hare, E.H., Moran, P.A.P., Macfarlane, A. The changing seasonality of infant deaths in England and Wales 1912–78 and its relation to seasonal temperature. *J Epid Comm Hlth* 1981; **3:** 77–82.

36 Elwood, J.H. Anencephalus in the British Isles. *Dev Med Child Neurol* 1970; **12:** 582–91.

37 Office of Population Censuses and Surveys. *Occupational Mortality: Childhood supplement 1979–80, 1982–83.* Series DS no 8. England and Wales. London: HMSO, 1988.

38 Anderson, H.R. Respiratory disease in childhood. In: Alberman, E.D., Peckham, C.S., eds. Childhood epidemiology. *Br Med Bull* 1986; **42:** 167–171.

39 Butler, N.R., Alberman, E.D. *Perinatal Problems: the second report of the 1958 British Perinatal Mortality Survey.* Edinburgh: Livingstone, 1969.

40 Miller, D.L., Ross, E.M., Alderslade, R., Bellman, M.H., Rawson, N.S. Pertussis immunisation and serious acute neurological illness in children. *Br Med J* 1981; **282:** 1595–1599.

41 Atkins, E., Cherry, N.M., Douglas, J.W.B., Kiernan, K.E., Wadsworth, M.E.J. In: Mednick, S.A., Baert, A.E., eds. *The 1946 British Birth Cohort Survey: an Account of the Origins, Progress and Results of the National Survey of Health and Development. An Empirical Basis for Primary Prevention: Prospective Longitudinal Research in Europe.* London: Oxford University Press, 1980.

42 Fogelman, K. (ed). *Britain's Sixteen Year-Olds.* London: National Children's Bureau, 1976.

43 Golding, J., Butler, N.R. *From Birth to Five: a Study of the Health and Behaviour of a National Cohort.* Oxford: Pergamon, 1986.

44 Ross, H.R., Bland, J.M., Patel, S., Peckham, C. The natural history of asthma in childhood. *J Epidemiol Community Health* 1986; **40:** 121–29.

45 Tibbenham, A.D., Peckham, C.S., Gardiner, P.A. Vision screening in children tested at 7, 11 and 16 years. *Br Med J 1978;* **1:** 1312–1314.

46 Peckham, C.S., Logan, G.S. Cytomegalovirus infection in pregnancy. In: Cosmi, E.V., Di Renzo, G.C., eds. *Proceedings of XI European Congress of Perinatal Medicine.* London: Harwood Academic Publications, 1988: 225–60.

47 Department of Health and Social Security. *Reports on Public Health and Medical Subjects no. 122.* The fluoridation studies in the United Kingdom and the results achieved after eleven years. London: HMSO, 1969.

48 Carpenter, R.G., Emery, J.L. Identification and follow-up of infants at risk of sudden death in infancy. *Nature* 1974; **250:** 729.

49 Royal College of General Practitioners, Office of Population Censuses and Surveys, Department of Health and Social Security. *Morbidity Statistics from General Practice: Third National Study, 1981–82.* London: HMSO, 1986.

50 McCormick, A., Rosenbaum, M. *Morbidity Statistics from General Practice.* RCGP, OPCS, DoH series MB5 no. 2. Third National Study: Socio-economic analyses. London: HMSO, 1990.

51 Skegg, D.C.G., Doll, R. Record linkage for drug monitoring. *J Epidemiol Community Health 1981;* **33:** 25–31.

52 Cancer Research Campaign. Factsheet 15, 1990. *Br Med J* 1990; **300:** 1673.

53 Central Statistical Office. *Family Expenditure Survey 1988.* London: HMSO, 1990.

54 Office of Population Censuses and Surveys. *Labour Force Survey 1987.* Series LFS no. 7. London: HMSO, 1989.

55 Department of Health. *The Diets of British Schoolchildren.* DoH Reports on Health and Social subjects no. 36. London: HMSO, 1989.

56 Goddard, E. *Smoking among Secondary School Children in England 1988: An Enquiry Carried Out by Social Survey Division of the OPCS on behalf of the DoH.* London: HMSO, 1989.

57 Marsh, A., Dobbs, J., White, A., *Adolescent Drinking: A Survey Carried Out on Behalf of the DHSS and the Scottish Home and Health Department by OPCS.* London: HMSO, 1986.

58 Bone, M., Meltzer, H. *The Prevalence of Disability Among Children.* OPCS Surveys of disability in Great Britain. Report 3. London: HMSO, 1989.

59 Coyne, A.M. *Schoolgirl Mothers.* Health Education Council Research Report No. 2. London: HEA, 1986.

60 Balding, J. *Young People in 1988: The Health Related Behaviour Questionnaire Results for 33,459 Pupils between the Ages of 11 and 16.* HEA Schools Health Education Unit and University of Exeter. London: HEA, 1989.

61 Hall, S.M., Glickman, M. Report of the British Paediatric Surveillance Unit. *Arch Dis Child* 1990; **65:** 807–809.

62 Evans, P., Elliott, M., Alberman, E.D., Evans, S. Prevalence and disabilities in 4 to 8 year-olds with cerebral palsy. *Arch Dis Child* 1985; **60:** 940–45.

63 King, K., Ball, D. A holistic approach to accident and injury prevention in children's playgrounds. London: London Scientific Services, 1989.

64 Walsh, S.S., Barton, S. Jarvis, S.N., Clark, W. *Children Injured in Road Traffic Accidents: A Collaborative Project with Northumbria police.* North East regional research laboratory research report 90/3, Centre for Urban and Regional Development Studies.

Newcastle-on-Tyne: University of Newcastle-on-Tyne, 1990.

65 Rigby, M. Child health comes of age – the completed national system. *Brit J Health Care Computing* 1985; **2:** 13–15.

66 Roche, S., Stacey, M. *Overview of Research on the Provision and Utilisation of Child Health Services in the Community*. Warwick: University of Warwick, 1984 and updates 1986, 1987, 1988 and 1991.

67 Department of Health and Social Security, Department of Education and Science, and Welsh Office. *Fit for the Future: Report of the Committee on Child Health Services* (Chairman Professor S.D.M. Court). London: HMSO, 1976.

68 Hall, S. Current epidemiology of childhood infections. In: Alberman, E.D., Peckham, C.S., eds. Childhood Epidemiology. *Br Med Bull* 1986; **42:** 127–130.

69 Office of Population Censuses and Surveys. Social Survey Division. *General Household Survey 1987*. London: HMSO, 1989.

70 Office of Population Censuses and Surveys. *Mortality Statistics 1987*. London: HMSO, 1989.

71 Department of Health and Office of Population Censuses and Surveys. *Hospital In-patient Enquiry 1984*. Summary tables. London: HMSO, 1986.

72 MacFaul, R. Much data but limited information in the NHS. *Arch Dis Child* 1988; **63:** 1276–1280.

73 Bewley, B.R., Walsworth-Bell, J. The inadequacy of adolescent health statistics. *Community Med* 1982; **4:** 97–99.

74 Carstairs, V. Multiple deprivation and health state. *Community Med* 1981; **3:** 4–13.

75 Cuckle, H., Wald, N. The impact of screening for open neural tube defects in England and Wales. *Prenat Diagn* 1987; **7:** 91–99.

76 Office of Population Censuses and Surveys. *Mortality Statistics, Cause 1988*. England and Wales. Series DH2 no. 15. London: HMSO, 1989.

77 Department of Transport. *Children and Roads: a Safer Way*. Government proposals for reducing the number of child casualties on our roads. London: DTI, 1990.

78 White, J., Leon, S. *Cover of Vaccination Evaluated Rapidly: 22* 1992, review no. 8, R 96, 97, 98, 104. Communicable Disease Report 1992. London: CDSC.

79 Begg, N.T., Noah, N.D. Immunisation targets in Europe and Britain. *Br Med J* 1985; **291:** 1370–1371.

80 Anderson, H.R., Bailey, P.A., Cooper, J.S., Palmer, J.C., West, S. Morbidity and school absence caused by asthma and wheezing illness. *Arch Dis Child* 1983; **58:** 777–784.

81 Stacey, M. Realities for change in child health care: existing patterns and future possibilities. *Br Med J* 1980; **280:** 1512–1515.

82 Department of Education and Science and Welsh Office. *Special Educational Needs*. Report of the Committee of Enquiry into the Education of Handicapped Children and Young People (Chairman H.M. Warnock). London: HMSO, 1978.

83 Butler, J.A., Rosenbaum, S., Palfrey, J.S. Ensuring access to health care for children with disabilities. *N Engl J Med* 1987; **317:** 162–165.

84 Kangesu, E., McGowan, M.E.L., Edeh, J. Management of epilepsy in schools. *Arch Dis Child* 1984; **59:** 45–47.

85 Hansard 12th March 1990, Cols. 26–29.

86 Rutter, M., Graham, P., Yule, W. A neuropsychiatric study in childhood. *Clinics in Developmental Medicine 35/36*. London: Heinemann, 1970.

87 Graham, P.J. Behavioural and intellectual development. In: Alberman, E.D., Peckham, C.S., eds. Childhood epidemiology. *Br Med Bull* 1986; **42:** 155–162.

88 Rona, R.J., Chinn, S. The National Study of health and growth: nutritional surveillance of primary school children from 1972 to 1981 with special reference to unemployment and social class. *Ann Hum Biol* 1984; **11:** 17–28.

89 Jobling, M. Anorexia nervosa: a review of research. *National Children's Bureau Highlight no. 63*. London: NCB, 1985.

90 Rutter, M., Cox, A., Tupling, C., Berger, M., Yule, W. Attainment and adjustment in two geographic areas: I, prevalence of psychiatric disorder. *Br J Psychiatr* 1975; **126:** 563–579.

91 Rutter, M., Tizard, J., Whitmore, K. *Education, Health and Behaviour*. London: Longmans, 1970.

92 Research and Statistics Branch of the Inner London Education Authority. *Children's Health: an Analysis of School Entrants' Medical Examinations*. RS 1139/89. London: ILEA, 1989.

93 Armstrong, N., Balding, J., Gentle, P., Kirby, B. Patterns of physical activity among 11 to 16 year old British children. *Br Med J* 1990; **301:** 203–205.

94 Goddard, E. *Smoking among Secondary School Children in England in 1988*. An enquiry carried out by Social Survey Division of OPCS on behalf of the Department of Health. London: HMSO, 1988.

95 British Medical Association, Board of Science and Education. *Young People and Alcohol*. London: BMA, 1986.

96 Havard J. Drunken driving among the young. *Br Med J* 1986; **293:** 774.

97 Ashton, C.H. Solvent abuse: little progress after 20 years. *Br Med J* 1990; **300:** 135–136.

98 Office of Population Censuses and Surveys. *Birth Statistics 1988 for England and Wales*. Series FM1 no. 17. London: HMSO, 1990.

99 Wells, N. Teenage mothers. *European Collaborative Committee for Child Health*. London: Children's Research Fund, 1983.

100 Pugh, G., De'Ath, E. *The Needs of Parents*. London: Macmillan, 1984.

101 National Council for One Parent Families and Community Development Trust. *Pregnant at School*. (Miles Report). London: NCOPF, 1979.

102 Lynch, M., Roberts, J. Early alerting signs. In: Franklin, A.W., ed. *Child Abuse*. Edinburgh: Churchill Livingstone, 1978.

103 Creighton, S.J. *Trends in Child Abuse. Research Briefings nos. 6,7,8*. London: NSPCC, 1984.

104 Baker, A.W., Duncan, S.P. Child sexual abuse: a study of prevalence in Great Britain. *Child Abuse and Neglect* 1985; **9:** 457–467.

105 Troyna, B., Hatcher, R. *Racial Harrassment in Schools*. Highlight no. 92. London: National Children's Bureau with Barnado's, 1990.

106 Commission for Racial Equality. *Learning in Terror*. London: CRE, 1988.

107   Samaranayake, L.P., Pindborg, J.J. Our children's teeth. *Br Med J* 1989; **298:** 272–273.

108   Downer, M.C. Time trends in dental decay in young children. *Health Trends* 1989; **21:** 7–9.

109   Dowell, T.B. The caries experience of five-year-old children in England and Wales. A survey co-ordinated by the British Association for the study of Community Dentistry in 1985–6. *Community Dental Health* 1988; **5:** 185–197.

110   Whitehead, M. *The Health Divide*. Harmondsworth: Penguin, 1988.

111   Balarajan, R. On the state of health in inner London. *Br Med J* 1986; **292:** 911–14.

112   Backett, E.M., Johnston, A.M. Social patterns of road accidents to children: some characteristics of vulnerable families. *Br Med J* 1959; **1:** 409–413.

113   Richman, N., Stevenson, J., Graham, P. *Pre-school to School: a Behavioural Study*. London: Academic Press, 1982.

114   Department of Health. Children's growth and nutrition. In: *On the State of the Public Health for the Year 1988*. London: HMSO, 1989: 74.

115   Hall, A.J., Barker, D.J.P., Dangerfield, P.H., Osmond, C., Taylor, J.F. Small feet and Perthes' disease. *J Bone Joint Surg* 1988; **70B:** 611–13.

116   Committee on Medical Aspects of Food Policy. *Third Report of the Sub-committee on Nutritional Surveillance: Executive Summary*. (Chairman: J.S. Garrow). Reports on health and social subjects; no. 33. London: HMSO, 1988.

117   Platt, S.D., Martin, C.J., Hunt, S.M., Lewis, C.W. Damp housing, mould growth, and symptomatic health state. *Br Med J* 1989; **298:** 1673–1678.

118   Lowry, S. Health and homelessness. *Br Med J* 1990; **300:** 32–34.

119   Constantinides, P., Walker, G. *Child Accidents and Inequality in a London Borough*. Unpublished Report to North East Thames Regional Health Authority. 1986.

120   Black, J. Child health in ethnic minorities. *Br Med J* 1985; **290:** 615–617.

121   Fuller, J.H.S., Toon, P.D. *Medical Practice in a Multicultural Society*. Oxford: Heinemann Medical, 1988.

122   Polnay, L. Research in community child health. *Arch Dis Child* 1989; **64:** 981–983.

123   Pharoah, P.O.D. Impairment, disability, and handicap. *Arch Dis Child* 1990; **65:** 819.

124   World Health Organization. *International Classification of Impairments, Disabilities and Handicaps: a Manual of Classification relating to the Consequences and Disease*. Geneva: WHO, 1980.

Further reading

Abramson, J.H. *Making Sense of Data: A Self-Instruction Manual on the Interpretation of Epidemiological Data*. Oxford: Oxford University Press, 1988.

Alderson, M. *An Introduction to Epidemiology*, 2nd edn. London: Macmillan Press, 1983.

Barker, D.J.P., Rose, G. *Epidemiology in Medical Practice*, 4th edn. Edinburgh: Churchill Livingstone, 1990.

Fletcher, R.H., Fletcher, S.W., Wagner, E.H. *Clinical Epidemiology: the Essentials*. Baltimore: Williams & Wilkins, 1982.

Gehlbach, S.H. *Interpreting the Medical Literature: Practical Epidemiology for Clinicians*, 2nd edn. New York: Collier, Macmillan, 1988.

Kirkwood, B.R. *Essentials of Medical Statistics*. Oxford: Blackwell Scientific Publications, 1988.

Riegelman, R.K., Hirsch, R.P. *Studying a Study and Testing a Test: How to Read the Medical Literature*, 2nd edn. Boston: Little Brown, 1989.

Rothman, K.J. *Modern Epidemiology*. Boston: Little, Brown and Company, 1986.

Chapter 3

Child development

Bridget Edwards and Martin Bellman

Development is defined as a process of revealing, unfolding, making progress or becoming complete, and child development is a term that is usually used by paediatricians to mean the process of maturation of brain function as distinct from physical growth. In contrast to the latter which clearly starts at conception, there is much debate about the point at which the infant has an independent mind. The neuroanatomical development of the brain is discussed in Chapter 10, but the origins and progress of development of neurological function in general, and thought in particular, are poorly understood. In this type of situation multiple hypotheses and explanations thrive and there are numerous theories associated with child development.

Theories of development

Neurological theory

Many paediatricians pay allegiance to the work of Arnold Gesell in the USA who mapped out the stages of child development by observing large numbers of children over several years.[1] He laid great emphasis on the progressive inevitable process of maturation of the central nervous system and related the achievement of *developmental milestones* to this. Gesell was also responsible for first classifying development into four major fields:

1 Motor behaviour – gross and fine movements
2 Adaptive behaviour – reactions to the environment
3 Language behaviour – speech and comprehension
4 Personal-social behaviour – feeding, dressing, toileting etc.

Gesell distinguished between temporary developmental activities, e.g. crawling and a palmar grasp, and permanent activities, e.g. walking and mature manipulation. Skills progress from an undifferentiated gross form to one that is specific and precise. He considered

that child development followed an invariable sequence and any deviation from this indicated abnormality. Because the developmental process is determined by the rate of central nervous system maturation it can be neither prevented nor advanced by artificial processes such as imposed restraints or training.

Well known British followers of the Gesell school include Dr Mary Sheridan[2] and Professor Ronald Illingworth.[3]

Learning theories

Although the neurological basis of child development, as described by Gesell, is undoubtedly a very important framework, the ways that children respond to environmental stimuli change as they accumulate experience. Humans have a great capacity for remembering these experiences and modifying their behaviour through learning. Some psychologists assert that all behaviour is learned. This depends to a large extent upon the experiences that the child encounters (nurture) but must also be affected by the child's genetic and physical constitution (nature).

The process by which humans learn is probably one of the most complex and intriguing natural phenomena. Many theories have been propounded but none can be proved or disproved, perpetuating the current confusion.

1 Stimulus-response theories

These are fundamental to the process of adapting to the environment as all organisms learn by experience; such knowledge as we have is largely derived from animal experimentation. This provides a basis for speculation but extrapolation to the human state must be tentative.

a   REFLEX CONDITIONING

A classical learning experiment was done by the Russian medical physiologist Ivan Pavlov at the end of the 19th century; he described the conditioned reflex of salivation in dogs when a bell was rung even when food with which it had originally been trained was not offered.[4]

The consistency and power of the reflex depends upon frequency and timing of the conditioned and unconditioned stimuli. There are many situations in human life when conditioned reflexes occur, for instance when school children hear the last bell before dinner time they too may start to salivate, even though it may be a considerable time before they get to the table.

b   INSTRUMENTAL CONDITIONING/OPERANT LEARNING

Under this theory, response to a stimulus occurs as a result of reinforcement, which may be positive by giving a reward or negative by giving punishment. The classical experiments in this field were done on rats in a box containing one or more levers. The rat relatively quickly learns to press the lever that delivers food and conversely not to press a lever that delivers an electric shock. Again, it is easy to think of human situations in which operant learning occurs, as a large part of the child development/learning process is based on experience. The principles of positive and negative reinforcement by reward and punishment are well used even if not consciously understood by all parents. They are also the basis for behaviour conditioning or modification therapy which may be carried out if a child has a behavioural disorder needing treatment.

Any conditioned behaviour, whether reflex or instrumental will be extinguished if the response ceases to happen after the stimulus is offered. Moreover powerful reinforcement of adverse behaviour occurs when the relation between the stimulus and response is variable and the anticipated response only happens inconsistently. An example of this is the child who is refused a treat on some occasions but not others and who therefore comes to know that if he makes his stimulus long, loud and frequent enough he will get what he wants. The most effective way for parents to maintain firm control is for them to be consistent in their management.

2   Piaget

A very important pioneer in the field of cognitive development was Jean Piaget, a Swiss zoologist who initially made detailed observations and descriptions of the development of his own children and then carried this technique into nurseries and schools. From precise notes on the behaviour of many hundreds of children functioning and interacting in everyday situations, he evolved a detailed account of development at progressive ages.[5,6]

a   SENSORI-MOTOR STAGE

During this period the child is experiencing sensations from the environment and learning to distinguish self from others especially the mother. The following phases are seen:

i) Reflex actions – in the first month of life there is virtually no voluntary control over responses.
ii) Habituation – from approximately 1 to 4 months of age the child develops schemata to repeat sequences of actions which produce pleasurable responses (primary circular actions). In the period from about 4 to 9 months of age, intention is introduced into the schemata in order to produce the most satisfying result (secondary circular actions).
iii) Coordination – between the ages of about 9 and 12 months, actions and schemata are coordinated through a trial and error type of process. Increasing mobility and memory for previous experiences allow more complex schemata to develop.
iv) Experimentation – the child actively tries out alternative actions from 12 to 18 months of age and modifies strategies (tertiary circular actions).
v) Internalization of schemata – at approximately 18 to 24 months of age the child thinks through ways of dealing with problems using rapidly increasing levels of experience and knowledge.

b   CONCRETE OPERATIONS STAGE

i) Realism and symbolism – between 2 and 4 years the child sees the world as unchangeable and related directly to self or personal thoughts. The child learns about models, pictures and eventually words as symbols of real life – which can be manipulated.
ii) Intuitive thought – from the age of 4 to 7 years language is rapidly expanding and social relationships with others (especially children in school) are developing. Thinking necessarily becomes more complicated and sophisticated.
iii) Concrete operations – between 7 and 12 years old the child begins to understand about sequences, comparisons and processes and to integrate thoughts into overall plans in order to deal with increasingly complex situations.

c   FORMAL OPERATIONS STAGE

From approximately 12 years onwards the child progressively develops understanding of concepts and abstract ideas. Learning includes adoption of systematic approaches to problem solving, deductive reasoning, hypothesis forming and testing.

Psychoanalytical theories

Interwoven with mental development is the development of the personality or *psyche*. This is an extremely important component of behaviour and is therefore a crucial factor in any child's development.

1 Freud

Probably the most famous psychoanalyst who worked in the field of child development was Sigmund Freud. He traced the origins of sexuality back to childhood and described three basic components of personality development: the *Id* which contains the unorganized unconscious drives; the *Ego* which is the organized rational part of the mind and the *Super-ego* which is akin to the conscience.[7] As these psychological areas emerge the child goes through several different stages of infant sexuality during which the personality can be affected by experiences and conflicts.[8]

a ORAL STAGE

During the first year of life gratification is gained mainly through the mouth via the mother. Satisfaction leads on to optimism, but dependence and conversely dissatisfaction to pessimism and resentment.

b ANAL STAGE

From 1 to 3 years, pleasure comes from faecal excretion. Conflict and repression at this time can be a precursor of an obsessive personality who retains and hoards things.

c PHALLIC STAGE

Between 3 and 5 years of age, the child enjoys genital exploration and stimulation. The oedipal complex is a crucial part of this phase especially in boys. Inhibition during this stage may lead to sexual fears or alternatively exhibitionism.

d LATENT PERIOD

From 5 to around 12 years, there is a latent period followed by a genital stage up to approximately 18 years of age during which adult sexuality evolves.

Freud had many pupils and followers some of whom broke away and formed their own schools of analytic psychology. Two of the most eminent of these were Carl Jung who explored the primitive symbolic archetypes (anima/animus)[9] and Alfred Adler who described the concept of the inferiority complex.[10] Two other child psychoanalysts of particular significance were Anna Freud (Sigmund's daughter)[11] and Melanie Klein who developed further the method of *transference* of feelings held by the patient onto the analyst.[12] More recently an important practical contribution was made by Donald Winnicott who related child psychological theories to child rearing practices and problems.[13,14]

2 Erikson

Although Eric Erikson was trained in the Freudian school he described a psychoanalytical theory of child development which moved beyond the classical mother–father–child triangle to a dynamic personal–social model of a child coming to terms with changing situations and reality.[15] His theory covers development from birth to old age. Passage from one stage to the next depends on reaching an equilibrium between conflicting influences. Behavioural responses result from the state of the balance that has been achieved. Failure to reach equilibrium creates anxieties and stresses, which may last into adulthood.

a STAGE 1 – TRUST/MISTRUST

During the first months of life the infant is totally dependent for his needs. Satisfaction leads to confidence, trust and bonding with the carers. Failure may lead to difficult behaviour and poor emotional attachments and relationships.

b STAGE 2 – AUTONOMY/SELF-DOUBT/RESTRICTION

From 1 to 3 years old, the child becomes aware of his own strength and will, as well as the conflicting need to conform to authority which brings a sense of security. He needs to balance his will against the external restraints provided by the will of others. Failure to achieve an equilibrium may cause a lack of confidence or alternatively overconfidence and inability to conform.

c STAGE 3 – SENSE OF INITIATIVE AND GUILT

Between ages 3 to 5 years the child steps away from parental control and explores group situations. He experiences sharing as well as initiation of autonomous behaviour which may be in conflict with the needs of others. This can cause guilt feelings and conscience develops. It is also the age of emerging sexual curiosity.

d STAGE 4 – SENSE OF INDUSTRY AND COMPETENCE

During the primary school period (5 to 11 years) play becomes less important and the child develops drive and a competitive spirit. He starts to relate to adults other than his parents. The balance of success or failure may be a precursor of an inferiority/superiority complex which may cause learning and relationship difficulties.

e STAGE 5 – SENSE OF IDENTITY

In adolescence a readiness to face the world develops, with long-term perspectives of examinations and career prospects. Sexual identity also develops and understanding of the need for a leadership role. Self-doubt, uncertainties and identity difficulties may result from failure to achieve appropriate balances.

f STAGE 6 – ADULT VALUES

After adolescence personal emotions such as intimacy and love develop. An individual learns to care for others and becomes prepared for parenthood. The right balances in this stage lead to emotional satisfaction, integrity and wisdom.

Communication and language

These skills are crucial aspects of child development and cannot be separated from consideration of the developing mind and personality. High level language is one of the skills that is unique to humans (another is fine complex manipulation) and not surprisingly it has been studied in detail. A great deal of descriptive information is available but, for obvious reasons, there is little knowledge about the exact neurophysiological basis for language processing. Epidemiological studies of language development have allowed the construction of centile charts which enable a child's linguistic status to be defined and a prediction of likely future achievement to be made.[16] Charts for expressive and receptive language development are shown in Figure 3.1. Linguistic milestones can be plotted longitudinally and consistent attainment of milestones later than the 10th percentile indicates that the child is at risk of language and cognitive delay.

One of the major influences in the field of the theoretical basis of language development came from the work of Jean Piaget who argued that language developed in parallel with general cognitive development and could not be in advance of the child's conceptual understanding. Accordingly, language development goes through similar stages to those described above for cognitive development. Clearly, these processes must be interdependent as thought requires some form of language and vice versa. The interdependence is also true in relation to measurement of cognition, which is carried out by communication even if nonverbal since this also relies upon inner language.

The classical theory of language acquisition based on piagetian principles was that it is a behavioural process of listening, imitation and reinforcement. Children learn to talk by copying sounds that they hear, and by trial and error find that modifying their own vocalizations based on adult models will get them desired responses. However this theory was dis-

puted, in particular by the American linguist Noam Chomsky, who suggested that humans are born with an innate capacity for language development.[17] When the child is exposed to appropriate triggers this *language acquisition device* starts to operate. An analogy can be made to a microcomputer that contains a dedicated processor which is ready and waiting to be programmed before it can work. Evidence for this theory comes from studies of children who have been abusively deprived of language stimulation in early life. When they are exposed to normal language they develop the skill very quickly without going through the drawn out stages shown by normally developing children.[18]

The comparison with a computer can also be stretched to cover some specific language abnormalities such as dyspraxia or dyslexia, as well as motor disorders such as clumsiness. If the brain is considered to be a wired-up processor, the defects could be due to a bug in the system which prevents the use of a specific circuit. The function can then only be performed by following an alternative pathway which produces a less efficient or satisfactory result. These alternative circuits can be improved by practice (therapy), but the bug may not be eliminated.

The acquisition of communication and language is a good example of a skill dependent upon the competence of skills in other developmental fields. Reynell and Huntley[19] devised a model for verbal communication; Figure 3.2 shows this in a modified form and its various interactions with other abilities. From this it can be seen that impairment in virtually any developmental field may adversely affect communication.

Developmental progress

Neurodevelopment begins before birth and the newborn baby already has a wide range of well developed skills. For instance, fetuses move in utero, sometimes quite vigorously. Fetoscopy has shown that these movements can be fairly well coordinated and that the fetus also sucks, licks and swallows, opens its eyes, and can hear and startle to loud sudden noises. The birth process sets off a series of physiological changes and provided that the baby is at a suitable stage of development, it adapts almost immediately to extrauterine life. Schemes for determining gestational age at birth such as the Dubowitz score[20] are, in effect, methods of performing developmental assessment on newborn babies. This requires both observation of physical characteristics and of neurodevelopmental signs and reflex activity. Useful assessment techniques more neurologically orientated are the Brazelton behavioural score[21] and the Prechtl examination.[22] These are claimed to correlate with future neurodevelopmental progress.

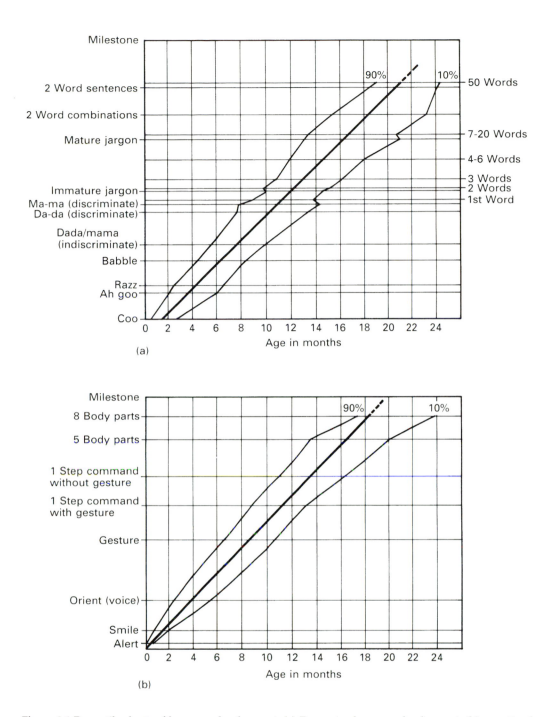

Figure 3.1 Percentile charts of language development. (a) Expressive language development; (b) receptive language development. 90th and 10th percentiles for normative population. Infants whose attainment of milestones is consistently later than the 10th percentile are at risk of language and cognitive delay.

Primitive and secondary responses

The normal newborn infant has a number of primitive or primary inherent responses most of which wane after 2–4 months so that their absence in the neonatal period or their presence after 6 months may be evidence of abnormal cerebral maturation. Most of these responses are mediated at subcortical level and some are even demonstrable in anencephalics. As the primary responses disappear, secondary inherent responses appear and persist in part in normal older children.

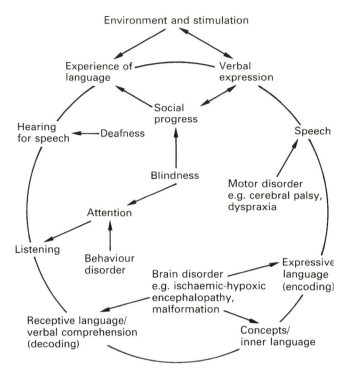

Figure 3.2 Verbal communication pathway: cycle of language processing shows interactions with other developmental factors. Modified from Reynell 1987.[19]

1 Primitive responses

a MORO REFLEX

This is evoked by a sudden movement of the head on the shoulders. It can be produced by jarring the cot, sudden extension of the head by dropping it through 2.0 cm, or holding and extending the arms and suddenly releasing them. Both arms are extended, then flex over the chest in an embrace type reaction (Fig. 3.3). The response may include flexing of the legs and crying; it should be symmetrical and the hands fully open. An asymmetrical response is suggestive of a hemiplegia or brachial plexus lesion. Absence of the Moro reflex in the mature neonate or persistence after 6 months strongly suggests cerebral dysfunction.

b THE EYE RIGHTING REFLEX

When the neck is flexed, extended or rotated (doll's eye manoeuvre) the eyes should move in the direction of rotation of the head. This is the oculovestibular eye-righting reflex; its emergence may be delayed for a few weeks in normal premature and full-term infants, so that its absence at this age (in which the eyes stay still or even appear to move in the opposite direction to rotation) may be part of normal development, but could signify brain stem damage. Persistent absence of the reflex is certainly pathological. Failure to

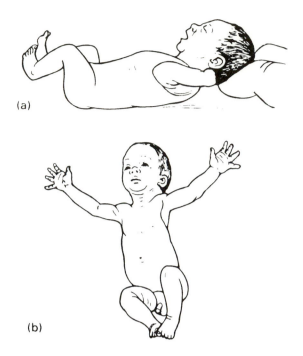

Figure 3.3 The Moro reflex: (a) one method of elicitation; (b) normal response.

demonstrate the reflex in a comatose patient is known as the doll's eye movement.

c THE TRACTION RESPONSE

When the baby is lying supine and the trunk is pulled upward by traction on the wrists, the head is pulled into the neutral position soon after the shoulders leave the couch.

d PLACING REFLEX

For this the infant is held vertically and the dorsum of the feet brought against the side of a hard surface. The baby lifts each foot up in turn and places it on the hard surface. This may be present in the newborn baby, is easily elicited at 6 weeks, usually disappears by about 4 months but may persist into the second year (Fig. 3.4).

e POSITIVE SUPPORTING REACTION

When the baby is lowered onto a surface and touches it, both legs are extended at the knees followed by trunk extension. There is usually some hip flexion (Fig. 3.5). The response disappears by 4 months. There is not much actual weight bearing to the reaction. In fact, if extension in the supporting reaction is very marked, and flexion in the placing response is very slight, it indicates increased extensor tone in the legs as seen in spasticity.

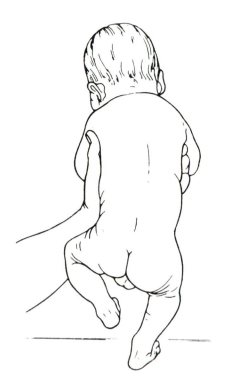

Figure 3.4 The placing reflex.

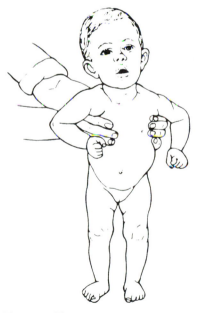

Figure 3.5 The positive supporting reaction.

f PRIMARY STEPPING RESPONSE

If the newborn infant is leaned forward in the vertically supported position, flexion of the legs and alternate stepping actions occur (Fig. 3.6). The response disappears by 2 months of age, but can be elicited for longer if leant forward to 45° and the head passively extended.

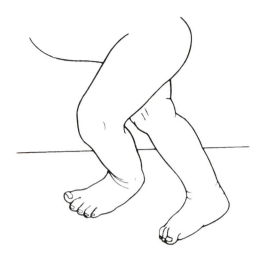

Figure 3.6 The primary stepping response.

g PALMAR AND PLANTAR GRASP REFLEXES

In the first 2 months the hands are tightly closed with the thumb under the fingers. The newborn infant will firmly grasp a small object placed in the palm and can support most of its body weight in this way (Fig. 3.7). The reflex is strongest in the first few weeks and may have declined in strength by 6 weeks. By 3–4 months it has usually disappeared, after which the hands are open more of the time and beginning to reach for objects in voluntary grasp. Persistent fisting after 2 months is abnormal and if unilateral suggests hemiparesis. Testing for the palmar grasp is conveniently combined with testing the traction response. In this the baby's hands firmly grasp the examiner's fingers and head control can be observed. As the baby is lifted forwards, the head is brought to the vertical position, though there is usually some head lag in the early stages. The plantar grasp is elicited by pressure with a finger at the base of the toes (Fig. 3.7). This response persists until 9 or 10 months but must disappear before standing or walking can be established, just as the grasp response has to disappear around 3 months before active prehension can develop.

h ASYMMETRIC TONIC NECK REFLEX (ATNR)

This is tested by rotating the head to either side in the supine position while keeping the shoulders flat. The limbs on the face side extend and those on the occipital side flex. It is usually present at birth but is more consistent at 6 weeks and becomes absent by the age of 6 months (Fig. 3.8).

2 Secondary response

These mainly emerge progressively from 4 months as the primary responses fade though a few are

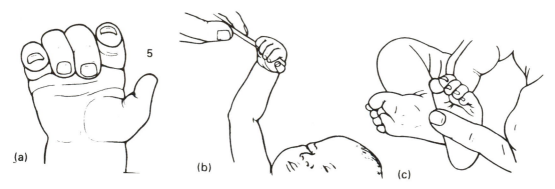

Figure 3.7 The grasp reflex: (a) sequence of finger flexion; (b) tonic component of the palmar grasp reflex; (c) plantar grasp reflex.

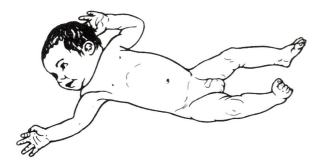

Figure 3.8 The asymmetrical tonic neck reflex.

demonstrable earlier. They form the basis for the subsequent development of locomotion.

a HEAD RIGHTING AND BALANCE REACTIONS

These occur in the *opposite* direction to the displacing force, and they keep the head and body properly orientated in space. If the body is tilted, the head is righted with the mouth and the eyes horizontal and the head vertical. The body then comes in line with the head (Fig. 3.9). Head control or head balance is the first necessity for sitting and walking. The extension of the head seen at 10 weeks with the infant in vertical suspension is a head righting response. Sideways balance is tested by holding the infant vertically and then tilting slowly to one side. From 4 months the head will be brought back to the vertical if the trunk is tilted through 30°. Later the lower limbs are also brought back to the vertical in order to keep centre of gravity of the baby vertically above its base. These reactions are demonstrable from 4 months but are only used later as the baby adjusts to sitting, crawling and standing.

b ROLLING

In this the trunk, on neck righting response, changes so that the pelvic and pectoral girdles respond separately.

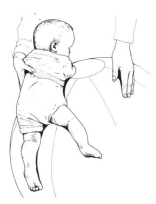

Figure 3.9 The head righting reaction.

If the head is turned, the hips and legs turn, followed by the shoulders. Or if the pelvis is rotated, the head turns followed by the shoulders. This is how the infant learns to roll.

c THE PROTECTIVE REACTIONS

Unlike the balancing reactions, these occur in the *same* direction as the displacing force. Under the age of 4 months, an infant held vertically and moved suddenly downwards reacts with a Moro reflex, over the age of 5 months infants displaced forwards and downwards usually extend and abduct the lower limbs. Their arms simultaneously show sideways, then forward and backward extension. This is the downward parachute (Fig. 3.10). If the legs adduct in the downward parachute, the child may have spastic diplegia. Sideways propping reactions appear in a sitting position at 7–8 months, and backwards propping at 10–12 months (Fig. 3.11). Severely delayed children may appear to walk with trunk and hands held, but until they have good balancing and propping responses, they cannot walk alone.

Examination of the primitive and secondary responses should be an integral part of the neurodevelopmental assessment of any infant at birth, 6 weeks and later in the first year of life.

An abnormal child will usually show several abnormal features and the combination of the neurological signs with the developmental profile can give good diagnostic information. The value of the responses lies in several ways; they correlate with gestational age regardless of birthweight. They allow comparison of one side of the body with the other since they are mainly bilateral responses. Persistence of the primary responses beyond the prescribed time, abnormal extensor tone or failure of emergence of the secondary responses is very suggestive of neurodevelopmental abnormality, of which the most common is cerebral palsy. The primitive responses each imply a defect along that pathway, e.g. as seen in the asymmetrical Moro reflex of a child with a hemiplegia or in disorders of the fourth and fifth lumbar roots supplying sensation to the dorsum of the feet.

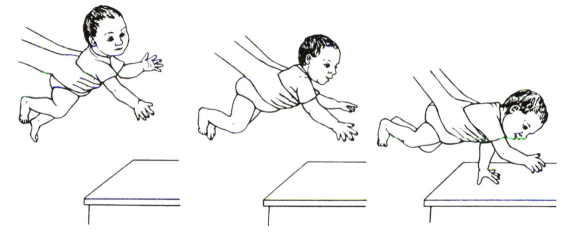

Figure 3.10 The protective reaction of downward parachute.

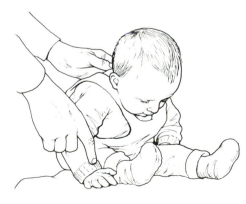

Figure 3.11 Sideways propping response.

Individual variations and patterns of development

In studying infant and child development, Illingworth's advice,[3] that children are different, should be remembered. To this could be added the fact that nearly all children are normal and very few are completely average in all respects.

Developmental progress is not a simple matter of reaching milestones in a uniform and predictable manner. It should be viewed as a continuous process that reflects the maturation of a child, but which also varies between individuals with regard to the rate of progress, and the specific developmental pattern (or normal variant) followed. The latter is particularly relevant in gross motor development.

Holt used the terms 'initial age' and 'limit age' to describe either side of the mean age at which an ability is acquired.[23] This is a useful concept, particularly the limit age for the acquisition of a skill, as delay in acquisition beyond this age will indicate the need for further assessment (Table 3.1). The limit age also denotes the time by which certain activities should have ceased, and their persistence beyond the stated age is a definite warning sign that development is not progressing normally. In addition, the rate of progress may vary greatly over time, unlike physical growth whose velocity normally follows a smooth curve. This is particularly true of the development of language. A lull of some months when few new words have been uttered may be followed by a rapid increase in words and sentences.

Robson[25-27] described the different locomotor patterns that children show in their progress towards independent walking. The majority (83%) proceed direct to crawling and then to walking; 1% roll and 1% creep before walking with only a short period crawling before standing and walking; 9% bottom shuffle prior to walking, and 6% 'just stand up and walk'. Individuals in both these last two groups rarely crawl, and often exhibit similar locomotor patterns to other family members, suggesting locomotor patterns are an expression of a familial non-crawl tendency. Robson[25] compiled initial, mean and limit ages of normal motor milestones for children with the different locomotor patterns (Table 3.2) demonstrating that the limit age for achieving independent walking in creepers is 27 months, in shufflers 28 months while for crawlers it is 15 months. Crawlers and the 'just stand up and walk' group sit significantly earlier than shufflers, creepers and rollers. This wide variation in the rate of progress makes it important in judging the normality of an individual's progress to use the norms for a specific locomotor pattern and not total population norms.

Individual fields of development, gross motor, fine motor and vision, hearing and language, social and emotional, will usually progress in parallel. When this does not happen, and one field lags considerably behind the others, a child is said to have a specific developmental delay. If development in all fields is occurring more slowly than the norm, the child is said to be showing global developmental delay. Isolated delay or advancement in one field, especially motor, does not necessarily correlate with subsequent overall progress. A child who walks relatively early may later prove to have significant learning difficulties. Advanced language development is however common in bright children while delayed language development is often found in slow learners. An abnormality in one area may also have a very profound effect on an otherwise normal area, for example

Table 3.1 Limit ages

Age	Ability which should be present	Activity which should have ceased
4 weeks	Noticing things	
6 weeks	Responsive smile	
3 months	Good head control	
4 months		Fisting of hands
5 months	Reaching for objects	Hand regard
6 months		ATNR
7 months	Purposive grasp of objects	
10 months	Sits unsupported	
18 months	Walks alone	Casting, mouthing and drooling
	Says single words with meaning	

ATNR: asymmetric tonic neck reflex
Modified from table 12.3 in Holt 1991.[24]

Table 3.2 The influence of early motor patterns on ages for sitting, crawling, standing and walking*[25]

Motor activity	Early walkers (approx. 85–95% of children)		Late walkers (approx. 10–15% of children)		
	'Just stands and walks'	Crawlers	Rollers	Creepers	Shufflers
Sitting	5–7–11	5–7–9	6–8–10	6–9–12	7–12–15
Crawling	–	6–9–12	11–14–17	12–15–19	–
Shuffling	–	–	–	–	7–12–16
Getting to standing	8–10–13	7–10–13	12–15–20	11–19–24	10–18–26
Walking	8–11–14	11–13–15	14–18–26	15–20–27	12–19–28

*The figures refer to ages in months and are given in the order: initial–mean–limit ages.

the delayed motor progress seen in a child who is blind.

In assessing a child's development, it is essential to take into account all those factors known to affect it. Thus, a thorough history must always be taken including perinatal and family history and details of the environment within which the child is being reared. Prematurity delays the chronological age at which developmental stages are reached; and they should therefore be considered in relation to the gestational age at least during the first year of life.[28] The greater the degree of prematurity the longer some allowance must be made for it, and if there have also been perinatal problems a decision as to whether these have produced additional sequelae can be difficult to assess.[29]

Familial patterns of late walking and talking are seen but, in addition, parental attitudes, expectations and abilities will have a considerable influence on the child's developmental progress. Information about the child's environment may be best obtained from the health visitor, general practitioner or from home visits. This is particularly true when the social circumstances of the family are likely to be affecting the child's progress. The way in which one family can surmount the problems of living in crowded temporary accommodation may be very different to that of another family, and it should never be assumed that such conditions are inevitably disadvantageous.

The profile a child presents will reflect the test environment and also the state of both the parents and the child. A young child who is hungry or tired and who would normally be having sleep at the time of the assessment, is not likely to perform well. Recent bad experiences in an accident and emergency department, ill health, parental conflict, or anxiety may all make the assessment of a child's development very difficult. The attitude of the doctor is extremely important as well as the environment provided for the assessment. Time spent just observing a child, and gaining the confidence of the parents before approaching the child is always well spent.

Stages of development

Developmental progress is described here in four main stages, the choice being influenced principally by the work of Gesell,[30] together with the later interpretations and additions made to his observations by Illingworth,[3] Holt[24] and Brett.[31] The appropriate chapters in their works are much recommended for further reading, together with the accounts they give of the European and American workers involved in the study of the neonatal period.

The first and fourth stages are further subdivided into three sections and in each part there is an overall picture of the infant or child, describing social behaviour and interaction with family, peers and the examiner. A short account of the development in each field follows and also shows how development in the different fields is interrelated. Each stage is summarized in a table, which shows the age range over which particular milestones or abilities can be expected to appear.

The stages of development chosen are:

1 From birth to 16 weeks   see Table 3.3
2 From 4 to 10 months   see Table 3.4
3 From 12 to 24 months   see Table 3.5
4 From 2 to 5 years   see Table 3.6

1 Birth to 16 weeks (Table 3.3)

a From birth to 6 weeks

Gesell described the human infant as being 'not fully born until about 4 weeks of age' and it is true that the activities of a newborn are predominantly sleeping, waking, crying for feeds and feeding.[30] A lot of activity at this stage is reflex in nature but studies since Gesell have also shown that, in addition to primitive reflexes, the newborn infant also possesses considerable visual, auditory and perceptual abilities. These are seen in the infant's close visual attention to the mother's face, the quietening and calming that occurs in response to a soothing low voice and to the physical comfort that results from being held and cuddled. Feeding is one of the earliest situations when signs of pleasure are seen, with spreading and small twitching movements of the fingers and toes often occurring during feeding. Occasionally a responsive smile is seen in the first days or week but more often after 3 or 4 weeks of age. Responses to sound are usually by a startle reaction, crying or stilling if previously crying. It is some time before the baby can turn its head towards the source of the sound but looking towards sounds is occasionally seen in the early weeks.

The natural posture for the newborn, and indeed for some weeks to come, is flexion (Fig. 3.12). Lying on the side is the most usual position for babies, initially with the arms and legs flexed, but if laid supine with the head to the side, the asymmetric tonic neck reflex (ATNR) posture will be seen. The limbs are also flexed in the prone position so that the pelvis is raised high from the couch with the knees drawn up under the abdomen. The head cannot be raised against gravity in this position but will turn to the side to avoid suffocation, and in ventral suspension or when pulled to sit from supine the baby's head will hang down limply or loll backwards. Posture, tone and movements should be symmetrical and spontaneous movements will often be quite tremulous and jerky with occasional sudden extensions in the absence of any provocation. Symmetry of movement is also well seen at this age by eliciting the Moro reflex. The palmar and plantar grasp reflexes are demonstrable and also the

Table 3.3 Summary of development: birth to 16 weeks

	0–4 Weeks	6–8 Weeks	12–16 Weeks
Social	Watches mother and may smile	Responsive smile by 6 weeks and vocalizes	Recognizes family, shows pleasure
Motor			
Ventral Suspension	Head hangs down until 3–4 weeks then up momentarily	Head held in horizontal plane, and briefly up by 8 weeks	Head maintained well above plane of body by 12 weeks
Prone	Head to side, pelvis high, knees drawn up under abdomen	Chin up intermittently at 6 weeks, well up at 8 weeks. Pelvis flat	Head and shoulders up, and chest by 16 weeks. Weight on forearms
Supine	Head to side, limbs flexed or ATNR posture	ATNR posture common but head to midline by 8 weeks	ATNR declining. Head and hands now to midline
Pull-to-sit	Complete head lag	Less head lag	Slight head lag
Held sitting	Very round back. Head drops forward	Back rounded. Head briefly up	Back straighter and head up
Held standing	Walking and placing reflexes present until 6 weeks	Sags at hips and knees, getting head up by 8 weeks	Increasingly bears weight on legs
Hands	Strong grasp reflex. Hands often closed	Grasp reflex present but slight by 8 weeks. Fingers extend more often	Grasp reflex fades between 12 and 16 weeks. Can hold rattle briefly
Vision	Blink and pupil reflexes. Eye righting reflex. Random movements but can fixate	Smoother conjugate eye movements. Fixates on face /objects and follows through 45°–90°	Follows through 130°. Hand regard common. (12–20 weeks)
Vocalization/hearing	Cries, stills or startles to sounds	Eyes turn to sounds. Starts vocalizing	Varied coos, squeals and laughs. Turns to sounds

ATNR: asymmetric tonic neck reflex

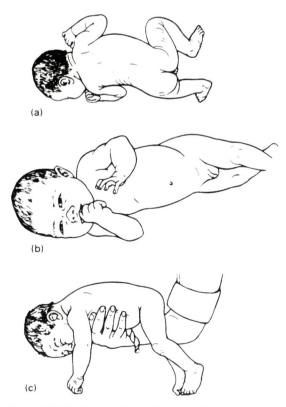

(a)

(b)

(c)

Figure 3.12 Newborn baby in (a) prone, (b) supine and (c) ventral suspension.

traction response. At rest the hands are often in a closed position but the thumb should not be adducted across the palm. The fingers increasingly open in the first 3 or 4 weeks and the stepping and placing reflexes are present.

b 6–8 weeks

At 6 weeks the normal baby's ability to fix its gaze on the mother's face, visual awareness and ability to smile are very notable features. Smiling usually develops a little earlier than this and if not present until after 6 weeks this raises suspicion of developmental delay. Between 6 and 8 weeks the baby who is talked to starts to respond with smiles accompanied by vocalizations.

The flexed posture and reflex responses still predominate but spontaneous movements start to become a little smoother. Head lag is decreasing on traction, though still considerable at 8 weeks, and the head can certainly be held up against gravity in both ventral suspension and prone positions. The ATNR is still often seen at rest in the supine position but, by 8 weeks, the head is starting to come to the midline intermittently (Fig. 3.13). The stepping reflex begins to wane but the palmar grasp reflex is still present at 6 weeks though lessening at 8 weeks, and the hands

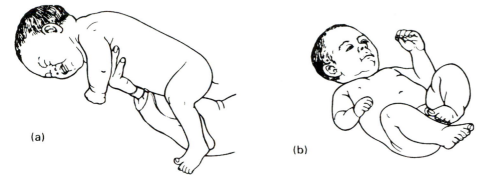

Figure 3.13 Six-week-old baby in (a) ventral suspension and (b) placed in supine position.

are becoming more frequently open. The Moro reflex is still easily elicited for some weeks yet.

c 12–16 weeks

By this age the baby is able to recognize the mother and other members of the family, show a lot of interest in events going on around and recognize familiar situations. The infant loves being propped up to look at everything that is going on, and being chatted to; observing meal preparations may cause huge excitement with wild movements of all limbs and an increased respiration rate. Vocalizations increase and are made in response to being spoken to, and they include cooing and gurgling noises, squeals of pleasure and laughing aloud.

In the motor field, the infant is gradually emerging from the predominantly flexed position so that the head, then the shoulders and then the chest can be raised up from the prone position and supported on the forearms by 16 weeks (Fig. 3.14). The pelvis is also lying quite flat by then with the legs extended. Complete head control has not developed but there is only very slight head lag at the start of pulling a 16 week old to sit. In the sitting position the head is erect but a little wobbly, and the back is also straightening up though still rounded in the lumbar region. Held stand-

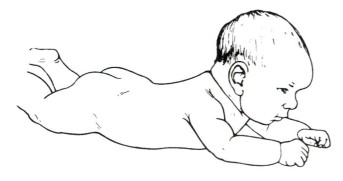

Figure 3.14 Three-month-old baby in prone position.

ing, the sagging knees of the 6–8 week baby are now straightening though full weight bearing is not possible yet.

The ability to use the hands to explore and hold objects is still at a very early stage but needs to be considered along with both gross motor progress and visual development. By 3 months the baby can focus and follow near objects. The eyes can move vertically and horizontally from side to side through 180° and can converge on near objects such as the feeding bottle. The baby looks at the hand stretched out to the side in the ATNR posture, but when the hands start to come more often to the midline, so too the gaze focuses on them. This stage of hand regard is very characteristic of the supine infant from 12 to 20 weeks, but should not persist after that age.

Visual awareness is now intense and the baby will often scrutinize small objects such as a cube or a pellet as small as 8 mm in size. It is another 3 or 4 weeks before the hand can successfully reach out and grasp an object. This purposive grasping cannot develop until the grasp reflex disappears, which occurs gradually between 12 and 16 weeks. By 16 weeks the hands can be brought together and will hold an object like a rattle if it is placed in them.

2 Four to 10 months (Table 3.4)

After 4 months the infant becomes increasingly responsive and able to initiate actions such as raising arms to get picked up, and enjoys attracting attention by vocalizing or shaking his rattle. Differentiation between family and strangers starts to occur but may not include the latter until about 9 months. Interest in others includes own mirror image to whom he may smile and vocalize. At this age the infant will also start to wave goodbye, but really just as an imitative game rather than a proper farewell, and play pat-a-cake or clap hands.

After 4 months when the primitive responses have largely faded, the secondary responses essential for the attainment of mobility start to appear. The labyrinthine head righting reflex develops from 2 to 3

Table 3.4 Summary of development: 4–10 months

	4–6 Months	6–8 Months	8–10 Months
Personal and social behaviour	Responsive to all comers	Discriminates between family and strangers	Wary of strangers
	Smiles at self in mirror	Attracts attention	Waves bye-bye
	Excited at approach of food	Hand feeds biscuit	Attempts to use spoon
Gross motor	No head lag in traction	Lifts head up in supine	Sits steadily, pivots and leans
	Rolls prone to supine	Rolls supine to prone/creeps	Can get from prone to sitting
	Back straight in supported sitting	Sits without lateral support. Bears weight on feet (5–8 months)	Pulls self to stand and crawls
Fine motor and vision	Reaches and grasps toys (4–6 months). Plays with toes	Transfers cube hand to hand (5–7 months). Can hold two cubes	Pincer grasp of pellet (8–12 months). Releases object and looks for it (7–11 months)
	Very alert visually	Any squint reported after 6 months is abnormal	Points at 1 mm sweet
Language and hearing	Varied sounds and squeals. Consonants such as ba or da	Starts to babble da-da. Turns to sounds (4–8 months)	Varied babble ma-ma, ba-ba, da-da. Indicates and understands 'No'. Locates sounds well

months, and this is followed and reinforced by the neck righting and then the body righting reflexes, from about 7 months. Other protective reactions are also developing – the downward and forward parachute, and the propping or saving reactions in sitting. This sequence with the ability to control the position of the head against gravity, and to balance, is essential for the development of the basic motor skills of rolling, crawling, sitting and then standing and walking.

It is at this age that different locomotor patterns, or locomotor variants, influence the rate of motor progress. Before these normal variants were so well described by Robson,[26] they were often a cause of anxiety both to parents and doctors. This is particularly the case with bottom shufflers who tend to be hypotonic in the lower limbs, have a great dislike of being placed in a prone position, and when held up to bear weight on their legs tend not to do so, but flex the legs at the hips so that they are in a position known as sitting on air. These less common but normal variants must be well understood and distinguished from motor disorders which are the cause in about half of the 3% of children who are still not walking at the age of 18 months.[32] The distinction is difficult but important when for example cerebral palsy occurs in a child who is also a shuffler. A more detailed review of these late-walking children, both normal and abnormal, has been made by Chaplais.[32]

In the prone position, prior to crawling, the ability to raise the chest and abdomen gradually increases (Fig. 3.15) until the weight is supported on the hands with extended arms (24 weeks) and on just one hand a month or so later. At the same ages the baby can roll

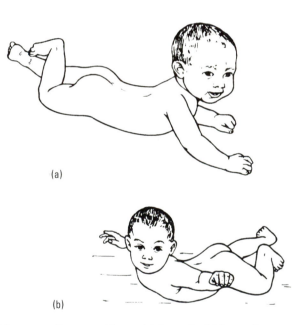

Figure 3.15 Prone position at (a) 6 months (b) 8 months.

first from prone to supine, and then in the reverse direction. Crawling on hands and knees with the abdomen off the floor is usually preceded for a few weeks by creeping, often backwards at first, before pulling himself forwards (also known as hauling or scooting).

By the age of 5–6 months the baby can sit quite well, supported just at the back, and from this position can reach out and grasp objects voluntarily and soon transfer them from hand to hand. These skills can also be

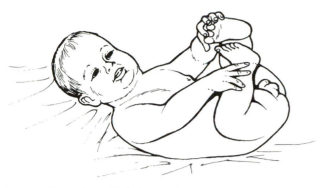

Figure 3.16 Playing with feet in supine.

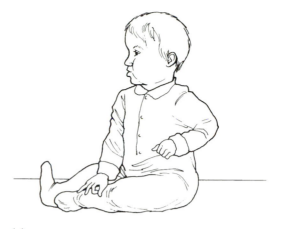

(a)

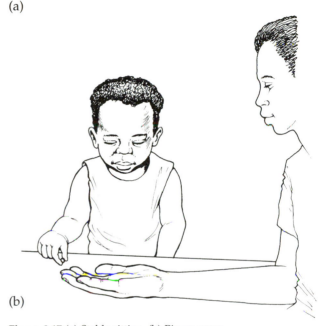

(b)

Figure 3.17 (a) Stable sitting. (b) Pincer grasp.

used for feeding with a piece of bread or biscuit. When lying supine at this age, the infant will also bring the feet up and grasp them with his hands (Fig. 3.16), and both the feet and objects may be put into the mouth. Persisting hand regard at this age, instead of these exploratory manipulative activities, is abnormal.

Sitting gradually becomes entirely stable (Fig. 3.17a) and the manipulation of objects increasingly accurate and adept. The palmar grasp using the ulnar side of the hand at 6 months gradually becomes more radial and the neat pincer grasp between the finger and thumb should be well developed by 9 months (Fig. 3.17b). The permanence of objects is now established so the baby will look for a fallen toy. However, it is not until around 10 months that an object can be released voluntarily though still not with any control over where it is placed. Vocalization increases with babble starting at 5–6 months and at this age there is some definite pre-verbal communication, though not with any real understanding of words as such, but more of social expression and tone of voice. By 9 months the babble is polysyllabic and often very tuneful and by then the baby may both understand 'no' or shake the head to indicate 'no', and will certainly recognize his name.

Eight to 9 months is the age commonly chosen for a distraction hearing test; this test is also a useful, quick screen of the child's development as a whole. The child must be able to sit stably in order to turn the head and shoulders round to each side and accurately and quickly locate the position of the sound, whether it is on a level with the ear or somewhat above or below. Two months earlier, the child would have required two stages to locate sounds which were not at the ear level, first turning to the side and then downwards, rather than the one diagonal movement which should be seen at 8–9 months. A sound made directly above the infant's head at this age would be quite puzzling for another month or so. The distraction hearing test needs to be carried out quickly and skilfully before the child gets bored and wants to interact to show how he too can wield the rattle.

3 Twelve to 24 months (Table 3.5)

At the end of the first year of life, the child has become very much a member of the family, liking to be near a parent or sibling, both to watch intently what is happening and also to imitate and show off. He likes to sit exploring toys in detail with his hands and eyes with very little mouthing, and soon he will start to cast toys vigorously on the floor to get them picked up again. This repetitive activity will go on from 12 to 13 months through until 15 months. After this age, certainly by 18 months, both mouthing and casting are signs of developmental delay except when toys are thrown on the floor, at 18 months, in anger or more deliberate play.

The majority of 15-month-old children are mobile, can explore a wide environment with great curiosity and are in need of very close supervision and protection from dangerous objects in cupboards and drawers

Table 3.5 Summary of development: 12–24 months

	12–15 Months	18–24 Months
Personal and social behaviour	Shows affection and may be shy	Becoming egocentric, clinging and resistant
	Indicates wants, points, claps hands (10–18 months)	Loves domestic mimicry
	Mouthing stops (12–15 months)	Definitely stopped mouthing and casting (by 18 months)
	Enjoys casting (12–15 months)	Helps undress
	May manage cup and spoon with spills (10–17 months)	Independent with cup and spoon (15–24 months)
Gross motor	Walks holding on (8–12 months)	Walks well (12–18 months)
	Walks alone (11–15 months)	Climbs stairs, kneels (14–22 months)
Fine motor and vision	Fine pincer grasp. Bangs bricks together (8–14 months)	May show hand preference (after 15 months)
	Holds two cubes.	Builds 2 to 3 cubes.
	Scribbles (12–18 months)	Turns pages (15–24 months)
Language and hearing	Mama, Dada, with meaning (9–15 months)	Can point to 3 parts of body, has 6 to 20 words and jargon (15–24 months)
	Three to four clear words (12–18 months)	

which they will be able to open. The 18-month-old child plays more constructively, liking to imitate domestic tasks. They also play contentedly alone with toys on the floor. They are often still very emotionally dependent on their mother, but there is also the start of resistant or negative behaviour. Self-help skills progress from the first attempts at spoon feeding at around 11–12 months, with still a lot of spilling at 15 months as the spoon gets turned over, to a great deal more control and accuracy by 18 months.

Similarly, drinking from a cup needs supervision at 15 months but can be fairly independent by 18 months. At this age also they can start to take simple clothing off and a few will start to indicate their toilet needs.

Although quite a number of children take some steps unsupported at about 12 months, the majority need to have one hand held or are just cruising around furniture. However independent mobility is almost within reach in the upright position and in the next few months all but a few will be walking independently. At first, walking is on a very wide base but gradually with better control the child walks without the need to raise the arms up to maintain balance, and can now use hands to carry toys around. This combined activity is much more difficult but not impossible for a bottom shuffler of the same age (Fig. 3.18a, b). By 18 months, many children can go upstairs with one hand held and are quite controlled in their movements on the level, being able to squat and rise without help and easily sit down in a small chair. Coming down stairs is far more difficult and is usually by bumping down on the bottom.

By a year, very small objects can be picked up between the tip of the forefinger and thumb in a neat pincer grasp and this ability becomes more precise in the following months. Cubes however will still be picked up with a tripod or intermediate grasp (Fig. 3.19) and the cubes will be scrutinized, compared and often banged together spontaneously and in imitation.

In addition to casting bricks or toys and looking to see where they have gone, the child likes putting them in and out of boxes and containers. A little later, two bricks can be held in one hand and may be placed one on top of the other on a table. By 18 months, a tower of

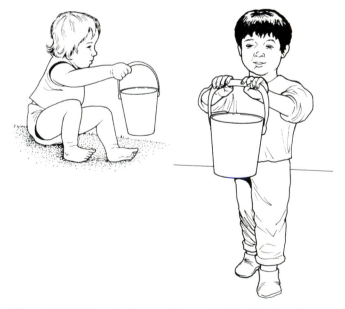

Figure 3.18 (a) Carrying toys as a bottom shuffler. (b) Carrying toys as a walker.

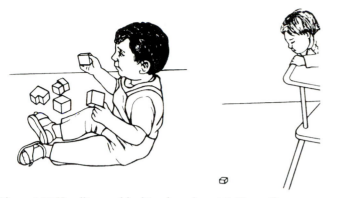

Figure 3.19 Handling and looking for cubes at 9–12 months.

three bricks can be achieved but releasing one cube to place it on top of another still requires intense concentration. At this age, children like scribbling on paper (or anything else), and also looking at a book, still often turning more than one page at a time. At about this age handedness is usually established.

An understanding of language is developing very definitely by one year. In addition to knowing their name, they will usually understand names of people in the family and simple everyday commands. They may hand one or two objects on request and demonstrate understanding of the use of everyday objects such as a hairbrush. Babble progresses into meaningful 'mamma' and 'dadda' and perhaps two or three

Table 3.6 Summary of development: 2–5 years

	2–2½ years	3–4 years	5 years old
Personal and social skills	Enjoys solitary play, alongside peers, not sharing. Possessive: tantrums if thwarted	Plays with peers, sharing toys. Enjoys make-believe play. Shows concern and sympathy for others, and able to take turns by 4 years	Plays complicated cooperative games. Makes friends. Comforts playmates and siblings in distress
	Feeds quite neatly, using spoon and fork or fingers. May be clean and dry by day, with supervision, or may refuse to cooperate	Easily manages spoon and fork and then knife. Mostly dry day and night. Can wash hands, dress and undress by 4 years, except fastenings	Almost completely independent in self help-skills now. Can carry out simple domestic tasks and run errands
Gross motor	Now very mobile. Runs, kicks ball, tries to throw. Walks up and down stairs two feet to a step. Propels tricycle by pushing with feet on floor	Up stairs one foot per step at 3, and down by 4 years. Can walk, then run on tip-toe, and hop, by 4 years. Enjoys climbing, pedals a tricycle skilfully	Enjoys running, jumping, climbing, swings and slides, and starting to play ball games. Can stand on one leg, hop 10 times and heel-toe walk a narrow line.
Fine motor and vision	Neat prehension, and controlled release. Tower of 6–8 bricks. Holds pencil in fist. Circular scribble [24 months] copies vertical line, imitates circle, [30 months]. Simple puzzles and can thread large beads	Tower of 9–10 and imitates 3 cube bridge at 3 years, steps or gate by 4 years. Awkward tripod grasp of pencil at 3 years – copies circle and imitates cross. Dynamic tripod after 4 years; draws man with head, trunk and legs	Can write name, copy a square and a triangle. Draws man with detailed features and limbs. Can fold paper and use scissors to cut out shapes
	Difficult age to test vision. Recognizes two-dimensional symbols and may match letters at 30 months	Can do letter-matching vision tests, using linear charts, each eye separately, by 3½ to 4 years	Performs Snellen chart type of vision test
Language and hearing	Listens to simple stories and understands two-part instructions. Can say 50–100 single words and join two to three: [Daddy gone car]. Many questions – what? & who? Long monologues, still some jargon, enjoys nursery rhymes and jingles	Intelligible but immature speech, 3–5 word sentences, knows name and sex, at 3 years. Long stories, constant more abstract questions, grammar mostly correct, and speech clear, by 4 years. Knows age and address, 6+ colours and can count to 4+	Enjoys riddles and jokes. Understands negatives and complex questions and instructions. Gives long descriptions and explanations. Speech easily intelligible with few errors.
	Toy tests of hearing or may point to named pictures	Can do cooperative (conditioned) hearing tests	Manages full audiometry and speech discrimination now

other words. By 18 months communication is by both gesture and sound with a vocabulary of perhaps six to 20 words. Comprehension can be demonstrated by the child pointing on request to eyes or nose and other parts of the body, or to toys, shoes or other common objects. Inability to show some verbal comprehension at this age is of greater concern than the inability to say more than a few words, since comprehension develops well in advance of expressive ability.

4   Two to 5 years (Table 3.6)

a   The 2–3 year-old child

By the age of 2 years, most children are very mobile and able to run. They enjoy practising these skills and need careful supervision to prevent them from wandering away. They enjoy kicking and trying to throw a ball (Fig. 3.20). In order to negotiate stairs, the child starts to walk up and down rather than crawling and this

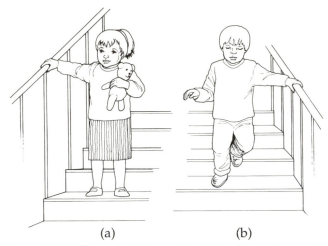

(a)   (b)

Figure 3.21 (a) Two and a half year old walking downstairs two feet to a step. (b) Four year old walking downstairs alternating steps.

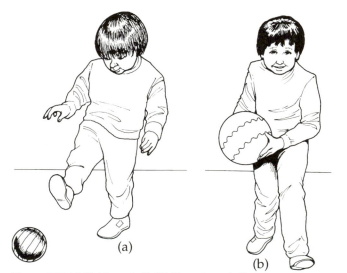

(a)

(b)

Figure 3.20 (a) Kicking a ball. (b) Throwing a ball.

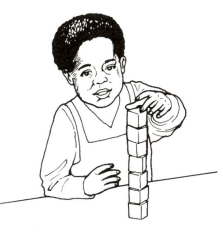

Figure 3.22 Building a seven brick tower.

ability steadily improves from the slow process of putting both feet on each step to an adult type of stair walk putting alternate feet on successive steps (Fig. 3.21a,b).

At 24 months the child has a precise finger-thumb grip and can grasp tiny objects. Pencil grasp is still somewhat immature but by 3 years it is tripod in nature between thumb and fingers. Drawing becomes steadily more sophisticated and at 2 years the child may try to imitate a circle by producing circular scribble and by 3 years a cross. He enjoys building with bricks and constructs an increasingly high tower of bricks up to seven or eight by the age of $2\frac{1}{2}$ (Fig. 3.22).

At 2 years the child can recognize a number of miniature toys by name (Fig. 3.23) and can understand and point to named objects in pictures. At $2\frac{1}{2}$ or sometimes a little older, many children are able to perform a simple shape matching test of visual acuity such as a letter matching test.

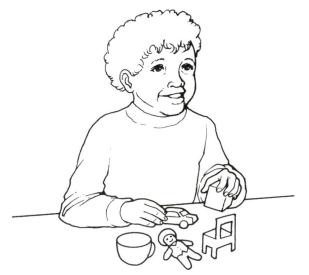

Figure 3.23 Recognizing miniature toys by name.

Symbolic play becomes more complex and by 30 months comprehension has developed to the level of understanding following first one idea and later, two. The vocabulary of 2 year olds is often greater than 50 single words and they are starting to put words together to make phrases and short sentences.

However the normal range of vocabulary is very wide indeed and some children do not say any clear words until 21 to 24 months. The child listens attentively and does much imitation of words and sounds and is often able to recite short rhymes heard frequently from family or the television. At $2\frac{1}{2}$ old, the child often talks to himself at length using personal pronouns and some prepositions. Speech becomes increasingly intelligible and fluent though stammering may occur in up to 5% of children but in these it is usually a normal developmental stage.

b   The 3–4 year-old child

The 3-year-old child is becoming more adventurous, sociable and cooperative (Fig. 3.24). He likes playing with other children and is willing to share. Relationships become more important and complicated. He likes to please adults and help with simple tasks. Play becomes more complex involving many toys and objects, both real and imaginary.

The 3 year old can use a spoon and fork and drink from a glass without spilling. Most children are clean and dry at night as well as by day, but some continue to wet the bed. He can pull pants up and down and generally take easy clothes like socks, shorts and T-shirts on and off. Dressing skills improve steadily and by 4 years he can manage most clothes without complicated fastenings.

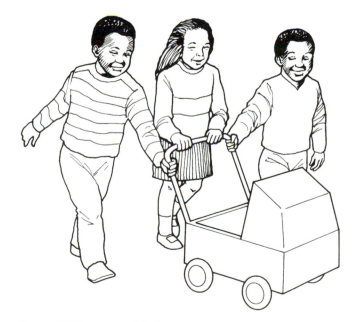

Figure 3.24 Three year old play.

At 36 months most children are very agile and energetic and like to climb and balance on suitable apparatus in a playground or nursery. They can walk on tip-toe and by the age of 4 years, they can usually run on their toes and stand briefly on one foot (Fig. 3.25). Between 3 and 5 years the child is joining in more with other children particularly in physical and interactive games which involve complex motor manoeuvres (Fig. 3.26).

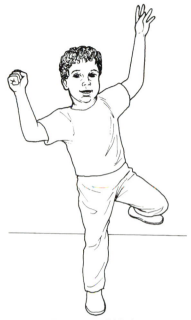

Figure 3.25 Four year old balancing on one leg.

At this age many children can copy a bridge of three bricks and the pencil or crayon is now held with a mature tripod grasp which, over the next year, becomes dynamic, allowing more precise and fluent control for drawing shapes (Fig. 3.27). At 3 years they can copy a circle and imitate, if not copy, a cross; and by 4 will try to imitate a square with some difficulty, and when asked to draw a man can produce a recognizable picture with head, body and limbs. This can be used as a test of increasing developmental skill by scoring the number of features in the Goodenough-Harris test.[33] Also by 4 years children enjoy doing jigsaws of increasing complexity and are able to cut out simple paper shapes. All these skills become progressively more accurate through the fifth year of life.

At 3 years of age, a linear letter matching test can usually be administered at 6 metres. Primary colours are recognized and matched at 3 years and named by 4 years. Visual acuity at distance is very good often with recognition of objects and people in the far distance.

At 3 years of age children love listening to stories and often ask for them to be repeated again and again. Speech is easily intelligible and conversations are

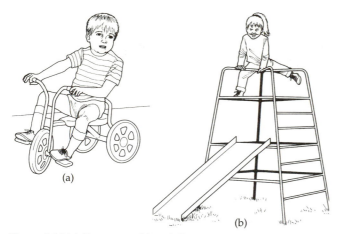

Figure 3.26 (a) Four year old pedalling tricycle. (b) Three to four years: enjoying climbing.

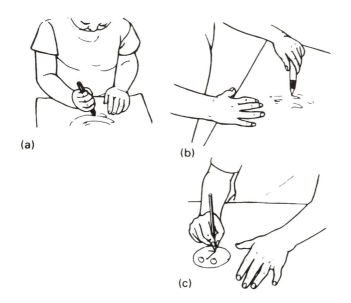

Figure 3.27 Development of pencil control. (a) Cylindrical grip; (b) early thumb-finger grip; (c) dynamic tripod.

carried on with sentences of four to five words. He will ask more complicated and abstract questions by the age of 4, making longer sentences with only minor errors of pronunciation and grammar. The complexity of questions asked increases and at this age many parents find the child's insatiable appetite for information quite wearing.

Comprehension has now progressed to the stage of easily understanding and following instructions containing two ideas. This can be made use of in hearing tests which for this age group take the form of conditioned or cooperative play audiometry.

5 Five years old

On school entry most children are very sociable and soon enjoy participating in team and group activities.

They acquire the concepts of rules, fair-play, turn-taking and the need for sharing. From about 6 years, they start to understand the feelings of others and show emotions such as sympathy or pleasure in relation to the experiences of others. This social competence goes on developing through the school age years. In infant school, children start to choose their own friends and form alliances. The competitive spirit often develops strongly at 6 to 7 years and may be encouraged according to social attitudes in school and at home.

Most 5 year-old children are very competent at feeding themselves without any help and begin to prepare simple foods such as bread and butter at 7 years of age and may enjoy cooking under supervision from 8 years old. They are able to perform all normal toilet manoeuvres efficiently and can dress and undress alone, though parents may need to help if speed is a factor. By 5 most children can manage zips and press-studs, by 6, buttons and by 7 years, tie shoe laces.

At school entry children are very agile and competent at physical activities. They can skip, hop, jump and play hand and foot ball games well (Fig. 3.28a,b). Gross motor coordination steadily improves and they have good balance. With practice, children become increasingly skilful at many physical activities such as swimming, dancing and team sports.

Pencil skills improve and children should be able to copy several geometric shapes including a triangle at about $5\frac{1}{2}$ years, and a diamond at about 6 years. They first copy letters mechanically but as concept of written language begins they start to use letters in a symbolic way to form words. Many children of 5 to 6 years old are able to write their names and other simple words, and reading and writing skills should develop rapidly from the age of 6. This requires sound teaching at school and also benefits from help at home. Other manipulative skills also increase and the child is able to perform intricate manoeuvres with building materials, bricks, cardboard and scissors, nuts and bolts.

By school entry most children are visually very observant and their acuity can be tested easily with a linear letter chart at 6 metres with each eye covered in turn. They can usually pick out detail in complex pictures and photographs and name at least four colours and match ten or more by 5 years old.

The development of visual skills in the young child is related to that of perceptual skills and the tests applied, once visual acuity has been measured and found normal, assess the cognitive interpretation of visual stimuli. The same situation applies to the relation between hearing skills and understanding.

Pure tone audiometry with head phones should be easily performed now. Speech audiometry also becomes progressively easier through and beyond the age of 6 years. The verbal understanding of school children becomes rapidly more sophisticated and jokes and riddles of increasing complexity are understood

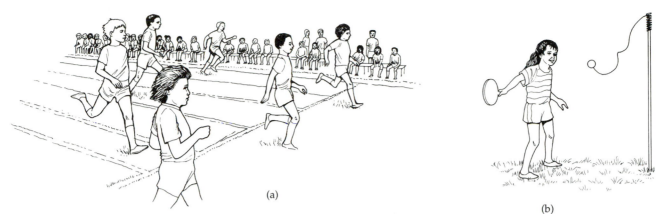

Figure 3.28 (a) Five to six year olds running in school sports; (b) 6 year old skilled with bat and ball.

and enjoyed. Comprehensive tests of hearing skills at this age should measure the child's verbal comprehension, auditory perception, attention and intellect rather than just the sense of hearing.

Many children aged 5 years have speech that is nearly perfect from a grammatical point of view, except for some irregular constructions. Pronunciation is very good with only a few remaining immaturities which disappear with time and practice. The incessant stream of repetitive questions usually slows down as the inner language and general knowledge build up, though the depth of the questions asked may be a problem for the parents who are expected to know everything!

References

1 Gesell, A. *Studies in Child Development*. New York: Harper and Row, 1948.
2 Sheridan, M.D. *Children's Developmental Progress from Birth to Five Years: the STYCAR Sequences*. Windsor: NFER Nelson, 1976.
3 Illingworth, R.S. *The Development of the Infant and Young Child*, 9th edn. London: Churchill Livingstone, 1980, 169–193.
4 Pavlov, I.P. *Conditioned Reflexes*. New York: Dover Publications, 1960 (originally published 1927).
5 Piaget, J. *The Grasp of Consciousness* (translated by Wedgewood S). London: Routledge and Kegan Paul, 1977 (originally published 1974).
6 Hobson, R.P. Piaget: on the ways of knowing in childhood. In: Rutter, M., Hersov, L., eds. *Child and Adolescent Psychiatry: Modern Approaches*. Oxford: Blackwell Scientific Publications, 1985, 191–203.
7 Freud, S. The ego and the id. In: Strachey, J., ed. *The Standard Edition of the Complete Psychological Works of Sigmund Freud*, vol XIX. London: Hogarth Press, 1975, 13–66 (originally published 1923).
8 Freud, S. Three essays on the theory of sexuality. In: Strachey J., ed. *The Standard Edition of the Complete Psychological Works of Sigmund Freud*, vol. VII. London: Hogarth Press, 1975, 125–245 (originally published 1905).
9 Jung, C.G. *Dreams*. Princeton: Princeton University Press, 1974.
10 Adler, A. *The Neurotic Constitution*. London: Kegan Paul, Trench and Trubner, 1918.
11 Freud, A. *Normality and Pathology in Childhood*. Harmondsworth: Penguin Books, 1973.
12 Segal, H. *Introduction to the Work of Melanie Klein*. London: Hogarth Press, 1973.
13 Winnicott, D.W. *The Child, the Family and the Outside World*. Harmondsworth: Penguin Books, 1964.
14 Winnicott, D.W. *The Maturational Processes and the Facilitating Environment. Studies in the Theory of Emotional Development*. London: Hogarth Press, 1976.
15 Erikson, E.H. *Identity: Youth and Crisis*. London: Faber and Faber, 1971.
16 Capute, A.J., Palmer, F.B., Shapiro, B.K., Wachtel, R.C., Schmidt, S., Ross, A. Clinical linguistic and auditory milestone scale: prediction of cognition in infancy. *Develop Med Child Neurol* 1986; **28:** 762–771.
17 Chomsky, N. *Aspects of the Theory of Syntax*. Cambridge, Mass: MIT Press, 1965.
18 Skuse, D. Extreme deprivation in early childhood II. Theoretical issues and a comparative review. *J Child Psychol Psychiat* 1984; **25:** 543–572.
19 Reynell, J., Huntley, M. *Reynell Developmental Language Scales*. Windsor: NFER-Nelson, 1987.
20 Dubowitz, L.M., Dubowitz, V., Goldberg, C. Clinical assessment of gestational age in the newborn infant. *Paediatrics*, 1970; **77:** 1–10.
21 Brazelton, T.B. Neonatal behavioural assessment scale. *Clinics in Developmental Medicine 88*. London: Spastics Int Med Pub, 1984.
22 Prechtl, H. Continuity and change in neural development. *Clinics in Developmental Medicine 94*. London: Spastics Int Med Pub, 1984.
23 Holt, K.S. *Developmental Paediatrics*. London: Butterworths, 1977; 243–252.
24 Holt, K.S. *Child Development*. London: Butterworths 1991; **12:** 163.
25 Robson, P. Prewalking locomotor movements and their use in predicting standing and walking. *Child Health Care Devel* 1984; **10:** 317–330.

26   Robson, P. Shuffling, hitching, scooting or sliding: some observations on thirty otherwise normal children. *Devel Child Neurol* 1979; **12:** 608–617.

27   Robson, P. Screening for children. *R Soc Health J* 1978; **98:** 231–237.

28   Duden, L.D., Rijken, M., Brand, R., Verloove-Vanherick, S.P., Ruys, J.H. Is it correct to correct? Developmental milestones in 555 'normal' preterm infants compared with term infants. *J Pediatr* 1991; **118:** 399–404.

29   Miller, G., Dubotwitz, L., Palmer, P. Follow-up of preterm infants: is correction of the developmental quotient for prematurity helpful? *Early Hum Devel* 1984; **9:** 137–144.

30   Gesell, A. *The First Five Years of Life.* London: Methuen, 1950.

31   Brett, E.M. *Paediatric Neurology.* Edinburgh: Churchill Livingstone, 1983; 4–**13**, 24–35.

32   Chaplais, J. The late walking child. In: MacFarline, J.A. ed. *Progress in Child Health,* vol 1, Edinburgh: Churchill Livingstone, 1984.

33   Harris, D.B. *Children's Drawings as Measures of Intellectual Maturity.* Harcourt: New York, 1963.

Chapter 4

Growth and puberty

Helen Spoudeas and Charles Brook

Growth lasts from conception to maturity. Thereafter, a recurring cycle of cell growth, death and replacement continues in adult life. Growth and pubertal maturation are complex, continuous and carefully regulated processes. Height is but one easily accessible measure of growth; the acquisition of secondary sexual characteristics is the first manifestation of puberty. Normal growth and the eventual attainment of reproductive capability are dependent on harmonious interactions of regulatory hormones.

Their disharmony results in an abnormal pattern of growth, rate of maturation, loss of the normal consonance of puberty and possible infertility. Careful monitoring of these processes forms a reliable and simple screening procedure of general health and also for the detection of disease, since all disease processes, not just endocrine ones, affect growth.

Normal growth

Prenatal growth

Prenatal growth is due mainly to cell division (multiplicative growth). After birth, the emphasis is principally on enlargement (auxetic growth) and specialization of already existing cells and laying down of intercellular matrix (accretionary growth). An unfavourable intrauterine environment (e.g. intrauterine malnutrition or hypoxia) may result in a profound growth deficit which is irreversible postnatally.

Fetal growth curves compiled from data obtained at antenatal ultrasound show that there is relatively little variation in fetal size until the last trimester of pregnancy.[1] Thus, early ultrasound (before 20 weeks' gestation) is useful in dating pregnancies whereas later measurements of abdominal and head circumference and their ratio may detect up to 90% of growth-retarded babies. A decrease in abdominal circumference is the first indication of slow growth; head circumference also becomes reduced if the growth failure is severe.

The placenta grows faster than the fetus at first, but from about 30 weeks the placental/fetal ratio falls. At 34–36 weeks' gestation there is a dip in fetal growth velocity, probably resulting from the constraints of limited space within the maternal uterus. Multiple births slow down earlier than singleton pregnancies. Those infants most restrained in the uterus demonstrate a period of 'catch-up' growth postnatally, the peak velocity of which continues the smooth curve of the prenatal velocity 2–3 weeks earlier before the antenatal dip occurred.[2]

The most important constraining influence on neonatal size is the size of the mother herself,[3] although the subsequent postnatal growth of that infant will conform to his or her genetic potential. The correlation between length at birth and adult height is only 0.3, but this increases sharply during the first year so that by the age of 2 years the correlation is nearly 0.8.[4]

Unlike the maximum rate of growth in height, the maximum rate of growth in weight is not achieved until shortly after birth, but then rapidly declines. Birthweight is more variable than birth length and reflects the maternal environment more than heredity.[3,5] Individual weight curves fluctuate more within the centiles than height, and this is more evident in the first few months of life.

Adverse maternal factors compromise the intrauterine environment; maternal illness, smoking or hypertension result in low birthweight babies, whereas uncontrolled maternal hyperglycaemia stimulates fetal hyperinsulinism and results in a tall, overweight baby with a tendency to hypoglycaemia.

Postnatal growth

Not all parts of the body grow at the same rate throughout childhood. The skeleton, body weight, thoracic and abdominal organs follow the general curve (Fig. 4.1). The pattern of muscle development is similar to that of bone but is particularly laid down in puberty, especially in the male. The gonads and external genitalia develop constantly but very slowly in infancy and early childhood and rapidly increase in size with puberty. Conversely, the uterus and adrenal glands are relatively large at birth, subsequently decrease in size, and do not regain their weights at birth until just before puberty. The pituitary gland is also relatively large at birth but subsequently grows like the thyroid gland at a fairly steady rate. The anterior lobe of the pituitary is noticeably larger in the female from early childhood and this difference is emphasized at puberty and even more so in pregnancy. The growth rate of the nervous system (and hence head circumference) is so rapid in early life that the structures involved attain 90% of their adult size by 5–6 years of age.

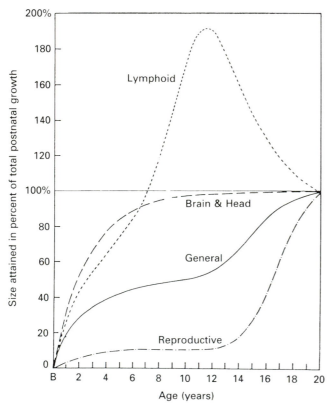

Figure 4.1 Growth curves for different parts of the body. (Redrawn from Tanner, J.M.[61])

Techniques of growth assessment

Height is the best single index of growth as it is a measure of the growth of a single tissue, bone. Weight increase in children is sometimes taken as an indicator of satisfactory growth but as it is a measure of all tissues, including fat and muscle as well as body water, it is a much less useful long-term indicator.

Satisfactory estimates of subcutaneous fat may be made by caliper measurement of skinfold thicknesses[6] (Fig. 4.2) and those of the triceps correlate well with body density and can be used as an index of total body fat. The change in the distribution of subcutaneous fat with puberty may also be useful in estimating maturity.[7]

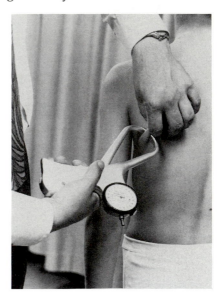

Figure 4.2 Measurement of subscapular skinfold with Holtain caliper. The width of a pinch of skinfold is measured with the calipers at right angles to the skin.

Without good measurement techniques and suitable equipment the error margins involved in auxological assessment are unacceptably great. Careful use of purpose-built precision equipment (Fig. 4.3a–d) by the same trained observer reduces measurement error to 1 mm in standing heights and to 1.5 mm in supine lengths (representing a coefficient of variation of <1%).[8] Too often, however, this basic skill is considered unimportant; measurements generated by untrained personnel operating with inadequate equipment are frankly inadequate for proper assessment.

Height distance curves and height velocity

The amount of growth achieved depends on both duration and speed of growth. The age at which sexual maturity is reached determines the duration of growth; the nutritional influences in utero and early postnatal life and the hormonal factors operative in childhood and puberty determine the speed of growth. The longitudinal progress of an individual is represented by the height distance curve (Fig. 4.4a) which flattens out to a plateau as maturity is reached. The variations in an individual's speed of growth with time are shown in velocity curves, which tend to zero as growth ceases. The velocity

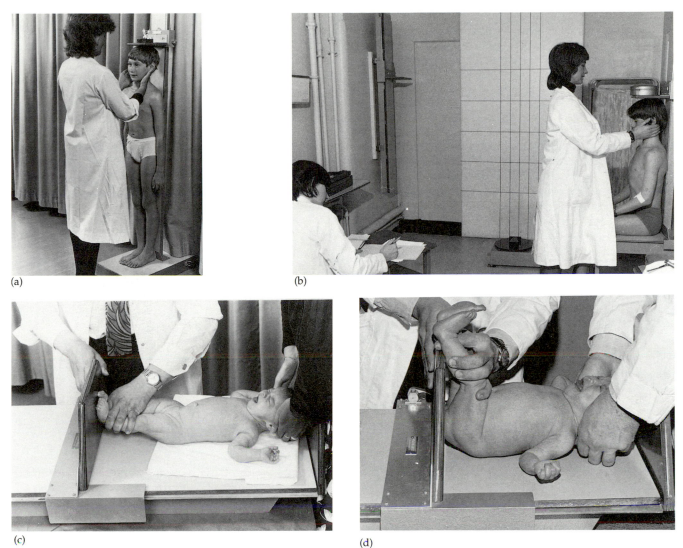

Figure 4.3 Harpenden stadiometer for standing and sitting heights. (a) A child's height should be taken standing without shoes, heels together on the ground and in contact with an upright wall. The head is held with the external auditory meatus and the outer angle of the eye in a horizontal (Frankfurt) plane. While pressure is upwardly applied under the mastoid processes, the child is encouraged to stretch against a weighted, moving horizontal surface thus eliminating the shrinking which occurs in upright posture as the day goes on and which may be as much as 2 cm. (b) Sitting height is similarly measured, ensuring that the child sits with the angle of the knees at the edge of the stadiometer and is not pushing upwards with hands or feet which should rest on the lap or a lower bar respectively. (c,d) Measurement of supine length and crown-rump distance. In children less than 2 years of age, measurement of supine length or crown-rump measurements are undertaken. One examiner holds the head in contact with a fixed board and a second person stretches the child and then brings a moving board into contact with the heels or bottom. This method averages about 1 cm more than the standing height measurement of the same child, hence the break in the centile charts at 2 years of age. (Equipment available from Holtain Ltd, Crosswell, Crymych, Dyfed SA42 3VF. A variety of cheaper instruments may be obtained from Child Growth Foundation, 2 Mayfield Ave, London W4 1PN.)

curve in Fig. 4.4(b) demonstrates the three principal phases of childhood growth: the rapid but rapidly decelerating growth of infancy, the slow deceleration of mid-childhood and the pubertal spurt. A small mid-childhood growth spurt between the ages of 6 and 8 years is also evident from this chart.

The height centiles (Fig. 4.5) are simply a measure of the percentage of children in that particular study population who reached a given height at a given age and there is a considerable spread because of individual variation.[9] Thus 3% of children will have a centile position on or below the third centile and similarly, 3% will fall on or above the 97th centile. Similar centile charts exist for other anthropometric measurements: sitting height; subischial leg length; weight; triceps and subscapular skinfold thickness; head, arm and calf circumference; and bi-iliac and bi-acromial diameter (they can be obtained from Castlemead Publications, Castlemead, Hertford SG14 1LH).

Height velocity curves computed from averages of cross-sectional data[9] do not allow for differences in the age at which adolescence begins and result in an

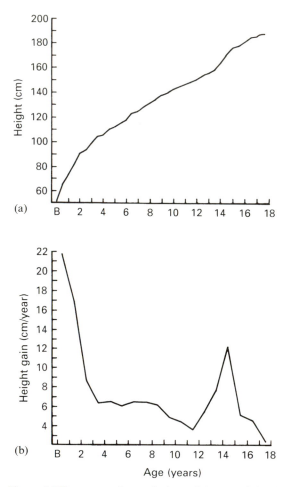

(a)

(b)

Age (years)

Figure 4.4 The postnatal growth chart of the son of the Count Phili-bert Gueneau de Montbeillard 1759–1777. The upper portion is a height–distance curve constructed from 6-monthly height measure-ments while the lower graph is a velocity curve showing the annual increments in height plotted at the midpoint of that year. (From Brook, C.G.D.[8])

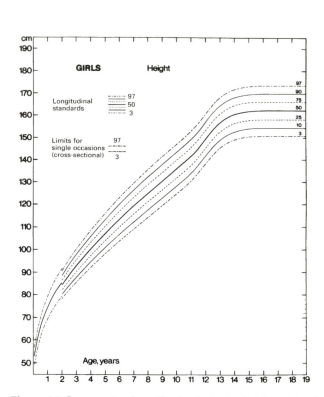

Figure 4.5 Cross-sectional centile standards for height attained at each age in girls.

uncharacteristic smoothing of the individual peak growth spurt over the time axis (Fig. 4.6a). To avoid this distortion, curves have been constructed, the 50th centile of which is an average of all the peak height velocities arranged so that they coincide;[10] these now accurately represent the actual growth of a typical individual (Fig. 4.6b). The absolute values for begin-ning and end were obtained from large cross-sectional surveys. The result[9] is, as before, a mixed longitudinal standard (Fig. 4.6c). Limits are also given for early and late maturing individuals, i.e. those maturing within two standard deviations (approximately 2 years either side) of average. It can be seen from these charts that children with an earlier puberty achieve a higher peak velocity than those maturing later. Those with puber-tal delay will experience a continuing prepubertal deceleration in height velocity and may even appear to stop growing, but will achieve a normal growth

spurt eventually. Girls have a growth spurt occurring at an earlier stage of puberty than boys. The extra 2 years of slow prepubertal growth and the greater max-imum peak velocity in boys[10] accounts for the average 12.5 cm difference in adult heights between the sexes (Fig. 4.7a,b).

In order that a child does not lose or gain height with respect to his peers, his height velocity must oscillate about the 50th centile. Thus while a 25th cen-tile stature may be quite normal, a 25th centile height velocity is potentially abnormal and will result in extreme short stature if that growth rate is maintained over more than one year; a child growing at a 3rd centile velocity for one year has only a 3% probability of being normal but would have to exhibit a 97th centile 'catch-up' velocity the next year to remain on the same distance centile line.[11] To facilitate the screen-ing of children who require further assessment and investigation, the Middlesex height velocity chart has been devised (Fig. 4.8).

The mid-childhood growth spurt evident on the individual longitudinal data is also smoothed out on height velocity curves. This phase of growth once thought to be absent in females[12] is, as yet, incomple-tely understood but features more prominently in males[13,14] and is probably attributable to the influence of adrenal androgens at adrenarche.

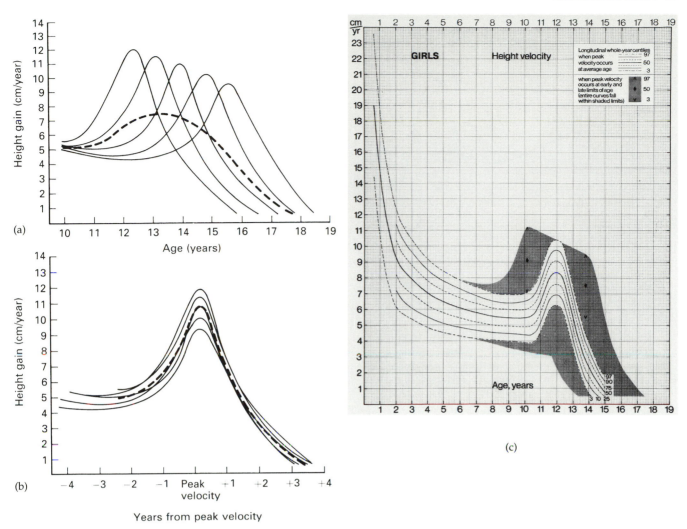

Figure 4.6 The relationship between individual (solid lines) and mean (dashed lines) velocities during the adolescent spurt. (a) Shows the mean constructed by averaging their values at each age. (b) Shows the mean of the same curves all plotted according to their peak height velocity. (From Tanner, J.M. *et al.*[10]) (c) Height velocity curve for girls giving range for early and late maturing individuals. (From Tanner, J.M. and Whitehouse, R.H.[9])

The Infancy-Childhood-Puberty (ICP) model for growth

The human growth curve has proved a mathematical challenge to many.[15,16] The most recent of these analyses[16] divides what at first appears to be a single continuous line of growth into three mathematically distinct phases each corresponding to the three phases of growth observed in height velocity curves (Fig. 4.9).

The infancy component is a continuation of intrauterine growth and accounts for about 70 cm of adult height. Although both growth hormone (GH)[17] and its hypothalamic regulatory hormones are present in the fetus well before birth, their role in prenatal and early postnatal life is controversial. It appears, however, that this phase of growth is largely nutritionally determined, insulin and insulin-like growth factors possibly playing a contributory role.[18] Overfeeding

during this period results in growth advance, and underfeeding in growth retardation.

By the end of the first year, the infancy component tails off but, superimposed on this, is the onset of the childhood component, the point at which this begins being particularly important to final height. This phase's contribution of 70 cm in girls and 80 cm in boys to final height will be less effective if the take-off is delayed and from a lower baseline. This appears to be the most frequent cause of short stature in developing countries in which the nutritionally determined early phase of growth is compromised.[19,20]

With the onset of the childhood component, there is a change from nutritional control to dependency on the amplitude of pulsatile GH secretion. There is an

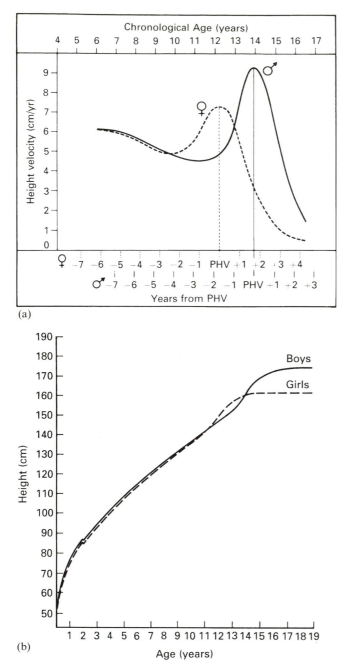

(a)

(b)

Figure 4.7 (a) Typical height velocity curves in average girl and boy. (b) Typical individual height-attained curves for boys and girls. (From Tanner, J.M. et al.[10])

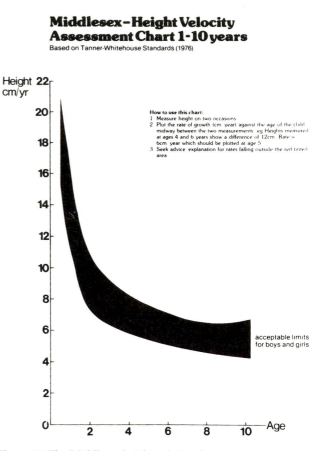

Figure 4.8 The Middlesex height velocity chart.

asymptotic relationship between the amount of growth hormone secreted and the rate of growth (Fig. 4.10). Tall children become tall by growing consistently faster than small children and secreting more growth hormone.[21] This explains why the growth centiles widen with increasing age.

Further support for the theory of a GH-regulated childhood phase comes from the demonstration that

receptors for GH only appear after the first 200 days of life.[22] This is the period during which children with deletion of the GH gene or GH deficiency present with growth failure and a growth pattern which simply follows the infancy curve. Thyroid hormone and cortisol are necessary for the transcription of the GH gene,[23] so deficiencies of these hormones will similarly result in pituitary GH depletion and growth failure. The earlier the problem occurs, the greater the deficit, so prompt diagnosis and therapy are paramount to attainment of a satisfactory adult height.

There are important differences in growth between the sexes at puberty.[24] The female pituitary-gonadal axis appears more sensitive to the pulsatile secretion of gonadotrophin-releasing hormone (GnRH) than the male, this accounting for the greater tendency to precocious puberty in girls and to constitutional delay in boys. Oestrogens augment growth hormone secretion at puberty which is achieved in boys by chemical conversion of testosterone to form oestradiol at hypothalamic level once adequate testosterone concentrations have been reached. Thus the peak of the pubertal growth spurt in girls is seen as soon as oestrogen levels rise with the onset in breast development (Fig. 4.11a) whereas in boys this occurs later in the course of

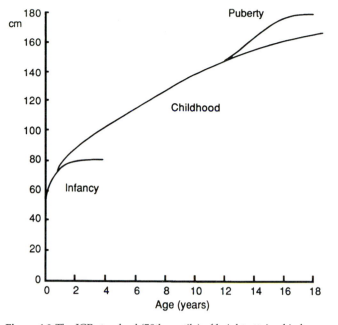

Figure 4.9 The ICP standard (50th centile) of height attained in boys. (From Karlberg, J. *et al.*[16])

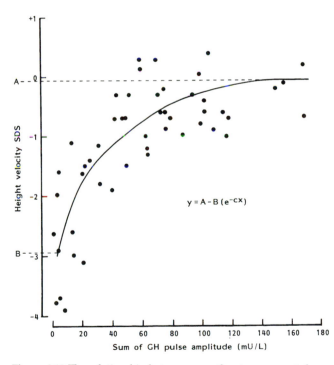

Figure 4.10 The relationship between growth rate, represented as a standard deviation score (SDS) and the sum of GH pulse amplitudes over a 24 hour period. (From Hindmarsh, P.C. *et al.*[21])

puberty when the testes have reached a volume of 10–12 ml (Fig. 4.11b).

The greater magnitude of the spurt in boys is due to the anabolic effects of testosterone. Pubertal growth

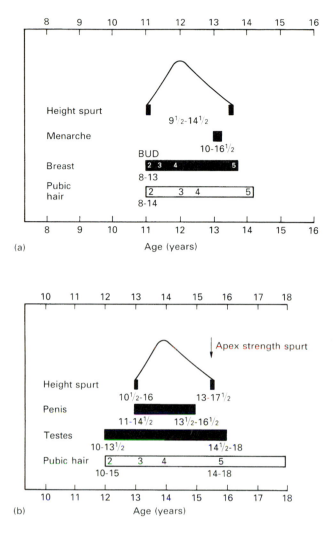

Figure 4.11 The relationship between the growth spurt and other pubertal events (average and age range) in (a) girls and (b) boys. (From Marshall, W.A., Tanner, J.M.[9])

provides about 25 cm of height beginning from about 140 cm in girls and 150 cm in boys.

Assessment of skeletal maturity

The rate of maturation varies from individual to individual and this has important implications for growth assessment. The maturation of the epiphyseal centres in the skeleton follows a sequence of radiographic changes from their first appearance in infancy to their fusion at the end of puberty. Estimates of skeletal maturation may be made from radiographs of epiphyseal centres, frequently those of the hand and wrist using either the atlas method of Greulich and Pyle[25] or by the more detailed scoring system of Tanner and Whitehouse.[26] It should be noted that the two methods are not directly comparable without a correction being made.[27] The main purpose of estimating bone age is to define the amount of growth which has already taken place, and that which is yet to come. It is helpful in predicting adult height[26,28] but not of great benefit in pointing a diagnosis.

Dental age

The times of appearance of the primary and secondary dentitions may be used to supplement bone age in the estimation of maturity. The simplest method of obtaining dental age requires nothing more than enumerating the secondary teeth present, although difficulties occur if eruption is not consistently defined.[29] Staging by the radiographic appearances of the developing jaws and teeth is more accurate and takes into account such factors as calcification and the completion of crown, cusps, and roots in addition to tooth eruption.[30]

Factors influencing growth

Ethnic differences[31] and secular trends[32,33] as well as genetic[34] and environmental[35] factors may influence a child's position on a centile chart. Thus the progress of any given child is a complex interaction of many different factors.

Genetic factors

Heredity has perhaps the strongest influence. Parental heights (which should be measured in the clinic) are invaluable in assessing a child's centile position. Parents' heights and centile positions adjusted for sex should be plotted on the child's growth chart; 95% of normal children will reach a final height within a range defined by the midparental centile ±9 cm.[28]

Ethnic differences

Although there are genetic and environmentally determined ethnic differences in the growth pattern and timing of puberty,[31] these are not as great as those variations within races; thus British standards are usually quite satisfactory for assessing children of Asian parents even though these adults are generally smaller, provided that the principles of growth assessment, and in particular growth velocity, are adhered to. Most ethnic differences are differences in body build rather than rates of growth.

Skeletal ossification in African children is ahead of Caucasians at birth and their permanent teeth erupt earlier. In good economic circumstances this advancement is maintained in all aspects of growth and development and African-descended Americans end up as tall as or taller than their European-descended counterparts. Well circumstanced Chinese and Japanese grow up even faster, though their adult height is less.[31]

Seasonal variations

Children do not grow at the same rate throughout the year. Instead, seasonal variations occur which are particular for each child.[36] Thus, height velocity (the increment in height over two successive points in time), is traditionally calculated using a decimal calendar at yearly intervals, in order to minimize the variations in individual growth and the errors inherent in measurement. Caution must be taken when interpreting velocities over shorter periods of time[37] or over periods longer than one year.

Socioeconomic differences

Socioeconomic differences have, in the past, also been shown to influence height, children of professional parents being 2 cm taller than those of unskilled labourers at the age of 3 years and almost 5 cm taller at adolescence.[36] Part of this difference must be due to nutritional influences, fewer siblings and earlier maturation of the more socially disadvantaged children, but the height differential between the classes is maintained by a system of social mobility in which tall people tend upwards and short people tend downwards. Interestingly, however, data from a generally more affluent and taller Swedish population suggest that these socioeconomic differences no longer exist.[38]

Secular trends

Over the last 100 years there has been a marked secular trend towards a greater height (1.3 cm every 10 years between 1880 and 1950) at all stages of childhood and, to a lesser degree, a greater final adult height. Most of this trend (interrupted during periods of war and famine) is due to an earlier maturation and only minimally due to a greater ultimate size.[33,34] The trend, which is still continuing in Europe, is relatively greater in the postnatal period and up to the age of 5 years than subsequently; however, prosperous Americans appear to have reached their optimal growth potential.

Nutrition

Adequate nutrition is essential for normal growth particularly during the infantile phase. Infants born small for gestational age as a result of relatively recent placental failure often demonstrate catch-up growth after birth and seldom pose a problem to the paediatrician.[39] However, those whose growth has been progressively impaired over many weeks of pregnancy, have a cellular deficit which has been demonstrated in adipose tissue, and they have the same percentage deficit in length at maturity as they did at birth.[40] Thus, the effects of intrauterine growth retardation or severe malnutrition during the nutrition-dependent early phase of growth may be profound and persistent.[19,20,39]

Conversely, overfeeding in the first few months of life results in tall stature, obesity and growth advance, implying an earlier puberty and acquisition of adult height. However, children who become obese after the age of 1 year are not significantly taller than controls.[41] Because the childhood phase of growth is largely growth hormone dependent the role of nutrition at this time is relatively small.

Disorders of growth

Growth is the most sensitive indicator of well-being in children and abnormalities in growth rates may often pre-date the symptoms of systemic disease. All illnesses of childhood affect growth, but the immediate period of 'catch-up' which occurs on recovery means that only after a prolonged illness does the reduction in growth velocity become manifest in short stature.

Assessment of the short child

Growth assessment requires the accurate measurement of stature on at least two occasions (preferably 6 or more months apart) and the calculation of height velocity. If the growth rate is normal (see Fig. 4.8) an explanation for the current height attained may be necessary (e.g. constitutional short stature with short parents, mild forms of skeletal dysplasia or intrauterine or infantile malnutrition), but no further investigation is necessary since, by definition, the child is normal. Bone age estimates may be helpful in calculating a height prediction but these hold true only where normal growth continues.

Differential diagnosis of short stature (Fig. 4.12)

All those dealing with children suffering from chronic conditions are aware that their growth is often stunted. As therapeutic possibilities increase, more children will be long-term survivors of previously lethal renal, cardiac or respiratory diseases and maintaining their growth rate becomes an important future aim.[42] Others surviving treatment for childhood malignancies may be suffering the growth and puberty-related consequences of the intensive irradiation or chemotherapy regimens with which they have been treated.[43]

Short stature in infancy

In general terms, children with short stature can be divided into those who look normal and those who do not. The former group will include some premature and low birthweight infants and those suffering from protein-energy malnutrition, all of whom have incurred a deficit which cannot be corrected later on. The latter group will comprise a proportion of low birthweight infants who have lost out on intrauterine growth as a result of multifactorial influences (e.g. Cornelia De Lange and Silver Russell syndromes) or whose short stature or low birthweight is the result of a chromosomal imbalance (e.g. Turner syndrome) or genetically inherited conditions (e.g. the skeletal dysplasias). If the dysmorphic features of the latter group are not identified at or around the time of birth then their growth problem may only become manifest later on in childhood or in puberty. Although congenital hypopituitarism may present at birth, it does so more frequently because of other endocrine effects (e.g. hypoglycaemia or prolonged jaundice), before it results in growth failure.

Short stature in childhood

Measurement of sitting height is helpful in assessing the child who is short for his parents' height and in whose birth and infantile history there is no aetiological factor identified. This can then be compared with stature on a standard chart and any body disproportion diagnosed (Fig. 4.13). Some of the milder skeletal dysplasias, largely autosomally dominant in inheritance (e.g. hypochondroplasia or spondylo-epiphyseal dysplasia), may be difficult to diagnose both clinically and radiologically unless one has some expertise in this field and, as a consequence, are much more prevalent than previously recognized.

Such children may grow at a relatively normal rate in infancy and early childhood, but their pubertal growth spurt is blunted.[44] Since one or other parent may also have the condition (thereby affecting the mid-parental target height), these children may remain undiagnosed until too near the end or after the completion of their growth, when it is too late for potentially therapeutic intervention with GH.[44]

It is also now becoming clear that the short stature of girls with the Turner syndrome,[45] the commonest sex chromosomal disorder affecting at least 1:5000 female births, is due to a combination of factors which include intrauterine growth retardation, a gradual decline in height velocity in childhood and the absence of a pubertal growth spurt.[46,47]

Differential diagnosis of tall stature (Fig. 4.14)

Overfeeding in infancy may result not only in obesity but also in an increase in lean body mass and the height of children obese from infancy.[41]

Tall children growing at a normal rate are very unlikely to have a pathological cause for their tall

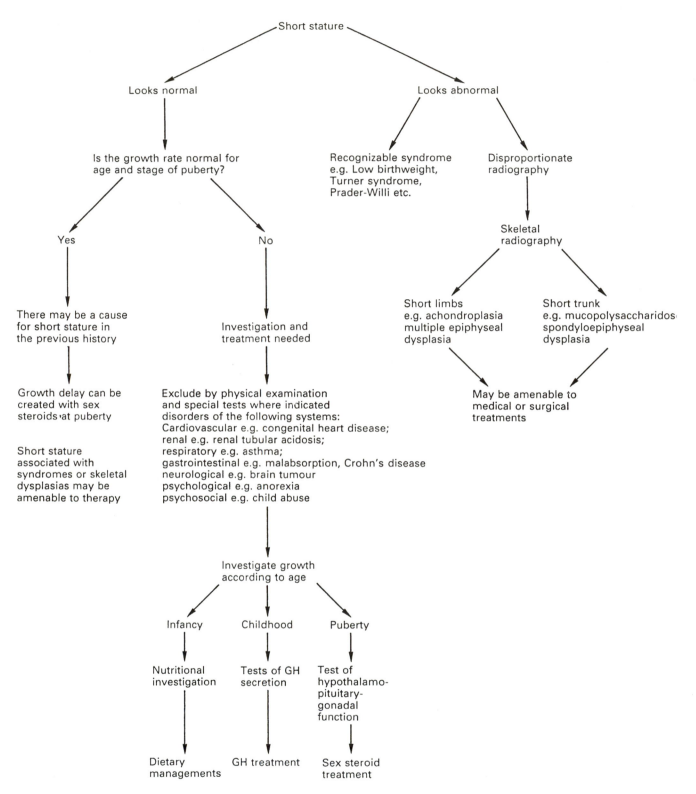

Figure 4.12 Algorithm for the differential diagnosis of short stature.

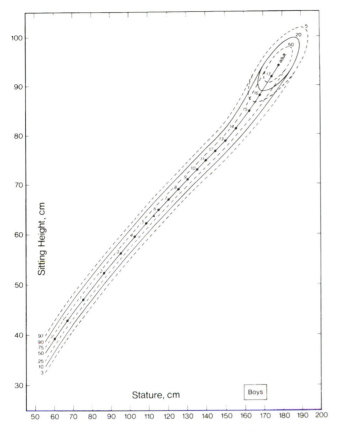

Figure 4.13 Centile chart for sitting height in relation to stature. Children with short-limbed dwarfism and normal trunks (e.g. achondroplasia) fall above and to the left of the standards while those with short backs and normal limbs (e.g. spondylo-epiphyseal dysplasias) fall below and to the right.

stature which is therefore often appropriate for their mid-parental target height.

Those children with an increased growth velocity inappropriate for their age are, most frequently, in precocious puberty which dictates its own differential diagnosis and treatment; an increased growth velocity may be the first and only sign of adrenal disease. Rarely, tall stature is caused by pituitary giantism (GH-secreting pituitary tumours) or thyrotoxicosis.

Treatment in those growing with a normal velocity is reserved for those whose predicted final height is unacceptable. Until recently, this was in the form of large supraphysiological doses of sex steroids to induce premature fusion of the epiphyses. This carries the disadvantages of inducing an early puberty and, in girls, risking the thromboembolic complications of excessively high oestrogen doses (300 mg/day), a consideration which precludes their use in cases such as Marfan Syndrome. For these reasons, alternative methods of reducing the velocity seen in the childhood component of growth, by pharmacologically inhibiting growth hormone secretion with somatostatin[48] or anticholinergics[49] are being tried with some success.

Normal puberty

Puberty is defined as the acquisition of reproductive capability. Its onset is heralded by the appearance of secondary sexual characteristics. The age at onset of puberty, as defined by the appearance of breast development in a girl and increase in testicular volume in a boy, is similar in both sexes with more than 50% of children showing pubertal characteristics by their 12th

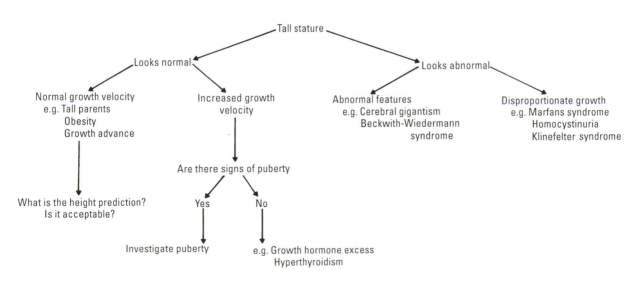

Figure 4.14 Algorithm for the differential diagnosis of tall stature.

birthday. The sequence of events between the sexes differs only in the timing of the adolescent growth spurt, the duration of which is about 2–3 years. This occurs in boys at a testicular volume of 10–12 ml at a time when most girls have already reached breast stage 3–4 and have begun to decelerate. It is this difference and the more obvious manifestation of breast development which explains the apparent earlier pubertal onset in girls and their apparent tallness at this time.

From its onset to its completion, puberty may span as little as 18 months (3rd centile) or as much as five (97th centile), and occasionally more, years. Variations in both time of onset and duration of the pubertal process will naturally cause those children falling at the outer limit of normality to present to physicians. Differentiating these otherwise normal children, who may nevertheless require therapeutic assistance, from those with true pathology requires an intimate understanding of the sequential phenotypic changes which occur at this time and, to a certain extent, the factors which control them.

The physical characteristics of puberty

The age at onset of puberty is very variable, but the appearance of secondary sexual characteristics before the age of 8 years or the lack of development after the age of 14 years in any child requires serious consideration. The bone age at which puberty begins varies just as much as the chronological age and is not a helpful indicator of the timing of puberty.[50]

The first physical sign of puberty in a boy is usually a change in the external genitalia and an increase in testicular volume from 2 to 4 ml. The equivalent in a girl is the onset of breast development. The appearance of pubic hair then follows but axillary hair and the secretion of apocrine sweat glands develops relatively later and, in the male, is usually coincident with the peak of the adolescent growth spurt and deepening of the voice. Facial hair in the male rarely appears before genital development is complete. The change in body shape and muscular development which also occurs is more marked in boys than in girls, but there is a change in the limb to trunk fat ratio in both sexes as measured by skinfold calipers.[7] Less commonly, the appearance of pubic hair may precede the onset of breast or genital development; it may develop (as may axillary hair) in girls with gonadal dysgenesis since it is primarily mediated through adrenal androgens. Thus, children with ACTH deficiency are unable to develop pubic hair.

There is also some increase in the areolar diameter of the male breast in puberty which is associated with an enlargement of the underlying breast tissue in most boys.[51] This rarely persists for longer than a year but occasionally the gynaecomastia is severe enough to warrant surgical treatment; 36% of normal young males have residual palpable breast tissue, usually <4 cm in diameter.[52]

Menarche

Menarche occurs in girls after their peak height velocity has been achieved and their growth is decelerating. Although usually occurring after the attainment of breast stage 4, it occurs at breast stage 3 in 25%. Ninety-five per cent of girls in Western Europe experience menarche between the ages of 11 and 13 years,[53] this being under both genetic[54] (identical twins differing by only about 2 months) and environmental influence; poor children[55] and those from large families[56] being relatively delayed.

Although better nutrition is one of the many environmental factors believed to be influential in the trend towards an earlier age at menarche,[33] the theory that menarche occurs at a critical body weight[57] has been largely disproved.[58] However, there is an association of menarche with skeletal maturation and >80% of girls will menstruate when their bone ages are between 13 and 14 years.[59] A girl who is otherwise fully developed pubertally but complains of primary amenorrhoea is unlikely to menstruate spontaneously if she has a bone age greater than 14.5 years and therefore needs investigation.

Spermarche

Sperm have been detected in the early morning urines of boys with testicular volumes less than 10 ml, sometimes at 6 ml,[60] usually during their 13th year (range 12–15.7 years).[60,61] It therefore occurs at a similar age as menarche in girls but is much earlier in the sequence of their pubertal changes.

Pubertal assessment

This is performed using a number of clinical criteria detailed by Tanner[62] and which are described below (Fig. 4.15a,b). Testicular volumes are measured with the aid of a Prader orchidometer (Fig. 4.16) (obtainable from Holtain Ltd., Crosswell, Crymych, Dyfed, UK SA41 3UF).

Control of the onset of puberty

The mechanisms controlling the onset of puberty have been the subject of much controversy. The hypothalamo-pituitary-gonadal axis is fully functional in the fetus[63] and elevated gonadotrophins have been documented in both normal[64] and agonadal[65] newborns and infants. It has been postulated that, in childhood, some inhibitor with a changing sensitivity must act at either gonadal or hypothalamic level,[63,66] thereby

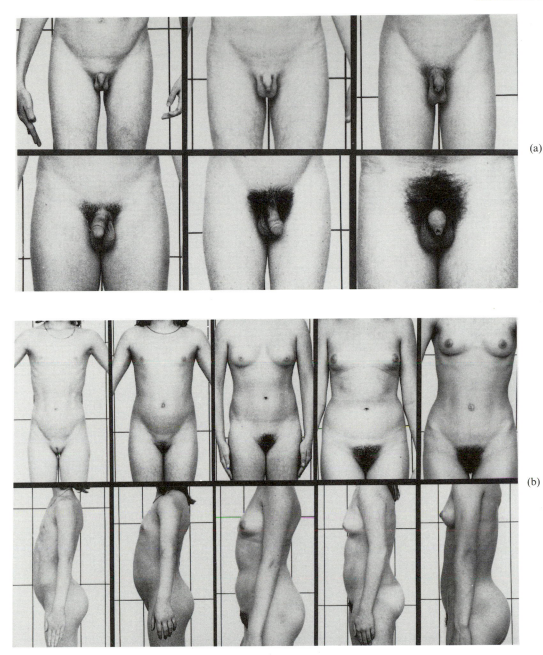

Figure 4.15 (a) The stages of male genital and pubic hair development. (b) The stages of breast and pubic hair development in a female. (a) Boys: genital development: **Stage 1**: Preadolescent: testes, scrotum and penis are of about the same size and proportion as in early childhood. **Stage 2**: Enlargement of scrotum and testes. Skin of scrotum reddens and changes in texture. Little or no enlargement of penis at this stage. **Stage 3**: Enlargement of penis, which occurs at first mainly in length. Further growth of testes and scrotum. **Stage 4**: Increased size of penis with growth in breadth and development of glans. Testes and scrotum larger; scrotal skin darkened. **Stage 5**: Genitalia adult in size and shape. (The volume of the adult testis varies in size from 12 to 25 ml). (b) Girls: breast development: **Stage 1**: Preadolescent: elevation in papilla only. **Stage 2**: Breast bud stage: elevation of breast and papilla as a small mound. Enlargement of areolar diameter. **Stage 3**: Further enlargement and elevation of breast and areola, with no separation of their contours. **Stage 4**: Projection of areola and papilla to form a secondary mound above the level of the breast. **Stage 5**: Mature stage; projection of papilla only, due to recession of the areola to the general contour of the breast. (This last stage may not be reached in women until after their first pregnancy.) (a,b) Both sexes: pubic hair: **Stage 1**: Preadolescent. The vellus over the pubes is not further developed than that over the abdominal wall, i.e. no pubic hair. **Stage 2**: Sparse growth of long, slightly pigmented downy hair, straight or slightly curled, chiefly at the base of the penis or along the labia. **Stage 3**: Considerably darker, coarser and more curled. The hair spreads sparsely over the junction of the pubes. **Stage 4**: Hair now adult in type, but area covered is still considerably smaller than in the adult. No spread to the medial surface of the thighs. **Stage 5**: Adult in quantity and type with distribution of the horizontal (or classically feminine) pattern. Spread to medial surface of thighs but not up linea alba or elsewhere above the base of the inverse triangle (spread up linea alba occurs later and is rated Stage 6). Both sexes: axillary hair: **Stage 1**: Preadolescent. No axillary hair. **Stage 2**: Scanty growth of slightly pigmented hair. **Stage 3**: Hair adult in quality and quantity.

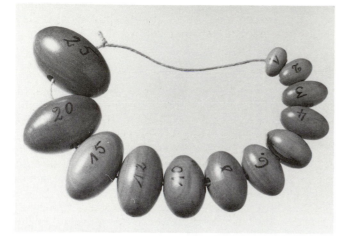

Figure 4.16 The Prader orchidometer. The testis is differentiated from the epidydimis and palpated gently between the thumb and first two fingers of one hand and compared with the models which are similarly palpated with the other hand.

causing the nadir in gonadotrophin values between 6 months and 2 years in normal infants and between 4 and 11 years in agonadal patients. However, the search for such an inhibitor has proved fruitless.

The current view is that a gradual increase in the pulsatile amplitude of hypothalamic GnRH with advancing age is the most likely controlling mechanism of puberty.[67] Occasional short-lived bursts of gonadotrophin secretion are seen in early childhood, but the onset of regular nocturnal luteinizing hormone (LH) pulses[68] induces a nocturnal rise in testosterone or oestradiol, the latter[69] occurring at a later time during the night than the former.[70] As puberty progresses, an increase in the amplitude of gonadotrophin secretion occurs and eventually this is present during the day as well as the night. The observation that sleep-associated enhanced LH secretion also occurs in agonadal patients during the prepubertal period suggests that this pattern does not depend on gonadal function.[71] In normal and simple precocious puberty, LH concentrations always predominate over those of follicle-stimulating hormone (FSH) which is in direct contrast to the situation after puberty.[72] To induce an LH surge lasting 36 hours and subsequent ovulation, 24-hour LH pulsatility together with oestrogen-mediated positive feedback is ultimately necessary[67] and is not usually established in the female until about 18 months after menarche.[73]

Adrenarche

The increase in adrenal androgen secretion (predominantly dehydroepiandrosterone sulphate, DHEAS) which occurs as the zona reticularis appears in the adrenal cortex in mid-childhood, results in the growth spurt and may be accompanied in some children by the appearance of pubic hair without other genital or

breast development. Adrenarche is an entirely physiological process whose regulation is as yet poorly understood,[74] but it needs to be differentiated from pathological conditions, such as congenital adrenal hyperplasia or androgen secreting tumours. Its timing does not seem to predict the timing of the onset of puberty.

Disorders of puberty

Disorders of pubertal maturation divide themselves into those in which the normal sequence of pubertal events proceeds harmoniously, but where the onset is delayed or precocious, and those in which this harmony is disturbed (Fig. 4.17). The latter require investigation as pathology is highly likely; the former may still contain children who have a significant endocrinopathy, but will also contain some normal children who simply fall two standard deviations (SDs) outside the mean.

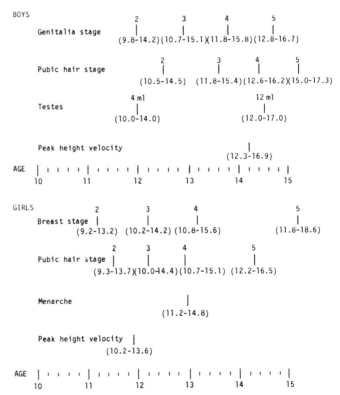

Figure 4.17 The timing of the events in puberty in years.

The classification of pubertal disorders (Table 4.1)

Puberty is precocious when signs of sexual maturation appear before 8 years and delayed when there are no such signs in a 14 year old.

Table 4.1 Classification of disorders of puberty according to presence or absence of normal controlling mechanisms

Precocious puberty
Gonadotrophin-dependent
  Central precocious puberty
    idiopathic
    secondary to:
      central tumour
      infection
      Raised intracranial pressure
      Cranial irradiation
Gonadotrophin-independent
  Adrenal disorders
    Cushing's syndrome
    Congenital adrenal hyperplasia
    Primary tumours (adrenarche)
  Gonadal disorders
    Primary tumours
    McCune Albright syndrome
    'Testotoxicosis'
  Primary hypothyroidism[75,76]
  Isolated premature
    thelarche and variants
Delayed puberty
Gonadotrophin-dependent
  Constitutional delay of growth and puberty
  Hypogonadotrophic hypogonadism
    idiopathic
    secondary to hypothalamic or pituitary disease

Precocious puberty

Central or gonadotrophin-dependent (true) precocious puberty

Central precocious puberty (Table 4.2) may be idiopathic (more commonly girls) or secondary to an intracranial[77,78] lesion (more usually boys) but it is always a consequence of premature activation of the hypothalamo-pituitary-gonadal axis and hence results in the normal sequential appearance of pubertal characteristics excepting that the growth spurt in boys may occur at a smaller testicular volume than normal.[79]

Gonadotrophin-independent precocious puberty

Secondary sexual characteristics caused by adrenal or gonadal sources of sex steroids result in the loss of the normal consonance of puberty.[80] The commonest cause is congenital adrenal hyperplasia (most usually 21-hydroxylase deficiency), in which the adrenal spillover to androgen production causes virilization (with small testes) in boys, an increased growth rate and a rapidly advancing bone age (Figs. 4.18 and 4.19).[81]

By means of differentiation, malignant adrenocortical tumours tend predominantly to result in severe virilization whereas benign adenomas are usually distinguished by their cushingoid features. Twenty-four-hour urinary steroid excretion patterns as measured by gas-liquid chromatography[82] may be a helpful diagnostic pointer in the differentiation of adrenal disorders.

More recently, the familial syndrome of 'testotoxicosis' has been described in boys.[83,84] Interestingly, although gonadotrophin pulsatility is absent, the sequence of phenotypic changes is identical to normal puberty. By contrast, the equivalent in girls occurs in association with the McCune Albright syndrome[84–86] but, in this case, puberty is usually atypical.[87]

Isolated premature thelarche (Table 4.2) is a form of incomplete pubertal maturation in young female infants consisting of isolated and typically cycling breast development without any of the other sequelae of precocious puberty.[88] Its main distinguishing feature from early central precocious puberty is a normal growth velocity and uncompromised final height (i.e. no advance in bone age). Although subsequent puberty usually progresses normally at the appropriate age, future fertility may be compromised.[67]

More recently, the condition of thelarche variant has been recognized[89] in which some features of central

Table 4.2 Distinguishing clinical features of central precocious puberty (CPP) and isolated premature thelarche (IPT) and variants

Feature	CPP	IPT	Thelarche variant
Age of onset	<8 years	Usually <2 years	
Breast development	Progressive	Minor (B2 or B3) cycling	Cycling
Pubic and axillary hair	Progressive	Absent	Absent
Menses	Appropriate	Usually absent	Absent
Bone age	Advanced	Appropriate	Appropriate
Height velocity	Accelerated	Normal	Accelerated
Final height	Compromised	Normal	?Compromised
Duration	Continues	Resolves	?Resolves
Fertility	Normal	?Compromised	?Compromised
Ovaries	Multicystic	Large cysts (1–3)	Intermediate
Predominant gonadotrophin	LH	FSH	LH and FSH unsynchronized

LH: luteinizing hormone; FSH: follicle stimulating hormone

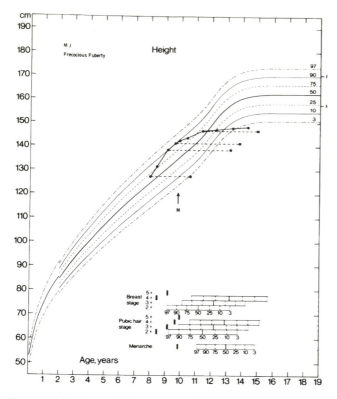

Figure 4.18 Resultant adult stature may be significantly reduced in a boy with untreated precocious puberty

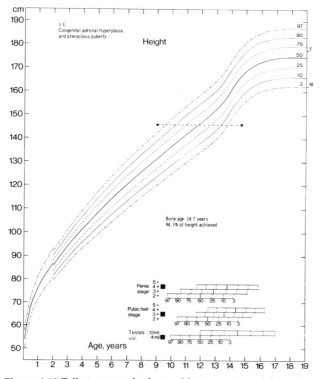

Figure 4.19 Tall stature and advanced bone age in a child with uncontrolled congenital adrenal hyperplasia. The growth potential is significantly reduced.

precocious puberty (abnormally increased growth velocity) coexist with features more typical of isolated premature thelarche (breast cycling and an appropriate bone age).

Delayed puberty

A girl with absent breast development and a boy with no testicular enlargement at the age of 14 years or more requires investigation and appropriate treatment in every case. Even if ultimately no pathology other than constitutional delay or associated chronic disease is found, it is unnecessary to risk extra emotional disturbance in these children as they enter their teens by further delaying their adolescence.[90]

Investigation of delayed puberty

Although increased serum gonadotrophins will identify the child with gonadal failure (when a karyotype should always be performed), differentiating those with constitutional delay of growth and puberty from those with hypogonadotrophic hypogonadism and abnormal endocrine function is often impossible and it may be necessary to institute therapy first, the diagnosis only becoming clear in retrospect. In general, however, those with constitutional delay are short for their chronological age (this is the commonest cause of short stature in boys presenting to growth disorder clinics), but of appropriate height for their bone age which is usually delayed; those with hypogonadotrophic hypogonadism usually demonstrate normal stature with eunochoidal proportions (longer limbs than trunk) and a bone age usually arrested around 13 years.

In either sex, the pituitary gonadotrophin response to an intravenous bolus of native GnRH is generally unhelpful in distinguishing the aetiology of the pubertal delay[91] and should probably be abandoned in this context. Similarly, tests of GH secretion which are performed without prior priming with sex steroids may be very misleading.[79] In boys, a human chorionic gonadotrophin (HCG) test with testosterone measurements before and after stimulation will distinguish between constitutional delay and hypogonadotrophic hypogonadism in the majority of cases.[92]

The secretion of both GH and gonadotrophins is affected early by tumours of the hypothalamo-pituitary area and both basal unstressed prolactin measurements (elevated in prolactinomas) and high resolution computerized tomography (CT) or magnetic resonance imaging (MRI) pituitary scans may be necessary to exclude such a tumour. However, some germinomas and craniopharyngiomas are so slow growing that it is only many years after clinical symptoms occur that they are anatomically identifiable.[93] Gonadotrophin deficiency after cranial irradiation for tumours distant to the hypothalamo-pituitary axis does occur but is much less frequent by comparison.[94]

Hypogonadotrophic hypogonadism

Penny *et al.* first showed that the onset of puberty was characterized by a progressive increase in the amplitude of LH pulses[95] presumably in turn regulated by a hypothalamic GnRH pulse generator. Since then it has become increasingly recognized that idiopathic hypogonadotrophic hypogonadism comprises a spectrum of disorders, most probably hypothalamic in origin, in which the gonadotrophin secretion is abnormal (in terms of pulse frequency or amplitude) or altogether absent.[96] Thus, the clinical presentation may vary from delayed or arrested puberty to secondary amenorrhoea and infertility depending on the degree of deficiency. It is hardly surprising, therefore, that pharmacological tests of pituitary gonadotrophin reserve do not always accurately diagnose this predominantly hypothalamic disorder or distinguish it from constitutional delay.[91,97] Associated distinguishing clinical features in boys include anosmia (Kallman syndrome), colour blindness, cryptorchidism[98] and micropenis.[99]

Treatment of delayed puberty

The aim of treatment, regardless of the aetiology, is to induce secondary sexual characteristics and a growth spurt over an appropriate time span (at least 2 years), since this results in a better physical and psychological outcome (Fig. 4.20). This may be achieved in both girls and boys by the administration of the appropriate sex steroid commencing in low doses and increasing gradually (Table 4.3).

Oral testosterone is not recommended in boys because its absorption is unreliable. HCG is an alternative therapy in boys and can also be used to achieve

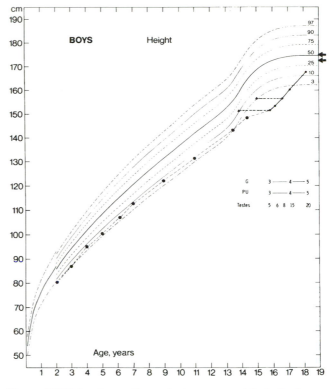

Figure 4.20 Delayed growth spurt at an appropriate testicular volume in a boy presenting with short stature due to constitutional delay.

fertility, but is not recommended in girls because it causes a hyperstimulation syndrome. Transdermal methods of delivering natural oestrogens to girls are currently being developed[100] in an attempt to avoid the problems of first pass metabolism in the liver and the thromboembolic complications of oral synthetic oestrogens in a population which may be most at risk of such problems (e.g. Turner syndrome patients).

Table 4.3 Treatment regimens for delayed puberty

Females	Males
Ethinyl oestradiol	Oxandrolone
2 μg daily × 3 months	2.5 mg daily × 3–6 months
5 μg daily × 3 months	Depot testosterone
10 μg daily × 6 months	50 mg monthly × 3–6 months
15 μg daily × 6 months	In cases of hypopituitarism:
20 to 30 μg daily thereafter with cyclical progesterone on 7/28 days per month	incremental increase in dose;
	100 mg monthly × 6 months
	150 mg monthly × 6 months
	200 mg monthly × 6 months
	200 mg 2–3 weekly (adult)
	HCG injection
	1500 IU i.m. weekly increasing to twice weekly

HCG: Human chorionic gonadotrophin

Pulsatile GnRH therapy is the only treatment which can induce both normal puberty and fertility in a patient who otherwise has functional gonads. Doses at first must be small since the use of adult doses rapidly causes desensitization in children.[101] Because of the difficulties in its administration, it is usually reserved for cases in which fertility is immediately required, although in males its success in this purpose is inversely related to the age at which it is administered. Whether inducing testicular maturation by pulsatile GnRH improves the chances of fertility, when GnRH is re-introduced later in life, remains to be seen.

In boys with constitutional delay, inducing puberty by the administration of a 3-month course of low-dose testosterone (50–100 mg by monthly depot injection) results in a sustained growth spurt but tends to advance bone age perhaps thereby decreasing final height. It also causes a rapid advance in puberty which may produce psychological difficulties in the emotionally immature, counterproductive to the original problem. However, testosterone-derived anabolic steroids such as oxandrolone in a daily dose of 2.5 mg for 3–6 months administered when the testicular volume is 4–6 ml will, at this low dose, accelerate growth without advancing bone age or causing hepatic side effects which are dose dependent.[102] The growth spurt is sustained once the treatment is stopped,[103] the mechanism by which this occurs still being far from clear, but an increase in growth hormone secretion[104] may play a contributory role.

Polycystic ovaries

Polycystic ovaries (PCO) are larger than normal, exhibit numerous circumferential small cysts around an increased amount of central stromal tissue[105] and need to be differentiated from the normal multicystic ovary which is indicative of early puberty.[106] It now appears that PCO is not an uncommon finding in prepuberty and puberty and that in many cases it is responsible for menstrual irregularities and delayed menarche.[107] As well as the typical ovarian appearance on ultrasound, women with the PCO syndrome have characteristically raised serum LH concentrations and increased LH/FSH ratios[108] at all times of the cycle, probably secondary to a primary abnormality within the ovary.

Conclusion

Childhood growth may be divided into three phases each with separate controlling mechanisms. Failure of these mechanisms at any stage is manifest early as a decreased growth velocity; if it remains undiagnosed or untreated, the resultant height loss may be irretrievable.

Growth after the age of 8–9 years is intimately linked with puberty and, at this time, the two processes cannot be considered independently. Accurate assessment relies exclusively upon a knowledge of the normal consonance of sexual maturation and its relationship to the peak height velocity in each sex, as pharmacological tests are more often than not unhelpful in the differential diagnosis of disorders.

Treatments for the disorders of growth and puberty are still developing and in some cases, as in treating the skeletal dysplasias with GH, experimental. However, there is now no case for withholding therapy that has been proven to be beneficial on both psychological and physical grounds.

The measurement of height, and its relationship to pubertal status forms the basis of health surveillance in childhood and the importance of such measurements and their accuracy, should never be underestimated.

References

1 Tanner, J.M. *Foetus into Man*. London: Open Books, 1978.

2 Tanner, J.M. Physical growth and development. In: Forfar, J.O., Arneil, G.C., eds. *Textbook of Paediatrics*, 3rd edn. Edinburgh: Churchill Livingstone, 1984: 279–329.

3 Miller, H.C., Merritt, T.A. *Fetal Growth in Humans*. Chicago and London: Year Book Medical Publishers, 1979: 65–75.

4 Tanner, J.M., Healy, M.J.R., Lockhart, R.D., MacKenzie, J.D., Whitehouse, R.H. Aberdeen growth study: 1. the prediction of adult body measurements from measurements taken each year from birth to 5 years. *Arch Dis Child* 1956; **31:** 372–81.

5 Yates, J.R.W. The genetics of fetal and postnatal growth. In: Cockburn, F. ed. *Fetal and Neonatal Growth*. Chichester: Wiley Medical Publications, 1988: 1–10.

6 Tanner, J.M., Whitehouse, R.H. Revised standards for triceps and subscapular skinfolds in British children. *Arch Dis Child* 1975; **50:** 142–45.

7 Hindmarsh, P.C., Stanhope, R., Brook, C.G.D. Changes of skinfold thickness during puberty induced by pulsatile gonadotrophin-releasing hormone therapy. *Pediatrician* 1987; **14:** 234–36.

8 Hindmarsh, P.C., Brook, C.G.D. Normal growth and its endocrine control. In: Brook, C.G.D., ed. *Clinical Paediatric Endocrinology*, 2nd edn. Oxford: Blackwell Scientific Publications, 1989: 57–73.

9 Tanner, J.M., Whitehouse, R.H. Clinical longitudinal standards for height, weight, height velocity and weight velocity and the stages of puberty. *Arch Dis Child* 1976; **51:** 170–79.

10 Tanner, J.M., Whitehouse, R.H., Takaishi, M. Standards from birth to maturity for height, weight, height velocity and weight velocity, British children, 1965. *Arch Dis Child* 1966; **41:** 454–471, 613–35.

11 Brook, C.G.D., Hindmarsh, P.C., Healy, M.J.R. A better way to detect growth failure. *Br Med J* 1986; **293:** 1186.

12 Gasser, T., Kohler, W., Muller, H.G., Largo, R., Molinari, L., Prader, A. Human height growth: correlational and multivariate structure of velocity and acceleration. *Ann Hum Biol* 1985; **12:** 501–15.

13 Tanner, J.M., Cameron, N. Investigation of the mid-growth spurt in height, weight and limb circumferences in single-year velocity data from the London 1966–67 growth survey. *Ann Hum Biol* 1980; **7:** 565–77.

14 Molinari, L., Largo, R., Prader, A. Analysis of the growth spurt at age 7 (mid-growth spurt). *Hel Paediatr Acta* 1980; **35:** 235–334.

15 Preece, M.A., Baines, M.J. A new family of mathematical models describing the human growth curve. *Ann Hum Biol* 1978: **5:** 1–24.

16 Karlberg, J., Engstrom, I., Karlberg, R., Fryer, J.G. Analysis of linear growth using a mathematical model. *Acta Paediatr Scand* 1987; **76:** 478–88.

17 Kaplan, S.L., Grumbach, M.M., Shepard, T.H. The ontogenesis of human fetal hormones: 1. growth hormone and insulin. *J Clin Invest* 1972; **51:** 3080–93.

18 Hindmarsh, P.C., Brook, C.G.D. Hormonal control of infant growth in the first year. In: Cockburn F., ed. *Fetal and Neonatal Growth.* (*Perinatal Practice*; vol 5). Chichester: Wiley Medical Publications, 1988: 195–210.

19 Karlberg, J., Jalil, F., Lindblad, B.S. Longitudinal analysis of infantile growth in an urban area of Lahore, Pakistan. In: Karlberg J. *Modelling of Human Growth* [PhD thesis]. Goteborg: University of Goteborg, 1987: 113–26.

20 Costello, A.M. de L. Growth velocity and stunting in rural Nepal. *Arch Dis Child* 1989; **64:** 1478–82.

21 Hindmarsh, P., Smith, P.J., Brook, C.G.D., Matthews, D.R. The relationship between height velocity and growth hormone secretion in short prepubertal children. *Clin Endocrinol* 1987: **27:** 581–91.

22 Waters, M.J., Bernard, R.T., Lobie, P.E. *et al.* Growth hormone receptors: their structure, location and role. *Acta Paediatr Scan* [suppl] 1990; **366:** 60–72.

23 Evans, R.M., Birnberg, N.C., Rosenfeld, M.G. Glucocorticoid and thyroid hormones regulate gene expression. *Proc Natl Acad Sci USA* 1982; **79:** 7659–63.

24 Stanhope, R., Brook, C.G.D., Pringle, P.J., Adams, J., Jacobs, H.S. Induction of puberty by pulsatile gonadotrophin releasing hormone. *Lancet* 1987; **ii,** 552–55.

25 Greulich, W.W., Pyle, S.I. *Radiographic Atlas of Skeletal Development of the Hand and Wrist,* 2nd edn. California: Stanford University Press, 1959.

26 Tanner, J.M., Whitehouse, R.H., Cameron, N., Marshall, W.A., Healy, M.J.R., Goldstein, H. *Assessment of Skeletal Maturity and Prediction of Adult Height (TW2 Method),* 2nd edn. London: Academic Press, 1983.

27 Buckler, J.M.H. Comparison of systems of estimating skeletal age (letter). *Arch Dis Child* 1977; **52:** 667–68.

28 Bayley, N., Pinneau, S.R. Tables for predicting adult height from skeletal age revised for use with the Greulich-Pyle hand standards. *J Pediatr* 1952; **40:** 423–41 (correction 1952; **41:** 371).

29 Buckler, J.M.H. Dental development. In Buckler, J.M.H. *A Reference Manual of Growth and Development.* Oxford: Blackwell Scientific Publications, 1979: 74–75.

30 Demirjian, A., Goldstein, H., Tanner, J.M. A new system of dental age assessment. *Hum Biol* 1973; **45:** 211–27.

31 Eveleth, P.B., Tanner, J.M. *Worldwide Variation in Human Growth.* London: Cambridge University Press 1976.

32 Tanner, J.M. Earlier maturation in man. *Sci Amer* 1968; **218:** 21–27.

33 Tanner, J.M. Trend towards earlier menarche in London, Oslo, Copenhagen, The Netherlands, and Hungary. *Nature* 1973; **243:** 95–96.

34 Hawk, L.J., Brook, C.G.D. Family resemblances of height, weight and body fatness. *Arch Dis Child* 1979; **54:** 877–79.

35 Goldstein, H. Factors influencing the height of seven-year-old children. *Hum Biol* 1971; **43:** 92–111.

36 Marshall, W.A. The relationship of variation in children's growth rates to seasonal climatic variations. *Ann Hum Biol* 1971; **2:** 243–50.

37 Marshall, W.A. Evaluation of growth rate in height over periods less than a year. *Arch Dis Child* 1971; **46:** 414–20.

38 Lindgren, G. Height, weight and menarche in Swedish urban school children in relation to socio-economic and regional factors. *Ann Hum Biol* 1976; **3:** 501–28.

39 Fancourt, R., Campbell, S., Harvey, D. Follow-up study of small-for-dates babies. *Br Med J* 1976; **i:** 1435–37.

40 Brook, C.G.D. Evidence for a sensitive period in adipose-cell replication in man. *Lancet* 1972; **ii:** 624–27.

41 Brook, C.G.D. *Obesity in Children* (MD thesis). Cambridge: University of Cambridge, 1972.

42 Preece, M.A., Law, C.M., Davies, P.S.W. The growth of children with chronic paediatric disease. *Baillière's Clin Endocrinol Metab* 1986; **15:** 453–77.

43 Shalet, S.M. Endocrine consequences of treatment of malignant disease. *Arch Dis Child* 1989; **64:** 1635–41.

44 Appan, S., Laurent, S., Chapman, M., Hindmarsh, P.C., Brook, C.G.D. Growth and growth hormone therapy in hypochondroplasia. *Acta Paediatr Scand* 1990; **79:** 796–803.

45 Varrela, J., Vinkka, H. The phenotype of 45X females: an anthropometric quantification. *Ann Hum Biol* 1984; **11:** 53–66.

46 Brook, C.G.D., Murset, G., Zachmann, M., Prader, A. Growth in children with 45XO Turner's syndrome. *Arch Dis Child* 1974; **49:** 789–95.

47 Ranke, M.B., Stubbe, P., Majewski, F., Bierich, J.R. Spontaneous growth in Turner's syndrome. *Acta Paediatr Scand* 1988; **343** [suppl]: 22–30.

48 Hindmarsh, P.C., Pringle, P.J., Di Silvio, L., Brook, C.G.D. A preliminary report on the role of somatostatin analogue (SMS 201–995) in the management of children with tall stature. *Clin Endocrinol* 1990; **32:** 83–91.

49 Hindmarsh, P.C., Pringle, P.J., Brook, C.G.D. Cholinergic muscarinic blockade produces short-term suppression of growth hormone secretion in children with tall stature. *Clin Endocrinol* 1988; **29:** 289–96.

50 Marshall, W.A. Interrelationships of skeletal maturation, sexual development and somatic growth in man. *Ann Hum Biol* 1974; **1:** 29–40.

51 Neyzi, O., Alp, H., Yalcindag, A., Yakacikli, S., Orphon, A. Sexual maturation in Turkish boys. *Ann Hum Biol* 1975; **2:** 251–59.

52 Nuttall, F.Q. Gynaecomastia as a physical finding in normal men. *J Clin Endocrinol Metab* 1979; **48:** 338–40.

53 Marshall, W.A., Tanner, J.M. Variations in pattern of pubertal changes in girls. *Arch Dis Child* 1969; **44:** 291–303.

54 Tisserand-Perrier, M. Etudes comparatives de certain processus de croissance chez les jumeux. *J Genet Hum* 1953; **2:** 87–102.

55 Neyzi, O., Alp, H., Orphon, A. Sexual maturation in Turkish Girls. *Ann Hum Biol* 1975; **2:** 49–55.

56 Roberts, D.R., Dann, D.C. Influences on menarcheal age in girls in a Welsh college. *Br J Prev Soc Med* 1967; **21:** 170–71.

57 Frisch, R.E., Revelle, R. Height and weight at menarche and a hypothesis of menarche. *Arch Dis Child* 1971; **46:** 695–701.

58 Billewicz, W.Z., Fellowes, H.M., Hytten, O.A. Comments on the cortical metabolic mass and the age of menarche. *Ann Hum Biol* 1976; **3:** 51–59.

59 Marshall, W.A., De Limongi, Y. Skeletal maturity and prediction of age at menarche. *Ann Hum Biol* 1976; **3:** 235–43.

60 Schaefer, F., Sceidel, C., Marr, J., Tilgen, W., Vecsei, P., Scharer, K. Spermaturia as an indicator of gonadal maturation – a study in healthy schoolboys (Abstract). *Horm Res* 1989 (Suppl); **70:** 18.

61 Nielsen, C.T., Skakkebaek, N.E., Richardson, D.W. *et al.* Onset of the release of spermatozoa (spermarche) in boys in relation to age, testicular growth, pubic hair, and height. *J Clin Endocrinol Metab* 1986; **62:** 532–35.

62 Tanner, J.M. *Growth at Adolescence*, 2nd edn. Oxford: Blackwell Scientific Publications, 1962.

63 Reiter, E.O., Grumbach, M.M. Neuroendocrine control mechanisms and the onset of puberty. *Ann Rev Physiol* 1982; **44:** 595–613.

64 Winter, J.S.D., Faiman, C., Hobson, W.C., Prasad, A.V., Reyes, F.I. Pituitary-gonadal regulations in infancy: 1. patterns of serum gonadotropin concentrations from birth to four years of age in man and chimpanzee. *J Clin Endocrinol Metab* 1975; **40:** 545–51.

65 Conte, F.A., Grumbach, M.M., Kaplan, S.L. A diphasic pattern of gonadotropin secretion in patients with the syndrome of gonadal dysgenesis. *J Clin Endocrinol Metab* 1975; **40:** 670–74.

66 Bourguignon, J.P. Time-related neuroendocrine manifestations of puberty: a combined clinical and experimental approach extracted from the 4th Belgian Endocrine Society Lecture. *Horm Res* 1988; **30:** 224–6234.

67 Brook, C.G.D., Jacobs, H.S., Stanhope, R., Adams, J., Hindmarsh, P. Pulsatility of reproductive hormones: application to the understanding of puberty and to the treatment of infertility. *Baillière's Clin Endocrinol Metab* 1987; **1:** 23–41.

68 Boyar, R.M., Finkelstein, J., Roffwarg, H. *et al.* Synchronisation of augmented luteinising hormone secretion with sleep during puberty. *N Engl J Med* 1972; **287:** 582–86.

69 Boyar, R.M., Rosenfeld, R.S., Kapen, S. *et al.* Human puberty – simultaneous augmented secretion of luteinising hormone and testosterone during sleep. *J Clin Invest* 1974; **54:** 609–18.

70 Boyar, R.M., Wu, R.H.K., Roffwarg, H. *et al.* Human puberty: 24-hour estradiol patterns in pubertal girls. *J Clin Endocrinol Metab* 1976; **43:** 1418–21.

71 Boyar, R.M., Finkelstein, J.W., Roffwarg, H., Kapen, S., Weitzmann, E.D., Hellman, L. Twenty-four hour luteinizing hormone and follicle stimulating hormone secretory pattern in gonadal dysgenesis. *J Clin Endocrinol Metab* 1973; **37:** 521–25.

72 Dickerman, Z., Prager-Lewin, R., Laron, Z. Response of plasma LH and FSH to synthetic LHRH in children at various pubertal stages. *Am J Dis Child* 1976; **130:** 634–38.

73 Dewhurst, J. *Female Puberty and its Abnormalities*. Edinburgh: Churchill Livingstone, 1984.

74 Kelnar, C.J.H., Brook, C.G.D. A mixed longitudinal study of adrenal steroid excretion in childhood and the mechanism of adrenarche. *Clin Endocrinol* 1983; **19:** 117–29.

75 Pringle, P.J., Stanhope, R., Hindmarsh, P., Brook, C.G.D. Abnormal sexual development in primary hypothyroidism. *Clin Endocrinol* 1988; **28:** 479–86.

76 Laron, Z., Karp, M., Dolberg, L. Juvenile hypothyroidism with testicular enlargement. *Acta Paediatr Scand* 1970; **59:** 317–22.

77 Kitay, J.I. Pineal lesions and precocious puberty: a review. *J Clin Endocrinol Metab* 1954; **14:** 622–25.

78 Brauner, R., Rappaport, R. Precocious puberty secondary to cranial irradiation for tumors distant from the hypothalamo-pituitary area. *Horm Res* 1985; **22:** 78–82.

79 Stanhope, R., Brook, C.G.D. Disorders of puberty. In: Brook, C.G.D. ed. *Clinical Paediatric Endocrinology*, 2nd edn. Oxford: Blackwell Scientific Publications, 1989: 189–212.

80 Stanhope, R., Brook, C.G.D. The clinical diagnosis of disorders of puberty: the loss of consonance. *Br J Hosp Med* 1986; **35:** 57–58.

81 New, M.I., Speiser, P.W. Congenital adrenal hyperplasia. In: Brook, C.G.D., ed. *Clinical Paediatric Endocrinology*, 2nd edn. Oxford: Blackwell Scientific Publications, 1989: 441–62.

82 Honour, J. The adrenal cortex. In: Brook, C.G.D. ed. *Clinical Paediatric Endocrinology*, 2nd edn. Oxford: Blackwell Scientific Publications, 1989: 341–67.

83 Rosenthal, S.N., Grumbach, M.M., Kaplan, S.L. Gonadotrophin independent familial sexual precocity with premature Leydig and germinal cell maturation (familial testotoxicosis): effects of a potent luteinising hormone-releasing factor agonist and medroxyprogesterone acetate therapy in four cases. *J Clin Endocrinol Metab* 1983; **57:** 571–79.

84 Wierman, M.E., Beardsworth, D.E., Mansfield, J. *et al.* Puberty without gonadotrophins: a unique mechanism of sexual development. *N Engl J Med* 1985; **312:** 65–72.

85 McCune, D.J., Bruch, H. Osteodystrophia fibrosa: report of a case in which the condition was combined with precocious puberty, pathological pigmentation of the skin and hyperthyroidism, with a review of the literature. *Am J Dis Child* 1937; **54:** 806–48.

86 Albright, F., Butler, A.M., Hampton, A.O. *et al.* Syndrome characterised by osteitis fibrosa disseminata, areas of pigmentation and endocrine dysfunction with precocious puberty in females, report of five cases. *N Engl J Med* 1937; **216:** 727–46.

87 Foster, C.M., Feuilan, P., Padmanabhan, V. *et al.* Ovarian function in girls with McCune-Albright syndrome. *Pediatr Res* 1986; **20:** 859–63.

88 Stanhope, R., Adams, J., Brook, C.G.D. Fluctuation of breast size in isolated premature thelarche. *Acta Paediatr Scand* 1985; **74:** 454–55.

89 Stanhope, R., Pringle, P.J., Adams, J., Brook, C.G.D. Premature thelarche variant. A new syndrome of precocious sexual maturation. *Pediatr Res* 1988; **24:** 540.

90 Brook, C.G.D. Management of delayed puberty. *Br Med J* 1985; **290:** 657–58.

91 Job, J.C., Chaussain, J.L., Garnier, P.E. The use of luteinizing hormone-releasing hormone in paediatric patients. *Horm Res* **1977; 8:** 171–87.

92 Perheentupa, J., Dessypris, A., Adlercreutz, H. Plasma testosterone levels in boys following gonadotrophin stimulation. *Acta Paediatr Scand* 1972; **61:** 265.

93 Sherwood, M.C., Stanhope, R., Preece, M.A., Grant, D.B. Diabetes insipidus and occult intracranial tumours. *Arch Dis Child* 1986; **61:** 1222–35.

94 Livesey, E.A., Darendeliler, F., Hindmarsh, P.C. *et al.* Endocrine disorders following treatment of childhood brain tumours. *Br J Cancer* 1990; **61:** 622–25.

95 Penny, R., Olambiwonnu, N.O., Frasier, S.D. Episodic fluctuations of serum gonadotrophins in pre- and post-pubertal girls and boys. *J Clin Endocrinol Metab* 1977; **45:** 307–11.

96 Stanhope, R., Adams, J., Jacobs, H.S., Brook, C.G.D. The induction of puberty by low dose pulsatile GnRH. *Pediatr Res* 1984; **18:** 1210.

97 Stanhope, R., Adams, J., Brook, C.G.D. Disturbances of puberty. *Clin Obstet Gynaecol* 1985; **12:** 557–77.

98 Santen, R.J., Paulsen, C.A. Hypogonadotrophic eunochoidism: clinical study of the mode of inheritance. *J Clin Endocrinol Metab* 1973; **36:** 47–54.

99 Laron, Z., Kaushanski, A., Josefsberg, Z. Penile size and growth in children and adolescents with isolated gonadotrophic deficiency. *Clin Endocrinol Metab* 1977; **6:** 265–70.

100 Massarano, A.A., Spoudeas, H.A., Holownia, P., Honour, J.W., Brook, C.G.D. Transdermal oestrogen for the induction of puberty in girls (Abstract). *Horm Res* 1989 (Suppl); **240:** 60.

101 Stanhope, R., Abdulwahud, N.A., Adams, J., Jacobs, H.S., Brook, C.G.D. Problems in the use of pulsatile GnRH for the induction of puberty. *Horm Res* 1985; **22:** 74–77.

102 Stanhope, R., Brook, C.G.D. Oxandrolone in low doses for constitutional delay of puberty in boys. *Arch Dis Child* 1985; **60:** 379–81.

103 Stanhope, R., Buchanan, C.R., Fenn, G.C., Preece, M.A. Double blind placebo-controlled trial of oxandrolone in the treatment of boys with constitutional delay of growth and puberty. *Arch Dis Child* 1988; **63:** 501–05.

104 Stanhope, R., Hindmarsh, P., Pringle, P.J., Honour, J., Brook, C.G.D. Oxandrolone induces a sustained rise in physiological GH secretion in boys with constitutional delay of growth and puberty. *Pediatrician* 1988; **14:** 183–88.

105 Adams, J., Polson, D.W., Abdulwahid, N.A. *et al.* Multifollicular ovaries; clinical and endocrine features and response to pulsatile gonadotrophin releasing hormone. *Lancet* 1985; ii: 1375–78.

106 Stanhope, R., Adams, J., Jacobs, H.S., Brook, C.G.D. Ovarian ultrasound assessment in normal children, idiopathic precocious puberty and during low dose pulsatile GnRH therapy of hypogonadotrophic hypogonadism. *Arch Dis Child* 1985; **60:** 116–19.

107 Brook, C.G.D., Jacobs, H.S., Stanhope, R. Polycystic ovaries in childhood (editorial). *Br Med J* 1988; **296:** 878.

108 Rebar, R., Judd, H.L., Yen, S.S.C., Rakoff, J., Vandenburg, G., Naftolin, F. Characterisation of the inappropriate gonadotrophin secretion in polycystic ovary syndrome. *J Clin Invest* 1976; **57:** 1320–29.

Chapter 5

Child health service

5.1 An overview

Stuart Logan

Introduction

Separate medical services for children are a relatively recent development. It is easy to forget that our modern view of childhood is itself a new concept. In medieval iconography, and even in some 18th century painting, children are depicted as miniature adults, a reflection, it has been suggested,[1] of how they were seen by their society. Children participated in all aspects of life; they played the same games as adults and were expected to work from an early age. Part of the reason for the different way children were regarded in earlier times was that a large proportion did not survive infancy: it is said that in the middle of the 18th century less than half the children born in London survived to the age of 5 years. It is not surprising that parents may have invested rather less emotion in their young infants than we would think normal today.

The modern concept of childhood developed in western society during the 18th and 19th centuries. A discussion of the reasons for this discovery of childhood is beyond the scope of this chapter, but it is interesting that the idealization of childhood among the middle class in Victorian times coincided with some of the most inhumane treatment of poor children ever seen. One consequence of the interest in childhood was increasing attention to the health and diseases of children. The first recorded children's clinic was started by Dr George Armstrong in London in 1769, although it closed some 12 years later on his retirement. A similar clinic was opened in Vienna in

1781 and, gradually, others were established in many of the cities of Europe. The lead in the development of paediatrics was taken in Germany where the first paediatric journal was established in 1834, the first chair of paediatrics in 1845, and the first association of paediatricians in 1883.

Child health services in the UK before the 1942 Beveridge Report

Curative services

The development of paediatrics in Britain was slower than in some other parts of Europe; the first separate ward for children was opened in Guy's Hospital, London in 1833 and in 1852 the Hospital for Sick Children, Great Ormond Street, London was founded. Similar hospitals were soon established in other parts of the country and gradually most general hospitals developed facilities for children. Paediatrics was not, however, established as a separate discipline in the UK until well into the 20th century; before this, most paediatric care was provided by doctors who also looked after adults. The foundation of the British Paediatric Association in 1928 led to a sustained campaign for the establishment of consultant posts in paediatrics and for greater training opportunities for young paediatricians.

There were four types of hospital in the 19th century: voluntary hospitals, which included the famous teaching hospitals, which depended on endowed funds and public charity; public hospitals which had developed out of poor law institutions dealing with the destitute sick; fever hospitals which were set up by local authorities because the voluntary hospitals did not accept infectious cases; and asylums for pauper lunatics. An Act of Parliament in 1867 provided for the construction of infirmaries specifically designed as hospitals. These hospitals provided a better standard of care, but tended to exclude people with chronic conditions and mainly admitted those with acute illnesses other than fevers. In 1929 all the poor law hospitals were transferred to the local authorities which meant that all except the voluntary hospitals were under one administrative structure. Nonetheless, by the time of the Second World War it was obvious that reform was urgently needed; many of the hospitals were too small to be viable and there was no planning to match provision with need. The need for coordination of emergency medical services during the Second World War was one of the spurs which helped create a general acceptance of the need to bring all hospital services into one system.

Primary care for children in the late 19th and early 20th centuries was provided partly by the developing general practice service, by hospital outpatient departments and by the local authorities. General practitioners (GPs) were originally private practitioners whose services were only available to those who could pay their fees. For some adults the situation changed after the National Health Insurance Act of 1911, which funded medical services for certain groups of compulsorily insured workers, but did not extend cover to their dependants. Gradually, however, it became the norm for general practitioners to provide primary care for all age groups, a position eventually institutionalized by the National Health Service Act of 1946. GPs have traditionally provided curative services for children as well as being the source of referral to specialist paediatric services, but until very recently preventive services remained, for the most part, outside their remit. In contrast, most other countries in Europe and in North America developed systems where primary care functions for children were largely delivered by specialist paediatric doctors.

Community services

In large part, the community child health services in the UK have been built around the work of specialist nurses: health visitors for the under-fives; school nurses for older children. In 1867 the Manchester and Salford Ladies Sanitary Reform Association provided for the employment of the first health visitor, initially a 'respectable woman' rather than a trained nurse. Similar schemes began to appear in other parts of the country, first established by charitable groups and later taken on by the local authorities. It was hoped that these women, who visited mothers in their homes

to provide advice on the feeding and management of their infants, would help to decrease the very high infant mortality rates in British cities at that time. The setting up of the first certificated training course in health visiting in Buckinghamshire in 1891 was the beginning of attempts to set the discipline onto a more professional footing. National training regulations for health visitors were laid down in 1919 and, after responsibility passed from the Board of Education to the Ministry of Health in 1925, these required that they first be trained in midwifery as well as in general nursing. Around the turn of the century, many local authorities began to open centres providing free sterilized milk for mothers and infants, a practice that was then widespread in Europe. Gradually, health visitors came to be based in such centres where they met mothers and dispensed advice.

In 1918, the Maternity and Child Welfare Act empowered local councils to provide free antenatal and postnatal care for mothers, and health care services for children, official recognition of what was already widespread practice. Medical services for the non-working population were then still not covered under the National Health Insurance scheme.

As well as new services for mothers and young children, there was the gradual development of services for school children. The beginning of compulsory education in 1870 helped to expose the appalling state of health of children in Britain. Malnutrition was the most obvious problem and many education boards and charities began to supply meals for poor children in schools. School medical officers were appointed and systematic medical inspections instituted. The evidence that a large proportion of men enlisting for service in the South African war were unfit to serve, provided a further impetus for the development of the service as the bad health of the poor came to be seen as a threat to the future of the Empire. The existence of widespread malnutrition continued to be seen as the major problem and the provision of school meals the solution. As one member of a government board of enquiry into the health of the population in 1904 commented, 'we must face the question whether the logical culmination of free education is not free meals in some form or other, it being cruelty to force a child to go and learn what it has not strength to learn'.[2] At the same time the continuing power of the ideology underlying the old Poor Law is illustrated by the many comments made by other members of this committee stressing the importance of forcing parents to pay wherever possible so as not to weaken 'self-respect'. One witness to the committee, the Bishop of Ross, argued that no free meals should be provided as it was worse to weaken people's self reliance than to allow their children to starve.[2] The view of the State's responsibilities towards children expanded over subsequent years and some local authorities appointed school nurses and began to offer treatment for minor ailments. In 1907, after much debate and considerable opposition, the Education Act gave local authorities the power to inspect and to attend to the health of all children in elementary schools, a power extended to include secondary school children in 1918.

The role of the school doctor developed from simply examining children to include the provision of advice to school authorities on the appropriate educational services for children with special needs. In the 1890s, education boards had been empowered to provide special schools for children with handicaps; by 1908, 17 000 children were attending special schools. In 1913, Sir Cyril Burt was appointed as psychologist to the London County Council to advise on the placement of such children. This type of support spread and by the mid-1930s most local authorities employed psychologists and many had established child guidance clinics for children with behavioural problems.

In the years leading up to the Second World War there was tremendous development of community services for women, the under fives and for schoolchildren. By the 1930s, local authorities had been obliged by the Department of Health to provide antenatal and obstetric services for all women and virtually all had established infant welfare provision based in child health centres. Similarly, school health services had extended provision for treatment and preventive care for older children. In retrospect, it seems amazing that not only were community services separate from general practitioner services, but even the two branches of community care for children, both provided under the aegis of the local authorities, remained for the most part separate.

From Beveridge to the modern National Health Service

The Second World War provoked great changes in British society. Nowhere is this more evident than in the reforms which resulted from the Beveridge report of 1942. There had already been great improvements in the health of the population since the turn of the century. The infant mortality rate which had remained virtually constant at around 150 per 1000 livebirths between 1840 and 1900 had fallen to 50 per 1000 by 1940.[3] The death rate in children aged 5–9 years had fallen more steadily, from 8.69 per 1000 population in 1840 to 4.12 in 1900 and 1.84 in 1940.[3] These changes are reflected by an increase in life expectancy at birth for females from 47.8 years at the turn of the century to 71.5 years by 1950–52.[4] There remained, nonetheless, widespread poverty, deprivation and ill health. A consensus developed within the political establishment that the situation could not continue without leading to discontent and social disruption, coinciding with a general view among the population that the sacrifices of the war entitled them to a fairer share of society's wealth. In 1941 the wartime coalition government appointed a commission under the chairmanship of Sir William Beveridge to examine the question of social and health services for post-war Britain.

The recommendations of this commission were perhaps more radical than had been envisaged by the politicians who had appointed it. Beveridge talked of the five giants – Want, Disease, Ignorance, Squalor and Idleness – which stood on the road to reconstruction and must be thrown down if the society was to be just and successful. The report proposed a number of measures to tackle these problems including a new system of social security which would guarantee a basic minimum income for all citizens, partly by the payment of a universal child benefit irrespective of income; changes to the education system making schooling compulsory till 15 years (to rise to 16 years as soon as possible); the provision of free meals and milk to schoolchildren and great extension of the scope of the school health service; the provision of a national health service funded from taxation which would be available to all. Virtually all the benefits of this system were to be universally available as of right and not means tested. This, thought Beveridge, would help to avoid both the effects of the 'poverty trap' which could mean people were worse off if they worked, and also to avoid the stigma attached to accepting charity. This represented a new philosophy of welfare provision; the poor law system explicitly used stigma as a deterrent and as a punishment for the destitute.

Commentators often imply that the implementation of these proposals was accomplished with little opposition. There was indeed a degree of social consensus at the time, but considerable opposition had nonetheless to be overcome, both from those who felt that the changes were too radical, and from special interest groups such as doctors who feared the loss of privilege. Although the basic thrust of the report was translated into legislation, many compromises, including rights of private practice for consultants and independent contractor status for GPs, had to be accepted before the changes could be implemented.

The central aim of the 1946 National Health Service Act was to provide a comprehensive health service for the whole population which would be free at the point of use. The new health service was to consist of three arms. Each National Health Service registered patient would have a general practitioner who would provide acute primary care for the whole family and would refer patients on to specialist services when required. All hospitals, public and voluntary, were brought under the control of the Ministry of Health and would provide specialist and inpatient services. The local authorities retained the responsibility for public health, first vested in them by the 1848 and 1875 Public Health Acts and for preventive services for under-fives and schoolchildren. In 1974 the system was reorganized and the local authority services were brought into the National Health Service, though retaining their separate staff.

Community paediatrics into the 1990s

We have seen that the National Health Service institutionalized the tripartite system of health care which had developed in the UK. This separation has come to be seen as both unnecessary and not in the best interests of children. The report of the Court committee on child health services published in 1976 after 3 years of deliberation[5] was particularly influential in persuading both paediatricians and policy makers of the need for the integration of all aspects of paediatric care. Inevitably there has been opposition to attempts to produce a truly integrated service; however, considerable, though slow, progress has been made.

The need for an integrated service is perhaps most obvious in the management of children with disabilities or chronic disease. These children are likely to require the services of a large number of different sub-specialities. A child with spina bifida for instance may well be seen by a developmental paediatrician, a physiotherapist, a speech therapist, an orthopaedic surgeon, a neurosurgeon and a urologist, in addition to the GP and health visitor. Optimum management demands that the activities of these professions be carefully coordinated. Equally important is the realization that most of the child's time is spent not with these professionals, but at home and in school, and that the family and teachers must be fully involved in their management. In recent years it has come to be accepted that good paediatric care is not just the efficient treatment of disease, but also includes working with families to help children achieve their full potential. One of the benefits of this change has been the development of multidisciplinary teams for the management of children with special needs. Most districts now have such teams working with children with disabilities and those who have been abused.

One of the changes envisaged by the Court committee was the creation of a new type of paediatrician, a consultant community paediatrician, with special skills in developmental, educational and social paediatrics. After a slow beginning there has been a rapid expansion of such posts. In 1990 a census by the British Paediatric Association identified 140 consultant community paediatricians undertaking five or more sessions in community paediatrics. It is envisaged that a further substantial number of such posts will be established over the next few years. The British Paediatric Association has recommended that there should be at least one consultant community paediatrician in each district health authority, although a lack of suitably trained people remains a problem. These doctors are of equivalent status with their hospital-based colleagues and work closely with them. Their role has not yet been fully defined and varies greatly from district to district: some are essentially clinicians working with children with disabilities and dealing with child abuse, while others fulfil a role much closer to that of a public health doctor for children, being responsible for the planning, organization and evaluation of services for children in a defined population. Many are expected to encompass both sets of responsibilities. A joint report[6] of the Faculty of Public Health Medicine and the British Paediatric Association has highlighted the implications of this dual role for the future training of community paediatricians.

Most of the routine work in community paediatrics has traditionally been performed by clinical medical officers. Under the terms of the new GP contract, it is envisaged that the bulk of this work will in the future be undertaken by general practitioners. The integration of primary acute and preventive care for children in a general practice setting has been generally welcomed. There are however a number of concerns. Although clinical medical officers were not required to have either formal training or higher qualifications in paediatrics, fears have been expressed about the effects of the loss of their skills and experience on the quality of child health surveillance. Most general practitioners have had little experience or training in paediatrics and will require considerable back-up if they are to provide an effective service. District health authorities will retain overall responsibility for child health surveillance, but the issue of how they will monitor the service provided by the independent contractor GPs has not yet been fully addressed. The future of doctors presently employed as clinical medical officers is unclear. It seems likely that many will continue to run the school health service and to provide a service in areas where GPs do not wish to be involved in surveillance for the under-fives, while others will develop a more specialized role providing advice and training for GPs.

This discussion of the changes in the type of doctor responsible for community paediatric services should not obscure the fact that the system continues to rest largely on the work of health visitors and school nurses, much as it has done since its inception. It seems likely that the role of health visitors in particular will expand as GPs take more responsibility for child health surveillance for their patients. Health visitors will generally have more experience than the GPs both in child development and in the management of feeding, sleep and behavioural problems which are so common in young children. Where health visitors and GPs are not working as partners in a primary care team, there may well be problems over the division of responsibilities and possibly over the rewards as well. It is to be hoped that school nurses will take on a wider role in health promotion and also increase their involvement in counselling. It is obviously necessary that if school nurses and health visitors are to take on more responsibilities that appropriate training is made available.

Child health services in other countries

This section concentrates on the services in the rich countries of Europe, North America and Australasia. There are however common principles which underlie the provision of services in any country and there is much to learn from the experience in the poorer parts of the world.

There is a remarkable diversity of systems of health care finance and of health care delivery for children in the rich countries. Common to all, however, are the provision of primary and referral services for acute illness and some form of child health surveillance. In some countries, including the USA, both primary acute paediatric care and child health surveillance are carried out by specialist paediatricians; others follow the UK model of separating acute and preventive services. The frequency of visits for child health surveillance varies greatly in different countries as does the type of professional involved. In Denmark and New Zealand specialist nurses take a leading role, whereas in the Netherlands child health surveillance involves eleven visits to a paediatrician in the first year of life and a further six visits between one year and school entry just before 4 years of age. All surveillance programmes include the examination of children at intervals by professionals, with the aim of detecting abnormalities, but many have broader aims as well. These include advice on the management of minor problems, the sharing of knowledge about child development and health prevention and health promotion. In recent years the efficacy of the screening functions has been questioned, with the result that more attention is being paid to these other activities. In Sweden, for example, in 1969 the aim of the preventive service for children was defined as 'a complete health surveillance and a handicap-finding activity': in 1979, the wording was changed to read 'to support and activate parents in their parenthood and thereby create favourable conditions for a comprehensive development of children.'[7]

Perhaps the central issue confronting health care planners in all countries is that of access to services for those most in need. There is compelling evidence that, the poorer you are, the worse your health, and that this health gradient is apparent even in very rich countries where the poorest have adequate food and shelter. In 1971 Tudor Hart suggested that, 'the availability of good medical care tends to vary inversely with the need for it in the population.'[8] Unfortunately, this appears to remain true today in most parts of the world. Although most rich countries offer services to all, poor people not only have the greatest need but are generally least likely to use the services. The barriers to the utilization of services by the poor may include a lack of perception of the benefits of preventive services or alienation from officialdom, in addition to the direct costs of health care and indirect costs such as transport or loss of income from time off work.

While this inverse care law is often quoted, the second of Tudor Hart's conclusions is referred to less frequently: he also suggested that the greater the exposure of medical services to market forces the more completely did this law apply.[8] Although the balance between state funding and private or state-run insurance schemes varies, virtually all countries have systems which attempt to provide access to acute and preventive care for all children. It remains true however that, even in rich countries, the most deprived groups probably have the worst services as a result of these informal barriers. The country which best illustrates the problems that can arise with predominantly private provision is the USA. For most Americans health care is funded by a system of private health insurance with the poorest being entitled to services provided by state funding through Medicaid. In 1981 the report of the Select Panel for the Promotion of Child Health to the United States Congress highlighted the gaps in the system.[9] They argued that strict criteria for eligibility to the Medicaid programme and variations from state to state in the adequacy of provision resulted in seven million children, defined as poor by federal criteria, receiving no benefits from the programme. Overall they suggested that American health funding systems provide health services, 'that collectively are unresponsive to a significant part of patient needs, especially those of children and pregnant women.'[9] They recommended that the interests of these groups would be best served by a national health financing programme that ensured universal entitlement to health care and included comprehensive health care for children from birth to 5 years. The political climate at the time this report was published meant that the recommendations were ignored; with the election of a new president, however, interest in a national health system has increased and it appears likely that the proposals will be revived.

In our search for the most effective ways of organizing health care for children, we should take note of the lessons learned by attempts to set up services in poorer parts of the world. In the 1960s pioneers such as David Morley in Nigeria and David Werner in Mexico began to argue that transplanting high technology western medicine to poor countries simply ate up their resources without improving the health of the population. Instead they proposed community-based primary health care which concentrated on prevention. Since that time vast numbers of primary health care projects have been set up; some have succeeded but many have failed. The common thread which runs through the successful projects is community involvement. Although there can be no guarantee of success when working in areas of great poverty and often inadequate infrastructure, the lack of community participation is an almost certain remedy for long-term failure. Unfortunately it may be virtually impossible to gain real community participation in modern European cities where the population is mobile and often has little sense of community. We must at least be sure however that health services are sensitive to health needs as perceived by the consumers and not simply what professionals think is good for them.

Conclusions

The National Health Service in the UK has been successful in making available health services for the whole population and in allowing the beginnings of rational planning. Unfortunately, the inherited, uneven distribution of facilities remains an unresolved problem. A major weakness of the original plan was that Beveridge failed to anticipate the rapid escalation in health care costs which followed, expecting instead that demand would decline as the population became healthier. Although the National Health Service has been more successful than most health care systems in providing low cost services, the best method of rationing resources has yet to be established. The distribution of resources within the National Health Service, particularly between acute and community services, remains a contentious issue. There has been a tendency for the more glamorous acute services headed by powerful, high-status consultants to absorb the lion's share of resources.

Child health services developed in this country in a context of high child mortality and morbidity and widespread poverty. Although the standard of living has risen rapidly since the Second World War there remains a great deal of poverty and there is much evidence that the poor have become relatively worse off in the last decade. It is true that mortality and illness in children have both declined in the 40 years since the establishment of the NHS, but this is more likely to be the result of socioeconomic changes than of any effect of the health service. Paediatricians have yet to define their role in this new environment. Little effort has been devoted to the question of what the aims of child health services should be, particularly community child health services. Our services are not the result of rational planning but, like Topsy, 'just growed'. Most community paediatricians, if asked what the service hopes to achieve, would probably focus on the need for early detection of abnormality, although in practice they fulfil a much wider role. In the face of demands for the evaluation of services it becomes imperative that we clearly set out the aims of our work so that we can be judged accordingly. The time has come for a more specific statement of aims which reflects the developing perception that the central role of child health services should be to provide support for children and their carers.

References

1 Aries, P. *Centuries of Childhood*. Harmondsworth: Penguin, 1973.
2 *Report of the Select Inter-Departmental Committee on Physical Deterioration*. London: HMSO, 1904 (no. C2175).
3 Office of Population Censuses and Surveys. *Mortality Statistics, Perinatal and Infant: Social and Biological Factors*. London: OPCS, 1983 DH3 no. 15, table 2.
4 Office of Population Censuses and Surveys. *Demographic Review*. London: OPCS, 1977 DR no. 1, table 2.5.
5 Committee on Child Health Services (Court, D. Chairman) *Fit for the Future*: London: HMSO, 1976 Cmnd. 6684.
6 Faculty of Public Health Medicine and British Paediatric Association. *Together for Tomorrow's Children: the Interface Between the Work of Consultant Paediatricians (Community Child Health) and Public Health Physicians*. London: BPA/FPHM, 1990.
7 Köhler, L., Jakobsson, G. *Children's Health and Wellbeing in the Nordic Countries*. Oxford: MacKeith Press, 1987: 6.
8 Tudor Hart, J. The inverse care law. *Lancet* 1971;i: 405–412.
9 Select Panel for the Promotion of Child Health. *Better Health for Our Children: a National Strategy*. Washington: United States Dept of Health and Human Services (PHS Publication); 79–55071, 1981.

5.2 Primary care aspects of community child health

Colin Waine

The overriding aim of any system of medical care must be to improve on its present state. The starting point must be an assessment of the problem areas which need to be tackled.

In July of 1982, using the World Health Organization (WHO) definition of health which includes both physical and emotional health of children, the Royal College of General Practitioners published *Healthier*

Children – Thinking Prevention.[1] The report concluded that the environment and deficiencies in medical services were the main areas to be addressed if improvement in child health were to be achieved.

Environmental problems

Social class

The report highlighted the effect on infant mortality of social class difference. In 1931 twice as many babies died in the first year of life in social class V compared with social class I.

By 1951 the picture was no better; although the infant mortality rate had almost halved, the death rate in social class V had only improved to the level in social class I recorded 20 years previously.

In 1980 the Black Committee reported that, 'A child born to professional parents, if he or she is not socially mobile, can expect to spend over five years or more as a living person than a child born to an unsheltered manual household.'[2] The same report made it clear that in 1970 the infant mortality ratio in social class V compared with social class I had widened further to 2.5:1.

The social class divide is unfortunately not diminishing with time.

Poverty and disadvantage

For large numbers of children material conditions have deteriorated in the following respects: the proportion living in poverty has increased – nearly one-third in the lowest income groups are families with children; many more children live in families deemed homeless; more children live in families where the parents are unemployed and many children face unemployment in the future.

The incidence of racism and violence seems to be rising in the inner cities and increasing numbers of children are from ethnic minority groups. These are often among the most disadvantaged and they present a special challenge to the health services.

Accidents

Accidents remain the single major cause of childhood death between the ages of 6 months and 15 years and many occur in the home.

Unemployment

Unemployment levels are falling but unemployment acts as a major stress on families and therefore has a substantial impact on children. Beale and Nethercott have carefully documented the effects of unemployment on health.[3]

Deficiencies in the medical services

Although successive governments have acknowledged the importance of primary care and despite the fact that the British government signed the WHO declaration of Alma-Ata,[4] the proportion of NHS resources devoted to primary care has fallen.

Lack of resources is not the only problem. For too long prevention has not been given a high enough priority.

Primary child health care

Four key principles affect health and the health services:

- Environment
- Prevention
- Accessibility
- Cost-effectiveness.

Environment

The health of children depends on the provision of shelter and food by caring parents. The biggest single factor affecting death and disease in childhood is the environment which for the child is home and the family.

General practitioners were among the first clinicians to study the relationship between home and health.[5-8] Their studies showed the adverse effect of an unfavourable environment. Pollak[9] showed that children's development was influenced more by the type of mothering they received than by the standard of housing – emphasizing the importance of a secure emotional environment.

Because the health of children is so substantially influenced by the environment – the children's home and family – it is logical that the primary responsibility is with the general practitioner (GP) who regularly enters this environment. The GP's knowledge of the parents and often the grandparents as well adds to the opportunity for good primary care.

Prevention

'Prevention is better than cure' is a statement with which few would disagree. Indeed Pereira Gray[10] quoted Thackrah that it was 'the supreme activity'.

Prevention is particularly important for children. 'The rewards of prevention in childhood are unique because the benefits may last a whole lifetime.'[11]

If the importance of prevention is recognized it follows that it should be provided by those who know the child and home best – the general practitioner and practice-based team. Furthermore, primary care provides the ideal vehicle for bringing together prevention, surveillance and therapeutic care. This has been well demonstrated by Stott and Davis who have described a four-point framework designed to achieve greater breadth in each GP consultation (Table 5.1).[12]

Table 5.1 The potential in each primary care consultation

A	B
Management of presenting problems	Modification of help-seeking behaviour
C	D
Management of continuing problems	Opportunistic health promotion

Source: Stott and Davis.[13]

Accessibility

The WHO declaration 'Health for all by the year 2000' emphasized the importance of reaching the whole population.[4]

The social class divide in health has been previously mentioned and here it is reassuring to quote the General Household Survey which showed that general practitioners are more in touch with the lower social classes than with those in the upper social classes and that the NHS has achieved equality in terms of access to primary care.[13]

Since general practitioners have more consultations with people in social classes IV and V, this gives them and primary care teams a unique chance to be in contact with those children whose needs are greatest.

Cost-effectiveness

No country can afford to commit unlimited resources to health care. Careful choices have to be made to secure the best value for money. Generalist-based primary health care has emerged as the most cost-effective. The cost of general practitioner care (including expenses) is now about £23 per year per individual (including bank holidays) and is substantially less than the cost of a single outpatient appointment.

It has previously been shown that the main causes of mortality and morbidity in children are associated with the environment. Thus, if health services are to have a significant impact they must be sensitive to the child's:

1 Socioeconomic circumstances
2 Home
3 Family.

General practitioners and health visitors have a long tradition of caring for children and their families, often in their homes. They are accessible and cost-effective and general practice offers an ideal opportunity to bring together prevention, surveillance and therapeutic care. This is the greatest strength of primary care.

Approach to surveillance in primary care

'Children are the basic resource for all human endeavour.' (Wedgewood R.J. 1992)

As children thrive, so does mankind, because children represent our access to the future. Primary care is about recognizing that children are the resource for all that the human race seeks to achieve and it is about seeking the means by which our child population – our most precious inheritance – can be allowed to realize their full potential by seeing that they enter adulthood at an optimal state of development physically, mentally and socially.

Child care is about the continued growth and development of its subjects and, in this respect, is different from other parts of medical care.

The recognition of the importance of children for the future is nothing new. Galen (130–200) emphasized a need for special consideration of the nurture of children. Rhazes (850–932) devoted an entire treatise to children's diseases.

The first printed medical text book in the middle ages was devoted solely to child rearing and the diseases of children (Bagellardus, Libellus, Deegritudinibus Infantium, 1472). In the 16th century Pare, Gesner and Mercurialis provided abundant evidence about the unique importance of maternal and child health.

Over the years there has been no lack of published works relating to the upbringing and the well-being of children. But, all too often, this has resulted in acceptance of what has been handed down rather than the development of a programme of surveillance which has been critically evaluated. More recently a programme has been agreed by professionals in the UK who regularly practise child health surveillance.[14]

The aims of any child health surveillance programme are defined elsewhere in this book (Chapter 6.3).

Since the 19th century, the main improvements in the health of the population have resulted from better nutrition, sanitation, housing and contraception.[15]

In the case of children, the main determinants of childhood mortality and morbidity are nutrition and housing, parental care and genetic factors. Accidents are the main cause of death between the ages of 6 months and 15 years in the UK. This factor is intimately related to the child's environment – the home, the family and the peer group. The home provides the physical environment; the family the emotional environment; yet nowadays one in three marriages ends in divorce with the resulting necessity for children to adjust not only to the break-up of their parents' relationship, but often to adapt to a new parent also.

Interventions

Primary care teams should bear in mind that there are six well validated interventions which can make a major impact on the health of their child population:

1 Encouraging family planning
2 Encouraging antenatal care
3 Encouraging breast feeding
4 Advising against smoking
5 Advising on the responsible use of drugs and alcohol
6 Promoting health.

Encouraging family planning

Rutter[16] showed that pre-school children in larger families are less likely to do well at school, have a higher incidence of conduct disorders and are in fact more likely to die.

In 1980 in England the postneonatal mortality rate for children born to mothers with four or more children was 50% greater than the national average. In addition, Forssman and Thuwe[13] showed that children born of unwanted pregnancies are more likely to be disturbed emotionally and Kempe and Kempe[18] showed that such children are more likely to be physically abused.

Encouraging antenatal care

Antenatal care lends itself to team work between the general practitioner, midwife, health visitor and secondary care services led by the consultant obstetrician and gynaecologist. Antenatal patients are usually very receptive to information about the importance of good nutrition of both mother and infant, and the importance of immunization. Pregnancy is a good time for anti-smoking advice, the reasonable use of alcohol and drugs and checking on general health and nutrition. If necessary, genetic counselling can be offered.

Encouraging breast feeding

While breast feeding is clearly the optimum method of feeding children, those mothers who fail must not be made to feel inferior. Encouraging breast feeding is most likely to succeed when primary and secondary care teams deliver consistent advice.

Advising against smoking

There is no doubt that smoking is the greatest single preventable health hazard (WHO). Colley[19] demonstrated that the children of smokers have more respiratory problems and that discouraging smoking is likely to improve the health of both parents and children. Russell[20] showed that general practitioners are a major source of anti-smoking advice and that their advice was likely to be the most effective.

Children of non-smoking parents are less likely to smoke as teenagers and adults. The recommendations detailed in the RCGP Report of 1982, are as relevant now as when they were first produced.[1]

Advising on the responsible use of drugs and alcohol

Evidence is accumulating which underlines the importance of human behaviour. In 1975 Lalonde, a minister in the government of Canada, found that the main causes of death and hospital admission in Canada arose from environmental factors, especially human behaviour. Encouraging families to take a responsible attitude to the use of alcohol and abstention from the taking of drugs is a highly important part of preventive medical care.

Promoting health

Stott and Davis,[12] in their work on the consultation, showed that it could be used to deal with presenting problems and to encourage health promoting behaviour. Child surveillance should not be merely about the identification of abnormality; it should equally emphasize the importance of adopting a healthy lifestyle and the contribution which this can make to future health and well-being. Later in the chapter, suggestions are made of topics which can be raised at each of the surveillance examinations.

Delivery of child health care within primary care

'Growth and development are the essence of childhood. Parents find endless satisfaction in watching and discussing the development of their children and, in most cases, quickly become concerned when the child lags behind their idea of what is normal. Books and magazines, radio and television are increasing both knowledge and anxiety about the growth and development of children and the family doctor must know the facts and see that there is a time and a place to pass them on to the young mothers of his practice. For many doctors this will mean turning their minds to a subject which received scant attention in their training and seems far removed from the concept of the doctor's work with which they left their medical school. We feel that this subject should not be left wholly to the health visitor and the child welfare clinic. The facts can be learnt by any doctor willing to watch and record the development of the young children in his practice and such knowledge must strengthen his relationship with the parents of young families and, at the same time, assist him to detect abnormality at an early age.' (Court[21])

Increasingly, general practitioners are moving towards a proactive role to promote the healthy growth of children protected from hazards of the environment.

A system based on a series of check-ups at key ages in a child's development can aid this but, to be successful, certain principles must be borne in mind. They are:

- The need to develop good and effective relationships with patients and within the primary care team.
- Good practice organization.
- Sound knowledge and skills in the handling and examination of children.

It is heartening to report that Cartwright and Anderson have generally found good relationships between patients and their doctors.[22] Introducing a programme of child health surveillance into general practice can improve these relationships.

Because general practitioners have extensive contact with families, surveillance provided by a general practitioner who knows the family is likely to be more effective than that done by a doctor who is a stranger and who may never have visited the family home. (The average patient sees his doctor 3.7 times each year.[13] Thus the average nuclear family of two parents with 2.1 children would see a general practitioner $4.1 \times 3.7 = 15.2$ times every year.)

In addition, the average NHS patient stays with the average NHS general practitioner about 9 years; 35% have the same general practitioner for over 10 years and 30% for over 15 years.[23]

Parents need to be supported in the difficult task of rearing children. It is important to note the work of Cox et al. in Hounslow,[25] who found that approximately 30% of parents who brought their children to child health surveillance clinics thought that abnormality existed when this was not so. Reassurance about normality is as important as detecting abnormality.

Time should be allowed to consider a family holistically. It is important to try to find out what the child means to each parent. Efforts must be made to see problems as they present through the child's eyes. Problem children are not trying to create problems, but merely trying to solve them.

There has long been in general practice a strong tradition of family-based care, and practitioners are now increasingly trained to see their patients in the context of their home and social environment. The importance of the home and the family must be reflected in the organization and delivery of health services for children.

Primary health care team

In addition to an effective relationship between the primary care team and children and parents, there is the necessity for good relationships to develop within the team itself. Team work is the key to providing comprehensive care for children.

The care provided by a group of professionals pooling their skills should be much more effective than that provided by professionals working in isolation. Each primary care team will work in different ways to make the best use of its members' interests and skills. There is evidence that a joint approach by general practitioners and health visitors has a beneficial effect on the uptake of primary care services and immunizations. Equally, high profile team work must always function in a way which maximizes the role of the family. The aim should be to encourage the family's strengths, not to diminish them.

Practice organization

Although the practical elements of a primary child health care programme will be delivered by professionals, i.e. general practitioners and health visitors, the back-up of practice managers, receptionists and secretaries is fundamental.

Records

A parent-held record card is now available. The use of this will aid the sharing of information between general practitioners, health visitors, community health doctors, the school health service, specialist services and other professionals. While such a development should be welcomed, there will remain the need for individual professional workers to keep records as required.

Coverage

The aim of every practice should be to see that the whole of their child population benefits from a systematic programme of child health care and surveillance. It is essential that each general practice develops its own system to identify and chase up defaulters. Failure to attend on one occasion should lead to the offer of another appointment. Failure to attend on two occasions should result in a home visit by the practice health visitor. It is essential that general practitioners within each health district transmit information about their child health care programmes to district health authorities to promote recording of health trends and needs and planning of new approaches uniformly for the future.

Personnel and equipment

A suggested list of equipment of use in child health surveillance appears in Appendix 5.I. It is important that the doctor and health visitor undertaking this work are able and willing to listen and observe the mother and child. They must give the mother ample time to express any anxieties that she may hold. It is essential that the waiting area be made attractive for children with a variety of toys and books. Much can then be learned from observing the ways in which they play and behave.

Time

Primary health care teams need to make their own arrangements how they carry out their work but protected time to do this in is necessary. Protected time allows the coming together of different professionals; general practitioners and health visitors and, where appropriate, practice nurses and staff. It also allows them to discuss findings and to decide what action should be taken.

There are many views about when are the best times to check on children and their development. The programme described below takes account of the recommendations made in *Health for All Children*[14] and is a consensus view of representatives including general practitioners, paediatricians, nurses, and community physicians. There should be a first examination shortly after birth. Thereafter, reviews or examinations should occur at 6–8 weeks, 7–9 months, between 18 and 24 months, and around 39 months. Many people would also recommend an examination at or about school entry.

Neonatal examination

See Table 6.3 for details.

Every infant should be examined soon after birth. The parents should be given the chance to voice any concerns before commencing the physical examination.

Any indication from the history that the baby is in a high risk category for a hearing defect should be noted and consideration given to specialist referral. At 10 days, it is useful to recheck the hips.

Examination at 6 to 8 weeks

See Table 6.3 for details.

A sense of how the parents are coping and enjoying the baby should be sought and whether they have any areas of concern. Then it is necessary to perform a full physical examination again. Enquiries should elicit any concerns for the child's hearing or vision.

Each of the structured examinations gives the health professionals the opportunity both to receive and give information and discuss issues with parents.

If breast feeding is occurring, encouragement should be given for its continuation. It is appropriate to check whether the parents need any advice in respect of family planning and to confirm that the mother has had her postnatal check. The doctor should check that he has written confirmation of the results of chemical screening for phenylketonuria and hypothyroidism.

A record should be made of the feeding method and any associated difficulties.

Things to look for include:

- Mothering behaviour and her general emotional attitude
- Major anxiety in the mother
- Restricted abduction of the hip(s)
- Unusually large or small head
- Excessive head lag on pulling to a sitting position
- Asymmetry of tone
- Inadequate visual response
- Inadequate weight gain

Constructive discussion appropriate to this stage:

1 Advice about preventing hypothermia or over-heating the baby.
2 Information concerning the importance of vaccination/immunization procedures for the baby. It is useful to note the mother's attitude and beliefs about vaccination/immunization.
3 Advice about the effects of passive smoking on babies, young children and others. The smoking status of mother and close family members should be reviewed.
4 Encouragement to continue breast feeding if relevant.
5 Confirm mother's postnatal check.
   Establish her rubella status.
   Establish adequacy of family planning advice.

Examination at 7–9 months

See Table 6.3.

By this age most babies have adequate sitting balance and can locate sounds well enough to make it possible to screen hearing using a distraction test performed by two trained health professionals.

Initially there should be a review of the history since the last examination and the mother asked if she is enjoying the baby and whether she has any specific worries. Feeding and any associated difficulties should be reviewed and the immunization status of the child considered.

Things to look for include:

- Major anxiety in the mother
- Limited abduction of the hip(s)
- Abnormal posture or movements of the baby
- Squint
- Nystagmus
- Failure to fixate properly
- Delayed social and language development
- Inadequate weight gain

Constructive discussion appropriate to this stage:

1 Confirm immunization uptake and reinforce advice about the importance of the vaccination/immunization programme.
2 Establish current smoking status of mother and immediate family.
3 Discuss nutritional progress of baby.
   Give special attention to vegetarian weaning.

4 Home safety is of vital importance. Advise on ways to prevent:
   (a) Inhalation of food, airway obstruction and suffocation.
   (b) Mechanical suffocation by plastic bags etc.
   (c) Scalds/burns.
   (d) Falls, e.g. from sofas, prams, stairs, mobile toys.
   (e) Poisoning, e.g. medicinal tablets, household cleaning fluids, etc.
   and give advice on:
   (f) Legal requirements for fireguard for *all* types of fire or other heating appliances, e.g. very hot radiators.
   (g) Provision of safety gates.
   (h) Safe toys.

Examination at 21 months (range 18–24 months)

See Table 6.3.

The history since the last check should be reviewed and, once again, the parents allowed the opportunity to express concerns. It is important to ask particularly about concerns regarding vision or hearing. It should be confirmed that the child is walking with a normal gait, is understanding phrases when spoken to and is beginning to say words.

Things to look for include:

- Major anxiety in the mother
- Inability to take six steps
- Limited abduction of the hip(s)
- Abnormality of grasp, e.g. failure to develop fine pincer grasp and to manipulate fine objects
- Visual defect or squint
- Lack of interest and responsiveness: failure to look at the mother or failure to play meaningfully with toys
- Failure to make spontaneous vocalizations
- Casting, mouthing and drooling
- Heart murmur, but note this could be benign
- Undescended testes

Constructive discussion appropriate to this stage:

1 Again reinforce the importance of the vaccination/immunization programme.
2 Establish and advise about the current smoking status of mother and immediate family.
3 Reinforce home safety advice; the child is now mobile and more at risk from all forms of home accident. Check on provision of fireguards, safe toys and play equipment.
4 Discuss nutritional patterns and ability to feed and drink independently.
5 Foot health education, e.g. suitability of footwear to permit growth without deformity.
6 Dental health education.
7 Toilet training.
8 Language development.

9 Temper tantrums and behaviour in general.

Examination at 36–42 months

See Table 6.3.

Again the history since the last examination should be reviewed with specific enquiry about vision, squint, hearing, behaviour and general development. Measure the child's height and plot this on the appropriate centile chart and in boys recheck testicular descent. If there are reasonable concerns about vision, squint or hearing, referral to the specialist clinic for more detailed assessment will need to be arranged.

Things to look for include:

- Major anxiety in the mother
- Clumsiness in performing simple tasks
- Suspected defect of vision or hearing
- Indistinct speech or stuttering, immature language
- Problems of behaviour
- Lack of reasonable concentration span (the child should be directable and show concentration on a given task)

Constructive discussion appropriate to this stage:

1 Remind mother of need for pre-school vaccination/immunization.
2 Establish and advise about the current smoking status of mother and immediate family.
3 Continue with:
   (a) Dental health education
   (b) Foot health education.
4 Continue with advice about:
   (a) Nutritional patterns
   (b) Exercise/sleep patterns
   (c) Play opportunities
   (d) Home safety. This age group is fully mobile but has not yet learnt caution. Maintaining safety at home and on the road is of prime importance. Accidents are the commonest cause of death among toddlers and older children. Advice, support and encouragement for mother to promote safe independence of the young child cannot be overstated.

Further consideration

It is important when carrying out primary child health care examinations to bear in mind factors in the history which may influence the child's development. These may be genetic factors, psychiatric history, epilepsy, relative infertility, severe pre-eclamptic toxaemia, infections or consumption of drugs in pregnancy and intrauterine growth retardation.

There are specific risk factors relating to vision. These are:

- Family history of visual problems
- Rubella in early pregnancy

- Severe prematurity
- Ophthalmia neonatorum
- The presence of nystagmus
- The presence of squint

There are also specific risk factors in respect of hearing. These are:

- Dysmorphic features
- Familial deafness
- Rubella in pregnancy
- Severe pre-eclampsia in pregnancy
- Maternal drug consumption in pregnancy (e.g. streptomycin, quinine, gentamicin, kanamycin, neomycin)
- Extreme prematurity
- Hyperbilirubinaemia in the neonatal period
- Cerebral palsy
- Cerebral anoxia
- Intrapartum bleeding
- Maternal AIDS
- Down syndrome
- Birth trauma
- Meningitis at any age

If any of these risk factors are present, it is advisable that there is detailed assessment at the earliest opportunity.

The mother's opinion should always be taken seriously as should any opinion expressed by relatives or friends. Doubt in the mind of the mother at the end of an examination is often an indication that:

1 The situation has not been handled well or
2 There is the need for a further opinion.

Assessments of children should never be carried out when the child is tired, bored or hungry. The doctor should always look for treatable problems. Assessments are made on what has happened up to the present time and therefore on what is known. Conclusions are based on how the child has developed so far and it does not always follow that future development will necessarily occur at a similar rate.

It is necessary to remember that there are dangers and pitfalls in assessing the development of children. Indeed, detailed developmental assessment is a function of secondary and not primary care.

If an abnormality is suspected the doctor should be sure that this is so before sharing concern with the parents and should never refuse a further opinion.

Since the publication of the Court Report[24] over 15 years ago, there have been some distinct advances in the health care of children. Despite these advances, we still cannot view the health and social conditions of many children with anything but deep concern. Yet, as Philip Graham wrote in June of 1987, 'Politicians, businessmen, health professionals and above all parents, must surely be united in one belief; there can be

no better form of investment for the future than a healthy child.'[26]

General practitioners and primary care teams can make a tremendous contribution to such an investment by seeing that their services enable parents to care for their children with prevention as the main thrust and with close links between the preventive and curative elements.

Child Health Surveillance Lists: The pre-school health surveillance of children has increasingly moved into general practice and this has been encouraged by the new contract for general practitioners which became operative on 1st April 1990. While any general practitioner can carry out child surveillance, only those accredited to do so by the Family Health Service Authority can be remunerated. Guidelines for the accreditation and training of those doctors were issued jointly by the Royal College of General Practitioners, British Paediatric Association, General Medical Services Committee and the Joint Committee on Postgraduate Training for General Practice, in 1991.[27]

There have been anomalies in the past in that a GP in contract with adjoining Family Health Service Authorities has been accredited by one and not the other. Guidelines were formulated to try to avoid such anomalies but mainly to achieve national standards. Family Health Service Authorities should expect accredited general practitioners to operate a programme of child surveillance based on that outlined in *Health for All Children* and in the departmental circular.

While district health authorities are perfectly entitled to develop their own programmes of child surveillance, it is expected that they base them on the programme which was developed after widespread consultation with all the professional groups concerned with the welfare of children.

Appendix 5.I Equipment for the doctor undertaking primary child health care work

Elaborate equipment is not necessary but the following basic equipment is recommended.

General

Accurate height measuring equipment
Baby scales
Stand on scales
Auriscope
Ophthalmoscope
Tape measure (non-stretch)
Pencil light
Stethoscope

The choice of equipment for use in screening procedures is influenced by the items included in the local child health surveillance programme and personal preference.

Acknowledgements

I would like to acknowledge with gratitude the permission of the editor of publications of the Royal College of General Practitioners to use material from *Healthier Children – Thinking Prevention and the Handbook of Preventative Care for Preschool Children* (2nd edn).

I would also to acknowledge the help of Mrs Wendy Robertson, who has read drafts of the text and made many helpful suggestions.

My special thanks to Mrs Susan Spence who has typed the several drafts which led to the production of this chapter.

References

1 Royal College of General Practitioners. *Healthier Children – Thinking Prevention*. Report from general practice No. 22. London: RCGP, 1983.

2 Black, D. (Chairman). *Inequalities in Health. Report of a Research Working Group*. London: Department of Health and Social Security, 1980.

3 Beale, N., Nethercott, S. The nature of unemployment morbidity. *Roy Coll Gen Practit* 1988, **38:** 197–202.

4 World Health Organization. *Declaration of Alma-Ata. Lancet 1978; ii: 1040–1041*.

5 Hodgkin, G.K.H. Caravans as homes. *Br Med J* 1960; **2:** 854–855.

6 Carne, S.J. Housing in London. *Br Med J 1961;* **2:** 1556–1559.

7 Goodman, M. The pathology of planning. *J Roy Coll Gen Practit* 1974; **24:** 223–235.

8 Richman, N. Depression in mothers of pre-school children. *J Ch Psychol* 1976; **17:** 75–78.

9 Pollak, M. Housing and mothering. *Arch Dis Child* 1979; **54:** 54–58.

10 Pereira, J., Gray D. The care of the handicapped child in general practice, Gold Medal Essay. *Transact Hunterian Soc* 1971; **28:** 121–125.

11 Joseph, M., Mackeith, R.C. *A New Look at Child Health*. Tunbridge Wells: Pitman Medical, 1966.

12 Stott, N.C.H., Davis, R.H. The exceptional potential in each primary care consultation. *J Roy Coll Gen Practit* 1979; **29:** 201–205.

13 Office of Population, Censuses and Surveys. *General Household Survey* 1978. London: HMSO, 1980.

14 Hall, D.M.B. (ed.) *Health for All Children: A Programme for Child Health Surveillance*. Oxford: OUP, 1991.

15 McKeown, T. A sociological approach to the history of medicine. *Medical History* 1970; **14:** 342–357.

16 Rutter, M., Tizard, J., Whitmore, K. *Education, Health and Behaviour*. London: Longmans, 1970.

17 Forssman, H., Thuwe, I. One hundred and twenty children born after application for therapeutic abortion refused. Their mental health, social adjustment and educational level up to the age of 21. *Acta Psychiatr Scand* 1966; **42:** 71–88.

18 Kempe, R.S., Kempe, C.H. In: Bruner, J., Cole, M., Lloyd, B., eds. *Child Abuse in the Developing Child*. London: Fontana Open Books, 1978.

19 Colley, J.R.T., Holland, W.W., Corkhill, R.T. Influence of passive smoking and parental phlegm on pneumonia and bronchitis in early childhood. *Lancet* 1974; ii: 1031–1034.

20 Russell, M.A.H. *et al.* Effects of general practitioners' advice against smoking. *Br Med J* 1979; **2:** 231–235.

21 Court, S.D.M. (ed). *The Medical Care of Children*. London: Oxford University Press, 1963, 211.

22 Cartwright, A., Anderson, R. *General Practice Revisited*. London: Tavistock, 1981.

23 Cartwright, A., Anderson, R. Patients and their doctors 1977. *J Roy Coll Gen Practit* 1979; occasional paper no. 8.

24 Court, S.D.M. (Chairman). *Fit for the Future*. Report of the committee on child health services. London: HMSO, Cmnd 6680, 1976.

25 Cox, C.A., Zinkin, P.M., Grimsley, M.F. Aspects of the six-month developmental examination in a longitudinal study. *Dev Med Child Neurol* 1977; **19:** 149–159.

26 National Childrens Bureau. London: National Childrens Bureau, 1987.

27 Royal College of General Practitioners, British Paediatric Association, General Medical Services Committee and Joint Committee on Postgradudate Training (General Practice). *Training and Accreditation of General Practitioners in Child Health Surveillance*. London: RCCP, 1991.

5.3 Secondary child health care

Diane Smyth

The aim of every health district should be to have a child health service that enables children to reach their potential with as little adverse effect from illness, environmental hazards and unhealthy lifestyle as possible. The service needs to be accessible, well-coordinated and available in such a way as to promote rather than hinder family life. Children constitute about 20% of the resident population and need health care services that are both hospital and community based but which are part of a single, combined service.

Primary health care is one function of the community child health service: child health surveillance is increasingly provided by general practitioners (GPs) with a complementary contribution from community child health doctors. The service offered depends upon local policies and parental choice but it should include immunization and child health surveillance programmes for the under fives, health promotion, school health services, referral when a child has a problem which requires specialist input, shared care of children with complex problems, collaboration with other agencies on child protection, identification of children in need in accordance with the Children Act 1989, and attention when a child falls ill or is thought to be ill. GPs need to be registered on the child health surveillance list for this part of their work which comes under the auspices of the consultant community paediatrician from whom they may seek guidance.

Secondary health care services complement the primary care service by providing speciality health care for children within the context of the family, home, school or hospital; they are divided into community and hospital based services. The community services should include:

1 Services for the disabled or chronically sick child.
2 Secondary referral clinics in collaboration with other specialist resources such as audiology, opthalmology, clinical psychology, child psychiatry.
3 Identification and management of children in need of protection, including participation in court proceedings.
4 Professional advice on health surveillance, health promotion, and counselling services.
5 Clinical and policy forming advice to local education authorities and social services.
6 Clinical and policy forming advice on adoption and fostering.
7 Services to special schools and children with special educational needs.
8 Consultative service to GPs.

The hospital services should include:

1 An acute service (medical, surgical, psychiatric) able to respond immediately to the needs of the acutely ill or injured child and newborn infant.
2 Medical contribution to home care services.

The secondary health care services are accessed by direct referrals from the primary health care team, though departures from this practice do occur with self-referral to accident and emergency departments, through child surveillance at some community child health clinics, and by some open door child health clinics.

Some conditions in children are so unusual or complex as to require care by *tertiary health care services* specializing in all aspects of a disorder including its effect on growth and development of the child in home and school. Tertiary services are a regional or supra-regional resource, accessed mainly by district consultants at secondary care level, but sometimes by GPs, and are usually located in a regional children's centre or teaching hospital but may be locally delivered by visiting consultants carrying out combined clinics. The nature of the service varies with the disorder. Such specialities include cardiology, clinical genetics, clinical immunology, complex disability, endocrinology, gastroenterology, infectious diseases, metabolic disorders, neonatal intensive care, nephrology, neurology, oncology, paediatric surgery, respiratory diseases and rheumatology.

A single combined child health service

In the child health service, integration describes both the inter-dependent working relationship of the hospital and community services as originally advocated by the Brotherston Report, the Maternity Services Advisory Committee, and the Court Report, and the inter-dependency between the primary and secondary health care services.[1] To avoid confusion or failure to recognize the separate importance of each concept, it is now recommended that the integrated hospital and community child health service is known as the combined child health service. Such a service has the support of the medical and nursing professions (British Paediatric Association, Royal College of Physicians, Royal College of Nursing, Health Visitors Association) and the National Children's Bureau, and its concept was incorporated into the NHS and Community Care Act 1990.[2]

Since the late 1980s there has also been general agreement that this combined child health service should be consultant led and that district paediatricians should have varying degrees of complementary expertise to provide for the needs of children and their families for whom they are responsible. The part of the service responding to acutely ill children should be led by hospital-based general paediatricians, working largely in comprehensive children's departments though sometimes with additional duties in the community, while services for the disabled, disadvantaged or chronically ill child should be led by a consultant paediatrician with special expertise in community child health (CPCCH), working largely in the community but sometimes with duties also at the hospital. The balance of this combined consultant service should vary according to local circumstances; consequently posts may differ considerably one from another and the skill mix will need to be tailored to the particular local requirements. The larger the area served and the greater the developmental, social and educational problems of the child population, the less likely it is that CPCCHs will participate in the on-call rota for acute services, but they may have on-call duties relating to their responsibilities in the field of social paediatrics such as child abuse.

The hospital based paediatric service has long been consultant led, but agreement for a consultant led community child health service followed the deliberations of working parties of the Child Health forum of the British Medical Association (BMA) including representation from the British Paediatric Association (BPA), Faculty of Community Medicine of the Royal College of Physicians, and Department of Health.[3,4] As far back as 1984 the BPA's document *Paediatric manpower; towards the 21st century* indicated that on average a district should have three general paediatricians and between two and three CPCCHs.[5] Their further recommendation in 1991 was that there should be an absolute minimum of one CPCCH to each health district with further posts being required in larger districts approximating to 100 000 total population, so that many districts will require two or three such posts.[6] Clearly the degree of overlap of work within various consultant posts in a district will influence overall provision and content of CPCCH posts. CPCCHs will also have more variable work patterns than hospital-based general paediatricians, and this has implications when identifying administrative support.

Thus the consultant paediatrician is providing secondary specialist expertise and support to the primary care services. For a CPCCH, this is reflected in the range of skills expected: organization of services, experience of social and epidemiological aspects of child health, normal growth and development, preventive medicine, educational medicine, various types of handicap, child abuse, nutrition, liaison with social services, education authorities, and provision of clinical care. Computer literacy is an advantage in order to advise on information systems.

Areas of responsibility for the CPCCH will include:
1 Oversight of the health district's surveillance, illness prevention, health promotion and counselling services:
   a Pre-school surveillance
     Professional advice and monitoring in conjunction with general practitioner and Family Services Authorities. In some districts, service provision of these functions has to be undertaken by the community child health care service. This will decrease as primary care teams take on this activity.
   b Health promotion
     Monitoring and improvement in public health issues, such as smoking, substance abuse, and accident prevention
     Health advocacy
     Accident prevention

     Liaison with director of public health/production of annual report
     Interface work with consultants in public health medicine
   c Counselling
     Services to meet the health and developmental needs of adolescents.
   d Immunization and infectious disease advice in the role of immunization coordinator.
2 School health and educational medicine
   a Provision of a surveillance programme for school children.
   b Services for children with special educational needs including services to special schools.
   c Liaison with local education authorities with one CPCCH to be the designated contact doctor as stipulated in the Education Act 1981.
   d Professional advice to schools and local education authorities, and statutory service obligations under the provision of the Education Acts 1981 and 1993.
3 Special needs
   a Assessment and monitoring of children who are chronically sick or who have impaired development or disabilities. This will often be through a child development centre and will include early recognition, comprehensive assessment, regular review and coordination of care including therapy. Where appropriate it will also involve collaboration with other agencies such as education authorities and social services departments over statutory assessments in accordance with the provisions of the Children Act 1989, Education Acts 1981, 1986 and, 1993 and Chronically Sick and Disabled Persons legislation 1979.
   b Service planning, audit, and evaluation. This may include maintaining a register of children with special needs and auditing the care of individual children to ensure defined needs are being met.
   c Input to services for children at social disadvantage including identification of children in need.
   d Professional advice and liaison with social service departments for work arising from Children Act 1989.
   e Advice to the adoption and fostering agencies including health status and health care needs of children in foster homes, children's homes and day nurseries; input as medical adviser to adoption and fostering panels.
   f Advice to children undertaking employment with particular support for those with physical difficulties.
   g Cot death coordinator.
4 Child protection service
   a Collaboration with other agencies such as the local authority social services department and

the local education authority with regard to children in need of protection. This will include identification, assessment, investigation and management.

b   Participation in case conferences and court proceedings on emergency protection orders, child assessment orders, and care and supervision orders under the Children Act 1989, and work with the area child protection committee.

c   Liaison with police and social services, with one CPCCH to be the designated doctor for child protection.

d   Preventive work including support to families with children in high-risk groups due to social and economic deprivation.

e   Inter-agency collaboration on planning and operational issues.

5   Clinical specialities

a   Secondary referral clinics sometimes in collaboration with hospital paediatricians or other specialists for the assessment of hearing and vision, and the assessment of development or disability resulting from disorders such as cerebral palsy, primary muscle disease, epilepsy, severe learning difficulties, developmental delay, chronic illness.

b   Collaboration with child psychiatry, clinical psychology or psychotherapeutic services on care and support to families and children.

6   General paediatrics

A hospital or community based consultation service for children with general or developmental problems or behavioural disorders. This may be as part of the secondary care service or together with general practitioners.

The CPCCH must also be mindful of service provision and ensure there is adequate accommodation for clinical work (nurseries, schools, child protection, child development), for teaching and training activities, and for professional, management and clerical staff. Standards required for community child health services have been described[7] and should be met. Accommodation for community based child health services can be located within or outside the hospital. Shared accommodation for use of the combined child health service as a whole has many advantages. In particular, contact and communication is facilitated between all the staff of the combined service; consequently there is more efficient use of time and simpler record keeping. For the child and the family there is better coordinated care and a less confusing service. CPCCHs together with representatives of social services departments and local voluntary organizations are also concerned in ensuring that there is adequate local respite care available for families and carers of children with severe chronic disability, multiple handicap and life-threatening illness who require a high level of continuous medical and nursing care.

Areas of responsibilities for the hospital-based general paediatrician will include:

1   A general inpatient and outpatient service including sessions at peripheral clinics, day care, emergency care and some specialist medical services.

2   General paediatric support to the surgical services for children such as in orthopaedics, ophthalmic, ENT and general surgery, and care in the accident and emergency department.

3   Resuscitation and treatment for all healthy new born, sick or premature infants who require special care.

4   General paediatric support to the child psychiatric service and to services for children with learning difficulties.

5   Children's intensive care, neonatal intensive care and general paediatric support to the specialized tertiary services.

6   Medical contribution to home care and community nursing services.

7   Collaboration with the primary health care team and other staff or agencies monitoring children with chronic illness, disability or life-threatening conditions.

As part of the wider brief to children and families, the general paediatrician must ensure adequate and appropriate inpatient accommodation for children (cots in cubicles to be 40% of total bed number), intensive care, close proximity of neonatal and maternity services, a rehabilitation department for children, adequate accommodation for teaching, training, professional management, clerical staff and a paediatric social services department.

Wherever they are working all the medical staff of the combined child health service should also be involved to varying degrees in some or all of the following duties:

1   Information collecting and evaluation (epidemiology).

2   Service development, achieved by establishing standards of practice, clinical protocols, targets and assessment of outcome measures.

3   Audit and quality control of clinical work, service provision and resources.

4   Undergraduate and postgraduate teaching, and training programmes for medical, nursing, social services and education staff.

5   Clinical research.

6   Joint planning with other agencies to identify and provide services for children.

7   Management roles such as personnel, budget holding, administrative and committee work, resource management, advice to the health authority.

In the field of health promotion, planning, management roles, service and policy development, the CPCCH will normally collaborate and share responsibility with the specialist in public health and community medicine.

A service for children with special needs, aged 0–19 years

In 1967, the report of a Ministry of Health sub-committee on child welfare centres[8] recommended that hospital authorities be asked to review their present arrangements relating to assessment centres for handicapped children. Following a conference to consider this situation, a working party chaired by Sir Wilfred Sheldon was established 'to consider what guidance should be given to hospital authorities in the setting up of comprehensive assessment centres for handicapped children including their relationships with local authority and general practitioner services'. The working party reported in 1968 and recommended the establishment of Child Assessment Centres for assessment of and therapeutic input to handicapped children.[9] Over succeeding years it was recognized that most of these children have evolving clinical problems not static conditions. With the knowledge that therapy could modify functional difficulties and therefore severity of the handicap, it became clear that regular reappraisal of the children's needs and progress was required, not single assessments as had been the initial approach following Sheldon's recommendations. Increasing emphasis was placed on regular monitoring through newly titled Child Development Centres.

In 1976 the Court Report[10] on paediatric services recommended that the professionals involved in the care of handicapped children should organize themselves into District Handicap Teams. The suggested composition of the team was: paediatrician, social worker, educational psychologist, senior nurse and teacher, but the report stopped short of recommending that the members should provide all the clinical care, supervision and organization of services for handicapped children or how a coordinated service should be provided when health, education and social services' boundaries were not co-terminous. This last situation is a particular problem in inner city areas. In practice, most health districts have resolved the situation by their own modification of the Court proposals. Most districts now have a multidisciplinary Child Development Team (CDT) working from a Child Development Centre (CDC) whose aim is to provide diagnostic and assessment services with ready access to other specialist clinics for children with complex handicap, developmental delay (specific or global), learning difficulties, severe sensory (vision and hearing) problems, autism, physical disability and sometimes chronic illness.

The aim of the professionals within a CDT is to help the child make the most of his abilities however limited, and to help the family come to accept and cope with their child's limitations.

Membership of the CDT has also moved on from the original suggestions of the Court Report. Most CDTs consist of a core group of professionals from the clinical disciplines of paediatrics, physiotherapy, speech therapy, occupational therapy, clinical psychology, health visiting and sometimes child psychiatry. Some teams also include representation from local educational psychology and social services' departments. Teams vary in whether they offer a purely clinical service, exist to monitor the care of individual children, maintain a register of children with special needs, plan and implement local service policies, or a combination of all or several of these activities. For monitoring and planning purposes it is important that team professionals are senior managers of their clinical services. They meet to review the care of individual children at regular intervals, to take action where necessary and to look for gaps in service provision which need to be corrected. These meetings are sometimes known as Special Needs Review Groups. The clinical care of children is often devolved to other members of each clinical discipline who come together at regular, often weekly, intervals (business meeting of the CDT) to discuss particular children's current progress and problems. Health visitors in the community can share care with the CDT by visiting each family of a special needs child to ensure the parents receive all the correct information at the appropriate time. A check list (Table 5.2) is useful for all clinicians caring for special needs children but particularly for the health visitor.

Referral criteria to the team and the process of referral should be defined and this information made available to the district primary care team. Most districts adopt the practice whereby a child with a suspected developmental problem or established handicap is seen first in a child development clinic in the Child Development Centre by the CPCCH who will then seek involvement from members of the CDT as appropriate. The method of multidisciplinary assessment varies between districts and depends on local resources, personal styles, family constraints and so on. There is no evidence that any one method of assessment is superior. In some units, assessment may last a week, in others an afternoon. Most multidisciplinary assessments lead on to individual appointments with therapists. Throughout, the service is mainly supervised by the CPCCH. Diagnosis and management programmes are of little use unless they are communicated to those in services the child uses outside the CDC. Communication of information is of great importance for all children with special

Table 5.2 Health care check list for special needs children

1	Do the parents understand who you are and how you come to know their child has a problem? Have you checked personal details, diagnosis and functional needs? Does the child need regular reviews or the parents a case discussion?
2	Do the parents know what is wrong with the child? Do they have any report in writing to read themselves or show relatives? If the child is on medication, do they know what, how much and why? Have they a child development team leaflet indicating the names and telephone numbers of the professionals involved? Do they have a parent held record card with medication details entered?
3	Do *you* understand what is wrong? If any doubt, check with the child's consultant paediatrician or GP. Remember that in many conditions there are additional later complications as well as those obvious at initial diagnosis.
4	Check the child is getting regular medical care from a specialist service, including vision and hearing. Make sure that routine surveillance considerations are not neglected such as growth and behaviour. Are there other worries? Remember that specialist clinics can miss wider health problems.
5	Has there been appropriate dental advice? If not, can you link the child with a dental hygienist or suitable dentist?
6	Have the parents been offered genetic advice? If not, and they want it, contact the consultant paediatrician involved.
7	Does the child have significant behaviour probems? Are there sibling or family difficulties as a result of the child with special needs? Would the family like advice from a clinical psychologist?
8	Is the planned therapy input occurring? Is there a need for therapists from other disciplines to be involved?
9	Does the family want books or leaflets on the child's problem? The child development centre is an information resource.
10	Does the family want help from a social worker? Would they like to meet another family with similar problems? Be careful, this can be helpful but also painful. Do the parents know about relevant self-help groups or voluntary organizations? If not, can you tell them or ask?
11	Does the family qualify for financial help such as the Disability Living allowance, Mobility allowance, Invalid Care allowance? Do they have a need for support from the Family Fund? Do the family know how to claim?
12	Would the family like day care from a nursery school or day nursery? Would the child benefit from more peer group or structured input?
13	Is the family's housing appropriate to the child's needs now or within the forseeable future? If not, should you ask the social worker or occupational therapist to become involved to assess the situation?
14	Does the child need a referral to the Education Authority? Has this already happened? Explain about the 1981 Education Act and the rights this gives the child and family. Should a pre-school liaison teacher or teacher for the hearing or visually impaired be involved? Would a home based learning programme (Portage) be appropriate for the child?
15	Is there a need for respite care? Some parents are upset at this suggestion so it needs careful timing and handling. Should you discuss it with the social worker?
16	Explain about the special needs register as a means of improving services for children with special needs. Is the child on the special needs register?
17	Are there any unmet needs? If you think so, tell the consultant paediatrician.

needs. A coordinator for the CDT is vital to the service though the importance of this post is seldom appreciated by managers. CDCs are variably located; some are on hospital sites in close proximity to other specialist services, others are in the community. Both locations have advantages and disadvantages.

Children referred to the CDC are generally under 5 years old but older children moving into a district or presenting late can also be assessed. They may continue to be seen in the CDC, regardless of their age, if this is in the child's best interests; but normally once the child goes to school, either mainstream or a special school, health overview and intervention will come from a school based special needs service. This is simply an extension of that offered for pre-school children at the CDC. Membership of the school based team should continue to include a paediatrician, physiotherapist, speech therapist, occupational therapist, and psychologist with the addition of the school nurse. In many cases these are the same individuals who offered the pre-school service. The school nurse takes the role previously filled by the health visitor and for special schools there is often an attached social worker. Together the teachers, school doctor, and therapist should work closely with the child and parents to encourage development and learning. When the child leaves school, relevant health, social and educational information should be formally handed onto agencies such as the Learning Disabilities Team (with its associated mental handicap register) or a Physical Disabilities Team, if support continues to be needed after school leaving. In practice, it is the pre-school special needs team that tends to be known as the CDT, but in reality both this and the school based team are simply part of a single special needs service for all children aged 0 to 19 years. Team membership and individual professional involvement vary according to the stage of the child's life.

At any point, both before and in school, it may be necessary for multidisciplinary case discussions to be held between parents and professionals; after starting school these meetings take the form of the statutory annual review for children with special needs. It is good practice to nominate a key worker from those professionals involved with a child, to whom the parent may always readily turn for information and advice. This is normally a health professional, often a therapist or health visitor, but for pre-school children maybe the CPCCH; the key worker concept is less often practised for school-aged children. The CDC should also be seen by parents as a resource for information on benefits, voluntary agencies, respite care, incontinence aids, equipment and general support.

Multidisciplinary work is difficult, demanding and time consuming. Many roles overlap. A respect and understanding for the contribution of other disciplines, flexibility in allocating tasks and adequate time for discussion are essential components. The CPCCH has to steer a leadership path through this that both encourages the child and parents, and selects appropriate moments for clinical intervention or liaison with other professionals.

Service delivery is often complicated by health, education and social services boundaries not being co-terminous; also by lack of an identified senior health manager to take development of the multidisciplinary team as a whole forwards and ensure adequate funding of the component clinical disciplines. Without this, reduced input from one clinical discipline may not be addressed, and its impact on multidisciplinary team work and service care ignored or not appreciated. Service delivery is compromised by too little administrative support requiring clinicians to spend an inappropriate amount of their time on organization.

Joint planning teams with senior professionals/managers from health, education and social services are being increasingly established to plan services for children with special needs, both immediate and long term. Insufficient resourcing of parts of the multidisciplinary service should be taken to these planning teams as well as to individual senior managers of each service. The special needs registers that many health districts maintain have moved from being lists of children with a labelled handicap to information on children with their functional needs defined; this transition has greatly facilitated checking that the children's needs are met. Social services are now also required by the 1989 Children Act to maintain a register of children with disabilities to improve provision of care; in the future it seems likely that these two registers will become more closely linked.

Future developments

The philosophy of a combined child health service has thus been developed but some districts still lack an adequate number of consultant led posts both for hospitals and community based services. Secondary care community paediatric work is undertaken in such districts by the CPCCH sharing clinical responsibility with doctors currently working as associate specialists, senior clinical medical officers (SCMOs) and clinical medical officers (CMOs) in the community child health service. As these posts fall vacant they are likely to be replaced either by training posts (senior house officer, registrar or senior registrar) or career grade posts (staff grade or associate specialist) in community based paediatric services. Any of these appointments may or may not incorporate an on-call responsibility for the acute paediatric service or neonatal care. Some SCMO posts will be replaced by consultant posts. In recent years a few SCMO posts have been specifically recognized as training SCMO posts – with status equivalent to senior registrar – as preparation for CPCCH applicants. CMOs and SCMOs are clinically responsible to the CPCCH and they may also be managerially responsible to the CPCCH. Training is achieved through supervised modules of work which specifically reflect the responsibilities of a CPCCH. The Joint Committee for Higher Medical Training (JCHMT) produces guidelines for higher specialist training which are upgraded on a regular basis. Before being appointed, a CPCCH would have been expected to have had 4 years of higher medical training in approved posts (2 years in general paediatrics and 2 years in community child health).

The increasing use of doctors in training, in rotating posts between the hospital and community paediatric services, is another step towards achieving a combined child health service.

General practitioner involvement in child health surveillance of the under 5 year olds is still being developed and there is considerable variation from one district to another in the general practitioner's contribution. It is unfortunately low in areas of social deprivation where children and their families have greatest need of community child health services. It is also clear that there are considerable community child health needs (both at a primary and secondary level) beyond the resources of either general practitioners or doctors in training; this work is particularly concerned with the assessment and support of children with special educational needs, child protection, adoption and fostering, and the school health service. It is still too early to determine the full effect of the implementation of the general practitioner contract and 1989 Children Act in terms of the resources available and demand on time. For this reason the Joint Working Party on Medical Services for Children[11] has recently recognized that for a foreseeable period there will continue to be a need, within the combined child health service, in many districts, for basic level career grade posts (staff grade) other than consultant paediatricians. The Joint Working Party has also accepted that similarly there will be a need for some districts to have or continue to have senior level career grade posts (associate specialist) below consultant level in the community based paediatric services. Holders of these posts would:

1 Assist in the teaching and supervision of doctors in training (rotating hospital appointments, general practitioner vocational posts, general practitioners undergoing child health surveillance training and basic level career community child health posts).
2 Provide the secondary care input into the specialist community child health clinics – audiology, child development, child protection – together with continuity in collaborative working with families and staff by the health service, local education authorities, social services departments, voluntary agencies and schools.
3 Staff specialist clinics at centres to which secondary referrals can be made by general practitioners and other members of the primary health care team involved in surveillance and child health duties. In some instances this may avoid referral to a hospital based service and the stress that involves for most families.

After some time, it may be possible for greater interchange of work between the hospital and community elements of the child health service, thus further strengthening the development of a combined child health service.

References

1 Department of Health. *Integrating Primary and Secondary Care*. London: HMSO, 1991 (EL (91)) 27.
2 National Health Service and Community Care Act 1990.
3 British Medical Association. *Report of the Child Health Working Party: supplementary report of Council*; 1988–1989, 3–5.
4 Faculty of Community Medicine. *An Integrated Child Health Service: a Way Forward*. London: Royal College of Physicians, 1987.
5 British Paediatric Association. *Paediatric Manpower: Towards the 21st Century*. London: BPA, 1984.
6 British Paediatric Association. *Paediatric Medical Staffing for the 1990s*. London: BPA, 1991.
7 British Paediatric Association. *Community Child Health Services: an Information Base for Purchasers*. London: BPA, 1992.
8 Report of the Sub Committees of the Standing Medical Advisory Committee, Ministry of Health. *Child Welfare Centres*. London: HMSO, 1967: paragraph 143.
9 British Paediatric Association. *Commentary on the DHSS's Memorandum on Comprehensive Assessment Centres for Handicapped Children*. Chairman Sir Wilfrid Sheldon. RP68. London: BPA, 1968.
10 Court, S.D.M. (Chairman). *Fit for the Future*: report of the Committee on Child Health Services. London: HMSO, 1976.
11 Department of Health and British Medical Association. *Report of the Joint Working Party on Medical Services for Children*. London: DoH and BMA, November 1992.

5.4 Management of child health services in the community

John Mitchell and Judith Riley

Introduction

The word management often induces very strong negative connotations amongst doctors; control, constraints and restrictions are words that come to mind and managers, those people who carry out these duties, are perceived as 'the enemy'. This section outlines an alternative perspective, arguing that well managed health services are essential if professionals are to provide high quality services to patients. Also that it is the responsibility of all senior professionals to contribute to the leadership and management of

their units, departments and hospitals. Further that this contribution to the managerial process depends in essence on an attitudinal and behavioural change, rather than more skills or a raft of new knowledge, although these can often be assets!

There is no *right* way to manage. Rather, management is about continually trying to improve outcomes for those who use services, particularly by exploring the different ways that things can be done. However, it is a common tendency to think that there really might be a *right way*, and questions often posed are whether this or that structure is the right one, in the expectation that if only the structure can be got right then things will work better. The answer is often a disappointment. Explanation is needed that structures are simply a way in which organizations arrange themselves to carry out their purpose more effectively.

The National Health Service has been particularly vulnerable to the myth that structure is the essence of organizational performance. Any person appointed to a senior position in the service is likely to be overwhelmed by the complexity of the challenge, be frustrated by their inability to influence the organization and be easily tempted to create some order and security by designing a new structure. This seldom produces the expected benefits; these materialize when the culture, style and communication begin to shift and these issues are addressed later in this section.

Another common experience has been the myth of the *new discovery*. Community care and health gain are good examples and another is resource management. There are usually politically or managerially inspired initiatives which are given a new name, a launch, a glossy brochure, which contain little of substance. The illusion is created that something new has materialized which has a unique body of knowledge and requires special expertise. Many doctors enquire about resource management as if somebody had discovered how to manage first hospitals and then community units. In the event resource management was the extension and devolution of general management throughout the service, required major attitudinal and cultural change, some gentle organizational realignment and was accompanied by capital to facilitate the change and provide for the management information systems. Resource management and similar initiatives are, at best, an opportunity to be exploited, but not an answer. There are no quick fix solutions to complex managerial issues.

This section has been written with the senior clinician in mind and, in particular, the complexity and multiplicity of their roles and responsibilities. As an example, one consultant community paediatrician working in a non-teaching rural health authority ana-lysed her work activity for two randomly selected months (Carter, J. personal communication) (Table 5.3). In a teaching authority more time might be spent in research and teaching, but the most striking aspect was the proportion of time spent in managerial activities and how varied those responsibilities were.

The more senior the clinician, the greater the involvement with management. Attempts by consultants to ignore management issues, in order to concentrate on the more traditional clinical or academic roles, can often result in their departments lacking leadership and being isolated from management. Crucial decisions are left to managers outside the department, who cannot be expected to make appropriate, considered and well-informed decisions about either service improvements or resource development. This is not to say that all doctors should become managers; indeed many should and will continue to work primarily as clinicians. They should, however, contribute actively to leadership of the service, not just by a greater commitment of time, but more in terms of approach, attitude and understanding of what management is about.

This section examines some of the managerial challenges which face all public sector organizations, using examples from the National Health Service and child health services. How those challenges might be addressed is explored, emphasizing the role of the community paediatrician.

Key managerial challenges

While every clinic and department has its own problems, some issues are common to most parts of the service and can usually be traced to a few linked themes:

1 Difficulty in identifying the business one is in and the values which should drive it.
2 Identifying priorities.

Table 5.3 Work activities of a community paediatrician for selected months

Type of work	1st month (hours)	2nd month (hours)
Management meetings (with groups and individuals)	39	36
Clinical work	32.5	29
Combined clinics with teams	8.5	7.5
Child abuse (clinical)	3	2.5
Training (personal)	7.5	–
Training (others)	2.5	20
Time with secretary	10	10
Travel	8	8

In addition there is a miscellaneous group of activities: dictating, reading, writing reports and letters, seeing visitors, etc. which are not included.

3 Managing the tension between those who guide the service and those who are focused on service delivery.
4 Managing clinicians who need both freedom and to be held to account.
5 Professionals in a managed organization.
6 Working with a variety of organizations and professions.
7 A fast pace of change.

Challenge 1: difficulty in identifying the business one is in and the values which should drive it

While many manufacturing organizations can readily describe what business they are in, their range of products or services, their customers and their markets, public sector services are less clearly focused and have been characterized by ambiguity. On the one hand, all-embracing statements such as: 'to improve the health of the whole community', allow everyone to justify their own contribution. On the other hand, reality is rather different; those who work in a teaching hospital, for example, might see their role as being primarily concerned with education or research, rather than responding to local community needs. Some cynics claim that many doctors see the NHS as primarily a means for them to secure interesting employment, while the public sector unions recognize that it has a crucial role in providing one million jobs for a poorly paid, predominantly female, workforce.

This ambiguity about the role of the NHS is further complicated by the contribution of other agencies to health. Is the NHS simply a repair service, or has it a responsibility to work for children's social, psychological and physical well-being? If the latter is the case, then do child health services have wider responsibilities to secure housing status, parental income or road safety?

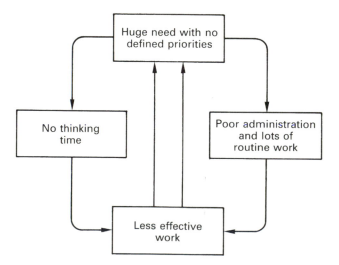

Figure 5.1 The downward cycle of morale and effectiveness.

Decisions are difficult to reach since the benefits of the service have not been precisely defined and clinicians differ on the emphasis they would give to prevention and surveillance, compared to services for children with chronic disability or those with acute illness.

Challenge 2: identifying priorities

Many community paediatricians have described a sense of being caught in a downward cycle of morale and effectiveness (Fig. 5.1).

The cause for this downward cycle is apparently obvious: lack of funding, and the ready availability of someone to blame. It could be 'the managers' or 'the region' or 'the purchasers'. The problem about this approach is that it does not help; blaming others, however justified it might seem, colludes with the status quo and the downward cycle. It can prevent those who are responsible for providing the service from reviewing and evaluating the quality of the service delivery, agreeing what is essential, and most importantly, agreeing what should not be provided.

The real challenge, therefore, lies not in the increasing problem of dividing up a cake that feels too small, but rather in continuously rethinking the priorities in a positive way. When every service has benefit, it is very hard to put services into an order of priority and even more difficult to withdraw an established one. When a difficult challenge has been faced and accepted by staff, it is even harder to change again as needs and opportunities alter.

Case study

In one district health authority the role of the school nurse has changed over the past 5 years to a proactive one of health promotion with responsibility for health inspection. The new role was welcomed by the nurses as it gave them much more responsibility. However, it also resulted in the nurses being much less involved in the day-to-day health of the children and spending less time at each school.

These changes coincided with the introduction of the 1981 Education Act[1] which resulted in children with a variety of disabilities being admitted to mainstream education. The headteachers' response was to demand the reinstatement of nurses in order to have a qualified person on site to deal with any health emergency or eventuality. The consequences of this would be significant. The cost would result in a service reduction elsewhere and the school nurses would not be able to carry out their new role. Neither the interest of the majority of children nor the nurses would be served.

Meanwhile the headteachers were able to generate support for their position from parents, teachers and parent/teacher associations and they persuaded the education committee of the local authority to pressurize the health authority to provide nurses in every school. The community paediatrician who was the lead manager had few possibilities for action; either to brazen it out or succumb to the pressure, reintroduce the nurses and manage the consequences.

Instead she came up with an alternative: to train the ancillary staff in each school to manage the immediate health needs of the children with disabilities, with the understanding that the school nurses would visit regularly and would provide the necessary advice and support. The plan was implemented, it worked satisfactorily and had an added bonus: the ancillaries felt more involved and valued. For a minimal cost it was possible to alleviate the anxiety of parents and teachers, while ensuring that health support for all of the children was safeguarded and other services were not reduced.

Challenge 3: the tension between guidance and delivery

All larger organizations suffer from continuing tension between two essential managerial tasks: guidance and delivery.[2] Guidance management ensures that services are provided equitably, appropriately (to the wider community) and efficiently, thereby meeting the needs of the whole population. It deals with the complex political, social and economic environment which organizations have to operate within. It ensures that the organization remains viable and successful despite a variety of adverse effects which include a diminished buying power of the falling pound, the health authority having to fund a centrally agreed wage settlement which exceeds the rate of inflation, or the bottom falling out of the property market.

Delivery management on the other hand is about the day-to-day provision of services for individuals which are effective, appropriate to the needs of those individuals, accessible, and provided in an acceptable style.

Successful organizations manage the tension between these two functions explicitly and the providers and guiders negotiate to reconcile the different pressures that each feel. In the NHS, however, this process of reconciliation is harder to achieve. Doctors and other professionals align themselves on the delivery side of the fence while general managers and finance directors are perceived as being on the guidance side. This polarization leads to 'them and us' attitudes and organizational dislocation.

Organizations which do not reconcile the guidance and delivery tension will be imbued with distrust, acrimony and adversarial behaviour. It would seem, certainly in the short and medium term, that doctors need to share the responsibility for the guidance management decisions so that they can ensure that the delivery of services is of the highest standard.

Case study

The management (guiders) of an acute hospital is faced with a significant projected overspend at the year end. To reduce its amount they decide to close two wards for the last 4 months of the financial year. However the expected savings are not realized, because the consultants (deliverers) have not reduced their case load but simply increased their throughput in the remaining wards. The interests of the guidance managers (to provide the range of care and remain within the cash limit) and the interests of the deliverers (to treat as many of their individual patients as possible) have not been reconciled, the overspend is not controlled and the deliverers are now determining the priorities of the organization, which are not necessarily in the interests of the wider community.

Case study

A trust board agrees to implement an equal opportunities policy following considerable pressure from the local Labour councillors, the community health council, local women's groups, and the muslim women's association.

A month later a non-executive director, a strong supporter of the policy, fulfils a long-standing arrangement to chair an appointments committee for a registrar in general surgery at the local district general hospital. Eight people have been short listed, all are men, six were born in the UK, one in Australia and one in South Africa. Their names do not suggest that any come from an ethnic minority group.

The non-executive director enquires as to whether the shortlisting procedures, contained within the policy, have been followed. The personnel officer looks uncomfortable and the two consultant surgeons on the panel deny any knowledge of the policy. However, they go on to say that this post is highly regarded, attracts excellent candidates and the holders always move on to very desirable jobs in teaching hospitals. They think that an equal opportunities policy has nothing to contribute to this appointment and, indeed, might exclude some of the excellent candidates who have been short listed.

Again the guiders (the trust board in this case) have attempted not only to give equality of opportunity to women, but also to achieve a cultural and ethnic workforce (including senior managers and professionals) which mirrors the multicultural population of the local community. The consultants however live predominantly in the white male world of surgery which they are keen to sustain; they therefore discriminate against both women and people from black and ethnic minority communities, arguing that white male UK graduates are technically more competent.

Challenge 4: clinical freedom and accountability

This challenge is also related to the tensions between guidance and delivery but is such an important subset that we have separated it. It stems from the dependence which the NHS has on the commitment and decisions that doctors make for their patients; clinical judgement is a crucial factor in securing both the quality of the service and the trust of patients. Yet there is also a need for audit and accountability if all practice is to be raised to the highest standard and scarce resources are to be used most fairly and efficiently.

Balancing these two opposing forces can never be easy. When faced with the individual baby's needs the clinician will want to ensure that the baby receives the highest quality care and will not want to be constrained by other considerations. However, a process will need to be evolved whereby the benefits that the individual accrues are in the interest of the wider community. The days of pure clinical freedom have long since gone[3] but a too radical swing to the doctor as an accountable technician is equally undesirable. Instead we have to find a middle position where the ability of doctors to make sound judgements is safeguarded, while there is an area of discretion in which those judgements can be made.

Challenge 5: managing professionals

The professions have always been essential to the functioning of the health service and members of our society look to the professions for the definition and solution of their problems, granting them rights, privileges and power. However, the benefits of this relationship can be threatened particularly if the professionals misappropriate their specialist knowledge in their own interest.

Mintzberg describes professionals as 'trained and indoctrinated specialists' who work independently of their colleagues but closely with the clients, and they function by using a process which he describes as 'pigeonholing'.[4] This operates by first categorizing the client's needs in terms of a contingency (the diagnosis), thus indicating which standard programme to use and second by applying that programme. The consequence is that the organization seeks to match a predetermined contingency to a standard programme or protocol, an increasingly common development in the NHS of the 1990s. However, considerable discretion remains in the application of these protocols and many judgements are made, often on less explicit criteria. Clearly the professions have become essential to the functioning of the NHS and society has granted professionals, particularly doctors, rights, privileges and power. Others[5,6] have been concerned about the role and see it as 'the mystique of technical expertise' which acts as an instrument of social control by an elite. Medical professionals are at risk of using their superior knowledge and skill to control, disempower and make their patients dependent on them. The challenge is to create a relationship whereby the doctor is seen to serve the patient, enabling and empowering the individual to be in control.

The professional use of expertise is not necessarily restricted to the doctor–patient relationship but is manifest within the service itself. Sometimes this use of power is exercised subtly, but often it is more explicit. For example the doctor who uses fictitious data with authority or the numerous occasions when shroud waving is used to manipulate or block decisions. Work with doctors in the NHS has shown that they have some characteristic behaviour patterns. For example, they find it enormously difficult to praise each other and to celebrate success; they behave as if they were totally invulnerable; and finally they are reluctant to experiment and take risks as this may suggest that they do not know all the answers. Coates (personal communication) argues that these patterns stem from a desire of doctors to be perfect; unfortunately they contribute to an NHS which has difficulty in creating an effective learning culture.[7] Schon[8] proposes a shift of the role of the professional from an expert to that of a 'reflective practitioner'. He describes the benefits as follows: 'when practice is a repetitive administration of techniques to the same kind of problems, the practitioner may look to leisure as a resource of relief, or to early retirement; but when he functions as a researcher in practice, the practice itself is a source of renewal'. Handy[9] personalizes and thereby popularizes these concepts, promoting a challenging vision of a future which is achieved through a process of continual learning and development both at work and in society more generally.

Challenge 6: working with other professionals and other organizations

Managers are likely to fail if they isolate their concerns and work solely within the boundaries of their own organization. Instead they work with a range of different professionals and staff in their own organization while continually collaborating and negotiating with many others in the attempt to make services comprehensive and seamfree. Overlapping responsibilities lead to boundary disputes and take managers into the arena of political power and influence. In the child health services the number of other organizations is particularly problematic: local authorities, especially education and social services departments, a range of voluntary organizations which represent differing views, Community Health Councils as well as Family Health Services Authorities G.P. fundholders and the health authority.

Community paediatricians find themselves in the midst of this on a day-to-day basis, often leading multidisciplinary teams. Not only must they work with their own junior doctors and health service managers but also with general practitioners (GPs), dentists, district nurses, health visitors, the professions allied to medicine, and non-clinical professions such as headteachers, educational psychologists and social workers. Working in multidisciplinary teams is often difficult as differences in values, understanding, cultures and practices undermine an effective collective effort. One of the most difficult challenges is to escape the prejudice that each profession holds about another. For example, when we asked a group of senior community paediatricians for their views of NHS general managers, they produced a largely negative list of stereotypes which included the following:

- Always talking and never doing.
- Power-seeking personalities, who are ambitious and self-interested.
- No idea what it is like for a family to have an ill child and do not try to find out.

Similarly, when we asked them what they felt might be managers' views of community paediatricians, they expected the stereotypes to be equally negative and include the following:

- Worried about trivia, moaners and inefficient.
- Empire-building, protecting our overpaid status.
- Unrealistic and out of touch with what is possible and realistic.

In work with managers, professionals and staff working in child health, it has been found that these very strongly held stereotypical feelings about other colleagues and the organizations in which they work, effectively block collaborative working and efficient service delivery.

Challenge 7: the pace of change

In the UK during the last 10 years it would be natural to lay the blame for the pace and degree of change at the feet of politicians. We have seen a radical and assertive government questioning the principles of the welfare state. In the NHS this began with the 1982 reorganization, Patients First,[10] continued with the implementation of the Griffiths Report[11] in 1985 and with the changes stemming from three White Papers (Promoting Better Health,[12] Working for Patients[13] and Caring for People[14] in 1987, January 1989 and November 1989 respectively).

However, change has always been a feature of the health service and much of the change is internally generated. For example, medical and technological advance has been led by the medical profession, while those who work in the service aspire to develop and improve service delivery. Then there are external pressures; demographic change, the increasing number of people over the age of 75 years, and the appearance of new health challenges demand that services are modified. Finally there is the changing expectation of the public which will increasingly influence the pattern of services. Indeed it can be argued that the measures which the government has taken over the last decade are partially an attempt to control the escalating costs of health care that these changes imply.

The child health service has seen its full share of such changes; North West Thames Regional Health Authority[15] in their Regional Strategy pointed out:

'Over the last decade or so, there have been significant advances in the relatively rare diseases for which treatment is more complicated. Some of these advances are likely to develop further – for example, in the antenatal diagnosis of certain inherited diseases, the treatment of premature babies, the management of children with cancer and the care of children with mental and physical handicap to ensure that they are able to achieve their maximum potential.'

These changes must be set within a wider context which includes public concern on child abuse including sexual abuse, the effects of the 1981 Education Act,[1] the particular implications of the recent White Papers[12] on the role of GPs in child surveillance and immunization, and, more widely, a growing awareness of the rights of children and their families, coupled with a desire to make services demand rather than supply driven.

Powerful managerial approaches

While every manager must find a style that builds on their own strengths and preferences, and every situation calls for a unique response, there are some approaches that seem particularly powerful and widely applicable. Leaders of flourishing child health services will often be found to utilize several of these:

1 Establishing a vision and distinguishing ends from means.
2 Using the concept of transition.
3 Making sure the organization is being led.
4 Accepting that change is beneficial: the learning organization.

Approach 1: establishing a vision and distinguishing ends from means

It is all too easy to fall into the trap of confusing ends and means, to think that the way things are done, the organizational structure or the introduction of an information system, are an end in themselves and forget what one is trying to achieve. For example during the acrimonious debate surrounding the 1990 NHS legislation, the point was made that the changes were essentially about means, leaving the ends to which the reorganization was to be put to local determination.[16] Yet many managers (and professionals) became for a while obsessed with the tasks: internal markets, creating NHS Trusts, business plans and the contract. They lost sight of their own responsibility for determining what these changes were to achieve, what ends they were to serve.[17]

The concept of ends is not itself simple. As Ellwood points out: 'The centrepiece and unifying ingredient of outcome management is the tracking and measurement of function and wellbeing or quality of life.' This sounds like a hopelessly optimistic undertaking but he goes on to argue, 'that we already have the ability to obtain crucial, reliable data on quality of life at minimal cost and inconvenience.'[18]

Perhaps it is more the medical profession's reluctance to explore and test, rather than any inherent difficulty which is the major block to progress.

Most of the work has focused on adults, but there are good reasons why these concepts should be applied to children as they embody important dimensions. A clinical service functions as an interrelated series of processes, each of which produces intermediate or final outputs. But the outcome of each medical care process or subprocess is the combination of the physical result obtained (the output) and the users' evaluation (as opposed to professional). Further, beneficial outcomes have to be balanced against the risk of any intervention which usually rises exponentially with volume and the cost which parallels the rise in risk.[19]

Nor is the distinction between ends and means always clear. For example, when it is said that child health services must be integrated,[20] is that a statement about ends: that the services need to avoid overlaps and gaps; or about means: that various organizational arrangements must be brought together, under a single child health service? There are some excellent child health services in which both the acute hospital service and the community services for children, community paediatricians, health visitors, school nurses, speech therapists and other professionals are all managed as a single entity. However, there are equally good services (in terms of outcome) where the hospital service is managed as part of the other acute services and the community is further divided into neighbourhood patches. In essence each district should have its own unique way of delivering services; what is appropriate for Brixton is unlikely to work in Devon, although the intended outcomes might be identical.

A key element in moving towards this greater clarity about ends is to define the values which underlie the service. This is a continual process of reconciling the different individual values of the various people and groups who use, provide, manage or influence the service. Once these corporate values, or vision, have been defined and are owned by those who work in the service, they will then act as a clear guiding framework which will govern and help to prioritize the ends.

Maxwell[21] has suggested that these values might have six dimensions:

1 Is the pattern of provision relevant to the overall health needs of the local childhood population?
2 Are services provided equitably? Children with the same health needs should receive the same provision and there should be no discrimination on gounds of religion, class or ethnic background.
3 Are services accessible? Children should be able to receive services locally without waiting.
4 Are services (technically) effective and appropriate to the need of the individual child? Is the expertise, competence and judgement of the professionals producing a result which is in the particular interest of the child?
5 Are the services socially acceptable? Are children and their families being provided with services which promote dignity, choice and control in sympathetic and pleasant physical environments?
6 Are services being delivered efficiently? The efficient use of resources is as important as the other five dimensions because, as stewards of public money, managers and professionals are responsible for ensuring that it is spent wisely.

It will be clear that these six dimensions throw up contradictions. For example it would not be desirable to provide easy geographical access to highly specialized cardiac surgery for children by establishing a unit in every local hospital, not only because the cost would be prohibitive, but for a more important reason. The small number of cases would not accumulate enough experience or provide adequate numbers to achieve outcomes which would compare favourably with high volume units.[22] Instead a trade-off might be agreed whereby the surgeon does outreach consultations in local hospitals, children are investigated locally, and have to travel to the specialist centre only for the operation. However, the specialist centre is provided with accommodation so that parents can stay and be part of the treatment and rehabilitation.

If there is a clarity among managers and professionals about the vision and the health outcomes, then organizations will be well positioned not only to take advantage of externally imposed change, but also to protect the service from inappropriate proposals which do not serve its best interests.

Approach 2: using the concept of transition

Another powerful aid to coping with change is to develop the idea of a desirable transition state for a service rather than focusing on some ideal end-state. Unfortunately, in work with professionals and their organizations, it is found that the advantage of the learning opportunities which this approach affords can be undermined by disagreements about the exact nature of the perfect but unachievable service.

Managers who can identify what would be good progress one or two years ahead will be more able to take advantage of change and less likely to get lost in the enormity of their task. The transition state needs to be detailed in terms of what can be achieved and what might prevent achievement. Then attention can be given to managing the shift from the present to that transition state.[23]

Working in this way means that managers have constantly to review progress and rethink their aims. Their long-term strategy emerges from a series of over-lapping transition states, each developed to accommo-date events.[24] This is very different from the traditional NHS planning system, which was focused on specified long periods of years ahead.

Approach 3: making sure the organization is being led

Leadership is an essential component of effective man-agement but leading is tough and takes courage. Man-agers have different styles of leadership but there are a number of methods and activities which can assist managers in leadership.

Continual re-evaluation of priorities

Just as focusing on a too ideal and far-distant goal can be disabling, so trying to do everything at once can weaken managerial effectiveness.

Powerful leaders are often those who are able to identify a few crucial priorities from the multitude of desirable changes that might be addressed. They see the trade-offs between the values that drive their ser-vice and are willing to sacrifice good objectives for crucial developments. Then they can help their staff to escape from being mice on a treadmill of routine and overwork.

They are also able to see what is deliverable: what may be achieved in the immediate context of resources, balance of power and attitudes. They do not waste their efforts struggling for the impossible and they can recognize what progress is essential to gain the support of other key people. They focus on doing the right things rather than on doing things right. Given this sense of realism as a context, staff can be praised for what they do achieve, rather than working in a constant atmosphere of failure.

Working with others

Most effective managers are good at working with their colleagues, with other professionals and with members of different organizations. They listen, hear, manage by walking around,[25] delegate, support and so on. They couple this approach with having insight into their own strengths and weaknesses and are able to surround themselves with colleagues who have complementary rather than similar strengths. Often gaining insight can be a painful process of self devel-opment but it does help managers to work more effec-tively in teams. Fortunately each person has different strengths and weaknesses. It is the team's ability to use the strengths of all the participants to the full which will enable it to perform better than the sum of its members working independently.[26]

Countering negative feelings

It has been observed that senior managers and profes-sionals in the health service commonly have negative perceptions about themselves. Community paediatri-cians express feelings of being weak, disempowered, dispirited and ineffectual which must have a major influence on their attitudes. For example they pro-pound an extremely cynical view of the organization, blame others or fall into the trap of holding over-simple beliefs such as, 'all would be well if only we had a larger budget' or 'different structure' or 'more therapists'.

The reasons for these negative feelings are complex and multifactorial, but there are a number of helpful ways to counter them. For example it is essential for community paediatricians to review their own work and the work of the team they are leading both to celebrate what has gone well, however small that might be, but also to explore what has been difficult and tough, to feel the frustrations, the stresses and the anxieties and to be able to do this honestly in a safe, trusting environment. This process acts as a powerful catharsis which enables both individuals and teams to rejuvenate, to make visions and values explicit and to inform the priority setting process.

In addition, successful managers develop other support mechanisms. Networking, mentoring and using colleagues as co-consultants[27] are ways in which to make enormous contributions to the effec-tiveness of people who are undertaking complex and demanding jobs.

Community paediatricians are often surprised by the extent of the control and influence they have. It is possible for them to make and implement better informed decisions about priorities. An increasing sense of purpose allows them to consider how to influ-ence decisions outside their immediate sphere with greater confidence.

Approach 4: accepting change as normal

When the pace of change is fast and staff are over-worked, it is easy to see change as a threat to service delivery. When change is externally imposed and appears likely to harm the service it may be essential to resist the threat. However, in securing gains for child health, a negative approach does not seem as powerful as a stance of looking for opportunities within change. It does not help to label change as unfair, or to complain about changes or of moving the goal posts. The NHS will always change for the reasons set out above, and that is why management is essential.

In order to make use of the opportunities that change can bring, it is important to have a clear strategy and to identify priorities for desirable changes, as outlined above. Another essential in this approach is to re-evaluate all aspects of the service continuously, rather than allow precedent to protect some areas from scrutiny. The third essential is to recognize that while the clinician–manager may be able to cope with change, more junior staff may need leadership to adopt a positive attitude and to find ways to adapt work without adding to stress.

Continual change is inevitable and should not be resisted as a matter of principle. Instead, senior professionals and managers should relish the uncertainties and ambiguities which change brings, take advantage of the opportunities it affords and safeguard the services if they are being threatened.

Managerial culture

What has been recommended in these six managerial approaches involves a shift of the clinician's managerial culture within the NHS. In the past many doctors have seen management as bureaucracy, an unpleasant business of manipulation, boring meetings, unnecessary paperwork and cuts to budgets. There has been little time for mature reflection or the wise use of creativity to achieve better patient care in that task-oriented culture. The accepted attitude has been cynical, distrusting and blaming.

For example, one key idea can be seen in the contrast drawn between the static and the innovative organization by Temporal and Boydell.[28] In their terms a static child health service would be managed in order to control the staff who are of fixed and known ability. Change would be unwelcome and risks to be avoided. On the other hand an innovative child health service would be managed to support and develop its staff in a flexible, experimental style.

This latter positive innovative culture has been well elaborated by a study of public sector organizations in Canada,[29] which identified five key attributes of well-performing organizations:

- *Emphasis on people*: junior staff are challenged, encouraged and developed, and feel confident that they can deliver a good service to children and face any challenge, despite the difficulties that surround them.
- *Participative leadership*: the senior community paediatrician is not authoritarian but rather fosters communication and commitment at all levels among the whole child health team.
- *Innovative work styles*: there is intelligent problem-solving and real learning from the experience of working with local children and their parents.
- *Strong client orientation*: the service is supported by local parents and has a strong focus on serving their children rather than on a community unit or the profession of community paediatrics.
- *A mindset that seeks optimum performance*: clinic staff share values about the child's right to health, and have a clear vision of what that means in practical terms. When conditions change, they adjust their methods rather than their values.

We believe that clinical and general managers can collaborate in providing local leadership, clear purpose and innovation in facing the key managerial challenges that we have identified. By using the powerful approaches outlined above, their ability to safeguard and develop good child health services will be greater than is often the case in the UK. There is much that can be achieved at local level if community paediatricians accept the challenge of management.

References

1   Department of Education and Science. *Special Education Needs*. London: HMSO, 1978.
2   Best, G., Schaeffer, L.D. *Managing Health Care: the Guidance Delivery Tension*. King's Fund International Seminar Introductory Paper, 1990.
3   Hampton, J.R. The end of clinical freedom. *Br Med J* 1983; **287:** 1237–38.
4   Mintzberg, H. *The Structuring of Organisations*. Englewood Cliffs: Prentice Hall, Inc. 1979: 348–379.
5   Illich, I. *Deschooling Society*. Harmondsworth: Penguin, 1973.
6   Larson, M. Professionalism: rise and fall. *Int J Health Serv* 1979; **9:** 4.
7   Coates, R., Evans, K. In: Stocking, B., ed. *The Learning Organisation & In Dreams Begins Responsibility*. London: King Edward's Hospital Fund for London, 1987: 90–96.
8   Schon, D.A. *The Reflective Practitioner*. London: Maurice Temple Smith, 1983; 287–353.
9   Handy, C. *The Age of Unreason*. London: Business Books Limited, 1989: 44–63.
10 Department of Health and Social Security and Welsh Office. *Patients First*. London: HMSO, 1979.
11 Department of Health and Social Security. *NHS Management Inquiry*. London: DHSS, 1983.
12 *Promoting Better Health*, CM. 249. London: HMSO, 1987.
13 *Working for Patients*, CM. 555. London: HMSO, 1989.
14 *Caring for People*, CM. 849. London: HMSO, 1989.
15 North West Thames Regional Health Authority. *Towards a Strategy for Services for Children*. London: NWTRHA, 1987.
16 Mitchell, J. Local management in the limelight. *King's Fund News* 1989; **12:** 2–3.

17 Best, G. The white paper challenge to local strategist. *Health Service J* 1989; **99:** 686–687.

18 Ellwood, P.M. A technology of patient experience. *New Eng J Med*, 1988; **318:** 1549–1556.

19 Donabedian, A. *Explorations in Quality Assessment and Monitoring*. Michigan Ann Arbor: Health Administration Press, 1980.

20 British Paediatric Association. *The Mechanism for Integrating Child Health Services: a policy statement*. London: BPA, 1985.

21 Maxwell, R.J. Quality assurance in health. *Br Med J*, 1984; **288:** 1470–72.

22 Johnston, A., Black, N. *Volume and Outcome in Hospital Care: a Review of the Literature*. London: North West Thames Regional Health Authority, 1989.

23 Beckhard, R., Harris, R.T. *Organisational Transitions*. Wokingham: Addison-Wesley, 1987.

24 Mintzberg, H. Crafting strategy. *Harvard Business Review* 1987; **65:** 66–77.

25 Peters, T., Ansim, N. *A Passion for Excellence*. London: Collins, 1985; 8–83.

26 Belbin, R.M. *Management Teams*. London: Heinemann, 1981.

27 Barlow, A. *Transitions Book III*. Luton: Local Government Training Board, 1990.

28 Temporal, P., Boydell, T. *Helping Managers to Learn*. Sheffield: Sheffield City Polytechnic, Dept of Management Studies, 1981.

29 Dye, K. *Attitudes of Well Performing Organisations*. Ottawa: Auditor General of Canada, 1988.

Chapter 6

Child health surveillance

6.1 Introduction

Angus Nicoll

The history of surveillance in the UK

At both local and national levels, the UK has one of the longest traditions of systematic screening and surveillance within child health services. The origins of this may be traced back to the end of the 19th century to the time of the Boer War with attempts to improve the health of the working class in general and military recruits in particular.[1] These early developments concentrated on the school-age child. However, the next important initiative arose from the work of developmental psychologists (notably Gesell) and paediatricians in the 1920s and 1930s.[1,2] These workers developed a rationale of detecting developmental delays and abnormalities in the pre-school child with a view to treatments and recommended that all children should be screened for such anomalies at set ages as a form of secondary prevention.[3] A mass screening programme for pre-school children followed in the 1960s. Prescriptive texts were written[4] and a national recording card developed (the MCW-46). There were substantial problems with this programme, many stemming from its architects being practitioners rather than programme managers. It was unlikely that whole populations could be covered by the ambitious schedules (complex test arrays applied at seven set ages before the fifth birthday).[4] Individual components of the arrays were unevaluated and some were hard to administer accurately except in well-trained hands; yet training for field staff scarcely existed. Despite these deficiencies the programme was widely implemented under local authority medical services and it came to be known as *developmental screening* and this was considered synonymous with surveillance. Its popularity among the public and health professions alike represented a consensus that child health surveillance was a valid activity.[1]

In the 1970s similar schemes began to appear in general practice.[5,6] Usually the general practitioners (GPs) organized separate clinics for pre-school children outside of normal consultation hours which were known as well-baby clinics. However, the service was delivered in a more patchy manner[7] than that of the local authority clinics. With some exceptions[8,9] the distribution of general practice based services broadly followed the prediction of Tudor Hart's inverse care law,[10] so that child populations with greater health problems were less likely to have GPs running well-baby clinics. Stimulus for these developments in general practice arose from the Sheldon[11] and the Court[1] Reports. However, neither report captured the confidence of GP representatives[12] and by the late 1980s only 20–40% of GPs were actively involved in surveillance.[7]

The late 1970s and 1980s saw an acceleration of surveillance activity with parallel developments in 10 important areas.

1 Scepticism grew concerning the validity, usefulness and cost-effectiveness of screening tests of children, either for developmental of other childhood disorders.[13,14] Possible demerits of screening processes were recognized and thinking in developmental

paediatrics and education advanced with the appreciation that the complexity of many anomalies made simple pass/fail criteria undesirable.

2 Careful research looked at the validity and performance of many components of the earlier screening programme and its overall performance.[7,15]

3 It was realized that there was an important distinction between screening[16] and surveillance[15] and that most of what was happening in pre-school child health services fell in the province of surveillance.[7,17] At the same time emphasis moved from the detection of anomalies to *health promotion* and there has been more critical attention to screening programmes in general with an appreciation that screening has substantial costs as well as potential benefits.[15]

4 Surveys of service organizations were undertaken revealing major differences across the country with regard to what was being done, who was doing it and staffing levels.[15,18,19] Action-based research was carried out to explore new ways of organizing surveillance which involved professionals other than doctors.[20–22] There was recognition that health visitors could provide much of surveillance at lower cost and often higher quality.[17,20,23]

5 Emphasis was placed on training, appropriate procedures and materials.[24]

6 There was a rediscovery of the family and parents as caregivers and their role in surveillance in partnership with professionals. Parent-held records were developed and used on an increasing scale.[25–27]

7 Development in immunization information systems laid a basis for population-based computerized child registers which then could be utilized for surveillance.[28]

8 There was a trend towards better management of health services including the evaluation of their effectiveness and cost. In relation to this, central requirements for information on community health services (including surveillance) intensified and moved towards standardization.[29]

9 A statutory need for early identification and documentation of educational problems was consolidated in the 1981 Education Act.

10 An intense political debate developed between five different groups, general practitioners, community child health doctors, consultant paediatricians, health visitors and specialists in public health medicine all seeking roles and resources.[7]

Arguably the most important development in this period was the publication in 1989 of a white paper *Working for Patients*[30] and the ensuing contract which included child health surveillance among the services provided by general practitioners.[31] Thus after years of argument and indecision government support for surveillance was declared.

The position of child health surveillance in the mid 1990s is dynamic but fragile. Opportunities for progress exist[32] and with the support given to general practice the debate over who ideally should carry out surveillance has been resolved. Two major reviews about the process of surveillance have been published; one historical,[7] the other technical and prescriptive.[15] The latter was of political significance since it was produced by a carefully balanced working party with representatives from the concerned professional groups and observers from the Department of Health.

However, enactment of government policy remains incomplete. Responsibility has been given to district health authorities (DHAs), as purchasers, to determine what constitutes an adequate surveillance programme[33] and to family health service authorities (FHSAs) to administer accreditation procedures for GPs. However, decisions about accreditation vary widely.[34] General practice is the preferred base for surveillance but the roles and coordination of other professionals involved is unclear. Health visitors undertake much of surveillance; community paediatricians provide secondary level care and participate in surveillance training; consultants in public health medicine manage data systems for DHAs in collaboration with community paediatricians and FHSAs. Procedures whereby these different contributions can be harmonized have yet to be identified. Training procedures and materials remain to be developed and evaluated, though the Nottingham Community Child Health Training Programmes provide examples of the way forward. Resources for implementing training and data systems are scarce and the 1991 NHS reforms are encouraging fragmentation of the population base needed for optimal surveillance and public health purposes. There is a danger that short-term economic considerations or lack of managerial and professional imagination may determine the future of child health surveillance rather than the needs of children.[32]

Framework

The debates about child health surveillance have been handicapped by poorly defined terminology and a poorly understood framework. Indeed it is not easy to produce a simple definition of surveillance since it covers a range of activities. The best published framework is that offered by John Butler (Fig. 6.1).[7] This divides *preventative child health care* into four categories. *Primary prevention* aims to promote good health by reducing the incidence of disease through community efforts,[3] some would call this *health promotion*. The best examples from surveillance are immunization and the promotion of good nutrition. *Secondary prevention* aims to detect disease and other

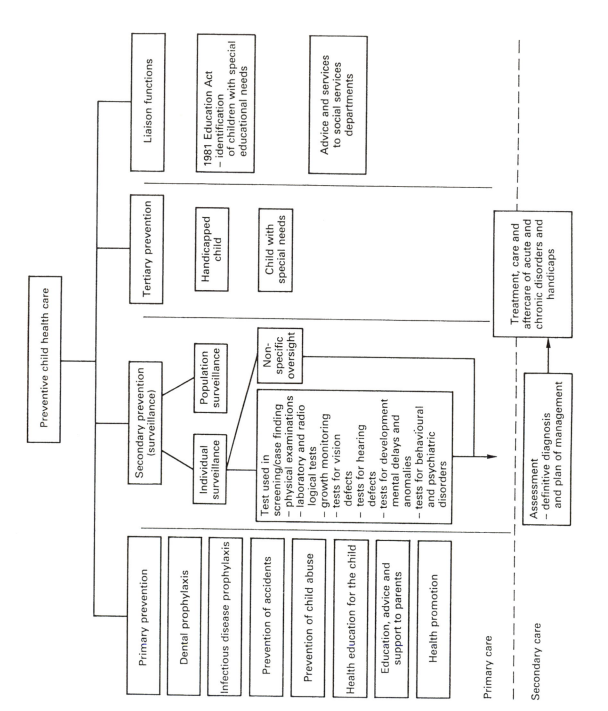

Figure 6.1 The preventive health care of pre-school children: a definitional framework. (From Butler[7] reproduced with permission of the author and Controller of Her Majesty's Stationery Office.)

departures from good health at an early stage, when treatment or remedy is possible, and so reduce disease duration or severity.[3] Here lies surveillance in Butler's view, and within it are all screening tests. Next is *tertiary prevention*, the care and amelioration of established handicapping disorders.[3] Finally child health care is concerned with professional *liaison*. But Butler's model is not conclusive. It has two obvious deficiencies, reflecting the terms of reference given to its author.[7] These are lack of:

1 The holistic perspective

From the point of view of the child, parents and service providers it is unsatisfactory merely to look at prevention. There are advantages to taking a holistic outlook (such as the Court Report attempted), in what has been recently called green paediatrics.[35] Butler's framework should be completed by adding *treatment*, both medical and social within primary and secondary care, and *epidemiological surveillance*, the population based aspects of preventative service (see below).

2 The parental perspective

A number of surveillance programmes now recognize a more active role for parents in prevention and early detection (see Section 6.3).[23] This can be acknowledged in a framework as *pre-primary care*, i.e. before the family approaches the primary health care professions.

Process

It is useful to consider different activities which may be components or are closely associated with surveillance. They include examination, assessment, non-specific oversight, parental detection and screening.

Examination/developmental examination

This is a clinical procedure or set of procedures used to detect abnormalities and disease. It includes developmental history, observation of the child's behaviour and the administration of various tests in order to establish the state of development of an individual child and to recognize deviations from the normal.[7] It is usual to include tests of special senses (vision and hearing). It should be noted that specific components of developmental examinations can be applied as screening tests.

Assessment and developmental assessment

This is an examination performed by highly trained personnel with a view towards diagnosis and treatment. It is essentially a secondary health care procedure (see Fig. 6.1).

Non-specific oversight

This is the vigilant supervision of all aspects of the health and well-being of children whenever they come into contact with health care professionals.[7]

Parental detection

This refers to concerns and problems identified within the family.

Screening

Screening is part of surveillance. It is the presumptive identification of unrecognized disease or defect by the application of tests, examinations and other procedures, which can be applied rapidly. Screening tests sort out apparently well persons who may have a disease from those who probably do not. A screening test is not intended to be diagnostic.[36] It is applied on whole populations at fixed ages or intervals. The World Health Organization (WHO) has issued clear criteria for evaluation.[16]

Using these criteria it can be seen that surveillance is more broadly based than screening, which is a small, but important, component of surveillance. Neonatal screening for phenylketonuria and hypothyroidism fulfils the WHO criteria,[37] although much else does not.[16] For example, developmental screening[38] is rarely applied to even a majority of those eligible,[17] the tests used are neither standardized nor readily reproducible and the abnormalities detected are frequently already known to the parents[39] or other practitioners.[13] Some findings were normal variants and many were not demonstrably treatable.[15] Hence developmental screening is not a recommended term since it does not meet conventional screening criteria[16]. If used, however, a suitable definition might be the application of developmental examinations at set ages as in published developmental screening programmes. This form of screening is further considered with surveillance below.

Opportunist screening is in one sense a contradiction in terms, since screening must be applied to whole populations.[16] However the term is used to mean the application of screening tests at times outside those at which they were planned, for example if a GP applies a missed hearing test to a child seen for another reason.[40]

Surveillance

An important distinction must be made between epidemiological or population surveillance and individual child health surveillance. Population level surveillance is a public health function.[41] It is of wider significance to the consultant community paediatrician and the public health specialist than to the practitioner within primary health care and will be defined and discussed further below.

Individual child health surveillance needs to be considered under definition, content and practice.

Individual child health surveillance

Definition

Surveillance involves a set of activities which are initiated by professionals. It includes the oversight of the physical, social and emotional health of all children; measurement and recording of physical growth; monitoring of developmental progress; prevention of disease by immunization and other means and health education.[15]

Content

Surveillance is sufficiently complex that content lists are now more useful than a definition. Butler's framework (see Fig. 6.1) offers a list within secondary prevention, namely:

1   Non-specific oversight.
2   Tests used in screening and case finding:
     physical examinations
     laboratory and radiological tests
     growth monitoring
     tests for vision defects
     tests for hearing defects
     tests for developmental delays and anomalies
     tests for behavioural and psychiatric disorders.
   To this should be added:
3   Parental detection.

The Court Report offered a similar view: 'oversight of health and physical growth of all children; monitoring the developmental progress of all children; providing advice and support to parents and treatment and referral of the child; providing a programme of effective infectious disease prophylaxis and participation in health education and training in parenthood' (para 9.6).[1]

Narrower definitions of the content of surveillance now represent minority or historical viewpoints.

Practice: comparing developmental screening and surveillance

Developmental screening has been the application of fixed tests which were limited by their over-ambitious content.[17] The frequency with which they were applied reduced the time available for more general overview and consideration of parent-initiated concern.[14] It was often the children with problems who did not attend appointments.[17] Some vision screening procedures for pre-school children have been shown to be of limited use.[42,43] Screening for hearing loss can be effective if staff are well trained and motivated.[44] However, when performed badly[45] it may be of less value than parental detection,[46] although surveillance by parents alone is inadequate.[47]

In contrast, *surveillance*, as recommended by the Joint Working Party, consists of 'doing better by doing less', with reduction of tests to a core programme in which only a minority of examinations are expected to meet screening test criteria.[15] In this programme some tests need to be applied at recommended dates, e.g. '6–8 months . . . carry out distraction tests of hearing'. Greater emphasis is placed on undertaking more general surveillance within broader age bands: e.g. 'At 39 months (range 36–48 months) pre-school examination the aims are: to ensure that the child is physically fit and that there are no medical disorders or defects which may interfere with education; to ensure that the immunizations are up to date; and to determine whether there are problems with development, language or behaviour which may have educational implications. The review can be shared between health visitor and doctor . . .'[15] This approach recognizes that some tests require rigorous, standardized performance applied to whole populations; such as hearing tests and examination for hip dislocation, while other examinations call for different skills, flexibility and experience, such as examinations for language skills. In this way, professionals are encouraged to use and develop their clinical skills to a greater degree.[15]

Persons involved in child health surveillance

The main enactors of specific examinations are general practitioners, health visitors and community child health doctors.

Those concerned with a more general overview of the child are: parents, nursery nurses, e.g. in day nurseries, nursery class teachers, speech therapists and social workers.

Other professionals involved in providing secondary or tertiary care or administratively are: consultant paediatricians, consultants in public health medicine and community health service managers.

These groups may act too independently[7] with the result that child health surveillance becomes 'many persons' business but nobody's responsibility'.

The question of who should do what has been difficult and controversial. To a large extent the issue has been decided with surveillance being based in general practice. However, important issues remain to be considered.

General practitioners

Professor Butler concluded that in the late 1980s one-half to two-thirds of all general practitioners were prepared to be involved in surveillance. He considered the proportion could be higher if financial incentives were introduced. However, uptake is unlikely to reach 100% and the issue remains of who will perform surveillance where GPs choose not to do so. Presently, many GPs have not received sufficient training to do this work. Hospital paediatric posts in vocational training schemes rarely address surveillance. In-service training is becoming available but problems remain over maintenance of clinical standards, data transfer to responsible authorities for population level surveillance and identification of handicapped children.

Health visitors

Health visitors potentially give excellent coverage. They exist in relatively large numbers reasonably spread across the country and they see child health surveillance as part of their recognized activities.[20,23] They have a statutory role to see all children and hence they are a significant force able to reach children that other professionals cannot. Their training for child health surveillance is variable but can be enhanced by in-service courses. Finally they have a management structure which facilitates supervision and data collection. Many GPs have developed team-work arrangements with practice health visitors, the latter undertaking most of the developmental surveillance and the GPs confining themselves to medical aspects. An issue to be resolved is whether health visitors should be attached to a GP and focus on the children registered with the practice or on a geographical caseload.

Community child health doctors and consultant community paediatricians

Community child health doctors are fewer in number than GPs.[7] Coverage of population is variable and dependent on local policy.[18] In the past, little training has been expected or given. Through structured training programmes and in-service training the situation is improving.

Currently, these doctors are becoming more highly trained, undertaking secondary care and tertiary prevention, and they have developed a career structure to consultant level, leaving the primary surveillance of pre-school children to GPs and health visitors.

Given the differing perspectives of the three groups and the lack of guidance from the Department of Health, the wide variations in staffing levels and service organization found across the country are not surprising.[18,20] However, in the more progressive areas a close relationship has developed between all three groups through the formation of community paediatric teams.[48]

Population level surveillance, communication, information transfer and evaluation

Population level information from surveillance should meet many objectives. Measurements of health outcome are necessary to inform judgements on priorities and they are required to check the effect of interventions. Data gathered from surveillance are essential for contractual and medical audit, giving vital information for programme management and professionals.

Broadly speaking, surveillance can provide two types of aggregate information: health outcomes, e.g. level of disease, for epidemiological purposes; and service processes, for example coverage of the population, for management purposes.

An important distinction must be made between individual and epidemiological surveillance. *Epidemiological surveillance* is defined as 'ongoing scrutiny; generally using methods distinguished by their practicability, uniformity and frequently their rapidity, rather than by complete accuracy. Its main purpose is to detect changes in trend and distribution in order to initiate investigative or control measures.'[3] In addition, surveillance data have occasionally and unexpectedly supplied valuable information for research on the longitudinal genesis of medical conditions.[49]

The Department of Health has encouraged the development and use of health outcome measures and indicators[29] which are, however, limited. Similar criticisms have been made of the government's targets in *The Health of the Nation*[35] and community paediatricians have developed their own package.[50]

Child health outcome measurements[50]

1   Outcome and death

To include the following and others:

- Perinatal mortality rate
- Birthweight specific perinatal mortality rate
- Neonatal mortality rate
- Post-neonatal mortality rate
- Infant mortality rate

2   Outcome and acute illness

To include the following and others:

- Immunization cover (diphtheria, tetanus, pertussis, polio, HiB, measles/mumps/rubella)
- Measles notifications
- Pertussis notifications
- Status asthmaticus admissions (requiring drip, intravenous bronchodilators and steroids)
- Gastroenteritis admissions (requiring drip)

3   Outcome and chronic illness, disability

PRIMARY PREVENTION

To include the following and others:

- Incidence of spina bifida
- Incidence of acquired severe mental handicap (intelligence quotient less than 60, unlikely to lead an independent life)
- Any case including elective surgical, dental or medical procedures, accidents, encephalopathy, child abuse, meningitis, etc.
- Prevalence of cerebral palsy
- Prevalence of severe hearing impairment

SECONDARY PREVENTION

To include the following and others:

- Cancer survival
- Periodic survey of asthma in the community – school loss, under diagnosis, under treatment
- Periodic survey of glycosolated haemoglobin in children with diabetes
- Prevalence of children with amblyopia on school entry – worse than 6/12
- Average age at diagnosis of children subsequently needing operative treatment for congenital dislocation of the hip

TERTIARY PREVENTION

- Average age at diagnosis of severe hearing impairment
- Average age at diagnosis of children subject of a statement of special educational need for specific developmental language delay
- Number of children subject of a statement before age 6 years, who were not recognized to have a problem before age 4 years, 3 years and 2 years

4   Outcome and adverse psychological consequences of disability or chronic illness for the family and child

- Rates of marital breakdown in families with a handicapped child
- Number of handicapped children living in mental handicap hospitals, community homes or with foster parents

5   Outcome and psychological and behavioural disturbance

- Number of children subject of a statement of educational need for behaviour difficulties
- Number of children suspended from schools, aged 4–11, 12–15
- Number of children, aged 12–15 years, admitted to hospital for poisoning
- Number of children under 13 years admitted to non-paediatric wards

6   Outcome and healthy lifestyles in children

- Number of conceptions in girls under 16 (births and terminations)
- Periodic survey of alcohol and smoking behaviour in school children
- Periodic survey of diet and exercise behaviour in school children

7   Outcome and optimal development of children

- Trends in height and weight
- Trends in birthweight
- Rates of breast feeding at age 6 weeks

8   Outcome and social and geographical inequality in health

- Local Authority ward-to-ward variation in birthweight
- Local Authority ward-to-ward variation in immunization cover
- Local Authority ward-to-ward variation in smoking behaviour in children
- Social class variation in prevalence of dental caries

This package was very ambitious and was curtailed in a more formal report by a group with a wider remit.[51] It also aggregates measures of professional performance, socially determined outcomes and epidemiological data. However, it provides a useful starting point and deserves further development.

References

1 Committee on Child Health Services. *Fit for the Future* (Court Report). Cmnd 6684. London: HMSO, 1976.

2 Gesell, A., Amatruda, C.S. *Developmental Diagnosis.* New York: Hoeber, 1941.

3 Last, J.M. *A Dictionary of Epidemiology.* Oxford: Oxford University Press, 2nd edn, 1988.

4 Egan, D., Illingworth, R.S., MacKeith, R.C. *Developmental Screening 0–5 Years.* London: Spastics International Medical Publications, 1969.

5 Bain, D.J.G. The results of developmental screening in general practice. *Hlth Bull* 1974; **32:** 189–93.

6 Curtis Jenkins, G., Collins, C., Andren, S. Developmental surveillance in general practice. *Br Med J* 1978; **1:** 1537–40.

7 Butler, J.R. *Child Health Surveillance in Primary Care: A Critical Review.* London: HMSO, 1989.

8 James, J., Clark, C. Well baby clinics. *Lancet* 1988; i: 61.

9 Crouchman, M.R., Gazzard, J., Forrester, J. A joint child health clinic in an inner London general practice. *Practitioner* 1986; **230:** 667–672.

10 Tudor Hart, J. The inverse care law. *Lancet* 1971; **1:** 405–13.

11 Central Health Services Council. *Child Welfare Centres* (Shelton Report). London: HMSO, 1967.

12 Anonymous. Court Report on Child Health Services: GMSC view. *Br Med J* 1977; **1:** 1551–53.

13 Hendrickse, W.A. How effective are our child health clinics? *Br Med J* 1982; **284:** 575–77.

14 Roberts, C.J., Khosla, T. An evaluation of developmental examination as a method of detecting neurological, visual, and auditory handicaps in infancy. *Br J Prev Soc Med* 1972; **26:** 94–100.

15 Hall, D.M.B. (ed.) *Health for All Children: Report of the Joint Working Party on Child Health Surveillance*, 2nd edn. Oxford: Oxford University Press, 1991.

16 Wilson, J.M.G., Junger, G. Principles and practice of screening for disease. Public Health Papers No. 34. Geneva: World Health Organization, 1968.

17 Development surveillance (editorial). *Lancet* 1986, i: 950–52.

18 Macfarlane, J.A., Pillay, U. Who does what, and how much in the preschool child health services in England. *Br Med J* 1984; **289:** 851–52.

19 Davies, L.M., Bretman, M.D. What do community health doctors do?: Survey of their work in the child health services in Nottinghamshire. *Br Med J* 1985; **290:** 1604–6.

20 Connolly, P. An enquiry into child health surveillance procedures undertaken by health visitors in England. In: *Health Visiting Principles in Practice*, ch 7. London: Council for the Education and Training of Health Visitors, 1982.

21 Nicoll, A., Mann, S., Mann, N., Vyas, H. The child health clinic: results of a new strategy of community care in a deprived area. *Lancet* 1986; i: 606–8.

22 Colver, A.F., Steiner, H. Health surveillance of preschool children. *Br Med J* 1986; **293:** 258–60.

23 Health Visitors' Association. *The Health Visitor's Role in Child Health Surveillance: a Policy Statement.* London: Health Visitors' Association, 1985.

24 Baird, G., Hall, D.M.B. Developmental paediatrics in primary care: what should we teach. *Br Med J* 1985; **291:** 583–86.

25 O'Flaherty, S., Jandera, E., Llewellyn, J., Wall, M. Personal health records: an evaluation. *Arch Dis Child* 1987; **62:** 1152–55.

26 Spencer, N.J. Parents' recognition of the ill child. In: Macfarlane, J.A. (ed.) *Progress in Child Health*, Vol. 1. Edinburgh: Churchill Livingstone, 1984.

27 Saffin, K., Macfarlane, A. How well are parent held records kept and completed? *Br J Gen Pract* 1991; **41:** 249–51.

28 Ross, E., Begg, N. Child health computing. *Br Med J* 1991; **302:** 5–6.

29 Health Service Indicators Group. *Report of the Working Group on Indicators for the Community Health Services.* London: HMSO, 1988.

30 Secretaries of State for Health, England, Wales, Northern Ireland and Scotland. *Working for Patients.* Cmnd 555. London: HMSO, 1989.

31 Department of Health. *National Health Service General Medical Services: Statement of Fees and Allowances Payable to General Medical Practitioners.* London: HMSO, 1990.

32 Hall, D.M.B., Prendergast, M. An integrated child health service. *Br Med J* 1990; **301:** 1341–42.

33 Bain, J. Child health surveillance. *Br Med J* 1990; **300:** 1381–82.

34 Waine, C. Child health surveillance lists. *Br Med J* 1991; **303:** 202.

35 Hull, D. The health of the nation: responses: children's health. *Br Med J* 1991; **303:** 514–15.

36 Commission on Chronic Illness. *Chronic Illnesses in the United States*, Vol. 1. Cambridge, MA: Harvard University Press, 1957.

37 Grant, D.B., Smith, I. Survey of neonatal screening for primary hypothyroidism in England, Wales and Northern Ireland 1982–4. *Br Med J* 1988; **296:** 1355–58.

38 Development screening (editorial). *Lancet* 1975; i: 784–86.

39 Mayall, B. *Keeping Children Healthy.* London: Allan and Unwin, 1986.

40 Houston, H.L.A., Harvard Davis, R. Opportunistic surveillance of child development in primary care: is it feasible? *J Roy Coll Gen Practit* 1985; **35:** 77–79.

41 Allsop, M., Colver, A., McKinlay, I. *Measurement of Child Health.* London: British Paediatric Association, 1989.

42 Hall, D.M.B., Hall, S.M. Early detection of visual defects in infancy. *Br Med J* 1988: **296:** 823–24.

43 Hall, S.M., Pugh, A.G., Hall, D.M.B. Vision screening in the under-5s. *Br Med J* 1982; **296:** 823–24.

44 McCormick, B. *Screening for Hearing Impairment in Young Children.* London: Croom Helm, 1988.

45 Stewart-Brown, S., Haslum, M.N. Screening for hearing loss in childhood: a study of national practice. *Br Med J* 1987; **294:** 1386–88.

46 Hitchings, V., Haggard, M.P. Incorporation of parental suspicions in screening infants. *Br J Audiol* 1983; **17:** 71–75.

47 Watkin, P.M., Baldwin, M., Laoide, S. Parental suspicion and identification of hearing impairment. *Arch Dis Child* 1990; **65:** 479–85.

48 Polnay, L. The community paediatric team: an approach to child health services in a deprived inner city area. In: Macfarlane L.J.A. (ed.) *Progress in Child Health*, Vol. 1. Edinburgh: Churchill Livingstone, 1984.

49 Barker, D.J.P., Osmond, C., Golding, J., Kuk, D., Wadsworth, M.E.J. Growth in utero, blood pressure in childhood and adult-life, and mortality from cardiovascular disease. *Br Med J* 1989; **298**: 564–67.

50 Working Party of the Executive Committee of the Community Paediatric Group. *Measurement of Child Health*. London: British Paediatric Association, 1989.

51 Outcome Measures Working Group for the British Paediatric Association Health Services Committee. London: British Paediatric Association, 1990.

Further reading

Hall, D.M.B. (ed.) *Health for All Children: Report of the Joint Working Party on Child Health Surveillance*. 2nd edn. Oxford: Oxford University Press, 1991.

Butler, J.R. *Child Health Surveillance in Primary Care: A Critical Review*. London: HMSO, 1989.

6.2 Screening

Sarah Stewart-Brown

Introduction

'Prevention is better than cure', so the saying goes and many an enthusiastic clinician has been inspired by these words to set up a screening programme to prevent disease and disability in childhood. The possibility that the programme might do more harm than good is seldom considered and potential detrimental effects on other services are ignored. Yet the evidence that these programmes can do harm is now incontrovertible and their potential for wasting large amounts of public money is also well recognized.[1] On the other hand, some programmes do contribute very significantly to population health and are highly cost-effective. Deciding whether a programme is likely to be valuable or not can be complex. This section outlines the principles of evaluating screening programmes and looks at some of the costs and benefits of those currently in use in child health.

All new screening programmes need to be carefully evaluated, usually in large randomized controlled trials before their introduction. Even when this is done, some uncertainty may remain as to how well the programme will work in practice; efficacy in clinical trials does not equal effectiveness in everyday practice and the need for monitoring and evaluation is not eliminated by trials. The situation in community child health is complicated because many of the current programmes were introduced before the epidemiological principles of screening had been clearly established. Many were based on clinical examinations or tests whose efficacy as population screening instruments was simply not investigated. Definitive evaluation requires the comparison of a screened population with an unscreened one. Once a programme has been running for a while and has been shown to bring some benefit to some children (however little to however few) ethical objections are likely to be raised to studies which require an unscreened control group.

Thus the legacy of our predecessors' enthusiasm for prevention is a programme of child health screening which many health professionals believe makes a vital contribution to the health and well-being of children and about which many others are extremely sceptical.

Definition of screening

Screening was defined in a classic World Health Organization (WHO) monograph in 1968[2] as 'the presumptive identification of unrecognized disease or defect by the application of examinations or other procedures which can be applied rapidly'. The definition is still sound. It emphasizes the important point that screening programmes are not diagnostic; they only sort out apparently well people who probably have a disease from those who probably do not. False-positive and false-negative cases are inevitable consequences of screening and problems arising from these cases cannot be ignored. The definition does not include reference to individual benefit, and there are good examples of programmes which do not have this goal.

Models of screening

Public health benefit

Mass radiography for tuberculosis (TB) was a screening programme set up to protect the health of the public by reducing the spread of disease; benefit to the cases was not the primary aim. Screening a group of school children to trace a suspected carrier of diphtheria is another example of this type of public protection screening; screening teachers for TB before starting teaching is a third.

No health benefit

Occasionally screening may be undertaken without any intention to benefit anyone's health. The insurance companies which insist on HIV testing before issuing life insurance policies do this screening to exclude high-risk individuals from their clientele. School medical examinations were originally introduced only to assess the prevalence of debilitating disease and disability in the child population.[3] School health clinics, where these children might receive treatment, followed later.

Individual health benefit

Most screening programmes (all those currently practised in child health surveillance) do aim to provide health benefits to detected cases or their families. The remainder of this section is concerned with this type of screening.

Different types of programme

All child health screening is targeted in the sense that it is confined to children, but some programmes are targeted at *selected groups* within this population. For example neonatal screening for haemoglobinopathies is best confined to communities with a high proportion of genetically susceptible ethnic minority groups. Impedance audiometry screening is not considered justifiable for all children,[4] but may be valuable for groups at high risk of conductive hearing loss (children with cleft lip and palate or with Down syndrome).

Screening programmes may be undertaken for either *secondary or tertiary prevention* (see Chapter 7.1). Screening for neonatal congenital dislocation of the hip is a good example of the former since it detects an early stage of a reversible disease process. Most child health programmes are designed to achieve tertiary prevention. Here, as in screening for sensorineural hearing loss, the disease process is not reversible but intervention can reduce the resulting disability and handicap. A fourth category *quaternary prevention* might perhaps be useful to describe programmes which are intended to reduce the impact of disability and handicap on all members of the family. Much of the benefit of early detection of severe learning disability is derived by the child's family; the child of course also benefits secondarily because a well-informed, well-adjusted and supported family is more likely to be able to cope with the problems presented by a child with severe learning disabilities.

Some screening programmes have become so much incorporated into clinical practice that they are no longer recognized as such. Urine testing in children admitted to hospital and routine antenatal care are good examples of this type of screening.

Principles of screening

The steps required to evaluate screening programmes were clearly elaborated in the 1968 WHO monograph.[2] They fall into three categories: those related to the disease, those related to the test and those related to treatment.

The disease

The disease must be important; either it must be common or it must be severe. Child health surveillance programmes include examples of both; phenylketonuria is a very rare but very serious condition; amblyopia causes only very mild disability, but is very common. Exactly how common or how severe a disease needs to be before screening is justified is a value judgement that should only be taken in the light of knowledge about the test, the effectiveness of treatment, and the cost of the programme.

The disease must have a recognizable latent or presymptomatic stage, and early treatment during this stage must confer some benefit. It is not useful to identify in the presymptomatic period conditions which can be effectively treated when they present clinically or those in which presymptomatic treatment does not improve prognosis. The early screening programmes for cancer were thought to be effective because they prolonged survival; but when the outcomes were examined in relation to the natural history of the disease it was found that this apparent effect was due to earlier diagnosis; the programmes had made no impact on survival times. Their only effect had been to make people aware that they had cancer sooner than they would otherwise have done; not everyone was grateful! This phenomenon is known as lead-time bias.

The natural history of the disease must be clearly understood. The effectiveness of intervention as a result of screening can only be assessed in the light of this knowledge. Screening for conditions which get better on their own is not a worthwhile activity. Many child health screening programmes are hampered by a lack of knowledge about the natural history of disease.

Although parts of the puzzle have been identified, we do not have a complete understanding of the natural history of secretory otitis media and its relationship with language development. If this extremely common condition does interfere with language development at what level of severity is intervention justified? It seems likely that some of the effect on language is only temporary and that complete catch up occurs. If this is the case should children be submitted to the risk of an anaesthetic and ill-advisedly prevented from swimming because of a mild self-limiting disability? The only way to answer these questions would be to do a randomized controlled trial with long-term follow up and measurement of a range of outcomes including educational and sporting achievement, behaviour and family relationships. Such a study would be difficult to do now, but would have been possible when the tests were first introduced.

Lack of knowledge of the natural history of congenital dislocation of the hip is one of the factors which makes this screening programme of doubtful value. The currently recommended screening programme requires examinations on three occasions after the newborn period. The arguments in favour of these late examinations are first that they will allow the identification of children whose dislocated hips have been missed in early examinations, and second that they detect hips which were stable at birth but dislocate at a later date. The first argument is untenable; the solution to missed cases is to improve the quality of the primary screen, not to subject the entire population to further examinations. The second is based on anecdotal clinical observation as the incidence of late dislocation is unknown. If, as seems likely, the incidence is negligible, children should not be subjected to repeat examinations which could in themselves be damaging. The considerable resources devoted to repeat screening could then be diverted to support more effective services.[5]

The test

The screening test needs to be both safe and acceptable, quick and easy to perform, and relatively cheap. Safety is a criterion that most of the child health screening tests meet and their acceptability is only a problem if parents perceive the tests to be a waste of their time. The failure rate on *quick and easy to perform* is rather higher. Tests like the performance and speech discrimination tests for hearing loss are essentially clinical investigations; while they are valuable in the assessment of children with clinical problems, they are neither quick nor easy to perform. Because the interpretation of the child's response to the test is very skilled requiring highly trained health professionals these tests are expensive in terms of manpower. The battery of orthoptic tests used in $3\frac{1}{2}$ year vision screening and the developmental screening tests, which used to be almost universal at all surveillance contacts, demand much professional time.

The other criteria on which screening tests are assessed are their validity and reliability. *Validity* is

the ability of a test to separate those who have a condition from those who do not; it is best illustrated by reference to a two-by-two table (Table 6.1).

Table 6.1 shows four different categories of screened individuals:

true positives	a
false positives	b
false negatives	c
true negatives	d

$\frac{a+b}{T}$ is the proportion of people the test identifies as positive or its yield. Some authors[6] have refined this definition to include only the positive cases whose prognosis is improved by early detection.

a + c may or may not be equal to the total number of children with the disease in the screened population, depending on whether all those with the disease would benefit from treatment. Screening for hearing loss identifies children with self-limiting conductive losses as well as those with permanent sensorineural loss. The former are *diseased* at the moment they are screened; but as they may not need treatment, they are false-positive cases. Because tests based on hearing cannot discriminate between the different causes of deafness their validity is bound to be limited.

The *sensitivity* is a measure of the test's ability to detect all those who would benefit from treatment and is defined as

$$\frac{a}{a + c} \times 100$$

The *specificity* is a measure of how well the test leaves alone those who would not benefit from treatment; it is defined as

$$\frac{d}{b + d} \times 100$$

The ideal screening test would have a sensitivity and specificity of 100%. In practice, tests which achieve 90% specificity and 80% sensitivity are usually good value. These two measures are interrelated and it is possible to increase one at the expense of the other by changing the criteria used to identify positive cases.

In Figure 6.2 the solid line represents the population distribution of a variable measured by a screening test in a normal population, for example neonatal thyroid stimulating hormone (TSH); the hatched line shows the distribution of the variable in the diseased population, for example babies with hypothyroidism. If the two distributions were distinct, that is they did not

Table 6.1 Categories of screened individuals

	Would benefit from treatment	Would not benefit from treatment	Total
Test positive	a	b	a + b
Test negative	c	d	c + d
Total	a + c	b + d	T

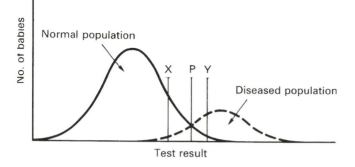

Figure 6.2 Distribution of screening test results in normal and diseased populations.

overlap at all, the test could achieve 100% sensitivity and specificity, but as is usual they are not. Test values between X and Y are borderline, some of these babies will be normal and some need treatment. The test value P gives the best balance between sensitivity and specificity; but if it was considered unacceptable to miss any cases of the disease the cut off point for positive cases could be set at X. This would make the sensitivity 100% but the specificity would decrease considerably and the number of false positive cases increase. The problems caused by underdiagnosis always have to be balanced against the problems caused by overdiagnosis; the optimum solution will depend both on the consequences of missing a case and on the consequences of false positive diagnosis.

The *predictive value* of a test is the proportion of positive cases who would benefit from treatment ($\frac{a}{a+b} \times 100$). This value may also be called the positive predictive value; its converse, the negative predictive value, is the proportion of negative cases who would not benefit from treatment. The positive predictive value falls as the prevalence of disease falls. If the prevalence is very low (as for example in phenylketonuria) a test with a specificity of over 99% may still have a predictive value of less than 30%. A screening programme with the same characteristics applied to a commoner condition would have a very much higher predictive value.

The test's *reliability* is a measure of its repeatability and is made up of a number of components. As the tests used in child health screening are very frequently based on clinical observation the most important component is observer variation; both inter-observer (between observers) and intra-observer (within observer) variations are common. Regular training for screeners and audit of performance is important and effective in keeping unreliability to a minimum, but the problem cannot ever be entirely eliminated.[7]

The child is another potential source of unreliability; tests which depend on a child's concentration and cooperation such as visual acuity may give variable results at different times of day and on different days. Finally, instruments may affect the performance of a test. Inaccurate weighing scales are a common cause of this type of unreliability. Clearly a test which is unreliable increases the number of false-positive and false-negative cases and is unlikely to provide the basis of an effective screening programme.

The treatment

The requirement that the disease being screened for can be effectively treated seems almost too obvious to state. Yet it is this criterion on which so many of the child health screening programmes fall down. Many of the therapies offered to disabled children have never been properly evaluated in randomized controlled trials and it is therefore impossible to say how much good they do; physiotherapy for cerebral palsy, speech therapy for language delay, patching for amblyopia and grommets for glue ear are all good examples of interventions which are now so much part of clinical practice that it has become very difficult to find out exactly how much good they do.

It is not enough to have demonstrated that the disease being screened for can be effectively treated, it is also necessary to show that it can be treated in practice. Screening programmes that are worthwhile uncover previously undetected disease and inevitably increase the demand for treatment; it is for this reason that screening needs to be carefully coordinated with secondary assessment and treatment services. Screening to detect language delay in districts which have too few speech therapists to treat all the children who present clinically cannot be justified. Many hearing screening programmes for 3-year-old children have been set up with no thought given to the additional requirements of the local hearing and speech centre. The inevitable increase in waiting time for audiological assessment has made some of these programmes unacceptable.

The costs and benefits of screening

The costs of screening need to be calculated both in financial and in human terms; of the two the latter are the most important.

Financial costs

The financial costs include the cost of the primary screen, the cost of secondary assessment and the cost of treatment.

The cost per screened individual needs to be low for a programme to be viable, but even with apparently cheap screening tests there may be pitfalls. In community child health it is not uncommon for an additional test to be added to an existing battery of tests in a single surveillance contact. In this situation the additional financial costs of the primary screen may be no more than a few minutes of health professional time and the screening programme may appear to be a very good buy. If, however, the existing tests are of doubtful value the addition of a new test may be used to justify retaining a surveillance contact which would otherwise have been discontinued. In this situation the test may be more costly than it would appear.

If, in addition, the test has a low specificity and secondary assessment is required for a large number of children who turn out not to have the disease the additional costs will also be high. Because the health professionals instituting primary screening are rarely the same as those who have to bear the brunt of assessments, these costs are frequently forgotten.

Human costs

Inappropriate reassurance of false-negative cases

Children who pass a screening test even though they are in need of treatment for a disease may be doubly disadvantaged; not only does the test fail to detect their problem, but the negative result may persuade parents that their worries about the child's performance were not justified. This can lead to long delays in diagnosis. This is most commonly reported after a distraction hearing test in the first year of life,[4] but it also occurs in children with other problems, for example developmental delay.

Generation of anxiety

Positive screening examinations do create anxiety.[8,9] For true positive cases such anxiety is a small price to pay for identification of a previously undetected problem, but for the false-positive cases there are no benefits. Although the cost may not seem to be great, the nuisance value of tests with a low specificity where large numbers of false-positive cases require secondary assessment should not be underestimated.

Development of false morbidity

Early in the history of school health surveillance in the USA an interesting study was undertaken on children found to have innocent murmurs. Morbidity in these children, who falsely perceived themselves as having heart disease, was actually greater than morbidity in children with organic lesions.[10] Such problems are, it is to be hoped, uncommon today, but the study is an important one to bear in mind.

Generation of true morbidity

Just occasionally, a screening programme may have unwanted side effects that cause serious problems. The screening programmes used during pregnancy in the 1980s for Down syndrome provide one example.

Amniocentesis at 16–18 weeks causes the abortion of a few normal viable pregnancies. When the programme was offered to women aged 35 years or more the number of miscarriages the procedure caused was greater than the number of Down syndrome babies detected by a figure of 3:2.[11] If a higher maternal age limit for screening is chosen the ratio becomes more favourable so that above 40 years the number of fetuses identified with Down syndrome would be greater than the number of miscarriages caused. Chorion villous sampling at 12 weeks' gestation causes similar problems; the post-sampling abortion rate is twice that after amniocentesis but about half of these abortions would occur spontaneously.[11] New approaches to screening for Down syndrome have increased the specificity of the test and have reduced this problem to some extent.

Another very different but potentially serious side effect occurs in screening for haemoglobinopathies. The problem is that the test can and does reveal illegitimacy. The social consequences of this revelation may be considerable for the families concerned. Whether the benefits of screening all babies in high-risk communities, as opposed to screening those for whom paediatricians and parents think the test is indicated, outweigh these potentially serious costs is debatable. Certainly all such programmes should include counselling for the mother about this possibility before testing.

Another potential human cost arises in programmes where it is impossible to distinguish children who would benefit from treatment from those who would not; this problem is illustrated by the congenital dislocation of the hip screening programme. Between five and nine babies receive treatment for hip instability for every one that would go on to develop a dislocation. If the treatment is relatively innocuous, as splinting appears to be, this may be no great problem. However, if there were some side effect of splinting which only manifested itself later in life and if this occurred in say one in three treated cases then there would be a serious possibility that the programme would do more harm than good.

Opportunity costs

Health services are now rationed in the UK. Therapies which have been proven to be effective cannot be offered to all, as and when they are needed. Rationing more frequently presents a problem for older age groups and people with physical and learning disabilities than for children; it is therefore more likely to be ignored by paediatricians and other health professionals caring for children. However, for these other groups opportunity costs are very real. Screening programmes consume resources which could be used elsewhere in the health service. If the health benefits of the programme are not commensurate with the costs (in relation to the costs and benefits of other health care programmes), the programme cannot justifiably be provided until additional resources are made available to the service.

A different type of opportunity cost is that for parents who have to attend both screening examinations and secondary assessments. Increasing numbers of families are headed by two working parents, and in these families one or other parent has to take time off work to attend clinics. In families where one parent is at home, time may also be difficult to find. These costs may seem trivial to health professionals in the face of potential benefit for children with problems, but for parents with no transport, several other children, or a job from which it is difficult to take time off, the benefits may appear small in comparison to the costs. There can be little doubt that these costs are considered by parents and that they account for a proportion of failed attendances at child health clinics.

Benefits

Prevention of disease, disability and handicap

For a few diseases early detection permits almost complete reversal of the effects of disease. Phenylketonuria and hypothyroidism screening in the neonatal period fall into this category. Although very rare, these diseases are extremely disabling and the benefits of screening clear.[4]

The detection and correction of congenital heart disease before irreversible circulatory changes occur is also effective in preventing disease and disability and prolonging life.[4]

However, for most child health programmes the goal of early diagnosis is not to reverse the physical or mental impairment but to reduce the resulting disability or handicap. The evidence that this happens in, for example, sensorineural hearing loss or cerebral palsy is based mostly on clinical observation, rather than more formal studies; but the great majority of clinicians believe that intervention is effective.

Parents' concerns

The evidence that parents welcome early diagnosis is now well documented[12,13] and there is also evidence that early diagnosis, combined with sensitive counselling and support, facilitates parental adjustment.[14]

Genetic counselling

The early detection of genetically determined conditions creates the opportunity for genetic counselling and possible prenatal detection in subsequent pregnancies.

Service provision

Knowledge of the numbers of children with particular problems is important for service provision. Education authorities need to be able to plan the number of places for children with special educational needs. This information also assists health authorities with forward planning.

Prevention of health service expenditure

In theory, the prevention of disease should reduce the need for health service provision and thus conserve scarce resources. In practice, current child health screening programmes rarely have this effect; it is much more common for them to increase service demand by uncovering disability and handicap which cannot be prevented and can only be ameliorated by costly interventions of one sort or another.

Cost effective screening programmes in community child health

The information necessary to make a full economic appraisal of current community child health screening is available for only a minority of programmes. Yet it is still possible to agree a best buy on the basis of the studies that have been done. A joint working party from the parent bodies of key health professionals involved in child health has considered all the evidence and reported on the programmes which seem to be worthwhile.[4] These are shown in Table 6.2 together with comments about any problems the programmes present.

Alongside the description of the recommended programmes the Hall report commented on a number of programmes which might prove beneficial in future when further research had been undertaken; these programmes included:

At birth
  inborn errors of metabolism
  cystic fibrosis
At 1–3 years
  iron deficiency anaemia

Among the more controversial of the working party's recommendations were the discontinuation of screening for squint using the cover–uncover test at any age, and screening for both conductive hearing loss and amblyopia in the fourth year of life. Reference has

Table 6.2 Summary of screening procedures recommended in the Hall report[4]

Condition and screening procedure	Age	Treatment for positives	Special groups	Comments
Clinical examinations *Congenital dislocation of hip*				Specificity of test at birth low (10–20%). Sensitivity unknown
Ortolani/Barlow manoeuvre Classic signs Classic signs	Birth 10 days	Splint Splint	Breech deliveries, multiple births, positive family history	10% of cases occur after the neonatal examination. The programme requires treatment for all unstable hips although only 1 in 5 would progress to full dislocation without treatment. Ultrasound examination may eventually replace Ortolani/Barlow manoeuvre. Treatment in neonate is non-invasive and inexpensive
Classic signs	6–8 weeks	Splint, traction or surgery		Most late presentations are detected by child health surveillance before walking. Yield uncertain. Research still needed
Classic signs (asymmetrical creases, limited abduction and leg shortening)	6–9 months	Surgery	Incidence in children with neurological disease is higher, so particular attention to hips needed in this group	
Classic signs and late walking	18–24 months	Surgery		Yield uncertain and likely to be very low. More research still needed
Congenital heart disease Clinical examination Tachypnoea	2–10 days and 6–8 weeks	Specialist monitoring Surgery	Down syndrome children are at high risk and all need ECG and echocardiography	Importance of auscultation in identification is over emphasized. Specificity of the test in non-specialist hands is poor. Need for better training recognized. Pre-symptomatic detection improves prognosis.
Clinical examination Tachypnoea	Once between 8 weeks and 5 years.	Specialist monitoring Surgery	Down syndrome children (as above)	Specificity very low.
Undescended testes Clinical examination of genitalia	2–10 days	Surgery	Do not neglect in the mentally handicapped. Higher incidence in low birthweight babies	Three out of four testes undescended at birth are normally descended by 3 months
Clinical examination of genitalia	8–9 months	Surgery	As above	Treatment before 18 months may improve prognosis for fertility
Clinical examination of genitalia	3–5 years	Surgery	As above	Testes fully descended at birth do not later ascend, but partially descended testes do and may be missed (incidence unknown)

Table 6.2 *Cont'd*

Condition and screening procedure	Age	Treatment for positives	Special groups	Comments
Laboratory and radiological tests				
Phenylketonuria Guthrie	7 days	Exclusion diet	None	–
Hypothyroidism T4/TSH	7 days	Thyroxin	Increased incidence in some ethnic groups and in Down syndrome children	7% of cases are missed by neonatal screening but a second screen would not be cost effective. Clinical awareness continues to be an important means of detection
Haemoglobinopathies All ethnic groups other than northern Europeans	Birth		Only advocated for appropriate ethnic minorities	Need for skilled counsellors; difficult ethical problems involved
Sickle cell disease Sickle test	6 months	Penicillin prophylaxis		Cost effectiveness of programme dependent on ethnic population size. The service is not appropriate in all districts
Thalassaemia Haemoglobin analysis		Prenatal screening in subsequent pregnancies. Early institution of treatment		Screening should be seen as part of a wider programme of prevention diagnosis and care. Neonatal screening without adequate support facilities is not desirable
Growth monitoring *Failure to thrive* Weighing	Birth. All clinic visits 0–1 years and on request	Advice on management. Investigation of pathology. Care of children with psychosocial problems	Children with physical disease such as congenital heart disease need careful monitoring	Under-evaluated, but popular with parents. Sensitivity of detection of treatable disease poor. Special recommendations made about procedures and about the management of abnormal weight gain
Failure to grow* Height monitoring	3–5 years and 5 years	Investigation and early treatment	Growth in selected children needs monitoring more closely, e.g. coeliac disease	Value of measurement at all other ages uncertain. Specific recommendations about how measurement should be done, and about the management of the abnormal child
Abnormally large or small head** Head circumference measurement	2–10 days 6–8 weeks	Ultrasound and neuroradiological investigation		Optimum timing of second test uncertain. Specific instructions needed on how to manage abnormal cases. Potential for creating unnecessary anxiety among parents high
Vision *Congenital cataract* Red reflex	Birth	Surgery	None	–

*Treatable conditions include: growth hormone deficiency, hypothyroidism, Turner syndrome and psychosocial dwarfism.
**Treatable conditions include: hydrocephalus and subdural effusion.

Table 6.2 *Cont'd*

Condition and screening procedure	Age	Treatment for positives	Special groups	Comments
Other causes of partial sight and blindness Family history and observation	Birth and 6–8 weeks	Various	Children in families with genetically determined visual disorders, children with severe neurological handicap and preterm infants all need ophthalmological examination	Parents and professionals can detect this problem without a formal screening test. Each visit for child health surveillance should include an enquiry about visual ability and an inspection of eyes
Amblyopia Visual acuity testing, eg Snellen chart	5 years	Occlusion. Spectacle correction		Value of screening at younger ages still uncertain. Acuity testing at $3\frac{1}{2}$ years has a poor specificity and treatment is not universally successful. Photo refraction in infancy may be useful in future
Refractive error Snellen visual acuity chart	5 years 8 years 11 years 14 years	Spectacle correction	None	Referral criteria need to be carefully specified to cover prescription of spectacles
Colour vision Several different tests available	11 years	Career advice	Sex-linked condition. Screening could be limited to boys	Programme value needs researching
Hearing *Sensorineural hearing loss* Distraction test	7–9 months	Educational guidance, hearing aids, genetic advice	Children born to families with genetically determined hearing loss, those with a history of intrauterine infection or meningitis and those at risk because of neonatal problems need special attention	Inadequately performed this test is positively harmful. Parental suspicion must be taken seriously and parental awareness should be increased by use of aids, given at 6 weeks, eg check lists. Parents should be asked about hearing at all contacts. Test picks up more conductive hearing loss than sensorineural (40:1) but treatment unnecessary for most conductive losses at this age. Tests at older ages remain of uncertain value because of poor specificity of test. Uncertainty about long-term disability and possible adverse effects of treatment

been made to problems with these programmes several times in this chapter and the evidence that they do good is very incomplete.[4,15] However, many health professionals believe on clinical grounds that they are very important. It is to be hoped the effect of the working party's recommendations will be to stimulate proper trials of their effectiveness so that the debate about their benefits can be resolved.

Monitoring screening programmes

Screening programmes that have been shown to be effective in clinical trials are not necessarily so when they are introduced in routine practice. Problems like high social mobility, poor uptake of surveillance contacts, and high staff turnover can confound the most cost effective programme. The first two problems mean that the most socially deprived members of the community are likely to be omitted from the programme. Since disease and disability tend to be commoner among this group the prevalence of problems in the screened group will be reduced and the programme become less efficient. Staff turnover is a problem because most of the child health screening tests rely heavily on clinical skills and experience to achieve validity.

Two recently published studies on hearing screening in the first year of life illustrate these problems clearly.[16,17] In the first study population coverage by screening was less than 60%, and none of the three children with sensorineural hearing loss, presenting during the study period, were identified by screening. In the second study considerable effort had been put into health visitor training before the study; but, although the effectiveness of the programme improved, six out of the 12 children with sensorineural loss presenting during the study passed the screening test. However effective screening programmes appear to be in theory, it is therefore very important that they are routinely monitored. Monitoring takes time and consumes some resources, so it is important that a balance is struck between what could be done and what is appropriate and practical on a routine basis.

The basic monitoring package

This should be carried out in all districts every year and includes the following:

Programme coverage

The proportion of eligible children screened in the previous year. This information should be made available general practice by general practice and clinic by clinic.

Referral rate

The proportion of children referred to each of the different services at each surveillance contact. This should also be available as above.

Secondary monitoring

Every few years it is important to do some more time-consuming evaluation including:

False-positive referral rate

This requires collection of information on referrals to the relevant clinics and documentation of the outcome of the initial assessment. The information is less likely to be routinely available but can be gathered without too much difficulty.

Attendance rate for secondary assessment

The number of children who do not attend following referral to a specialist clinic for assessment is an important statistic.

Waiting time for secondary assessment

Waiting for assessment is a time of considerable anxiety for parents; if the screening programme and the secondary assessment and treatment services are properly coordinated it will be kept to a minimum. In practice, waiting times for assessment of some of the conditions detectable in child health may exceed 6 months, which is unacceptable.

Assessing the accuracy of the child health register

The accuracy of this register is fundamental to efficient screening. Children who no longer live at their registered address are not likely to respond to invitations for surveillance. Accuracy is also extremely important in assessing both coverage and referral rates. Accuracy can be checked by comparison with other population registers like those held by general practitioners and Family Health Service Authorities.

Tertiary monitoring

To assess the false-negative referral rate and the sensitivity and specificity of the programme, it is necessary to have a system for identifying children whose health problems were not found on screening. This requires the district to have a special needs or disability register which holds details of all children with problems regardless of how they presented. It is probably sufficient to undertake such in-depth analysis of the programme's effectiveness every 5 years.

The final stage in monitoring these programmes is assessment of the outcome of intervention. This form of monitoring is expensive, but should be carried out for all current screening programmes at national level. The British Paediatric Association (BPA) recommends a set of outcome measures for child health services to be used at local level.[18]

Feedback

Monitoring is essential but on its own it is not enough. It is vital that the results of the exercise are fed back to the people performing the screening tests and discussed with them. Most of the more disabling conditions detectable through child health surveillance are rare and are likely to be seen by most screeners less than once in a lifetime. It is therefore important that the results of the more in-depth studies, particularly of false-negative and false-positive referrals, are discussed locally. For rare conditions quality assurance will always depend on primary screeners learning from other people's failures.

Conclusions

Screening is a complex activity and the costs and benefits are not easy to assess. In clinical practice, where patients present asking for help with a problem, it is sometimes legitimate to try interventions or treatments which have been only partially evaluated on the grounds that they might do that individual some good. In screening programmes such an approach is unethical. In these programmes, parents who believe their children to be healthy are presented with the possibility that they might have a problem which they had not detected. If the screening programme cannot identify the health problem with a reasonable degree of accuracy, provide prompt diagnostic assessment, and offer an intervention which will significantly benefit most of the children and their families then the programme cannot be justified on ethical grounds. These criteria are the critical ones to consider in deciding whether a new programme should be introduced or an old one discontinued; they hold good whatever the cost of the test and however important it would seem to be to do something to minimize the disability and distress caused by health problems in childhood.

References

1 Bergman, A.B. Menace of mass screening. *Am J Pub Hlth* 1977; **67:** 601–602.
2 Wilson, J.M.G., Junger, G. Principles and practice of screening for disease. *Public Health Papers* 34. Geneva: World Health Organization, 1968.
3 Ministry of Education. *The Health of the School Child. Fifty Years of the School Health Service. Report of the Chief Medical Officer of the Ministry of Education for the years 1956–1957.* London: HMSO, 1958.
4 Hall, D.M.B. *Health for All Children: a Programme for Child Health Surveillance.* Oxford: Oxford Medical Publications, 1989.
5 Knox, E.G., Armstrong, E.H., Lancashire, R.J. Effectiveness of screening for congenital dislocation of the hip. *J Epidemiol Commun Hlth* 1987; **41:** 283–289.
6 Rose, G., Barker, D.J.P. Epidemiology for the uninitiated: screening. *Br Med J* 1978; **2:** 1417–1418.
7 McCormick, B. Hearing screening by health visitors: a critical appraisal of the distraction test. *Health Visitor* 1983: **56:** 449–451.
8 Sorenson, J.R., Levy, H.L., Mangione, T.W., Sepe, S.H. Parental response to repeat testing of infants with 'false positive' results in a newborn screening programme. *Pediatrics* 1984; **73:** 183–187.
9 Marteau, T. The psychological costs of screening. *Br Med J* 1989; **299:** 527.
10 Bergman, A.B., Stamm, S.J. The morbidity of non cardiac disease in school children. *New Engl J Med* 1968: **276:** 1008–1013.
11 Royal College of Physicians. *Prenatal Diagnosis and Screening: Community and Service Implications.* London: Royal College of Physicians, 1989.
12 Quine, L., Pahl, J. First diagnosis of severe handicap: a study of parental reactions. *Dev Med Child Neurol* 1987; **29:** 232–42.
13 McConachie, H., Lingham, S., Stiff, B., Holt, K.S. Giving assessment reports to parents. *Arch Dis Child* 1988; **63:** 209–10.
14 Springer, A., Steele, M.W. Effects of physician early counselling in rearing children with Down's syndrome. *Am J Mental Deficiency* 1986; **85:** 1–5.
15 Stewart-Brown, S.L. Preschool vision screening: a service in need of rationalization. *Arch Dis Child* 1988; **63:** 356–359.
16 Brown, J., Watson, E., Alberman, E. Screening for hearing loss. *Arch Dis Child* 1989; **64:** 1488–1495.
17 Scanlon, P.E., Bamford, J.M. Early identification of hearing loss: screening and surveillance methods. *Arch Dis Child* 1990; **65:** 479–485.
18 British Paediatric Association. *Outcome Measurements for Child Health.* London: BPA, 1990.

6.3 Surveillance programmes

Aidan Macfarlane

Introduction

The functions of the child health services are confused because clear definitions for the words used to describe these functions are lacking. The definitions in this section are those suggested by David Stone[1] which are the most useful devised so far.

Surveillance

Child health surveillance is the systematic and ongoing collection, analysis, and interpretation of indices of child health, growth and development in order to identify, investigate and, where appropriate correct deviations from predetermined norms. Surveillance may be of two kinds: *clinical surveillance*, which focuses on the individual child, and *population surveillance*, in which data are recorded on a group, community or entire population of children. Clinical surveillance enables an early diagnosis to be reached when an abnormality is identified, regardless of whether or not the abnormality is treatable, while population surveillance provides the database for the early formulation of a community diagnosis.

Monitoring

Monitoring is synonymous with surveillance.

Screening

Screening is not intended to be diagnostic, but is the presumptive identification of unrecognized disease or defects by the application of tests, examinations, and other procedures designed to facilitate early diagnosis followed by prompt and effective treatment.

Assessment

Assessment is the systematic, detailed, and multidisciplinary examination of the physical, emotional, and social health of a child with suspected or established disability or disadvantage.

The part that each of the two kinds of surveillance (which overlap to a certain degree) plays within the maintenance of children's health within a population is shown in Figure 6.3 where population surveillance modifies the child health services provided.

Clinical child health surveillance programmes

The part of clinical surveillance carried out by health professionals is usually done alongside a number of other activities, which include giving immunizations; giving a wide variety of advice on such subjects as family planning, feeding, safety and minor illnesses; assessment of risk factors for child development such as housing, history of child abuse, single unsupported parent, and educational background. These other activities do not in themselves represent any part of surveillance.

The term surveillance, as used in any common English form, can only represent the types of activity used in the definition above and it would greatly aid debate in the field if this was recognized.

Even defined in this way, health surveillance involves a large number of people – parents, teachers, childminders, playgroup leaders, nurses, doctors, relatives and neighbours – all of whom are involved to different degrees in different places, at different times and in different ways.

Though the term health surveillance seems appropriate for some of the observations done by parents as part of their routine day-to-day, hour-to-hour, minute-to-minute caring for a child, the term *clinical surveillance programme* does not. A health surveillance programme suggests a more formalized activity with

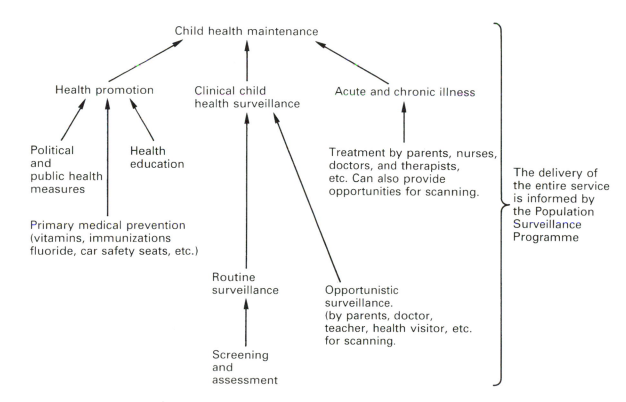

Figure 6.3 The role of clinical and population surveillance in child health maintenance.

specific aims, organized by health professionals but in some cases only partly carried out by them. Thus a programme might include parental observations via a questionnaire, or formalized training for teachers in recognition of certain problems. It would also include the concept of routine periodic health examinations by health professionals and encourage opportunistic screening when a child is seen by a doctor or nurse for some other problem, e.g. listening to the heart for congenital cardiac abnormalities when a child presents with ear trouble.

A review of the child health surveillance programmes from around the world indicates that concerns about the value of clinical child health surveillance are, if not universal, certainly widespread. Furthermore, the countries where there is no concern have often not looked critically at the value of what they are recommending. A further complication is that many countries who are looking critically at the theoretical value of surveillance are not then going on to examine the actual practice of surveillance (in terms of frequency, type of testing and method of carrying out the test) and what actually happens when a child is examined at their routine check (audit and quality control).

Looking at every clinical surveillance programme available would be an impossible exercise of little benefit. However, some of the present problems concerned with child health surveillance in the UK come from the British habit of ignoring research findings in general, and especially if the findings come from a country outside the UK – a ridiculously isolationist position in which it is assumed 'we know best' in the face of all facts.

International experience in the field is undoubtedly useful, there being many problems (but by no means all) which are universal to the periodic examination of any child whether the child lives in Sweden, England, Canada or China. The selection of countries chosen here is based mainly on the availability of literature and the personal contacts of the author. The range of different practices in the various countries examined is more likely to reflect the lack of sound research than differences in pathology in the child populations observed.

The UK

Much is written about the UK child health surveillance programme elsewhere in this book. The major step forward has been the publication of *Health for All Children: A Child Health Surveillance Programme* in 1989.[2] A brief outline of the recommended programme is given in Table 6.3.

Table 6.3 Summary of recommended screening procedures and assessments

Neonatal examination
- Review of family history, pregnancy and birth.
- Discuss any concerns expressed by the parents.
- Full physical examination, including weight and head circumference.
- Check for congenital dislocation of the hips.
- Check for testicular descent.
- Inspect eyes.
- Examine eyes for red reflex.
- If high risk of hearing defect – refer for further testing. Blood tests for phenylketonuria and hypothyroidism.

At discharge or within 10 days of birth
- Check for congenital dislocation of the hips again.

Six to 8 weeks
- Check history and ask about parental concerns.
- Physical examination, weight and head circumference.
- Check for congenital dislocation of the hips again.
- If status of testicular descent not known from birth information, or if not fully descended at birth – check again.
- Specifically enquire about parental concerns regarding hearing and vision.
- Inspect the eyes
- Consider giving parents a checklist or questionnaire for detection of hearing loss.

Seven to 9 months
- Enquire about parental concerns regarding health and development.

- Ask specifically about vision and hearing.
- Check weight if indicated or parents wish it.
- Check for congenital dislocation of the hips.
- Check testicular descent if testes not previously recorded as being fully down.
- Observe visual behaviour and look for squint.
- Carry out distraction test for hearing.

Eighteen to 24 months
- Enquire about parental concerns, particularly regarding behaviour, vision, and hearing.
- Confirm that the child is walking with a normal gait.
- Confirm that the child is beginning to say words and is understanding when spoken to.
- No formal testing of vision and hearing but arrange detailed assessment if there is any doubt about either being normal.

Thirty-six to 42 months
- Ask about vision, squint, hearing, behaviour and development.
- If any concerns, discuss with the parents whether the child is likely to have special educational needs and arrange further action as appropriate.
- Measure height and plot on centile chart.
- Check for testicular descent unless previously fully descended at birth.

The significance of this programme is:

1 that it covers some activities required from routine visits, as well as surveillance
2 that it is based upon available research evidence
3 that it provides a gold standard for professionals in the UK carrying out child health surveillance
4 that the recommendations were put together by a joint working party including nurses, paediatricians and general practitioners
5 that it is not seen as final but rather that it should develop as new evidence becomes available
6 that it recognizes the essential role played by parents.

The USA

The latest American recommendations for child health surveillance were put forward in 1988 by the Committee on Practice and Ambulatory Medicine of the American Academy of Pediatrics (AAP).[3] These recommendations serve as guidelines for general paediatricians carrying out the majority of office-based care, including preventive care, of children in the USA. There are 12 recommended routine visits between early infancy and 5 years of age and these are outlined in Figure 6.4.

The programme again nicely shows how some of the clinical surveillance procedures (e.g. vision and hearing testing, height and weight measurements) are combined with primary prevention procedures (e.g. immunizations and anticipatory guidance) at routine visits.

One of the most comprehensive recent reviews of this American child health surveillance programme was written by Professor Paul Dworkin, when comparing the American and English recommendations.[4] Much of his review concentrates on *developmental* surveillance, a term he uses to cover 'all the activities relating to the detection of developmental problems *and the promotion of development* during primary child care' (my italics). He goes on to suggest that developmental surveillance has a new emphasis, that of 'skilfully observing children and identifying parental concerns, rather than on administering tests. In contrast to screening at fixed ages, it is a flexible, continuous process, involving input from health professionals, parents, teachers, and others.'

He compares the English working party's recommendations concerning developmental surveillance, '. . . skilled health professionals, possessing a detailed knowledge of child development and an awareness of the various factors that may adversely affect it, observe children longitudinally during the course of child health care. Instead of developmental testing, emphasis is placed on eliciting and attending to parental concerns, making accurate and informative observations of children and obtaining a relevant developmental history.'[4] With the AAP recommendations 'development should be assessed by history and appropriate physical examination during the course of child health supervision.'[4] Both statements, he feels, are reconcilable if one accepts that in essence development is continually monitored within the context of the child's overall well-being, rather than viewed in isolation during a testing session. All encounters between the child and health professional are possible opportunities for such surveillance. During opportunistic surveillance observations of children's development and behaviour are not restricted to encounters during routine well-child visits but also are performed during visits for illness or other matters.

Sweden

More than any other country, Sweden has a long history both of having a detailed child health surveillance programme, and of researching its value. Although the reasons behind this are complex, two interlinked factors are outstanding. One is the presence in Sweden of the Nordic School of Public Health, and the other is its director Professor Lennart Kohler's long-standing interest in evaluating surveillance programmes. He has continuously highlighted the fact that although many programmes have been analysed in terms of their structure – who did what, and how much – almost no evaluation has been done in terms of outcome or result.

In Sweden, the formal programme, introduced in 1982, recommended examination by a physician at 2, 6, 10 and 18 months, and at 4 and $5\frac{1}{2}$ years. On average, each child in their first year is seen in child health clinics five times by a doctor and three times by a nurse. On top of this the nurse also makes three house calls. The types of screening examinations carried out are much the same as those in the UK: for phenylketonuria, galactosaemia and hypothyroidism at birth; congenital dislocation of the hip, vision, hearing, speech and general development at various intervals. Screening for anaemia and bacteriuria have been abandoned because anaemia is almost non-existent in Sweden (something the UK might like to examine) and because asymptomatic bacteriuria was no longer considered to be a threat.

In the mid-1970s, Sweden introduced a formal special health examination at 4 years of age. This age was chosen as a compromise between the need to identify handicaps early and the desire to use reliable and simple methods. On evaluation of the results of the new programme on long-term outcome, the conclusion was '. . . the measurable, direct impact of the screening on the health of the children is marginal. The programme seems to have contributed very little to the prevention of most problems, with the possible exception of visual screening and dental problems.' In

RECOMMENDATIONS FOR PREVENTIVE PEDIATRIC HEALTH CARE
Committee on Practice and Ambulatory Medicine

Each child and family is unique: therefore these Recommendations for Preventive Pediatric Health Care are designed for the care of children who are receiving competent parenting, have no manifestations of any important health problems, and are growing and developing in satisfactory fashion. Additional visits may become necessary if circumstances suggest variations from normal. These guidelines represent a consensus by the Committee on Practice and Ambulatory Medicine in consultation with membership of the American Academy of Pediatrics through the Chapter Presidents.

The Committee emphasizes the great importance of continuity of care in comprehensive health supervision and the need to avid fragmentation of care.

A prenatal visit by the parents for anticipatory guidance and pertinent medical history is strongly recommended.

Health supervision should begin with medical care of the newborn in the hospital.

	INFANCY						EARLY CHILDHOOD					LATE CHILDHOOD					ADOLESCENCE[1]			
AGE[2]	By 1 mo.	2 mos.	4 mos.	6 mos.	9 mos.	12 mos.	15 mos.	18 mos.	24 mos.	3 yrs.	4 yrs.	5 yrs.	6 yrs.	8 yrs.	10 yrs.	12 yrs.	14 yrs.	16 yrs.	18 yrs.	20+ yrs.
HISTORY Initial/Interval	•	•	•	•	•	•	•	•	•	•	•	•	•	•	•	•	•	•	•	•
MEASUREMENTS Height and Weight	•	•	•	•	•	•	•	•	•	•	•	•	•	•	•	•	•	•	•	•
Head Circumference	•	•	•	•	•	•														
Blood Pressure										•	•	•	•	•	•	•	•	•	•	•
SENSORY SCREENING Vision	S	S	S	S	S	S	S	S	S	S	O	O	O	O	S	O	O	S	O	O
Hearing	S	S	S	S	S	S	S	S	S	S	O	O	S3	S3	S3	O	S	S	O	S
DEVEL./BEHAV.[4] ASSESSMENT	•	•	•	•	•	•	•	•	•	•	•	•	•	•	•	•	•	•	•	•
PHYSICAL EXAMINATION[5]	•	•	•	•	•	•	•	•	•	•	•	•	•	•	•	•	•	•	•	•
PROCEDURES[6] Hered./Metabolic[7] Screening	•																			
Immunization[8]		•	•	•			•	•	•			•					•			
Tuberculin Test[9]	←	—	—	—	—	•	→	←	•	→	←	—	—	•	—	→	←	—	•	→
Hematocrit or Hemoglobin[10]	←	—	—	—	•	—	→	←	•	→	←	—	—	•	—	→	←	—	•	→
Urinalysis[11]	←	—	—	•	—	—	→	←	•	→	←	—	—	•	—	→	←	—	•	→
ANTICIPATORY[12] GUIDANCE	•	•	•	•	•	•	•	•	•	•	•	•	•	•	•	•	•	•	•	•
INITIAL DENTAL[13] REFERRAL										•										

1. Adolescent related issues (e.g., psychosocial, emotional, substance usage, and reproductive health) may necessitate more frequent health supervision.
2. If a child comes under care for the first time at any point on the schedule, or if any items are not accomplished at the suggested age, the schedule should be brought up to date at the earliest possible time.
3. At these points, history may suffice: if problem suggested, a standard testing method should be employed.
4. By history and appropriate physical examination: if suspicious, by specific objective developmental testing.
5. At each visit, a complete physical examination is essential, with infant totally unclothed, older child undressed and suitably draped.
6. These may be modified, depending upon entry point into schedule and individual need.
7. Metabolic screening (e.g., thyroid, PKU, galactosemia) should be done according to state law.
8. Schedule(s) per Report of Committee on Infectious Disease, *1986 Red Book.*

9. For low risk groups, the Committee on Infectious Diseases recommends the following options: ① no routine testing or ② testing at three times—infancy, preschool, and adolescence. For high risk groups, annual TB skin testing is recommended.
10. Present medical evidence suggests the need for reevaluation of the frequency and timing of hemoglobin or hematocrit tests. One determination is therefore suggested during each time period. Performance of additional tests is left to the individual practice experience.
11. Present medical evidence suggests the need for reevaluation of the frequency and timing of urinalyses. One determination is therefore suggested during each time period. Performance of additional tests is left to the individual practice experience.
12. Appropriate discussion and counselling should be an integral part of each visit for care.
13. Subsequent examinations as prescribed by dentist.
N.B.: Special chemical, immunologic, and endocrine testing are usually carried out upon specific indications. Testing other than newborn (e.g. inborn errors of metabolism, sickle disease, lead) are discretionary with the physician.

Key: • = to be performed: S = subjective, by history: O = objective, by a standard testing method.

September 1987

Figure 6.4 Recommendations for preventive paediatric health care. (Reproduced from American Academy of Pediatrics[3] by kind permission.)

reviewing the early detection and screening programmes for children in Sweden, Kohler concludes: 'After careful evaluation in admittedly limited areas and on selected populations, it is safe to conclude that only a few of the screening methods have been shown to fulfil the criteria of a proper screening test, i.e. with high sensitivity and specificity, detecting a decent number of cases where effective and efficient treatment is available. These tests usually belong to the area of physical health. The value of formal screening for mental, behavioural, linguistic or social development in small children has still not been convincingly proved and therefore tests have not generally been introduced. It is not reasonable or probable that the complicated biological and social background of developmental retardation should be easily revealed by simple questionnaires or tests. Nor is it realistic to expect that the findings at a very early age will predict with certainty problems later in childhood and adulthood, because this disregards the complex interplay between inherited tendencies and environmental influences and underestimates the adaptive capacities of the growing mind and body. However, pilot research studies in this field are being, and should be, undertaken.'[5]

Canada

The Canadian programme of child health surveillance is to give 5 routine checks in the first year, and a further four between the first and fifth years.[6] The programme is kept under review by the Canadian Task Force on Periodic Health Examination. This was established in 1976 to develop recommendations regarding the efficacy and effectiveness of preventive interventions based on a scientific review of medical literature.

The Task Force defined the routine periodic health examination 'as an early detection procedure in asymptomatic, ostensibly healthy persons; specifically a group of tasks undertaken to determine the risks of subsequent illness or to identify illness in its early symptomatic state. These tasks include history taking, physical examination and laboratory tests.'

The Canadian Task Force reporting in 1979 and 1989 reviewed the various components of the routine preschool examination and nicely highlighted the arguments that continue to surround the field due to lack of good research work. In 1979, they came to the conclusion that there was no justification for routine screening for visual defects among asymptomatic children, but that there was fair justification for doctors to actively identify children with hearing impairment.[7]

Reviewing this statement again in 1989, the Canadian Task Force, after a further literature review, suggested: there was fair evidence to include testing of visual acuity in the periodic health examinations of pre-school children; and there was insufficient evidence to recommend the inclusion or exclusion of screening for hearing impairment among pre-school children.[6]

In 1989, they had a clear opinion about developmental screening: '(1) There is good evidence to recommend the exclusion of the Denver Developmental Screening Test (DDST) from the periodic health examination of preschool children. (2) There is insufficient evidence to support either the inclusion or exclusion of other screening instruments. Caution is advised, however, since problems exist with all current assessment tools, and no interventions have been conclusively proven to be effective. Large-scale community programmes to prevent poor school performance in high-risk or disadvantaged groups have also given mixed and controversial results.'[6]

There is little or no mention by the Task Force of the role of parents within the Canadian child health surveillance programme. This omission probably reflects that consideration of the parental role was not included in the Task Force's brief.

The Netherlands

The Netherlands have undertaken a major review of their child health surveillance programme, questioning every aspect of their present provision. This provision is, compared with English standards, comprehensive. The programme, directed at children aged 0–7 years, was prepared by a joint national committee of state representatives, health professionals and parents in 1981. It includes, among the usual screening tests, a systematic longitudinal investigation of a child's development (revised Van Wiechen scheme) containing 37 items spread over seven sessions when the child is aged 0–15 months and a further 39 items spread over six sessions between 8 and 54 months.

The general opinion from the Dutch working party is that the scheme needs more evaluation and their review paper on the subject concludes: 'In general one pleads to make more use of information supplied by the child's parents in developmental surveillance. This would compensate the problem of method validity, as well as encourage the competence of the parents.'[8]

The Dutch working party is organized by Professor Micha de Winter of the Centrum voor Onderzoek en Ontwikkeling van Jeugdggezondheidszorg en jeughdhulpverlening, in Utrecht. He has a particular interest in the involvement of parents in surveillance programmes and observes, of the present changes of increasing parental involvement:

'This convergence of different interests resulted in what has been a shift from a "passive, expertocratic" health system towards an "active, democratic" one. The new images of clients, parents and professionals played an important role in this process. Parents could consider themselves responsible, competent citizens in spite of their increasing call for professional support, professionals could part with the negative image of self-interest and tutelage, and the government could support its health and population politics by pointing out the demands of the parties involved.

It would be too simple to analyse this development as a new and subtle control system. Parents and patients have gained something from it: they have become emancipated with respect to their own and their children's health. The question, however, is whether the concept of the responsible active parent will be as emancipating as it seems.

The parent as an active partner in the process of medicalization and professionalization is a concept which implies two paradoxical messages: you (parent and patient) are responsible for looking after your own child, but we (professional and the state) want to keep an eye on the way you do it.'[9]

New Zealand

In 1989 the Plunket Society in New Zealand was contracted by the government to take on overall national responsibility for child health surveillance.

The Plunket nurse visits the home regularly for 3 months after the birth of a child, according to the needs of the family (negotiated between the nurse and family) and in some places a positive emphasis is put on identifying 'priority families' on the basis of background factors including history of child abuse, prematurity, postnatal depression. Routine visits to child health clinics are at 6 weeks, 9 months, 18 months and 3 years. These are mainly strictly on appointment because of staff shortages. However, there has been a national movement towards having infrequent 'open clinics' where any parent can bring a child whom they feel concerned about. These clinics are staffed by dieticians, doctors, psychologists, speech therapists, nurses and others. They are well received and attended by parents but are seen as an expensive facility by management.

Routine distraction testing for hearing problems has been abandoned in favour of responding to parental concern about hearing difficulties. A recent survey of height, weight and head circumference norms has led to the development of new centile charts for New Zealand children. A specified percentage of the children measured were from the Maori population, but no separate centiles have been developed for this group.

Increasing emphasis has been put on parental participation in the programme and for the last 5 years parents have held their own health and development record given to them by the Plunket nurse on the visit to the home after the child's birth. Both GPs and hospitals have shown increasing use of the book.

(General acknowledgement: I am most grateful to Jenny Black, Senior Plunket nurse, for this information.)

Conclusions from review of international surveillance programmes

As already suggested, a comprehensive review of various child health surveillance programmes would be impossible. Nevertheless as more and more countries undertake major reviews of their child health services a gradual consensus appears to be emerging:

1 that there need to be clearly agreed definitions of certain key words which are regularly used and concerned with various activities carried on in the field of child health
2 that the term 'child health surveillance' should be used in the sense given at the beginning of this section
3 that clinical 'child health surveillance programmes' are usually embedded with other activities either at routine visits, or opportunistically at other times
4 that many child health surveillance activities need urgent review and a great deal of further research
5 that a very wide range of carers are involved in child health surveillance – the health professionals being only one variety
6 that the central role of parents is beginning to be recognized
7 that parents cannot always recognize health problems in their child at an early stage, and that they need to be supported in surveillance by other professionals
8 that overall child health surveillance serves a useful purpose, but this purpose needs better definition to ensure that the outcomes of the activity are improved by the processes involved.

Population child health surveillance programmes

The essential importance of a *population child health surveillance programme* is only just beginning to be realized. Yet it is basic to the provision of effective health services to a population. The recognition that in all countries at all times resources for health care will lag behind health needs as perceived by the population and the professionals, means that optimal distribution of resources must rest on a systematic approach to health problems in the community. Such a strategy contains a number of interlinked elements, each one reliant on the others.

1 The identification of the main medical problems of the population and an order of them in priority in terms of the mortality and morbidity that they cause.

2 The identification by research (which includes looking at all existing evidence as well as researching new intervention programmes) of effective interventions, whether these be political, social, educational, medical, environmental etc.

3 A decision on which programmes to put into place in the light of
   a) available resources
   b) priority of the health problem to be tackled
   c) the effectiveness of the intervention.

4 Monitored outcomes in terms of the health problems being tackled using the population health surveillance programme.

Unless the health problems within a population are monitored (in the case of this section a population of children), it is impossible to distribute efficiently the necessary resources to deal with the problems.

It is obvious that information concerning population surveillance can come from many different sources, not just clinical surveillance. Thus information about accidents, the single most common cause of death in children over the age of one year, might come from the police, accident and emergency departments, the county council safety officer, hospital admissions and surveys of homes etc.

A report by the Outcome Measures Working Group of the BPA Health Services Committee forms a good basis for the beginning of a population based child health surveillance programme.[10]

Their suggestions include:

1 For care of the newborn:
   mortality on the first day of life and neonatal mortality.

2 Screening for congenital impairments and developmental problems:
   congenital deafness
   congenital dislocation of the hip
   congenital hypothyroidism
   developmental problems
   notification of children with measles and pertussis
   immunization cover

3 Acute and chronic illness
   number of children admitted to hospital with asthma
   management of children with insulin dependent diabetes.

Concerning the specific health status of a population they recommend that each district health authority collect the following health status measurements:

1 Perinatal and infant mortality rates

2 Rates of low birthweight
3 Children less than the third centile for height on starting school
4 Deaths and hospital admissions of children due to road traffic accidents
5 Extent of fluoridation cover
6 Smoking in school children.

There are considerable problems with many of these outcomes. Some are measurements of health status, others, such as fluoridation of water supply, are interventions. Further, many of the outcomes measured are so rare that several years of cumulative data would need to be collected before any significant change in outcome would be recorded. Nevertheless the suggestions represent a move towards developing outcome measures that are valid.

However, a second reason for having total population surveillance is to identify individual cases that have been missed by the clinical surveillance system. These can then be reviewed and any factors that have resulted in the problem identified and rectified. For example, if a child with congenital dislocation of the hip is only identified when aged 9 months, then the case should be reviewed to see if the child had been through the normal screening programme, or had for good reason missed out on the routine checks. If the child had been checked, were the procedures carried out correctly? If they were then this provides further information concerning the overall false-negative rate of the screening test.

Auditing clinical and population surveillance

One further essential aspect of both clinical and population child health surveillance that has been sadly lacking both nationally and internationally is the question of audit. Again the term *audit* can mean different things to different people. In the sense used here it means a process of systematically looking at:

1 the resources needed to carry out surveillance
2 the processes involved in carrying out surveillance
3 the outcomes of surveillance
4 the feedback of information concerning resources, processes and outcomes to those responsible for the surveillance programmes.

It is this process of audit which allows the resources (equipment, staff, etc) continuously to be applied most effectively to achieve specified outcomes.

References

1 Stone, D. Terminology in community child health: an urgent need for consensus. *Arch Dis Child* 1990; **65**: 817–818.

2 Hall, D., ed. *Health for All Children: a Programme for Child Health Surveillance*. Oxford: Oxford Medical Publications, 1989.

3 American Academy of Pediatrics, Committee on Practice and Ambulatory Medicine. Recommendations for preventive pediatric health care. *Pediatrics* 1988; **81**: 466.

4 Dworkin, P.H. British and American recommendations for developmental monitoring: the role of surveillance. *Pediatrics* 1989; **84**: 1000–1010.

5 Kohler, L. Early detection and screening programmes for children in Sweden. In: MacFarlane, J.A., ed. *Progress in Child Health*. Vol 1. Edinburgh: Churchill Livingstone 1984, 230–242.

6 Canadian Task Force on Pediatric Health Examination 1989. Update 3: preschool examination for developmental, visual and hearing problems. *Can Med Assoc J* 1989; **141**: 1136–1140.

7 Canadian Task Force on Periodic Health Examination: The periodic examination. *Can Med Assoc J* 1979; **121**: 1193–1254.

8 Working paper 001 UK to Dutch working party on preventive child health care, 1991.

9 de Winter, M. Early detection of abnormality in Dutch children. In: MacFarlane, J.A., ed. *Progress in Child Health*. Vol 2. Edinburgh: Churchill Livingstone, 1985; 77–78.

10 Report of the outcome measures working group of the BPA Health Services Committee. Feb 1990. Available from the BPA, 5 St Andrews Place, London, NW1 4LB.

6.4 Children who may need special attention

Neil Marlow, Elizabeth Bryan and Alan Emond

Biological, genetic and environmental factors may conspire to place certain children at particular risk of neurodevelopmental and medical problems. Particular attention needs to be directed at the identification and prospective follow up of such children. This section deals with specific risks attributable to biological, perinatal and certain socioeconomic factors, and is followed by discussion of the risks found among ethnic minorities.

The low birthweight child

Over the past 20 years there have been dramatic improvements in survival for low birthweight children (LBW: <2500 g), particularly for very preterm (<30 weeks' gestation) or very low birthweight (VLBW: <1500 g) children, set against a background of falling overall perinatal mortality. Seventy per cent of neonatal mortality occurs in the VLBW group, who comprise 1% of total births. Morbidity among LBW children is high and comprises a range of neurodevelopmental and medical problems. Lower birthweights (<1250 g) are associated with particularly high frequencies of impairment and more complex disabilities.[1] Much of the morbidity among heavier LBW children may be accounted for by the action of subtle socioenvironmental influences,[2] and the birthweight itself may just be a marker for such problems. It is uncertain whether the same is true for major impairments or the excess of problems found among the lowest birthweight groups, who are at particular risk of brain injuries[3] and more subtle neurological influences such as the quality of nutrition[4] or hypoglycaemia.[5]

Most newborn nurseries provide a follow-up service for infants considered to be at high risk. That this is usually provided by hospital based services may pose problems for the transfer of children with impairments to the community team, and close liaison between the two is necessary. However, it is desirable that the hospital service provides surveillance for several reasons. Neonatal intensive care results in the disruption of the normal relationship between mother, child and the family. The dependence on psychological support given during a neonatal illness is valued highly by parents who frequently relish the continuity provided by subsequent contact. There are many areas in which health care professionals find difficulty in adapting practice for the VLBW group (e.g. immunizations, feeding, growth and development), which may confuse the parent further. Finally, the practice of neonatal medicine cannot be refined without long-term data on the effects of various neonatal interventions. Combined clinics with professionals from both hospital and community teams, although difficult to organize, may provide the best option.

Neurodevelopmental impairments in VLBW children

Major motor impairments

Approximately 5% of children with birthweights 1251–2000 g develop cerebral palsy and 30% of those <1250 g[1] or <28 weeks' gestation.[6] There is little evidence that the latter frequency has declined significantly over the last 5–10 years.[6] Spastic diplegia has long been associated with prematurity, but spastic quadriplegia and hemiplegia are found equally frequently among very low birthweight children. More complex disability with mental, visual or auditory impairment is found in handicapped extremely low birthweight (ELBW) children compared to LBW children with heavier birthweights[1] or other children with cerebral palsy.[7]

Motor impairment was initially ascribed to the perinatal occurrence of intraventricular haemorrhage. More recent evidence suggests that cortical lesions, usually in the region of the internal capsule, presenting as periventricular leucomalacia are better markers for later impairment,[8] with or without associated intraventricular haemorrhage. Such lesions may be detected using serial high resolution ultrasound scanning.

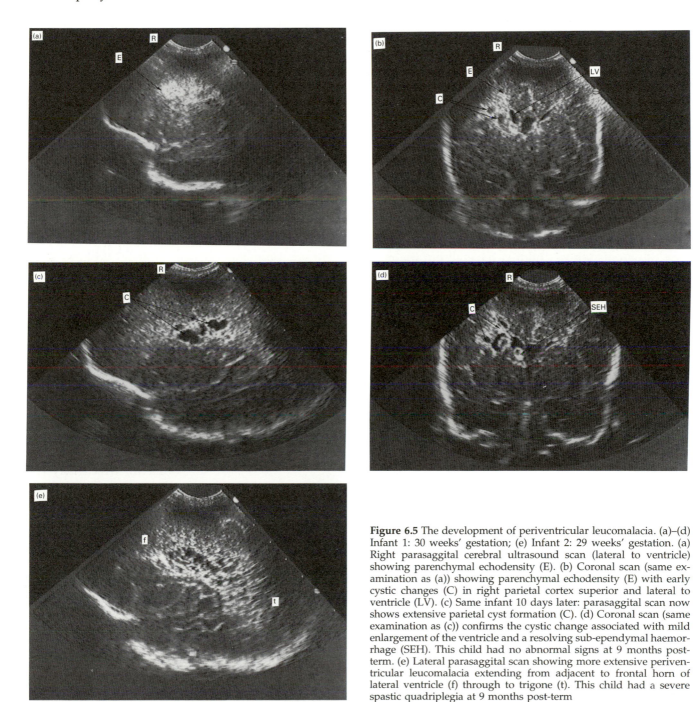

Figure 6.5 The development of periventricular leucomalacia. (a)–(d) Infant 1: 30 weeks' gestation; (e) Infant 2: 29 weeks' gestation. (a) Right parasaggital cerebral ultrasound scan (lateral to ventricle) showing parenchymal echodensity (E). (b) Coronal scan (same examination as (a)) showing parenchymal echodensity (E) with early cystic changes (C) in right parietal cortex superior and lateral to ventricle (LV). (c) Same infant 10 days later: parasaggital scan now shows extensive parietal cyst formation (C). (d) Coronal scan (same examination as (c)) confirms the cystic change associated with mild enlargement of the ventricle and a resolving sub-ependymal haemorrhage (SEH). This child had no abnormal signs at 9 months post-term. (e) Lateral parasaggital scan showing more extensive periventricular leucomalacia extending from adjacent to frontal horn of lateral ventricle (f) through to trigone (t). This child had a severe spastic quadriplegia at 9 months post-term

The aetiology of periventricular leucomalacia (PVL) is obscure. Hypotension, asphyxia and hypocarbia have all been implicated. Pathologically, it may represent an arterial ischaemic injury or a venous infarction. On ultrasound scanning, PVL appears initially as echodensities in the periventricular region (Fig. 6.5a and b). These may then regress to normal appearances or progress to form cysts which on occasions coalesce (Fig. 6.5c and d) to form what is termed a porencephalic cyst on later imaging in childhood. The normal multicystic appearances (Fig. 6.5e) may be confined to the frontal, parietal or occipital regions or be more extensive. With time these cysts are resorbed and the end result on scanning with CT in later childhood is often mild irregular ventricular enlargement.

Motor deficits are more common with the more posterior or more extensive lesions and may be associated with developmental impairment.[8] As yet the uncertainty over the outcome of particular areas of PVL precludes the association of other specific impairments with PVL.[6,9]

Prediction of the probability of major impairment from clinical or ultrasonographic data is relatively imprecise,[6,10] although in some studies it appears better.[9] The use of somatosensory evoked potentials has been found to be a better predictor.[11] However, such techniques are not widely available and the counselling of parents whose children have all but the most severe periventricular leucomalacia must remain imprecise. Close surveillance is thus necessary for all VLBW children and early referral for support and developmental therapy essential.

Visual impairment

Visual problems encountered among LBW children are especially common in the very preterm or VLBW child. Because of the high frequency and the urgency of intervention consequent on the critical period of visual development, close attention must be paid to visual function during surveillance.

Retinopathy of prematurity (ROP) is the best recognized aetiology and most neonatal units provide a screening service for preterm children to facilitate early identification and therapy if necessary. Serial eye examinations by an ophthalmologist, using indirect aspheric ophthalmoscopy, are made around 33–37 weeks' gestation to identify children with all degrees of retinopathy.[12] In most children, the changes of ROP regress with no discernible retinal sequelae. Such children may have a high frequency of later myopia.[13] In those with cicatricial ROP there is a risk of retinal detachment and blindness. Cryotherapy has been shown to be of benefit in these children and will be instigated by the ophthalmologist.

In North America, severe ROP occurs in approximately 10% of children with birthweights under 1000 g.[14] Data from Trent region suggest that cicatricial ROP with significant sequelae is less common in the UK.[15] When ROP was initially recognized 40 years ago, its occurrence was clearly related to the administration of oxygen and the population affected were heavier and more mature newborns. It is no longer certain that ROP is simply due to oxygen therapy[16] and many other factors, even hypoxaemia,[17] have been implicated. Attempts at prevention with high dose vitamin E therapy have been unsuccessful. Careful attention to arterial oxygen tension, close surveillance and early intervention remain the mainstay of current management.

Squints are found more frequently among preterm than term children.[18] Squints may be related to mild cases of ROP with refractive errors, injuries to the optic tracts as part of periventricular leucomalacia or hydrocephalus, or damage to the occipital cortex (central visual loss). Early referral for ophthalmic assessment is necessary.

Auditory impairments

Later *sensorineural hearing loss* may be found in about 2% of babies weighing less than 1000 g at birth,[19] and with decreasing frequency in heavier LBW children. The aetiology remains obscure. Bilirubin-induced neural injury, hypoxic-ischaemic injury secondary to recurrent postnatal apnoea, aminoglycosides, frusemide, incubator noise and even direct middle ear involvement in intraventricular haemorrhage have been postulated.[1] All infants are managed to minimize the risk from these areas. Aminoglycosides and frusemide remain in use because of their clinical efficacy, although aminoglycoside levels must be frequently monitored and the simultaneous administration of frusemide should be avoided.

The developing preterm child may be particularly vulnerable to *secretory otitis media*, for reasons that are obscure. The observation from one study that verbal skills were particularly associated with poor school performance[20] would suggest that early intervention for such chidren may have important long-term implications.

Some units provide screening for hearing impairment in VLBW or very preterm babies prior to discharge, using brainstem auditory evoked responses (BAER), or more recently click evoked acoustic emissions[21] or an acoustic cradle.[22] Hearing assessment, nonetheless, must form an integral part of surveillance and early recourse to BAER is recommended when there is doubt. At later examinations impedance audiometry may be of value in the assessment of impairment from glue ear.

Post-haemorrhagic hydrocephalus

Hydrocephalus may complicate recovery from intraventricular haemorrhage. Although this usually presents during the initial hospitalization, delayed presentation after a period of 'arrest' may occur. The outcome for children with shunted hydrocephalus primarily depends upon the presence and results of any cortical injury, rather than the hydrocephalus per se.[23]

Other neurodevelopmental impairments

In addition to major motor and sensory impairments, the VLBW child may exhibit other less disabling but nonetheless problematic impairments. Over the first postnatal year up to 25% VLBW[24] or preterm (<35 weeks' gestation[25]) children may develop transient neurological abnormalities (transient dystonia). Although such children do not go on to develop cerebral palsy there may be early confusion. Transient dystonia is a marker for learning impairments at school age[24,26] and such children are frequently considered as overactive, distractible or inattentive over the second and third postnatal years.[24] As to whether this comprises a true attention deficit disorder[27] or an expression of intermediate degrees of impairment awaits confirmation.

The pre-school VLBW child may be regarded as clumsy, with poor scores on formal motor testing in early school age.[28] These motor scores may be predictive of later schooling difficulties[3] despite IQ scores which are in the normal range, once those with major motor and sensory impairments are excluded. Reviewing the pattern of school problems among various studies reveals no particular association with VLBW, emphasis being on motor,[28] verbal[20] or visuospatial problems[29] depending on the study concerned. In one cohort[3] of very low birthweight (less than 1251 g) infants only 50% of 8 year olds were performing well at school compared with 80% of controls. Furthermore, 30% of the VLBW group were failing in two or three of the three main scholastic areas. These data are similar to those reported from the USA and confirm the high risk nature of this population.

The neurological maturity of VLBW children lags behind that of term children. An excess of minor neurological signs are observed[30] which are independent of maturity and perinatal course[28] and may cloud the assessment of fine motor skills and developmental testing. Many studies assess behaviour in VLBW children and record differences compared with controls, most of which are related to those areas already mentioned. The VLBW child additionally is more likely to be anxious, a trait which may reflect parental anxiety that they may have a particularly 'vulnerable' child.

Despite this recorded morbidity, the majority of VLBW or preterm children do not have significant sequelae ascribable to perinatal problems.

Respiratory morbidity

Approximately 5–6% of *ventilated* preterm children remain oxygen dependent at term with chronic lung disease or bronchopulmonary dysplasia (BPD). The frequency is highest at lowest gestations. After discharge many of these children will require continuing domiciliary oxygen and close medical support. Ongoing therapy with diuretics and aminophylline may need to be supplemented with bronchodilators.

Children with BPD are at great risk of developing life-threatening episodes of respiratory failure, secondarily to intercurrent infections, and prompt use of antibiotics with early referral for specialist care is usually recommended. Close cooperation between the neonatal and the community teams is necessary to ensure coordinated multidisciplinary support for the family. Many children with chronic lung disease will have associated neurodevelopmental impairments. Attention to nutrition, parental support and immunization are thus particularly important for this group.

The frequency of rehospitalization with respiratory symptoms is highest in this group over the first two postnatal years and many will go on to develop reversible airways disease, although it seems that such children have more frequent family histories of asthma. Despite this most children with bronchopulmonary dysplasia recover well and appear to grow out of their symptoms by early school age, although respiratory function tests continue to show abnormalities.[31] There are no long-term data concerning adult outcome.

In contrast children who have had respiratory distress syndrome seem in the main to make a full recovery with normal school age lung function in the majority of survivors.[32]

Immunization

Preterm infants should receive their first immunization 2 months after birth, irrespective of the degree of prematurity.[33] Generally the same cautions apply as do for term infants, and the occurrence of cerebral injuries should not encourage delay or non-immunization against pertussis. Indeed for the child who has chronic lung disease it is imperative that full immunization be completed as soon as possible, in light of the dangers associated with intercurrent infection during infancy.

Children who were small for gestational age

It is widely held that small for gestational age (SGA) children have an impaired neurodevelopmental outcome. Careful reviews of the literature, however, fail to produce consistent findings for the group of children whose birthweight lies below the 10th centile for their gestational age, although there may be differences in outcome for preterm SGA and term SGA children. Reviews of preterm SGA children reveal conflicting results in contrast to term SGA children who have been observed to have poorer long-term outcomes than controls in terms of behaviour, intellectual and school outcomes.[34,35] The contribution of socioenvironmental factors to these outcomes may outweigh that of the growth retardation itself.[36]

Within the SGA group there is an excess of children with a spectrum of minor dysmorphic features who appear to be at risk of impaired outcome.[24,37] Children whose growth is severely compromised (<3rd centile[1]) and children whose head growth retardation has its onset before 26 weeks[38,39] may have impaired growth and intellectual outcome. Delivery upon recognition of poor growth may be associated with better outcome than allowing the pregnancy to continue to term[40] and short-term neonatal morbidity is worse if intrauterine growth retardation progresses to be associated with abnormal fetal umbilical blood flow velocity or abnormalities of biophysical profile.

However, 10% of normal children will have birthweights below the 10th centile and many other external factors may influence birthweight but not necessarily outcome (e.g. multiple pregnancy, maternal height). The effect of growth retardation is not an 'all-or-none' phenomenon and it is not surprising that the choice of an arbitrary definition, such as the 10th centile, produces conflicting results. Consideration of the integral between birthweight and gestation as a continuous variable and weighting this by known influences, such as parity, parental size and sibship size, may lead to a clearer picture.

Children who have neonatal seizures

In contrast to older children, the newborn infant is frequently observed to have seizures, which may be as common as 3% of neonatal ICU admissions.[41] Such seizures must be regarded as symptoms of an underlying disturbance, the cause of which should be sought. The prognosis for these children is dependent upon the aetiology rather than the seizures themselves, although the duration of seizures may be an important variable.[42,43] The outcomes studied have been mainly severe impairments. Prognosis varies between excellent for those children with neonatal hypocalcaemia or promptly treated hypoglycaemia, to poor for those where seizures are associated with hypoxic-ischaemic encephalopathy or underlying CNS malformations. For the whole group, normal survival may vary from 47% for term infants with seizures to only 15% for very low birthweight children.[43]

Children with perinatal asphyxia

Children may make astonishing recoveries after severe perinatal asphyxia,[44] but generally moderate and severe perinatal asphyxia are associated with significant neurodevelopmental impairment. Clinical staging of such children has proved most useful in predicting outcome,[45–47] in contrast to biochemical markers or physiological measures, such as Apgar scores. Children with grade 1 (mild) encephalopathy, who exhibit irritability, hypertonus and wakefulness in the immediate postnatal period, tend to settle quickly and long-term sequelae are unusual. Children with grade 3 (severe) encephalopathy, who are comatose, needing ventilatory support and often with intractable seizures, have a high mortality and most long-term survivors have major neuromotor impairment. Children with the intermediate grade 2 encephalopathy have less certain outcomes. A significant proportion will have later major impairment and among the remainder scores on cognitive testing may be significantly reduced,[48] implying a spectrum of affectation. The presence of neonatal seizures which are difficult to control is usually regarded as an ominous sign, although discrete and infrequent seizures are not uncommon, and probably not associated with significant long-term impairment.

Twins

Approximately one in 50 children born in the UK is one of a multiple birth. In the UK, the proportion of twin births fell from about 1 in 80 maternities in the early 1950s to about 1 in 100 in 1980. The twinning rate is now rising again and a much more rapid rise has been seen among higher order births.[49] The number of triplets has doubled in the last 10 years, due to the increasing use of new techniques to assist reproduction.

Twinning rates vary greatly in different ethnic groups due wholly to variations in dizygotic (DZ) twinning, although the monozygotic (MZ) twinning rates remain at 3–4 per 1000 maternities worldwide. The highest rates of DZ twins are found among black Africans and the lowest among East Asians. Caucasians and Asian Indians lie between. Among Caucasians approximately one-third of twins are MZ and two-thirds DZ.

Twins tend to be disadvantaged in many ways. The incidence of twinning increases with parity so they are likely to be born into large families and the known disadvantages of close sibling spacing are compounded by having a sibling of the same age.

One-third of twins are born preterm and half are of low birthweight (<2500 g). Poor intrauterine growth is frequently observed – the average birthweight of a twin infant being nearly 1000 g less than that of a singleton.[50] Marked intrapair discrepancies in birthweight are not uncommon particularly in monozygotic pairs. There are also intrauterine hazards peculiar to twins[51] such as the feto–fetal transfusion syndrome.

Sudden infant death syndrome

About twice as many twins as singletons die unexpectedly in infancy.[52,53] This higher incidence may be partly due to prematurity/low birthweight but twinship as such appears to be a factor, possibly only twins under 2500 g.[54] DZ pairs appear at similar risk to MZ and both groups have an unexpectedly high concordancy rate. One study found that both babies died within days of each other in 8% of cases.[55] The risk to the second baby is increased for about one month but the greatest risk is during the first 4 days. It is therefore recommended that the survivor should be admitted to hospital immediately for observation.[56]

Emotional factors

Parents of twins need particular understanding. Few are prepared for the emotional in addition to the practical and financial stresses involved in caring for two babies at once. Relating to two babies at the same time can be difficult at first and this may delay the development of a close mother–infant relationship with one or both of the twins. This may be further delayed if the mother is unable to tell the babies apart or if one baby proves more attractive to her than the other.

Mothers are more likely to have a strong preference for one baby if they are of very different size at birth,[57] most mothers favouring the larger baby. Mothers find dividing their attention difficult if one baby is more demanding than the other. They feel guilty that they are unable to give their twins equal attention and frustrated that they can so rarely just quietly enjoy giving undivided attention to one baby.

Identity and individuality

Although most parents intend to treat their children as individuals there are enormous social pressures to dress them alike and therefore make them harder to distinguish. This must inhibit individual development. Moreover, once a pattern of similar dressing is established, it can be very difficult to break. Clothes of the same style but different colours seem to be a useful compromise. Different hairstyles can make a remarkable difference.

Even MZ twins may have very different personalities and these differences should be respected. The constant drawing of comparisons and contrasts however should be avoided as these can lead to a reinforcement and exacerbation of what may start as only slight differences in character.

Language

It has long been recognized that twins are slower in their language development than singletons. Many children whose overall intelligence is normal will have significant deficit in their verbal performance.[58–61] Twins have to develop a complicated form of interaction – triadic communication. Their mothers are also likely to talk less to them, to use shorter sentences and to offer fewer explanations.[62,63] Mittler[64] studied 200 4-year-old twins and found that they were on average 6 months behind in language development. Performance was influenced neither by zygosity nor birth order. In the nine subtests, twins performed less well in all with the exception of the one concerned with the speed of reaction to speech. Constant competition may have led to the more rapid development of this particular skill.

The main model for speech for twins is also different. A single child's model is usually their mother or at least someone who speaks better than themselves. The person a twin communicates most with is someone who talks as badly as they do – their twin. Thus speech is likely to be immature and deviations from the normal will often be reinforced by their twin. This is probably the origin of the twin language phenomenon, known as cryptophasia or idioglossia. This is quite common among twins, probably in the order of 40%.[65] As long as normal speech is developing at the same time it is probably harmless.

Speech delay in twins is neither inevitable nor irremediable and parents should be made aware of this as another important reason for having time alone with each child from the start.

Discipline

Many parents have been surprised by the difficulty they encounter in disciplining twins compared with previous single children. There are probably a number of reasons for this difference. A child responds to discipline because he wants the respect and love of the person who is exerting it. If the respect of his twin, however, is to be gained by continuing with the misdemeanour, it is no surprise that greater parental pressure is needed to get the same effect. Misdemeanours may also be more extreme because one child will goad the other child on way beyond the limits that a child on its own would normally risk or have the perseverance for.

Mental development

Earlier studies have shown that twins tend to have a level of intelligence a few points lower than singletons. However, more recent studies have shown that this deficit is reduced, or has disappeared, by late childhood.[66] Furthermore, when allowance is made for close sibling spacing the difference is anyway reduced.[66]

Few studies have differentiated between MZ and DZ twins but it appears that not only are MZ more alike in their mental development than DZ but that they tend to have their spurts and lags in parallel.[67]

Since mental and physical disability are more common among twins than single children, it is not unusual to find pairs with one disabled and one normal child. Such families need support not only in coping with the disabled child but with the reactions of the healthy twin who often suffers profound guilt and even jealousy.[68]

Starting school

Twins often settle into school more easily than single children. They have the reassurance of having their twin with them, even though separated from their mother. However to encourage the twins' long-term independence of each other, most authorities recommend that the twins should be in separate classes at least by secondary school.

The timing of the separation should depend on both the children themselves and on the facilities available. But if it appears that a child is not performing to his or her full potential then the separation may need to take place sooner rather than later.

The many advantages of separation include the chance for the child to be thought of as an individual without comparisons, the chance to have privacy without a brother or sister telling tales at home.

A child who is being dominated by his twin may unexpectedly blossom when separated. Some twins strive to perform similarly and this may actually hold back the more able child. In other pairs, the less able twin may be discouraged and opt out altogether and stop trying.

In a mixed sex pair, the girl will tend to develop faster in the early school years and may start mothering her twin brother. The boy may need to be separated in order to find his own strengths.

Finally twins may need separating for the sake of the rest of the class. Such a powerful (and sometimes conspiratorial) unit can have a very disruptive effect on the other children, particularly if the teacher is unable to tell who is who.

Social deprivation

Although increasing standards of living during this century have been associated with a reduction in childhood mortality rates, poverty, overcrowding and poor housing remain important factors prejudicing children's health in the 1990s. The Black Report[69] confirmed that rates of perinatal, neonatal and infant mortality are still considerably higher in children of manual workers than among those of professionals. There is no evidence[70] of any narrowing of the social class differences in childhood mortality and morbidity.

Children from economically deprived families have higher rates of chronic illness, respiratory infections, hearing loss, nutritional and growth problems and accidents. Socioeconomic status has consistently been shown to be the single most important factor in determining a child's developmental attainments.[71] Poverty affects children not just in material terms, such as diet, housing, play facilities but also in terms of the quality of their emotional environment, for example their mothers are more likely to be depressed.

Children from large families are particularly vulnerable to the effects of socioeconomic deprivation; they consistently underachieve compared to their peers[72] and are more likely to show disturbed behaviour.[73] In an impoverished large family, material and personal resources are more thinly spread, resulting in a poor quality home environment and little parental time for individual children. Clinicians need to be aware of the ways in which children of different ages in a family are vulnerable. The infant may fail to thrive, while the toddler shows language delay and the school child has behaviour problems. To improve the health and help fulfil the developmental potential of socially deprived children, doctors and health visitors are required to utilize a range of strategies – health promotion, primary and secondary prevention, and treatment – and also be prepared to act as the child's advocate if required, to improve his environment and facilitate access to health and social services.

Other groups of children whose health, growth and development are particularly susceptible to the effects of social deprivation may require increased surveillance and support from health workers. These include: children born to first-time parents, children from one-parent families, and children in homeless or traveller families.

First-born children

Few couples realize what is ahead of them when their first child is born: no amount of information from books, TV and videos, or advice from professionals, friends and relatives can be a substitute for the experience of looking after a child 24 hours a day. In a society based on small, nuclear families it is unusual for a young adult to have acquired the necessary practical experience of childcare within their own family of origin. However, although first-born children may be vulnerable because of their parents' inexperience or immaturity, they also have a developmental advantage by being first.

First-borns receive greater adult attention and more varied stimulation than is possible when there are several young children in the family.[74] Observational research has shown that first-borns receive more verbal, social and object stimulation from the care giver.[75] Second and subsequent children suffer from relative developmental impoverishment, due to a progressive decrease in parental attention, and an increased reliance on immature siblings for their social interaction as families grow larger.[76] Studies have repeatedly shown that first-born and only children obtain higher scores on measures of intelligence than do later born children. These effects are also found in economically disadvantaged children,[77] in whom the provision of intensive pre-school education does not override the effect of birth order. The increased parental attention given to first-born children results in better verbal skills, particularly vocabulary, so that verbal tests are more likely to affect birth order differences than non-verbal tests. However, although birth order has been shown to have the effect of reducing IQ by one point for each birth within the family,[76] within a population these effects account for less than 2% of overall IQ variation.[78]

In spite of this advantage, some first-born children may need special attention because of inexperienced or poor parenting. The first child of young parents may be vulnerable because of the parents' shortage of experience, lack of role models and poor understanding of children's needs. Young parents may still be growing up themselves and may find it difficult to place the child's needs before their own. A young couple will have to come to terms with their change of status as the arrival of the first baby inevitably stresses the relationship between the adults. In addition, if a young mother has moved away from her own family, she may be isolated from her support at the time she needs it most. All these problems are particularly difficult for single parents from socially deprived backgrounds.

First-born babies were found in the British Child Health and Education Study[79] to be more likely to have feeding and sleeping problems, to be perceived to cry more frequently, and to have more reported temper tantrums. Parents' anxiety and concern about their first-born resulted in an increased reporting of minor somatic symptoms (e.g. stomach ache). First-borns are also more likely to be subject to child abuse and neglect, and are vulnerable to nutritional problems and failure to thrive.

All health professionals need to understand the particular problems of first-time parents, spend time with parents discussing their concerns, and provide appropriate health promotion (e.g. nutrition, accident prevention). Parenting skills are more likely to be encouraged by an approach based on partnership with the parents rather than that of an expert giving instructions.

The philosophy of empowerment of parents is behind the Child Development Programme (CDP),[80] which aims to improve parenting skills in first-time mothers by modifying health visiting practice. The First Parent CDP visitors use a structured programme of home visiting to encourage parental skills and awareness of preventative health care, and early development. It is now in use in many districts in England and Wales and claims to improve immunization rates and uptake of surveillance services, to reduce hospital admissions and to provide parents with the skills and confidence to promote their child's development. It remains to be seen whether targeted initiatives such as the Child Development Programme will result in a reduction in the need for costly interventions for child abuse and neglect, behavioural problems and educational failure in vulnerable first-born children.

Single-parent families

The number of one-parent families has been steadily increasing over the last 20 years, and it is estimated that one in six children in the UK are now brought up by one parent. The majority (85%) of such families are headed by women, with contact from the child's father varying from a regular visiting relationship to none at all. One-parent families are formed in a number of ways – the majority through separation or divorce, an increasing minority from single motherhood (whether planned or unplanned), and a few through death of a partner.

It is possible to meet a child's physical, emotional and developmental needs within a one-parent family, and successful families often have the support of one or more strong adult figures (e.g. grandparent). A detailed developmental study in New York[81] found that the presence in the child's life of such an adult figure was the strongest predictor of successful adaptation and behavioural and developmental maturation. Unfortunately, children in one-parent families do not always have the consistent presence of such an adult, and must look to a lone mother to provide for their needs while struggling to meet her own.

Children in one-parent families are often brought up in relative economic deprivation, in poor housing, by a stressed and emotionally unsupported parent. Poverty is an important factor restricting a child's potential and a large number of single parents and their children live close to the poverty line. As many as 85% of divorced women claim benefits at some time, and over 60% of all single parents need income support from the state. Many single parents would rather work than live on state benefits, but are hampered by the lack of suitable day care and nursery provision at a realistic cost. The 1983 Family Expenditure Survey revealed that the average income of one-parent families had fallen over the previous few years, and this poverty trap has been exacerbated in the late 1980s by changes in benefit regulations and the freezing of child benefit. Recent initiatives by the British government to force absent fathers to pay maintenance for their children will not alleviate this poverty, as any money paid over to the mother will be deducted from her benefits.

The effects of poverty on a child's health and development are undisputed. Socioeconomic status remains the most important influence on almost all measures of health in children and adults,[81] and also has a strong effect on child development. The effects of economic deprivation are greatest on language development, and least on motor development,[81,82] but are also strongly associated with behavioural problems.[73]

One-parent families are more likely than two-parent families to live in poor housing or in overcrowded conditions shared with relatives or friends. The crisis in rented accommodation in the UK has resulted in many single-parent families being placed in unsuitable bed and breakfast accommodation in hotels, with severe consequences for the health, development and behaviour of the children.[83] Children living in temporary accommodation have difficulty accessing primary care, preventative and surveillance services, are more vulnerable to accidents, and are more likely to be admitted to hospital. When rehoused, one-parent families often have little choice but to accept accommodation far from friends and relatives and the resulting isolation may contribute to maternal depression and emotional and social deprivation for the children.

Looking after young children is demanding and hard work; the stresses on both parent and child are increased in one-parent families. The incidence of depression among single mothers is high[84] and emotional problems in parents are reflected in emotional and behavioural problems in children. The Child Health and Education Study[79] found that children from young single parents performed below average on language tests and were more likely to have behaviour problems at 5 years old. Many studies have shown relationships between stress (adverse life events) and adult ill health, and single parents often have higher malaise scores and more somatic symptoms than couples. Morbidity in childhood is also related to family stress, through a reduction in maternal coping ability and a difficulty in meeting the child's needs.[85,86]

Single parents are particularly vulnerable to adverse life events, which on top of chronic economic difficulties and lack of support can result in family break-up and the children being taken into care. Such a failure is rarely due to lack of maternal love or commitment and professionals working with single parents must be sensitive to the pressures on these families and be careful not to make hasty judgements.

In spite of the dramatic changes in family structure over the last 20 years, British society remains centred around the two-parent family. The advantages of a stable family with two parents are that the child is provided with two positive role models, that the parents can share tasks and support each other, and that it is easier for the parents to earn an adequate income and run a household. However, the two-parent nuclear family is not the only model to provide the necessary love and security and stimulating environment for children to thrive physically and emotionally. Children need a range of different adult caretakers to meet their needs, and benefit from strong relationships with adults (e.g. grandparents) outside the immediate family. These conditions can be provided in the context of a one-parent family, but such children may need special attention and priority for day care and nursery places to ensure that they are not disadvantaged.

Travellers

Travellers are a heterogeneous group of families who share a nomadic way of life, but there are marked differences in culture and income between different traveller groups, e.g. Irish, Scots, Romany, New Age travellers. These different groups have a common difficulty in gaining access to health care, and a flexible approach is required to provide health surveillance to children from these mobile families.

There are at least 12 000 traveller caravans in Britain[87] containing more than 20 000 children under 16 years. Less than half the families in Britain are living on official sites, the majority living illegally and in fear of eviction and suffering hostility from the settled population. Many studies have shown that the health of families is poor, partly due to the poor facilities and environmental conditions of the sites, but also due to low uptake of preventative health services.[88] Lack of toilets, hot and cold running water, electricity and regular rubbish collection results in an increased risk of waterborne and gastrointestinal infections, chronic infestations and other infectious diseases.[89] Immunization rates in children and adults are low, and outbreaks of polio, pertussis, measles and hepatitis have been reported.[90] Children who live on both official and unofficial sites have an increased rate, and follow up of injuries treated in accident and emergency departments is problematic, resulting in unnecessary complications.

Lack of access to pre-school surveillance results in treatable impairments (e.g. hearing loss) not being identified, with subsequent disability and learning difficulties.

Frequent changes of school may result in little surveillance from the school health service, so that potential problems are not identified or treated. Levels of literacy and numeracy are low among many travellers, and children with learning difficulties may not be identified and are unlikely to receive the help they need.

The GP contract, setting targets for uptake of preventative measures such as immunization and cervical cytology, does not encourage GPs to register travellers and mobile families. In addition, some practices will not take travellers onto their list as the doctors do not wish to, or cannot, provide a full range of general medical services including home visits on site. Mothers and children subsequently often use accident and emergency departments for primary care. Moreover, even if travellers are seen by primary care teams, delivering effective treatment and arranging referral is problematic as travellers have difficulty in keeping appointments. Continuing surveillance and follow up of non-urgent conditions is often impossible.

The health of travellers would be improved by the provision of permanent sites across the country, but current public attitudes make this unlikely. In the mean time, if the health of traveller children is to be improved, access to surveillance clinics must be facilitated and appropriate screening and preventative measures supplied with culturally sensitive health promotion. Reports from the King's Fund,[91] Save the Children Fund[92] and Maternity Alliance,[93] recommend that health authorities have a coordinator to liaise with travellers, local authorities, family health service authorities and general practitioners, to encourage families to register with GPs and use health and social services.

Many districts now have a nominated health visitor for traveller families, and some provide a mobile clinic facility.[94] The introduction of parent-held records has improved the continuity and documentation of both primary and secondary health care, and will encourage the necessary opportunistic approach to immunization and surveillance.

The way forward in improving child health for travellers must commence with improving access to antenatal and maternity services, to identify high-risk pregnancies and promote maternal and infant health.[93] In the neonatal period, good communication is required between hospital staff, community midwives and health visitors to give good quality care to mothers and babies in the community. Professionals involved in assessment of the infant must be aware of the increased risk, through intermarriage, of congenital malformations and recessive conditions. Where screening is possible (e.g. phenylketonuria) active follow up is needed to ensure that babies do not slip through the net.[95]

Promotion of breast feeding should be encouraged to improve infant nutrition and reduce gastrointestinal infections. However, many travellers are resistant to breast feeding, and to achieve these ends it will also be necessary to ensure water purity and improved standards of hygiene with formula feeding.

A very positive approach to immunization is necessary to overcome lack of awareness of its benefits, and a cultural prejudice towards immunization among travellers. In most districts BCG is recommended in the neonatal period, and the introduction of an accelerated schedule will facilitate the completion of the primary course of immunization in mobile families. It may be necessary to immunize parents at the same time as their children, particularly with oral polio vaccine.

Most pre-school surveillance will have to be opportunistic, with appropriate positive advice about accident prevention and health promotion. The identification of hearing loss is particularly difficult in travellers' children as it is often not possible to undertake distraction testing on site, and mothers and children will have to attend clinics at an appropriate time. Positive action will be necessary to ensure follow up and treatment of children with hearing problems. Whenever and wherever young children are brought to health services, special attention should be given to growth and nutritional status, dental health, developmental assessment and the identification of chronic problems such as asthma and glue ear.[96]

For school-age children, collaboration and good communication between community health services and education authorities is necessary for effective health surveillance and the identification of special educational needs. By moving around, travellers' children have enough problems learning to read and write without being further disadvantaged by their special needs being neglected. The recognition and treatment of sensory impairments and the management of disorders of growth and development require positive action from education authorities and school health services. Given the high incidence of infectious diseases among travellers, it is particularly important to ensure that young women are rubella immune by immunizing pre-pubertal girls against rubella.

Travellers have different cultural perceptions of health and illness from most health workers,[97] and to be effective primary care professionals and paediatricians need to approach travellers with a respect for and understanding of their lifestyle, culture and beliefs about health. However, the recognition of the special needs of travellers must not merely label and increase discrimination but result in imaginative positive action to ensure that their children enjoy the same standards of health and the same equality of opportunity as the rest of the population.

The bereaved child

Despite the awful reality of death, as portrayed in daily newspapers, television and films, death is a subject which rarely needs to be discussed within the family group. Death in childhood and therefore loss of a sibling is now rare in contrast to the past. Children may come across death in a parent or relative or, less frequently, in a sibling through accidents, sudden infant death syndrome, malignancy or perinatal loss, as the major causes. The reaction of a child to bereavement must be understood in context of the child's age, the circumstances surrounding the bereavement and the reaction of the child's parents.

Death is perceived very differently by children at different ages.[98,99] To the pre-school child death represents simple separation and is in all probability temporary. It provokes the transient anxieties with respect to separation which are often quickly forgotten in conceptual terms. In the young school age child, death is often perceived as part of the natural order of things, but something that happens to other people and does not intrude beyond separation in the child's life. From 10 years onwards the true meaning of death becomes more apparent to the child, but within this framework it is overlaid with the classical peripubertal fantasies. These concepts allow an understanding of the child's response to his own impending death as well as to the death of a close relative.

The circumstances surrounding death and the events which follow are important to the child in terms of the response to the loss. The child may witness for example the finding of a sudden unexplained death. In this situation parental grief, guilt and anger may spill over into an initial blaming of the parent or the child. The child may see the events surrounding bereavement as events which result in separation for long periods from their parents. The management of parental grief has been helped by an understanding of the necessity for the parents, and indeed siblings, to see and hold their dead family member. It is important for the child that the death be discussed openly and truthfully without too many euphemisms, which can lead to misunderstanding.[100]

The parental reaction to the loss of a baby from sudden infant death may be to blame either themselves or the sibling for the death. Parents find the period after loss a difficult period in which to communicate both with each other and with other family members, although young children may be often seen comforting their parents through periods of particular stress. Subsequent to their recovery from the initial stages of grief parents may either under or over-react to the sibling, becoming under or over-protective, which may in itself generate its own problems.

The child may cope with loss in many ways. Frequently a lack of understanding may be perceived by others as uninterest in the loss, whereas among adults and young children denial of a traumatic event is an important defence mechanism. Children may respond to bereavement from sudden infant death with the development of sleeping disorders. It often amounts to fear that the child is not going to wake up (in the same way as a sibling) or fear that some other awful event may happen during the sleep periods. These may be compounded by the development of fantasies in both young and older children about joining the dead individual or being snatched from the conscious world like the dead person. Occasionally loss and stress in the child are translated into aggression which may manifest within the home setting or at school. Bereaved children may also have problems in relating and discussing the events with other children. It is often important for children to act out their thoughts in play, such as mock burials or accidents, which may be distressing for adults to watch.

These items emphasize the importance of whole family support for bereavement and for due consideration to be given to siblings when counselling bereaved parents. Children should not be excluded from the family's grief and the needs of bereaved children need to be understood by the family and other carers, such as teachers or nursery staff.

There are many children's books which deal with death which can be used as a basis for discussion with the individual child. Other publications may deal with metamorphosis as an aid to understanding the cycle of life, such as *The Very Hungry Caterpillar*[101] for very young children and *Water Bugs and Dragonflies*[102] for older ones.

References

1 Marlow, N., Chiswick, M.L. Neurodevelopmental outcome in extremely low birthweight survivors. In: Chiswick, M.L., ed. *Recent Advances in Perinatal Medicine*, Vol II. Edinburgh: Churchill Livingstone, 1985: 181–205.

2 Illsley, R., Mitchell, R.G., eds. *Low Birthweight: a Medical Psychological and Social Study*. Chichester: John Wiley, 1984.

3 Casaer, P., De Vries, L., Marlow, N. Perinatal risk factors for psychosocial development. In: Rutter, M., Casaer, P., eds. *Biological Risk Factors for Psychosocial Development*. Cambridge: Cambridge University Press, 1991.

4 Lucas, A., Morley, R., Cole, T.J. Adverse neurodevelopmental outcome of moderate neonatal hypoglycaemia. *Br Med J* 1988; **297**: 1304–1308.

5 Lucas, A., Morley, R., Cole, T.J., *et al*. Early diet in preterm babies and developmental status in infancy. *Arch Dis Child* 1989, **64**: 1570–1578.

6 Cooke, R.W.I. Outcome and costs of care for the very immature infant. *Br Med Bull* 1988; **44**: 1133–1151.

7 Hagberg, B., Hagberg, G., Olow, I. von Wendt, L. The changing panorama in Sweden. *Acta Paediatr Scand* 1989; **78:** 1–8.

8 Fawer, C.L., Diebold, P., Calame, A. Periventricular leucomalacia and neurodevelopmental outcome in preterm infants. *Arch Dis Child* 1987; **62:** 30–36.

9 Graham, M., Trounce, J.Q., Levene, M.I., Rutter, N. Prediction of cerebral palsy in very low birthweight infants: prospective ultrasound study. *Lancet* 1987; **ii:** 593–596.

10 Stewart, A.L., Reynolds, E.O.R., Hope, P.L., *et al*. Probability of neurodevelopmental disorders estimated from ultrasound appearance of brains of very preterm infants. *Dev Med Child Neurol* 1987; **29:** 3–11.

11 Klimach, V., Cooke, R.W.I. Short-latency somatosensory evoked responses of preterm infants with ultrasound abnormalities of the brain. *Dev Med Child Neurol* 1989; **30:** 215–221.

12 Fielder, A.R., Ng, Y.K., Levene, M.I. Retinopathy of prematurity: age at onset. *Arch Dis Child* 1986; **61:** 774–778.

13 Zacharias, L., Chisholm, J.F., Chapman, R.B. Visual and ocular damage in retrolental fibroplasia. *Am J Ophthalmol* 1962; **53:** 337–345.

14 Phelps, D.L. Retinopathy of prematurity: an estimate of vision loss in the United States. *Pediatrics* 1981; **67:** 924–926.

15 Ng, Y.K., Fielder, A.R., Levene, M.I. Retinopathy of prematurity in the UK. *Eye* 1987; **1:** 386–390.

16 Lucey, J.F., Dangman, B. A re-examination of the role of oxygen in retrolental fibroplasia. *Pediatrics* 1984; **73:** 82–96.

17 Phelps, D., Rosenbloom, A.L. The effect of marginal hypoxaemia during the recovery period in oxygen-induced retinopathy in the kitten. *Pediatrics* 1984; **73:** 1–6.

18 Kushner, B.J. Strabismus and amblyopia associated with regressed retinopathy of prematurity. *Arch Ophthalmol* 1982; **100:** 256–261.

19 Yu, V.Y.H., ed. Survival and neurodevelopmental outcome of preterm infants. In: *Prematurity*. London: Churchill Livingstone, 1989.

20 Michelsson, K., Noronen, M. Neurological, psychological and articulatory impairment in five-year-old children with a birthweight of 2000 g or less. *Eur J Pediatr* 1983; **141:** 96–100.

21 Stevens, J.C., Webb, H.D., Hutchinson, J., *et al*. Click evoked otoacoustic emissions compared with brain stem electric response. *Arch Dis Child* 1989; **64:** 1105–1111.

22 Bhattacharya, J., Bennett, M.J., Tucker, S.M. Long term follow up of newborns tested with the auditory response cradle. *Arch Dis Child* 1984; **59:** 504–511.

23 Cooke, R.W.I. Early prognosis of low birthweight infants treated for progressive post-haemorrhagic hydrocephalus. *Arch Dis Child* 1983; **58:** 410–414.

24 Drillien, C.M., Thomson, A.J.M., Burgoyne, K. Low birthweight children at early school age: a longitudinal study. *Dev Med Child Neurol* 1980; **22:** 26–47.

25 De Vries, L.S., Regev, R., Pennock, J.M., Wigglesworth, J.S., Dubowitz, L.M.S. Ultrasound evolution and later outcome of infants with periventricular densities. *Early Hum Dev* 1988; **14:** 225–233.

26 PeBenito, R., Santello, M.D., Faxas, T.A., Ferretti, C., Fisch, C.B. Residual developmental disabilities in children with transient hypertonicity in infancy. *Pediatr Neurol* 1989; **5:** 154–160.

27 Astbury, J., Orgill, A., Bajuk, B. Relationship between two-year behaviour and neurodevelopmental outcome at five years of very low-birthweight survivors. *Dev Med Child Neurol* 1987; **29:** 370–379.

28 Marlow, N., Roberts, B.L., Cooke, R.W.I. Motor skills in extremely low birthweight children at the age of 6 years. *Arch Dis Child* 1989; **64:** 839–847.

29 Klein, N., Hack, M., Gallagher, J., Fanaroff, A. Preschool performance of children with normal intelligence who were very low-birth-weight infants. *Pediatrics* 1987; **75:** 531–537.

30 Hertzig, M.E. Neurological 'soft' signs in low birthweight children. *Dev Med Child Neurol* 1981; **23:** 778–791.

31 Heldt, G.P. Pulmonary status of infants and children with bronchopulmonary dysplasia. In: Merritt, T.A., Northway, W.H., Beynton, B.R., eds. *Bronchopulmonary Dysplasia*. Boston: Blackwell Scientific Publications, 1988: 421–438.

32 Heldt, G.P., McIlroy, M.B., Hansen, T.N., Tooley, W.H. Exercise performance of the survivors of hyaline membrane disease. *J Pediatr* 1980; **96:** 995.

33 Department of Health. *Immunisation Against Infectious Disease*. London: HMSO Publications, 1990.

34 Allen, M.C. Developmental outcome and follow up of the small for gestational age infant. *Semin Perinatol* 1984; **9:** 123–156.

35 Tegberg, A.J., Walther, F.J., Pena, I.C. Mortality, morbidity, and outcome of the small-for-gestational age infant. *Semin Perinatol* 1988; **12:** 88–94.

36 Neligan, G.A., Kolvin, J., Scott, D.M., Gardide, R.F. Born too small or born too soon: a follow-up study to seven years of age. *Clinics in Developmenal Medicine*, no. 61: Spastics International, 1976.

37 Largo, R.H., Pfister, D., Molinari, L., Kundu, S., Lipp, A., Duc, G. Significance of prenatal, perinatal and postnatal factors in the development of AGA preterm infants at five to seven years. *Dev Med Child Neurol* 1989; **31:** 440–456.

38 Fancourt, R., Campbell, S., Harvey, D., *et al*. Follow up of small for dates babies. *Br Med J* 1976; **1:** 1435–1437.

39 Parkinson, C.E., Scrivener, R., Graves, L., *et al*. Behavioural differences of school-age children who were small-for-dates babies. *Dev Med Child Neurol* 1988; **28:** 498–505.

40 Ounsted, M., Moar, V.A., Scott, A. Small-for-dates babies, gestational age, and developmental ability at 7 years. *Early Hum Dev* 1989; **19:** 77–86.

41 Ment, L.R., Freedman, R.M., Ehrenkranz, R.A., Neonates with seizures attributable to perinatal complications. *Am J Dis Child* 1982; **136:** 548–550.

42 Holden, K.R., Mellits, E.D., Freeman, J.M. Neonatal seizures I: correlation of prenatal and perinatal events with outcome. *Pediatrics* 1982; **70:** 165–176.

43 Watkins, A., Szymonowicz, W., Jin, X., Yu, V.Y.H. Significance of seizures in very low birthweight infants. *Dev Med Child Neurol* 1988; **30:** 162–169.

44 Scott, H. Outcome of very severe birth asphyxia. *Arch Dis Child* 1976; **51:** 712–716.

45 Sarnat, H.B., Sarnat, M.S. Neonatal encephalopathy following fetal distress. *Arch Neurol* 1974; **33**: 696–705.

46 Amiel-Tison, C., Ellison, P. Birth asphyxia in the full term newborn: early assessment and outcome. *Dev Med Child Neurol* 1986; **28**: 671–682.

47 Levene, M.I., Sands, C., Grindulis, H., Moore, J.R. Comparison of two methods of predicting outcome in perinatal asphyxia. *Lancet* 1986; i: 67–69.

48 Robertson, C.M.T., Finer, N.N., Grace, M.G.A. School performance of survivors of neonatal encephalopathy associated with birth asphyxia at term. *J Pediatr* 1989; **114**: 753–760.

49 Botting, B.J., Davies, I.M., MacFarlane, A.J. Recent trends in the incidence of multiple births and associated mortality. *Arch Dis Child* 1987; **62**: 941–50.

50 Campbell, D.M., Samphier, M. Birthweight standards for twins. In: MacGillivray, I., Campbell, D.M., Thomson, B., eds. *Twinning and Twins*. Chichester: John Wiley, 1988: 161–178.

51 Bryan, E.M. The intrauterine hazards of twins. *Arch Dis Child* 1986; **62**: 941–950.

52 Carpenter, R.G. Sudden death in twins. *MOH Rep Pub Hlth Med Subjects* 1965; **113**: 51–52.

53 Kraus, J.F., Borhani, N.O. Post-neonatal sudden unexplained death in California: a cohort study. *Am J Epidemiol* 1972; **95**: 497–510.

54 Beal, S. Some epidemiological factors about sudden infant death syndrome in South Australia. In: Tildon, J.T., Roeder, L.M., Steinschneider, A., eds. *Sudden Infant Death Syndrome*. New York: Academic Press, 1983: 15–28.

55 Spiers, P.S. Estimated rates of concordancy for the sudden infant death syndrome in twins. *Am J Epidemiol* 1984; **100**: 1–7.

56 Emery, J.L. Welfare of families of children found unexpectedly dead: (cot deaths). *Br Med J* 1972: **1**: 612–5.

57 Spillman, J. The role of birthweight in maternal–infant relationships. [MSc Thesis]. Cranfield Institute of Technology, 1984.

58 Koch, H.L. *Twins and Twin Relations*. Chicago: University of Chicago Press, 1966.

59 Zazzo, R. The twin condition and the couple effect on personality development. *Acta Genet Med Gemellol* 1979; **25**: 343–352.

60 Watts, D.A., Lytton, H. *Twinship as Handicap: Fact or Fiction? A Longitudinal Study*. Calgary: The University of Calgary, Canada, 1980.

61 Hay, D.A., Prior, M., Collett, S., Williams, M. Speech and language development in preschool twins. *Acta Genet Med Gemellol* 1987; **36**: 213–222.

62 Lytton, H., Conway, D. The impact of twinship on parent–child interaction. *J Pers Social Psychol* 1977; **35**: 97–107.

63 Lytton, H. *Parent–Child Interaction: The Socialization Process Observed in Twin and Singleton Families*. New York: Plenum Press, 1980.

64 Mittler, P. Language development in young twins: biological, genetic and social aspects. *Acta Genet Med Gemellol* 1976; **25**: 359–365.

65 Mittler, P. Biological and social aspects of language development in twins. *Dev Med Child Neurol* 1980; **12**: 741–757.

66 Zazzo, R. *Les Jumeaux: le Couple et la Personne*. Paris: Press Universitaire de France, 1960.

67 Wilson, R.S. Mental development in the pre-school years. *Dev Psychol* 1974; **10**: 580–588.

68 Bryan, E.M., ed. The growth and development of twins. In: *The Nature and Nurture of Twins*. Eastbourne: Baillière Tindall, 1983: 141–155.

69 Department of Health and Social Security. *Inequalities in Health*. London: HMSO, 1980.

70 Whitehead, M. *The Health Divide: Inequalities in Health in the 1980s*. London: Health Education Authority, 1987.

71 Siegal, L.S. Reproductive, perinatal and environmental factors as predictors of the cognitive and language development of preterm and full term infants. *Child Dev* 1982; **53**: 963–973.

72 Wedge, P., Prosser, H. *Born to Fail*. London: National Children's Bureau, 1973.

73 Osborn, A.F., Butler, N.R., Morris, A.C. *The Social Life of Britain's Five Year Olds*. London: Routledge and Kegan Paul, 1984.

74 Hunt, J. McV. *Intelligence and Experience*. New York: Ronald, 1961.

75 Jacobs, B.A., Moss, H.A. Birth order and sex of sibling as determinants of mother–infant interaction. *Child Dev* 1976; **47**: 315–322.

76 Zajonc, R.B., Marcus, G.B. Birth order and intellectual development. *Psychol Rev* 1975; **82**: 74–88.

77 Boat, B.W., Campbell, F.A., Ramey, C.T. Preventative education and birth order as co-determinants of IQ in disadvantaged families. *Child Care Hlth Dev* 1986; **12**: 25–36.

78 Falker, D.W., Eysenck, H.J. Hereditary and intelligence. In: Eysenck, H.J., Falker, D.W., eds. *The Structure and Measurement of Intelligence*. Berlin: Springer-Verlag, 1979.

79 Butler, N.R., Golding, J., eds. *From Birth to Five*. Oxford: Pergamon Press, 1986.

80 Barker, W.J. *The Child Development Programme*. Bristol: Early Childhood Developmental Unit, School of Applied Social Studies, University of Bristol, 1989.

81 Escalona, S.K. *Critical Issues in the Early Development of Premature Infants*. New Haven and London: Yale University Press, 1987.

82 Taylor, D.J., Howie, P.W., Davidson, J., *et al*. Do pregnancy complications contribute to neurodevelopment disability? *Lancet* 1985; i: 713–716.

83 Conway, J., ed. *Prescription for Poor Health: the Crisis for Homeless Families*. London: London Food Commission, Maternity Alliance, SHAC and Shelter, 1988.

84 Wolf, S. *Children Under Stress*. Harmondsworth: Penguin, 1981.

85 Richards, M.P.M. *Children and Divorce*. In: McFarlane, J.A., ed. *Progress in Child Health*, vol 1: Edinburgh: Churchill Livingstone, 1984.

86 Wadsworth, J., Taylor, B., Osbourn, A., *et al*. Teenage mothering: child development at 5 years. *J Child Psychol Psychiatr* 1984; **25**: 305–313.

87 Department of Environment. *Count of Gypsy Caravan Sites 1989*. London: DoE, 1989.

88 Hussey, R.M. Travellers and preventative health care. *Br Med J* 1988; **296**: 1098.

89 Golding, A.M.B. The health needs of homeless families. *J R Coll Gen Practit* 1987; **37**: 433–434.

90 Pahl, J., Vaile, M. *Health and Health Care Among Travellers*. Canterbury: University of Kent Health Services Research Unit, 1986.

91 Cornall, J. *Improving Health Care for Travellers*. London: King's Fund Centre, 1984.

92 Luthanate, P. *Health and Health Care in Traveller Mothers and Children*. London: Save the Children Fund, 1983.

93 Durnand, L., ed. *Traveller Mothers and Babies: Who Cares for their Health?* London: Maternity Alliance, 1990.

94 Streeting, A. Health care for travellers: one year's experience. *Br Med J* 1987; **294**: 492–4.

95 Tyfield, L., Meredith, A.L., Osbourn, M.J. Identification of lapotype pattern associated with mutant PKU allele in the gypsy population of Wales. *J Med Genet* **26**: 499–503.

96 Feder, G. Traveller gypsies and primary care. *J R Coll Gen Practit* 1989; **39**: 425–429.

97 Oakley, J. *The Traveller Gypsies*. Cambridge: Cambridge University Press, 1983.

98 Yudkin, S. Children and death. *Lancet* 1967; i: 37–41.

99 Koochen, G.P. Talking with children about death. *Am J Orthopsychiatr* 1974; **44**: 404–411.

100 Burton, L. *Care of the Child Facing Death*. London: Routledge and Kegan Paul, 1974.

101 Carle, E. *The Very Hungry Caterpillar*. London: Hamish Hamilton, 1970.

102 Stickley, D. *Waterbugs and Dragonflies*. London: Mowbray, 1984.

6.5 Ethnic minorities

Nellie Adjaye

Definition

Ethnic minorities may be defined as groups of people who consider themselves separate from the general population and are seen by the general population at large to be distinct because of their racial origin, skin colour, language, religious beliefs, cultural practices or dietary customs. Many people when they think of ethnic minorities in the UK, refer mainly to the Afro-Caribbean and Asian populations, probably because they are the largest groups of the ethnic minorities distinguishable by their colour. The UK Office of Population Censuses and Surveys endorsed this practice by adopting the terms non-white and white in their Annual Labour Force Surveys 1983–85 and includes Chinese, Arabs and peoples of mixed origins when describing the main demographic features of ethnic minority populations resident in Great Britain.[1] However this definition excludes significant white ethnic minority groups notably the Greek and Turkish Cypriot population of approximately 179 900; the Italian population of approximately 202 000[1] and the Jewish population of about 350 000.[2] The history of colonization during the era of the British Empire, and the political stance subsequently adopted has attracted immigration into the UK from countries with whom it has had long association. The result is that Britain is now a multiracial or multi-ethnic society. The population includes people from several ethnic groups of varying sizes as shown in Table 6.4.

It is estimated that non-white ethnic minorities comprise 4.3% of the UK population. Seven per cent of young people under 16 years are non-white (Table 6.5). Most ethnic minority groups have migrated and settled in the UK for a variety of reasons which include the direct recruitment of skilled labour for employment in British industries, hotels and restaurants, the National Health Service and London Transport, especially when Britain had a reduced labour force. Others have migrated into the UK as political refugees and there is regularly a large student population from all parts of the world. The ethnic minority groups have tended to settle in the large metropolitan counties and are not evenly distributed through the UK (Tables 6.5 and 6.6).

Table 6.4 Ethnic minority populations in Great Britain 1983–85 average[1]

Ethnic group	Number (thousands)	Percentage which is UK-born
West Indian or Guyanese	530	50
Indian	760	35
Pakistani	380	40
Bangladeshi	90	30
African	100	35
Chinese	110	20
Arab	60	10
Mixed Origin	220	75
Other	100	25
Total non-white group	2350	40

Table 6.5 Percentage of the population of Great Britain which is non-white, by age, 1983–85 average[1]

	Age group					
	Under 16 years	16–29 years	30–44 years	45–64/59* years	65/60 years and over[†]	All ages
Non-white						
Born overseas	1	4	4	3	1	2.5
Born in UK	6	2	–	–	–	1.8
Total	7	6	4	3	1	4.3
Numbers (thousands)	810	660	480	340	60	2350

*45–64 for males; 45–59 for females.
[†]65 and over for males; 60 and over for females.

Table 6.6 Population resident in metropolitan counties by ethnic group, Great Britain 1983–85 average[1]

Ethnic group	Metropolitan county of residence						
	Greater London	Greater Manchester	West Midlands	West Yorkshire	Other metropolitan counties	Resident outside metropolitan counties	Great Britain
Total population	12	5	5	4	7	67	100
West Indian or Guyanese	57	4	14	3	2	19	100
Indian	39	4	19	5	1	32	100
Pakistani	14	10	24	16	4	31	100
Bangladeshi	54	5	12	5	3	22	100
African	64	3	2	2	5	24	100
Chinese	33	4	3	2	8	49	100
Mixed	36	7	7	3	6	42	100
Other (incl. Arab)	51	3	4	2	4	36	100
Total non-white group	41	5	15	6	3	30	100
Percentage which non-white group forms of total population of area	14	5	13	7	2	2	4

Cultural differences in child care, language and religion

The two strong determinants of cultural beliefs, language and religion, also influence health beliefs and practices and child rearing practices are not excluded. All the world's major religions are represented within the ethnic minority groups of the UK. They include Christianity, Islam, Sikhism, Judaism, Hinduism and Buddhism. Thus, for example, it would be expected that most immigrants from Bangladesh and Pakistan, (the Punjab, North-West frontier and the Mirpur district) would practise the Islamic religion or at least be influenced by that religion, while those from the Indian subcontinent and Sri Lanka would be mostly Hindus. The Chinese population in Britain tends to practise Buddhism, and Sikhism is observed by most people from the Punjab or by East-African Asians. African immigrants usually practise the Christian religion, but a substantial number may be Muslims. Most of the Arabic people observe strict Islamic practice. People of West Indian, Guyanese and mediterranean origins usually observe Christianity, but sometimes Muslim or Hindu practices may be found in these groups, depending on their ancestry. Where distinct ethnic minority groups exist, it is good practice for doctors and other health workers to explore the health beliefs and attitudes within the community before imposing any major changes designed to ensure conformity with the standard health care provisions (Fig. 6.6 and Table 6.7).

Table 6.7 Main Asian ethnic groups in Britain[3]

Origin	Name	Religion	First language and subsidiary languages	Dietary customs
India – Gujarat (Kutch and South Gujarat)	Gujaratis	Hindu	Gujarati (Hindi)	No beef Usually vegetarians
India – Punjab State	Sikhs	Sikh	Punjabi (Hindi)	Usually no beef Pork rarely No halal meat Some vegetarians
India – Bombay, Delhi and other major cities	Indians (or name of state)	Hindu	Hindi (English)	No beef Usually vegetarians
East Africa – Kenya, Malawi	Gujaratis	Hindu	Gujaratis (Hindi, Swahili, English).	No beef Usually vegetarians
Tanzania Uganda, Zambia	Sikhs	Sikh	Punjabi (Hindi, Swahili, English)	Usually no beef Pork rarely No halal meat Some vegetarians
Pakistan – Punjab Province	Punjabis	Muslim	Punjabi (Urdu)	No pork Halal meat
Pakistan – Mirpur District (Azad Kashmir)	Mirpuris	Muslim	Mirpuri (Punjabi dialect, Urdu)	No pork Halal meat
Bangladesh – Sylhet District	Sylhetis Bengalis or Bangladeshis	Muslim	Sylheti (Bengali dialect, Urdu)	No pork Halal meat

Reproduced with kind permission of author and publishers.

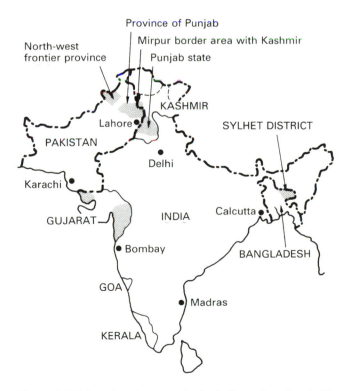

Figure 6.6 Main emigration areas in the Indian subcontinent. (Reproduced with permission from Henley, A. *Asian Patients in Hospital and at Home* London: Pitman Medical, 1979.)

Once settled in a host country a migrant group may marry and reproduce. During the period of settlement, acculturation frequently occurs. Thus the adoption of the new lifestyle of the host country, improved education, and social mobility may affect some of the cultural beliefs originally held. The differences become evident in the second generation immigrants who may not strictly adhere to their cultural beliefs or retain their ethnicity. Often this is a source of friction between the first and second generations, particularly in areas of marriage and child rearing practices. Ethnic minority groups display a diversity of social classes; like their host country, there is considerable mobility within their social strata. The temptation to adopt an attitude that treats all ethnic minority groups as one group must, therefore, be rejected by health workers, particularly when addressing issues like child care and child health surveillance.

Marriage and naming

Marriage is a sacrament in the Hindu and Sikh religions. Most parents from these groups approve of arranged marriages and their children generally accept them. Dissent from the second generation may be met with strong disapproval, sometimes resulting in the couple being ostracized. This is relevant since the help they may otherwise receive from the extended family on the arrival of children may not be forthcoming. This in turn may put the parents under further stress.

Hindus have a first or personal name, a middle or complementary name and a family or subcaste name. The latter is equivalent to the surname in Britain. The wife and children adopt the husband's/father's subcaste name (Table 6.8).

Table 6.8 Hindu naming system[4]

	First name (personal, usually different male and female names)	Middle or complementary name (different male and female names)	Subcaste name
Female	Arima	Devi	Patel
Male	Naresh	Lal	Chopra

Reproduced with kind permission of the author and publishers.

The Sikh naming system is based on the Hindu system. Although subcaste names have been abandoned in rural India, they are sometimes readopted on settlement in the UK. The wife and children adopt the husband's/father's subcaste name. All male Sikhs have Singh (meaning lion) as their middle names and women have Kaur (meaning princess) as their complementary or middle names. When the subcaste name has been abandoned, Singh or Kaur may appear on the child's health records as the 'surname' with subsequent reference to the mother as Mrs Kaur (Mrs Princess). This must sound ridiculous to the Sikh woman and is very puzzling to the uninformed health worker who may be surprised to find she has several Singhs or Kaurs on her case load. An attempt should be made to identify the subcaste name and use it (Table 6.9).

Table 6.9 Sikh naming system[4]

	First name (personal name, male and female names usually the same)	Middle or complementary (religious) name	Subcaste name
Female	Jaswinder	Kaur (all women)	Gill
Male	Armarjit	Singh (all men)	Bamra

Reproduced with kind permission of author and publishers.

In the Islamic or Muslim religion, marriage is a civil contract. Contrary to the popular belief that most Muslims adopt polygamy, it is apparently rare for a Muslim man from the Indian subcontinent to have more than one wife. This is not necessarily true of other Muslim groups of Arabic or middle-east origins. Muslims from different parts of the world have different

Table 6.10 Muslim naming system and way of recording it[4]

Name	Record as:
Husband	
Mohammed Habibur Rahman	(Mohammed) Habibur RAHMAN
Wife	
Jameela Katoon	Jameela Katoon, wife of Mohammed Habibur RAHMAN
Son	
Shafiur Mia	Shafiur Mia, son of Mohammed RAHMAN
Daughter	
Shameema Bibi	Shameema Bibi, daughter of Mohammed Habibur RAHMAN

Reproduced with kind permission of author and publishers.

naming systems. Generally, the wife and children do not adopt the husband or father's name. The men have two or more names; one is personal and the other usually has religious associations such as Mohammed or Ali. The clan names such as Chaudhury or Khan may be used as the surname. A woman may also have a personal name followed by her title, Begum or Bibi which is equivalent to Ms or Miss in the British naming system. Child health records giving the name of a girl child as Shameema Bibi for instance, will often refer to the mother as Mrs Bibi, thus giving rise to the situation already described. To avoid confusion, all record clerks and health workers should be trained to ask for the husband or father's family name and record information as shown in Table 6.10.

Getting the name right from the beginning will help to ensure a good relationship with one's patient.

The Jewish or Christian religious marriage is both a sacrament and civil contract. Jews have a long relationship with the UK and are well assimilated into British culture, though a substantial proportion continue to observe their own religion. Naming is not often a problem. Christianity may be observed in all the ethnic groups, but more so in the Mediterranean, African and Caribbean groups of people. The African groups, particularly the west and central Africans, adhere to their traditional marriage. In addition, the couple may opt for a civil contract or religious blessing. In the traditional marriage the woman retains her maiden name though the children take the father's name. If there is a religious blessing or a civil contract, then the woman adopts the husband's surname or family name.

The family and attitudes to children

Children have always been regarded as assets in most societies of the world. The ethnic minority groups in the UK would share this philosophy. However, an understanding of the different family systems and family lifestyles is essential for successful child health surveillance since family and family relationships can influence health care. Doctors, nurses and other health workers in the community should avoid imposing their own cultural expectations on families who live differently. For example, in most Afro-Caribbean societies, the desire for a woman to demonstrate parenthood may take precedence over marriage. Children born out of wedlock are fully accepted into the family in its wider sense. The term illegitimacy is not recognized. Although this attitude may be reflected by the high proportion of single parents among this group today, the influence of secularism cannot be entirely ignored. The strong matrilineal influence in this group means that the maternal grandmother may be the most influential person in her grandchild's upbringing. She is the centre of the family. The family in this case would consist of mother and baby, maternal grandmother with or without a maternal grandfather, with or without the siblings of the mother plus any other relative that might be staying in the household at the time. Depending on the size of the accommodation, overcrowding may result with all the associated effects, but at the same time the child receives love and attention from many carers in the household.

The extended family support may break down in some groups of ethnic minorities. This pattern is seen in young African or Arabic couples who have initially come to the UK to pursue further education or to advance their career and improve their social standing by having children. When there are no other family members to help with child care, the couple or the woman may opt to place the child with a daily childminder or in voluntary private foster care which may be outside the area in which the child was born and registered. The implications of this for child health surveillance are obvious and they may have adverse consequences on the child's development.[5]

The minority groups from India, Pakistan, West Africa, Bangladesh, China, Hong Kong, or Vietnam also look to the extended family members for support, but the extent to which this is achieved depends on whether or not the community is a migrant or settled population. The family unit may be very large. It may contain three or four generations with several adult couples. The children may be brought up by all the adults and grow up to regard them all as parents. The older family members may have final authority rather than their biological parents. There is usually a hierarchy of responsibility and authority. Thus older children may have authority over, and expect respect from, younger siblings. The family unit consisting of four or more generations may live under one roof with, or without, adequate accommodation or be split up into the nuclear units to which the British health worker is more accustomed, depending on the socio-economic circumstances. However, because of the common cultural background, close bonds of support and responsibility may be maintained between the units either in the UK or from the original country. In some families it is the norm for children to be brought up by other relatives, including uncles and aunts. This concept is often difficult for British health workers to accept. It can be a source of anxiety to the health worker who may take a disapproving view of the situation and it calls for mutual understanding to effect successful child health surveillance.

Childlessness is often regarded as unfortunate, even calamitous. Couples may go to great lengths to have investigations and treatments to achieve successful parenthood. Investigations and treatment may be along the lines of conventional western medical practice or couples may seek the help of the traditional medical practitioner. However, although the more settled and westernized members of the community may not pursue the traditional beliefs and practices with much zeal, pressure from the closely knit and extended family system may be difficult to resist. It is important to realize that the traditional medical practitioner may be consulted for a variety of illnesses in adults and children while undertaking western medical treatment, especially if the medical condition is a chronic one.

Most of the ethnic minority groups (particularly the men), regard formal adoption as alien to their culture. The informal kin-fostering system described above is preferred. Immigration regulations have made kin-fostering of children from relations overseas more difficult, so this practice will be less prevalent in the UK in the future. Attitudes to fostering and adoption among black ethnic minorities are also changing towards acceptance of legally defined fostering and adoption.

General child care

Support is expected from an older member of the family, usually the grandmother, particularly if it is the first in the family. Within the West African community, the child's maternal grandmother if available and able, is called upon to help the young first parents. The benefits derived from the grandmother's nurturing and the help she gives her daughter far outweigh the cost incurred by the journey to the UK. The mother of the child learns to take instructions in child care in this way.

In the Islamic and Jewish religions, routine male circumcision is performed, on the eighth day in the cases of Jews. Since this is not offered on the National Health Service (NHS), some parents may opt to have this done privately by surgeons or by their respective religious practitioners – Imam or mohel respectively. In the Hindu, Sikh and Chinese communities circumcision is undertaken by custom rather than for religious reasons. Similarly, in the non-Muslim Afro-

Caribbean groups, circumcision may be customary depending on the parents' cultural background. Parents often expect this procedure under the NHS and are disappointed when it is not forthcoming without a medical indication.

Among the immigrants from the Indian subcontinent and East African Asians, black eye make-up is put round the eyes and inside the eyelids of babies as protection against infection. Since this surma was shown to cause lead poisoning through conjunctival absorption of the lead sulphide contained in the preparation,[6-8] its importation has been officially banned. However, it may still be available for use through non-commercial channels. Health workers should make discreet enquiries about the origin of the black eye make-up in families who use it on their children and suggest non-lead containing alternatives.

In the Hindu, and to a lesser extent, Muslim religions, the baby's hair may be shaved after 28 days to allow for more healthy hair growth. The opposite practice is observed in the Sikh religion where head and body hair is not cut. Boys wear a comb to secure the hair on the head and initially cover the knot of hair with a small muslin cloth called rumal until they reach the age of 12 years, when they are allowed to wear the now familiar Sikh turban. Just as Christians may wear the cross as a necklace, a metal bracelet worn on the right wrist by a Sikh child has its religious importance and must never be removed without the express consent of the parents. Similar religious ornaments like a bead on black string may be found round the wrist or neck of a Hindu child to protect the child.

In general terms, assiduous cleanliness is observed in the babies by most of the ethnic groups. Babies are bathed twice a day in the Asian and African communities. In the latter, care is taken to part the labia majora and minora in girls and clean the area thoroughly. In the present climate of concern about child abuse, this practice could be misinterpreted.

Hair plaiting in Afro-Caribbean children is a well established art. Both boys and girls may have their hair plaited though it is more common in girls than boys, but the pure African boys do not have the hair plaited. There is a need to caution parents not to pull too tightly on the hair roots around the temporal hairline as it can lead to permanent alopecia in early childhood.

Attitudes to child rearing and discipline

It is difficult to generalize about all the ethnic minorities mentioned in this paper. Child rearing practices vary within the same ethnic group. Social class mobility, acculturation education, expectations of the child health, education, and social services, influence people's attitudes to child rearing – notwithstanding discipline. On the whole, people from the Asian culture, including India, Pakistan and Bangladesh, and from West African cultures, expect instant unquestioning obedience from their offspring. The same might be said for the Chinese. In traditional West Africa it is disrespectful for a child to answer back to an adult or look the adult directly in the eye when being spoken to. The Asian culture also observes similar attitudes to children. Physical punishment is expected and used on disobedient children. It comes as a cultural shock to the immigrant when the young child defiantly answers back and does not avoid the adult's gaze. More punishment may be meted out. Apart from physical punishment there are other unsavoury punishments that some families still practise, such as inserting pulped ginger anally or vaginally to 'teach the child a lesson!' Similarly, multiple pin-pricks of the tips of the fingers are used to deter children from pilfering. Since these signs may initiate a child abuse inquiry the need to be familiar with cultural practices within different ethnic groups cannot be overemphasized.

Developmental differences and nutrition

Breast-feeding patterns in the ethnic minorities vary according to traditional weaning practices and the extent of acculturation of the minority groups in the host country. Socioeconomic factors also play a role. A research survey established in 1983 by the Department of Social Medicine in Birmingham University[9] collected nutritional data about 131 Afro-Caribbean women aged 18–41 years. It revealed that although 91% started to breast feed this figure dropped to 78% after 8 weeks, with 35% ceasing to breast feed before one month. The main predictor of breastfeeding continuing beyond one month was being an owner-occupier, an indirect reflection of social class. It is interesting to note that traditional West Indian weaning practices were continued in the Afro-Caribbean households by mothers born in the UK who had adopted British patterns of infant feeding. In the traditional Afro-Caribbean households semi-solid foods in the form of corn meal may be introduced around the age of one month. Other weaning foods may be mashed sweet potato, cooked green bananas, and plantain. Health visitors and health promoters need to be aware of this.

In the Chinese and Vietnamese immigrant communities with traditional breast feeding and weaning practices, breast feeding up to or beyond 3 months is more common. The child may be weaned on to congee (rice porridge mixed with chopped meat and vegetable). Families who have come from rural areas are more likely to breast feed longer. This is particularly true of the Bangladeshi communities. Many proprietary baby foods are unsuitable for people who observe dietary restrictions, for example the vegetarian Hindus and Sikhs, Muslims and Jews. Some mothers will continue breast feeding for as long as possible to avoid the prohibited foods. They may only buy products that they know contain no meat at all, such as puddings or custards. Alternatively, there may be early introduction of unfortified cow's milk containing little iron and vitamin D. Sugar may be added to the milk and the feeding bottle kept for up to 2 years. If solids are not introduced by 9 months there may be increased difficulties in establishing full mixed feeding. This combination of late weaning and high carbohydrate intake can lead to relative obesity in infancy. In the Birmingham study of groups of Muslims, Sikhs, and Hindus in the Asian community, the mean age of introduction of solids was 23–25 weeks.[10] Although mothers should be encouraged to give the family diet, mashed up, this has been found not to be the case in the Asian community (Indian, Pakistani, Bangladeshi).[11] In the nutritional survey of Bangladeshi children carried out in Tower Hamlets,[12] it was found that very few Bangladeshi children eat the family foods by one year, but 91% do so by the age of 2 to 3 years.

Growth and developmental differences

Jivani has shown that some Asian immigrant children are undernourished and may show faltering growth at the time of weaning.[13] The Tower Hamlets study[12] also showed a slight reduction in mean growth between the ages of 1 and 3 years. Bengali parents often show concern and anxiety about the poor stature of their child[14] but in many cases the parents are small and the child is growing at a normal rate. It has been suggested that special centile charts are not required for these children.[15] However Rona and Chinn[16] have advised that the use of British standards of height, based on caucasian children, to assess growth of another ethnic group in England should be interpreted with caution. The first National Anthropometric Survey of children of the major ethnic groups in Britain which looked at both social and biological background of each of the ethnic groups by first language spoken at home: Afro-Caribbean, Urdu, Gujarati, Punjabi (other Asians including a small number of Bengali-speaking people) showed very large differences in height between the ethnic groups.[16] Using multiple regression analysis, ethnic background explained 5% of the variation in height. The Afro-Caribbean children were the tallest; and the Gujarati and other Asian groups the shortest. In most age groups the Afro-Caribbean group was on average 3–4 cm taller, and the other ethnic groups between 0.5 and 3 cm shorter than the representative sample. Within most ethnic groups children in social class V were much shorter than other social classes. The same was true of the sample of caucasian children examined. Parental height and the child's birthweight were positively associated with the child's

height in most ethnic groups. However, differences were evident between the ethnic groups when certain selected variables were examined. For example, household overcrowding and the child's height were negatively related in most of the Asian groups while in the Afro-Caribbean group there was a significant positive association with the child's height. Mother's education was an important factor in the Asian group, good education being positively associated with the child's height.

Afro-Caribbean children usually achieve earlier motor milestones than those from other ethnic minority groups or caucasians. However, language development will vary according to the social background of each ethnic group. Parental insecurity, stress and the use of more than one language in the household may all be factors which might mitigate against appropriate language development in ethnic minority groups. Poor language development is frequently associated with behaviour difficulties. It can be very difficult to diagnose in a child whose family is bilingual or where no English is spoken in the household. The use of a link worker or interpreter in such cases is invaluable.[17]

Disorders occurring in certain ethnic groups

A knowledge of certain diseases or disorders which occur in the main ethnic groups under discussion is helpful for child health surveillance purposes.

Jaundice

Prolonged neonatal jaundice may be difficult to diagnose in the dark-skinned baby.[18] Examination by blanching the skin of the soles of the feet, palms, or gums or examination of the hard palate may be a helpful method of clinical diagnosis of jaundice in the newborn, but this is not very reliable when performed by clinicians unused to working with dark-skinned people, and scleral examination may then be more reliable. Among the usual causes of prolonged non-obstructive jaundice in the newborn (jaundice after the first 2 weeks of life) glucose-6-phosphatase (G6-P) deficiency should be considered in Chinese babies from Hong Kong and South China (oriental form), mediterranean and Afro-Caribbean children all of whom may present up to 6 weeks of age. This inherited enzyme deficiency is common in these ethnic groups and may be a cause of unexplained anaemia.

Anaemia

Anaemia in a dark-skinned person is easily missed. It is important to examine the oral mucosa, nail beds, palms and soles of the feet.

Hereditary anaemias

The ethnic minority groups described in this section may present with the most common of hereditary anaemias; sickle cell anaemia in Afro-Caribbeans and thalassaemia major, in the mediterranean and Asian populations. Homozygous sickle cell anaemia (Hb SS) usually presents from 3–4 months of age with the hand/foot syndrome (dactylitis) or anaemia but can now be detected by screening tests on blood taken in the neonatal period. The heterozygous form (HbAS) is symptomless. The combination of HbS with other hae-moglobin variants, for example HbC or B thalassemia trait, gives rise to Hb SC usually with mild symptoms or HbSTThal with moderate to severe symptoms of anaemia, bone pain and hepatosplenomegaly. Thalassaemia major presents with anaemia, and from about 6 months of age hepatosplenomegaly; it requires regular blood transfusions and iron chelation to keep the children alive. Detailed description of these anaemias is given in Chapter 16.

Acquired anaemias

Iron deficiency anaemia, by far the commonest of all the acquired anaemias, is more prevalent in Asian children[19] and responds favourably to treatment by oral replacement. Increase in weight gain and improved psychomotor development have been observed in a group of Asian children treated thus in Birmingham.[20] The Afro-Caribbean groups may also display iron deficiency anaemia in childhood.[21] When iron deficiency anaemia is resistant to treatment it is worth examining the stools for evidence of helminthiasis, particularly in immigrant children who have recently arrived in the country from India, Pakistan, Bangladesh and Africa. Hookworm infestation and ascariasis (round worm) may often be the cause of chronic hypochromic, microcytic anaemia.

Rickets

Nutritional rickets in Asian children has been highlighted in several studies since the mid 1970s: Glasgow,[22] Bradford,[23] Edinburgh[24] and Brimingham.[10] It would appear that children on vegetarian diets tend to have suboptimal 25 (OH)D concentrations compared to their white peers. The main contributory factors to the lack of vitamin D are inadequate exposure to sunlight, and vegetarian diets, particularly in the strict Hindu families (see Table 6.7), the use of door-step milk for infant feeding and maternal deficiency of vitamin D during pregnancy and lactation. In 1981 an attempt to eradicate rickets was spearheaded by the Department of Health and Social Security (DHSS) in conjunction with Save the Children Fund. The Stop Rickets campaign was designed to inform and educate Asian communities and health workers about the causes, prevention and detection of nutritional rickets. However, it was soon discovered that Asian families were often unable to make full use of health services because of lack of information and cultural and language barriers. The lessons learned from that campaign gave rise to the more successful Asian Mother and Baby Campaign in 1984 which employed link workers with a good knowledge of English and Asian languages. Their role was to act as interpreters in antenatal clinics, to explain procedures to Asian mothers, and to advise on diet. In Afro-Caribbean groups nutritional rickets is less common although it may occur in the Rastafarian subgroup, some of whose members may be strict vegetarians. Others may avoid processed or canned foods preferring natural foods and may develop vitamin D deficiency.[25] Vitamin supplements are recommended from the age of 1 month to 5 years.

Hepatitis B

About 10–12% of adults in South-East Asia and China are asymptomatic, potentially infective, carriers of hepatitis B virus. In sub-saharan Africa, the Indian subcontinent and the mediterranean area, the carrier rate is about 3–10%. Women who have the e antigen are more likely to infect their children at the time of delivery.[26] Although the children are usually asymptomatic they contribute to the pool of persistent carriers in the community.

Congenital rubella

Asians from India, Pakistan, Bangladesh, Sri Lanka, and East Africa have been found to have higher susceptibility to rubella than non-Asians.[27,28] This is probably because they miss contact with the rubella immunization programme offered by the school health service by arriving in the UK after the ages at which immunization is usually given. The incidence of notified congenital rubella was found to be two to three times higher in Asian than non-Asian births in England and Wales during the period 1974–1983.[29] Reasons for this high figure include underdiagnosis of rubella in the Asian mother during pregnancy and different attitudes of Asian women to termination of pregnancy for an affected child. It is likely that this trend will change for the better in future as the preventive health services improve their coverage of the susceptible populations and as MMR vaccination increases herd immunity.

Other conditions often associated with the ethnic minority groups

Tuberculosis

There is a large variation in incidence of the disease among ethnic minority groups, but there is no evidence to suggest that there is a genetic susceptibility to the disease or that it is a racial problem. Social and environmental factors are major contributory factors to its spread. Highly susceptible groups, such as immigrants into more prosperous countries, show a progressive fall in incidence, and rates come to resemble that of the host country.[30,31]

Umbilical hernia

This is more common in the Afro-Caribbean and African children under the age of 5 years. It may rarely require surgery if very large or persisting longer than 6 years.

Keloid formation

This is more likely to develop in the Afro-Caribbean skin after surgery or burns than in other racial groups.

Premature thelarche (premature breast development)

This may occur as early as 4–5 years in Afro-Caribbean girls. If there are no other signs of puberty, the condition does not require further investigation, and parents only need reassurance. Premature pubarche (development of pubic hair) may also be an isolated finding in Afro-Caribbean girls under 6 years and needs no investigations unless associated with breast development.

Education

There is considerable concern within education circles about the academic underachievement of immigrant or minority group children in mainstream schools. Rutter and Madge in a review of the literature reported that children from immigrant families, especially West Indian, were more likely to be in lower streams in school and less likely to be selected for academic programmes in secondary schools.[32] Other studies have also highlighted the poor achievement of West Indian pupils compared with indigenous children. When Yule and colleagues tested a sample of West Indian and indigenous British school children aged between 10 and 12 years in a London borough, they found that the former achieved lower scores than the indigenous children, using non-verbal reasoning, SRA Reading Test, WISC shortform, and Neale Analysis of Reading.[33] The black people's Progressive Association and the Redbridge Community Relations Council also found that white indigenous 10 and 11 year olds scored higher than West Indians and Asians using the silent reading B Test. The more recent reports by Rampton[34] and Swann[35] reaffirm the same findings of underachievement of black ethnic minority children

compared to their white peers. Although the Rampton Report indicated that when socioeconomic status is taken into account the achievement of West Indian or Afro-Caribbean children appears to rise by 50% in relation to their white peers, the survey did not standardize the children's performances for such factors as parental education or social class, all of which have important influences on children's educational achievements.

The study of Scarr and others[36] elegantly charts the cumulative deficit in the achievements of West Indians compared with other groups from birth to 18 years in a British midlands town, without attempting to draw conclusions about possible reasons for this state of affairs. Among the many reasons advanced to explain underachievement of West Indian school children there is some evidence that racism, both intentional and unintentional, may have a direct and important bearing on the performance of West Indian children in schools.[37] Driver has suggested that factors such as gender, socioeconomic status, the ethnic composition of the school and the school ethos in relation to academic work affect pupils' performance at 16 plus examinations.[38] In his ethnographic study of five secondary schools in England, his overall findings were that:

1 Afro-Caribbean girls obtained better results than Afro-Caribbean boys with the exception of mathematics and physics.
2 Asian and Afro-Caribbean girls showed a higher level of persistence through examinations than English girls.
3 The only school in which Afro-Caribbean pupils performed *less* well than Asian and white pupils was a school where Afro-Caribbeans comprised between 5% and 8% of the total school population. In the other four schools, the Afro-Caribbean population was 25%–30%.

Thus it would appear that there is a differential educational performance between the boys and girls and the composition of the minority group in the schools, but this would need to be examined in a larger number of schools. Factors such as parental education, attitudes to education and parental expectation of *teachers* would be very important factors to correlate with school performance of ethnic minorities. It has been observed that the attitude frequently adopted by first generation West Indian parents is to leave discipline and educational matters to school teachers. The expectation from schools is usually quite different. Active participation of parents in helping children with homework is expected by some. Parents may be expected to attend open days in the schools to discuss their children's progress. The relevance of this activity may not be appreciated or given a high priority by the West Indian parent, and this attitude may be regarded by the teacher as negative and uncaring about the child's education. This perpetuates the pre-judice that may already exist; the negative attitudes thus created do not help to advance the West Indian child's education.

The Swann Report concludes that because there is no single cause for underachievement there can be no single solution. In contrast, children of Asian and African groups may be under considerable pressure to succeed. This happens more commonly in the middle classes who have high financial and educational expectations. The child may react to this pressure with psy-chosomatic illness, abdominal pains, headaches or school refusal. The problem may be compounded if the child's school progress is being hampered by lin-guistic difficulties and he may elect to be mute. Children may be expected to help with housework or in the shop or restaurant owned by the family. Clearly the long hours may interfere with the child's alertness in school with resulting tiredness. The school doctor and nurse need to be aware of the family expectations, lifestyle and the child's school progress when fatigue or inattention is noted by the school staff.

Conclusion

The ethnic minority population in the UK is not homo-geneous. It is composed of diverse groups of people characterized by different cultural practices, lan-guages, religious beliefs and skin colour, though the latter is *not* necessarily true of all ethnic minorities. Within the sub-groups of the ethnic minorities the usual social class structures also exist.

Paediatric surveillance within the community depends on mutual understanding of practitioner and patient (client group). The greater the cultural distance between practitioner and patient, the more difficult communication becomes. Communication problems are time-consuming and may lead to reduced compliance, and ineffective treatment and health education. Failure to understand lifestyles, naming systems, logic behaviour and language diffi-culties can lead to irritation on both sides. Non-white minority groups who face racial discrimination in society at large may read this impatience as an uncar-ing or racist attitude.

Problems can be minimized if health professionals give consideration to the following:

1 Migration – first or second generation migrants.
2 Social and cultural background of the group.
3 Family lifestyles.
4 Language, communication and naming systems.
5 Child-rearing practices.
6 Dietary customs.
7 The availability and use of the health service and other local amenities by ethnic minorities.

In recent years, some health authorities have taken initiatives to improve communication between health care workers and ethnic minorities and have intro-duced link worker schemes, a list of which is available at the Department of Health. Information on general health care, in appropriate languages, which is cultu-rally acceptable, has been prepared and made avail-able in several health districts, including Bolton and West Birmingham, Brent, North Manchester, Coven-try, Lewisham and Wandsworth and Central Manche-ster Health Authorities. Through inner city partnership funds, various projects are being pursued to improve health care provisions in the ethnic mino-rities. Notable examples are to be found in speech therapy projects in central Birmingham and the City and Hackney Health Authorities. In the latter, the sig-nificant language delay in children who do not have English as their first language has been tackled by re-examination of existing services, and their suitability for ethnic minorities. In central Birmingham, the health authority has an interpreter for the speech therapy unit who assists in counselling and the adaptation of treat-ment procedures for the ethnic minorities.[17] Efforts to improve paediatric surveillance in ethnic minority groups will be enhanced by implementation of the Children Act 1989.

References

1 Population Trends No. 46 UK Office of Population Censuses and Surveys. Ethnic minority populations in Great Britain. London: HMSO, 1986.
2 Japhet, R. *The Jewish Yearbook*. London: Jewish Chron-icle Publications, 1989.
3 Black, J.A. Paediatric problems in the Asian commu-nity. *Update* 1987; **35:** 1300–1309.
4 Black, J.A. *The New Paediatrics – Child Health in Ethnic Minorities*. London: *Br Med J*, 1983.
5 Ellis, J. Foster kids in the culture gap. In: J. Cheetham, *et al.* eds. *Social and Community Work in a Multi-Racial Society*, London: Harper and Row, 1981.
6 Green, S.D.R., Lealman, G.T., Aslam, M., Davis, S.S. Surma and blood lead concentrations. *Public Health* 1979; **93:** 371–6.
7 Fernando, N.P., Healy, M.A., Aslam, M., Davis, S.S., Hussein, A. Lead poisoning and traditional practices: consequences for world health. A study in Kuwait. *Public Health* 1981; **95:** 250–60.
8 Warley, M.A., Blackledge, P., O'Gorman, P. Lead poi-soning from eye cosmetics. *Br Med J* 1968; **1:** 117.
9 Kemm, J., Douglas, J., Sylvester, V. A survey of infant feeding practices by Afro-Caribbean mothers in Bir-mingham. *Proc, Nutr Soc* 1986; **45:** 87a.
10 Grindulis, H., Scott, P.H., Belton, N.R., Wharton, B.A. Combined deficiency of iron and vitamin D in Asian toddlers. *Arch Dis Child* 1986; **61:** 843–848.
11 Dawar, A. Food for thought in work with immigrants. *Nursing Mirror* 1979; **149:** 27–30.

12 Harris, R.J., Armstrong, D., Al, R., Loynes, A. A nutritional survey of Bangladeshi children under 5 years in the London Borough of Tower Hamlets. *Arch Dis Child* 1983; **58:** 428–432.

13 Jivani, S.K.M. The practice of infant feeding among Asian immigrants. *Arch Dis Child* 1978; **53:** 69–73.

14 Black, J. Paediatrics among ethnic minorities. Asian families II: conditions that may be found in the children. *Br Med J* 1984; **290:** 830–833.

15 Aukett, A., Wharton, B. Nutrition of Asian children; infants and toddlers. In: Cruikshank, J., Beevers, D., eds. *Ethnic Factors in Health and Disease*. London: Butterworths, 1989.

16 Rona, R.J., Chinn, S. National study of health and growth: social and biological factors associated with height of children from ethnic groups living in England. *Ann Hum Biol* 1986; **13:** 453–471.

17 National Association of Health Authorities and Trusts. *Action not Words. A Strategy to Improve Health Services for Black and Minority Ethnic Groups*. London: NAHAT, 1988.

18 Tarnow-Mordi, W.O., Pickering, D. Missed jaundice in black infants; a hazard. *Br Med J* 1983; **286:** 463–464.

19 Ehrhardt, P. Iron deficiency in young Bradford children from different ethnic groups. *Br Med J* 1986; **292:** 90–93.

20 Aukett, M.A., Parks, Y.A., Scott, P.H., Wharton, B.A. Treatment with iron increases weight gain and psychomotor development. *Arch Dis Child* 1986; **61:** 843–848.

21 Oppe, T.E. Medical problems of coloured immigrant children in Britain. *Proc R Soc Med* 1964; **57:** 321–323.

22 Groell, K.M., Sweet, E.M., Logan, R.W., *et al*. Florid and subclinical rickets among immigrant children in Glasgow. *Lancet* 1976; i: 1141–1148.

23 Ford, J.A., McIntosh, W.B., Butterfield, R., *et al*. Clinical and subclinical vitamin D deficiency in Bradford children. *Arch Dis Child* 1976; **51:** 939–943.

24 O'Hare, A.E., Uttley, W.S., Belton, N.R., *et al*. Persisting vitamin D deficiency in the Asian adolescent. *Arch Dis Child* 1984; **59:** 766–770.

25 Ward, P.S., Drakeford, J.P., Milton, J., James, J.A. Nutritional rickets in Rastafarian children. *Br Med J* 1982; **285:** 1242–1243.

26 Zukerman, A.J. Perinatal transmission of hepatitis B. *Arch Dis Child* 1984; **59:** 1008–9.

27 Peckham, C.S., Tookey, P., Nelson, D.B., Coleman, J., Morris, N. Ethnic minority women and congenital rubella. *Br Med J* 1983; **287:** 129–130.

28 Crawford, C.M. Congenital rubella in babies of South Asian women in England and Wales. Letter. *Br Med J* 1987; **294:** 1099–1100.

29 Miller, E., Nicoll, A., Rousseau, S.A., *et al*. Congenital rubella in babies of South Asian women in England and Wales: an excess and its causes. *Br Med J* 1987; **294:** 737–739.

30 Sutherland, I., Springett, V.H., Nunn, A.J. Changes in tuberculosis notification rates in ethnic groups in England between 1971 and 1978/9. *Tubercle*, 1984; **65:** 83–91.

31 Nunn, A.J., Darbyshire, J., Fox, W., *et al*. Changes in annual tuberculosis notification rates between 1978/79 and 1983 for the population of Indian subcontinent ethnic origin resident in England. *J Epidemiol Comm Hlth* 1986; **40:** 357–363.

32 Rutter, M., Madge, N. *Cycles of Disadvantage*. London: Heinemann Educational, 1976.

33 Yule, W., Berger, M., Rutter, M., Yule, B. Children of West Indian immigrants II: intellectual performance and reading attainment. *J Child Psychol Psychiatr* 1975; **16:** 1–17.

34 Rampton, A. *West Indian Children in our Schools: Interim Report of the Committee of Inquiry into the Education of Children from Ethnic Minority Communities*. London: HMSO, 1981.

35 The Swann Report. *Education for All. The Report of the Committee of Inquiry into the Education of Children from Ethnic Minority Groups*. London: HMSO, 1985.

36 Scarr, S., Caparulo, B.K., Ferdman, B.M., Tower, R.B., Caplan, J. Developmental status and school achievements of minority and non-minority children from birth to eighteen years in a British midlands town. *Br J Devel Psychol* 1983; **1:** 31–48.

37 Mares, P., Henley, A., Baxter, C. *Health Care in Multiracial Britain*. Cambridge: Health Education Council and National Extension College, 1985.

38 Driver, G. *Beyond Underachievement*. London: Commission for Racial Equality, 1980.

6.6 Record systems

Mario Cordeiro

I have six faithful serving men,
they taught me all I knew.
Their names were What and Why and When
and Where and How and Who.   Rudyard Kipling

In this chapter the word *information* is used many times. How should it be defined? Possibilities include 'the content of a message that is able to trigger an action' (Rosnay)[1] or 'a representation of reality' (Knox)[2]. The first definition, being longitudinal and prospective, allows us to think in terms of the future whereas the second, being transverse, is limited to the description of the present. On the other hand, the first definition agrees with the principles of the communication theory which states that the only information which actually exists is that in which reality can be described in the Kiplingesque terms of *what, who, when, why, where* and *how*.[3]

Historical background

Evidence of events, ideas, facts and fiction predates written history. Even before the introduction of writing, man left his fingerprint on rocks, stones and the walls of caves, being surely conscious of the importance of this act for future generations.

Medical records and data have been available for thousands of years. Acts of sorcery, description of illnesses, therapeutic measures are widespread in prehistorical graphic representations.

The invention of writing produced a boom in data registration. In the Bible, for instance, one can find many references to diseases, epidemics, forms of prevention and treatment and also data on some population characteristics.

Vital statistics are the maps and milestones of public health; as early as 1250 BC in Egypt, Rameses II's kingdom first developed an organized registration system. The implementation of this sytem is believed not to have been universal throughout the kingdom but where the system did apply, births and deaths were probably fully recorded. In Rome, five centuries BC, citizens were required to give account of newly born children within 30 days of birth and officials were appointed throughout the provinces to record the relevant facts on births, adolescents and deaths. In the eighth century AD these registrations became compulsory in Japan, and in 1532 in England an ordinance required weekly records of burials containing data on the number of deaths from plague. Soon after, all weddings, baptisms and burials began to be systematically recorded. The Church played an important role in these first systems of data collection, which soon spread to other countries and were broadened to keep a wider spectrum of data.

Although the amount of information that has been stored throughout the centuries is enormous, nowadays the amount of data that one single person can collect on a single day is also vast.

In the medical profession, the collection and storage of data have become a routine procedure, accompanying the increasing importance of epidemiology and research into scientific validation of procedures, and in monitoring and evaluation of programmes of health care (audit). These are constant requirements from those who care about honest work and quality of services.

In modern societies, a huge percentage of the working population produces information every day. It has been estimated that every year there is an increase of 10% in the amount of information produced worldwide. However only 3 to 4% of this new information is considered to be even minimally useful.

The possibilities of data collection are ever increasing, one might even say endless. However, it is an old saying, that 'quantity spoils quality'.

Why collect data?

We may collect data for two main reasons: (1) for the care of the individual child; (2) for the care of children in general through more efficient and efficacious use of resources.

So, we must bear in mind that data collection in child health, independent of *how*, *where* and *when* we do it, should always aim to benefit the child and his or her family.

It is very difficult to define what kind of data should be collected, as problems vary from child to child and from one region or country to another. However, there are certain standard indicators shared by almost all countries, which allow the comparison of health status and trends so far as sex and age groups, years, areas, occupational groups and social classes are concerned, either within a single country or between countries. This obviously implies not only a standardization of methods of data collection, namely as to how the numerators and denominators are chosen, but also strict definitions concerning the 'nature' of the data to be collected. The World Health Organization has issued recommendations and guidelines for international use, related to how several health indicators should be collected. The *International Statistical Classification of Diseases, Injuries and Causes of Deaths* (ICD), the *International List of Causes of Death* and the various mortality rates are good examples of this.[4]

Although we may collect data just for fun or for very personal purposes, this should never be the main reason. On the contrary, any system of information should be devised according to the aims that have been established for the child health services and professionals. Table 6.11 shows some goals for improvement of services for all children based on which we can then choose health indicators and systems of data collection and storage.

Table 6.11 Aims of child health services

1	To decrease mortality
2	To decrease acute morbidity
3	To decrease chronic morbidity
4	To decrease inequalities in health
5	To promote and support parenthood
6	To promote health and healthy lifestyles
7	To increase primary prevention (by increasing immunization uptake rates, fluoride supplementation, accident prevention, etc)
8	To increase secondary prevention (by making an early diagnosis through screening and early and correct sign and symptoms evaluation, referral and therapy)
9	To increase tertiary prevention (by diminishing the consequences of disease and hospitalization, supporting chronically ill children and their families, etc)
10	To increase educational achievement, professional choices and fulfilments, quality of life and the role of each individual in society.

Using another perspective, data can be collected in order to:

- Measure and analyse problems and trends.
- Look for causes.
- Predict needs and plan services.
- Monitor and audit services.
- Compare the cost and benefits of programmes.
- Serve as a tool for professional training.
- Serve as a tool for research.

How to collect information

The first steps necessary for collecting information are to define:

1 What sort of items or health problems we want to have information about and our reasons.
2 What sort of health indicators we want to use, based on the items and problems in 1.
3 How these indicators can best be collected, so that minimum standards of quality, reliability and feasibility are assured. This standardization of procedures, methods, regular assessment and evaluation of their quality and pertinacity are fundamental.[5]

A further step of utmost importance is the sharing and the feedback of information to those who collected it. People responsible for collecting information must be involved in, and understand, the importance to them and the children they look after, of the information being collected. One reason for a decrease in the quality of the data collection process is the lack of motivation which can result from performing a routine, unimaginative activity without fully comprehending its aims and without knowledge of its results and consequences.[6]

Following data collection it is then necessary to take a critical approach to the data that have been registered, in order to detect any mistakes or misunderstanding and to avoid the consequences of, for instance, official publication of wrong data or the planning of activities based on incorrect information.

Data can be obtained systematically in three ways:

1 By registration which may be defined as the continuous and permanent recording of the occurrence and the characteristics of events, either for their value as legal documents or for their usefulness as a source of information.
2 By enumeration represented by the census of population or by surveys.
3 By special returns such as the notification of infectious diseases or the use of hospital case records.

In some countries, like the UK and most other European countries, the ultimate responsibility for this task of data collection rests with the state. Registration is usually organized in a pyramidal way, from the local to the district and national levels.

However, at each level one can identify structures, procedures and outcomes, which are integrated both vertically and horizontally. The evaluation of each level is closely related to evaluations performed at other levels. So, the degree of quality at each level can determine the success or failure of the whole system and consequently lead to incorrect assessments and decisions. The individuals responsible for each of the levels of decision have to concern themselves with the production and the trustworthiness of the health care procedure data. This will be improved if procedure data are closely connected with result data.

Information storage

Generally speaking, in most hospitals and clinics data are still kept in manually designed individual files. Being relatively scarce these data can be pooled together at a regional or national level at least according to minimum criteria of reliability. In every country, professionals are overwhelmed by their daily work and by the burden of clinical activities, and most data which are collected are designed only to profit the individual patient and the individual doctor or nurse.

Population registers, developed according to the local district or country, hold basic information on mortality (figures and causes), preventive measures (immunizations, fluoride supplementation, screening procedures), use of services (attendance rates, hospital admissions), households and families, marriage and divorce, education, employment, income and wealth, expenditure and resources, health and professional services, housing, environment, leisure and social participation.

The essential question is whether we need more data to perform our tasks or, on the contrary, we are still underusing the information that is already available. It seems wise that before trying to define and implement new data and develop information systems to hold these, we should have a full knowledge of what is already available, its degree of reliability, and how well we are using it for our objectives.

It is well known that data suffer a process of loss of quality due to errors and failures which occur all the way up from the initial source to its final user. Nevertheless, any change in the present record system should prove either its need or that it represents a better alternative to what already exists.

Moreover, the more information we collect the more space we need for its storage, and the more organized and practical the storage system must be.

Computers

Computers have almost overnight become an indispensable tool and their importance parallels the importance of the information revolution. They can store and manipulate information and hold lists of complex instructions and perform them sequentially and automatically; they are capable of doing comparisons and logical operations with data from various sources; they can link data from various sites within a real-time network and can also perform other tasks, like word-processing, statistical analysis or drawing. Computers can do nothing that the human brain and hands cannot, but perform in seconds the same task that would consume an entire lifetime when done manually. They may, however, also suffer from 'virus infections', and although this is part of a very particular end-of-cen-

Table 6.12 Shows some of the applications for computers in health services:

Patient registration and identification
Immunization call and recall
Screening procedures call and recall
Screening procedures monitoring and evaluation
Surveillance of at-risk groups and default monitoring
Surveillance of chronically ill children and default
monitoring
Prescription printing
Total medical record and summary
Personal medical attendant's report
Referral letters
Patient instructions
Appointments scheduling and recording
Standard personalized letters
Drug interactions and contraindications
Problem classification and code
Research, audit and workload studies
Business administration
Communication with other health or educational facilities

tury biological war which falls beyond the scope of this section, it has to be considered as it may cause the loss of entire sets of data if preventive back-up measures are not taken. Here, like in so many other fields of paediatrics and child health, prevention is better than cure.

So far as information collection and storage are concerned, we have to ask 'Why do we want to use a computer?' This relates closely to 'Why do we want information?'

The main use of computers is for rapid and complicated calculations on a large number of pieces of information. They are of less use for recording general clinical observations and data on individual cases.[7]

Therefore, computers can be used for:

- Basic registration information.
- Clinical practice information such as repeat prescribing, disease and follow-up registers, clinical summaries, morbidity and prevention measures.
- Research and evaluation of structures, processes and outcomes.
- Professional training and research.[8]

Computers also represent a huge temptation for collecting useless data. When designing a study using for instance a questionnaire, there may be a trend to add more and more questions in order to get the maximum information from the study, ending up with a decrease of quality and reliability of the answers and resulting in much harder work when coping with and analysing the data. In fact, the more important pieces of information and parameters may disappear completely among all the spurious, useless data that an uncontrolled curiosity forced us to collect. This problem is worse when using computers, because, on the one hand input and output of data are much easier but, on the other hand, the drawing of conclusions is still work done by the human mind, not the computer.

The problem of confidentiality

The problem of confidentiality has increased as the use of computers has become more widespread. It is possible that a person might sometimes be suspicious of computers, almost as if they could use the stored information for their own (evil) pleasure or purposes. Computers are, *hélas*, harmless. HAL 9000, Kubrick's computer in *2001 – a Space Odyssey*, is only a character of science fiction. Problems that may actually arise, like the breaking of confidentiality, are alas products of human culpability rather than the 'perverted mind' of hardware and software. Computers are after all only information processors, and left to themselves they will do nothing! The misuse of information by people for unethical or even malicious purposes can happen not only with computers, but with all types and systems of information storage. It is well known, for example, that access to a patient's clinical non-computerized record – such as those which exist in most hospitals and clinics – by a non-professional person, is extremely easy both at hospital or primary care levels. Computer information, on the contrary, is more likely to be well protected from foreign eyes if the software is cautiously programmed with codes for different levels of access. Data protection is in reality far easier when dealing with computers.

Another point about which there are sometimes arguments concerns the question, 'to whom does the data belong?' No matter if we store it in clinical files, videotape recorders or computers, this question has only one answer. So far as child health is concerned, the parents and the child himself should be considered as the legal owners of information which they obviously have to share with the professionals, not the contrary. Professionals remain the users of information as a means for child health promotion and maintenance, not as a goal in itself.

The British Data Protection Act,[9] which ensured that people have full access to any computer information held on them or their dependants, is an example of a necessary step in the right direction. So is the EC proposal for community action on advanced computers in medicine in Europe (pilot project 87/C 356/05), in which human dignity and the right to a humanized medical/patient relationship is stressed and warnings are given concerning the 'robotization of medicine' and the dangers of 'telemedicine'.

The access of parents (or the child) to computer registers is perhaps today not as easy as we should like it to be. However, a system should be devised where all information is always actively shared with the parents, so as to ensure both that data are correct and to get permission to pass appropriate information to those other professionals (e.g. in the educational or social services) also responsible for the care of the child.

In order to overcome naturally suspicious attitudes towards these 'evil machines', it is advisable to assure patients that:

- All personal data held about their child on the computer are confined specifically to the needs of the child.
- No unauthorized person can gain access to it at any time.
- At no time is the computer system connected to telephone or other network system that allows the transmission of the patient's pesonal data out of the service without permission.
- When data are transmitted out of the service – for a population basic database, at a regional or nationwide level, or within a research project – they are anonymous and lack information by which the individuals can be identified.
- At no time will data be transferred to a third party without fully informed written consent of the parents.

Computerization of a service or of an institution represents an important investment, which must be performed in logical steps according to a previously planned programme. This should be based on known needs, demands and resources. This economic investment is still a limiting factor in countries where health budgets are small. Nevertheless, it can be anticipated that the use of computers will continue to rise even at a local level, and that professionals will progressively acquire the necessary expertise to take on most computerized systems of information. Specialists in programming will also develop new and better user-friendly software programmes, easier to deal with and less subject to errors in the data-input process.

Finally, when deciding to buy or use a computer, the subject should be first fully discussed with a specialist, to ensure optimal choice of hardware and software, both in economic terms and as to whether it can adequately and fully achieve the aims for which it is being purchased.

Parent-held child health records

Philosophically, parent-held child health and development records must be a desirable step forward, notwithstanding that there will always be a need for a certain amount of information to be held by professionals. However, there is no reason why even this information should not be shared[10] and from November 1991 the Access to Health Records Act gave individuals the right of access, subject to certain exemptions, to information recorded in manually held records.[11]

This kind of record already exists in many countries, where there is a large overlap with the clinical files. In spite of the differences in relation to quantity and quality of information stored, design and attractiveness, they all share the most important fact that they are held by the parents, belong to them and implicitly recognize their right, as primary care givers to their children, to be informed about their child's health status and to be the main owner of this information. This conceptual aspect is extremely important.*

The theoretical advantages of a parent-held child health record are the following:[12]

1 The record is available whenever and wherever a child is seen, at home, at the surgery, at the child health clinic, at the hospital outpatients or in the emergency room. This point is particularly interesting in countries where child health is carried out by several systems and subsystems, public and private, forcing the child to be seen by a multiplicity of doctors and other professionals.
2 The parents, as the primary health care givers to their children are involved in recording their own observations on their child's health and development. The fact is that only 20% of children's health symptoms are actually referred to a doctor or a nurse, the rest being dealt with by the parents without the aid of doctors or nurses.

*We have obviously to consider the amount and content of information that is given as well as the way information is transferred from the professionals to the parents or the child.

3 The document acts as an active discussion document, rather than passively sitting in child health clinics between visits. Child health warrants a multidisciplinary approach, especially when children suffer from longstanding illnesses or any form of handicap. This implies observations by multiple agents, health, educational and social, who are not confined to child health clinics or hospitals.

4 Confidentiality rests with the parents so they can show the record to whomever looks after their child, childminder, playgroup leader or granny. Data and information should belong to the individuals and not to professionals or services.

5 When the parent and child move from one area to another the child health record is immediately available to the new health care professionals. This prevents gaps and avoids duplications and overlaps, so far as, for example, child health surveillance, screening procedures and referrals are concerned.

6 The document can act as a reminder as to when the child needs to be taken for a child health check. This improves parents' responsibilities and duties, a counterpart to their rights relating to their children.

7 Parents are able to correct any misinformation on their child's record card. Medical observations and routine checks, especially in the developmental and behaviour areas, may give rise to a significant number of false-positives and false-negatives. As parents or carers spend much more time with the child in its own normal environment, they can more readily perceive problems or suspect disturbance earlier than a professional in a 10 or 15 minute annual examination in a child health clinic, no matter how competent and trained that professional might be. On the other hand, parents are able to refute suspicions that may incorrectly arise about the child's development.

8 The access to useful medical information by other appropriate services, including educational and social services is easier. It can also serve for legal purposes to demonstrate that a programme of child care was delivered, or in court to support care proceedings.

9 Useful medical information can be translated into other languages, in countries where ethnic minorities are significant.

The hypothetical disadvantages could be:

1 Records might get lost more frequently than when held in child health clinics.

2 Sensitive information concerning such subjects as non-accidental injury, convulsions or developmental delay, being recorded in the child-health record could indelibly label the child and his family before society.

We have carried out research on the Portuguese parent-held child health record and our findings agree with those from other authors: parents very rarely lose their records and the reasons for not taking them to health facilities are closely related to professionals' attitudes. These attitudes include underestimating or even deprecating the importance of the record, exemplified by situations in which the record has simply not been asked for by the doctor or the nurse. This lack of interest shown by some of those who should fill them in and ask for them at every consultation is a painful but no less evident reality. This is undoubtedly associated with the loss of power that sharing information represents. Information means power, especially when it is not shared with anyone and is used as a trump card in human relationships. Doctors and other health professionals should recognize that this attitude is neither ethical nor justifiable, as sharing information will not lead to a decrease in the need for professional's help or underestimation of the professional's roles. Parents should be regarded as partners in child health, linked by the needs of the child, and the medical attitude of humbleness and availability will, no doubt, result in greater efficiency and professional satisfaction.[13]

Conclusions

Information collected by careful research serves to provide a full knowledge of needs and demands, to draw up programmes, to audit, monitor and evaluate these programmes and to validate scientifically medical activities, procedures and methods. It can also serve training purposes.

Data collection is a common, routine task but unless performed within certain guidelines using a lot of common sense it can end up as a flood of data that turns out to be useless. Therefore, information has to have its relevance selected and its quality filtered.

Some standard data are internationally recognized as useful and their collection is routinely performed in most countries. International cooperation is very likely to be enhanced as a result of increased political and economic cooperation between countries.

At a local level or for research purposes, it is necessary to define objectives before building up any new information system. At the same time, information already available should be gathered and approached in a critical way.

Quantity spoils quality and worse than having no information at all is to base our activities on incorrect or inaccurate data.

Computers are very helpful tools to deal with the amount of information that is required nowadays. However, the benefits of their use should be optimized. This is only achieved by using a cautious, multidisciplinary approach and not losing sight of the objectives that were originally set. The boom in the use of computers will continue for many years.

We need to take into account the increased concern about the issue of confidentiality, as ethics and the rights of citizens gain more importance. Computers do not threaten confidentiality, if they are well programmed and properly used. Moreover, confidentiality can be broken with any information system.

Information represents power so that children and their parents should be considered as the legal owners of this power so far as information related to them is concerned. Parents, as primary health care givers to their children, should be considered as partners in child health and have full access to information that is held on their children.

The implementation of parent-held child health records, either as a registration tool or associated with various other clinical records, is an important step in the right direction and has been proved in those countries where its use is routine to be feasible and very advantageous.

Every national health policy should include an organized information policy.

Efforts should be primarily concentrated on a critical approach to the use of information and to increasing the reliability of data that have already been collected. New data collection and storage systems imply expenditures and all options should be carefully considered in relation to the persons – in this case the children and their families – that our work aims to benefit.

References

1 Rosnay, J. *Le macroscope. Vers une vision globale.* Paris: Editions du Seuil, 1975.

2 Knox, E.G. *Epidemiology in Health Care Planning.* Oxford: Oxford University Press, 1979.

3 Briz, T. Os cuidados de saúde primários e a microinformática: o que se está a passar e o que há a esperar. (Primary health care and computers: what is going on and what is to be expected.) *Rev Port Clin Geral* 1989; **6:** 258–65.

4 Logan, W.P.D., Lambert, P.M. Vital statistics. In: Hobson, W., ed. *The Theory and Practice of Public Health.* 4th edn. London: Oxford University Press, 1975: 8–29.

5 Polnay, L., Hull, D. *Community Paediatrics.* Edinburgh: Churchill Livingstone, 1985.

6 Macfarlane, A. The use of computers in child health. Paper presented to the First Seminar on Community Paediatrics, Lisbon, May 1988.

7 Willis, A., Stewart, T. *Computers – a Guide to Choosing and Using.* Oxford: Oxford Medical Publications, 1989.

8 Justo, C. Justificação e objectivos do sistema de informação em saúde. (Reasons and objectives for a health information system) *Rev Port Clin Geral* 1989; **6:** 251–7.

9 Data Protection Act 1984.

10 Joint Working Party on Child Health Surveillance. *Health for All Children – a Programme for Child Health Surveillance,* Hall, D., ed. Oxford: Oxford University Press, 1991.

11 Access to Health Records Act 1990.

12 Saffin, K., Macfarlane, A. Parent-held child health and development records. *Matern Child Hlth* 1988; **13:** 288–291.

13 Cordeiro, M.J.G. Boletim de Saúde Infantil – sua utilização na urgência de Pediatria de três hopitais de Lisboa (Parent held child health record – its use in the paediatric A & E departments of the three central hospitals of Lisbon). *Saúde Infantil* 1990; **2:** 143–51.

Acknowledgements

I would like to express my gratitude to Dr Aidan Macfarlane for all his pertinent ideas and commentaries and for the English revision of the original draft.

Chapter 7

Preventive medicine

7.1 Prevention

Sue Jenkins

Prevention is a key component of community paediatrics, underpinning the aims and philosophy of most aspects of the service.

Efforts to promote child and family health are set against a background of government policies, with a growing body of evidence confirming what has long been known, that material and structural factors such as income and housing affect health far more than medical services.[1] Currently, in the UK, policies do not demonstrate a commitment to supporting families with young children. Housing policies contribute to the problems of homelessness. There is underfunding of education services and day care facilities, child benefits are inadequate, and the numbers of families living in poverty are increasing.[2] Against this background it is clear that prevention in many broad areas remains an uphill struggle.

This can be compared with, for example, Scandinavian countries where government priority is given to supporting healthier lifestyles, anti-poverty policies, and pre-school day care.[3] It should prove possible to monitor the effects of such policies (or lack of them) on markers of the health of the child population, particularly on the reduction of inequalities in health between different sectors of the population.[4] Policies for prevention need to recognize the link between social conditions and behaviour and health rather than focusing solely on the individual.

There is a wide spectrum of prevention to consider, from specifically focused medical aspects such as fetal screening for a biochemical abnormality to broad approaches such as accident prevention which will involve many other agencies in addition to health services. Many aspects of prevention will be discussed in detail later in this chapter in relation to specific issues.

The aim of all children's services, particularly community paediatric services, should be to promote optimal health and well-being in childhood in order that children grow up to fulfil their maximum potential. Clearly medical services and health workers can only play a small part in this, and most strategies for prevention and health promotion involve government and other agencies, of which the key ones include social services, education authorities, the voluntary sector, and housing, environmental health and leisure departments of local authorities.

There are specific areas where considerable progress in prevention has been made, and some of these will be considered here. Prevention can be considered under several headings and some definitions may be useful.

Primary prevention: the prevention of the occurrence of disease or injury.
Secondary prevention: halting the development or progress of a disease or disorder by early detection and intervention.

Tertiary prevention: impeding the progress of established disease or disability by appropriate treatment or management.

Examples of primary prevention

Probably the most well established and cost effective example of primary prevention is the programme of immunization against the infectious diseases of childhood, which aims to eliminate diphtheria, tetanus, pertussis, polio, rubella, congenital rubella, measles and mumps by the year 2000. The setting of specified targets, and monitoring of immunization uptake both nationally and locally has had a positive effect both on uptake rates and notification of infectious diseases.[5] Immunization is a good example of primary prevention where cooperative working at all levels of staff within district health authorities is taking place within a framework of national policy and guidelines and supported by a media campaign orchestrated by the Health Education Authority.

Another good example of primary prevention is the prevention and reduction of injury by use of car seat belts and children's car restraints, now made compulsory by legislation after many years of campaigning by professionals and politicians concerned with accident prevention.

A third example is the prevention of iron deficiency anaemia in young children by appropriate nutritional advice and dietary education to parents in the first 2 years of life. This has been shown to be both practical and effective within a primary care setting,[6] and if widely applied by motivated staff could reduce the need for iron supplementation.

Examples of secondary prevention

A good example of this is the well established programme of screening for phenylketonuria and hypothyroidism in the neonatal period, using the Guthrie test. These screening procedures have been subjected to critical evaluation and are examples of carefully organized screening programmes known to be cost effective.[7]

The tests are done on over 95% of the newborn population, currently organized on a regional basis, with careful recording and follow up of all positive results. By early detection of these disorders, treatment is started before clinical signs of disease are manifest, thus preventing or reducing the likelihood of mental retardation in affected children.

In the near future it is likely that screening for other genetic disorders such as cystic fibrosis and galactosaemia may be introduced in order to initiate early and effective management of these diseases.

Screening for haemoglobinopathies particularly sickle cell and thalassaemia by cord blood analysis has been introduced in some districts with large populations at risk of these disorders. Overall in the UK the population at risk of having an abnormal haemoglobin is approximately 3.3%; several districts with large Afro-Caribbean populations have neonatal sickle cell screening programmes which aim to reduce morbidity and mortality among affected infants by early medical management and counselling of families.[8,9] The support of the local community is essential and must clearly be established before the introduction of such screening programmes in any district.

Another good example of secondary prevention would be screening all children for growth limiting disorders by ensuring that height measurement was included in routine pre-school surveillance programmes, as advocated by the Joint Working Party on Child Health Surveillance.[10]

The aim is to permit the early detection of conditions which limit growth, such as growth hormone deficiency (incidence 1 in 3–5000) and Turner's syndrome (incidence 1 in 2500 females), so that prompt treatment can ensure these children achieve optimal growth.

Examples of tertiary prevention

Here we can include many examples of good clinical management of established chronic diseases or disability which aim to prevent further complications, deterioration of functioning, or secondary handicaps. Within this one should of course include psychosocial aspects of management and approaches that support families and children in healthy psychological adaptation to the disease or disorder.

Physiotherapy for children with cerebral palsy has as one of its aims the maintenance of function and prevention of contractures and is one example of prevention in this category. Another is the use of regular prophylactic antibiotics for children with recurrent urinary infections and evidence of vesico-ureteric reflux, in order to prevent further infection and renal scarring.

On the psychosocial side, there is good evidence that the quality of relationships within the family is a major determinant of diabetic control, and in skilled hands good outcome is seen both in better control of the illness and improvements in family functioning.[11] This can be considered another example of tertiary prevention.

Prevention of brain damage

The main causes of manifestations of brain damage are well described in Chapter 10. The topic of prevention of brain damage is best approached by considering the preconceptual, antenatal, natal and postnatal periods and factors operating in these periods which may be modified.

Cerebral palsy is perhaps the commonest manifestation of brain damage and there has been much debate about prevention, with obstetric management for many years being considered the key to prevention. Despite improved obstetric standards and neonatal care, there has been little evidence of any decline in recent years in the incidence of either cerebral palsy or mental retardation, and it has become increasingly evident that prenatal causes are responsible for the majority of cases.[12,13]

Recent epidemiological research now supports the view that the importance of perinatal factors in causing cerebral palsy has been overestimated in the past.[14] There are associations between abnormal labour, birth asphyxia and cerebral palsy, but many infants with cerebral palsy have other malformations indicating prenatal causes.[15] Thus a major challenge remains for researchers and clinicians working in the field of prevention.

The antenatal period

Causes of brain damage early in the antenatal period include genetic, infective and environmental.

Genetic causes have long been recognized as potentially preventable, although the ethical issues involved are complex and difficult. Down syndrome is the commonest genetic cause of mental handicap, and is potentially preventable if one assumes that termination of an affected pregnancy is acceptable.

The main difficulty is that in order to be cost effective, screening for Down syndrome by amniocentesis or chorionic villus sampling is only offered in most places to mothers over the age of 36 years. While the risks of having an affected offspring rise with maternal age, justifying this approach, only one-third of children with Down syndrome are born to older mothers. However, there is now encouraging evidence that a combination of biochemical screening, using maternal alphafetoprotein and oestriol levels (which are low in the first and second trimester in pregnancies with a fetus with Down syndrome) as well as maternal age, can predict which mothers should be offered further investigation in the form of amniocentesis.[16] This biochemical screening approach is now being developed in relation to the first trimester of pregnancy, when chorionic villus sampling could subsequently be offered, reducing the physical and emotional consequences of late termination of pregnancy.[17]

Early prenatal diagnosis is also offered to parents where there has been a previously abnormal fetus or confirmed genetic disease in an older sibling. Recent advances in ultrasound techniques have also increased the range of antenatal diagnoses, including some such as disorders which may be associated with brain damage of the central nervous system. The first routine ultrasound examination of the fetus is usually performed at 16–18 weeks.

An increasing number of enzyme defects (around one hundred) can now be diagnosed antenatally. Prenatal diagnosis of an enzyme defect is generally only carried out for pregnancies known to be at high risk of a severe disorder for which there is no effective treatment. Either chorionic villus samples or amniotic cell cultures can be used.[18,19] Amniocentesis for high risk pregnancies is performed at 15–16 weeks' gestation; cells from the amniotic fluid are then cultured, and examined for suspected enzyme abnormalities or for karyotyping and chromosome analysis. Chorionic villus sampling, normally by the transvaginal route under ultrasound guidance, is performed at 9–11 weeks' gestation. Indications for this are maternal age, previous child affected with chromosome abnormality or metabolic disorder, and gene probe assessment. The results are usually available between 2 and 7 days from sampling, hence first trimester termination where appropriate can be performed.

Table 7.1 illustrates some of the advantages and disadvantages of chorionic villus sampling and amniocentesis. Amniocentesis may be carried out earlier (11–12 weeks) in experienced hands, but carries a fetal loss rate of 2% which is normally considered unacceptably high.

As with most investigations or interventions, the complication rate relates to the experience of the operator, and must be weighed against the risk to the fetus. Counselling of families is an essential prerequisite before embarking on any of these procedures.

Infective causes

The most common infective agents which can affect the developing fetus in the antenatal period are rubella, cytomegalovirus (CMV), toxoplasmosis and herpes simplex. All can cause brain damage.

Congenital rubella is an important cause of handicap and remains one of the major causes of congenital sensorineural deafness. It is preventable by

Table 7.1 Advantages and disadvantages of chorionic villus sampling and amniocentesis

	Chorionic villus biopsy	Amniocentesis
Age preformed	9–11 weeks	16 weeks
Results available	2–7 days	0–14 days
Termination	1st trimester	2nd trimester
Fetal loss rate	1.1–2%	0.5–1%
False positive result	1–1.8%	< 1%
False negative result	0.1%	0.06%

immunization, and the introduction of measles, mumps and rubella (MMR) vaccine for children between 12 and 18 months, in addition to the schoolgirl rubella immunization programme, aims to eradicate congenital rubella by the year 2000.

Congenital cytomegalovirus infection has an incidence in the UK of 0.3%, but only a very small proportion of babies are symptomatic and brain damaged in the neonatal period. Where primary infection is acquired during pregnancy, virus is transmitted to the fetus in only 30–40% of cases, and in only 10% of these will the fetus be damaged by the virus.[20,21] In asymptomatic babies, sensorineural deafness may occur, sometimes becoming progressive in the first 2 years of life. Prevention of CMV infection is not yet possible, since termination of infected pregnancies would result in the loss of many normal babies.

Congenital toxoplasmosis can affect infants when primary infection occurs in pregnancy. The risk of transmission to the fetus rises from 20% in the first trimester to 70% in the third trimester, and is often associated with severe mental and physical handicap. Chorioretinitis is also common. It is estimated that four-fifths of pregnant women in the UK are susceptible to toxoplasma infection, hence screening is not justified.[22]

Human infection occurs most commonly from eating undercooked meat (beef and lamb) or from cats, asymptomatic human infection being widespread in most communities. Prevention is theoretically possible by education, particularly advice to pregnant women regarding hygiene in relation to animal contacts, and adequate cooking of meat and meat products.

Herpes simplex infection is only rarely acquired transplacentally; most congenital infections are acquired during birth when the mother has had genital herpes. When there is a maternal history of herpetic vulvo-vaginitis, the favoured route of delivery is by elective caesarean section to prevent the baby acquiring infection.

Prenatal environmental causes of brain damage

1 ALCOHOL

The largest potentially preventable cause of mental handicap worldwide is the fetal alcohol syndrome (FAS). The teratogenic effects of alcohol are well documented, with the severity of damage being correlated with the extent of maternal alcoholism. The fetal alcohol syndrome includes prenatal growth retardation, central nervous system dysfunction, microcephaly and dysmorphology.[23] Mild to moderate learning difficulties become evident over the first few years of life.

The effects of alcohol on the fetus can almost certainly be compounded by effects of nutritional deficiencies and by smoking. Estimates of the incidence of fetal alcohol syndrome vary according to the population studied, being around 1 in 2500 births in the UK, 1 in 1000 in France and around 1 in 600 in Sweden and some parts of the USA. A particularly high incidence has been reported for North American Indians living in reservations.[24]

More recently reports from Sweden and the USA suggest that the incidence is decreasing, probably as a result of health education and wide media publicity around the issue of alcohol and pregnancy. In Sweden, concern over the incidence of FAS resulted in strategies for prevention being developed in many centres alongside a well developed system of antenatal care. Early detection and counselling as part of the antenatal programme has reduced the number of new cases of FAS being diagnosed.[25] Alcohol abuse during the second and third trimester appears to have greater consequences for growth and mental and behavioural development than abuse during the first trimester,[26] underlining the potential for intervention early in pregnancy.

Alcohol consumption among the young remains worryingly high, with recent studies indicating that children are beginning to use alcohol earlier, and drinking more heavily at younger ages than previously. Strategies for prevention need to be directed towards school children from primary age onwards.

2 NUTRITION

Optimum nutrition both in the preconceptual period and antenatally is generally believed to be important to the welfare of the developing fetus. Poor maternal nutrition has been found to be associated with lower birthweight and increased likelihood of pregnancy complications.[27] Attention is increasingly being focused on the role of fatty acids and trace minerals; it is hoped that a better understanding of their role at a cellular level may contribute to the prevention of premature delivery with its consequent risks to the health and development of the newborn.

Central nervous system malformations such as spina bifida are particularly thought to be related to deficiencies in folic acid and vitamins, and to be preventable by preconceptual vitamin supplementation.[28]

Preconceptual nutritional status is of crucial importance, due to the rapid growth in the nervous system of the developing embryo in the first 28 days of the conception, long before dietary advice in pregnancy will be given.

There is now a considerable literature around the topic of diet in the preconceptual period and its importance, with evidence that consumption of fresh fruit and vegetables is beneficial not only for the vitamin and mineral content but also for their antimutagenic qualities.

The groups most at risk are those on low incomes, and several studies by Maternity Alliance and The London Food Commission have shown the correlation between diet and income and the true cost of eating the healthy diet which is recommended during pregnancy.[29] Health education advice on dietary changes is unlikely to be effective unless it can be backed by very practical individual counselling on adapting shopping and cooking strategies within a low budget.

3 DRUGS

A number of drugs have for a long time been known to be teratogenic to the developing fetus, of which thalidomide is perhaps the best known example. In relation to congenital malformations, the period at greatest risk from drug effects is from the third to the eleventh week of pregnancy, although drugs may have harmful effects on the fetus at any stage of pregnancy. Advice is normally to restrict drug usage to those that are essential to the health of the mother.

Women with central nervous system disorders are at particular risk, as there are recently established links with the use of both sodium valproate[30] and benzodiazepine[31] with congenital malformations. Other antiepileptic drugs particularly phenytoin have long been known to be associated with an increased risk to the fetus, but clearly the risk to the mother of stopping or changing drugs must be weighed against the risk to the fetus. It is now estimated that congenital abnormalities occur in 7% of babies born to mothers taking anticonvulsants.

Certain antibiotics are contraindicated in pregnancy, particularly streptomycin and kanamycin which can cause eighth nerve damage and deafness. Tetracyclines are contraindicated due to the likelihood of causing discoloration of deciduous teeth and enamel hypoplasia. A full list of drugs which should be avoided during pregnancy, or used with caution, can be found in the British National Formulary.

Self-administered drugs in pregnancy can be harmful to the developing fetus and in some cases are associated with intrauterine growth retardation and with high rates of pregnancy complications. Substance abuse is however frequently compounded by poor nutrition, by alcohol and tobacco use, by poor antenatal care and other lifestyle factors. Prevention needs to take a broad approach and cessation or reduction of drug taking in pregnancy alone may be insufficient to protect the child. There is however encouraging evidence that withdrawal programmes for people who misuse drugs can be successfully managed in general practice.[32]

Drug effects on the fetus and child include congenital abnormalities, fetal and neonatal growth retardation, initial drug dependency and withdrawal effects, and neurobehavioural abnormalities.

Later damage may be inflicted by child abuse and neglect, and it is of interest and concern that in New York City in 1987 half the cases of child abuse which were dealt with were found to be associated with drug abuse in a parent or caretaker.

Prevention of brain damage at birth

For a long time it was thought that improving obstetric care, particularly the management of labour and delivery, together with optimal care of the newborn, would result in a significant decrease in the numbers of children with cerebral palsy. This has been shown to be overoptimistic, as rates of cerebral palsy have remained largely static in the past decade and, as stated earlier, there is increasing evidence that genetic and prenatal causes predominate.

However, hypoxia in full-term neonates is still associated with significant mortality and morbidity, and fits due to hypoxic ischaemic encephalopathy carry a poor prognosis. Research continues into the optimal management of hypoxia, and newer techniques such as cerebral blood flow imaging are proving helpful. The overall contribution of perinatal hypoxia to cerebral palsy is now thought to be in the order of 8–10%.

The rate of major disability and handicap among survivors of very preterm births is however increasing with better survival rates and emphasis is now more focused on preventing or delaying premature labour with the aim of reducing the numbers of very low birthweight survivors.

Major disabilities including cerebral palsy, blindness, deafness, and severe developmental delay occur in around 10% of extremely low birthweight children (below 1000 g) when these children are followed up to school age,[33] and there are also high rates of attention deficit and behavioural disorders among these children. Even very low birthweight (below 1501 g) children have high rates of major handicap, learning difficulties, and speech and language delay when assessed at school age and compared to controls.[34]

Premature delivery and low birthweight are strongly correlated with lower social class, illustrating again that efforts at prevention should focus on social, economic and environmental rather than predominantly medical factors.

Postnatal prevention of brain damage

The three most common causes of postnatally acquired brain damage are accidents, infections, and child abuse. There are social class differentials in the incidence of all these; in particular for accidents, where children of unskilled workers are ten times more likely to die in childhood from accidents than children of professional workers.

Serious head injury resulting in brain damage occurs particularly in pedestrian and road traffic accidents, also from falls and near drownings. Prevention lies in strategies to reduce accidents as well as educating children in road safety and wearing appropriate protection such as cycle helmets.

Meningitis particularly in early childhood not infrequently has long-term sequelae, including deafness, neurological impairment and developmental delay. *Haemophilus influenzae* B is the most common causative organism of meningitis in the first two years of life. *Haemophilus influenzae* B vaccine was introduced in 1992 nationally in the UK as part of the childhood immunization programme.[35]

Meningococcal vaccine against groups A and C organisms is also available but it is not recommended for routine vaccination, as the risk of meningococcal disease is very low, and the major cause of the disease in the UK is from group B organisms.

The proportion of postnatal acquired brain damage caused by child abuse has never been quantified but is probably substantial, and includes children who already may have some degree of developmental delay or disability. It is in this area that one of the greatest challenges in the field of prevention lies, not just for community child health professionals but for the whole of society.

References

1 Wilkinson, R.G. Income and mortality. In: Wilkinson, R.G., ed., *Class and Health*. London: Tavistock, 1986.

2 Bradshaw, J. *Child Poverty and Deprivation in the UK*. London: National Children's Bureau, 1990.

3 Kohler, L., Jakobsson, G. *Children's Health and Wellbeing in the Nordic Countries*. London: Mackeith Press, 1989.

4 Whitehead, M. *The Health Divide: Inequalities in Health in the 1980s*. London: Health Education Council, 1987.

5 Department of Health. *Immunisation against Infectious Disease*. London: HMSO, 1990.

6 James, J., Lawson, P., Male, J.H. Antecedents of cerebral palsy. *New Engl J Med* 1986; **315**: 81–86.

7 Lindsay, G., ed. *Screening for Children with Special Needs*. London: Croom Helm, 1984.

8 Griffiths, P.D., Mann, J.R., Darbyshire, P.J., Green, A. Evaluation of eight and a half years of neonatal screening for haemoglobinopathies in Birmingham. *Br Med J* 1988; **296**: 1583–85.

9 Evans, J.P.M. Practical management of sickle cell disease. *Arch Dis Child* 1989; **64**: 1748–1751.

10 Hall, D.M.B., ed. *Health for All Children: a Programme for Child Health Surveillance*. Oxford: Oxford Medical Publications, 1989.

11 Lask, B. Psychosocial factors in childhood diabetes and seizure disorders – the family approach. *Paediatrician* 1988; **15**: 95–101.

12 Paneth, N. Birth and origins of cerebral palsy. *New Engl J Med* 1986; **315**: 124–126.

13 Hall, D. Birth asphyxia and cerebral palsy. *Br Med J* 1989; **229**: 279–282.

14 Blair, E., Stanley, F.J. Intrapartum asphyxia: a rare cause of cerebral palsy. *J Pediatr* 1988; **112**: 515–519.

15 Nelson, K.B., Ellenberg, J.H. Antecedents of cerebral palsy. *New Engl J Med* 1986; **315**: 81–86.

16 Wald, N.G., Cuckle, H.S., Densem, J.W. *et al*. Maternal serum screening for Down syndrome in early pregnancy. *Br Med J* 1988; **197**: 883–887.

17 Cuckle, H.S., Wald, N.J., Barkal, G. *et al*. First trimester biochemical screening for Down's syndrome. *Lancet* 1988; ii: 851–852.

18 Winchester, B. Prenatal diagnosis of enzyme defects. *Arch Dis Child* 1990; **65**: 59–67.

19 Cleary, M.A., Wraith, J.E. Antenatal diagnosis of inborn errors of metabolism. *Arch Dis Child* 1991; **66**: 816–822.

20 Best, J.M. Congenital cytomegalovirus infection. *Br Med J* 1987; **294**: 1440–41.

21 Pearl, K.N., Preece, P.M., Ades, A., Peckham, C.S. Neurodevelopmental assessment after congenital cytomegalovirus infection. *Arch Dis Child* 1986; **61**: 323–326.

22 Best, M., Sutherland, S. Diagnosis and prevention of congenital and perinatal infection. *Br Med J* 1990; **301**: 888–889.

23 Poskitt, E.M. Fetal alcohol syndrome and fetal alcohol effects. In: Macfarlane A., ed. *Progress in Child Health*. Edinburgh: Churchill Livingstone, 1984.

24 Gase, J.M. The fetal alcohol syndrome in American Indians: a high risk group. *Neurobehaviour Toxicol Teratol* 1981; **3**: 153–156.

25 Larsson, G., Bohlin, A. Fetal alcohol syndrome and preventative strategies. *Paediatrician* 1987; **14**: 51–56.

26 Aronson, M., Olegard, R. Children of alcoholic mothers. *Paediatrician* 1987; **14**: 57–61.

27 Crawford, M., Doyle, W., Craft, I.C., Lawrance, B.M. A comparison of food intake during pregnancy and birthweight in high and low socio-economic groups. *Prog Lipid Res* 1986; **25**: 249–54.

28 Smithells, R.W., Sheppard, S. Possible prevention of neural tube defects by periconceptional vitamin supplementation. *Lancet* 1980; i: 647.

29 Durward, L. *Poverty in Pregnancy: the Cost of an Adequate Diet for Expectant Mothers*. London: Maternity Alliance, 1988.

30 Anon. Sodium valproate and spina bifida. *Drug Ther Bull* 1990; **28**: 59–60.

31 Laegrid, L., Olegard, R., Couradi, N., Hagbern, G. Congenital malformations and maternal consumption of benzodiazepines: a case control study. *Dev Med Child Neurol* 1990; **32**: 432–441.

32 Cohen, J., Schamroth, A., Nazareth, I., Johnson, M., Graham, S., Thomson, D. Problem drug use in a central London general practice. *Br Med J* 1992; **304**: 1158–1160.

33 Marlow, N., Roberts, B.L., Cooke, R.W.I. Motor skills in extremely low birthweight children at the age of 6 years. *Arch Dis Child* 1989; **64**: 839–847.

34 Michelsson, K., Lindahl, E., Parre, M., Helenius, M. Nine year follow up of infants weighing 1500 g or less at birth. *Acta Paediat Scand* 1984; **73**: 835–841.

35 Booy, R., Moxon, E.R. Immunisation of infants against *Haemophilus influenzae* type B in the UK. *Arch Dis Child* 1991; **66**: 1251–1254.

7.2 Health promotion

Margaret Ayton

How health promotion can be ensured for children and their families

Health promotion in relation to children and their families can be considered from two perspectives; the creation of a healthy and safe environment during the childhood years and as a preparation for the future. Before addressing the issue of how health promotion can be ensured, the multifaceted nature of this topic is considered. In attempting to translate principles into practice, emphasis is given to those promulgated by the World Health Organization (WHO) on the grounds that they have provided the impetus for much of the current activity in health promotion. The process of health promotion is discussed in general terms but from a practical perspective.

Health promotion: definitions and principles

Any discussion of health promotion is usually of necessity preceded by an attempt to define the concept of health. Definitions of health are numerous and range from the World Health Organization's positive approach of 'physical, mental, and social well-being and not merely the absence of disease or infirmity' to those which as Pierret describes give emphasis to social connotations and relate it to man's ability to cope with his environment.[1] It is interesting to note that Pill in her study of health beliefs and behaviour in the home, using a sample of working class women, found a tendency to define health in negative terms.[2] It appears that whereas illness has implications for action on the part of the individual or his carers, the maintenance of health is widely considered not to require action.

Health promotion is often regarded as being synonymous with health education, but there are numerous definitions and the concept of health promotion has undergone changes in interpretation over the years. If health promotion were to consist only of health education there is a danger of assuming that the potential for adopting a healthy lifestyle lies entirely within the remit and responsibility of the individual. In reality health is not influenced only by the actions of the individual but also by the environment in which he lives, for example, the Black Report noted that social and economic factors affect health and favour those more socially and financially advantaged.[3] In addition, relationships with families, neighbours, and those at school or work can lead to ill health.[4]

Until comparatively recently health promotion was not a high priority for the majority of health care professionals (with the exception of health visitors) and in competition for resources was, and still is, often sacrificed to the more pressing needs of the palliative and curative services. The relief of actual pain and disability will always appear a more pressing need than the prevention of future pain and disability which may never happen. There are many happy smokers who live to a ripe old age.

In 1978 the Declaration of Alma Ata (WHO) brought health promotion to the forefront of the WHO's agenda for action.[5] This was followed by a series of WHO publications including the Ottawa Charter for health promotion in 1986.[6] The latter's statement on health promotion extends the remit of health promotion beyond the health sector to make it everyone's concern:

> the process of enabling people to increase control over, and to improve, their health. To reach a state of complete physical, mental and social well-being, an individual or group must be able to identify and to realise aspirations, to satisfy needs, and to change or cope with the environment. Health is, therefore, seen as a resource for everyday life, not the objective of living. Health is a positive concept emphasising social and personal resources, as well as physical capacities. Therefore, health promotion is not just the responsibility of the health sector, but goes beyond healthy lifestyles to well-being. (Reproduced by kind permission of WHO.[6])

Underpinning this definition of health promotion are principles identified in an earlier WHO discussion document.[7]

1 Health promotion involves the population as a whole in the context of their everyday life, rather than focusing on people at risk for specific diseases.
2 Health promotion is directed towards actions on the determinants and causes of ill health.
3 Health promotion combines diverse, but complementary, methods or approaches (including communication, education, legislation, fiscal measures, organizational change, community development and spontaneous local activities against health hazards).

4 Health promotion aims particularly at effective and concrete public participation.

5 Health professionals – particularly in primary health care – have an important role in nurturing and enabling health promotion. (Reproduced by kind permission of WHO.[7])

It can be seen that the above definition and principles are positive in their approach, avoid the dangers of victim blaming and extend health promotion beyond the realms of health care into the political arena by taking action against the determinants and causes of ill health. It acknowledges that the way to make health promotion acceptable to the population is to let it be seen as a resource to benefit everyday life, rather than it being viewed as a case of trying to prevent something which might never happen.

Health promotion is threefold in its aims: the maintenance and improvement of health and the prevention of ill health. It can operate at three levels:

- By modifying an individual's behaviour.
- By changing environmental factors and raising a consciousness of health aspects of many facets of life.
- By influencing social relationships which can affect health.

The modification of an individual's behaviour is achieved through health education in either a 'one to one', group or community setting. The challenge of health education is to motivate individuals to maintain or improve their health and to take steps when appropriate to seek medical advice.

Maslow's theory of motivation[8] seems to have particular relevance for health promotion as seen by the WHO. The Ottawa Charter referred to the need of individuals to identify and realize aspirations. Maslow's premise in constructing his hierarchy of social needs was that humans have wants but these are dependent upon those wants or needs that have already been gratified. It is only unmet needs which are motivators. This hierarchy is usually depicted in pyramidal form, the base being 'physiological needs', those which are necessary for the body to function, namely food, warmth, sleep. The hierarchy then progresses: safety, love (social needs), esteem (self-respect) and then self-actualization (the development of one's potential). The theory has been criticized but, as Mullins[9] points out, Maslow himself recognized its limitations suggesting that the hierarchy would not necessarily have a universal application nor would individuals necessarily attribute values to these needs in the same order; he wished it to be regarded as a basis for research. Within the context of health promotion it serves as a useful reminder to exert caution and negotiate with clients what their priorities are when defining needs.

The other two scenarios of health promotion pose problems because they affect the general structure of society and can have cost implications. On the whole, modification of an individual's behaviour does not involve public expenditure; if expense is incurred it is contained within the family budget. However, in the second scenario involving environmental changes, there is often an inherent conflict of interest and wide disagreement about priorities; for example, it is known that lead in the atmosphere is harmful to children but to remove lead from petrol increases motoring costs. Likewise the adverse effects of smoking are well documented but success in the campaign against smoking would mean unemployment in the tobacco industry and a loss of revenue for the government from the taxes currently raised on tobacco.

As regards the third scenario, social relationships are difficult to modify but the task facing the health promoter is the provision of alternative support networks or referrals to relevant agencies such as RELATE, or the Samaritans.

Implicit in the principles of health promotion there are three key concepts worthy of further note and all of which have been the subject of lengthy academic debate: community, need and participation. It is not the intent of this discussion to repeat such debates but merely to draw attention to the multidimensional nature of these concepts which tend to be used so freely by people on the assumption that there is an agreed understanding and definition.

Community

Geographical definitions of community can be restrictive if they ignore the variety of social and cultural influences that exists within society. Ashton raises the issue of definitions of community in his discussion of health promotion and the concept of community[10] and noted that Phillips and Le Gates identified over 90 definitions of 'community' in sociology.[11]

Need

Bradshaw's taxonomy of social need usefully highlights the diversity of interpretations:[12]

- Normative (needs which are generally agreed and usually professionally defined).
- Felt (needs which are felt by clients but have not been expressed).
- Expressed (felt needs which have been expressed by clients).
- Comparative (needs experienced by individuals comparing themselves with others in similar circumstances and realizing that they are not in receipt of the same services).

Participation

The issue of consumerism and participation has had a very high profile in health care in the UK in the last decade, with the publication of numerous government reports.[13,14] However, participation has a variety of definitions and is best perceived as a continuum covering the spectrum of a token consultation (usually after the decisions have been made) to the total involvement of clients at every stage of the planning process and their involvement in decision making. Participation in health care involves a shifting of the balance of power; too often in health care the relationship between professional and patient/client tends to polarize between the active professional and the passive client.[15] In health promotion the latter scenario is not feasible because of the need to work at the client's pace. The Ottawa Charter recognizes this when it refers to the enablement process required.

Practice

In preparing a strategy for the translation of principles into practice, a useful format is that of structure, process and outcome.

a   Structure

Within structure one is examining what are the resources for carrying out health promotion. Here one is considering not only financial resources but resources in terms of who are the key personnel to be involved and what locations/settings can be used.

It must be remembered that health promotion is dynamic for not only does the potential content (nutrition, exercise, avoidance of substance abuse, home safety, dental hygiene, foot health, coping with stress strategies) vary at different stages of the child and adult's life, but the relative importance of those who will be able to exert an influence will vary at different stages. Methods of intervention should respond accordingly. For example, in the teenage years the power of peer group influences is well documented and thus any strategies developed will have a greater chance of success if the child/adolescent does not have to oppose peer pressure.

Depending upon what health promotion is going to be undertaken and with what client group, any one of a range of personnel might be considered to be able to play a key role, for example, general practitioner, health visitor, community paediatrician, school nurse, midwife, dietician, dentist, teacher, housing officer, environmental health officer, health education officer.

As regards locations and settings for health promotion, there are probably no limits to potential venues, providing that they form part of everyday life and are easily accessible. Obviously one is considering not just health care facilities but nurseries, schools, leisure facilities, shops, markets, business premises and job centres. It must be ensured that the settings are compatible with the particular health promotion message being delivered.

Another aspect to consider under structure is access to health education materials; leaflets, posters, aids and equipment. Usually health education departments can supply these or have information about materials which have been developed to suit the requirements of particular campaigns, for example, the translation of health education material into other languages to meet the needs of non-English speaking residents.

b   Process

The process of health promotion consists of four stages: assessment, planning, implementation and evaluation.

1   ASSESSMENT

Assessment of local health issues can be addressed in two ways: by conducting research (formal and informal) on a local basis and/or by referring to national surveys and acting upon their findings.

National surveys have highlighted the problems of children smoking and of childhood accidents – the decision facing local health practitioners is whether to reproduce research locally to assess the magnitude of the problem or to act upon that information.

There is a range of factors to be considered in the assessment of local health issues. What are the local facilities to provide a healthy lifestyle? Are there leisure and sports facilities accessible to all irrespective of income or residence? Is it an economically deprived or wealthy area; what are the levels of unemployment; what is the access to wholesome food? It is a common phenomenon in inner city areas that the family on a low income with no transport is often reliant on the high prices charged by local shops whose choice of healthy foods is limited. Is the healthy choice the easy choice? What food policies do local schools and businesses have? What are local council policies on housing/housing repairs? Are there any local sources of pollution such as industrial waste or effluents? What agencies already exist which could be approached for their support? Just by raising these questions it is obvious that a multidisciplinary approach involving the local population is required when assessing what are the health promotion issues.

When working at an individual level a key part of the assessment process is to establish the current values and beliefs held and what is the client's knowledge base; this should also be reflected in assessments at group or community level.

2 PLANNING

Planning means determining priorities, goal setting, and making a range of decisions covering target setting, time scales to be used, methods to be employed and key personnel to be involved. At community and individual level it is essential that client(s) be involved. Practical issues should be considered, for example, the timing and venue of activities – will they be accessible to the client group being targeted?

3 IMPLEMENTATION

Implementation of the proposed programme of health promotion can be considered by examining the skills to be used. Obviously health educational skills will be at the forefront of any health promotion programme but there is a range of skills necessary to carry out the wider remit of health promotion, for example negotiating/advocacy, facilitating and lobbying skills.

Health education skills   Health education is concerned with enabling individuals by giving them information to make informed decisions and creating an awareness of their needs to motivate action. It is an umbrella term for a range of skills: basic communication skills including non-verbal communication, listening skills, helping people to talk, feedback; teaching in formal and informal settings; working with the media; and developing health education material.[16]

Negotiating/advocacy skills   In order to effect health promotion there may be a necessity for professionals to be involved in local political issues, become an advocate for health in the area, negotiate with local agencies and encourage mobilization of resources. A common complaint from council house tenants is inadequate repairs – how can home safety have any impact if the child is being reared in a damp, draughty house with broken windows and no fences around the garden? How can anti-smoking policies succeed if local shopkeepers are selling cigarettes to children?

Facilitating skills   Facilitating skills are probably the most important skills in health promotion as they result in enabling clients to participate in decision making processes. By acting as a facilitator the professional is acting as a resource to clients who develop their own activities or strategies. Examples might include a local women's group running its own health interest group and regarding the local health visitor or dietician as a resource to be consulted as necessary.

Lobbying skills   A classic example of lobbying skills in health promotion occurs when campaigners attempt to promote dental health through fluoridation of the water supply. Campaigners lobby the local health authority who then requests the local water company to fluoridate their supply. Other examples might include lobbying for the creation of new posts such as nutritional facilitator.

A key point to note in the implementation of health promotion programmes is the need for consistency in any information given by health care professionals. A common criticism levelled at health care professionals is that of conflicting advice being given. Newcastle Health Authority as part of its coronary heart disease prevention campaign attempted to overcome this problem by producing a policy statement which was circulated to all members of staff involved in health promotion. This included not only clinical staff but teaching staff based within the health authority, local university and polytechnic. In addition, a primary health care kit was made available to all general practitioners within the city.

4 EVALUATION

Whatever health promotion has been carried out it requires evaluation of the process and the outcomes (see below).

c   Outcome

What are the outcomes of health promotion? How can they be measured? What sort of indicators can be used? In curative and palliative health care where problems have been identified as reasons for intervention outcomes are relatively easy to define. This is not the case in health promotion where it is largely the healthy population who is targeted. In many spheres of health promotion the impact of strategies on the health of a population might only be apparent in the long term so there is a need to develop proxy indicators and short-term measures such as a reduction in the number of childhood accidents, the success of smoking cessation clinics, the improved uptake of immunization and local screening programmes. Where strategies have been aimed at creating change in the environment as in development of food or smoking policies in public places one can look at the outcomes in terms of whether the immediate objective has been achieved. However, such outcomes do not show the effect on the health of the population in the years to come.

Conclusion

This brief overview of health promotion has attempted to show the multidimensional nature of the topic. It is dubious whether it can ever be said that a health care professional can ensure good health for all children and their families because, although advice and education can be given, clients have the right to choose whether or not they respond. This raises issues of state intervention, the freedom of the individual and the responsibility of the individual which are part of health promotion's ethical debate.[17]

However, the potential of health promotion is now recognized by the government.[18–20] The challenge facing all health care professionals will be to deliver health care services which have an emphasis on health, not illness.

References

1 Pierret, J. What social groups think they can do about health. In: Anderson, R., Davies, J.K., Kickbusch, I., McQueen, D.V., Turner, J., eds. *Health Behaviour Research and Health Promotion*. Oxford: Oxford University Press, 1988, 45–52.

2 Pill, R. Health beliefs and behaviour in the home. In: Anderson, R., Davies, J.K., Kickbusch, I., McQueen, D.V., Turner, J., eds. *Health Behaviour Research and Health Promotion*. Oxford: Oxford University Press, 1988, 183–194.

3 Department of Health and Social Security. *Inequalities in Health. Report of a Research Working Group*. Chairman: Sir Douglas Black. The Black Report. London: DHSS, 1980.

4 Blaxter, M. *Health and Lifestyles*. London: Routledge, 1990.

5 World Health Organization. *Primary Health Care*. (Declaration of Alma Ata). Geneva: WHO, 1978.

6 World Health Organization. *Ottawa Charter for Health Promotion*. Geneva: WHO, 1986.

7 World Health Organization. *Health Promotion. A Discussion Document on the Concepts and Principles*. Copenhagen: WHO Regional Office for Europe, 1984.

8 Maslow, A.H. *Motivation and Personality*, 2nd edn. New York: Harper and Row, 1970.

9 Mullins, L.J. *Management and Organisational Behaviour*. London: Pitman, 1985.

10 Ashton, J. Health promotion and the concept of community. In: Anderson, R., Davies, J.K., Kickbusch, I., McQueen, D.V., Turner, J., eds. *Health Behaviour Research and Health Promotion*. Oxford: Oxford University Press, 1988, 140–153.

11 Phillips, E.B., Le Gates, R.T. *City Lights: an Introduction to Urban Studies*. New York: Oxford University Press, 1981.

12 Bradshaw, J. The concept of social need. *New Society* 1972; **30:** 640–43.

13 Department of Health and Social Security. *Health Services Management*, Implementation of the NHS Management Inquiry Report (Griffiths Report). London: HMSO, 1984.

14 Department of Health and Social Security. *Neighbourhood Nursing – A Focus for Care*. London: HMSO, 1986.

15 Dowling, S. *Health for a Change. The Provision of Preventative Health Care in Pregnancy and Early Childhood*. London: Child Poverty Action Group, 1983.

16 Ewles, L., Simnett, I. *Promoting Health: A Practical Guide to Health Education*. Chichester. John Wiley & Sons Ltd. (H.M. and M. Nursing Publications), 1985.

17 Knowles, J.H., ed. The responsibility of the individual. In: *Doing Better and Feeling Worse: Health in the United States*. New York: W.W. Norton and Co. Inc., 1977.

18 Department of Health and Social Security. *Promoting Better Health. The Government's Programme for Improving Primary Health Care*. Cmd. 249. London: HMSO, 1987.

19 Department of Health. *Working for Patients*. Cmd. 555. London: HMSO, 1989.

20 Department of Health. *The Health of the Nation. A Strategy for Health in England*. Cmd. 1986. London: HMSO, 1992.

7.3 Childhood immunization

Euan Ross

1991 was the first year in which there were no deaths from measles and whooping cough in England and Wales. This achievement has not been easy. This section addresses current trends in paediatric immunization practice with an emphasis on pertussis control, because it so well illustrates many aspects of vaccine policy and development.

All the individual requirements of an international readership cannot be covered; for schedules and administrative policy, reference must be made to local documents. There is far more variation in practice between countries than science requires; child health would be greatly improved if policies were harmonized and the lessons and vaccines available in the west were transferred to developing countries.[1] The 1990 New York declaration, the Children's Vaccine Initiative, makes the point: although 70% of children in the developing world are being immunized against the common preventable diseases, this achievement still leaves scope for preventing 2–3 million deaths annually through global immunization. Development of new vaccines against diseases (based on work already in progress) could save another 5–6 million lives annually during this decade and reduce morbidity and handicap in survivors.

Immunization against diphtheria, pertussis, tetanus and poliomyelitis was established as a non-controversial medical routine in most developed countries during the 1950s and 1960s.[2] The global eradication of smallpox in 1979 proved that it was possible to bring the benefits of immunization to even the most rural areas and led to the World Health Organization's (WHO) initiative *Health for all by the year 2000* which is attempting to bring immunization against the major preventable diseases to at least 90% of the world's children. Complacency over immunization has been disturbed by a series of problems. An early killed polio vaccine was contaminated by live virus giving rise to cases of paralytic polio; and the initial killed measles vaccines were soon found to have toxic side effects – they were withdrawn and replaced with live attenuated vaccines. The safety of pertussis vaccine was questioned and became the subject of much adverse media publicity. There were occasional reports of paralytic polio-like disease in the contacts of those children who had recently received oral polio immunization, and outbreaks of polio among the unimmunized in countries that used killed vaccine. The effectiveness of BCG vaccine particularly in developing countries began to be doubted. At the same time, there was an overwhelming case to introduce new vaccines such as measles, mumps and rubella (MMR) and *Haemophilus influenzae* b (Hib) as they became available. To some extent the controversies over the safety and effectiveness of existing vaccines stimulated new interest in harnessing advances in microbiology and genetic engineering towards the development of new generations of vaccines that are likely to become available during the 1990s.

Main types of vaccines

1 Bacterial vaccines

Whether it is possible to develop a useful vaccine against a bacterial organism depends on the organism's ability to produce discrete antigens. Early in the 20th century it was appreciated that bacteria greatly differed in this property. To this day it remains impossible to produce an effective vaccine against many organisms especially those that have the capacity to change their essential genetic characteristics or exist in vast numbers of serotypically different forms.

There are four main types of vaccines against bacteria:

a Toxoided

Certain bacteria, such as diphtheria and tetanus, produce a clearly characterized antigen which can be harvested and chemically altered to a non-toxic form known as a toxoid. The immunogenic properties remain as the basis for a vaccine. Modern vaccines such as HiB are made by bonding capsular antigens from the target organism onto carrier toxoids derived from other bacteria.

b Whole cell vaccines

Many organisms produce a series of toxic substances which may or may not act as antigens, the toxoiding process however may result in an ineffective vaccine. For this reason the traditional means of producing vaccines against bacterial infections such as cholera, typhoid or pertussis has involved preservation of the cell wall. Such vaccines are prepared by killing the organism with heat and denaturing with formalin.

c Component vaccines

Increasing understanding of the components of the intracellular contents of pertussis and other organisms is now making it possible to produce highly characterized or component vaccines. Such pertussis vaccines are in use in Japan and under intensive investigation elsewhere.

d Live attenuated bacteria

The basis of protection against tuberculosis through the development of a non-virulent mutant strain of mycobacteria known as BCG (Bacille Calmette – Guérin).

2 Viral vaccines

There are two types:

a Killed viral vaccine

The only example now in widespread use is Salk polio virus which is used in some Northern European countries. Killed virus vaccines against measles were used in the early 1960s but were soon abandoned in favour of live vaccines.

b Live attenuated virus vaccine

The first example of the use of such a vaccine was against smallpox. This followed the observation that infection from a comparable illness seen in cows gave protection against the antigenically related human disease, smallpox. Live attenuated virus vaccines currently in use include measles, mumps, rubella, hepatitis A and B and oral polio.

Pseudo-vaccines

In some countries unofficial preparations are sold as vaccines. These should not be used. As an illustration, there is a substance marketed in the UK as a homeopathic pertussis vaccine which does not carry the endorsement of the Faculty of Homeopathy who advise the use of conventional vaccine programmes.

Doctors working in some parts of the world have to be alert against the practice of selling fake medical preparations and the non-availability of disposable sterile syringes and needles. They must take personal charge of the sterilizing of non-disposable items.

Introduction of new vaccines

The development of new vaccines is extremely complex. First, it is necessary to decide whether it is desirable to produce such a vaccine. As an illustration, a dental caries vaccine has been developed but with the falling prevalence of caries its introduction was felt to be unjustified. While all infectious illness can be regarded as a hazard to some, there is probably no benefit in developing vaccines against minor infections such as common colds. With all vaccines there has to be a positive relation between cost, benefit and risk; the vaccines currently in large-scale use justify their costs and result in savings for the health service.

Other effective vaccines are available which it has not yet become policy to use. An example is varicella vaccine, and a rationale for its use has been made.[3] Others are in active development and their introduction depends on completion of the statutory licensing processes and being adopted nationally as part of a recommended immunization programme. In some cases, promising candidate vaccines, such as rotavirus, have failed when subjected to large-scale field trials. It takes about 15 years from theoretical concept and early animal studies to develop a vaccine to the stage of product licence.

Quality of information about infectious disease

There are considerable differences in vaccine policy between countries. Most of these differences have historical reasons rather than a solid basis in science. The quality of data about uptake, effectiveness and side reactions varies greatly. Information about the prevalence of infectious diseases is collected in varying ways. In the UK, it is estimated that only 20–25% of incidents of notifiable infectious disease are actually reported to the authorities.

Every country needs a reliable network of informed doctors who are up to date about immunization and infectious diseases. In England and Wales where the health service is based on population districts of about 250 000 people, a system of district immunization coordinators has been developed. One individual, usually a doctor, is given the task of promoting immunization and is expected to attend regular updating meetings where national policy is reviewed and explained and new developments are discussed. District targets for immunization uptake are set and monitored. Many districts offer special immunization advisory clinics or telephone advisory services. Local and regional immunization uptake statistics are sent out to each district every quarter.

Compulsory or voluntary immunization?

Attitudes vary greatly around the world. Immunization was compulsory in Soviet countries; it now appears that both vaccine coverage and the quality of vaccines administered were nothing like as satisfactory as previously claimed. The return of epidemic diphtheria in Russia to both adults and children exemplifies this; the seriousness of the situation cannot be over emphasized – the main adult infectious disease hospital in Moscow was admitting at least one serious case a day in late 1993. The author visited Estonia in 1993 where immunization rates were around 70%; inconsistent advice from doctors and unreliable availability of vaccines is reducing their efforts to get all children immunized. In many developed countries, immunization is seen by the population as a desirable necessity and high uptake rates are achieved without compulsion, as in Northern Europe, Australia, New Zealand and Japan. In the USA, immunization is not compulsory but admission to a state school requires a completed vaccination certificate resulting in a rush of immunization prior to school entry. The UK has long paid a penalty for being the pioneer country to use vaccination; there has always been an ambivalent attitude and a long history of people including doctors opposed to vaccination who receive much attention. This makes it harder to achieve a national sentiment as favourable to immunization as in neighbouring countries. The attitude of the British public as a whole appears to be one of cautious good sense; the Peckham report[4] studied professional and parental attitudes and found that both groups favoured compulsory immunization. Most parents of unimmunized children indicated that they would have their child immunized if it were made compulsory.

It has been repeatedly found in the UK, that doctors and clinic nurses often give conflicting or unofficial advice about immunization. It is important that all who promote and give immunizations receive regular training.[5]

Practical issues

Ensuring that patients are immunized depends on an effective record system. It is necessary to monitor closely the local population, in order to know when children have been immunized, and to pass on the information if they move away. In the UK this is achieved by the use of computer-based schemes.

About two-thirds of the health districts in England and Wales use the National Child Health Computing System which records immunization histories, generates appointments and handles vaccine ordering and doctors' payments. This system forms the basis of a complete child health system which also stores information about child health surveillance and details of handicaps and health at school.[6] McKinney *et al.*[7] showed how often parents and general practitioners disagreed over immunization histories and demonstrated the importance of computer-held immunization data.

Vaccine handling and storage

Not infrequently, even in temperate climates, there are complaints that the vaccine 'did not take'. Vaccines are fragile products that readily lose their potency if subjected to extremes of temperature. They must be kept at a stable temperature in the range 2°–5° C from leaving the factory to administration. Checks in the UK have shown how easy it is to exceed these temperatures. Transit in unrefrigerated vans, leaving supplies out of the refrigerator for whole clinic sessions and then returning the unused portion can drastically reduce potency.[8] The problem is far greater in tropical countries especially where field staff are poorly trained. The most elementary mistakes can readily be made.

What injection site?

Diphtheria, tetanus and pertussis (DTP), HiB, and measles, mumps and rubella (MMR) vaccines must be injected into muscle and BCG intradermally. Which site to use has been the subject of continuing discussion.[9] The use of the upper outer quadrant of the buttock is not supported by the medical defence organizations. In babies, the author advises the outer lateral thigh which is out of the napkin area and where there is far more muscle than in the commonly used deltoid region. The skin should be visibly clean; if not it should be washed with soap and water and allowed to dry prior to immunization. The syringe must be disposable and not reused. For infant immunization, a 25 gauge needle is advised. It should be inserted at 90° to the skin and inserted for about three-quarters of its length.

If a live and a killed or toxoided vaccine are to be given on the same occasion they should be injected via separate syringes to opposite sites. It is also necessary to give DTP and HiB in separate syringes on opposite sides. Since MMR vaccine is less painful than other vaccines it is sensible to give it first.

Anaphylaxis and immunization

All who undertake infant immunization must be trained in the treatment of anaphylactic shock and have an appropriate resuscitation kit to hand which must contain 1/1000 adrenalin and the correct syringes. Anaphylaxis following infant immunization is exceedingly rare. Most teenagers and adults who collapse while having immunizations have fainted through fear.

Schedules

Most countries give DTP vaccine in combination. Some add a killed Salk polio vaccine. Others give oral Sabin vaccine on the same occasion. Denmark gives plain pertussis vaccine at 5 weeks. Increasingly the tendency is to start DTP at 2 months and complete the primary course of three injections by 6 months or earlier thus protecting infants from pertussis during the period when most deaths from the disease occur. There are considerable differences in the scheduling of immunizations. Since these tend to change from time to time, it is important to keep to the current local policy; there must be compelling reasons before departing from it. Immunization can become a litiginous area and it is better not to develop a personal system. Policies about booster immunizations in later life vary considerably between countries. The UK does not schedule a pertussis booster while many countries, for example USA and Hungary, give two. The UK advises a booster diphtheria and tetanus dose plus oral polio at school entry and exit. National authorities give very varying advice about the intervals between booster doses of tetanus toxoid and local sources must be consulted.

Most developed countries advise a single MMR immunization after the first birthday. The optimal date was discussed by Preston.[10] There is some anxiety that this protection might not be life long and policies may change.

For the UK immunization schedule see Appendix on p. 697.

Immunization and travelling abroad with children

Increasing world travel makes immunization ever more important. Parents must appreciate that while serious disorders such as polio and diphtheria are rarely seen in developed countries which have achieved high levels of immunization uptake these conditions are common in much of the world. Travel agents and embassies are rarely good sources of advice. On occasions, unscrupulous people in some countries indulge in malpractice at airports and make illegal demands for unnecessary immunization certificates against conditions such as yellow fever, even though these certificates are not required by local law. People have been tricked into accepting such injections at airports with unsterilized equipment for a fee.

The primary immunization course should be commenced as early as possible before travel so that adequate immunity has been built up. There is nothing to stop newborn infants starting their DTP course early though advice will be needed about later boosters. MMR can be started at about 8 months with a repeat dose at about 18 months. Individual advice must be sought over the indications for typhoid, cholera and yellow fever. The protection given by these vaccines varies and their side effects have a degree of notoriety. The role of the new oral and component typhoid vaccines in childhood is still emerging. In developed countries advice is usually best obtained from university tropical health institutes. It is also necessary to get up-to-date advice about anti-malarial drugs. In developed countries, hepatitis B vaccine is usually recommended for hospital workers and for the protection of children of parents who have come from high-risk populations where the condition is endemic.

Protection and vaccines

1 Diphtheria

This is now a largely forgotten condition in developed countries and few doctors remain in practice with experience in its recognition, diagnosis and treatment. This is the result of immunization. In many parts of the developing world, the disease remains a major hazard. Occasional cases are brought into developed countries and there is an ever present possibility of outbreaks in the poorer parts of inner cities where immunization uptake rates are particularly low.

The incubation period is up to 5 days. Initial features tend to be non-specific – there is a low-grade fever, irritability and debility. A mild sore throat develops leading to an exudative grey-coloured membrane which may cover the entire pharynx and tonsils. Attempts to remove the membrane cause bleeding. Occasionally the membrane occludes the larynx leading to suffocation, so tracheostomy is required. The greater danger is the effect of the toxin particularly on the myocardium which can lead to sudden death – this is one of the few conditions where strict bed rest is needed. A peripheral neuropathy resulting in palatal and diaphragmatic paralysis may develop. Diphtheria

is part of the differential diagnosis of pharyngitis. If suspected, an immediate culture, performed by microbiologists who have been informed that diphtheria is a possible diagnosis, is needed; and expert advice about the use of anti-toxin from a physician experienced in the condition must be obtained.

The organism, *Corynebacterium diphtheriae*, was first cultured by Loeffler. Later Ramon described a toxoided diphtheria vaccine which was soon introduced in the USA though its use in Europe was much delayed. As a result, diphtheria remained a common disorder for much longer than necessary. By this time however initial problems due to impurities in the vaccine had been largely solved. Currently diphtheria vaccine can be regarded as having an extremely high benefit/risk ratio. A course of three injections is needed to gain adequate immunity. Side effects with the vaccine increase with age and for those over 10 years of age a special low-dose toxoid should be used.

2 Tetanus

Tetanus is unique among the diseases against which immunization is routinely offered because it is only spread by spores and cross infection between patients does not occur. The author has seen over 30 infants with neonatal tetanus in a ward in Pakistan measuring no more than six by six metres. It is believed that the disease is spread via unsterile knives used for cutting the umbilical cord; in some communities dung is put on the umbilical stump. While high degrees of skill have been developed which can rescue up to 70% of these infants through prolonged tube feeding and deep sedation this is a disease that could be prevented. Immunization of mothers with at least two doses of vaccine provides a safeguard though teaching hygienic birth practices is the key to prevention. Unfortunately this can be a difficult message to transmit to traditional birth attendants.

In western societies, tetanus is mainly seen in the older generations born before widespread tetanus immunization. The causal organism, *Clostridium tetani*, lives in the lower mammalian bowel. Spores can survive for up to 50 years and are resistant even to boiling and weak disinfectants. Adequate cleansing of cuts and judicious use of penicillin are the key to prevention of infection. Even a contaminated rose thorn prick can be enough to cause tetanus. This condition requires exceedingly skilled intensive care nursing. The fatality rate for the type of case seen in developed countries remains high; all these cases could be prevented through immunization.

In Europe, deaths from tetanus are now few; in the UK, about 10 cases are reported every year, of whom some survive thanks to intensive care. Most are in elderly people who were never vaccinated.

Contraindications to diphtheria and tetanus vaccination

In practice true contraindications to diphtheria and tetanus vaccination in infancy and young childhood are confined to those occasional children who have had an excessive red swelling around the immunization site following a previous immunization. This is more likely if the injection was given subcutaneously. It is assumed, although it cannot be proven, that the child shares some naturally occurring immunological factor with the vaccine. Such swellings seem to be as common whether DT or DTP vaccine is used. DT vaccine was studied in the course of the National Childhood Encephalopathy Study in the UK.[11] While some cases of time-associated encephalopathic conditions were reported there was no significant excess. Occasional cases of fever, myalgia and headache and even more rare peripheral neuropathy have been reported in adults. These side effects appear to be more common in those who had excessive immunizations.

3   Whooping cough

Whooping cough or pertussis (serious cough in Latin) is a worldwide disorder confined to humans. At the turn of the 20th century, it was second only to measles in the league of the most common lethal infectious diseases of children in European countries. As the century progressed, the number of recorded deaths from whooping cough declined greatly. The most rapid drop was before the introduction of immunization. This occurred at the time when vitamins were being understood, slum clearance was accelerating, and the benefits of fresh air and family spacing were recognized. For most of the world, where these benefits have not occurred, whooping cough remains a major killer of infants. It is estimated – admittedly from rather poor data – that about half a million children die from whooping cough in the world each year. The impact of immunization in the control of the incidence of whooping cough must not be underestimated. Most developed countries had introduced pertussis immunization by the end of the 1950s, with the exception of Italy. Those countries with high levels of immunization, particularly those in the Eastern bloc where it was compulsory, showed that the disease could be largely eliminated. In a number of countries, particularly Sweden (which abolished immunization in 1979),[12] the UK, and Japan,[13] where its use markedly declined following adverse publicity there was a very rapid return of epidemic illness. This did not occur in countries where immunization uptake remained high. Readers needing a major text on pertussis should refer to Wardlaw and Parton's book.[14] This section can only give an overview of a complex, litigious and at times acrimonious matter. Edwards and Kar-

zon[15] reviewed the microbiology of pertussis infection and the steps underway to develop new types of vaccine.

Although many bacterial and viral pathogens can make children cough, classical whooping cough only follows infection with the bacterial organism *Bordetella pertussis*, first cultured by Jules Bordet and Octave Gengou at the Pasteur Institute, Brussels. Although the disease is usually diagnosed on clinical findings the diagnosis can only be confirmed by culturing the organism. This must be done by experienced personnel; a special flexible wire swab is passed through the inferior nasal turbinates to the post-nasal space. The swab must be plated without delay on to a special medium. Although culture is the only way to confirm the diagnosis, rapid serological and enzyme-linked immunosorbent assay (ELISA) and DNA typing techniques are becoming available.

Pertussis is a highly infectious disease spread by those who are incubating or have the active disease. There is no firm evidence that symptomless carriers of the disease exist though subclinical cases can be found, particularly in older children and adults with waning immunity. Following an incubation period of 7–14 days the patient first develops a coryza, with fever and irritability; gradually, coughing usually with characteristic paroxysmal cough or whoop becomes more marked.

Although the disease can occur at any age it is particularly common and most lethal in the first 6 months of life, when it is less easy to diagnose than in the older child who is much more likely to develop the classic whoop. Young infants choke rather than whoop loudly and are at risk of inhaling vomit, particularly after a paroxysm.

The pathophysiology of pertussis has still not been fully worked out. The likely sequence is: that those with severe disease, particularly frail infants, get exhausted; this, coupled with poor nutrition, probably made worse by a tendency to pancreatic islet hyperstimulation, leads to inanition. The debility of whooping cough is due to the production of toxins. Ability to cope with infection is impaired because white cells cannot readily be released from the circulation; hence the presumably useless lymphocytosis characteristic of the disease.

The organism provokes the production of excess adenylate cyclase which interferes with the ability of the white cells to kill bacteria. At its worst fatal pneumonia results. Fortunately secondary infection can be treated with antibiotics and life can usually be maintained with intravenous therapy and ventilation. If antibiotics are to be of value in preventing the disease they must be given in the prodromal phase before the cough has developed. Giving them later will not stop the disease. Erythromycin, which *in vitro* at least is the most effective antibiotic against the organism, should be given as follows: children up to 2 years of age,

125 mg every 6 hours; children over 2 years of age, 250 mg every 6 hours. Treatment should be continued for 14 days to protect unimmunized symptom-free siblings.

There is no evidence that whooping cough as currently seen is a milder disease than in the past. Infants do not have significant passively acquired transplacental immunity from their mothers; breastfeeding may give some temporary protection though so far no specific antibody has been detected in mother's milk.

Mortality and morbidity

It is difficult to obtain a clear picture of the current pattern of morbidity. Lambert[16] found little chronic respiratory morbidity in the UK. Pertussis disease is significantly associated with encephalopathy. Cherry[17] found indirect evidence that pertussis associated deaths are underreported during pertussis epidemics. The disease became less common after the advent of immunization. Epidemics tend to occur in predictable 3–4 yearly cycles which, in the UK, were getting smaller every 4 years until 1977. Subsequently two large and two smaller epidemics occurred; by 1991 the vaccination level had risen to satisfactory levels and for the first time no pertussis deaths were reported.

The vaccine

Attempts to make pertussis vaccines began around 1912. Apart from Japan and several neighbouring islands where acellular vaccines are used, whole-cell vaccines are used. Although there were earlier reports, credit belongs to Madsen[18] who used a pioneering Danish vaccine in the remote Faroe Islands in the North Sea to quell an epidemic. The account included two deaths in recently vaccinated infants which started the controversy about the vaccine's safety that has persisted ever since. Madsen's vaccine however was a crude unstandardized substance far removed from present-day commercial products.

Whole-cell pertussis vaccine consists of a suspension of *B. pertussis* cells derived from the three pathogenic serotypes of the organism killed by exposure to heat or chemicals. During the 1930s pertussis vaccines were developed in the USA and generally were found to be effective, but their introduction to Europe was delayed by the war. During the period from the late 1940s to the mid-1950s, the British Medical Research Council (MRC) carried out a series of field trials of several pertussis vaccines; some gave excellent protection against naturally acquired whooping cough, while others were useless. The Michigan State Laboratories vaccine was selected as being both effective and safe and was adopted as the British standard. Preston[10,19] showed that vaccines need to include three serotypes. Failure to include them all in adequate titre explains why the vaccine used in the UK in the late 1960s was

losing its protectiveness; subsequently its potency was increased in line with WHO standards and modified to incorporate antigens against all three main serotypes. Most countries produce similar vaccines to WHO specifications though some, like Denmark, produce a weaker vaccine. The potency of the vaccine is assessed by a biological test (Kendrick test) which involves intracerebral injection of virulent strains of *B. pertussis* to unimmunized mice and the monitoring of subsequent weight gain. These tests, although far removed from the situation in human infants, gave results that correlated well with human protection in the MRC trials.[20,21]

Pertussis vaccine controversies – effectiveness

The effectiveness of pertussis vaccines has aroused considerable controversy.[22] Local studies summarized in a report from the Public Health Laboratory Service,[23,24] showed that far fewer immunized children than unimmunized developed pertussis in the recent British epidemics, confirming the protectivity of the present vaccine.

No immunizing procedure is likely to be 100% protective; vaccine potency can be damaged by incorrect storage; it may be incorrectly administered or, for unexplained reasons, fail to take presumably due to naturally occurring blocking antibodies. If any vaccine of known 90% efficacy is given to 90% of the population to be protected, half of the disease cases will occur among the immunized.

Unwanted effects of pertussis vaccine

Unlike the biologically simpler toxoid vaccines used against diphtheria and tetanus, pertussis vaccine contains whole dead bacterial cells. Several theoretically undesirable features can be demonstrated, mainly from animal work. These include: an islet-stimulating factor, though there is no evidence that newly immunized infants actually develop hypoglycaemia; a histamine-sensitizing factor; and potential haemagglutinins. When large amounts of the vaccine are mixed with brain extract and injected into rats, an auto-allergic encephalomyelitis can result.[25] This however is a far different situation from human use.

Whole-cell pertussis-containing vaccines are more pyrogenic than diphtheria-tetanus toxoid,[26] though a British study[27] found lower rates. The biological characteristics of vaccines from different manufacturers are comparable and for practical purposes the commercially available pertussis vaccines used in western Europe and the USA can be regarded as generic products, despite differences in manufacturing technique.[28]

Flight from vaccination

In Madsen's paper[18] there had been two fatalities among recently immunized children. In the subsequent literature there is sporadic mention of adverse neurological reactions.[29–34] Kulenkampff et al.[35] reviewed the literature and added 36 children with serious neurological disorders resulting in death or brain damage within 28 days of immunization against pertussis. The authors did not claim that these problems had been caused by the immunization but suggested a need for further studies. Ehrengut,[36] from Hamburg, questioned his country's pertussis vaccination policy on the grounds of neurological side effects.

In 1974, the British media picked up the Kulenkampff paper and used it as a case against pertussis vaccine. Pertussis immunization rates fell nationally from 70% to 35%, though in South Wales they fell to 9%.[37] Questions were asked in Parliament, the government reacted by commissioning a series of studies including the Dudgeon[38] and Meade[39] panels which demonstrated the difficulty of drawing meaningful conclusions from anecdotally collected series of cases.

In Sweden where there was similar concern following Ström's papers,[32,33] the strength of the vaccine was gradually reduced and then withdrawn in 1979.[12] Japan stopped pertussis immunization temporarily in 1976,[40] but there was soon return of serious disease and deaths and the vaccine was reinstated (though only for those over age 2 years) and subsequently replaced by acellular vaccines.

Controversy started later in the USA than in the UK, but by the early 1980s multimillion dollar law suits against manufacturers began. This resulted in many manufacturers withdrawing from the production of pertussis vaccine, consequently the price of a dose of DTP vaccine rose from a few cents to around $15 to cover the cost of liability insurance.

British vaccine safety studies

Serious neurological diseases in infancy commonly present between 6 and 9 months, the very age range when immunization was recommended. Many of these devastating illnesses still defy explanation though the proportion is falling as virology, immunology and brain scanning improve. Could the whole question of vaccine-associated neurological illnesses and brain damage be explained by coincidence? It was necessary to determine the background incidence of the alleged problems and find whether they occurred significantly more often in recently immunized than in non-immunized children. Such problems can be tackled by a cohort approach where an entire community is studied for a period of time, or a case-control approach where those identified as having a certain disease or condition (in this instance serious acute neurological disease) are compared with matched controls. Both types of study have been undertaken in the UK.

NORTH WEST THAMES STUDY[41]

An intensive study of vaccine reactions reported through a voluntary scheme involving the child health departments of a health region with a population of 3.5 million was undertaken from January 1975 to December 1981. With an annual birth rate of 44 000, of whom about 40% had a full course of three DTP immunizations, 12 children were reported to have vaccine-associated temporary or permanent neurological impairment. Five children developed their symptoms within 48 hours of immunization, though all had an acceptable alternative infectious cause for the problem over and above immunization (an identified virus in two, suspected virus in one and otitis media in two). The study concluded: 'we cannot rule out the possibility that some vaccines may on rare occasions cause brain damage but no convincing evidence of this has appeared during our study.'

THE NATIONAL CHILDHOOD ENCEPHALOPATHY STUDY (NCES)

This is the only nationally-based case-control study that has explored the risk of serious neurological illness following immunization.[11,42–44] All consultant paediatricians in England, Scotland and Wales took part in a 3-year study which started in mid-1976. They were asked to return a card each month saying whether or not they had admitted any children aged 2–35 months with:

1 Acute or subacute encephalitis, encephalomyelitis or encephalopathy.
2 Unexplained loss of consciousness.
3 Convulsions:
   a) with a total duration of more than half an hour or
   b) followed by a coma lasting one hour or more, or
   c) neurological sequelae lasting 24 hours or more.
4 Infantile spasms (West syndrome).
5 Reye's syndrome (acute encephalopathy with abnormal liver function tests).

Conditions explained by lead or other toxic encephalopathies were excluded as well as proven bacterial or viral meningitis, though all cases attributed to unspecified viral encephalopathy were included.

Referring paediatricians were asked to report without reference to vaccination histories which were sought separately from the child's local health authority and family doctor. Each health authority was asked to seek two controls matched by date of birth and sex. Paediatricians were asked to supply details of the child's medical history up to 15 days after admission.

Those children who had not fully recovered by 15 days, about half of the group, were examined by a paediatrician member of the study team. The remainder were followed through postal questionnaires completed by their hospital and family doctors. Local health visitors also visited them and the control children to gather information about current health and social background.

The findings from the first 1000 of the eventual 1172 in the study and their matched controls were reported in the *British Medical Journal* 1981,[11] and in a government publication.[44] Results of the analysis of the entire group do not differ significantly.[43,45] Using results from the whole group the main conclusions were:

1 A total of 39 children developed an illness of an encephalopathic nature within 7 days of a pertussis immunization.
2 These problems were equally common after first, second or third immunizations and were not confined to the product of any one of the British manufacturers then marketing vaccines in the UK.
3 No consistent type of neurological illness was found in these children.
4 Infantile spasms were not found to be associated with immunization significantly more often than expected by chance.[46]
5 There were thus 30 children with neurological problems (excluding those with infantile spasms) out of 904 who developed a serious neurological illness within 7 days of receiving pertussis immunization. Of these, four had a history of neurological illness prior to immunization, indicating the possibility of a pre-existing neurological abnormality.
6 In comparison with controls there was a statistically significant excess relative risk associated with receipt of pertussis vaccine. Four children, only one of whom was severely handicapped 12 months later, had no alternative cause found for neurological disability.

These findings need very careful and cautious interpretation. The numbers are small and statistically fragile. However, there are reasons to argue that error or bias in the conduct of the study could have led to both underestimation or overestimation of any possible risk associated with vaccination. Hence they have been used by both sides in legal actions. It is important to appreciate the nature of the study and the limits of epidemiological and other methods in settling disputes in complex biological issues. Further analysis does not lead to any change in the original conclusions. The authors of the report hold to their view that, while there was a significant association between pertussis immunization and onset of acute neurological illness, this does not prove causation and it seems likely that permanent damage as a result of pertussis immunization, if it occurs at all, is a very rare event

and attribution of a cause in individual cases is precarious.[44]

While there have been no comparable studies to the NCES, further information is available from the American Collaborative Perinatal Study where 54 000 births at eight teaching hospitals in the USA were studied in detail and followed up for seven years.[47] Ten children had at least one seizure within 2 weeks of pertussis immunization, though only one had persistent sequelae.

The British Child Health and Education Study,[48] has studied all children born in the UK in a week in April 1970. Of 12 692 followed to the age of 10 years, four compared with an expected 1.9 had a convulsion within 72 hours of pertussis immunization. None had persistent neurological sequelae; those children who had pertussis disease had poorer educational test scores on follow up. Those who had been immunized were doing better at school than the unimmunized.

AFTER THE NCES

Those prepared to read the 400 page legal judgement in Loveday v. Renton will find why pertussis vaccine became a *cause célèbre*. Griffen et al. reviewed the current situation.[49] Golden[50] concluded 'there is clearly an increased risk of a convulsion after diphtheria-tetanus-pertussis immunisation but no evidence that this produces brain injury or is a fore runner of epilepsy. Studies have also not linked immunisation with either sudden infant death syndrome or infantile spasms.'

Wentz and Marcuse[51] found that a significantly more powerful study than the NCES would require a study population of approximately 4 000 000 subjects and concluded that this might not be a wise use of public money. Reviewing the NCES and other studies, they said, 'we do not know if pertussis vaccine causes permanent brain damage. If it does, it occurs more rarely than it causes serious acute neurologic illness.' No convincing biological case has been made that pertussis vaccine is the cause of brain damage in infancy and few biological products have been scrutinized in such depth. The current consensus view is that the vaccine, despite its pyrogenic tendency, is safe, certainly in comparison to the natural disease and that there are no hard-and-fast circumstances when it should not be given. In view of the difficulty in proving a negative, it remains sensible not to give pertussis vaccine to a child who already shows signs of an evolving neurological disorder of unknown aetiology. There are no grounds for withholding it from children with known congenital or static neurological disorders.

Present situation

There is pressure to introduce the well-characterized toxoided vaccines which are already in use in Japan.[40]

In Sweden, two Japanese acellular vaccines were tested using plain whole-cell vaccine as a control. It was found that fewer fevers occurred in those children given the new vaccines and that they developed higher levels of antibody. In the subsequent phase II trials, controls were given dummy injections in a blinded study. The best of the acellular vaccines used only had a 69% protectiveness which compares poorly with British experience using whole-cell vaccine. Unfortunately adsorbed whole-cell vaccine was not used for control purposes. Matters were complicated by four deaths, probably from unrelated infections, in immunized but not in control children. The Swedish authorities decided not to adopt this vaccine pending further studies.[52,53] In France, Sweden, UK and USA, trials of acellular vaccines of differing types are in progress. It is clear that toxoided acellular vaccines give good antibody levels and little fever. The difficulty is to determine whether a new vaccine would be as protective and safe as existing whole-cell vaccine. The recent marked decline in pertussis following the return of a high pertussis immunization rate makes efficacy studies in the UK almost impossible. Until a licensed component pertussis vaccine is available the present whole-cell vaccine should be used; it is well proven, effective and safe. Alum-adsorbed preparations are associated with less fever, they are generally available either as a DTP or in monovalent form, though Gupta and Relyveld,[54] in a discussion on fever, advocate calcium-based adjuvants. In some countries other combinations are available including killed polio and *Haemophilus influenzae* B. The British contraindication advice was simplified in the 1992 Green book to:

1 If the child is suffering from any acute illness, immunization should be postponed until the child has recovered. Minor infections without fever or systemic upset are not reasons to withhold immunization.
2 Immunization should not be carried out in children who have a history of a severe local or general reaction to a preceding dose. (Local and general reactions are then defined in detail.) Earlier contraindications that included a personal or family history of stable neurological conditions have been withdrawn. A family or personal history of allergy has never been an official contraindication.

4 Poliomyelitis

The eradication of poliomyelitis through immunization is one of the greatest medical successes of the 20th century. The disease was first recognized as a clinical entity in the 19th century. Following heroic and sometimes misguided human experimentation, the principle of producing an effective vaccine was discovered but not acted upon in the 1940s. In the 1950s two highly effective types of vaccine were developed – the first was Salk's killed virus followed 5 years later by Sabin's oral vaccine.

There are three strains of polio virus each with a fixed antigenic structure. Failures have occurred when vaccines have not included all three antigens in sufficient quantity. Countries have polarized in their choice whether to use killed or live vaccine. For the UK where injections are unpopular, oral polio vaccine is an obvious choice. It produces a very complete protection and its use soon led to the eradication of endemic wild polio disease. The potential for reversion of the vaccine strain to wild paralytic virus presents a very small problem. The 1985 WHO estimate is one recipient case and one contact case per 4 million doses of vaccine distributed. These figures must be assessed cautiously, since other coincidental virus diseases cause paralytic states and the presence of wild type polio virus is not conclusive proof of vaccine reversion.[55]

The obvious way to prevent this is to ensure that adults who come into contact with children are immunized. Parents, particularly those born before 1958 when the British programme started, should have had a complete polio immunization course by the time their child is due to be immunized. The number of cases of contact polio declined markedly as the proportion of the immunized population rose.

Killed polio vaccine is favoured in Scandinavian and other North European countries and is administered in combination with DTP. The disadvantage is the lack of vicarious protection for the unimmunized, a point dramatically shown in Holland where a religious sect, who declined immunization, developed many cases of paralytic polio which spread to adherents of this sect in the USA and Canada. The importance of having optimal composition of the killed polio vaccine was shown in Finland where an epidemic of paralytic polio occurred following the long-standing use of a vaccine relatively deficient in type 3 antigen.

Poliomyelitis virus is easily transmissible with high infectivity, but the paralytic disease is relatively rare. The infection/paralysis rate is much higher in adults than in children. The importance of intact tonsils in protection against polio was demonstrated in the USA where, in pre-immunization days, recently tonsillectomized children had a markedly increased risk of the disease.

Poliomyelitis must be suspected in any child who develops a sudden and otherwise unexplained paralytic condition. In developed countries, doctors and parents now have little practical experience of the disease and it is vital that they understand that immunization is absolutely necessary to prevent its return. In many developing parts of the world, the disease is still endemic and it is wise to have booster immunization before foreign travel.

The oral vaccine is usually given as drops directly into the mouth of infants at the same visit as DTP immunization. Killed vaccine can also be given in conjunction with DTP vaccine. The oral vaccine is particularly unstable in extremes of temperature, it must be handled and stored between 2°–8° C.

Special circumstances

The oral vaccine should not be given to immunocompromised people. Those who are HIV-positive but free from symptomatic AIDS can be given oral vaccine. In neonatal nurseries it is sensible to give the first dose of oral vaccine at the door of the nursery when the babies leave, on the theoretical grounds that vaccine virus spread to premature infants might be undesirable.

5   Haemophilus influenzae b (called Hib vaccine)

Most bacterial meningitis in North European countries in infants after the neonatal stage is caused by one of three organisms: Neisseria meningitidis; Haemophilus influenzae b or Streptococcus pneumoniae. Although these diseases are treatable by timely antibiotics they are rapidly invasive and continue to cause appreciable mortality, and morbidity in survivors. Effective vaccination against these three diseases would prevent about 200 deaths per year in the British child population. Great efforts are underway to develop vaccines against these diseases. The first such vaccine commercially available is against H. influenzae b.

The original Hib vaccine only produced significant immunity in children over 18 months but a development which involved adsorption on to bacterial toxoids such as diphtheria, tetanus or meningococcus (these carrier toxoids however do not have useful immunogenic properties) has resulted in an effective vaccine for use in early infancy; this is a killed bacterial conjugate vaccine that contains capsular antigen. In some countries such vaccine is licensed as a combined preparation with DTP; but in the UK, at the time of writing, Hib is only available in a monocomponent form. This has to be administered in a separate syringe and site from DTP, though on the same occasion, starting at 2 months, followed by a further two doses at monthly intervals. Since nearly all the serious disease occurs in children under 5 years, British policy is to reserve it for this age group.[56]

Immediately before the introduction of Hib vaccine into the UK, it was estimated that each year one in 600 children under five developed some form of the disease of which over half had meningitic symptoms; among these were about 65 deaths annually from meningitis and a further 150 infants were left with postmeningitic damage including deafness; other serious manifestations include epiglottitis, osteomyelitis and pneumonia.

In Finland, where this vaccine was pioneered, the clinical disease has almost vanished. This vaccine has been extensively tested and experience is based on the administration of over 20 million doses. There are no reports of serious side effects; the main problem has been transitory redness and swelling around the immunization site, generally worst with the first rather than subsequent doses.

6   Tuberculosis

During the 20th century, the prevalence of tuberculosis (TB) has fallen dramatically in developed countries; in developing countries it remains a major health problem.[57–59] It is believed that half the world's population has active infection. In developed countries the greatest rate of improvement occurred before the event of either antibiotics or immunization showing that improved living standards are of the greatest benefit in protecting against this potentially lethal disease.

BCG immunization is based on a live attenuated form of mycobacterium tuberculosis: Bacille Calmette–Guérin (BCG), named after its developers. The vaccine was subcultured every 3 weeks over a 13-year period before its introduction by Weill-Halle. There is more variation between countries for practice of immunization against TB than for any other immunizing procedure. This stems from differing interpretation of studies of effectiveness. In the USA, BCG has never been in routine use; the prevalence of TB there fell greatly during this century until the recent arrival of human immunodeficiency virus (HIV) disease and rapidly declining health standards associated with narcotic drug use especially in the deprived inner cities.

In Asia and Africa there has been a lesser decline in tuberculosis. Large-scale studies of BCG vaccine have cast much doubt on its ability to influence immunity in these countries – is the appropriate antigenic strain of BCG being used? Has the vaccine been correctly handled? Is the vaccine intrinsically ineffective in countries where the level of exposure is very high?

The current British policy is to recommend that the vaccine should be offered in the newborn period to infants who come from families where a household member has a history of tuberculosis or where there is a major material risk of exposure from other sources. In the early 1970s the large refugee populations which came from Uganda and Kenya to the UK had a worryingly high prevalence of tuberculosis, mainly due to strains of mycobacteria specific to the UK. Intensive control campaigns using classic methods involving skin testing, mass radiography, universal neonatal BCG and contact tracing were set up and again proved their worth; currently only sporadic cases are seen in the UK child population.[60]

High-risk child groups

In the rare instances where a mother has active open tuberculosis it may be necessary for the child to be kept away from the mother while undergoing intensive treatment. The other main risk group in the UK are immune-suppressed children. In 1990 there was an outbreak of tuberculosis in a children's malignant disease unit.

The majority of British children, not considered to be at high risk, are offered tuberculin testing at school. A minority can be expected to have a healed infection and will be tuberculin positive. The strongly positive child will require examination and chest X-ray and the occasional case of active tuberculosis will be found. The majority can be expected to be tuberculin negative and will be offered BCG vaccination.

Medical opinion is divided whether the time has come for the programme to be abandoned. Because of the advent of HIV disease a decision has been postponed.

Practical aspects

TUBERCULIN TESTING: MANTOUX TEST

This is performed on the flexor surface of a forearm which must be dry and free from infection or other skin disorder. Using a 1 ml sterile syringe with a short bevel no. 25 needle 0.1 ml Tuberculin Purified Protein Derivative (PPD) is injected intradermally (half this dose is used for infants). This must be done by a skilled person and not delegated to the untrained. The size of the reaction has to be read 72 hours later. A raised, red, persistent lesion of 5 mm or greater is taken as a positive reaction.

HEAF TEST

The alternative test which involves the use of the Heaf multiple puncture gun is widely used in the UK. If the standard reusable Heaf gun is used it is important to ensure effective sterilization between patients. Use of the recently introduced disposable head apparatus ensures that there is no cross infection between subjects and is recommended.[61] The head for use for under 2 year olds is blue and for older children and adults is white. These heads have six needles and should not be confused with the red 18 needle head used to administer BCG vaccine. The Heaf test is performed on the flexor surface of the forearm using PPD of the correct dilution. The reaction is read between 3 and 10 days, graded 0–4 and recorded.[61]

BCG vaccination

BCG vaccine is supplied as a freeze dried preparation together with water for reconstitution in a separate vial. The injection (0.1 ml for all ages apart from babies under 3 months who should receive 0.05 ml) must be given intradermally raising an indurated surface about 7 mm in diameter. It must not be given intramuscularly. The preferred site is over the insertion of the deltoid to the humerus on the upper arm. BCG must not be given by jet injectors, though the redheaded multiple puncture gun can be used (a different vaccine is used under 2 years of age). A positive take will leave a small scar. If a scar does not develop a tuberculin test is indicated with a view to possible revaccination. A few of those immunized will develop a local abscess. Most settle spontaneously, though persistent abscesses may need treatment with isoniazid.

7 Measles, mumps, rubella vaccine

While monovalent modified live virus measles and rubella vaccines had been in use as separate preparations for two decades in the UK their uptake was vastly improved when they were reintroduced as a combined measles, mumps, rubella (MMR) vaccine in 1988. MMR had been used successfully elsewhere in Western Europe and North America during the previous decade and shown to be both safe and highly effective. With hindsight much morbidity could have been prevented in the UK if it had been introduced earlier. The reasons for the delay in its introduction were understandable. The image of immunization in the UK as a whole had been badly shaken by adverse publicity against pertussis vaccine. Older doctors whose memories stretched back to the original killed measles vaccines in the early 1960s remained unenthusiastic for any type of measles vaccine – although the live attenuated vaccine was a totally different type of product.

The public perception was that measles was a benign illness. It was not well appreciated that, worldwide, measles was one of the great child killing diseases and that in Europe 1 in 1000 children developed measles encephalitis leaving some with permanent brain injury and deafness. In addition there was a smattering of cases of subacute sclerosing encephalitis and measles can be an appreciable cause of death in immunocompromised children.

From a public health standpoint the introduction of MMR to the UK marked a shift towards the primary prevention of rubella by immunizing both boys and girls in infancy rather than the previous practice of vaccinating pre-pubertal girls only. Making this change lays open a potential risk that by eliminating wild rubella the whole nation would in future have to rely on vaccine-associated immunity for protection giving rise to the question – how long does immunity last? In the case of rubella would this protect potential mothers through their child-bearing years? There is now ample experience from the USA to be reassured that this occurs.

So far as measles and mumps are concerned there has been controversy that these immunizations might need repeating; this stems from the fact that the earlier live-attenuated measles vaccines were not as antigenic as present types. This situation is being carefully watched but experience so far is reassuring.[62]

The potential problem is among the older people who have never been immunized and who remain at risk. For reasons that remain unknown these illnesses tend to be more serious in older people. There has been concern that some people do not develop antibodies following immunization even if given repeatedly. This situation appears to be very rare. There is, however, evidence that the vaccine is protective even in the absence of demonstrable antibodies. The presumption is that the antibodies that can be measured demonstrate only part of the protective mechanism. There is now solid evidence that attenuated virus vaccines cannot spread by person-to-person contact unlike oral polio vaccine virus.

Contraindications to MMR

In the UK these include:[61]

1   Children with acute febrile illness when they present for immunization; this should be deferred.
2   Children with untreated malignant disease or altered immunity; those receiving immunosuppressive or radiotherapy or high-dose steroids.
3   Children who have received another live vaccine – including BCG – within the previous 3 weeks.
4   Children with allergies to neomycin or kanamycin.
5   If MMR is given to adult women, pregnancy should be avoided for one month.
6   MMR vaccine should not be given within one month of an injection of immunoglobulin.

When to immunize

Conventional advice in the UK is to give the immunization (once only) in the age range 12–15 months. Whether to start at 12 or 15 months has given rise to controversy. Preston[19] has drawn attention to the lower rates of vaccine failure against measles in children immunized at 15 months. On the other hand, the impression is that, the younger the child, the more likely they are to be brought up for their immunization.

Eggs and other allergies[63]

The single commonest worry about MMR seems to be a history of egg allergy. In recent years measles vaccine has not been grown on egg medium; mumps vaccine is grown on chicken embryo at an early stage though it is later transferred to chicken fibroblast cell culture which does not contain any egg protein. The actual amount of egg protein in the vaccine is exceedingly small and anxiety about this tends to get out of proportion. It is important to differentiate between anaphylaxis – choking and collapse after eating egg – and so-called egg allergy, which usually consists of blotchiness of the skin or often just dislike of egg.

Uptake of MMR vaccine

Since the introduction of MMR in the UK, the uptake rate has risen from 60% to over 90% coverage in most of the country and is still rising. There has been a steep decline in notifications of measles and mumps. For the time being the existing policy of administering monovalent rubella vaccine to girls aged 10–14 years is being continued in the UK; this policy will be reviewed when the cohort given MMR reach this age.

Safety of the vaccine

A number of anecdotal reports of problems in recently immunized children have appeared in the medical literature. The most common sequel is a minor systemic upset. A mild form of measles occurring about 5 days after immunization with a transitorily erythematous rash is well known. A smaller proportion of children develop a mild form of mumps about 21 days after immunization with transient swelling of the parotid glands. There is an occasional case of transient rubella-like rash at about 28 days. These are all self-limiting and acceptable problems. What is of more concern are the occasional reports of encephalitis about 14 days after measles immunization. This question was thoroughly explored in the course of the National Childhood Encephalopathy Study.[44] While such cases occurred with an attributable risk of about 1 in 10 000 of children immunized, these conditions subsided and there was no evidence of any cases of lasting neurological problems that could be attributed to the measles component. This compares to a figure of 1 in 1000 children developing encephalitis associated with clinical wild measles.[64] So far as the mumps component is concerned there have been a handful of reported cases of transitory encephalitis about 3 weeks after MMR immunization without lasting sequelae.[65–68]

Following further reports of mild meningoencephalitis the British authorities decided to withdraw MMR vaccines Urabe attenuated mumps virus strain and rely on the alternative Jeryl Lynn strain which has not shown this association.[66]

By 1992 measles and mumps came under control in the UK and the number of reports of congenital rubella continues to fall – most of the 20 cases currently detected annually in the UK are due to rubella contracted in women born and infected abroad.

While it is good news for children and their parents that these preventable diseases are disappearing, the benefits to the nations concerned are enormous in economic terms. The much feared secondary presentations of these diseases are already becoming rare; this includes subacute sclerosing panencephalitis (SSPE) of measles; deafness and pancreatitis associated with mumps and congenital rubella syndrome. Parents seem to appreciate the rationale of protection against three diseases with one shot of vaccine. Having a high level of herd immunity will protect those who were born abroad and were never immunized. These three diseases do not have a natural animal reservoir and it would be possible to eliminate them globally once very high levels of vaccine uptake are achieved.

Acknowledgements

I am grateful to my colleague Professor David Miller for checking the pertussis section and to the PHLS for use of their library.

Sources for further reading

Immunization has now become a major area of research interest. Most of the developmental work is published in relatively obscure publications or delivered at conferences. Information about infectious disease and its control through vaccination is carried in the regular bulletins from WHO and the national disease control agencies such as *Morbidity and Mortality Weekly Reports* (MMWR) in the USA; *Communicable Disease Report (CDR)* in England and Wales; *Communicable Diseases and Environmental Health* in Scotland; *Communicable Diseases Intelligence* in Australia; and *Communicable Disease New Zealand* (CDNZ). Many countries produce guidelines on immunization either sponsored by paediatric associations or health ministries. Examples include the Red Book of the American Academy of Pediatrics or the green *Immunisation against Infectious Disease* in the UK. France produces *Vaccination aujourd'hui* and Canada *Vaccination Canada*. There are international journals *Vaccine* and the newly started *Vaccine Research*. The US Center for Disease Control annual survey of recent research, *Immunization*, contains many hundred references and annotations. *The Lancet* carried a series of review articles on immunization in the first half of 1990.

References

1 Poore, P. A global view of immunisation. *J Royal Coll Phys* 1987; **21:** 22–27.
2 Hinman, A.R. What will it take to fully protect all American children with vaccines? *Am J Dis Child* 1991; **145:** 559–562.
3 Isaacs, D., Menser, M. Measles, mumps, rubella and varicella. *Lancet* 1990; i: 1384–1387.
4 Peckham, C.S., Bedford, H., Senturia, Y., Ades, A. *National Immunisation Study: Factors Influencing Immunisation Uptake in Childhood*. Horsham: Action Research, 1989.
5 Kinder, J., Teare, L., Roa, M., Bridgman, G., Kurian, A. False contraindications to childhood immunization. *Br J Gen Practit* 1992; **42:** 160–161.
6 Ross, E.M., Begg, N. Child health computing, *Br Med J* 1991; **302:** 5–6.
7 McKinney, P.A., Alexander, F.E., Nicholson, C., *et al.* Mothers' reports of childhood vaccinations and infections and their concordance with general practitioner records. *J Public Health Med* 1991; **13:** 13–22.
8 Bishai, D.M., Bhatt, S., Miller, L.T., Hayden, G.F. Vaccine storage practice in pediatric offices. *Pediatrics* 1992; **89:** 193–196.
9 Thompson, M.K. Needling doubts when to vaccinate. *Br Med J* 1988; **297:** 779–780.
10 Preston, N.W. Childhood immunisation issues in the new decade. *Br Med J* 1991; **302:** 966–967.
11 Miller, D.L., Ross, E.M., Alderslade, R., *et al.* Pertussis immunisation and serious acute neurological illness in childhood. *Br Med J* 1981; **1:** 1595–1599.
12 Romanus, V., Jonsell, R., Bergquist, S.-O. Pertussis in Sweden after the cessation of general immunization in 1979. *Pediatr Infect Dis J* 1987; **6:** 364–371.
13 Kimura, M., Kino-Sakai, H. Current epidemiology of pertussis in Japan. *Pediatr Infect Dis J* 1990; **9:** 705–709.
14 Wardlaw, A.G., Parton, R., eds. Pathogenesis and immunity in pertussis. Chichester: John Wiley, 1988.
15 Edwards, K.M., Karzon, D.T. Pertussis vaccines. *Pediatr Clin N Am* 1990; **37:** 549–566.
16 Lambert, H.P. The enigma of pertussis. *J Roy Coll Phys Lond* 1985; **19:** 67–71.
17 Cherry, J.D. The epidemiology of pertussis and pertussis immunization in the United Kingdom and the United States: a comparative study. In: Lockhart, J.D., ed. *Current Problems in Pediatrics*. Chicago: Year Book Medical Publishers, 1984; vol 14, no. 2.
18 Madsen, T. Vaccination against whooping cough. *J Am Med Assoc* 1933; **101:** 187–188.
19 Preston, N.W. Pertussis today. In: Wardlaw, A.C., Parton, R., eds. *Pathogenesis and Immunity in Pertussis*. Chichester: Wiley, 1988; 1–18.
20 Medical Research Council. Vaccination against whooping cough: relation between protection in children and results of laboratory tests. *Br Med J* 1956; **2:** 454–462.
21 Medical Research Council. Vaccination against whooping cough. *Br Med J* 1959; **1:** 994–1000.
22 Fine, P.E.M., Clarkson, J.A. Reflections on the efficacy of pertussis vaccines. *Rev Infect Dis* 1987; **9:** 866–883.
23 Pollock, T.M., Mortimer, J.Y., Miller, E., Smith, G. Symptoms after primary immunisation with DTP and DT vaccine. *Lancet* 1984; ii: 146–149.
24 Waight, P.A., Pollock, T.M., Miller, E., Coleman, E.M. Pyrexia after diphtheria-tetanus-pertussis and diphtheria-tetanus vaccines. *Arch Dis Child* 1983; **58:** 921–923.
25 Levine, S., Wenk, E.J. A hyperimmune form of allergic encephalomyelitis. *Am J Pathol* 1965; **47:** 61–88.
26 Cody, C.L., Baraff, L.J., Cherry, J.D., Marcy, S.M., Manclark, C.R. Nature and rates of adverse reactions

associated with DTP and DT immunizations in infants and children. *Pediatrics* 1981; **68:** 650–660.

27 Miller, C.L., Pollock, T.M., Clewer, A.D.E. Whooping cough vaccination: an assessment. *Lancet* 1974; ii: 510–513.

28 Hooker, J.M.H. A laboratory study of the toxicity of some diphtheria-tetanus-pertussis vaccines. *J Biol Stand* 1981; **9:** 493–506.

29 Byers, R.K., Moll, F.C. Encephalopathies following prophylactic pertussis vaccine. *Pediatrics* 1948; **1:** 437–457.

30 Toomey, J.A. Reactions to pertussis vaccine. *J Am Med Assoc* 1949; **139:** 448–450.

31 Berg, J.M. Neurological complications of pertussis immunization. *Br Med J* 1958; ii: 24–30.

32 Ström, J. Is universal vaccination against pertussis always justified? *Br Med J* 1960; ii: 696–697.

33 Ström, J. Further experience of reactions especially of a cerebral nature, in conjunction with triple vaccination: a study based on vaccinations in Sweden 1959–65. *Br Med J* 1967; iv: 320–323.

34 Malgren, B., Vahlquist, B., Zetterstrom, R. Complications of immunization. *Br Med J* 1960; ii: 1800–1801.

35 Kulenkampff, M., Schwartzman, J.S., Wilson, J. Neurological complications of pertussis inoculation. *Arch Dis Child* 1974; **49:** 46–49.

36 Ehrengut, W. Läßt sich die Reserve gegenüber der Pertussis-Schutzimpfung begründen? *Ped Praxis*, 1980; **23:** 3–13.

37 Royal College of General Practitioners; Swansea Research Unit. Effect of a low pertussis vaccination rate on a large community. *Br Med J* 1981; **282:** 23–26.

38 Dudgeon Panel Report. In: *Whooping Cough*. London: HMSO, 1981: 6–26.

39 Meade Panel Report. In: *Whooping Cough*. London: HMSO, 1981; 27–49.

40 Kimura, M., Harumo-Sakai, H. Developments in pertussis immunisation in Japan. *Lancet* 1990; ii: 30–32.

41 Pollock, T.M., Morris, J. A 7 year survey of disorders attributed to vaccination in North West Thames Region. *Lancet* 1983; i: 753–757.

42 Miller, D.L., Alderslade, R., Ross, E.M. Whooping cough and whooping cough vaccine: the risks and benefits debate. *Epidemiol Rev* 1982; 4: 1–24.

43 Ross, E.M. Reactions to whole-cell pertussis vaccine. In: Wardlaw, A.C., Parton, R., eds. *Pathogenesis and Immunity in Pertussis*. Chichester: Wiley, 1988: 375–398.

44 DHSS. *Whooping Cough*. London: HMSO, 1981.

45 Miller, D., Madge, N., Diamond, J., Ross, E. Pertussis immunisation and serious acute neurological illness in children. *Br Med J* 1993; **307:** 1171–1176.

46 Bellman, M.H., Miller, D.L., Ross, E.M. Infantile spasms and pertussis immunisation. *Lancet* 1983; i: 1031–1034.

47 Hirtz, D.C., Nelson, K.B., Ellenberg, J.H. Seizures following childhood immunization. *J Pediatr* 1983; **102:** 14–18.

48 Butler, N.R., Golding, J. Immunisations. In: *From Birth to Five*. Oxford: Pergamon, 1986; 295–319.

49 Griffen, M.R., Ray, W.A., Mortimer, E.A., Fenichel, G.M., Schaffner, W. Risk of seizures and encephalopathy after immunization with the diphtheria-tetanus-pertussis vaccine. *J Am Med Assoc* 1990; **263:** 1641–1645.

50 Golden, G.S. Pertussis vaccine and injury to the brain. *J Pediatr* 1990; **116:** 854–861.

51 Wentz, K.R., Marcuse, E.K. Diphtheria-tetanus-pertussis vaccine and serious neurologic illness: an updated review of the epidemiologic evidence. *Pediatrics* 1991; **87:** 287–297.

52 Ad hoc Group for the Study of Pertussis Vaccines. Placebo-controlled trial of two acellular pertussis vaccines in Sweden: protective efficacy and adverse effects. *Lancet* 1988; i: 955–960.

53 Storsaeter, J., Olin, P., Renemar, B. *et al.* Mortality and morbidity from invasive bacterial infections during a clinical trial of acellular pertussis vaccines in Sweden. *Pediatr Infect Dis J* 1988; **7:** 637–645.

54 Gupta, R.K., Relyveld, E.H. Adverse reactions after injection of adsorbed DTP vaccine are not due only to pertussis organisms or pertussis components in the vaccine. *Vaccine* 1991; **9:** 699–702.

55 Nkowane, B.M., Wassilak, S.G.F., Orenstein, W.A., Bart, K.J., Schonberger, L.B., Hinman, A.R., Kew, O.M. Vaccine associated paralytic poliomyelitis, United States: 1973 through 1984. *J Am Med Assoc* 1987; **257:** 1335–1340.

56 Booy, R., Taylor, S.A., Dobson, S.R.M. *et al.* Immunogenicity and safety of PRP – T conjugate vaccine given according to the British accelerated vaccination schedule. *Arch Dis Child* 1992; **67:** 475–478.

57 Smith, M.D.H., Marquis, J.R. Tuberculosis and other mycobacterial infections. In: Feigin, R.D., Cherry, J.D. *Textbook of Pediatric Infectious Diseases*. Philadelphia: Saunders, 1987; 1342–1387.

58 Fine, P.E.M., Rodriques, L.C. Mycobacterial diseases. *Lancet* 1990; i: 1016–1020.

59 Miller, F.J.W., Thompson, M.D. Decline and fall of the tubercle baccillus: the Newcastle story 1882–1988. *Arch Dis Child* 1992; **67:** 251–255.

60 Conway, S.P. BCG vaccination in children. *Br Med J* 1990; **301:** 1059–1060.

61 UK Departments of Health. *Immunisation against infectious disease*. London: HMSO, 1992.

62 King, G.E., Markowitz, L.I., Patriarca, M.D., Dales, L.G. Clinical efficacy of measles vaccine during the 1990 measles epidemic. *J Pediatr Infect Dis* 1991; **10:** 883–887.

63 Greenberg, M.A., Brix, D.L. Safe administration of mumps measles rubella vaccine in egg allergic children. *J Pediatr* 1988; **113:** 504–508.

64 Miller, D.L. Frequency of complications of measles, 1963. *Br Med J* 1964; **2:** 75–78.

65 Noah, N. Mumps: worthy of elimination? In: Morgan-Capner, P., ed. *Current Topics in Clinical Virology*. London: Public Health Laboratory Services (PHLS), 1991: 46–60.

66 Miller, E., Goldacre, M., Pugh, S., Colville, A., Farrington, P., Flower A., Nash, J., Macfarlane, L., Tettmar, R. Risk of aseptic meningitis after measles, mumps and rubella vaccine in UK children. *Lancet* 1993; **341:** 979–982.

67 Anon. Mumps meningitis and MMR vaccination (editorial). *Lancet* 1989; ii: 1015–1016.

68 Fujinaga, T., Motegi, Y., Tamura, H., Kuroume, T. A prefecture wide survey of mumps meningitis associated with measles, mumps, rubella vaccine. *Pediatr Infect Dis J* 1991; **10:** 204–209.

Further reading

The most important textbook is:

Plotkin, S.A., Mortimer, E.A. *Vaccines*. Philadelphia: Saunders, 1988. A comprehensive account of all vaccines in current use.
Also very useful:
Aicardi, J. Neurological complications of immunizations. In: *Diseases of the Nervous System in Childhood*. Oxford: Mac Keith Press, 1992: 719–731.
American Academy of Pediatrics. Report of the Committee on Infectious Diseases. 'The Red Book'. Evanston, Illinois: AAP.
Christie, A.B. *Infectious Diseases: Epidemiology and Practice*. 4th edn. 2 vols. Edinburgh, Churchill Livingstone. 1987.

Dudgeon, J.A., Cutting, W.A.M., eds. *Immunization: Principles and Practice*. London: Chapman and Hall Medical, 1991.
Feigin, R.D., Cherry, J.D. eds *Textbook of Pediatric Infectious Diseases*. 2nd edn. Philadelphia: Saunders, 1987.
Howson, C.P., Howe, C.J., Fineberg, H.V. eds *Adverse Effects of Pertussis and Rubella Vaccines*. Washington DC: National Academy Press, 1991.
Rudd, P., Nicoll, A., eds. *Manual on Infections and Immunizations in Children*. Oxford: Oxford Medical Publications, 1991.
UK Departments of Health. Immunisation against infectious disease. 'The Green Book'. London: HMSO, 1992.
Wardlaw, A.C., Parton, R. eds *Pathogenesis and Immunity in Pertussis*. Chichester: John Wiley, 1988.

7.4 Food and nutrition

Brenda Clark and Brian Wharton

Recommended daily amounts

Recommended daily intakes (RDAs) are defined as 'the average amount of the nutrient which should be provided per head in a *group* of people if the needs of practically all the members of the group are to be met.' Thus RDAs are not indicators for the diets of individuals but are often used incorrectly in this way. The recommended levels set for the various nutrients are well above physiological requirements in order to cover 'practically all members of the group'; only energy is set at the average requirement for the group.

Recommended daily amounts do not cover every essential nutrient. Non-essential nutrients such as carbohydrate and fibre are not referred to, nor is the quality of certain nutrients such as the type of fat. The use of these tables for children poses particular problems as age is used as the basis for the recommendations without regard to the considerable variations in body size which occur in children of the same age.

Table 7.2 is an amalgam of various recommendations[1–3] where age is used as the reference. In order to overcome the problem of variation in body size, we have found it more useful to relate advisable nutrient intakes to energy by expressing each nutrient per 100 kcal of energy intake. This allows an automatic adjustment for body size when considering the advisable intake of an individual child and the quality of a particular diet can be more readily assessed. Table 7.3 shows advisable nutrient intakes based on a per 100 kcal basis.

Dietary guidelines

It is important for health professionals in the community to be quite clear about the difference between RDAs and dietary guidelines. The figures for RDAs have frequently been set following metabolic balance studies or from observations of nutrient deficiency states in humans. Each country will have only one set of RDAs.

Dietary guidelines are a more recent and, in general, more highly publicized development aimed at promoting the health of the general population by reducing the adult degenerative diseases believed to be wholly or partly attributed to diet. Such diseases are arterial disease, obesity, dental decay, hypertension and various large bowel disorders. There have been many dietary guidelines published by such authorities as COMA,[4] WHO,[5] BMA,[6] AAP,[7] NACNE,[8] and AHA[9] and Table 7.4 gives examples, some of which specifically exclude children below certain ages. Although there are slight differences in 'target' intakes for dietary components such as fibre and fat, the new diet called a 'healthy' diet is one which is in general lower in sugar and fat (particularly saturated fat), and higher in fibre. Thus, unlike RDAs, dietary guidelines address the quality of the dietary components rather than the quantity and have not been based on physiological and biochemical studies in individuals but on analysis of adult population lifestyles, diets, morbidity and mortality statistics. These high fibre, low fat diets should not be indiscriminately advised for young children as weight loss and mineral deficiency may occur due to the low nutrient density and bulkiness of the food and poorer mineral absorption. The use of refined wheat bran to achieve the targets for fibre intake is not recommended for very

Table 7.2 Recommended daily amounts of food energy and some nutrients for population groups. Adapted from DH 1991 Dietary Reference Values for Food Energy and Nutrients for the UK,[1] NRC 1989[2] and WHO 1974[3]

Age range	Average expected body weight (kg)	Fluid ml/day for a full fluid diet	Energy mean[1] Age (months)	Mj	kcal	Protein (g)[3]	Thiamin (mg)[1]	Riboflavin (mg)[1]	Nicotinic acid equivalents (mg)[1]	B12 (µg)[2]	Ascorbic acid vit C (mg)[1]	Vitamin A retinal equivalents (µg)[1]	Vitamin D cholecalciferol (µg)[1]	Calcium (mg)[1]	Phosphorus (mmol)[2]	Iron (mg)[1]
Infants																
0–6 months		150[a]	0–3m	2.22	530	2.2[a,3]	0.3	0.4		0.3	25	350	8.5	525	9.7	1.7 0–3 months
			0–6m	2.79	667											4.3 0–6 months
7–12 months		150[a]	7–9m	3.32	795	2.0[a,3]	0.3	0.4		0.5	25	350	7.0	525	16.1	7.8
			10–12m	3.73	892											
Boys																
1	11.5	1100		5.15	1230	30.0	0.4 mg/1000 kcal →	0.6	6.6 mg/1000 kcal →	0.7	30	400	7.0	350	25.8	6.9
2	13.5	1300		5.15	1230	35.0		0.6		0.7	30	400	7.0	350	25.8	6.9
3–4	16.5	1500		7.16	1715	39.0		0.8		0.7	30	400	7.0	450	25.8	6.1
5–6	20.0	1700		7.16	1715	43.0		0.9		1.0	30	400	b	450	25.8	6.1
7–8	25.0	1800		8.24	1970	49.0		1.0		1.4	30	500	b	550	25.8	8.7
9–11	32.0	2200		9.27	2220	57.0		1.2		2.0	35	500	b	1000	38.7	8.7
12–14	44.0	2300		9.27	2220	66.0		1.2		2.0	35	600	b	1000	38.7	11.3
15–17	62.0	3000		11.51	2755	72.0		1.3		2.0	40	700	b	1000	38.7	11.3
Girls																
1	11.0	1050		4.86	1165	27.0		0.6		0.7	30	400	7.0	350	25.8	6.9
2	13.5	1300		4.86	1165	32.0		0.6		0.7	30	400	7.0	350	25.8	6.9
3–4	16.0	1450		6.46	1545	37.0		0.8		0.7	30	400	7.0	450	25.8	6.1
5–6	20.0	1700		6.46	1545	42.0		0.9		1.0	30	400	b	450	25.8	6.1
7–8	25.0	1800		7.28	1740	47.0		1.0		1.4	30	500	b	550	25.8	8.7
9–11	32.0	2000		7.28	1740	51.0		1.2		2.0	35	500	b	800	38.7	8.7
12–14	50.0	2200		7.92	1845	53.0		1.1		2.0	35	600	b	800	38.7	14.8[c]
15–17	56.0	2200		8.83	2100	53.0		1.1		2.0	40	600	b	800	38.7	14.8[c]

[1] DH 1991 Dietary Reference Values for Food Energy and Nutrients for the UK. Based on the Reference Nutrient Intake – an amount of a nutrient that is enough for almost every individual, even someone who has high needs for the nutrient.
[2] From NRC 1989
[3] From WHO 1974
[a] Value/kg actual body weight per day.
[b] No dietary sources may be necessary for children and adults who are sufficiently exposed to sunlight, but during the winter children and adolescents should receive 10 µg (400 i.u.) daily by supplementation. Those with inadequate exposure to sunlight, for example those who are 'housebound' may also need a supplement of 10 µg daily.
[c] About 10% of women with very high menstrual losses will need more iron then shown. Their needs are best met by taking iron supplements.

Table 7.3 Advisable intake of nutrients per unit energy

Nutrient/100 kcal	0–11 months	Age of child 1 year–1 year 11 months	2–10 years
Protein (g)	2.25–3.0	2.25–3.0	2.25–3.5
N_2(g)	0.36–0.48	0.36–0.48	0.4–0.56
Non-protein Kcal:N_2 ratio	160:1–238:1	193:1–228:1	194:1–175:1
Fat (g)	3.3–6.5	3.3–5.5	3.3–4.2
C8:0 % total fat	Maximum 20%		
C10:0% total fat	Maximum 20%		
C12:0% total fat	Maximum 15%		
C14:0% total fat	Maximum 15%		
Linoleic acid (g) C18:2	0.3–1.2	0.3–1.2	0.3–1.2
Total carbohydrate (CHO) (g)	7–14	10–15	12–15
Lactose	Min 3.5		
Sucrose	<20% total CHO		
Fructose	Not usually added		
Pre-cooked starch and/or gelatinized starch	<30% total CHO		
Minerals			
Iron (mg)	0.5–1.5	0.6–1.2	0.6–1.2
Calcium (mg)	Min 45	Min 45	Min 35
Phosphorus (mg)	25–90	50–100	50–100
Sodium (mmol)	1.0–2.6	1.0–3.0	1.0–3.0
Potassium (mmol)	1.6–3.8	1.6–5.7	1.6–5.7
Chloride (mmol)	1.4–3.5	1.4–3.5	1.4–4.0
Magnesium (mg)	5–15	10–20	10–20
Copper (μg)	60–120	Min 100	Min 100
Zinc (mg)	0.3–1.0	0.5–1.0	0.5–1.0
Manganese (μg)	2–8	Min 100	Min 100
Iodide (μg)	Min 5	Min 5	Min 5
Chromium (μg)	3–10	3–10	3–10
Molybdenum (μg)	5–15	5–15	5–15
Selenium (μg)	3–10	3–10	3–10
Fluoride (mg)	0.02–0.1	0.04–0.15	0.04–0.15
Vitamins			
Vitamin A (μg RE)	60–180	25–45	20–45
Vitamin D (μg cholecalciferol)	1–2	0.8–1.0	0.6–1.0
Vitamin E (mg)	Min 0.5	Min 0.4	Min 0.4
(mg/g PUFA)	Min 0.5	Min 0.4	Min 0.4
Vitamin K (μg)	2.5–15.0	1.5–15.0	1.5–15.0
Vitamin C (mg)	Min 5	Min 1.5	Min 1.5
Thiamine (mg)	0.04–0.09	0.04–0.09	0.04–0.09
Riboflavin (mg)	0.06–0.4	0.1–0.4	0.1–0.4
Nicotinic acid (mg equivalent)	0.250–1.25	0.6–1.25	0.6–1.25
Folic acid (μg)	4–10	8–20	8–20
B_{12}(μg)	0.1–0.5	0.15–0.5	0.15–0.5
Pyridoxine (mg)	0.035–0.16	0.08–0.16	0.08–0.16
Biotin (μg)	1.5–5.00	Min 5	Min 5
Pantothenic acid (mg)	0.30–0.75	0.20–0.75	0.20–0.75
Energy		110–(3 × age) × kg body weight	

Table 7.4 Examples of dietary guidelines

Professional body	Age groups excluded	%Total food energy as		Fibre (g/day)	Sugar (kg/head/day)
		Saturated fat	Total fat		
COMA[4]	<5 years	15	35		
WHO[5]		10	30		
BMA[6]		10	30	30	20
AAP[7]			30–40		
NACNE[8]		10	30	30	20
AHA[9]	<2 years	10	30		

COMA   Committee on Medical Aspects of Food Policy, UK.
WHO   World Health Organization.
BMA   British Medical Association.
AAP   American Academy of Pediatrics.
NACNE   National Advisory Committee on Nutrition Education, UK.
AHA   American Heart Association.

young children. Bran contains phytate which may bind minerals such as calcium, iron, zinc and copper, and limit their absorption from the gut. Fibre intake is better achieved with whole foods, such as wholemeal bread and pasta, whole grain rice and other cereals, starchy vegetables, peas, lentils, fruits and vegetables. It is then more likely that adequate amounts of both fibre and micronutrients will be achieved.

Normal diet

Infancy 0–12 months

Nutrition during the first 12 months of life can be divided into two stages:

  a the suckling phase
  b the weanling phase.

The suckling's diet

This phase covers the first 6 months of life when infants are either predominantly breast or bottle fed.

BREAST FEEDING

Breast milk, with its correct balance of nutrients and chemical constituents, is the nutritional ideal. It contains taurine and carnitine, not found in such high concentrations in the milk of other mammals and also lymphocytes, macrophages, secretory IgA and other non-specific immunological substances such as lactoferrin which help to confer immunological protection against potential pathogens.

Between 1975 and 1980, the incidence of breast feeding in the UK gradually increased but since then has remained static at around 65% of babies being put to the breast at birth but only 39% still being breast fed at the age of 6 weeks.[10] Mothers over 25 years of age living in the south of England, and from the higher social classes, are most likely to breast feed. Clearly

education about the benefits of breast feeding has to be targeted to poorer mothers from the lower social classes.

Community midwives can give enormous support and much practical guidance to breast-feeding mothers. Family doctors will find it useful to know the approach to breast feeding by community midwives working in their practices. This is explained in a publication of the Royal College of Midwives.[11]

There are few contraindications to breast feeding. Even mothers who have open (sputum positive) tuberculosis may breast feed so long as their babies are given isoniazid-resistant BCG vaccine shortly after birth and then receive isoniazid for 6 weeks.

Mothers who have AIDS are advised not to breast feed their babies and some maternal drugs may be a contraindication. An up-to-date list of these is given in the British National Formulary. Some other contraindications to breast feeding are if the baby is born with a rare condition such as galactosaemia or congenital lactase deficiency, where there would be an inability to digest or metabolize the lactose present in breast milk. Babies with some of the inborn errors of metabolism such as phenylketonuria, can now be safely breast fed so long as paediatric dietetic and medical supervision is available.

Occasionally some breast-fed babies require extra nutrients even when thriving:

i Haemorrhagic disease A rare occurrence seen almost exclusively in breast-fed babies due to vitamin K deficiency. Vitamin K should be given to all babies at birth. The British Paediatric Association recommends:

Oral vitamin K 500 μg as Konakion on the day of birth for all babies;
Then for breast-fed infants, 500 μg at 7–10 days and 500 μg at 4–6 weeks.

ii Rickets Due to maternal vitamin D deficiency: breast milk contains little vitamin D and the infant depends on the maternal supply of vitamin D to provide sufficient stores in utero. The Department of Health recommends vitamin D supplements for pregnancy and this will also reduce the risk of the mother developing osteomalacia during her pregnancy and her baby having hypocalcaemic convulsions around 7 days of age. Five drops daily of the Department of Health vitamin drops provide 7 μg vitamin D (also 200 μg vitamin A and 20 mg vitamin C).

BOTTLE FEEDING

Which feed?   Bottle feeding is a safe alternative to breast milk so long as an approved infant formula is used. The present infant formulas closely mimic the chemical composition of mature breast milk but cannot mirror its complex immunological and enzyme content. Table 7.5 summarizes the currently available infant formulas based on cow's milk which comprise two groups: whey-predominant or casein-predominant formulas. Casein-predominant formulas are essentially skimmed milk plus a fat blend and some other nutrients; the protein is 80% casein and 20% whey, that is the same as cow's milk. Whey-predominant formulas are based on demineralized whey plus a fat blend and other nutrients; the protein is 60% whey and 40% casein, as in breast milk although the source of the protein is still cow's milk. Generally we advise a demineralized whey formula but there are no objections to those based on casein.

Soya formulas   Although growth has been found to be generally satisfactory in babies fed formulas based on soya protein isolates, qualitatively their nutritional content is quite different to breast milk. Whether this will have implications for the child's future physical and neurological development is presently unknown. For this reason, unless there is a proven intolerance to cow's milk, the casual use of soya formulas should be discouraged. They are contraindicated for preterm and low birthweight infants and for those with impaired renal function because of their high aluminium content.[12]

When a soya formula is required, it is essential that a nutritionally complete formula designed for infants is used. Currently available formulas are: Isomil (Abbott); Infasoy (Cow and Gate); Ostersoy (Farley); Pro-

sobee, liquid and powder (Mead Johnson) and Wysoy (Wyeth).

Liquid soya drinks which are sold in supermarkets and health food shops are unsuitable due to their low energy and nutrient density.

HOW MUCH MILK?

The two yardsticks of an infant's nutritional health are the baby's satisfaction and growth. The assessment of growth is more objective and this is discussed in an earlier chapter. Healthy babies who are growing normally consume a wide range of volumes – anything between 110 and 200 ml/kg/day divided between five to eight feeds daily.

Mothers need reassurance that if their baby is thriving an adequate volume of feed is being consumed. This is particularly relevant to mothers who are breast feeding; as long as growth is adequate, there is no need for test weighings and they may cause so much anxiety as to be counterproductive. Both breast-fed and bottle-fed babies should be fed on demand and receive as much as they wish to take. This *ad libitum* policy does not lead to an excessive prevalence of obesity because, from about the age of 6 weeks, infants develop an internal sensor which enables them to control their energy intake (as long as the feed has been correctly reconstituted in the case of bottle-fed babies).

SWITCHING TO OTHER FORMULAS

The majority of bottle-fed babies receive a whey-based infant formula initially as most maternity units use these. Many studies have shown that at around the age of 6 weeks, 20–25% of babies have their formula changed.[13] Indeed, some health professionals advise mothers to give casein-predominant feeds from 3 months of age because they believe they are theoretically more satisfying. There is no evidence that this is true and the practice of switching milks should be discouraged, as this often causes unnecessary anxiety for mothers. In some cases, the diagnosis of disease may be delayed due to the misconceived idea that formula swapping may be the answer. The formula chosen at birth can be safely continued throughout the first year of life. However, if the mother insists on changing, little harm is done and it is pointless to continue with a particular formula if a mother is convinced (however mistakenly) that it does not suit her baby.

OTHER FLUIDS

Extra drinks of fruit juice or boiled water during the first 2 weeks of life may interfere with the establishment of breast or bottle feeding. Young infants normally require no additional fluids but bottle-fed

Table 7.5 Infant formulas available in UK

Whey-predominant formulas	Casein-predominant formulas	
Aptamil	Milumil	(Milupa)
Nutrilon Premium	Nutrilon Plus	(Cow & Gate)
Farley's first milk	Farley's second milk	(Farley)
SMA Gold	SMA White	(Wyeth)

infants may be thirsty in hot weather and can then be offered cool boiled water. Fruit juices and baby drinks contain glucose or fructose and may contribute to dental caries. They are expensive and not necessary in the suckling's diet; if given, they should always be well diluted.

FEED PREPARATION

Water from water softeners should not be used to prepare infant formulas as it may contain excess sodium. Similarly, some bottled (spring) waters contain high concentrations of sodium, nitrate, fluoride and sulphate. Repeatedly boiled water will concentrate the mineral content and should not be used. Making up a feed with boiling water will destroy some of the vitamin content as well as denaturing the protein; ideally, the water used to reconstitute a feed should be at 40–60°C, i.e. boiled and then allowed to cool for a few minutes.

Microwave ovens should never be used to warm feeds as the internal temperature of the milk may be much higher than the bottle feels. Burns and scalds around the baby's mouth have been occasionally reported with this practice.[14]

The weanling's diet

The Department of Health in its third report,[15] recommends that solid foods be introduced between the ages of 3 and 6 months. The reasons and principles of the weaning process are outlined in Table 7.6.

About 12 weeks after the introduction of solids, most babies will be able to cope, if supervised, with finger foods and manage soft mashed foods rather than a strained or puréed consistency. The British Dietetic Association's Paediatric Group produce an easy to read leaflet with good practical advice for mothers about weaning, details of which are in Appendix 7.1.

LIQUIDS FOR THE WEANLING

From the age of 6 months until one year, breast milk, infant formula or a follow-on milk should be used as summarized in Table 7.7. Follow-on formulas are manufactured in similar ways to infant formulas but have a slightly higher protein content. Like the infant formulas they have added vitamins and iron. Unlike infant formulas or follow-on milks, cow's milk contains relatively large amounts of saturated fats and sodium and only minimal amounts of iron. It seems prudent to recommend the more nutritionally appropriate infant

Table 7.6 Principles of weaning

Why?	• To add to or replace total energy received from liquid diet.
	• To provide certain micronutrients which may be required, particularly iron, vitamin D (depending on sunlight) and copper (if receiving ordinary cow's milk).
	• For development of chewing action as opposed to suckling only.
When?	Three to 6 months: very few will need anything other than breast milk or an infant formula before 3 months. Almost all will need extra solid foods after the age of 6 months.
What food?	1 Cereal-based weaning foods are most commonly used initially and the majority of the commercially available ones are gluten-free. Then proceed to baby meals, family foods, etc.
	2 Beware of weaning diets that contain fruit, puddings and vegetables only.
	3 Dishes containing meat are a good source of iron. The iron in green vegetables is more easily available if meat or poultry is included with them and/or there is a good supply of vitamin C, say, from a baby fruit juice at the same meal.
	4 Continue to breast feed or use an infant formula (or a follow-up milk) till age one year.

Table 7.7 The liquid part of the weanling's diet from 6 months

	Breast fed	*Bottle/cup fed*
What food	Breast milk	An approved infant formula or a follow-on milk such as Farley's follow-on milk, Progress (Wyeth)
Vitamin A,D,C, drops	Strongly recommended	Not essential since they are present in infant formulas, follow-on milk
Fruit juices	Not essential but helps the absorption of iron from green vegetables	Not essential but helps the absorption of iron from green vegetables
Extra source of iron	Some extra source of iron is increasingly necessary as the infant gets older – usually obtained from weaning foods	Adequate supply from infant formula or follow-on milk

formulas or follow-on milks which have reasonable amounts of vitamin D and iron and lower amounts of saturated fat and sodium.

Whole cow's milk can be safely given from the age of one year and the solid part of the diet should be similar to that of the family. Current recommendations are that semi-skimmed milk should not be introduced before the age of 2 years and skimmed milk not before the age of 5 years.[15]

The pre-school child

Many children under 5 years of age have small appetites and so should be encouraged to take foods which have a high nutrient and energy density. Milk is an important contributor of energy, calcium, riboflavin and vitamin A in the diet of many pre-school children and 500 ml daily should be provided. However, if children drink in excess of 1000 ml milk daily, this will compromise their appetite for solid food. Usually pre-school children will cope best with three small meals and two or three snacks. The Paediatric Group of the British Dietetic Association have produced a guide for mothers about feeding the pre-school child (see Appendix 7.1).

The pre-school child progresses through various stages in feeding from the messy finger feeding at one year of age, through the bowl and spoon feeding stage of the 2 year old to the competent eating (using child-sized cutlery) of the 4 or 5 year old.

Guidelines for pre-school child

It is difficult to make specific dietary recommendations for the pre-school child because we know little of what these children are actually eating since only a few studies of food intakes have been carried out. In any case, the chosen diet of healthy normally growing toddlers varies widely in quality and quantity.

The naturally high fat diet of the suckling and weanling (up to 55% of energy from fat) should be *gradually* shifted towards the current recommendation of around 35% fat for the adult population[4-9] from about the age of 2 years. However, this must be achieved without compromising the intake of energy and other nutrients necessary for normal growth. A suitable interim step is to advise the introduction of semi-skimmed milk from the age of 2 years by which time the child is usually able to consume a wide range of foods. However, if there is any doubt about the child's overall energy intake as in very fussy or picky eaters, then whole milk should be continued.

Toddler food refusal

Toddlers are often faddy eaters causing considerable parental anxiety. Reassurance is often required that this is a normal developmental stage. Advice to parents should be:

- To restrict sweets and snack foods such as crisps and not to substitute these for a refused meal.
- To be aware of fluid intake. Often toddlers will resort to staving off hunger by ingesting large amounts of fluid either as fruit juice or milk. If this is taken from a bottle it is a convenient form of food constantly on tap for the child. Drinks should be given at meal and snack times and a cup rather than a bottle should be used.
- To establish regular meal and snack times.
- To offer finger or bite-sized pieces of food on the plate and keep portions small.

The school child

The diet of children from the age of 5 years onwards can move towards our present concept of a healthy diet for adults; fat intake can be reduced and fibre increased. Fatty foods such as chips and fried foods and sugary or fatty snacks such as confectionery and crisps should not be eaten daily – once or twice weekly is acceptable. Fizzy drinks and squashes contain considerable quantities of sugar and should be avoided if possible in order to help prevent dental caries.

Meals

Fresh fruit and vegetables should be encouraged together with wholegrain cereals and wholemeal or high-fibre white bread. Pasta, rice and baked potato can substitute for chips. Confectionery should be kept for special occasions, so that dental decay may be minimized.

Snacks

Snack foods can consist of fresh fruit, nuts, dried fruit or crunchy bars rather than sweets and crisps. Lower fat varieties of foods such as low fat spreads, lower fat cheeses and reduced fat yoghurts can be used.

Drinks

Semi-skimmed or skimmed milk can be safely used. Low calorie fizzy drinks, squashes, spring water or fresh fruit juices can be taken.

The majority of school children in Britain grow well. Some from lower social groups, where there is financial hardship, rely on free school meals to provide a significant proportion of their nutritional intake.[16] However at weekends and during school holidays these children may receive a poorer diet. Health workers in the community can help these families with practical advice on basic cooking skills and budgeting.

The adolescent

At adolescence, weight increases in both sexes particularly in boys. Girls accumulate relatively more fat, boys more lean tissue (muscle and skeletal). Children who have chronic illness with nutritional implications such as cystic fibrosis will often show a marked delay and reduction in the pubertal growth spurt and delayed puberty due to an inability to meet their increased nutritional demands.

Most adolescents' appetites increase in proportion to their accelerating rate of growth and many adopt a grazing pattern of eating, consuming frequent snacks in addition to their meals, to meet the increased nutritional demands. However the two nutritional problems which can occur at this time in Britain are iron deficiency anaemia and rickets.

Iron deficiency anaemia

Iron requirements in boys increase substantially because of the new muscle tissue laid down but, as their growth velocity decelerates, their iron requirements fall to the low needs of adult man. Although girls put on less muscle, menarche increases their need for iron which continues throughout their reproductive life. The extra requirement for iron can be met by eating more lean red meat, but many teenagers become rebellious about foods traditionally considered as good for them, such as meat. If this is the case, or if the adolescent is vegetarian, iron-fortified breakfast cereals, pulses (peas and beans) and green vegetables should be included in the daily diet if possible. Ideally these should be eaten together with a rich source of vitamin C (such as fresh fruit juice) or, if acceptable, a source of animal protein such as eggs or fish. Further guidelines on vegetarian diets are given below.

Rickets

The pubertal growth spurt increases the demand for bone minerals, especially calcium, but this can only be efficiently absorbed if there is sufficient vitamin D. Inadequate intakes or an inability to utilize calcium and/or vitamin D will result in rickets. The vitamin D status of Asian pubertal girls is at risk, perhaps due to limited exposure to the sun because of wearing more covering clothes, playing less sport and living more of their lives indoors.[17]

An adequate calcium intake can usually be met if around 500 ml of milk (whole, semi-skimmed or skimmed) is taken. Alternatives to this are other dairy foods such as yoghurt, cheese, ice cream and flavoured milk drinks or shakes. In the UK, flour is fortified with calcium; so bakery foods such as bread, biscuits and cakes can contribute significant amounts to the diet. Two average-sized slices of white bread will supply about one-tenth of a child's recommended daily intake of calcium.

If none of these foods are eaten, for whatever reason, it may be necessary to prescribe a calcium supplement to provide about 20 mmol calcium daily.

Only a few foods contain significant amounts of vitamin D and exposure to sunlight is the most effective means of obtaining this vitamin. However, liver, oily fish and vitamin-fortified margarine do contain significant amounts. Butter and ghee contain little vitamin D. It may be necessary to prescribe a vitamin D supplement if exposure to sunlight is limited. Some authorities recommend that all Asian children should receive a vitamin D supplement (300–400IU/7.5–10 μg daily) until growth is over.

Many adolescents worry about their body image and this can lead to abnormal eating and exercise patterns. Anorexia nervosa and bulimia may result, but these are primarily psychiatric rather than nutritional disorders and are dealt with in a later chapter.

Some adolescents opt out of eating hitherto traditional foods and switch to alternative dietary regimens such as vegetarianism, often because some wish to rebel against conventional foods, and some because of their concerns regarding the environment and animal rights. Support should be given to the adolescent during these dietary dabblings, so that a nutritionally adequate intake may be ensured. The addresses of local and national self-help groups are available from libraries. Addresses of the Vegetarian and Vegan Societies are in Appendix 7.1.

Although food fads in adolescence can be bizarre, they are frequently short lived and a return to a normal eating pattern soon occurs. If helped and supported through the extremes of dietary regimens, they will often be more receptive to nutritional education, particularly if this can be shown to be associated with an improvement in physique and or appearance.

The vegetarian child

Vegetarians comprise an extremely heterogeneous group with innumerable dietary variations. Table 7.8 summarizes the different categories of vegetarian

Table 7.8 Types of vegetarian diets

Description of diet	Animal foods eaten	Animal foods excluded
'Semi'-vegetarian	Poultry, fish, eggs, milk	Red meat
Lact-ovo vegetarian	Eggs, milk	Meat, poultry, fish
Lacto-vegetarian	Milk	Meat, poultry, fish, eggs
Vegan	None	Meat, poultry, fish, eggs, milk

diets. Nutrition in ethnic groups has been discussed in a previous chapter but vegetarianism has been gaining popularity in western societies recently usually because of conservation, animal welfare, health and environmental issues rather than because of religion.

There are only limited published data on why people choose to become vegetarian and their attitudes, health knowledge and beliefs. In the UK, some information is available from a study carried out in Cardiff[18] showing that vegetarians tended to smoke and drink less and perceived themselves as being healthier than their non-vegetarian counterparts. Another recent study[19] which looked at the reasons for people adopting vegetarianism, showed that meat was seen as harmful and that organic foods were regarded as healthier and safer. Although these beliefs are without scientific basis, it appears that they are strongly motivated ideologies for many vegetarians. The food industry, food additives and processed food were viewed with great cynicism.

For the young child, vegetarian diets can be bulky and so sufficient food may not be able to be eaten to provide all of the energy and nutrient requirements. Toddlers, especially if they are faddy eaters, could be nutritionally disadvantaged by certain vegetarian practices, e.g. those based on Rastafarian, Zen Macrobiotic and Hare Krishna beliefs. Expert nutritional advice is essential otherwise severe clinical malnutrition is a very real risk.[20] However, many vegetarian and vegan diets can be nutritionally adequate for both children and adults,[21] particularly if dietary regimens are based on well-established, long-standing traditional practices. Some may even have health benefits for older children and adults due to their (generally) high fibre, low cholesterol and saturated fat content. Table 7.9 summarizes some religious food regimens.

For the first year of life, a moderately high intake (>600 ml) of breast milk, infant formula, follow-on milk or soya protein isolate feed (as listed in the section on soya milks) should be given. This ensures energy, calcium and protein intake are likely to be adequate.

When milk and eggs can be eaten, the risk of nutritional inadequacy for the child is minimal. If cow's milk is not acceptable, then a soya protein isolate formula should be used until the child is at least 2 years of age. Liquid soya drinks have a very low energy and nutrient content and so are inappropriate for children under 2 years of age and also for those under 5 years if food intake is limited for whatever reason.

Vitamins A and D should be given to all vegetarian children from weaning until at least the age of 2 years and preferably 5 years. The Department of Health vitamin drops are suitable.

Table 7.10 indicates the sources of various nutrients in total vegetarian diets, i.e. when no foods of animal origin are eaten. The Nutrition Committee of the British Paediatric Association have produced detailed guidelines for weaning vegetarian children and details of this are in Appendix 7.1.

Common dietary problems

Infants and young children often present with a wide range of symptoms which can be related to, or are thought to be related to, the digestive process or food. Although these symptoms are usually mild they can be a source of great anxiety to parents and take up a great deal of the health visitor's and doctor's time.

Posseting, vomiting and reflux

Milk feeds and liquids are frequently and effortlessly regurgitated. Most infants thrive normally and

Table 7.9 Guide to foods avoided by some religions and cults

Religion	Pork	Beef	Other meat	Non-scaly fish, shellfish	Eggs	Milk	Canned foods
Jewish*	x			x			
Hindu*	x	x			?		
Jain	x	x	x		x		
Skih*		x					
Muslim*	x						
Buddhist	?	?	?	?	?	?	
Seventh Day Adventist	x	x	x	x			
Rastafarian	x	x	x	x	x	?	x
Macrobiotic (Zen)	x	x	x	x	x	x	x
Hare Krishna	x	x	x	x	x		x

* Dietary restrictions may be greater if foods not prepared in acceptable way
x Food generally avoided
? Denotes considerable variation within religion over consumption of these foods

Table 7.10 Nutrient checklist for vegetarian diets assuming no animal products taken

Nutrient	Best sources	Practical suggestions
Protein	*Fortified soya milks High biological value protein by combining: beans pulses e.g. lentils } with cereals nuts tofu (soya bean curd)	Ground nut loaf or rissoles and breadcrumbs Baked beans on toast Lentils (dhal) and rice
Energy	Nuts, nut butters, coconut Margarine, cooking oils *Fortified soya milks Seeds – sunflower/sesame seeds	Incorporate into dishes. Sprinkle sunflower/sesame seeds into soups and stews. Margarine and cooking oils added to starchy weaning foods can moisten the food
Iron	Pulses, e.g. lentils, ideally take daily Wholegrain bread and cereals. Ideally take twice daily Small but useful sources: wheatgerm, nuts, dried fruit, green veg, cocoa, molasses, curry powder	A vitamin C containing drink or food should be taken at each meal to enhance absorption of iron. Sweeten foods with dried fruit or molasses instead of refined sugar. Avoid tea and coffee at meals as these inhibit iron absorption
Calcium	*Fortified soya milks Sesame seeds and spread (tahini) Almonds Millet Tofu	Add sesame seeds to soups, stews and desserts. Mix ground almonds with soya milk puddings. Use millet as an alternative to rice
'B' vitamins	Wholegrain cereals and bread Green vegetables Wheatgerm Yeat extract	Add yeast extract to soups and stews
Vitamin B_{12}	B_{12} fortified yeast extracts e.g., Barmene, Tastex *Fortified soya milks Grapenuts	
Vitamin D	*Fortified soya milks. Vitamin D fortified margarines. Breakfast cereals	Vitamin D intake should be adequate if there is good exposure to sunlight. NB Butter, ghee and most low fat spreads are *not* fortified with A and D

*Fortified soya milks. This denotes the soya protein isolate infant formulas, e.g., Isomil, Infasoy or liquid soya drinks, which have been fortified by the addition of energy or vitamins and minerals, e.g. Granose.

symptoms usually abate around the age of 6 months as solids are introduced. In the absence of other symptoms such as poor weight gain, blood or bile in the vomit, persistent or projectile vomiting or pain and discomfort with feeding, feed regurgitation is only rarely a sign of allergy. Nor is it an indication to switch milk formulas.

Views on the cause of this frequent symptom are varied.

Aerophagy (swallowing air)

This is considered by many to be a frequent cause of vomiting. The child swallows air as he feeds and when the air is brought up, some of the feed comes with it. The excessive air passing downwards causes intestinal distension and sometimes pain (colic). A definite cause of aerophagy and thence regurgitation is underfeeding. In this instance, the baby achieves a comfortable feeling of being full, not from food alone but from air and food. The questions are:

- Is the breast-fed baby suckling the nipple and areola rather than only sucking the nipple?
- Is the hole in the teat large enough? (the milk should drip at one drop per second from an inverted bottle).
- Is the baby's nose blocked, so that he breathes orally?
- Is the baby receiving a predetermined calculated volume of feed rather than allowing him to drink as much as desired? Occasionally the cause of the vomiting has been thought to be overfeeding so that less feed is offered.

- Is the feed too dilute?

Developmental

The oesophageal sphincter is said to be less mature than in later life.

Emotional

Some babies seem to enjoy the sensation of regurgitating food and chewing the cud since they are seen to smile immediately the food is returned to the mouth. Some paediatricians have suggested this is more common where there is a disturbed mother and child relationship.

Physical problems

Swallowing problems (incorrectly interpreted as vomiting) due to anatomical or neurological defects can arise. A true hiatus hernia and cow's milk protein allergy are also causes of vomiting.

After dealing with the possible cause of aerophagy and being reasonably confident that there is no physical problem, three approaches are commonly used:

1 To reassure the mother that the vomiting is within the acceptable range of normal and, like wet nappies, will gradually lessen and disappear.
2 To suggest sitting the baby up after each feed for about an hour.
3 To advise thickening the feeds either by earlier use of low protein, low sodium weaning cereals such as baby rice or the use of an instant gel thickener, e.g. Instant Carobel (Cow & Gate) or Nestergel (Nestlé). These thickening agents should be mixed with each feed.

It is doubtful whether 2 and 3 achieve anything other than a vehicle for reassurance to the mother. Time is usually the best curer of the condition.

Constipation

The bowel habits of normal infants show wide variation from eight times each day to once every two days. Constipation should mean not only infrequent bowel motions but also hard faeces perhaps associated with pain or difficulty on defaecation. A painful anal fissure may be a cause of constipation which will require treatment.

Infants

Constipation is more usually seen in bottle-fed rather than breast-fed infants. Often extra drinks of boiled water or diluted fresh orange juice will be a successful remedy. Alternatively, the addition of one teaspoon of sugar to the milk feed will have an osmotic effect of drawing water into the bowel and softening the stools.

Toddlers and older children

Toddlers and older children may become constipated due to a poor intake of fibre but frequently this is because of a poor overall food intake. Constipation can be seen in association with food refusal and commonly in children with picky appetites, particularly if meals are usually refused and the food eaten is mainly snacks taken at irregular intervals. The management is similar to that described for toddler food refusal. Often recommending an increase in fibre intake is inappropriate because high fibre foods are often disliked by children and so may lead to an even poorer food intake. However, the following are usually popular and it may be appropriate to recommend the daily inclusion of at least one serving of these high fibre foods:

> Baked beans
> Wholewheat breakfast cereals (e.g. Weetabix)
> Sweetcorn
> Peas
> Pineapple
> Nuts and raisins (for children over 5 years)
> Coleslaw
> Raw carrot

Unprocessed bran should never be used for children under one year as it can reduce the bioavailability of certain minerals such as iron and calcium and its use for older children should be carefully monitored.

Gastroenteritis

Acute gastroenteritis rarely affects the nutritional status of healthy children. Management should be aimed at preventing dehydration, correction of electrolyte loss and resumption of normal nutrition. Most infants and children can be treated at home but persistent vomiting, abdominal distension, hypothermia, altered consciousness and a fall in urine volume output are indications for hospital admission.

The recommendations in Table 7.11 for the management of gastroenteritis have been made by representatives of the British Paediatric Association and the British Society of Paediatric Gastroenterology.[22]

Toddler diarrhoea

This is a term applied to diarrhoea, often seen between 6 months and 3 years of age in an otherwise healthy and normally growing child without any other evidence of gastrointestinal pathology such as abdominal distension and blood in the stools. The symptoms may be associated with emotional disturbance but mostly the children are normal in all respects apart from their frequent watery stools.

Parents may suspect that their child is allergic to specific foods but this is rarely the case and complex dietary avoidance regimens are not indicated. If the child's growth is satisfactory, an assessment of foods eaten may reveal an excess of fibre-containing foods or a diet which is low in fat. A low fat diet will accelerate gastric emptying and this has been implicated as a reason for toddler diarrhoea.[23] Adequate healthy dietary fat can be ensured by the addition of polyunsaturated margarines into cooked vegetables, spreading these on to bread, using vegetable oils for cooking, and ensuring at least 500 ml of whole cow's milk is taken daily.

Occasionally an excessive consumption of fruit juices has been implicated as a cause of toddler diarrhoea because of their high sugar content. Rarely is the diarrhoea due to an inherited sucrase isomaltase deficiency.

Drugs such as cholestyramine and prostaglandin inhibitors (e.g. indomethacin) have been used for the condition but these are no longer recommended. Toddler diarrhoea does not usually respond to intestinal sedatives such as loperamide but in the occasional child it is helpful particularly if the diarrhoea is socially humiliating when a short trial may be justified.

Iron deficiency anaemia

Below the age of 2 years, it is reasonable to regard iron deficiency anaemia as due to a dietary deficiency. An iron supplement is prescribed and, if there is an adequate response, no further investigation is required. If the child is more than 2 years old, or the anaemia does not respond to a simple trial of iron therapy (rise in haemoglobin of at least 1 g per month on ferrous sulphate 60 g daily), then possible malabsorption or blood loss should be considered.

Thalassaemia can mimic the blood film appearances and red blood cell indices of iron deficiency. If the race of the child indicates that thalassaemia is a possibility, then ideally investigation should be performed before giving iron supplements.

Special diets

Obesity

In adults, the Quetelet or Body Mass index is used as an indicator of obesity:

$$\frac{\text{weight in kg}}{\text{height in m}^2}$$

In children, this is less useful because of the variation in size with their age. However, Poskitt[24] has suggested the following can be used in children:

$$\text{Calculation} = \frac{\text{child's weight}}{\begin{array}{c}\text{weight of a child on standard}\\ \text{growth chart who has the same}\\ \text{height centile as the patient}\end{array}} \times 100$$

then

90%	= underweight
90–110%	= normal weight
110–120%	= overweight
>120%	= obese

For example: a boy aged 13 years who weighs 70 kg (well over 97th centile) has a height of 155 cm (90th centile). On the standard growth chart, the 90th centile weight for a 13 year old is 50.1 kg.

$$\text{therefore calculation} = \frac{70}{50.1} \times 100$$
$$= 139\%, \text{therefore obese}$$

Obesity is a common problem in school children, often with its origins in the toddler years or in infancy. An excess weight must be due to energy intake from food being greater than expenditure on growth, exercise and maintenance, but genetic and environmental influences are important factors which appear to modify both intake and expenditure.[25] Fat parents often have fat children. A minority are obese secondary to some pathological condition such as Downs syndrome, Prader-Willi syndrome, adolescent hypothyroidism etc or some may be overweight as a

---

Table 7.11 Recommendations on the dietary management of gastroenteritis[22]

1 Home-made salt and sugar solutions and soft drinks should not be used in managing gastroenteritis.
2 Bottle-fed infants over 6 months who have only mild diarrhoea should return immediately to full strength feed after 24 hours of oral rehydration solution.
3 Bottle-fed infants below 6 months should be regraded in the conventional way after 24 hours of oral rehydration solution, that is, increasing from quarter strength (one part of made up formula to three parts of oral rehydration solution) through half strength and three-quarter strength to full strength.
4 Special infant formula or food need not be used when routinely managing gastroenteritis.
5 In those cases in which a special formula is needed use a nutritionally complete formula based on oligopeptides or amino acids.
6 Whole protein sources such as unmodified goat's milk or ewe's milk should not be used for either normal or ill babies.

Trials published subsequent to these recommendations have shown that many infants below 6 months of age are able to return to full strength feeds after 24 hours of oral rehydration solution as in 2 above.

result of drug therapy, e.g. corticoidsteroids, sodium valproate.

Treatment should aim to achieve a weight appropriate for the child's height while still allowing for normal growth. Both the child and parents must be strongly motivated and, if the obesity is familial, the whole family must change their eating habits.

A careful dietary assessment will usually highlight the foods contributing the excessive calories. Frequently fizzy drinks, crisps, chips, fried foods and sweets are eaten in large amounts. Rather than a formal diet the following advice should be given to children who are mildly to moderately obese:

1   Eat only at mealtimes. If desired, one piece of fresh fruit can be eaten at specified snack times.
2   Avoid taking sugar in drinks, fried foods (including chips) and puddings.
3   Use sugar-free (diet type) soft drinks. Fresh fruit juices should not be used for drinks throughout the day.
4   Avoid grazing on low calorie snack foods. This perpetuates the habit of constant between meal eating.
5   Promote the use of wholegrain bread and cereals as these tend to be more filling.

Children who are grossly overweight should be given a weight reducing diet sheet tailored to the individual. Bread, milk and starch foods should be limited and it may be necessary to indicate portion sizes of foods. Paediatric dietetic supervision should be sought for these children.

Weight loss should be slow, no more than 500 g weekly or, in some instances, the plan may be for weight maintenance so that the child grows into the weight. Although exercise alone will not reduce weight, children should be encouraged to take some because it will tend to promote a feeling of well being. Initially some children may be embarrassed and reluctant to participate so some initial weight loss may be appropriate before beginning an exercise programme.

Obese children require a great deal of support and close follow up if weight loss is to be achieved. Often regular weigh-ins and a star chart system can act as stimuli to continue their diet.

Very-low-calorie adult-type liquid slimming regimens which provide 300–600 calories daily are unsuitable for children as the balance of nutrients is inappropriate to sustain a normal growth velocity.

Poor growth or weight gain

Poor weight gain or growth can be caused by:

1   Not getting enough of the right food (Fig. 7.1)
2   Inability to suck or swallow (Fig. 7.2)
3   Poor retention of food (Fig. 7.3)
4   Malabsorption (Fig. 7.4)
5   An inability to utilize food (Fig. 7.5)

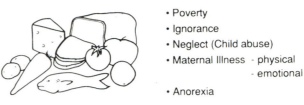

- Poverty
- Ignorance
- Neglect (Child abuse)
- Maternal Illness - physical
                   - emotional
- Anorexia

Figure 7.1 Reasons why there may be a lack of appropriate foods in a child's diet.

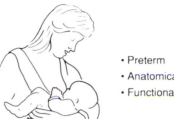

- Preterm
- Anatomical defect
- Functional (neurological defect)

Figure 7.2 Reasons why infants or children may be unable to ingest enough food.

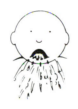

Any cause of vomiting

- Feeding problem
- Infection
- Mechanical
- Metabolic

Figure 7.3 Reasons why infants or children may be unable to retain food.

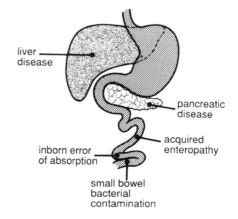

liver disease

pancreatic disease

acquired enteropathy

inborn error of absorption

small bowel bacterial contamination

Figure 7.4 Reasons why infants or children may be unable to absorb dietary components, (Intraluminal or Mucosal).

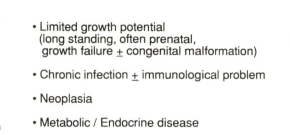

- Limited growth potential
  (long standing, often prenatal,
  growth failure ± congenital malformation)

- Chronic infection ± immunological problem

- Neoplasia

- Metabolic / Endocrine disease

Figure 7.5 Reasons why infants or children may be unable to utilize food efficiently, (usually anorexia as well).

The problems 2–5 are usually indications for further investigations and it is the reasons for 1 which are discussed.

Infants and children who are underweight or are failing to grow normally should have their dietary intake carefully assessed ideally by a paediatric dietitian. This assessment should carefully explore not only the type and quantities of foods and liquids taken but also the times these are given throughout the day. A simple way of taking a dietary history is to record the previous day's intake in detail starting with breakfast, working methodically through until bedtime, with some idea of quantities of food consumed each time. In the absence of any underlying disorder, a frequent cause of poor weight gain in pre-school children is lack of an adequate intake of milk. Drinks often consist mainly of fruit juice and the volumes taken may be such that appetite for foods is compromised. Not only will the energy content be inadequate, but it is likely that the intake of protein, iron, folic acid, calcium, other minerals and vitamins will also be insufficient. If the cause is failure to receive enough of the right food then the reason should be determined and treatment aimed at giving more of the normal food rather than instituting some special feed or dietary supplement. Often the management is similar to that for toddler food refusal.

Treatment of growth failure with special therapeutic diets such as omitting some possible offending nutrient (e.g. gluten), or adding some extra single nutrient (e.g. energy supplements or iron) should not be instituted until a provisional diagnosis is made.

Occasionally children from better off families are fed an adult healthy diet regimen of high fibre, low fat foods. While such diets are fine for adults who have ceased to grow, the food can be bulky, low in energy density and perhaps also low in nutrient availability and will not supply sufficient nutrition to allow for normal growth. These children have been labelled as suffering from Muesli Belt Malnutrition because of misguided parental beliefs that such diets are equally beneficial for adults and children. Adults in certain religious sects also follow a dietary regimen which is totally inappropriate for children.[26]

Children under 5 years of age should take at least 500 ml of milk daily and if there is concern about weight gain, whole cow's milk (not skimmed or semi-skimmed) should always be continued after the age of 2 years. If milk is disliked as a drink, children will often take it in milk puddings, flavoured milk shakes or yoghurt drinks. Fruit juice and soft drink intake in excess of 300 ml daily should be discouraged. A vitamin supplement such as the Department of Health vitamin drops may be beneficial. Usually parents need a careful explanation as to the relative merits of milk versus juices and the special nutritional needs of children in comparison to adults. It is important that all health professionals are consistent with advice. Dietary help and support in the home environment may be particularly beneficial.

Therapeutic diets

Therapeutic diets are an important aspect in the management and treatment of a number of diseases, but any child who requires a modified diet must have his or her growth regularly monitored and the diet continually reviewed for nutritional adequacy to take account of changing requirements. The use of some therapeutic diets must be combined with careful biochemical monitoring, e.g. diabetes mellitus and phenylketonuria.

Some conditions such as coeliac disease require lifelong dietary modification, but others need only a special diet for a short period of time, such as a temporary lactose intolerance. The continuing need for short-term diets must be assessed and no child should be put on to a special diet without some form of clinical and/or dietetic follow up.

Most of the more specialized therapeutic diet regimens will have been instituted when the child was an inpatient or an outpatient at a hospital and dietary progress and supervision is likely to be continued by the hospital. However, for many of the dietary regimens, general practitioners will be asked to prescribe specific dietary products and health visitors and other community workers may visit at home so a general overview of the dietary principles is desirable. Table 7.12 summarizes a few specific therapeutic diets but more detailed information can be obtained from books in the references list.[27,28]

Table 7.12 Summary of a few specific diets

Condition	Dietary information	Dietary principles	ACBS* products	General information
Diabetes	Carbohydrate	As a guide, base daily CHO allowance on 120–140 g + 10 g CHO for every completed year of life. Ideally, use high fibre CHO foods.	None	Generally 10 g CHO system used for diabetic children. Proprietary diabetic foods not recommended. Dietary management principles frequently reviewed.
Renal disease	The following may be increased or decreased: Protein Phosphate Calcium Potassium Sodium Calories Fluid	Diet tailored to the individual's biochemical parameters. Pre-dialysis Continuous ambulatory peritoneal dialysis (CAPD), continuous cyclatory peritoneal dialysis (CCPD) } Increased energy intake to promote growth. Continous ambulatory peritoneal dialysis (CAPD), continuous cyclatory peritoneal dialysis (CCPD) } Increased protein to counteract dialysate losses. Post transplant – usually restricted energy.	a Glucose polymer supplements b Milk-based supplements c Fat emulsion d Low-protein bread, flour, flour mixes, biscuits, pasta e Mineral mixtures	Dietary restrictions likely to vary depending on biochemical parameters. Water soluble vitamin supplements of the 'B' group and vitamin C usually required. 1 – Alpha vitamin D may be used.
Cystic fibrosis	Increased dietary intake	Energy and protein requirements may be up to 150% RDA. Nasogastric/gastrostomy feeding sometimes used.	a Infant formulas which have fat and/or protein source modified. b Enteral feed products c Glucose polymer supplements d Milk-based supplements e Vitamin supplements	Pancreatic enzyme replacement therapy essential. Reduced fat diets or diets based on medium chain triglyceride (MCT) fat rarely used.
Coeliac disease	Gluten-free diet and occasionally also oat free	Avoidance of foods based on or containing wheat, barley, rye (oats)	Gluten-free bread, biscuits, flour, flour mixes, pastas	Diet lifelong. Iron, folic acid and complete vitamin supplement required for few weeks/months following diagnosis. Many gluten-free foods *not* on prescription, but available for purchase in large chemists and health food shops. Coeliac Society address – see Appendix 7.1

Table 7.12 *(cont'd)*

Condition	Dietary information	Dietary principles	ACBS* products	General information
Cow's milk protein intolerance	Avoidance of cow's milk and products containing this, e.g. butter, margarine, yoghurt, ice cream, infant formulas	Check ingredients' labels for: casein whey caseinates milk, skimmed milk	a Infant formulas based on soya, e.g. Wysoy b Infant formulas based on casein hydrolysates, e.g. Pregestimil c Infant formulas based on whey hydrolysate, e.g. Prejomin	Most children with a gastrointestinal intolerance to cow's milk protein are able to tolerate cow's milk protein by two years of age. An immunological reaction to cow's milk protein, e.g. in eczema, is usually of longer duration. Goat's milk and sheep's milk unsuitable. Liquid soya drinks unsuitable as a milk substitute for children under 2 years of age.
Crohn's disease	Increased intake. Complete vitamin supplement	Elemental and hydrolysed protein nasogastric feeds often used during acute phases of the disease	a Whey/casein protein powders, e.g. Maxipro HBV super soluble b Glucose polymer powders and liquids, e.g. Hycal c Elemental feed products, e.g. Elemental 028 d Whole protein and hydrolysed protein feed products e Medium chain triglyceride (MCT) based feed products	Drugs and surgery often required. Complete vitamin supplement required. Supplements of magnesium, zinc and calcium may be required.
Galactosaemia	Exclusion of dietary lactose and galactose	Most dietary galactose derived from lactose so diet is essentially lactose free. Also avoid offal meats – these contain galactosides.	a Low lactose infant formulas, e.g. Galactomin 17 b Infant formulas based on soya, e.g. Wysoy	Diet lifelong. Care with medicines and artificial sweetners – lactose often used as a filler.
Epilepsy	Fat a Medium chain triglyceride (MCT) ketogenic diet b 4:1 Ketogenic diet	a 60% kcals in diet to come from MCT fat b 4 g of normal dietary fat : 1 g protein + CHO	a Liquigen (MCT emulsion) b Calogen (long-chain triglyceride (LCT) emulsion)	Urinary ketones to be monitored. Complete vitamin supplement required. Calcium and/or iron supplement may be required.
Eczema	Avoidance of the food(s) known to provoke reaction in sensitive individuals: eggs cow's milk nuts citrus fruits salicylates	Strict elimination diet may be required to identify multiple food allergies	a Infant formulas based on soya, e.g. Wysoy b Infant formulas based on casein hydrolysates, e.g. Pregestimil	Medication usually adequate treatment for most children. Only a few severe cases require dietary manipulation. Regular dietary supervision and evaluation required due to changing allergenicity to foods. Vitamin or mineral (especially Ca) supplement may be required for very restricted diets.

Table 7.12 *(cont'd)*

Condition	Dietary information	Dietary principles	ACBS* products	General information
Urticaria	Avoidance of the food(s) known to provoke reaction in sensitive individuals: nuts antioxidants eggs preservatives fish pork shell fish chocolate salicylates bananas Azo dyes strawberries		No	
Migraine	Avoidance of vasoactive-amine-containing foods: citrus fruits and juices, chocolate, coffee, tea, nuts, cheese		No	Relatively simple medication is often adequate treatment for most children – only a few will require dietary manipulation.
Phenylketonuria	Reduce dietary intake of phenylalanine to maintain plasma phenylalanine between 120–360 μmol/litre (N=40–100)	a Very low intake of natural protein from foods b Main source of protein from low phenylalanine-free amino-acid mixes for the toddler or older PKU c Limited phenylalanine, essential for growth, from measured amounts of natural foods, e.g. potato, breakfast cereals, normal infant formula d Fruits, fats, sugar, and limited vegetables allowed freely	a Low phenylalanine infant formulas b Mineral mixtures c Low-protein bread, flour, biscuits and pasta d Low-protein drink e Amino-acid mixes f Vitamin supplements g Fat emulsions	Regular blood phenylalanine monitoring done. Now recommended diet to be continued as long as possible. Young women with phenylketonuria who intend having a family must return to a strict low phenylalanine diet preconceptionally and throughout pregnancy.

*ACBS – Advisory Committee on Borderline Substances. This is a Department of Health Committee which reviews and determines whether special dietary products can be prescribed by general medical practitioners at NHS expense for specified medical conditions.

Appendix 7.1

The British Dietetic Association
7th Floor
Elizabeth House
22 Suffolk Street
Queensway
Birmingham B1 1LS

Vegetarian Society (UK) Ltd
Parkdale
Durham Road
Altrincham
Cheshire WA14 4QG

Vegan Society
33–35 George Street
Oxford
OX1 2AY

British Paediatric Association
5 St Andrew's Place
Regents Park
London NW1 4LB

The Coeliac Society (UK)
Dept 1
PO Box 220
High Wycombe
Bucks HP11 2HY

References

1   Department of Health and Social Security. Recommended daily amounts of food energy and nutrients for groups of people in the United Kingdom. Reports on health and social subjects: No 15. London: HMSO, 1979.

2   National Academy of Sciences. *Recommended Dietary Allowances* 10th edn. Washington DC: Food and Nutrition Board, National Research Council, 1989.

3   World Health Organization. *Handbook on Human Nutritional Requirements*. Monograph series No 61. Geneva: WHO, 1974.

4   Department of Health and Social Security. Diet and cardiovascular disease (COMA report). Reports on health and social subjects: No 28. London: HMSO, 1984.

5   World Health Organization. *Prevention of Coronary Heart Disease*. Technical Report Series No 678. Geneva: WHO, 1982.

6   British Medical Association. *Diet, Nutrition and Health*. Report of the Board of Science and Education. London: Cameleon Press Ltd, 1986.

7   American Academy of Pediatrics. Committee on nutrition recommendations. *Nutr Rev* 1976; **34**: 248.

8   National Advisory Committee on Nutrition Education (NACNE). *Proposals for Nutritional Guidelines for Health Education in Britain*. London: Health Education Council, 1983.

9   American Heart Association. Diet in the healthy child. *Circulation* 1983; **67**: 1411A–1414A.

10 Martin, J., White, A. *Infant Feeding 1985*. Office of Population Censuses and Surveys. London: HMSO, 1985.

11 Royal College of Midwives. *Successful Breastfeeding: A Practical Guide for Midwives*. London: Royal College of Midwives, 1988.

12 Freundlich, M., Zilleruclo, G., Abitbol, C., Strauss, J., Sangere, M.-C., Malluche, H.H. Infant formula as a cause of aluminium toxicity in neonatal uraemia. *Lancet* 1985; ii: 527–529.

13 Taitz, L.S., Scholey, R.E. Are babies more satisfied by casein based formulas? *Arch Dis Child* 1989; **64**: 619–621.

14 Sando, W.C., Gallagher, K.J., Rodgers, B.M. Risk factors for microwave scald injuries in infants. *J Pediatr* 1984; **105**: 864–867.

15 Department of Health and Social Security. Present day practice in infant feeding: 3rd report. London: HMSO, 1988.

16 Department of Health. The diets of British schoolchildren. (Report on health and social subjects No 36). London: HMSO, 1989: 1–289.

17 Belton, N.R. Rickets – not only the 'English disease'. *Acta Paediatr Scand* 1986; suppl. 323: 68–75.

18 Shickle, D., Lewis, P.A., Charny, M., Farrow, S. Differences in health, knowledge and attitudes between vegetarians and meat eaters in a random population sample. *J Roy Soc Med* 1989; **82**: 18–20.

19 Draper, A., Malhotra, N., Wheeler, E. Who are 'vegetarians' and what do they think about food? *Proc Nutr Soc* 1990; **49**: 61A.

20 Roberts, I.F., West, R.J., Ogilvie, D., Dillon, M.J. Malnutrition in infants receiving cult diets: a form of child abuse. *Br Med J* 1979; **1**: 296–298.

21 British Paediatric Association *Vegetarian Weaning*. London: BPA, 1987.

22 Wharton, B.A., Pugh, R.E., Taitz, L.S., Walker-Smith, J.A., Booth, I.W. Dietary management of gastroenteritis in Britain. *Br Med J* 1988; **296**: 450–452.

23 Lloyd Still, J.D. Chronic diarrhoea in childhood and misuse of elimination diets. *J Pediatr* 1979; **95**: 10–13.

24 Poskitt, E.M. Management of obesity. *Arch Dis Child* 1987; **62**: 305–310.

25 Poskitt, E.M.E., Cole, T.J. Nature, nurture and childhood overweight. *Br Med J* 1978; **1**: 603–605.

26 Gorodischer, R., Bar-Ziv, J. Multiple nutritional deficiencies in infants from a strict vegetarian community. *Am J Dis Child* 1979; **133**: 141–144.

27 Francis, D. *Diets for Sick Children*. Oxford: Blackwell Scientific Publications, 1987.

28 Bentley, D., Lawson, M. *Clinical Nutrition in Paediatric Disorders*. London: Baillière Tindall, 1988.

7.5 Dental health

James Hogan

Changing patterns of dental disease

The two main dental diseases, caries and periodontitis, can both be prevented, yet are endemic in industrial societies.

Two factors contribute to this paradox:

1 The conditions in their reversible phase are usually symptomless, and though dentists encourage individuals to attend regularly for check-ups to anticipate problems, only half the population in the UK takes this advice.[1]
2 Caries and periodontitis are caused by accumulation of plaque and sugar consumption. In theory, it would be possible to eliminate both diseases completely by efficient plaque removal and sugar control. In practice, though curative dentistry is unpopular and expensive, these preventive procedures are not widely followed.

Caries

Nevertheless, a substantial decrease in dental caries in children was observed in the UK in the 1970s.[2] Caries experience fell by half for children starting school, and by one third for school leavers. By 1983, over half of 5-year-olds were free of caries, though still only 7% of 15-year-olds (in 1993 it was 37%). A similar decline was recorded in most industrial societies (but offset in global terms by the rapid rise of caries among children in developing countries). This is mainly attributable to the wide availability of fluoride in toothpaste from the early 1970s onwards; though other factors also contributed, including water fluoridation, fluoride supplements and rinses, and changes in dietary preferences, particularly among middle-class families.

During the 1980s, however, the decrease in caries in English 5-year-olds halted.[3] Caries experience is measured by the DMF index, i.e. the sum of decayed (D), missing (M), and filled (F) teeth in the mouth. The filling (F) component continues to decline, and this is not so much due to fewer teeth being repaired, but rather to increased application by dentists of preventive alternatives to restorations, such as fissure sealants. Furthermore, it is now becoming increasingly evident that the class distribution of caries has markedly altered; and the nature of caries as a disease has undergone changes.

Class distribution

In the 1960s and 1970s, class was not considered a significant factor in the prevalence of caries,[4] and the benefit from the introduction of fluoride into toothpastes was shared by all. But once the effect of fluoride toothpaste reached its plateau at the turn of the 1970s, class differences in caries experience began to emerge.[5] A rise in caries in social classes IV and V (particularly marked among ethnic minority groups within these classes) has been evident in recent years. Only among the small proportion of the population (7%) with fluoridated water has the class equity in caries distribution been maintained.

The reason for this widening gap is a subject of some speculation in dental circles, but it is generally accepted that supplementary sources of fluoride and improvements in diet are less likely to be available to the socially disadvantaged. This emergence of high-risk caries groups within the community has at least helped to establish criteria for identifying target groups for concentrating preventive programmes for children (Fig. 7.6).

The nature of caries

In the last 15 years, the rate of progression of caries in teeth has slowed down.[7] This is due to the presence of more fluoride in plaque. Increasingly, carious lesions in children now occur in the pits and fissures of teeth, rather than the smooth surfaces. Pit and fissure caries tend to be smaller and slower to develop, and so easier to treat or reverse. This facilitates an up-to-date treatment philosophy of delayed intervention, combined with the preventive approach.

Periodontal disease

Tooth loss from periodontitis among adults has fallen: 20 years ago this was the main cause of extractions among people over 34 years of age. This is not because the incidence of the disease has notably decreased, but because of more positive attitudes to retaining natural teeth, held equally by patients and dentists. In the past, a fatalistic view of the prognosis of established periodontal disease (so-called pyorrhoea) prevailed. Now increasingly it is being shown that restoring the functional stability of periodontally damaged teeth, through dental treatment and careful

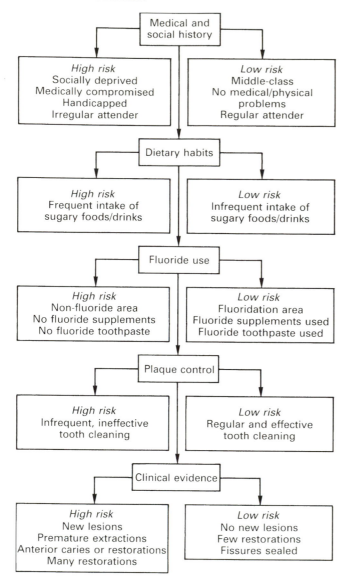

Figure 7.6 Flow diagram showing five types of data to be considered when assessing the caries risk of individual patients. Reproduced from Blinkhorn and Geddes.[6]

oral hygiene, is less a counsel of perfection than hitherto believed.[8]

However, there is no evidence that periodontal inflammation (gingivitis) is decreasing among children. In 1983, about half the 15-year-olds in the UK had established gingivitis. Since the prevention of periodontitis is rooted in oral hygiene habits acquired in childhood, this trend is disappointing.

Improvements in oral health

The conclusion to be drawn, therefore, is that although there have been considerable improvements in oral health over the last 20 years in the UK, these, despite considerable advances in preventive research, have been more the result of the commercial availability of fluoride in toothpaste and of a shift in attitudes to tooth loss, than better oral hygiene and dietary habits.

The normal dentition

Teeth

Most of the tooth buds of the deciduous (baby) and permanent (adult) dentitions are fully formed by the thirtieth week of fetal life. The deciduous teeth appear in the mouth between 6 months and 2 years in infants (Table 7.13). Delayed eruptions are more common than early ones. The variation from the norm is about 3 months for front and 6 months for back teeth. There are 20 deciduous teeth in all: each quarter has two incisors, one canine, and two molars. The lower central incisor is usually the first tooth to erupt. The majority of baby teeth come through without difficulty, but discomfort with one or two can be expected, even with a healthy child with reasonable oral hygiene.

The permanent teeth erupt between 6 years of age and early adulthood. The full complement is 32 teeth: each quarter has two incisors, one canine, two premolars, and three molars. The third molars or wisdom teeth usually erupt between 16 and 22 years of age. It is not uncommon for wisdom teeth to be retarded from coming through into the mouth because of lack of development in modern jaws.

The first permanent molars appear at 6 years of age behind the primary molars and are frequently mistaken by parents for baby teeth. Shortly afterwards the permanent incisors replace the deciduous incisors. Around 10 years of age the premolars replace the deciduous molars, and the permanent canines replace their deciduous precursors. By 13 or 14 years the permanent dentition, with the exception of wisdom teeth, is normally in place.

The teeth vary in shape according to their function. Incisors are spade-shaped for biting; canines are conical, pointed, and long-rooted to tear; premolars have two cusps to comminute food; and molars are multicusped to grind up food before swallowing.

Saliva

The main functions of saliva are:

1 To lubricate food and muscles (lips, cheeks, tongue) to facilitate swallowing
2 To cultivate the oral flora, and to produce dental plaque
3 To help maintain a stable alkaline environment in the mouth by its buffering action
4 To promote mineral exchange through calcium, phosphate, and trace elements, when enamel is demineralized by dietary acids.

Table 7.13 Chronology of tooth development

Tooth		Tooth germ fully formed	Dentine formation begins	Formation of crown complete	Appearance in mouth cavity	Root complete
Deciduous	Incisors	3–4 months fetal life	4th–6th month fetal life	2–3 months	6–9 months	1–1½ years after appearance in mouth cavity
	Canines			9 months	16–18 months	
	1st molars			6 months	12–14 months	
	2nd molars			12 months	20–30 months	
Permanent	Incisors	30th week fetal life	3–4 months (upper lateral incisor 10–12 months)	4–5 years	Lower 6–8 years Upper 7–9 years	2–3 years after appearance in mouth cavity
	Canines	30th week fetal life	4–5 months	6–7 years	Lower 9–10 years Upper 11–12 years	
	Premolars	30th week fetal life	1½–2½ years	5–7 years	10–12 years	
	1st molars	24th week fetal life	Birth	2½–3 years	6–7 years	
	2nd molars	6th month	2½–3 years	7–8 years	11–13 years	
	3rd molars	6th year	7–10 years	12–16 years	17–21 years	

Plaque

Plaque is a soft cream-coloured layer of bacteria, in a matrix containing glycoprotein and bacterial products, which adheres to the teeth and gum margins. The composition of plaque varies with different diets. For instance, in populations with a high sugar intake, cariogenic bacteria (*Streptococcus mutans* and *Streptococcus sanguis*) predominate. Stale plaque (over 48 hours old) generates anaerobic bacteria, which secrete the enzymes that cause periodontitis.

Popular myths about tooth development

In considering the development of the normal dentition, certain common misconceptions need to be discounted. It is frequently said that certain caries-prone children are 'born with soft teeth'. This is usually attributed to a vitamin D or calcium deficiency. Only in cases of extreme protein-deficiency, unknown in this country, or in very rare congenital conditions (amelogenesis and dentinogenesis imperfecta) do soft teeth occur.

Another popular fallacy is that breast feeding, because human milk contains lactose, causes dental caries. In theory this could happen, but it would take constant breast feeding prolonged into late infancy to induce any caries at all. Compared with bottle feeding with a sweetened liquid, it cannot be considered remotely a problem.

Common abnormalities of children's teeth

Pathological teething

The mild local irritation of normal teething occasionally spreads into more generalized inflammation of the gums. Sometimes a bluish ischaemic bulge forms over the erupting tooth and mouth ulcers, particularly those associated with primary herpes, may appear. These developments tend to occur when the child's resistance is reduced by complicating conditions such as influenza.

It is important not to let the oral problems mask the underlying systemic condition. The oral symptoms usually disappear when the tooth has erupted, though a severe primary herpes simplex infection may require systemic acyclovir in an elixir. Persistent teething problems may demand some local alleviation: a little teething gel (containing topical anaesthetic but not aspirin) rubbed around the erupting tooth before meals and at bed times, or a teething ring between meals, should suffice.

Thumb sucking

Most children engage in habitual thumb or finger sucking at some time or other. If the habit is frequent and prolonged the front teeth may begin to protrude. The effect is transient so long as the digit-sucking stops before 9 years, but if the habit persists into early adolescence an appliance may have to be fitted to realign the prominent front teeth.

Accidental damage to front teeth

About one quarter of children in the UK experience traumatic damage to at least one permanent incisor tooth by the age of 15 years. This can be prevented by the wearing of mouth-guards if the accident is sport related. However, only one in 10 fractures in children occur in organized sport. Playground and bicycle accidents are a more frequent cause. When the tooth is completely avulsed, if it is replaced in the socket as soon as possible the prognosis for replantation is greatly improved.

The majority (85%) of fractured front teeth observed in 15-year-olds in the UK remain untreated (1983), although over two thirds should probably have received dental attention. If the fracture is deeper than the enamel or causes discoloration, the tooth should be restored (with an acid-etch composite filling or a crown) to prevent further adverse consequences.

Malocclusions in children

The upper and lower teeth ideally occlude together to allow free vertical and lateral movements of the jaws, which are controlled by the temporomandibular joints. This permits mastication, and provides muscular support for facial expression. Normal variations in occlusion are inevitable, as a perfect set of 32 teeth is rarely achieved. The borderline between normal and abnormal dentitions is difficult to define: variations from the ideal are in different degrees acceptable on aesthetic grounds in different cultures and at different times. For instance, in the 19th century the prominent Habsburg jaw was a mark of aristocratic status. Only a few conditions (cleft palate, condylar hyperplasia and temporomandibular joint ankylosis) can be strictly speaking described as pathological. A malocclusion is more easily defined: when the occlusal variation could lead to a functional disability in eating or a temporomandibular dyscrasia.

Selection for orthodontic treatment

In the UK in 1983, nearly three-quarters of school children were regarded by dentists as needing orthodontic treatment. Parents, on the other hand, perceive the orthodontic need as considerably less. For example, less than half the children identified by dentists as having crowded dentitions were regarded by their parents as having crooked teeth. It is perhaps not surprising that only one third of children have had any orthodontic treatment at all by 15 years of age.

The following criteria for selecting children for treatment represent the likely basis of a dentist's decision to treat:

- Age to refer for an orthodontic opinion: 8 or 9 years of age (when the permanent incisors are through) is time enough for most initial assessments.

- The ugly duckling stage: as the deciduous teeth are shed (from 6 years on) the child's dentition goes through what is sometimes called the ugly duckling stage. The development of the jaws is not sufficient to accommodate all the erupting permanent teeth, and so the teeth look crowded or unevenly positioned. Parents frequently need to be reassured that room will probably be made for all teeth with jaw growth. The main orthodontic concern with the mixed dentition is to avoid the premature loss of deciduous molars, with subsequent loss of jaw space for permanent teeth.

- Dental status of the child: good oral hygiene with dental disease under control is essential.

- Medical status of child: children requiring antibiotic cover for dental procedures (valvular heart defects, etc), or with blood dyscrasias or severe epilepsy, need referral to a specialist for the assessment.

- Commitment of patient: the commitment of the child to orthodontic treatment is crucial to its success. The parent's enthusiasm is not enough. It is the child who has to wear the brace, accept extractions, and attend the dentist every month or so for two or more years.

Oral signs of eating disorders

Anorexia and bulimia nervosa usually show changes in the teeth. The commonest sign is the erosion of tooth enamel. The regurgitation of gastric acids in bulimia usually wears away the inner surfaces of all upper teeth, and the excessive citrus fruit consumption characteristic of anorexia frequently produces erosion of the outer surfaces of front teeth.

Non-accidental injury to children

The abuse of children by adults frequently manifests itself in facial and oral lesions. These have a consistent pattern: torn upper labial frenum, swollen lips, face bruises (finger-tip sized), burns (circular) in various stages of healing, bite-marks, fractured front teeth, fresh or healed jaw fractures or dislocations. Condyloma acuminatum (clusters of sessile papillomatous lesions) in the palate of a child or adolescent should raise serious concern about the possibility of sexual abuse.[9]

Oral sign of HIV infection in children

Oral candidosis is as frequently present in children infected with HIV as in adults. The majority of children infected perinatally with HIV develop mucocutaneous candidosis in the first year of life.[10] It is generally considered a warning sign of severe morbidity.

Preventing dental caries and periodontal disease

Most methods of preventing dental caries and periodontitis demand considerable motivation to obtain long-term results. The exception is the fluoridation of water supplies, but this only partly prevents caries (it halves the prevalence). Any approach must take into account the cultural and economic factors that militate against a combined regimen of day-to-day home care and preventive intervention by the dental team.

Four main steps can be taken to prevent dental caries and periodontal disease in children:[11]

1 Reduce the consumption, and especially the frequency of intake, of sugar-containing foods and drinks.
2 Clean teeth and gums thoroughly with a fluoride toothpaste.
3 Ensure adequate daily fluoride intake.
4 Ensure regular attendance at a dentist.

1 Sugar control

Within seconds of sugar consumption, acids are generated in plaque and enamel demineralization commences. After 20 minutes or so an alkaline pH is restored in the mouth, and remineralization begins. The timing and frequency of sugar intake determines whether teeth remain sound, or carious lesions form. At meals when other foods and drinks are consumed, the acid from sugar is diluted and largely neutralized. However with frequent sugar intakes between meals (snacks or sweet drinks) the demineralization is more likely to exceed the remineralization, and caries result.

In recent years the sale of sugar for household use has fallen sharply, but use of sugar by food manufacturers has risen: three-quarters of the sugar in the average UK diet is from sugar added to foods in processing. This hidden sugar, particularly in soft drinks and confectionery, is the main dietary cause of caries in children. Starchy foods, intrinsic sugars in whole fruit or lactose in milk, and sugar alcohols like sorbitol are harmless to teeth. It is the non-milk extrinsic sugars (sucrose, fructose, and glucose in fruit juices, honey, or added to processed foods or home cooking) that are cariogenic.

Sugar control is best achieved by discouraging an infant taste for sweetened foods and drinks. The following advice to parents of young children should be given:

- Do not add sugar to the feeding bottle.
- Avoid reservoir feeders, and sweetened dummies.
- Medicines or vitamins should be sugar-free.
- Snacks should be savoury rather than sweet – fresh fruit, raw vegetables, cheese, non-sugar-containing crisps.

- Soft drinks should be intrinsically (naturally) sweetened and fruit juices diluted.

2 Toothbrushing

Efficient plaque control prevents or reverses gingivitis (persistent periodontal inflammation). Gingivitis does not occur in children until the permanent teeth begin to erupt, and most frequently starts at the onset of puberty. Unless reversed by thorough daily plaque removal, periodontitis sets in, causing loss of tooth support tissues, including bone; teeth eventually become loose (this may take anything from several years to several decades, depending on oral hygiene standards).

Toothbrushing is the most satisfactory method of removing plaque from teeth and gums. Chemical plaque control (chlorhexidine gluconate mouth rinses, antibiotics) is usually only advised for short-term use (to reduce gingival inflammation) as it could lead to an unacceptable imbalance in the oral flora. Plaque reducing mouth rinses are no substitute for toothbrushing. Toothbrushing in itself only prevents caries if carried out within five minutes of every sugar intake. This is hardly practical.

> Dentists are generally agreed that of the two most widely taught toothbrushing methods, the roll and the scrub techniques, the scrub is more effective in plaque removal and is more easily taught and accepted. For this reason it is now the method of choice. It should be carried out with a small toothbrush for ease of access. The method is to place the filaments of the brush at the neck of the tooth and to use very short horizontal movements to dislodge plaque from the stagnation areas at the gum margins cervically and between the teeth interproximally. Emphasis should be placed on small movements and gentle pressure, together with an unhurried systematic approach to the cleaning of all surfaces. One method of toothbrushing is for the parent to stand behind the child and tilt the child's head upwards so that all tooth surfaces can be brushed using a gentle scrub motion.
>
> Reproduced from *The Scientific Basis of Dental Health Education. A Policy Document*, 3rd edn.[11] With permission of the Health Education Authority.

The toothbrush habit should be acquired as early in life as possible. Once teeth appear in the mouth, parents should start brushing the infant's teeth and gums with a baby brush, continuing until 6 or 7 years, when manual dexterity is usually sufficiently developed for self-care. A small-headed soft to medium brush (20 mm by 10 mm) with densely filamented nylon bristles is recommended. Dislodging plaque from the gum margins and between teeth is best accomplished with very short horizontal movements and gentle pressure. Toothbrushing should be performed at least once, preferably twice, a day (after breakfast, before bed). Disclosing tablets or dyes which colour plaque blue should be used from time to time to test the child's toothbrushing efficiency.

Gum infections periodically make toothbrushing difficult for most children. Anti-inflammatory toothpaste gels containing chlorhexidine gluconate used for a week or two will clear up local irritations. Persistent bleeding gums, particularly when the plaque removal is efficient, requires further investigation.

3   Fluoride

Water-fluoridation

The ability of fluoride to prevent caries and reverse early lesions has now been scientifically validated, after exhaustive research since the 1930s. Fluoride occurs naturally in the water supply, but in most communities the amount is insufficient to prevent caries. At a concentration of one part per million, water fluoridation is the most effective, efficient, and safe method of reducing dental decay.

The implementation of water fluoridation has been fraught with public controversy. The anti-fluoride lobby's objections are broadly that:

a   It is mass medication for a condition that does not affect everybody.
b   It is an 'infringement of human liberty'.
c   Fluoride itself is a 'poison'.

Only the mass medication argument need be taken seriously from a scientific point of view. Very few people are caries-free, and child-targeted alternative fluoride supplementation is more expensive and unlikely to be as effective in the most needy groups. The great advantage of water fluoridation is that it prevents caries in all ages and social classes, and does not require individual compliance.

However, the cost-effectiveness of water fluoridation compared to its alternatives depends not only on the size of the population served by the water supply, but also on local levels of caries. When the prevalence of caries falls below the WHO target goal of a mean of three permanent teeth with carious experience per 12 year old, alternative fluoride delivery may prove to be more cost-effective.[12]

Alternative fluorides

Fluoride drops and tablets have been shown to be as effective as water fluoridation in select highly motivated groups, such as dentists' children. The daily consumption of fluoride drops (up to 2 years of age) and tablets (up to 16 years) requires a degree of compliance from parent and child which is not easy to obtain without exceptional enthusiasm.[13] It can be strongly recommended for high-risk caries groups in non-fluoridated areas. Fluoride tablets can be distrib-

uted to groups of children in day-nurseries and infant classes in schools. Such teacher or nursery leader supervised programmes have proved a valuable method of caries control in deprived areas with high caries levels.

Fluoride mouth-rinses are arguably the cheapest way (next to water-fluoridation) of caries prevention when delivered by teachers to school groups of young adolescents (11–14 year olds). Fluoride rinses are most effective in protecting newly erupted teeth (and in remineralizing early lesions).

Fluoride gels or varnishes professionally applied to children's teeth are moderately effective in preventing caries. Like fluoride tablets, this is a long-term therapy (twice a year from 6 to 16 years of age) and continuity of care and patient compliance over such a long timespan is difficult to achieve.

Fluoride toothpaste (less than 1500 parts per million) can be used in combination with water fluoridation or alternative methods of delivering fluoride without altering the standard systemic dosage. The paste is usually spat out rather than swallowed.

Fluorosis

Fluoride in long-term dosages above the standard recommended (Table 7.14) can cause opaque white spots on enamel and in extreme cases a brown mottled staining. The British Dental Association in 1981 established minimum effective dosages. These take into account levels of fluoride in the water and the possibility of fluoride toothpaste ingestion by children. A pea-sized amount of toothpaste is advised for infants to avoid undue ingestion.

Table 7.14 Standard fluoride supplement dosage for children[14]

Age	Dosage daily (mg fluoride ion)
6 Months–2 years	0.25
2–4 years	0.5
4–16 years	1.0

4   Attending the dentist

Children should attend the dentist before they have a dental problem. Normally this should be at 3 years of age. Prevention can then be introduced and oral hygiene habits inculcated. The interval of recall should not be more than a year (twice a year at least) for caries high-risk children, particularly those living in city areas with high social mobility.

Care of handicapped children and those at special risk from dental problems

It is widely accepted that reorientating dental preventive resources to medically and socially disadvantaged children is the top priority for the dental profession in the UK. This can best be achieved by identifying these children and channelling them into dental care as early in life as possible.

Children with medical conditions that make future dental treatment difficult, even hazardous, should be the prime target for preventive dentistry. Such dentally significant medical conditions (Table 7.15) can usually be identified by doctors and health visitors at child health surveillance in the first or second year of life. The parent should then be put in contact with a dentist. Neglecting early pevention can cause needless complications: what is routine dental treatment for the normal child may only be possible for the at-risk child by attending a specialist dentist, and the dangers associated with bacteraemias, haemorrhage, general anaesthetics and so on are best avoided by prevention and early clinical intervention.

Table 7.15 Dentally significant medical conditions in preschool children

1 *Blood diseases*
  Haemophilia and other clotting defects
  Thalassaemia
  Leukaemia
  Sickle-cell disease
2 *Cardiovascular disease*
  Congenital septal and valvular defects
  Rheumatic heart disease
3 *Learning/communication disorders*
  Mental handicap
  Autism
4 *Central nervous system disease*
  Cerebral palsy
  Epilepsy
5 *Renal disease*
  Severe nephritis or nephrotic syndrome
6 *Congenital anomalies*
  Down syndrome
  Spina bifida
  Cleft palate or lip
7 *Orthopaedic*
  Osteogenesis imperfecta
8 *Viral carrier status*
  Hepatitis B
  HIV

Prevention

In the absence of water-fluoridation, fluoride supplements should be given from birth (but not before). In severely at-risk infants an optimum effective dosage can be prescribed under supervision (Table 7.16).

Table 7.16 Fluoride supplements dosage range for high-risk children[15]

Age	Dosage (mg/day)
Birth–6 months	0.25
6–18 months	0.25–0.5
18–24 months	0.25–0.75
Over 24 months	0.5–1.0

Sugar control should be introduced simultaneously (prenatal advice to parents on diet is provident). When teeth appear in the mouth fluoride varnish can be applied by a dentist or dental auxiliary. This is better accepted by handicapped children than fluoride gels or rinses.

Early clinical intervention

Fissure sealants are a key preventive measure against caries for handicapped and at-risk children, as well as 'high risk' caries groups (see Fig. 7.6). High impact resins seal off the pits and fissures of recently erupted permanent molar teeth which are the most susceptible sites of carious attack. If they are incipiently decayed, the seal starves the lesion, and the caries is reversed.

If sugar and plaque control in a severely at-risk child fails, and caries rates rise, the chemical reduction of cariogenic bacteria can be carried out as a last resort.[16] Chlorhexidine gel in vinyl trays is applied to the teeth for 5 minutes daily for 2 or 3 weeks. A nurse or parent can usually do this under the supervision of a dentist (in collaboration with a microbiologist).

Given good oral hygiene support and motivation, handicapped children can benefit from orthodontic care. Significant improvement in appearance, or of a speech defect, can be achieved by interceptive orthodontics (planned extractions and perhaps a simple removable appliance). An early orthodontic assessment (6 or 7 years of age) is recommended.

Mentally and physically handicapped people tend to lose their permanent teeth prematurely through periodontal disease. This is largely due to inadequate plaque control as a result of poor manual skills and oral hygiene support. Some conditions (Down syndrome) and medications (phenytoin sodium) predispose such children to periodontal disease. But a change of anticonvulsant and good oral hygiene can limit the damage substantially.

The future

Most dentally at-risk, and indeed caries high-risk, children should be able to benefit fully from advances in preventive and interceptive dentistry. However, this can only be realized if dentists can reach these signal target groups and their families by joining forces with paediatricians and other health professionals.

References

1 Bulman, J.S. Community health. In: Rowe, A.H.R., ed. *Clinical Dentistry*. London: Class Publishing, 1989: 1369–1372.

2 Todd, J.E., Dodd, T. *Children's Dental Health in the United Kingdom 1983*. London: HMSO, 1985.

3 Holt, R.D., Joels, D., Bulman, J., Maddick, I.H. A third study of caries in preschool aged children in Camden. *Br Dent J* 1988; **165:** 87–91.

4 Todd, J.E. *Children's Dental Health in England and Wales 1973*. London: HMSO, 1975.

5 Rugg-Gunn, A.J., Carmichael, C.L., Ferrell, R.S. Effect of fluoridation and secular trend in caries in 5 year old children living in Newcastle and Northumberland. *Br Dent J* 1988; **165:** 359–364.

6 Blinkhorn, A.S., Geddes, D.A.H. Assessment of caries risk and the potential for preventive management. In: Elderton, R.J., ed. *Positive Dental Prevention*. London: Heinemann, 1987, 27.

7 Ekanayake, L.S., Sheiham, A. Reducing rates of progression of dental caries in British school children. *Br Dent J* 1987; **163:** 265–269.

8 Burt, B.A. The status of epidemiological data on periodontal diseases. In: Guggenheim, B., ed. *Periodontology Today*. Basal: Karger, 1988: 68–76.

9 Lamey, P.J., Lewis, M.A. Oral medicine in practice: viral infection. *Br Dent J* 1989; **167:** 269–273.

10 Samaranayake, L.P. Oral candidosis: an old disease in new guises. *Dent Update* 1990; **17:** 36–38.

11 Health Education Authority. *The Scientific Basis of Dental Health Education: a Policy Document*. 3rd edn. London: HEA, 1989.

12 Andlaw, R.J. Fluorides and caries. In: Elderton, R.J., ed. *Positive Dental Prevention*. London: Heinemann, 1987: 52–56.

13 Hogan, J.I. Fluoride tablet distribution from maternal and child health centres: a feasibility study. *Health Visitor* 1982; **55:** 60–63.

14 British Association for the Study of Community Dentistry. *The Home Use of Fluoride for Pre-school Children: a Policy Document*. Cardiff: BASCD, 1988.

15 Stephens, K.W. Fluoride supplements: age related dosage. *Br Dent J* 1981; **151:** 40.

16 Krasse, B. Reducing cariogenic micro-organisms. *Caries Risk*. London: Quintessence: 1985: 63–65.

7.6 Accident prevention

Jo Sibert

Introduction

Accidents to children are an important area of work for the paediatrician working in the community. They are a common cause of death, handicap and presentation to hospital in childhood. If they are to be prevented there needs to be a clear community-based programme of environmental action in which the doctor should take a major role.

Mortality from accidents

Accidents are the most common cause of death in children in the UK. In 1987 688 children under 14 years died in England and Wales from accidents (Table 7.17).[1] Nearly twice as many children aged between 5 and 14 years died from accidents than from malignant disease (71 children to 37 children per million). Accidents account for about one third of deaths of children between the age of 1 and 14 years and even under the age of 1 year they account for a significant number of deaths, even when perinatal deaths are excluded.

Road traffic accidents remain the most common cause of accidental death in children, particularly to child pedestrians and children on bicycles or in cars. Deaths from conflagrations, and complications of burns and scalds have been highlighted with house fires due to foam furniture. They cause just under 100 deaths a year in England and Wales. Nearly 50 children die each year from drowning.

Morbidity from accidents

Accidents also cause significant handicap and suffering to children. A study of morbidity following childhood accidents in three health districts with a total child population of 210 000 by Avery in 1982[2] revealed four boys who had been permanently brain damaged by an accident. Head injuries, which may follow pedestrian, cycle or passenger road traffic accidents, falls or child abuse, are the major cause of handicap following accidents. Children are also brain damaged following near drowning or suffocation episodes. Cosmetic damage following burns, scalds and

Table 7.17 Fatal accidents by type. England and Wales 1987 Children 0–14 years

Transport accidents	
Vehicle occupants	80
Pedestrians	214
Pedal cyclists	63
Other	24
Total	381
Home accidents	
Burns and scalds	89
Suffocation	33
Drowning	20
Falls	11
Poisoning	7
Other causes	37
Total	197
Other locations	
Drowning	27
Falls	21
Other causes	62
Total	110
All accidents	688

Source OPCS, Deaths by Accidents and Violence. Quarterly Monitors DII4 Series 1988.

road traffic accidents may be very damaging psychologically to the child.

More minor accidents are very common in childhood and are a frequent cause of attendance at accident and emergency departments. Studies have demonstrated that one in five of the child population attends hospital because of an accident in a year. On the basis of such studies, it has been estimated that 2.33 million children attend an accident and emergency department annually. Although the majority of these injuries are relatively trivial, among them there are serious injuries. Twelve per cent of children attending an accident and emergency department have fractures.[3]

Accidents are also a frequent cause of children's admission to hospital.[4] Between 5 and 10% of the children who attend hospital require admission. In 1985 this proportion amounted to about 120 000 children in England and Wales.

Prevention

The prevention of accidents to children is increasingly recognized as an important public health concern.[5] Doctors who treat children and see the effects of accidents are in a unique position in society to alert the community to the problem and take action to prevent accidents. What is more difficult is how this can be achieved.

It is very tempting to think all that is needed is to alert the public to the dangers of accidents to children by education campaigns, but the evidence that this is effective is unconvincing. It is also tempting to look on accidents to children as a whole and think of general solutions to the problem. All the evidence however has pointed to accident prevention in children being most influenced by analysing types of accident, their epidemiology and then careful evaluation of preventive measures before their widespread introduction. Almost all cases where such measures have been effective have involved environmental change rather than education. The introduction of child-resistant containers (CRCs) is an example. Education campaigns have been ineffective in preventing accidental child poisoning,[6] the CRCs were evaluated on a small scale[7] and shown to be worthwhile and were then introduced more widely in the USA[8] and the UK.[9] This has resulted in a reduction in the numbers of children admitted to hospital with accidental child poisoning.[10]

Education campaigns

A number of studies have shown that education campaigns to prevent accidents to children are by themselves ineffective. A programme to prevent home accidents and directed at parents (the Rockwood County study) made no difference to accident rates between control and target families.[11] There was little evidence the *Play it Safe* television programmes made any impact on accident rates in children.[12] An education campaign with posters and literature in Cardiff only sensitized the population to trivial accidents.[13]

Education campaigns may be ineffective because psychosocial stress is involved in the aetiology of many childhood accidents and parents are unlikely to remember safety propaganda at these times. Stress has been found to be related to road traffic accidents[14] and accidental childhood poisoning in children.[15] In a study in South London,[16] the children of mothers who were psychiatrically disturbed had an accident rate nearly four times higher than control children. A study in New Zealand examining life events found accidents as a whole twice as common in families with a life-event score over twelve than those with a score under four.[17] There were larger differences if burns, scalds and poisoning were considered individually.

There is evidence, however, that health visitors visiting the home and giving specific attention to accident prevention can make differences in the way that families behave, in particular with regard to the installation of safety equipment.[18] Health education therefore must be directed either on a one-to-one basis by people such as the health visitor or general practitioner or to educate public opinion to institute environmental change.

Action on childhood accidents

Some accidents to children can be prevented by action at a national or even international level. Examples are the use of child-resistant containers and the seat-belt legislation to prevent accident to car passengers. In 1977, Professor Donald Court and Dr Hugh Jackson, paediatricians from Newcastle-on-Tyne, England, were instrumental in forming the Child Accident Prevention Trust (CAPT) (see address at the end of the chapter). The Trust brings many disciplines together to foster research and action on accidents to children.

Local action is also needed to reduce childhood accidents. To make road traffic conditions or playgrounds safer, local recognition and environmental action is required. Once an accident happens it can happen again. A dangerous balcony which allows a fall needs immediate repair. The paediatrician working in the community is ideally placed to know local statistics on child accidents and to initiate environmental change.

A number of local child accident prevention groups have been formed in the UK. Members have included health education officers, the police, home safety officers, park officials, educationalists, local councillors and paediatricians. The Child Accident Prevention Trust (1989) has brought together guidelines for local action and local groups and in Sweden their value has been documented. Schelp[19] described in Skaroborg County a reduction of 27% in home accidents following a group environmental intervention programme.

Check list for health care professionals to prevent accidents to children[20]

- Obtain accurate childhood accident statistics for locality.
- Form a local accident prevention committee.
- Establish links with councillors, parents' organizations etc.
- Analyse each type of accident separately.
- Establish a training programme for health care professionals.

Preventing road traffic accidents to children

Road traffic accidents (RTAs) are the commonest cause of accidental death in children. Their prevention remains a major challenge. In 1987, 381 children died from RTAs in England and Wales, of which 214 were pedestrians, 80 were vehicle occupants and 63 were pedal cyclists (see Table 7.17). RTAs are also a major cause of long-term disability.

Pedestrian road traffic accidents

Pedestrian road traffic accidents particularly occur in inner city children and those from socially deprived families. This has been shown in national death statistics, and in a study from Sheffield[21] where the fatality rate was related to the prosperity of the area. This is probably for two reasons. Poor families have features of their environment, such as front doors opening straight on to the road, which make accidents more likely to happen. Poor families are also often under considerable stress which will influence behaviour both of parents and children. Backett and Johnston[14] showed that psychosocial stress is also an important factor in road traffic accidents. The interaction of a poor environment with stress probably occurs in many accidents.

Boys are involved more than girls: those between 5 and 8 years are at maximum risk. Parents overestimate the ability of their children to handle traffic and let them go out on the road unsupervised. Primary school age children cannot judge the speed or dangers of traffic.[22] The spontaneous behaviour of these children is immature and marked by inability to anticipate dangerous situations.[23] Sharples and her colleagues[24] looking at deaths from head injury in the northern region found that 72% of these deaths occurred between 3 p.m. and 9 p.m. and mostly in boys playing after school.

A number of pedestrian children die each year after accidents in which a driver has had excess alcohol. The introduction of random breath tests has wide support in the community in particular from doctors and the police. Legislation on this matter is awaited.

Education and child pedestrian road traffic accidents

In Sweden, Sandels[25] showed that it was possible to teach some 6-year-old children basic traffic rules when they knew they were being observed. However, this approach would be unlikely to prevent accidents as a large number of children do not learn and indeed it may be just these children who have accidents. In the UK, it has been suggested that the Green Cross Code prevented accidents when it was introduced; however, careful analysis of the figures suggests this is not so.[26] Pease and Preston[27] found that kerb drill was not perceived by young children to detect traffic and was thought sufficient by itself to ward off the dangers of the road. Firth[28] concluded that adequate explanations of exactly what is involved in road safety could be given by very few children. Safety and traffic education are therefore not likely to prevent road traffic accidents by themselves.

Environmental change and child pedestrian road traffic accidents

The most important means of preventing pedestrian road traffic accidents is by modification of the environment. This can be done by redesigning residential areas to give priority to pedestrians and to separate them from traffic. The speed of traffic can be reduced by speed bumps and safe crossings can be provided. Sensitive schemes such as the Woonerf introduced in the Netherlands are good examples of what can be done.[29] A Woonerf is an area in which the residential function clearly predominates over any provisions for traffic. The provision of play areas and general improvement of the environment will reduce the number of children on dangerous streets. Local accident committees can help alter the local environment by encouraging councils to introduce such schemes and to provide more safe play areas for children. Community paediatricians need to work closely with traffic managers and local councillors on these issues.

Accidents to children in cars

Although fewer children die as passengers than as pedestrians, accidents to children in cars remain a serious problem. Improving the standard of road safety and driving generally will help but this may be difficult to achieve. However, there is good evidence that seat belts are effective in preventing death and serious injury to children travelling as passengers in cars. Much of the research on seat belts has been on adult car passengers. Educational campaigns to persuade people to wear seat belts were generally unsuccessful. Since 1983, when legislation was introduced into the UK to compel the wearing of seat belts in front seats of vehicles, serious injuries have fallen by as much as 20%. In America,[30] serious injuries have also been reduced after seat belt legislation.

There is good evidence that child restraint systems also prevent injury and death. The Transport and Road Research Laboratory[31] found that no child died in a 2-year period when in a restraint, whereas 264 non-restrained children were killed in that time. Scherz[32] found in Washington State, USA, that serious injuries were much less common in restrained children than non-restrained children. These differences were most pronounced in younger children. Child restraint systems also have the bonus of improving children's behaviour and thus probably improving driving standards.

Which restraint system to use?

The type of restraint system used for children depends on the age of the child. For babies, the safest way used to be the carry cot restraint but its value is limited because the cot and not the baby is restrained.

Recently a number of carriers for babies less than 10 kg have been developed. These are portable seats that can be fixed to the car with an adult safety belt. They have proved to be convenient and safe in use and do restrain the baby directly. Their wider use can be encouraged by loan schemes. A First Ride Safe Ride campaign encourages their use on the first ride home from the maternity unit. Community paediatricians are in an ideal position to initiate such a campaign.

Children between 10 and 18 kg need a child car seat. These can either be fixed directly to the car by two or four point anchorage or fitted with adult seat belts. Many good designs of all these types are now available. For children from 18 to 36 kg, adult seat belts should be used with a booster cushion. These are as safe as child harnesses. A survey in Cardiff[33] has shown that only 47% of children under 9 months and 26% of older children are appropriately restrained in cars. There has been recent British legislation requiring use for children of rear seat belts or safety seats in cars appropriately fitted.

Bicycle injuries

Most children use bicycles, particularly boys between 3 and 12 years. Injuries on bicycles cause about 5% of all child accidents presenting to hospital, and they also cause a significant number of serious injuries and death. Boys outnumber girls 3:1 in having bicycle injuries, and these injuries reach their peak at 8 years of age. Of particular concern are head injuries; one in 600 boys between 8 and 12 years have a serious enough head injury per year to be admitted to hospital under present criteria. Put another way, one in 100 boys have significant head injury while riding a bicycle during their childhood.[34]

There are factors in bicycle design which are vital to safety. For example the high-rise bicycle that was introduced into the UK in the early 1970s had features that made it more dangerous than standard models.[35] The centre of gravity was behind the back wheel when the rider was mounted, making the machine unstable, and the gear stick was placed in a way which caused severe genital injuries. Improvements in design have meant that this model has been superseded. More recently the widespread popularity of the BMX bicycle has caused concern, probably less because of intrinsic dangerous design factors than because the whole ethos of the bicycle encourages dangerous behaviour.

The prevention and reduction of severity of bicycle injuries may involve education, and environmental change. Children need to be taught to ride bicycles safely, by road safety officers, the Royal Society for Prevention of Accidents (ROSPA), and police officers. The courses organized by these agencies should also include proper maintenance of the bicycle chain, gear and brakes. Such training courses should begin as young as possible and parents should be encouraged to give thought to the type of bicycle they buy for their child or allow him to ride; also to the use of protective clothing and helmets. Head protection and helmets have been suggested as a way of reducing the severity of bicycle injuries. At present, this type of protection is not easily available and is expensive. A first step in their more widespread use would be to ensure that they are cheap and easy to buy, together with a publicity campaign to encourage their use. A British standard is now available.

Check list for health care professionals to prevent road traffic accidents to children[20]

- Encourage parents of children of 8 years of age and under to accompany them to school.
- Encourage councils to develop schemes to separate children from traffic.
- Encourage councils to provide play areas for children, particularly in inner city areas.
- Encourage local action in dealing with dangerous road situations, particularly near schools.
- Encourage use of car safety seats for children and acceptance of the law, also loan schemes to purchase child car restraints and 'First Ride Safe Ride' schemes.
- Encourage the use of bicycle safety helmets.
- Encourage parents to let their children attend bicycle riding instruction and maintain the bicycles adequately.

Preventing burns and scalds accidents in children

More children die accidentally from burns and scalds than any other cause apart from road traffic accidents. As well as being an important cause of death in childhood, burns and scalds cause significant morbidity from long-term scarring and psychological damage.

The majority of the children who die (81 out of 99 deaths in England and Wales in 1983)[36] die in conflagrations in private dwellings. Many of these children die from being overcome by gas and smoke rather than by direct heat. Many children under 5 years are scarred for life from scalds. This happens most commonly from hot fluids from a cup or a mug but significant numbers are scalded from teapots, kettles and in baths. In contrast to scalds, where younger children are commonly involved, the majority of children hurt by fire and flames are over 5 years of age.[37] Children are also burnt from small igniting sources such as matches, from outdoor fires, from space heating and from cooking equipment.

There has been a dramatic reduction in the number of deaths from the ignition of clothing which was a major problem in the immediate post-war years. In 1983, only five children died after accidents caused by ignition of clothing and only one from ignition by highly inflammable material. Firework accidents have also been reduced and are now a relatively small problem; only 320 firework accidents presented to hospital in children under 14 years in 1987.

Background factors to burn and scald accidents to children

Burn and scald accidents are most common in disadvantaged families. Mortality has been as much as fifteen times higher in social class V boys than social class I boys. When Chandler[38] looked at house fires there was a strong relationship between non-owner occupation, population density and children in care. National cohort studies have also confirmed heavy social class gradients in morbidity from burns and scalds, with poorer families being more liable to these accidents.[39] A study by Learmouth[40] found that thermal injuries strongly correlated with lack of hot water and overcrowding.

Disadvantaged families often live in an environment where smoking is common, where there are open fires and where there is inflammable furniture. They are also under psychosocial stress making supervision of young children difficult. Both factors make such families more liable to burns and scalds.

The prevention of burns and scalds accidents to children

There are a number of environmental measures which have helped or would help if introduced. Some of these need action by government or local councils; some need to be encouraged by health professionals visiting the home.

House fires, which cause the majority of burn deaths in childhood, could be reduced by stopping the source of the fire but also by reducing the flammability of the child's environment. Accidents involving open fires have fallen with the introduction of central heating but they still remain a problem, particularly with poor families. Fireguards should be used with young families and should conform with the British standard (BS 6539). Many conflagrations are initially started by cigarette smoking but it is unlikely that smoking will be reduced in disadvantaged families in the near future. A more practical approach is to reduce the flammability of the child's environment and to provide a warning if a fire takes place. Many children have died in house fires because of the flammability of upholstered furniture and from the toxic fumes produced when the foam burns. Pressure has now forced the government to insist on a new safety foam. The full effects of this legislation will take many years to come through because of the long life of furniture in homes. In the interim all those visiting the home can advise against this old foam furniture and they can also encourage the use of smoke detectors. These are widely used in the USA and are becoming more established in the UK. They have an important role in the prevention of conflagrations and their use should be encouraged both in public and private housing. Community paediatricians can encourage district councils to use them in their council houses and flats.

Injuries and deaths due to flammability of nightdresses have lessened with the Nightdress (Safety) Regulations in 1967. These injuries can be reduced further by extending the regulations on nightdress safety (BS 5722) and by reducing the number of open fires.

The prevention of scalds in children is a difficult problem. A wider use of mugs and elimination of unstable cups is to be encouraged. A number of children injure themselves from kettle spillage which can be avoided without large expense, by the use of coil or sprung electric flexes. Some children scald themselves by pulling saucepans down from cookers. Many of these incidents can be prevented by reducing access to the cooker and by cooker guards.

Firework accidents have been reduced with the discontinuation of certain types of fireworks, the restriction in the minimum age of people to whom fireworks are sold and the limitation of time fireworks are available in the shops to a few weeks before November the fifth.[41] The new British standard BS 7114 should further reduce this problem.

Check list for health care professionals to prevent burn and scald accidents to children[20]

- Encourage disposal of dangerous foam furniture.
- Encourage use of smoke alarms both by individuals and by local councils.
- Discourage open fires. If they have to be used, use fireguards.
- Emphasize dangers of hot liquids.
- Place kitchen units on either side of cooker or fit cooker guard.
- Use coiled flex electric kettles.
- Encourage safe use of fireworks.

Drowning and near drowning in childhood

Drowning is the third most common cause of accidental death in children in the UK; in 1988 and 1989, 306 children had confirmed submersion incidents. Of these 149 died and 157 survived after near drowning.[42] Drowning is an unusual accident, however, as unlike most other types it is an infrequent cause of presentation to an accident and emergency department. Many near drowning cases admitted to hospital are seriously ill and have to be admitted to an intensive care unit. A significant number of these children are left severely handicapped.[43] Many more boys drown than do girls which reflects the very different behaviour patterns of boys. There are also very major social class gradients, with disadvantaged children more likely to drown. One mode of drowning that does not follow this pattern is death in private swimming pools. The annual incidence in England and Wales of submersion accidents for children under 15 years of age was 1.5 per 100 000 with a mortality rate of 0.7 per 100 000. Boys under 5 had the highest incidence of submersion – 3.6 per 100 000.[42]

Warmer countries have a greater incidence of drowning than the UK. In the USA drowning death rates are as high as 1:8000 for boys aged 2–3 years in Los Angeles County.[44] Indeed much of the research on drowning and near drowning in childhood has been done in the USA and in particular Australia. The size of the problem of drowning and near drowning in the UK has been underinvestigated in the past. Recently however a nationwide UK study has been conducted through the British Paediatric Surveillance Unit (BPSU Study) (Table 7.18). The small number of serious incidents in public pools is most welcome.

Prevention

Drowning deaths and near drowning incidents in childhood can be divided into clear types with definite separate age ranges and epidemiology. Each site of drowning therefore has separate preventive measures that could be applied.

There is more evidence that education and training are effective for the prevention of drowning than for any other type of childhood accident. To be unable to swim increases the risk of drowning in childhood, and clearly it is advantageous if as many people as possible can swim. There is evidence that teaching children to swim may have reduced the number of deaths among 5–14 year olds.[45] Certainly, there has been an overall fall in the number of deaths in children from drowning, coinciding with better swimming training.

Bath drownings

Many drowning accidents occur with children too young to learn to swim. Bath drownings are seen in babies and toddlers and they can drown in shallow water. The problem occurs in families of low socioeconomic class and who are highly mobile[46] and sometimes there is evidence of neglect. Child abuse should always be considered in these children.[47]

The prevention of bath accidents in babies should be part of the health visitor's programme of education

Table 17.18 Cases of drowning in children under 15 years of age in UK 1988–1989 grouped according to site of incident. (141 notified 1988, 165 in 1989)[41]

Site (Mean age)	Survivors of near drowning	Drowning deaths	Total
Bath (1 year 2 months)	19 (1)*	25	44
Garden pond (1 year 10 months)	48 (4)*	11	59
Domestic pool (2 years 4 months)	15 (2)*	18	33
Private pool (5 years 9 months)	10	8	18
River, canal, lake (6 years 10 months)	17 (2)*	56	73
Public pool (7 years)	30 (1)*	2	32
Sea (7 years 10 months)	9	20	29
Other (4 years 2 months)	9	9	18
Total	157 (10)*	149	306

*Survivors who sustained severe neurological handicap

with mothers. It should be emphasized that it is unsafe to leave young children unsupervised in the bath, even for short periods.

Garden pond drownings

Garden pond drownings occur in toddlers. Children can drown in small, shallow ponds. The commonest story is of an unsupervised toddler wandering off when visiting friends or relatives. Most of these incidents occur in homes other than the child's home. A number of toddlers also can drown in pails, farm slurry pits, cattle troughs, and puddles.

Mothers should also be told about the dangers of drowning in garden ponds as part of the health visitor's programme of education with mothers. There are a number of environmental measures that could be used as well to prevent garden pond drownings. The ponds could be fenced and this is particularly important in parks and in garden centres. Another solution is the use of a grid just under the water to prevent children being able to immerse themselves. Garden ponds could also be brought under the building regulations.

Domestic swimming pools

Domestic swimming pools are a particular danger to toddlers. Drownings in these pools are a major problem in warm countries, particularly in the USA.[42] Nevertheless, they are a problem too in the UK.[48] In England and Wales in 1988–89, 18 children died and

15 were admitted to hospital after domestic swimming pool drownings.[44] These figures are much greater than public pool drownings, especially considering that many fewer children are exposed to domestic pools than public pools. Children wander off unsupervised and either fall into the pool or crawl under the covers.

There is good evidence that fencing which prevents children from having access to private pools with self-shutting gates can prevent drowning. Pearn and Nixon compared drownings from domestic swimming pools in Brisbane and in Canberra. In Canberra, swimming pools by law had to be fenced, but there was no such legal sanction in Brisbane at the time of the study: only one child died in Canberra from a swimming pool accident over a 5-year period, compared with 55 in Brisbane.[49] Fencing has been introduced by regulation in Australia, South Africa, New Zealand and parts of the USA. We still await any similar legislation in the UK.

Public pools

Deaths from public pool drownings have been reduced to a relatively minor problem in the UK following Health and Safety Regulations, introduced in 1985, which insist on a high level of supervision of children in pools.[50] Indeed only two children died in a public pool in the UK in 1988 and 1989.[42] Many of the children who are admitted to hospital after nearly drowning in public baths have had effective pool-side resuscitation.

The reduction in serious drowning in municipal public swimming pools incidents has been most welcome. Good supervision at the pool side should remain a high priority for local authorities and should be emphasized also in other public pools, such as those at holiday camps and private leisure centres.

Rivers, canals, lakes and sea

Drowning in rivers, canals and lakes is predominantly a problem in older boys. They play unsupervised and get into trouble in deep water. Many are non-swimmers. These boys correspond to the boys in Australia who drown in creeks. A number of children also drown in swimming parties in rivers which seem to be a dangerous activity.[42]

Studies in Australia and the UK have shown that a number of older children drown while swimming unsupervised in rivers, lakes and creeks: this unsupervised swimming should be discouraged.

Only six children drowned at sea in England and Wales in 1988. These are from a number of causes. Some children fall into docks, some are lost at sea in boating accidents and some drown swimming from the beach.

Life jackets and buoyancy aids are important for children using boats and canoes in helping to prevent drowning should they fall overboard.

Check list for health care professionals to prevent drowning accidents to children[20]

Bath
- Inform parents of the dangers as part of a child surveillance programme.

Garden pond
- Encourage fencing or draining of garden ponds.
- Inform parents of the dangers as part of a child surveillance programme.

Public pool
- Maintain high level of surveillance under the Health and Safety at Work Act 1974.

Private pool
- Extend a high level of surveillance to these pools.

Domestic pool
- Install fences (1.5 m) and self-locking gates around pools, if necessary by legislation.

Open water
- Supervise or restrict access for swimming in lakes and rivers.
- Youth organizations should not organize swimming parties in lakes and rivers.
- Extend lifeguard control to major beaches.
- Include water safety in the National Curriculum and in swimming programmes.
- Provide life jackets and buoyancy aids for use in boats and crafts.

Preventing accidents to children at play and recreation

Playground injuries

Playgrounds are dangerous places for children. In South Glamorgan, about one in 50 hospital attendances is due to injuries sustained in a playground.[3] The Leisure Accident Surveillance System (LASS) estimates that there are 24 000 such accidents each year in England and Wales.[51] Illingworth *et al*.[51] studied children with a variety of playground injuries, and found that fractures were three times more common in this group than in attendances overall at accident and emergency departments. A few children die each year in playground accidents. In Australia,[53] 14 deaths occurred in Brisbane during play and recreation over a 5-year period.

Prevention

The design of equipment in playgrounds is often contributory to causing accidents. Many can be prevented by attention to safe design. The type of surface of the playground is important if the severity of injuries to children falling onto it is to be reduced. Concrete is twice as hard as grass, and ten times as hard as sand. There are problems with sand, however, because of dog and cat fouling. The most satisfactory impact-absorbing surfaces commercially available are a granular bark compound, or a specially prepared, rubberized surface.

Swings can cause severe impact injuries and these can be reduced if the swing seats are made of an impact-absorbing substance, indeed, even an old tyre rather than metal. These impact injuries can also be reduced if by good playground design children do not need to rush past swings on the way to other equipment.

Falls from slides may be severe, especially from the old-fashioned type, where children climb a ladder to a platform 4.5 m (15 feet) or more from the ground. If the slide follows a contour of a hill there is just as much fun for children, and a much smaller fall if a mishap occurs. Severe falls can also occur from tall climbing frames. Design is again important, as it is as much fun to play horizontally as vertically, and much less far to fall. Impact-absorbing surfaces will again reduce injuries with climbing frames. Roundabouts of poor design may trap limbs and cause significant injury.

Influencing playground design

In England and Wales, most playgrounds for children are the responsibility of district councils but a few are managed by town and community councils. The Consumers' Association[54] found that in a sample of playgrounds there was evidence of bad design, poor maintenance, little safety surfacing and plentiful litter. Paediatricians will wish to influence playground safety in their districts by trying to influence the local authority, perhaps through a local accident committee. In many cases, parents and groups prove useful allies.

There is a British standard for playground design (BS 5696), although it is voluntary. However it can be used in an action for negligence against the local authority. Local councils have legal responsibility for playgrounds under the Consumer Safety Act, the Health and Safety at Work Act and the Occupiers Liability Act quite apart from their liability for negligence.

As well as influencing design, paediatricians will also wish to ensure adequate play facilities for children in their district. If these do not exist, children will be forced to play on the road and will be at risk from road traffic accidents.

Preventing sports injuries

All forms of sport and recreation have some risk and every year a few children die during sports and leisure activities. Children have died while playing cricket, karting, mountain walking, fishing and competing in athletics. Society cannot protect children from all risks in recreational activity, which is important in the development of personality and physical development. On the other hand, society should not expose children to unnecessary risk. Risks can be reduced by sensible supervision and other safety measures. For instance, hill and mountain climbing expeditions need careful supervision by experienced guides and teachers if disasters are to be prevented.

There has been little research on the risks of various sports, in particular whether rugby or soccer are dangerous for boys. A study in Wales[55] suggested that rugby may cause more injuries than soccer, particularly to the upper part of the body. There is also the danger of neck injuries, and paraplegia, with rugby.[56] Rugby injuries can be reduced if teams are not of different ages and ability; referees can also pay particular attention to collapse of a scrum and to mauls after tackles.

Dog bites

There has been much attention concerning danger to children of certain breeds of dog, such as rottweilers. Dog bites to children are however extremely common and as many as one in a hundred children a year present to an accident and emergency department with this problem.[3] In a study in America,[57] 20% of children were reported by their parents to have been bitten by a dog, the majority of whom were under 5 years of age. Many of the accidents occur in the home, or with dogs well known to the children. However a significant number of children are also bitten in public areas, particularly play areas. The majority of dog bites are minor, but severe lacerations, particularly facial lacerations, do occur. One in seven of the children in a study needed sutures.[57]

The health visitor has an important role in informing parents of the dangers of dogs. Small children should always be supervised when they are around dogs including family pets. Some areas have bylaws, insisting that dogs are kept on the lead in parks and should not be in playgrounds. This should be encouraged by health care professionals. Many people hope that certain breeds of dog will soon require a special licence to be kept. There is already limited legislation to control certain breeds of fighting dogs including pit bull terriers.

Horse accidents

Horse riding accidents are unusual as they are more common in girls than boys,[58] with the peak incidence in 10–14 year olds. Falls may cause head injuries, limb fractures and occasionally spinal injuries. Some children get kicked and some are crushed by horses falling on them. Horses sometimes bite, butt children and tread on their feet.

Many accidents to children on horses are caused by inexperience on the part of the rider particularly when the horse is startled in traffic. Injuries during competitions are rare. Good supervision and teaching are important in prevention as is matching the horse and rider. Good head protection is also vital in preventing serious head injury. Many traditional riding hats have in the past offered little protection for the rider. In April 1984, a new British standard, BS 6473 for protective hats for riders was introduced. The importance of wearing of such protection cannot be overemphasized.

Check list for health care professionals to prevent recreational accidents to children[20]

- Find playgrounds in the district and check on design and surfaces. Investigate any playground injuries.
- Influence safe design with local councils and accident committees. Campaign if necessary.
- Dangers of dogs as part of health visitor's accident prevention package.
- Keep dogs out of playgrounds.
- Supervise sporting activities in children.
- Teams to be of similar age and ability.
- Teach horse riding well.
- Head protection for horse riding: British standard, BS 6473.

Preventing accidents and falls in children by good architectural design

The design of homes where children live is important for their safety. Many falls, accidents associated with glass, and burns can be prevented by good design. Practical design guidelines are now available from the Child Accident Prevention Trust.[59] Discussion about safe design between architects and those treating accidents reduces accidents in the home.

Preventing falls in children

Falls are also the commonest cause of presentation to the accident and emergency department[3] and result in a significant number of deaths in childhood. They have a varied aetiology.

They may be on one level, such as falling on the pavement or in the school playground. These may occur as a result of unruly or poor behaviour and better supervision of play is perhaps the only answer to prevent these injuries which are rarely serious. Indeed falls on one level caused no deaths in an analysis of 253 fatal falls in children 0–14 years in England and Wales from 1975 to 1985.[60] In contrast, 19% of hospital presentations from falls due to home accidents were on one level.

Falls can also be from one level to another. Children may be dropped, fall from furniture, down stairs, from toys or windows. Falls down stairs are a particular problem for toddlers.[60] Much can be done to prevent them, by better stair design and stair-gates and health visitors can encourage the latter. Open stairs with wide gaps between balustrades may be fine aesthetically, but dangerous for young children. In 1985, building regulations were changed to ensure a 100 mm sphere could not be passed through any opening or guarding to a flight of stairs.

The danger of falls from baby walkers has been highlighted and they are no longer advised for children's use.[61] Older children fall from trees, cliffs, mountains, play equipment, and buildings.

Poor window catches and design cause a number of accidents, particularly in high-rise flats. The introduction of safety catches or window guards will reduce these accidents and in New York City a programme providing free window guards (The Children Can't Fly Program) has been successful in preventing window falls in a poor area of New York.[62]

Glass injuries

Glass may cause severe injuries to children. There may be lacerations to hands, wrists and arms, and occasionally the face. Glass may cause injury to arteries, nerves, tendons and internal organs. Scarring and permanent disability can follow. The child is usually injured by glass in doors or by low level glazing. A typical story would be a child falling downstairs into a glass door. The sharp jagged parts of the glass may cause severe lacerations to all parts of the body, particularly the upper limbs.

Most glass injuries in childhood could be prevented by the use of safety glass.[63] Safety glass may be either laminated, which absorbs impact and is resistant to penetration or toughened tempered glass, which shatters into small cuboid pieces. Other safe alternatives to annealed flat glass are polycarbonate sheet or plastic safety film. Laminated glass is only about 1.8 times more expensive than annealed flat glass. As yet there are no legal requirements for buildings to have safety glass, but only recommendations in codes of practice. The whole subject was reviewed by the Child Accident Prevention Trust in 1982.[64] A health visitor is in the ideal situation to find unsafe glass while visiting the home, and to suggest that safety glass should be used instead.

Check list for health care professionals to prevent accidents and falls to children by architectural design[20]

- Check design of stairs for child safety.
- Advise stair gates with toddlers in house.
- Advise against baby walkers.
- Check window and balcony design for child safety.
- Advise catches if necessary.
- Advise safety glass or safety film for low level glazing.

Preventing poisoning in childhood

There are a number of different types of poisoning seen in childhood: accidental child poisoning in under fives; deliberate poisoning in older children; non-accidental poisoning; iatrogenic poisoning.

Of these, accidental poisoning is the most common and the only type that can be correctly called an accident. This is an important problem for children under 5 years which has been prevented by a methodological approach. The epidemiology has been studied and education campaigns have been evaluated and shown to be ineffective. An environmental solution (child-resistant containers (CRCs)) has been evaluated on a small scale, shown to be worthwhile and then introduced more widely.

A very few children die from accidental poisoning each year.[65] As well as the few children who die each year, many more are admitted to hospital for treatment and observation, and more still present to hospital accident and emergency departments. The Home Accident Surveillance System[66] estimated that in 1986 37 000 children aged 0–4 years attended accident and emergency departments because of accidental poisoning. A cohort study in New Zealand showed that 19% of children had at least one incident of poisoning or suspected poisoning by the age of 3 years.[10] No medical help was sought in many of these incidents.

Aetiology of accidental child poisoning

Surprisingly availability of poisons does not appear to be a major factor in accidental child poisoning.[67,68] There is evidence that family psychosocial stress may be an important aetiological factor in childhood poisoning.[15,69] There may also be personality factors particularly hyperactivity that predispose towards child poisoning.[70,71] These family and personality findings have considerable importance for the prevention of child poisoning.

Preventing child poisoning

The two approaches tried to prevent accidental child poisoning have been education and changes in the environment. The link between accidental child poisoning and family psychosocial stress and hyperactivity make it unlikely on theoretical grounds that education would be effective. Families under stress are unlikely to remember safety propaganda.

Indeed a campaign in Birmingham to publicize the problem and to return medicines concluded, 'that publicity, storage and destruction of unwanted medicines have little preventive value'.[6] In New Zealand, an evaluation was made of placing Mr Yuk stickers on poisons together with a campaign to prevent child poisoning.[72] This again had no effect on poisoning admissions.

Child resistant containers

Dr Jay Arena from Durham, North Carolina first suggested the idea of child-resistant containers (CRCs) in 1959.[73] These containers were evaluated in a community in the USA by Scherz,[7] where poisoning cases were reduced from 147 to 17 cases per year by the use of child resistant closures. Following this success they were introduced into the USA for aspirin preparations in 1972 and reduced poisoning episodes by approximately 50%.[8] Reductions in accidental child poisoning numbers were found when CRCs were introduced for other medicines and household products in the USA under the Poison Prevention Act.[74]

Following the success of child-resistant containers in the USA, they were introduced by regulation in 1976 in the UK for junior aspirin and paracetamol preparations. This resulted in a fall in admissions of children under 5 years after salicylate poisoning in South Glamorgan and Newcastle-on-Tyne from 129 cases in 1975 to 48 cases in 1976.[9] Judged on a national basis, the Hospital In-Patient Enquiry (HIPE) estimated that before 1975, 7000 children were admitted in England and Wales per year because of analgesic poisoning. Admissions dropped to 2000 children in 1978 with the introduction of the safety regulations.[10]

In 1978 CRCs were introduced for adult aspirin and paracetamol tablets by regulation. In 1982 a voluntary agreement was made between the government and the Pharmaceutical Society whereby all prescribed solid dose medications would be placed in CRCs or safety packaging with the exceptions for the elderly and infirm. Experience since 1982 has not been entirely encouraging[75] and some pharmacists did not use CRCs.[76] However, since January 1989 the Royal Pharmaceutical Society has made it a professional requirement for pharmacists to use CRCs. In 1985 the Department of Trade and Industry agreed to put a number of household products, such as white spirit and turpentine substitute, into CRCs by regulation.

Other methods of preventing child poisoning

The use of lockable medicine cupboards has been suggested to prevent child poisoning. On theoretical grounds they are unlikely to be effective as parents under stress are unlikely to remember to put medicines away or lock medicine cabinets.

One possible solution to accidental poisoning from household products decanted into jars is to make them bitter with a suitable chemical agent, and thus unpalatable. A possible agent is Bitrex (denatronium bromide).

Serious accidental child poisoning can also be prevented by a reduction in the prescribing of drugs known to be seriously toxic to children. This has been done in the case of barbiturates and could be extended to such drugs as quinine and vaporizing solution.

Check list for health care professionals to prevent accidental poisoning in children[20]

- Encourage use of CRCs by pharmacists.
- Encourage storage of medicines and household products away from children.
- Discourage prescribing of quinine and barbiturates etc.

Useful addresses

Child Accident Prevention Trust
28 Portland Place
London W1N 2DE

Royal Society for Prevention of Accidents
Cannon House
The Priory
Queensway
Birmingham B4 6BS

References

1 Office of Population Censuses and Surveys. Deaths by accidents and violence. Quarterly Monitors DH4 Series. London: HMSO, 1988.
2 Avery, J.G. Child Accident Prevention Trust Occasional Paper. London: CAPT, 1982.
3 Sibert, J.R., Maddocks, G.B., Brown, M. Childhood accidents: an endemic of epidemic proportions. *Arch Dis Child* 1981; **56**: 226–226.
4 Department of Health and Social Security and Office of Population Censuses and Surveys. Hospital in-patient

enquiry main tables. Series MB4 No 27. London: HMSO, 1987.

5 Child Accident Prevention Trust. *Basic Principles of Child Accident Prevention*. London: CAPT, 1989.

6 Harris, D.W., Karindiker, D.S., Spencer, M.G., Leach, R.H., Bower, A.C., Mander, G.A. Returned medicines campaign in Birmingham 1977. *Lancet* 1979; ii: 599–601.

7 Scherz, R.G. Prevention of childhood poisoning. *Pediatr Clin North Am* 1970; **17:** 713–720.

8 Clarke, A., Walton, W.W. Effect of safety packaging on aspirin ingestion by children. *Pediatrics* 1979; **63:** 687–693.

9 Sibert, J.R., Craft, A.W., Jackson, R.H. Child resistant packaging and accidental child poisoning. *Lancet* 1977; ii: 289–290.

10 Jackson, R.H., Craft, A.W., Lawson, G.R., Sibert, J.R. Changing pattern of poisoning in children. *Br Med J* 1985; **287:** 1468.

11 Schlesinger, E.R., Dickson, D.G., Westaby, J., Logrillo, V.M., Maiwald, A.A. A controlled study of health education in accident prevention: the Rockland County child injury project. *Am J Dis Child* 1966; **111:** 490–496.

12 Sibert, J.R., Williams, H. Medicine and the media. *Br Med J* 1983; **286:** 1893.

13 Minchom, P., Sibert, J.R. Does health education prevent childhood accidents? *Postgrad Med J* 1984; **60:** 260–262.

14 Backett, E.M., Johnston, A.M. Social pattern of road accidents to childhood: some characteristics of vulnerable families. *Br Med J* 1959; **1:** 403–409.

15 Sibert, J.R. Stress in families of children who have injested poisons. *Br Med J* 197; **3:** 87–89.

16 Brown, G.W., Davidson, S. Social class, psychiatric disorder of mother and accidents to children. *Lancet* 1978; ii: 378–381.

17 Beautrais, A.L., Fergusson, D.M., Shannon, F.T. Life events and childhood mortality: a prospective study. *Pediatrics* 1982; **70:** 935–939.

18 Colver, A.F., Hutchinson, P.J., Judson, E.C. Promoting children's home safety. *Br Med J* 1982; **285:** 1177–1180.

19 Schelp, L. Community intervention and changes in accident pattern in a rural Swedish municipality. *Health Promotion* 1979; **2:** 109–125.

20 Sibert, J.R. Accidents to children: the doctor's role. Education or environmental change? *Arch Dis Child* 1991; **66:** 890–894.

21 Sunderland, R. Dying young in traffic. *Arch Dis Child* 1984; **59:** 754–759.

22 Howarth, C.I., Routledge, D.A., Repetto-Wright, R. An analysis of road accidents involving child pedestrians. *Ergonomics* 1974; **17:** 319–330.

23 Kohler, L., Ljungblom, B.-A. *Child Development and Traffic Behaviour: Traffic and Children's Health*. Stockholm: Nordic School of Public Health, 1987.

24 Sharples, P.M., Storey, A., Anysley Green, A. and Eyre, J.A. Avoidable factors contributing to death of children with head injury. *Br Med J* 1990; **300:** 87–91.

25 Sandels, S. *Children in Traffic*. London: Elek Ltd, 1976.

26 Grayson, G.B. The identification of training objectives: what shall we tell the children? *Accid Anal Prev* 1981; **13:** 169–173.

27 Pease, K., Preston, B. Road safety education for young children. *Br J Educ Psychol* 1967; **37:** 305–313.

28 Firth, D.E. *Roads and Road Safety: Descriptions given by 400 Children*. TRRL Supplementary Report 138UC. Crowthorne, Berkshire: Transport and Road Research Laboratory, 1975.

29 Royal Dutch Touring Club. Woonerf Club, PO Box 93200, Hague, Netherlands, 1977.

30 Partyka, S.C. Lives saved by seat belts from 1983 through 1987. *NHTSA Technical Report*. DOT HS 807 324. Springfield, Virginia: National Technical Information Service, 1988.

31 Transport and Road Research Laboratory. *The Protection of Children in Cars*. TRRL Leaflet 345. Crowthorne, Berkshire: TRRL, 1974.

32 Scherz, R.G. Restraint systems for the prevention of injury to children in automobile accidents. *Am J Public Health* 1976; **66:** 451.

33 Richmond, P.W., Skinner, A., Kimche, A. Children's car-restraints: use and parental atittudes. *Arch Emerg Med* 1989; **6:** 41–45.

34 Clarke, A.J., Sibert, J.R. Why child cyclists should wear helmets. *Practitioner* 1986; **230:** 513–514.

35 Sibert, J.R., Newcombe, R.G. Bicycle injuries in childhood. *Br Med J* 1974; **1:** 613–614.

36 Child Accident Prevention Trust. *Burns and Scald Accidents to Children*. London: CAPT, 1985.

37 Department of Trade. *Domestic Thermal Injury Study*. London: HMSO, 1983.

38 Chandler, S.E. The incidence of residential fires and the effect of housing and other social factors. BRE information paper 1 1979 P20/79. Watford: Building Research Establishment, 1979.

39 Butler, N.R. *et al. Britain's Five Year Olds*. London: Routledge and Kegan Paul, 1980.

40 Learmonth, A. Factors in child burn and scald accidents in Bradford 1969–73. *J Epidemiol Commun Med* 1979; **33:** 270–273.

41 Royal Society for Prevention of Accidents. *Firework Injuries Statistics, 1987*. Birmingham: ROSPA, 1987.

42 Kemp, A.M., Sibert, J.R. Drowning and near drowning in children in the United Kingdom: lessons for prevention. *Br Med J* 1992; **304:** 1143–1146.

43 Kemp, A.M., Sibert, J.R. Outcome for children who nearly drown: a British Isles study. *Br Med J* 1991; **302:** 931–933.

44 O'Carroll, P.W., Alkon, E., Weiss, B. Drowning mortality in Los Angeles County 1976 to 1984. *J Am Med Assoc* 1988; **260:** 380–383.

45 Graham, J.M., Keating, W.R. Deaths in cold water. *Br Med J* 1978; **2:** 18–19.

46 Nixon, J., Pearn, J., Wilkey, L., Corcoran, A. A fifteen year study of child drowning. *Accid Anal Prev* 1986; **18:** 199–203.

47 Nixon, J., Pearn, J.H. Emotional sequelae of parents and sibs, following drowning or near-drowning of a child. *J Psychol* 1977; **11:** 265–268.

48 Barry, W., Little, T.M., Sibert, J.R. Childhood drownings in private swimming pools: an avoidable cause of death. *Br Med J* 1982; **285:** 542–543.

49 Pearn, J.H., Nixon, J. Are swimming pools becoming more dangerous? *Med J Aust* 1977; **2:** 702–704.

50 Health and Safety Executive, Sports Council. *Safety in Swimming Pools*. London: Sports Council, 1988.

51 MacCleary, L. *Playgrounds: Leisure Accident Surveillance System (LASS)*. London: Consumer Safety Unit, Department of Trade and Industry, 1989.

52 Illingworth, C.W., Brennan, P., Jay, A., Al-Rawif, E.R., Collier, M. 200 injuries caused by playground equipment. *Br Med J* 1975; **4:** 332–334.

53 Nixon, J., Pearn, J., Wilkey, I. Deaths during play: a study of playground and recreation deaths. *Br Med J* 1981; **283:** 410.

54 Consumers' Association. Playground safety. *Which?* 1988; April.

55 Hughes, D.R., Evans, R.C., Sibert, J.R. Sports injuries to children. *Br J Accident Emerg Med* 1986; **1.4:** 13.

56 McCoy, G.F., Piggott, J., Macafee, A., Adair, I.A. Injuries to the cervical spine in schoolboy rugby football. *J Bone Joint Surg* 1984; **66B:** 500–503.

57 Lauer, E., White, W.C., Lauer, B.A. Dog bites: a neglected problem in accident prevention. *Am J Dis Child* 1982; **136:** 702–704.

58 Baker, H.M. Horse play: survey of accidents with horses. *Br Med J* 1973; **3:** 532–534.

59 Child Accident Prevention Trust. *Child Safety and Housing*. London: CAPT, 1986.

60 Nixon, J., Jackson, H., Hayes, M. *An Analysis of Childhood Falls involving Stairs and Bannisters*. London: Consumer Safety Unit, Department of Trade and Industry, 1987.

61 Glendill, D.N.S., Robson, W.V., Cudmore, R.E., Tavistock, R.R. Baby walkers: time to take a stand. *Arch Dis Child* 1987; **62:** 491–494.

62 Speyel, C.M., Linderman, F. Children can't fly: a program to prevent mobility and mortality from window falls. *Am J Public Health* 1977; **68:** 1143–1147.

63 Jackson, R.H. Lacerations from glass in childhood. *Br Med J* 1981; **283:** 1310–1312.

64 Child Accident Prevention Trust. *Architectural Glass Accidents to Children*. Occasional Paper 3. London: CAPT, 1982.

65 Craft, A.W. Circumstances surrounding deaths from accidental poisoning 1974–1980. *Arch Dis Child* 1983; **58:** 544–546.

66 Department of Trade and Industry. HASS Data Personal Communication. London: HMSO, 1988.

67 Baltimore, C.L., Meyer, R.J. A study of storage, child behavioral traits, and mother's knowledge of toxicology in 52 poisoned families and 52 comparison families. *Pediatrics* 1968; **42:** 312–317.

68 Sobel, R., Margolis, J.A. Repetitive poisoning in children: a psychosocial study. *Pediatrics* 1965; **39:** 641–651.

69 Bithoney, W.G., Snyder, J., Michalek, J. Newberger, E.H. Childhood ingestions as symptoms of family distress. *Am J Dis Child* 1986; **139:** 456–459.

70 Stewart, M.A., Thach, B.T., Freiden, M.R. Accidental child poisoning and the hyperactive child syndrome. *Dis Nerv Syst* 1977; **31:** 403–407.

71 Sibert, J.R., Newcombe, R.G. Accidental ingestion of poisons and child personality. *Postgrad Med J* 1977; **53:** 254–256.

72 Ferguson, B.A., Harwood, C.J., Beautrais, M.A., Shannon, F.T. A controlled trial of a poison prevention method. *Pediatrics* 1982; **69:** 515–517.

73 Arena, J.M. Safety closure caps. *J Am Med Assoc* 1959; **169:** 1187–88.

74 Walton, W.W. An evaluation of the Poison Prevention Act. *Pediatrics* 1982; **69:** 363–370.

75 Sibert, J.R., Clarke, A.J., Mitchell, M.P. Improvements in child resistant containers. *Arch Dis Child* 1985; **60:** 1155–1157.

76 Scottish Department. Drug testing in Scotland. *Pharm J* 1984; **233:** 55.

7.7 Health education in schools

Heather Richardson

Introduction

In 1990 it is the common expectation that a baby will survive to live a long life. Since the eradication or control of many of the infectious diseases children tend to die only in unforeseen tragedies. However, the media frequently bring to our attention problems of alcohol, drugs, and Aids that may reach epidemic proportions, with disastrous effects on our young people. Other significant issues interfering with the general health and well-being of the child population include housing, poverty, intrafamilial and extrafamilial violence, and poor nutrition, with the feelings of helplessness and powerlessness that these difficulties produce.

Heart disease, stroke, and cancer are the leading causes of death in middle and old age, and accidents in children and young people. Together these account for 400 000 deaths per year; over 70% of the total. Other major sources of suffering and ill health are chronic bronchitis, diseases of circulation, rheumatism and arthritis. Mental 'ill health', where men and women feel harassed and incapacitated by worry, anxiety, stress and strain, may result in physical ill health, and by and large will have its roots in unaddressed traumas and secrets of childhood, with unrelieved guilt, shame and emotional pain responsible for much of the symptomatology.

Man's environment is controlled by four factors.[1] Two are related to measures of public action, and can be divided into physical and social actions, and two are related to behaviour measures adopted by individuals, first those that affect themselves, and secondly those that affect others.

It might well be stated that major health improvements have been brought about by politicians and public health measures, rather than by actions of the individual. A reasonable hypothesis is that a planned national school health education policy, rather like the national curriculum, which included a no smoking, no alcohol policy, a balanced diet at school lunch, a tuck shop where only nuts and fruit were obtainable, a period of daily physical exercise, group meditation, an ethos of peer group counselling, and a commitment to involvement of family and community, would do more for the health of our children, than all other health education programmes put together.

Purpose

The purpose of health education in schools is to encourage health.

Health is a state of complete physical, mental and social well-being, and is not simply the absence of disease or infirmity.[2]

The focus of health education is on people and action. In general its aims are to develop health promotion whereby people adopt and sustain healthful life practices, use judiciously and well the health services available to them, and take their own decisions, both indirectly and collectively, to improve their health status and environment.[3]

There is much potential for the promotion of primary prevention through health education whereby people's attitudes towards smoking, alcohol, and exercise are altered. However, the onus of making the decisions in order to safeguard health must necessarily rest on the individual.

The kind of healthy society envisaged will determine the programme of health education. For the Navaho Indians,[6] health is symptomatic of a correct relationship between man and his environment, his supernatural environment, the world around him and his fellow man. Health is associated with good and blessing and beauty – all that is positively valued in life. Illness, on the other hand, bears evidence that one has fallen out of this delicate balance.

Although we know perfectly well with one part of our mind that smoking causes cancer, and that drinking causes road accidents, with another part of our mind we do not really believe it will ever happen to us. In short, shock approaches work for others, not for me.

In the context of human values health has a community basis, but closer to the heart of things is a poster issued by the Scottish Health Education Unit, based on one put out by Parents Anonymous Incorporated of the USA:

Children learn what they live

If a child lives with criticism she learns to condemn
If a child lives with hostility he learns to fight
If a child lives with ridicule she learns to be shy
If a child lives with shame he learns to feel guilt
If a child lives with tolerance she learns to be patient
If a child lives with encouragement he learns confidence
If a child lives with praise she learns to appreciate
If a child lives with fairness he learns justice
If a child lives with security she learns to have faith
If a child lives with approval he learns to like himself

If a child lives with acceptance and friendship he or she learns to find love in the world.

Philosophy

The priority given to health education is fundamentally a political one.[4] Some of the contributors in *Health by the People*[5] make the point that people want curative services first, and it is only later that preventive services are understood or requested. China, Cuba and Tanzania are countries which omitted the curative stage and adopted preventive policies from the start.[5] The advantages have been multiple, judged by health criteria and by economy over time.

History

In 1901–2 The director general of the Army Medical Services and the inspector general of recruitment indicated that more than 40% of all recruits examined in the period 1901–2 were unfit for army service. The report of the Interdepartmental Committee on Physical Deterioration (1904) gave the following as major defects: want of physical development, defective vision, diseases of the heart, and bad dentition. Schools were asked to give instructions about the effects of alcohol on physical efficiency; lessons in care of teeth, and systematic instruction for girls in the processes of infant feeding and management. The Education (Administrative Provisions) Act of 1907 enabled the regular inspection of school children by local authority medical officers. The findings and experience of 18 years, and the medical examination of 10 million school children, showed that physical impairment of these children was wide in its distribution and serious in its effect on adult life.[7]

It was said that Sir George Newman as Chief School Medical Officer during the period 1907–31 was unable, despite prodigious efforts, to get health education across to the schools.[8]

In 1928 after the setting up of the Central Council, the Board of Education issued a Handbook of Suggestions on Health Education for the consideration of teachers and others concerned in the work of public elementary schools. The purpose of the new handbook was summarized in the last paragraph. 'If children learn at school to keep themselves clean and tidy, to eat wholesome food, to keep their classrooms, corridors and playground free from litter, to keep the windows open, to see that the lavatories and closets are properly used, they are likely to carry these habits into practice when they leave school, and in this way will not only assist the Health Department in their task, but will also do much to build up the health and secure the wellbeing of the community.'

Health education thus remained, during the 1930s–50s, a subordinate matter, partly because few saw it as important, and partly because it became variously associated with different professional interests. In schools the subject was linked with physical education, religion, humanities, domestic science, and biology. In public health the medical officer of health counted the subject as one of his specialities. The health visitor from the beginning was recognized as the health educator of mothers and young children. In 1956 the Jameson report was the first government report that showed clearly that health education was important. In 1963 the Cohen Committee recommended the establishment of a strong central board in England and Wales that would promote a climate of opinion generally favourable to health education on selected priority subjects. A parallel board was recommended for Scotland. In 1968, The Health Education Council (England and Wales) was set up, and in Scotland, The Scottish Health Education Department.

In the 1960s and 1970s a narrow view of health education was prevalent in secondary schools, and it was linked mainly to hygiene and sex education. In the late seventies health education received a tremendous impetus. A health education programme was developed by the School Council Health Education Project. Programmes were developed for both primary and secondary school children. By 1982 the 13–15 year programme was in use in 15% of secondary schools, and by 1984 the 5–13 year material in 25% of primary schools. By 1983, 50% of secondary schools had assigned a teacher, usually of senior status, to be coordinator of health education in schools, and half the education authorities allowed senior school teachers to be released for health education training. In the 1980s a fair proportion of schools developed a broader, more positive concept associated with self-esteem, mental health, and relationships.[9] There was also active promotion of cooperation between health authorities, health education officers rather than school health personnel, and education authorities.

In 1985 the Scottish Education Department issued a circular to schools, stressing the importance of drug education, and even more importantly, paid for the in-service training for teachers in the subject in 1985–6. From this, a national programme of in-service training developed, and within 2 years virtually all secondary schools had a single member of staff trained in basic concepts of health education and to coordinate a drug and health education programme. In England and Wales the education authorities appointed advisers on drug education, and gave advice to hundreds of schools.

The 1986 Education (No 2) Act gave governors of individual schools the power to decide whether there should be any sex education at all in their schools, and if so what form it would take.[10] In addition, the national curriculum made no specific proposals for sex education. Also teachers were given much conflicting advice about sexual issues. The Department of Education and Science (DES) advised teachers that specific advice on contraception to girls under 16 would constitute a criminal offence; also major difficulties might occur in discussing homosexuality. Moral values were to be encouraged.

In 1987 national curriculum proposals did not include health education as a core subject, but felt it could be included in lessons such as biology. In 1989 drug coordinators advised governors that the basis of prevention comes from self-esteem programmes, and recommended the update of such programmes in the fight against alcohol, drugs, and AIDS.

In the last 20 years much has been learnt about the process and methods required for effective health education in schools. As a result general agreement has been reached on two key principles. The first and most fundamental was that total well-being and healthy behaviour are closely tied with self-concept and self-esteem, and this is an absolute prerequisite to any other health education strategy. Thus self-awareness programmes must be considered as the basic groundwork to any health education programme. It began to be realized that health education cannot succeed with a single lesson or talk on an isolated topic. It is still very popular for hard-pressed head teachers to invite an outside expert for a one-off lecture, e.g. police on drugs, so that particular subject can be ticked off as done. Schools come under much pressure, particularly from the police, but also from many other agencies who wish to spread their message to the children. These offers should be resisted, but the experts can be invited to advise and support teachers. In addition to the basic framework of on-going self-esteem programmes, themes such as sex, smoking, nutrition, and child care need to be repeated throughout the school years in ways which are matched to the child's stage of maturity. This is termed a SPIRAL curriculum, a phrase that often confuses doctors, but is beloved by health education officers and embraces the second key principle.

In 1985 Connel and others[11] evaluated a health education programme involving 30 000 American children in 1000 schools. This study confirmed the importance of the above principles, and showed that:

1 Knowledge gains could be achieved in a relatively few hours, but effects on attitude and behaviour

required a sizeable commitment of classroom hours (30 hours or more).

2 A programme conducted over 2 years was more effective than a 1 year programme.

3 In-service training and preparation of teachers greatly enhanced implementation and effectiveness of a health education programme.

4 The involvement of parents was influential.

5 The commitment of the school was fundamental to success.

6 A balanced comprehensive health education programme was important.

The basic concept of these programmes is that children are helped to identify and to talk about their feelings; to become self-aware; to become aware of their motives; to learn to listen and not to put others down. They must include strategies for resisting peer group pressure, assertiveness training, and training in relaxation and structuring time. In addition, the programme should offer the information necessary to make informed health decisions over a whole range of topics, such as smoking, alcohol, drugs, Aids, sex, healthy eating, and child care. Another fundamental concept of the programme is group work, and the underlying basic theme in terms of self-discovery and promotion of self-esteem are also core factors in therapeutic programmes for violent, delinquent, sexually abused and troubled youngsters.

One such programme was introduced to the UK, as well as throughout Europe, Australia and the USA, and has been received with unusual enthusiasm by teachers. It involves teachers, parents and children in secondary schools, and has resulted very speedily in improving the atmosphere both in and outside the classroom. It was evaluated by Dr Parsons of Christ Church College, Canterbury, UK and was recommended by the Department of Health to every district.[12] A similar programme is being developed at the present time for use in primary schools.

Health education for students is something that must be delivered primarily by teachers. The content of the programme will be influenced by government directives on the one hand, and what school governors perceive as necessarily right and proper on the other.

Health authority involvement

In many districts the community paediatrician may have the responsibility for advising schools about health education together with a health education department. There may be several health education officers assigned to assist schools with provision of ideas, courses, teaching aids, and evaluation of programmes. Coordination, liaison, and cooperation between all interested parties is mandatory for effectiveness.

The youngsters

Many young people view the future with concern, for example considering problems around pollution and HIV infection. Many consider that the adults in their lives deny, or do not wish to recognize, the youngsters' feelings, and do not, in their view, give time to listen to their problems. They appear to say 'No' to the very things that teenagers think would make them feel better: alcohol, cigarettes, cannabis, parties, driving too fast, binging, sweating out, and sex, activities which seem to hold promise for short-term happiness, or at least a way of coping with daily life that distances them from fears and from the unhappy events they expect in the future.

Youngsters also express their feelings about the choices they have to make. As one 16 year old said, one of the basic pressures is not knowing how to behave in specific situations. A girl describing a risk situation said: 'You want to do it so you are not left out, but inside you know you shouldn't do it, but you do it anyway because you don't want to lose your friends.' Comments like these can trigger discussions which get to the heart of behavioural choice analysis.

Teenage health problems are preventable, yet they continue to arise, in part because many teenagers do not know how to meet their personal needs in healthy ways. They begin smoking and drinking to be accepted; they get into fights because they have not learnt more constructive outlets for their anger; they overeat because they are lonely or bored; they become pregnant because they want attention, affection, escape, or a council house; and may do poorly in school because they have little self-esteem.

A health education programme must show children how to get what they want out of life without resorting to unhealthy habits. It must present a more positive view that marriage and family work, and that lifestyles can bring healthy exhilaration and satisfaction to their lives. The challenge is, therefore, to help young people to understand that when love (for the people to whom we are committed and for the ideas and beliefs that give our life meaning), and worth (the productive things we do to earn a living and help others) are balanced throughout life, then health is affected in a positive way. In other words, good health depends on actions of mind and body in a social context. This principle is based on the conceptual framework of effective health education of youngsters. Another central theme is care-giving, emphasizing the value of giving and receiving care from family members and friends throughout life.

Lifestyles and behaviour choices made during childhood can have far-reaching consequences. The health knowledge, skills and attitudes that children learn today can affect their health and the health of their families and friends in the community now and throughout their lifetime.

Suitable programmes are designed to develop skills in five basic areas:

1 Self-management
2 Communication
3 Decision making
4 Health management
5 Advocacy.

Schools

When schools, teachers or parents are asked what they perceive as important for health education they often reply the alcohol problem, and we must do something about smoking and sex, i.e. a subject rather than self-esteem. The Welsh Health Programme launched in Wales 1985, has taken on board that many of the life-style elements associated with increased risk of cardio-vascular disease have their elements in childhood and adolescence and have developed a youth health project which addresses itself to nutrition, smoking, physical activity and use and abuse of alcohol. The programme advocates a balanced educational approach to all these issues in schools, professional training, involvement of parents, youth clubs and addressing of environmental issues.

One of the most laudable parts of the project was to undertake surveys in 1986 to provide up-to-date relevant information for planning, monitoring and evaluation. The first, the Welsh Youth Health Survey, provided a wide range of information on the health and health-related behaviour, knowledge and attitudes of secondary school children. The authors comment that the information gained from the survey has been used in planning the health promotion programme, and the second survey specifically addressed the organization and health education policies in the school containing the pupils surveyed. It is only by such methods that we can devise and evaluate effective health promotion programmes.[13]

Programme examples

Each of the models presented below highlights both good and effective ways of delivery of health education, as well as strategies to be avoided.

Exercise

Five hundred children aged 10 and 11 years were divided into control and project groups. The P children did 40 minutes a day of either individual, team, or competitive sport, and these activities were discussed in the classroom. Control children did physical education twice weekly. Results showed the project children became more physically fit, and school attendance and self-confidence improved. In addition, school work improved and the children were more likely to be physically active outside school hours.[14,15] As a result, the local education authority planned to extend the scheme into local secondary schools.

Drugs

The long and stubbornly-held conviction that telling youngsters about drugs and associated dangers will actively stop them using them persists. It is a dangerous myth. In the mid-seventies the Netherland workers, De Haes and Schuerman, looked at the different approaches and their effectiveness in drug education. The approaches were:

1 Scare tactics
2 A factual approach
3 The personal relationship approach allowing pupils to talk about their own problems.[16]

The conclusion was that scare tactics and the factual approach increased drug experimentation.

These vitally important conclusions have influenced local and national policy.

Since then other studies, predominantly in the USA, have all reached the same general conclusion; that the methods aimed specifically at preventing drug abuse have at best been ineffective, and at worst counterproductive.[17-19] The most important single finding was the potential for programmes of self-awareness, enhancing self-esteem, and for learning to resist peer group pressure. Exactly the same remarks can be made for alcohol, smoking, pregnancy, AIDS, etc. Concentration on the subject at hand rather than the person in the social context is probably worse than useless.

AIDS

The HIV/AIDS Education Research Unit was set up in 1987 to organize research and health education in that field. They looked at schools in southern England, and found 22% of the fourth year, 34% of the fifth year, and 32% of the sixth formers claimed to have had full intercourse with a person of the opposite sex; 35% of those having sexual intercourse said they had used condoms, and 22% said they had never used them.

From their studies, the authors concluded that education on HIV disease must be conducted before youngsters become sexually active. There are other recommendations, such as that youngsters should be made aware that social contact with infected people does not carry a risk of infection; and that use of condoms is not a hundred percent guarantee of not getting AIDS. Also, many youngsters, particularly boys, have blaming attitudes towards those infected. The Unit suggests that education strategies should address the above issues in particular.[20] It is interesting to note that the International Planned Parenthood Federation wonder how to educate about AIDS without creating a generation of children who are afraid of sex, and who equate it with death. Judging by current attitudes, this seems remarkably unlikely.

Teenage pregnancy

It would appear that with intercourse so common among teenagers and relationships so tenuous, sex education, including biological information, contraceptive advice, and health advice clinics are an urgent necessity in health promotion. It should also be remembered that most of the major social health problems are found in the single mother and baby population, such as high infant mortality, poor immunization levels, delayed speech, and many childhood ailments such as wheezing and diarrhoea, poor school performance, behaviour problems, child abuse, teenage pregnancies, delinquency and unemployment. In later life there is increased risk of heart, chest and mental disorders.

As stated previously, if problems of poor self-esteem are not addressed, our efforts will not be successful.

It is possible to reduce accidental teenage pregnancy by school health education, and this evidence was presented by the Guttmacher Institute in 1985. They looked at the problem in three countries, and their studies concluded that the high rate of teenage pregnancy found in the USA was not only due to the high sexual activity rates in American teenagers, nor could it be accounted for by higher abortion rates in countries with low birth rates, nor at that time did the high rate of pregnancy correlate with high rates of deprivation, free availability of welfare benefit or actual provision of school/sex education. On the contrary, it was the more widespread availability of sex education, coupled with reasonable access to contraceptive advice and services in countries like England and Wales, which were the key factors helping to keep pregnancy rates lower than in the USA.[21]

Smoking

The 'My Body' project,[22] which is a programme for 10–12 year olds, was the first programme to be shown to influence smoking behaviour both in the children who were less likely to start, and in the children whose parents moderated their smoking habits. More excitingly, American studies have found that teenagers can be helped to develop and practice skills to resist social pressures.[20,23–25] Similar programmes have now been developed for use in British schools, and the Smoking and Me project is one such programme.[26] One of the major difficulties is that these programmes are frequently undermined by the fact that teachers smoke.

Nutrition

Healthy eating policies may well be addressed by co-operation with the school meal service in the provision of a healthy diet. Sussex Education Authority implemented an extremely effective policy when food was labelled with red, yellow and green markers – green being very healthy, and red the higher fat and sugar containing food. Also, many schools now have tuck shops where sugar free items are sold, thus being beneficial to both nutrition and teeth.

Child care

As will be abundantly clear, many of our teenagers are suffering from low self-esteem, and some will assuage their aching hearts by becoming pregnant. Some aspects of child care should be laid down in the curriculum, such as feeding, how to play with the child, early development, and the importance of communication. One programme asks all the class, boys and girls, to have a 'substitute baby', a sand bag, for 2 weeks so that youngsters can learn the difficulties of being responsible for 14 days, 24 hours a day, for an object. Visits to playgroups can be useful, but it is difficult to demonstrate effectively the changes that occur in lifestyles with a baby. Again involvement with local health visitors, and a programme such as the Child Development programme in Bristol – which is based on boosting the confidence of parents and empowering them to develop the parenting skills, and awareness of preventive health in relation to accident prevention, nutrition, communication, how to play, and the acquisition of language – would probably be the most valuable way forward for our youngsters.

Involvement of family

Many of today's current good health education programmes provide opportunities for transfer of information to parents, but most importantly workshops for parents and workshops for parents and children. These latter may be helpful in allowing children and parents to understand and listen to each other's attitudes.

Involvement of wider community

Ideally, major health education initiatives are more likely to succeed if school, family, village or town or city, are committed to such an endeavour. Certainly in the USA, although not yet in the UK, a major drug treatment centre will advise whole communities about drug education and prevention, and it is something which should be looked at in the UK.

Evaluation

The outcome indicators of effective health education can be difficult to measure, as so much depends on change of attitude and self-esteem. However, in the short term, the use of questionnaires for determining levels of smoking, alcohol use, drug use, and attitudes, should be used to monitor programmes, and The Schools Health Education Unit at the University of Exeter has a long and honourable reputation in providing well-researched questionnaires. In the longer term, of course, the success of health education programmes will be judged by such things as decreasing mortality rates, a drop in the number of referrals to psychiatric units and addiction units, and a falling prison population.

References

1 McKeown, T. *Medicine in Modern Society*, London: Allen and Unwin, 1965.
2 *Consultation of First Principle*. New York: WHO, 1946.
3 World Health Organization Expert Committee. Planning and evaluation of health education services. WHO Technical Report Series No. 409, 1969.
4 Society for Public Health Education. Health education policy issues. *Health Education Monographs* 1978; **6** Supplement 1.
5 Newell, K.W. *Health by the People*. Geneva, WHO, 1975.
6 Read, M. *Culture Health and Disease*. London: Tavistock, 1966.
7 Sutherland, I. *Health Education Perspectives and Choices*. London: Allen and Unwin, 1979.
8 Macintosh, J.H. *Trends of Opinion about Public Health 1901–51*. Oxford: Oxford University Press, 1953.
9 Brierly, J. Health education in secondary schools. *Hlth Educ J* 1983; **42**: 48–52.
10 Department of Education and Science. Education (No 2) Act. London: HMSO, 1986.
11 Connell, D., Turner, R.R., Mason, E.F. Summary of findings of the 'School Health Education Evaluations': health promotion effectiveness, implementation and costs. *J School Hlth* 1985; **55**: 316–321.
12 Burroughs, W.J. Skills for adolescence. Evaluation by Dr Parsons, Christ Church College, Canterbury. Department of Health Circular ED(89) P/63. 1989.
13 Pollatschek, J. 'The Linwood Project': a case for daily physical education. *Scot J Phys Educ* 1985; **13**(3): 12–15.
14 Nutbeam, D., Clarkson, J., Phillips, K. *et al*. The health-promoting school: organisation and policy development in Welsh secondary schools. *Hlth Educ J* 1987; **46**(3): 109–115.
15 Pollatschek, J. Physical education and beyond. *Edinburgh Scot Sports Coach* 1988; **7**: 3.
16 De Haes, W., Schuerman, J. Results of evaluation study of three drug education methods. *Int J Hlth Educ* 1975; **18**(4): Supplement 2.
17 Berberian, R., Gross, C, Lovejoy, J., Paparella, S. The effectiveness of drug education programmes: a critical review. *Health Education Monographs* 1976; **4**: 377–398.
18 Randall, D., Wong, M. Drug education to date: a review. *J Drug Educ* 1976; **6**: 1–21.
19 Swadi, H., Zeitlin, H. Drug education to school children: does it really work? *Br J Addiction* 1987; **82**: 742–46.
20 HIV/Aids Education Research Unit, Christ Church College, Canterbury, Kent. Before they begin . . . The HIV/Aids Education and Young People Project. *Aids Dialogue* 1989; **3**: 6–7.
21 Jones, E.F., Forrest, J.D., Goldman, N. *et al*. Teenage pregnancy in developed countries: determinants and policy implications. *Family Planning Perspectives* 1985; March/April (2): 53–63.
22 Health Education Council. *My Body*. Oxford: Heinemann Educational, 1983.
23 Evans, R.I., Hansen, W.B., Mittelmark, M.B. Social modelling films to deter smoking in adolescents: result of a three year field investigation. *J Appl Psychol* 1981; **66**: 399–414.
24 Aitken, P., Leather, D.S., Squair, S.I. Children's awareness of cigarette brand sponsorship of sport and games in the UK. *Hlth Educ Res* 1986; **1**: 203–211.
25 Perry, C., Killen, J., Telch, M. *et al*. Modifying smoking behaviour of teenagers: a school based intervention. *Am J Public Hlth* 1980; **70**: 722–725.
26 Gray, E.M. Smoking education for teenagers project. Smoking and me. A teachers' guide. London: Health Education Authority, 1988.

7.8 Volatile substance abuse

Joyce Watson[†]

Introduction

Solvent abuse, or volatile substance abuse (VSA), inhalant abuse and glue sniffing are all terms used to describe the deliberate inhalation of intoxicating substances. The practice is not a new phenomenon. It was reported as being part of the drug scene involving young adolescents in America from the 1950s. In the UK, headlines such as 'tragedy of the teenage sniffers', 'hairspray horror' and 'dangers of sniffing' appeared in local and national newspapers from the 1970s onwards. The reports of deaths from solvent abuse and of an adolescent problem of enormous proportions caused great concern among parents and professional

[†] Deceased

people alike and led to even more publicity. This in turn generated more public anxiety and fear.

Media reporting reached a peak in the mid-1980s. Solvent abuse is now less frequently headline news but the practice and its associated problems have not gone away. It is important that all professionals caring for adolescent and pre-adolescent children understand solvent abuse. They need to be familiar with details of practice and to consider it in the context of abuse of other substances by a wider section of the population.

The history of substance abuse

It is thousands of years since man first experimented with substances occurring naturally in his environment in an attempt to induce sleep, relieve pain, overcome anxiety or alter mood. Their use seems to depend on the availability of mind-altering substances and the desire to experiment. Opium, cannabis, mescaline and cocaine are all familiar names of drugs which are still used this way.

Any substance which alters an individual's behaviour, mental state, mood or physical functioning is a drug. Tea, coffee, cocoa and cola drinks all contain the drug caffeine which stimulates mental activity and affects mood and performance. The worldwide popularity of these drinks confirms the fact that their effects are enjoyed.

Cigarette smoking is an addiction which has world-wide appeal. This continues to be the case, despite the statistics which clearly show the morbidity and mortality associated with the habit.

Alcohol is also a drug which has been used by man for thousands of years. Originally perceived as a God-given gift, this is certainly not the prevailing current view.

These examples show a desire to try new experiences, find a happiness pill or alter one's mood or level of consciousness which reaches back into the distant past and continues today.

With the exception of opium and cannabis, which could be smoked, and cocaine, which could be sniffed, the drugs already mentioned were taken by mouth. More recently, some have been injected to produce a more immediate effect.

Another way of introducing substances into the body is via the lungs. This is a very effective route which ensures an onset almost as rapid as the intravenous injection of a drug. Volatile substance inhalation has a long and interesting history.

The earliest mention of vapour inhalation for the purpose of altering psychological state dates back to the Oracle at Delphi where some form of vapour inhalation is thought to explain the oracular pronouncements. Vapour inhalation was used in the religious cults of Assyria, Babylon, Egypt, Italy and many others over the centuries.

The ether *frolics* and chloroform *jags* indulged in by the student population of the 19th century were vividly described and widely reported at the time. It has become clear that nitrous oxide (laughing gas) and chloroform were first investigated because of their capacity to produce intoxication and this in turn led to their later use as anaesthetic agents.

During the present century the deliberate misuse of volatile substances by adults has not ceased but occurs only sporadically. The major concern has been about the abuse of volatile substances by adolescents and younger children.

The first cases to be described were those involving the inhalation of gasoline fumes by young people in remote rural parts of the USA in the late 1950s. The practice was not confined to America since there were reports published in the 1950s, 1960s and 1970s of sporadic petrol (gasoline) sniffing in Australia, India and the UK. Despite the ready availability of this product to young people, only 20–30 cases were reported worldwide over the years and involved young people who came to attention because of severe behaviour problems. These symptoms were investigated and found to show remarkable similarity to psychotic illnesses, but were actually due to petrol abuse.[1–4]

In November 1959, the *Denver Sunday Post* reported the arrests of children who were suspected of sniffing the fumes from glue. A tremendous amount of publicity followed and was accompanied by warnings about the dangers of such practice. The original reported incidents occurred in Tucson, Arizona and Pueblo, Colorado. However, some 10 months later, Denver was said to have an enormous glue sniffing problem involving mainly adolescents. The spread of the practice was thought to have been caused by all the publicity.

Although Denver was the first city in the world to suffer a serious glue sniffing problem, other American cities followed and by the mid 1960s glue sniffing was said to be occurring in every state in the USA. It is not clear whether the practice spread from one place to another or whether it started in many different places concurrently. It is also unclear whether the media reporting of the problem played a role in the spread after 1959.[5]

Products other than petrol and glue were misused, not on account of their smell but because their vapours caused intoxication. These products included nail polish remover,[6] anti-freeze,[7] paint thinners,[5] chloroform[8] and aerosol products of all kinds.

Surveys carried out among pupils attending schools in USA indicated that 3-30% had experimented with volatile substance abuse in the late 1960s and early 1970s.[9–11] Similar studies in Canada indicated an involvement of 3–8%. It was noted that the participants in glue sniffing episodes tended to be younger children which was unlike the general pattern of drug abuse.[6,12]

The prevalence of volatile substance abuse in Denmark was found to be less than 1%.[13]

A recent review of inhalant abuse in the USA demonstrated an increase at a time when other forms of drug abuse were in decline.[14] The National Household Survey of Drug Abuse revealed that annual inhalant misuse among the youth had increased from 2.9% in 1972 to 4.6% in 1979 and 5% in 1985.

Volatile substance abuse in the UK is now nationwide.

Definitions used

Volatile substance abuse involves inhalation of vapour from a substance which is normally a liquid but which evaporates easily at normal room temperature. This term would not include butane, propane, nitrous oxide or tobacco smoke, but would include petrol and all products containing volatile solvents. The word abuse is used to indicate that the substance is being used for other than its primary purpose.

The terms volatile substance abuse (VSA), solvent abuse, or inhalant misuse are used interchangeably in this section. It is much less important to get the name correct than it is to understand what is meant by the practice.

Process involved

During an episode of VSA, vapours from the various substances enter and leave the body via the nose, mouth and lungs, like oxygen and carbon dioxide. Most of the volatiles are breathed out in an unchanged form, but some are metabolized and excreted via the kidneys and some become attached to the fatty tissues of the brain.[15] The exact mechanism is not well understood. However, the immediate effect is to cause intoxication which develops very rapidly.

Products abused

Various products in common domestic and industrial use have been abused to cause intoxication. They include solvent-based adhesives and plastic cements, dry-cleaning fluids and spot-removers, paint thinners and strippers, industrial degreasing agents, pain relieving sprays, fire extinguishers, fuel gases including butane and propane, anaesthetic agents like ether, and aerosols of all kinds. The anthropologist, Karen Kerner, lists four kinds of inhalants:[16]

1 Volatile solvents such as those contained in glues and degreasing compounds.
2 Aerosols.
3 Anaesthetics, including ether and chloroform.
4 Volatile nitrites.

For the would-be sniffer, therefore, there is a whole range of products containing intoxicating chemicals. These are readily available and cheap to buy or easy to steal. If one product becomes unavailable for any reason, another suitable alternative can easily be found. However, products containing a high proportion of volatiles are preferred, therefore typewriter correcting fluids, butane gas and pain-relieving sprays are very popular.

The main volatile constituents of adhesives and cements are toluene, xylene, trichloroethane and ethylacetate.[17] Cleaning fluids usually contain one or more of the following, trichloroethylene, perchloroethylene and trichloroethane.[18,19] Nail polish remover contains acetone and esters.[6,20] Petrol is a volatile mixture of hydrocarbons. The components of an aerosol are its active constituents, a solvent system and liquefied gases.[21] It is the liquefied gas which is abused rather than the other ingredients.[22] All of these products are perfectly safe when used for the purpose for which they were designed and in accordance with the manufacturers' instructions. It is when the products are abused that problems arise.

Methods of abuse

Methods of abusing volatile substances have varied from time to time and from place to place. They have ranged from the extremely crude to the highly sophisticated. It is thought that information is passed along the juvenile grapevine.

The method of inhalation tends to vary according to the product type, but almost invariably involves deep breathing through the mouth or nose. Some researchers distinguish between inhalation by nose which they term *sniffing* and inhalation by mouth which they term *huffing*.[16]

With the early use of adhesives and plastic cements, the products were poured on to rags or handkerchiefs or sleeves and held over the nose and mouth. However, this led to irritation of the skin and ultimately to perioral and perinasal dermatitis. A later, more popular, method involved the use of a small polythene or plastic bag into which the individual breathed. A small potato crisp bag was found to be ideal, but suitable alternatives were readily available. Glue is squeezed or poured into the bag and the open end of the bag placed over the nose and mouth. The individual breathes deeply from the bag until the desired intoxicating effect is obtained. Sometimes other kinds of containers have been used.

Dry cleaning substances can be abused by direct inhalation of vapours from the tops of bottles. The liquid is also poured onto a rag, sleeve or handkerchief, which is held as a pad over the nose and mouth. Nail polish remover is used in the same way. These are not very efficient methods for achieving or maintaining the intoxicated state.

Fire extinguishers, butane gas and aerosols are often used in conjuction with larger bags from which the vapours are inhaled. Sometimes the contents are inhaled directly from their containers. Cigarette lighter refills containing butane gas are sometimes sprayed directly into the oropharynx causing cold burns with extensive and profound oedema. This results in profound respiratory difficulty while the chilling of the larynx may cause death by vagal inhibition.[22,23]

Sometimes adhesives have been heated on open fires, or larger polythene bags have been placed around the head and neck during sniffing sessions to produce enhanced effects. Cases of sexual masochistic hanging and related practices have been deliberately excluded from studies of solvent abuse since their primary purpose is sexual pleasure not intoxication and the population involved is very different.

Rebreathing

When glue vapours are inhaled from plastic bags the additional hazard of rebreathing occurs and can result in hypoxia and hypercapnia.

Who abuses solvents?

Despite an article which stated that abusers of volatile substances are a heterogeneous rather than a homogeneous group,[24] this view is not widely held by researchers in the field. It appears from worldwide literature that solvent abusers constitute a more distinct group than those who abuse other drugs, including alcohol. A variety of age ranges from 7 to 18 years has been quoted in America, Canada and the UK.[18,25,26]

It has been stated that the abuser of volatile substances is usually a young adolescent and typically male rather than female,[27,28] although Cohen has reported an increase in the number of females who are sniffers[29] and Swadi reported no sex differences among those who abused solvents.[30]

Early American reports of the practice indicated that adolescents living in areas of urban deprivation were more likely to be involved in volatile substance abuse. Later research indicated that the practice was by no means confined to areas of deprivation and that chil-

dren from every social class had been involved in solvent abuse at some time or another.[31]

It appears that most young people gained their knowledge about the practice from other members of their peer group. Friends at school and those who lived nearby were particularly influential in passing on information, and sometimes misinformation, about volatile substance abuse.

Reasons for solvent abuse

The two major reasons given by young people appear to be peer group pressure and curiosity, but following the example of older siblings, attempting to escape from the unpleasant realities of life and other less obvious reasons are also cited.

The main determinants seem to be the peer group pressure and the vulnerability of the individual at the time. Adolescents are particularly sensitive to peer group influence. The insecure adolescents are more likely to require the support of a peer group and conforming to the demands of that group is the price which has to be paid for the support provided. This can, and does, lead adolescents into difficulties.

A study of more than 800 solvent abusers seen over 12 years suggested that there were three categories of abuser.[31]

1 The experimental peer group user who was involved infrequently, sometimes alone and sometimes with friends.
2 The social or recreational user who indulges in the practice only when with the group and on a social basis.
3 The habitual abuser who may start sniffing in the peer group, but soon becomes a solitary sniffer because his needs are for the intoxication rather than for the company.

About 90% of all sniffers in Watson's study were in the first two groups and they matured out of the habit, coming to no serious harm in the process. The remaining 10% were the habitual sniffers and they needed expert help out of their difficulties.[31]

At a community rather than an individual level, various reasons have been offered in respect of VSA. Most prominent is that this is a drug-approving society and teenagers are merely imitating adults and finding a convenient form of intoxication. Other reasons put forward have included relief of boredom, desire for risk-taking, desire for parental disapproval and relief from emotional pain.[31,32]

The effects

Regardless of the substance involved, the early effects are similar to those of acute alcoholic intoxication.

These include fleeting stimulation of the central nervous system followed by depression of the central nervous system which varies in intensity. For the novice, a few deep breaths may induce intoxication in a matter of minutes; the chronic sniffer will require much more than this.

The stages of acute solvent intoxication are euphoria, blurring of vision, slurring of speech, incoordination of muscles, staggering gait and stupor. If the process continues, coma eventually supervenes.

Despite the similarity between intoxication due to VSA and that due to alcohol, there are some important differences. There is very rapid onset of intoxication with VSA which may take effect in a matter of seconds, and always less than 30 minutes. There is also very rapid recovery which normally takes between a few minutes and 2 hours and is much more rapid than recovery following alcoholic intoxication.[31]

There is very early disorientation in time and space with VSA unlike with alcohol and this factor is very hazardous in its effects.

Hallucinations occur in 30–50% of cases involving VSA. These hallucinations are usually visual, sometimes auditory and often frightening. According to Kerner,[16] the pharmacological effect of the substance cannot be isolated from the situation of use and the interaction of user, so that substance and situation is important. Verbal reports of group hallucinations would seem to confirm this statement and might help to explain why some sniffers have hallucinations and others with apparently similar practices and experiences do not.[31]

The combination of intoxication, disorientation and hallucination is very powerful and leads to accidents which occur in some VSA cases.[33]

Following an episode of VSA, the sniffer may suffer nausea, headaches, drowsiness, temporary disorientation and amnesia. The clinical state of any individual during or after any episode of VSA depends on the aggregate of a number of features:

1 Exact substance used.
2 Method used.
3 Amount of substance used.
4 Length of session.
5 Previous experience of VSA.
6 Presence or absence of hypoxia and hypercarbia.

Diagnosis

Acute episodes of VSA are characterized by intoxication, disorientation, a chemical smell on the breath, and signs of glue or other substance. The common picture is that of a drunk person and the specific sign is the smell of chemical from the breath.

The signs of longer term abuse are cracked lips, a history of nose bleeds, a vacant expression of the eyes, loss of appetite and weight, poor memory and poorly coordinated movements. Mothers of persistent abusers describe marked personality changes in their children dating from the start of VSA.

One uncommon sign is so-called glue sniffer's rash which appears round the nose and mouth of habitual sniffers. It is thought to result from repeated application of a plastic bag to the nose and mouth. It does not develop until a late stage of VSA. The rash disappears when the sniffing ceases.[31] The definitive diagnosis of VSA can be made by toxicological analyses of blood and body tissues and fluids.

It should be kept firmly in mind that all these signs and symptoms can be, and frequently are, due to some non-drug cause. However, VSA should be considered by professionals as a possible cause for changes in behaviour and deterioration in physical health occurring in adolescents and sometimes preadolescent children.

Solvent dependence and addiction

There is general agreement in the literature that repeated exposure to solvents results in tolerance. Some authors have stated that it could develop within 3 months of commencement of VSA. Psychological dependence is said to be common. Considerable doubt has been expressed about physical addiction to solvents. Some American and British psychiatrists have reported symptoms such as delirium tremens, irritability and headaches occurring among chronic sniffers on withdrawal of solvents,[34–36] while in Canada no such withdrawal symptoms were noted among chronic abusers of solvents.[37] Tolerance and psychological dependence have also been noted among chronic solvent abusers in Strathclyde,[31] but it is doubtful if physical dependence occurred and, if it did, no specific treatment was required.

Solvent abuse, alcohol and drugs

It has been reported that, after alcohol and tobacco, solvents are the next most abused products.[38,39] Mason reported that in the USA, the volatile solvents were not the first choice of most abusers but marijuana was.[40] In the UK, it has been reported that for some young people alcohol was their first choice, but solvents provided a cheap and reasonable alternative.[41] It has also been found that youngsters begin experimenting with alcohol and cigarettes at about the same time as they are experimenting with sniffing.

From American and British studies, there would appear to be an association between alcohol abuse by some parents and solvent abuse by their children. Two studies carried out in the west of Scotland showed that there was an association between early

VSA and subsequent alcohol and drug abuse.[31] While there was no evidence that solvent abuse caused subsequent drug abuse, it was concluded that vulnerable individuals involved in habitual VSA are more likely to change from one intoxicant to another. If this is so, then it is vital that those vulnerable individuals are identified so that early intervention can be offered.[18,31,42]

If there is any correlation it would surely be because, all too often, children are merely imitating their elders and choosing a form of intoxication which suits their pockets and their lifestyles at that time.

Morbidity

The most important risk associated with VSA is that of sudden sniffing death. However, there are quite a number of accidents associated with VSA which do not end fatally but may result in fractures from falls, burns and similar injuries during acute intoxication.[33]

Despite the fact that VSA is an old phenomenon, its long-term risks are not well known. However, there have been case reports of damage to liver, kidney and blood.[43–49] Neurological sequelae have also been reported.[50–55] There have been recent reports of cardiomyopathy associated with chronic solvent abuse.[56]

There has also been a report about a 16-year-old persistent glue sniffer who collapsed in a swimming pool. He was successfully resuscitated and it was postulated that the cause of his collapse had been due to either coronary artery spasm which led to anterior myocardial infarction and primary ventricular fibrillation or that he suffered an episode of primary ventricular fibrillation after solvent abuse.[57] This episode reflected acute toxicity rather than chronic toxicity.

Overall, the risk of an individual developing any organic damage due to VSA seems to be small and most abusers apparently come to no harm, regardless of the extent of their involvement in the practice.

Mortality

In 1970 Bass first reported an epidemic of sudden sniffing deaths in the USA. He attributed these deaths to a cardiac arrhythmia and hypothesized that volatile substances sensitized the heart to the arrhythmogenic effects of endogenous adrenaline. He thought that all volatile substances might be cardiotoxic and that any sniffer who became high during a sniffing session also risked developing an arrhythmia. This was thought to be particularly likely if the sniffer then took exercise.[58]

Deaths associated with VSA have been studied extensively over the last few years in the UK where the number of deaths has risen from two in 1971 to 111 in

1987 and since 1985 has averaged 100 per year. Although the age at death has ranged from 11 years to 76 years, the majority (72%) have been under 20 years of age with most of these in the 15–19 age group.[22] In 22% of deaths, there was apparently no previous history of VSA. Solvent-based adhesives accounted for 24% of deaths, other solvents for 29%, aerosols for 18% and gas fuels for 30%.

The exact mechanism of death is often unclear. However, in general terms, deaths from solvents in adhesives are more likely to be associated with trauma (52%) or direct toxic effects (26%) than plastic bag suffocation (19%) or inhalation of vomit (3%). Other solvent deaths are more likely to be due to direct toxic effects (64%) and inhalation of vomit (22%) than plastic bag suffocation (11%) or trauma (3%). Gas fuel and aerosol deaths are more likely to be due to direct toxic effects (68%) or inhalation of vomit (18%) than plastic bag suffocation (11%) or trauma (3%). Some of the reasons for disparity will lie in the different methods of use employed.

All deaths due to direct toxic effects or plastic bag suffocation will be sudden and unexpected. Sudden death from solvent abuse can be due to anoxia, vagal inhibition, respiratory depression, cardiac arrhythmias or trauma. Cardiac arrhythmias account for more than 50% of the deaths and the mechanism is thought to be sensitization of the myocardium to adrenaline and stimulation of the myocardium.[59,60] Once an arrhythmia develops it is often resistant to treatment. The risk of arrhythmia remains for some hours; any type of user is at risk, from the experimenter on his first session to the habitual abuser; each session is equally dangerous; exercise increases the hazard.

Just as Bass predicted years ago and other researchers noted,[61] the most alarming feature of solvent abuse is the risk of sudden unexpected death. It is disturbing that many of these occur in young people, some trying VSA for the first time. It is obvious from studying the distribution of the fatalities that all areas of the UK and all social classes have been represented.

Incidence and prevalence

A key issue in determining what strategy and policy to adopt in relation to any addiction is to have some idea of the size and nature of the problem. In the field of solvent abuse, this is of vital importance but hard data have been difficult to obtain.

A survey of the extent of solvent abuse in a Glasgow school (for boys only) found that the overall involvement in VSA was 10% in 1976, 14% in 1979 and 19% in 1982.[62]

Plant, in a study of over 1000 pupils in the fourth and fifth years of five secondary schools in Scotland, reported that 5% had tried VSA at least once.[63] The comparative figure from a survey to determine the prevalence of VSA among schoolchildren attending schools in one district in the north of England was found to be 6%.[64] A survey of secondary schoolchildren in a county in South Wales found that 6% overall had tried glue sniffing in the past but were not current users, and 9% of school leavers aged almost 16 years had tried glue sniffing at least once.[65]

Two surveys were carried out among fourth and fifth year comprehensive schoolchildren in 1985 and 1986. The purpose of the surveys was to estimate the incidence of drug and solvent misuse. It was found that this did not vary between the two surveys. Overall, 4% had used hard drugs at some time, 15% had used soft drugs and solvents and 10% had used solvents alone.[66]

A self-report survey carried out among more than 3000 adolescents attending six comprehensive schools in London established that 20% of those aged 11–16 years had tried solvents or drugs and one in 12 were repeated users. Two-thirds were found to have used alcohol, one ninth of them being possibly heavy drinkers and 20% smoked cigarettes. It was also found that VSA among girls was increasing.[30]

A more recent study suggested that between 4 and 10% of adolescents of both sexes in the UK had at least experimented with VSA and that between 0.5% and 1% were current users.[22]

Management of solvent abuse

This is divided into the treatment of emergencies and the management of non-emergency cases.

Intoxication due to VSA should be treated in the same way as other acute emergencies. It is important to ensure that the airway is clear. Any item used for VSA should be removed from the mouth or air passages. The person should be turned into the recovery position to prevent inhalation of vomit. Doors and windows should be opened to increase the flow of fresh air. The person's level of consciousness should be checked regularly while awaiting transport to hospital. If breathing stops, mouth-to-mouth resuscitation and external cardiac massage should be carried out. It is essential that anyone carrying out mouth-to-mouth resuscitation must take fresh breaths in between to avoid themselves becoming intoxicated.

In hospital, the treatment may include cardiopulmonary resuscitation, treatment of cardiac arrhythmias and supportive treatment.[60]

Most cases do not present as acute episodes of VSA. More likely the adolescent goes to the general practitioner with a definitive history of VSA, behavioural difficulties, family problems or, much less commonly, some form of morbidity such as renal failure. It is vital for doctors to take a good medical and drug history, with particular reference to the extent and duration of abuse, antisocial behaviour and family problems. This should be followed by physical and neurological examination. In most cases, there will be no physical damage but where it is found or suspected, patients can be referred to hospital for further investigation and treatment.

The anxieties of parents and adolescents can be allayed in the majority of cases involving VSA where abuse is sporadic and transitory. However, the management of chronic or habitual VSA is very difficult. In some cases it helps to improve the individual's reading or social skills or to provide recreational facilities. Family therapy, behaviour modification programmes, hypnosis, and individual counselling in conjunction with psychotherapy have been effective in some cases.[67]

General practitioners can play a major role in separating chronic abusers of volatile solvents from social abusers, by referring patients to the agency most able to provide appropriate facilities, and by supporting the family through a long and difficult time. Single-parent families need particular attention and support. Other professionals are likely to be involved with adolescents who habitually indulge in VSA, and include youth counsellors and social workers.

The various strategies for managing habitual VSA have not been evaluated, but there is no doubt that most adolescents who abuse volatile substances eventually mature out of the habit, given support, time and some expert help.

Prevention of solvent abuse by education

Prevention is not only better than cure but usually cheaper. Nowhere is this maxim more appropriate than in relation to VSA.

It is generally agreed that the best approach to VSA is through education and its widest sense. In a document dealing with solvent abuse recently produced by The Advisory Council on Alcohol and Drug Education (Tacade),* it was pointed out that, in the arena of education, the targets are the person, the drug and the environment. In relation to the person, the components which influence the drug-related behaviour are knowledge about drugs, attitudes about drugs, skills and relationships with peers and family. These components interact.

In relation to the drug, the vital components are composition, labelling and pricing and these factors also interact. In relation to the environment, the interacting factors are availability, sociocultural context, places used for sniffing sessions, promotion and advertising and legal sanctions.[68]

*Tacade. 1 Hulme Place, The Crescent, Salford, Greater Manchester, M5 4QA.

Health is not merely the absence of disease, disorder or disability. It involves a positive, dynamic aspect. Education has a responsibility to offer a programme to promote healthy behaviour and encourage healthy responses to situations rather than maladaptive ones including VSA.

Behaviour is said to be the result of interaction of several components.[69] These include knowledge, attitudes, relationships with peers and family, and skills including interpersonal skills. Educational endeavours at school level are, therefore, about addressing these issues to assist individuals in making informed choices about their behaviour and helping them acquire the skills they require to do so.

Education in its widest and most appropriate sense in the context of VSA involves parents and community as well as children and teachers. Community cooperation and a consistent approach to drug education are also required.

Re-Solv

Re-Solv is an independent national charity established in 1984. Originally funded for one year by the British Adhesives and Sealants Association, Re-Solv (Society for the Prevention of Solvent and Volatile Substance Abuse)* believes that VSA is a dangerous form of experimentation and that a broad educational programme offers the best hope of prevention.

Today, Re-Solv has nearly 150 corporate members representing local authorities, trade and industry associations, trade unions and other professional bodies. Re-Solv also has individual members who provide support and give input. Re-Solv produces educational material of all kinds including videos, pamphlets, newsletters and has sponsored books about solvent abuse as well as vital research on mortality data. It is a useful source of reliable information on all aspects of solvent abuse for anyone seeking assistance of this kind.

Re-Solv's future plans include sponsoring a study of incidence and prevalence of VSA, also a study of the morbidity associated with the practice and an international symposium.

Legislation

Scotland

It seems appropriate to set the scene regarding the law and VSA. Since Scotland has a different legal system from that applying to England and Wales and since Scotland was quicker to respond to a perceived need for appropriate action for VSA, the legal situation in Scotland is described first.

*Re-Solv. 30A High Street, Stone, Staffordshire ST15 8AW.

Juveniles under the age of 16 years who are in need of care and protection or who have offended against the law are usually dealt with informally by means of the children's hearing system rather than via the courts. This was made possible by the Socialwork (Scotland) Act 1968. There is no equivalent legislation in England and Wales. When VSA began to cause concern in some communities, the children involved in the practice were often declared to be 'outwith parental control' which came within the ambit of the Act while solvent abuse by itself did not. However, this policy was deemed to be inadequate, and pressure was exerted by means of a private member's bill to include VSA as a specific paragraph within the existing legislative framework. This resulted in the Solvent Abuse (Scotland) Act which came into effect in May 1983 and enabled the Reporter to the Children's Panel to exercise the same discretion for referral with regard to VSA as to the various other grounds.

Individuals over the age of 16 years have been successfully prosecuted in Scotland for causing a breach of the peace on account of their behaviour while under the influence of solvents.[31] Individuals have also been found guilty of driving under the influence of drugs under Section 5(1) of the Road Traffic Act of 1972, once it had been accepted that toluene in glue could be legally regarded as a drug within the meaning of the Act.[70]

In December 1983, the Crown brought a case against two Glasgow shopkeepers who were accused of wilfully, culpably and recklessly supplying to children solvents (and the means to misuse them) to the detriment of their health and their lives. The case was brought under common law, a decision having been taken earlier in 1983 by Law Lords that a crime of this sort could be brought to court in this way. The shopkeepers were found guilty and sentenced to 3 years' imprisonment which was reduced, on appeal, to 2 years.[71] Many prosecutions of this kind have followed in Scotland.

England and Wales

In England and Wales, there is no equivalent of the informal measures with respect to juveniles. However, successful prosecutions have been brought in relation to various aspects of VSA. There have been infringements of the Road Traffic Act 1972, successful prosecutions for breach of the peace, and infringements of both the Children and Young Persons Act 1969 and the Offences against the Persons Act 1861.[31]

Specific legislation regarding VSA was enacted in 1985 in England and Wales in the form of the Intoxicating Substances Supply Act which makes it an offence to supply or to offer to supply a substance other than a controlled drug to a person under the age of 18 years if he knows or has reason to suspect that it is likely to be used for the purpose of intoxication. The penalty can be up to 6 months in prison or a £2000 fine. This Act brought the law in England and Wales into line with existing legislation in Scotland and there have been several successful prosecutions to date.[72]

It is very difficult to assess whether this legislative activity has really made any impact on the problem but certainly legislation is better directed against the suppliers than against the sniffers.

Conclusions

Although much valuable information is now available about VSA, there are still gaps in our knowledge about certain aspects of the practice. More detailed information is required on the effects of different solvents on the body. This should be done at a national or even an international level. There should be evaluation of different treatment strategies for VSA so that it is possible to determine which strategies are most effective for different types of cases.

Educational programmes designed for children should also be evaluated to determine the best way of helping to promote health in its fullest sense and prevent negative behaviours, including alcohol abuse, VSA and smoking.

It is essential to remember that most adolescents will not experiment with substances containing volatile solvents and that those who do will regard it as a passing phase in their lives. Time, energy and enthusiasm are all required by professionals who help the unfortunate few who do become involved habitually or chronically in VSA.

There are three important aims when VSA problems arise:

1 To ensure that the professional people and the help they offer are widely known in the community.
2 To ensure that those involved and their families can find the help they require quickly and easily.
3 To put VSA in perspective along with the other problems present in each case.

Finally, it is vital to ensure that those in the caring professions respond with compassion as well as competence when approached by those who have problems with VSA.

References

1 Bethell, M.F. Toxic psychosis caused by inhalation of petrol fumes. *Br Med J* 1965; **2**: 276–277.
2 Black, P.D. Mental illness due to the voluntary inhalation of petrol vapour. *Med J Aust* 1967; **2**: 70–71.
3 Gold, N. Self-intoxication by petrol vapour inhalation. *Med J Aust* 1963; **50**: 582–584.
4 Tolan, E.J., Lingl, F.A. 'Model psychosis' produced by inhalation of gasoline fumes. *Am J Psychol* 1964; **120**: 757–761.
5 Corliss, L.M. A review of evidence on glue sniffing – a persistent problem. *J School Hlth* 1965; **35**: 442–449.
6 Gellman, V. Glue-sniffing among Winnipeg school children. *Can Med Assoc J* 1968; **98**: 411–413.
7 Guaraldi, G.P., Bonasegla, F. Su di un caso di tossicomania da tricloroetilene. *Riv Sperimentale di Freniatria* 1968; **92**: 913–920.
8 Weinraub, M., Groce, P., Karno, M. Chloroformism – a new case of a bad old habit. *Cali Med* 1972; **117**: 63–65.
9 Milman, H., Su, W. Patterns of illicit drug and alcohol use among secondary students. *J Paediatr* 1973; **283**: 314–320.
10 Gossett, J.T., Lewis, J.M., Phillips, A. Extent and prevalence of illicit drug use as reported by 56,745 students. *J Am Med Assoc* 1971; **216**: 1464–1470.
11 Strimbu, J., Sims, O.S. Jr. A university system drug profile. *Internat J Addict* 1974; **9**: 569–583.
12 Smart, R.G., Fejer, D. Six years of cross-sectional surveys of student drug use in Toronto. *Bull Narcotics* 1975; **27**: 11–22.
13 Boolsen, M.W. Drugs in Denmark. *Internat J Addict* 1975; **10**: 503–512.
14 Crider, R.A., Rouse, B.A. Inhalant overview. Research monograph series. *NIDA Research Monograph* 1988; **85**: 1–7.
15 King, M.D., Day, R.E., Oliver, J.S., Watson, J.M. Solvent encephalopathy. *Br Med J* 1981; **283**: 663–664.
16 Kerner, K. Current topics in inhalant abuse. Research monographs. *NIDA Research Monograph* 1988; **85**: 8–29.
17 Ackerman, H.E. The constitution of adhesives and its relationship to solvent abuse. *Hum Toxicol* 1982; **1**: 223–230.
18 Cohen, S. The volatile solvents. *Pub Hlth Rev* 1973; **2**: 185–214.
19 Malcolm, A.I. Solvent sniffing and its effects. *Addictions* 1968; **15**: 12–21.
20 Ackerly, W.C., Gibson, G. Ligher fluid 'sniffing'. *J Psychol* 1964; **120**: 1056–1061.
21 Roberts, D.J. Abuse of aerosol products by inhalation. *Hum Toxicol* 1982; **1**: 231–238.
22 Ramsey, J., Anderson, H.R., Bloor, K., Flanagan, R.J. An introduction to the practice, prevalence and chemical toxicology of volatile substance abuse. *Hum Toxicol* 1989; **8**: 261–269.
23 Watson, J.M. Solvent abuse: presentation and clinical diagnosis. *Hum Toxicol* 1982; **1**: 249–256.
24 Edeh, J. Volatile substance abuse in relation to alcohol and illicit drugs: psychological perspectives. *Hum Toxicol* 1989; **8**: 313–317.
25 Barnes, G.E. Solvent abuse: a review. *Internat J Addict* 1979; **14**: 1–26.
26 Press, E., Done, A.K. Solvent sniffing. *Paediatrics* 1967; **39**: 451–461, 611–622.
27 Giovacchini, R.P. Abusing the volatile solvents. *Reg Toxicol Pharmacol* 1985; **5**: 18–37.
28 Smart, R.G. Inhalant use and abuse in Canada. Research monographs. *NIDA Research Monograph* 1988; **85**: 121–139.
29 Cohen, S. Inhalant abuse: an overview of the problem. In: Sharp, C.W., Brehm, M.L., eds. *Review of Inhalants,*

Euphoria to Dysfunction. Rockville, Md: National Institute on Drug Abuse, 1977.

30 Swadi, H. Drug and substance use among 3,333 London adolescents. *Br J Addict* 1988; **83**: 935–942.

31 Watson, J.M. *Solvent Abuse: the Adolescent Epidemic?* London: Croom Helm, 1986.

32 Richardson, H. Volatile substance abuse: evaluation and treatment. *Hum Toxicol* 1989; **8**: 319–322.

33 Watson, J.M. Solvent abuse. *Med Sci Law* 1980; **20**: 137.

34 Wyse, D.G. Deliberate inhalation of hydrocarbons: a review. *Can Med Assoc J* 1973; **108**: 71–74.

35 Crooke, S.T. Solvent inhalation. *Texas Med* 1972; **68**: 67–69.

36 Merry, J., Zachariadis, N. Addiction to glue sniffing. *Br Med J* 1962; **2**: 1448.

37 Fornazzari, L., Wilkinson, D.A., Kapier, B.M., Carlen, P.L. Cerebellar, cortical and functional impairment in toluene abusers. *Acta Neurol Scand* 1983; **67**: 319–329.

38 Gossett, J.T., Lewis, J.M., Phillips, V. Extent and prevalence of illicit drug use as reported by 56,745 students. *J Am Med Assoc* 1971; **216**: 1464–1470.

39 Porter, M.R., Vieira, T.A., Kaplan, G.J., Heesch, J.R., Colyar, A.B. Drug use in Anchorage, Alaska. *J Am Med Assoc* 1967; **273**: 700–702.

40 Mason, T. *Inhalant Use and Treatment*. Rockville, Md: National Institute on Drug Abuse, 1969.

41 Watson, J.M. Solvent abuse. MD thesis, University of Glasgow, 1977.

42 Massengale, O.N., Glaser, H.H., Le Lievre, R.E., Dodds, J.B., Klock, M. Physical and psychologic factors in glue sniffing. *New Engl J Med* 1963; **269**: 1340–1344.

43 Baerg, R.D., Kimberg, D.V. Centrilobular necrosis and acute renal failure in 'solvent sniffers'. *Ann Intern Med* 1970; **73**: 713–720.

44 Clearfield, H.R. Hepatorenal toxicity from sniffing spot-remover (trichloroethylene). *Am J Dig Dis* 1970; **15**: 851–856.

45 Powers, D. Aplastic anaemia secondary to glue sniffing. *New Engl J Med* 1965; **273**: 700–702.

46 O'Brien, E.T., Yeomen, W.B., Hobby, J.A.E. Hepatorenal damage from toluene in a 'glue sniffer'. *Br Med J* 1971; **2**: 29–30.

47 Russ, G., Clarkson, A.R., Woodruff, A.J., Seyur, A.E., Cheng, I.K.P. Renal failure from 'glue sniffing'. *Med J Aust* 1981; **2**: 121–122.

48 Will, A.M., McLaren, E.H. Reversible renal damage due to glue sniffing. *Br Med J* 1981; **283**: 525–526.

49 Marjot, R., McLeod, A.A. Chronic non-neurological toxicity from volatile substance abuse. *Hum Toxicol* 1989; **8**: 301–306.

50 Knox, J.W., Nelson, J.R. Permanent encephalopathy from toluene inhalation. *New Eng J Med* 1966; **275**: 1494–1496.

51 Malm, G., Lying-Tunell, U. Cerebellar dysfunction related to toluene sniffing. *Acta Neurol Scand* 1980; **62**: 191–192.

52 Sasa, M., Igarashi, S., Miyazaki, K., Nakano, S., Matsuoka, I. Equilibrium disorders with diffuse brain atrophy in long term toluene sniffing. *Arch Oto-Rhino-Laryngol* 1978; **221**: 163–169.

53 Allister, C., Lush, M., Oliver, J.L., Watson, J.M. Status epilepticus caused by solvent abuse. *Br Med J* 1981; **283**: 1156.

54 Lolin, Y. Chronic neurological toxicity associated with exposure to volatile substances. *Hum Toxicol* 1989; **8**: 293–300.

55 Ron, M.A. Volatile substance abuse: a review of possible long-term neurological, intellectual and psychiatric sequelae. *Br J Psychol* 1986; **148**: 235–246.

56 Boon, N.A. Solvent abuse and the heart. *Br Med J* 1987; **294**: 722.

57 Wiseman, M.N., Banim, S. 'Glue sniffer's heart'. *Br Med J* 1987; **294**: 739.

58 Bass, M. Sudden sniffing death. *J Am Med Assoc* 1970; **212**: 2075–2079.

59 Shepherd, R.T. Mechanism of sudden death associated with volatile substance abuse. *Hum Toxicol* 1989; **8**: 287–292.

60 Ashton, C.H. Solvent abuse. *Br Med J* 1990; **300**: 135–136.

61 Watson, J.M. Morbidity and mortality statistics on solvent abuse. *Med Sci Law* 1979; **19**: 246–252.

62 Ramsay, A. Solvent abuse: an educational perspective. *Hum Toxicol* 1982; **1**: 265–270.

63 Plant, M.A., Peck, D.F., Stuart, R. The correlates of serious alcohol-related consequences and illicit drug use amongst a cohort of Scottish teenagers. *Br J Addict* 1984; **79**: 197–200.

64 Stuart, P. Solvents and schoolchildren – knowledge and experimentation among a group of young people aged 11–18. *Hlth Educ J* 1986; **45**: 84–86.

65 Cooke, B.R.B., Evans, D.A., Farrow, S.C. Solvent misuse in secondary school children – a prevalence study. *Comm Med* 1988; **10**: 8–13.

66 Diamond, I.D., Pritchard, C., Choudry, N., Fielding, M., Cox, M., Bushne, D. The incidence of drug and solvent misuse among southern English normal comprehensive schoolchildren. *Pub Hlth* 1988; **102**: 107–144.

67 Watson, J.M. Solvent abuse. *Update* 1989; **38**: 305–309.

68 *Dealing with Solvent Misuse – the Role of Education in a Prevention Strategy*. London: Tacade/Resolv Joint Publication, 1990.

69 Lee, J.T. Volatile substance abuse within a health education context. *Hum Toxicol* 1989; **8**: 331–334.

70 Duffy v Tudhope *Scots Law Times* 1984; 107.

71 HMA v Khaliq and Ahmed *Scots Law Times* 1984; 137.

72 Liss, B.I. Government, trade and industry and other preventative responses to volatile substance abuse. *Hum Toxicol* 1989; **8**: 327–330.

7.9 Smoking

Anne Charlton

Every day in the UK at present, between 300 and 400 people die of smoking-related diseases. Although most of these people are adults, many started smoking in childhood, probably thinking at that time that they could give up easily. Nicotine is a powerfully addictive drug and, once hooked on it, breaking free can be a difficult process. Smoking also causes health problems in childhood, sometimes related to the child's own smoking or to that of other people.

It is, therefore, especially important to prevent children from starting to smoke or to help them to stop if they have started. Equally it is necessary to be aware of parental smoking in relation to childhood health problems.

Smoking is not the only tobacco hazard to young people.[1,2] Chewed tobacco, snuff and specifically the little bags of tobacco for oral use, which are already popular with boys in Sweden and the USA, can cause oral cancers very quickly. They also increase the later risk of heart and digestive problems.

Tobacco use in children and their families is a very pertinent problem to community paediatricians.

Trends in prevalence of smoking

Statistics on cigarette smoking among adults from 16 years of age have been reported regularly every 2 years from the General Household Survey of England and Wales since 1972. During that period cigarette smoking among men has fallen from 52% in 1972 to 29% in 1992. In women, the decline has been less marked, namely from 41% to 28%. The trend is shown in Table 7.19. Two important elements are hidden in these statistics. First, smoking among adults is still far more frequent in the lower socioeconomic groups and secondly that the drop in smoking prevalence among women is largely in the older age groups, while in the 20 to 24-year-old women there was even a small increase, from 37% to 39% from 1988 to 1990. Many mothers of infants and pre-school children are in that age group.

Table 7.19 Current smoking by sex in persons aged 16 and over: 1972–1990 (Great Britain)

	1972	1976	1978	1980	1982	1984	1986	1988	1990	1992
Men (%)	52	46	45	42	38	36	35	33	31	29
Women (%)	41	38	37	37	33	32	31	30	29	28

From: Thomas, M., Goddard, E., Hickman, M., Hunter, P. *1992 General Household Survey. Series GHS no. 23*, London: Her Majesty's Stationery Office, 1994. (Crown Copyright)[3]

Table 7.20 Smoking behaviour (%) among secondary school children aged 11–15: 1982–1992 (England)

	1982	1984	1986	1988	1990	1992
Boys						
Regular smokers	11	13	7	7	9	9
Occasional smokers	7	9	5	5	6	6
Used to smoke	11	11	10	8	7	6
Tried smoking once	26	24	23	23	22	22
Never smoked	45	44	55	58	56	57
Girls						
Regular smokers	11	13	12	9	11	10
Occasional smokers	9	9	5	5	6	7
Used to smoke	10	10	10	9	7	7
Tried smoking once	22	22	19	19	18	19
Never smoked	49	46	53	59	58	57

From: Thomas, M., Holroyd, S., Goddard, E. *Smoking among Secondary School Children in 1992. An enquiry carried out by Social Survey Division of OPCS on behalf of the Department of Health, the Welsh Office and the Scottish Office Home and Health Department*, London: Her Majesty's Stationery Office, 1993. (Crown Copyright)

With regard to children's smoking, national surveys did not begin until 1982. These studies cover a sample of schoolchildren aged 11 to 15 years, from year 7 to year 11 at secondary school.[4] In the 1990 survey about a quarter of 15-year-olds were regular smokers (Table 7.20). In 1992, regular smoking among 15-year-old boys was 21% whilst regular smoking among the girls stayed at 25%. In recent years more girls than boys smoke in the mid-teen years, but the boy smokers tend to smoke more cigarettes than the girls do. No socioeconomic differences in prevalence have been shown in secondary school children.

Many children try a first cigarette before they go to secondary school. Boys tend to experiment slightly earlier than girls do.

Health problems of children's own smoking

Until recently, the health risks of smoking were seen to be something which manifested themselves in late adulthood. To a large extent this is still the case, but the foundations for many of these problems, and, indeed, some visible effects, are now known to begin in childhood smokers.

Foundations of future health problems

It has been clearly shown in large retrospective studies that the earlier regular smoking is started, the greater is the risk of that person contracting lung cancer.[5] The risk is particularly great when regular smoking begins in adolescence or childhood. This cancer risk may appear to the child to be a distant and meaningless one, but to the paediatrician it is something to be considered at this stage.

The early precursors of cardiovascular problems can be seen in young smokers. For example, atherosclerosis is already present in up to 30% of 20-year-old men,[6] and smoking is strongly related to this change. Regular smoking started between the ages of 15 and 19 years greatly increases the risk of premature death from coronary heart disease[7] and starting before 15 increases the risk even more.

After one year of smoking, lung function is impaired and precursors of adult chronic, obstructive lung disease develop.[8]

Immediate effects

It has been known for a long time that children who smoke are at increased risk of frequent coughs, phlegm production and other respiratory symptoms.[9-11]. As in adults, the cilia lining the trachea are paralysed and eventually destroyed by inhaled smoke, thus preventing the natural cleansing process from taking place in the respiratory system. Young smokers are more likely to have absence from school[12] for minor ailments which include coughs, colds, earache, tonsillitis, headaches and digestive disorders. Resistance to infections is lowered by smoking.

Lack of energy can result from reduced oxygen supplies to the muscles due to inhalation of carbon monoxide from the smoke, which replaces some of the oxygen transported by the haemoglobin.

The process of young people becoming smokers

A series of stages in the process has been identified and at each stage a different set of influences comes into play.[13]

Precontemplation and contemplation

At this stage the young person is receiving messages about smoking from family, friends and advertising and can begin to believe in certain positive values of cigarettes to him or herself. For younger children this is often related to appearance,[14] for example thinking that smoking looks grown up, tough or sophisticated. Older children tend to add more subtle beliefs such as smoking calms the nerves, gives confidence, controls weight and is enjoyable.

At first the child is not considering smoking but at the contemplation stage develops the intention to try smoking and is planning to get some cigarettes.

All these factors increase the likelihood that they will try a first cigarette, or at least a few puffs of one.

Initiation and experimentation

Initiation is the first trial of smoking a cigarette often urged on by peer group pressure or curiosity. Most children do not go beyond this stage, because they do not like it. Others persist with repeated experimentation. The longer experimentation goes on, the more frequently cigarettes are tried, and in due course the child could become a regular smoker.

Regular smoking and habituation

As more cigarettes are smoked the child develops the habit of regular smoking.

Maintenance, addiction or adult smoking

Smoking is both an addiction and a habit. The child who starts for social and psychological reasons can quite soon become physically affected by the drug, nicotine.[15] In small amounts it is a stimulant; in large amounts it is a tranquillizer. Many children claim to experience withdrawal symptoms if they are deprived of cigarettes. It is quite fashionable in the young people's world to claim to be addicted to something. Nevertheless true addiction *does* exist in children. Children often start to smoke in the belief that they can give up easily but then find it to be extremely difficult. There is evidence that 65% of 16 to 19-year-old smokers had already made at least one attempt to give up smoking, and most of them had had several tries.[16]

What influences a child's smoking?

At the precontemplation and contemplation stage, three sets of influences are in operation:

- The social background factors of family, peers, school etc.
- The child's own knowledge, beliefs, attitudes and intentions.
- The availability, accessibility and acceptability of cigarettes.

At the *initiation stage*, the same influences are still present, but may change in emphasis. For example, peers may become more influential than families and knowledge may be overridden or rejected. A new set of influences can develop based on self-image and personality of the young smoker.

The *habituation stage* maintains to some extent all the above influences but most of them are weaker in effect. The strongest at this stage are often peer influences and self-image, while a new influence comes into play – physiological reinforcement.

Finally, in the development of the maintenance, *adult smoking stage* the physiological reinforcement influence becomes very strong. Smoking is both an addiction and a habit.

Influences contributing to risk of smoking

Social background

Parents' smoking

It has frequently been shown that children whose parents are smokers are more likely to take up the habit themselves.[17] As the child becomes older this influence, not unpredictably, wanes. The influence is clearly strong in younger children who are at least twice as likely to be smokers if a parent smokes. It is unlikely that they see their parents as role models, but rather that cigarettes are more readily available in a smoking household, and smoking is the norm in the situation where primary socialization takes place. A baby born to a smoking mother has already received thousands of shots of the drug, nicotine, across the placenta while in the womb. When the baby cries, he or she smells smoke on the mother when she comes to tend to the needs and the baby sees a cigarette in mother's all-important face. In such households smoking is not only completely normal and acceptable, but it can also be a symbol of security. For some reason, as yet unexplained, children in single parent families are more at risk of smoking.[18,19]

Parents' opinions

If children perceive strong parental disapproval for their smoking, they have been shown to be considerably less likely to be smokers.[20] One study showed them to be up to seven times less at risk if they perceive parental disapproval than if they think their parents approve.[21]

Brothers' and sisters' smoking

The link between brothers' and sisters', especially older sisters', smoking has been shown to be even stronger than that of parents and children.[22] Again, it is probably the norm and the availability of cigarettes which play a part, but also the peer group relationship which can exist between siblings.

Friends' smoking

At school, friends become very important and replace parents in the key role with regard to influence.[23,24] It is far more important in the eyes of many children to conform with the peer group norm than to obey parents. In many studies of secondary school children, having a smoking best friend is the most significant risk factor.

School ethos and teachers' smoking

It is unlikely that many children see teachers as role models, but they do see them as authority figures. If a teacher smokes it can appear to a child that it is officially approved by someone who has special knowledge. It has been shown that in schools where teachers, especially the headteacher, smoke, there is a higher prevalence of smoking.[25] Not only the teachers' smoking, but also the policy with regard to smoking and the ethos of the school, have been shown to be associated with the prevalence of smoking. Stricter policies appear to lead to lower smoking prevalence later in life among those who attended them.[26]

The child's own knowledge, beliefs, attitudes and intentions

Knowledge

Knowledge of the health risks of smoking has been shown to have relatively little importance in influencing children to be non-smokers. It has been shown that some children deny the health risks just prior to the experimentation stage, so it is not clear whether it is lack of knowledge or lack of acceptance of knowledge which is associated with risk. Certainly there was some relationship between the increasing number of health risks named and the decreasing likelihood of trying smoking in the next few months.[27] Knowledge of health risks, however, often has little relevance to a child, either because the diseases are those of older people and appear to be irrelevant to children or because they cannot grasp what the diseases really mean.[28]

Beliefs, attitudes and intentions

A set of beliefs about smoking has been shown to exist in many children.[27] These beliefs are especially important for girls and are strongly related to experimentation with smoking. They include looking grown up, looking sophisticated or *cool*, calming nerves, giving confidence, controlling weight, being an enjoyable thing to do, relieving boredom, providing comfort in times of stress, being an enjoyable process with attractive objects such as a pretty cigarette packet associated with it, a means of making social contact, a friendly, sociable thing to do or it helps concentration. These and many more positive effects are attributed to smoking, and a child who believes several of them is at greatly increased risk of trying a cigarette.

Intention to smoke is a strong predictor. If a child expresses an intention to be a smoker in the future, it is very likely he or she will do so.

Availability, accessibility and acceptability of smoking

Availability of cigarettes

If a child can go into a shop or to a kiosk, ice cream van or vending machine and be sold cigarettes, whatever his or her age, it makes it much easier to choose to be a smoker. However, there is the school of thought which suggests that where there is a low age permitted from when cigarettes can be purchased, as there is in Britain of 16 years, that reinforces the adult image of smoking, thus making it more desirable to children. Purchase by children has been made easier by the tendency of some sales persons to split packets of cigarettes and sell them individually with a match. Recent legislation which imposes stricter fines might help to overcome this problem.

Accessibility

Availability, however, has little relevance if the child cannot afford the cigarettes. Among adults, it has been shown that, as the price of cigarettes rises, the amount smoked decreases and vice versa.[29] These changes are often linked to tax increases. Studies in America have shown that adolescents are even more price-sensitive than adults are.[30] When the price goes up, fewer smoke and those who continue smoke fewer cigarettes. Studies have shown that the majority of young smokers consider smoking to be a waste of money.

Acceptability

Even very young children are aware of advertising messages,[31] many like tobacco advertisements and those who do are more likely to see positive advantages to smoking.[32] Awareness of a cigarette brand was one of the most important factors in predicting onset of smoking during the next few months by 12 and 13 year olds.[27] Advertising can point out – sometimes very subtly – positive benefits of being a smoker and this influences the envisaged gains seen by the young decision-maker.

Self-image and personality of the young smoker

It has frequently been shown that smokers tend to be underachievers in the academic sense and that they are fed up with school.[33] There is also a strong element of rebelliousness in children who become smokers.[34]

Coping with stress[16,35] and lacking the self-efficacy to refuse cigarettes[36] are both elements which can increase a child's risk of smoking.

Physiological reinforcement

When a child reaches a state of frequent and regular smoking, his or her own body puts them at risk of continuing the habit. They become dependent upon the nicotine and also on the habit of smoking. Picking up a cigarette and taking it again and again to their mouth is done automatically by their hands. It acts as a comfort, a protective barrier in social situations and provides something to do with their hands. It is difficult to break the drug addiction and also difficult to break the habit.

Summary of risk factors (Figs 7.7 and 7.8)

The children who are most at risk of becoming smokers are those:

- whose parents smoke
- whose brothers or sisters smoke
- whose best friends smoke
- who cannot, or perhaps will not, name any health risks of smoking
- who have positive beliefs about what smoking will do for them e.g. make them look grown up, calm their nerves and help them to relax, give them

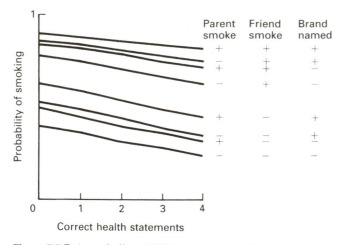

Figure 7.7 Estimated effects (GLIM) of predictors of smoking in girls with six positive beliefs about smoking. + = yes, − = no. Reprinted with kind permission from *Social Science and Medicine*, **29**: Charlton, A., Blair, V. Predicting the onset of smoking in boys and girls, copyright 1989, Pergamon Press PLC.

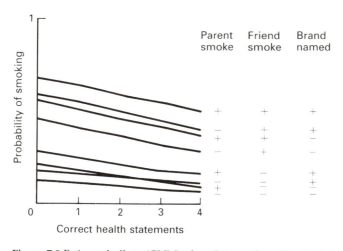

Figure 7.8 Estimated effects (GLIM) of predictors of smoking in the absence of positive beliefs about smoking. + = yes − = no. Reprinted with kind permission from *Social Science and Medicine*, **29**: Charlton, A., Blair, V. Predicting the onset of smoking in boys and girls, copyright 1989, Pergamon Press PLC.

confidence, look sophisticated, hard or cool, be enjoyable, control their weight etc
- who are underachievers academically or physically
- who are fed up with school; who rebel against authority
- children in single-parent families
- who can name a cigarette brand.

Socioeconomic status, although found to be important in the USA and in adults in the UK, appears unrelated to children's smoking prevalence in the UK at present.

At the time of writing, girls are more at risk than boys are of being smokers in the mid-teen years, but this has not always been so and may change in the future.

Health problems related to other people's smoking

For about 30 years, research findings have been showing links between parents' smoking and increased risk of numerous health problems in their children. It is, of course, important to bear in mind that other environmental factors will also play a part. Nevertheless, when factors such as ventilation of the home, cooking methods, socioeconomic status, general air pollution and other possibly related factors are taken into account, household smoking is often the one factor significantly related to increased risk of respiratory diseases in children.

Prenatal effects

The effect on the young child's growth and health can be considerable when the mother smokes in pregnancy. There are hundreds of papers on this subject and the ones referenced are examples, not an exhaustive review. Low birthweight,[37-39] increased risk of perinatal mortality,[40,41] reduced attention span,[42] effects on mental[43] and physical development[44,45] and sudden infant death syndrome,[46] to mention but a few examples, are more frequent in babies or infants of mothers who smoked in pregnancy. There is also now some evidence that father's smoking during his partner's pregnancy can also increase the risk of low birthweight.[47]

But by the time the infant reaches the paediatrician it is too late for these prenatal effects to be prevented. The least that can be done is to advise and help the mother not to smoke. At least she should not smoke if she is breast feeding the baby,[48] in the house, nor during future pregnancies.

Household smoking and diseases in children

It is in infancy and childhood that increased risks of numerous health problems have been unequivocally shown to exist as a result of parental, especially maternal, smoking. Again the papers referenced below must be taken as examples only and not an exhaustive list.

Respiratory problems

The first studies on this topic showed that infants of smoking parents were at greater risk of being admitted to hospital for pneumonia and bronchitis than were the children of non-smokers.[49,50]

Respiratory illnesses are all more frequent in the children of smokers. In almost all cases, maternal smoking is the most significant factor. Bronchitis,[51,52] wheezing,[53,54] and other diseases of the respiratory tract are more frequent in children of smokers. It appears that asthma in children, especially in boys, is exacerbated by maternal smoking.[55,56] The fact that the mother's smoking is more significant than the father's may be a prenatal effect which is carried over into infancy, or may be because the mother has much longer and closer daily contact with the child. Coughs[57,58] and general respiratory infections[59] are also more frequent.

Harmful chemicals

Breast feeding by non-smoking mothers is to be strongly recommended and has been shown to be protective against certain diseases, but if the nursing mother is a smoker, large quantities of cotinine, a product of nicotine, are present in the baby's urine.[60] It is therefore very important to advise a mother not to smoke during the lactation period. Raised concentrations of cotinine[61] and lead[62] have been found in the body fluids of children in smoking households.

Growth and development

Slower mental growth in the first few years,[63] and slower physical growth[64] and pulmonary growth[65] may occur in children of smoking parents.

Other effects

Smoking in pregnancy has been shown to be significantly related to an increased risk of sudden infant death syndrome (SIDS), but so has maternal smoking after the birth.[66]

Many minor and less minor ailments are more frequent in children of smokers. These include sore throats,[67] ear infections (particularly otitis media),[68] habitual snoring,[69] more frequent coughs and colds and alimentary upsets in babies.[70] Parental, especially maternal, smoking was shown to increase the risk of 12 and 13-year-olds being absent from school on a randomly selected day, whatever the children's own smoking habits.[12] There is also some evidence of increased risk of meningitis in children from a smoking household.[71]

Pre-existing diseases can be exacerbated by environmental tobacco smoke. Studies have shown this to be the case in children with cystic fibrosis,[72] and children with asthma.[56] Evidence is now also being collected in retrospective studies which indicates increased risk of cancer in adults who were subjected to 25 or more person-years of passive tobacco smoking during their childhood and adolescence.[73] A review of research studies on children and passive smoking was published in 1992,[74] however new evidence continues to be amassed.

Programmes and action for prevention

Health education approaches to prevent children from smoking

In view of the complex set of interrelated factors, it is not surprising that any programme aimed at preventing the onset of smoking cannot consist of a single focus. When the link between lung cancer and smoking was first publicized in the mid-1950s and the first report on smoking by the Royal College of Physicians followed in 1962, many teachers felt that this message alone would be sufficient to deter adults and children from the habit. The first health education programmes aimed at children took the health risks approach. Often in the form of lectures, these were illustrated with preserved black lungs from smokers, borrowed from the local hospital. Knowledge *is* needed as a basis for decision making. It must be relevant and understandable to the child. For example, blowing into a carbon monoxide monitor makes the problem very real to most young smokers. However, it soon became well-known that knowledge does not usually affect behaviour in the way it was once thought.

The next theme was that of personal decision making. People have a free choice and should be allowed to choose for themselves. This belief led to the development of packages which taught decision-making skills. This approach is sometimes called the educational model. Making decisions is fine, and must be done, but sometimes other influences, often outside the control of the decision-maker, create an impossible situation or push the decision in one direction or another. With regard to children and smoking, these factors have been discussed. Advertising, family or friends' norms with regard to smoking and many other forces are operating on a child's thinking. A broader approach, which attempts to remove the cause of a particular effect, is the radical model. It is vital. Children cannot be expected to make a decision to be non-smokers unsupported by the social environment.

All the three above models have their place in health education programmes to prevent the onset of smoking. Together they contribute to the best, and current approach which is the self-empowerment model. The external and internal attributes which enable the child to decide must be created. Internally, the children need self-efficacy to resist peer pressure to smoke; self-esteem and a good self-image so that they do not feel the need of smoking to build this part of their make-up; understanding of the ways in which advertising works as a persuader; self-confidence and social skills to relate to other people without needing cigarettes as a means of making contact. These skills and many more are needed by some children, especially by those most at risk. Outside factors are not in the hands of the children themselves. Advertising, the social acceptability of smoking among adults, the availability and price of cigarettes, family smoking and many other background elements need to be altered.

Current programmes are using one or more of these approaches. In 1989, the government allocated a large budget to the Health Education Authority for 5 years with the purpose of reducing smoking among teenagers, especially girls. A major programme has been developed which is not only focusing on schools, but is taking a wider approach as well. Among other things, they are using the media, including young people's magazines and advertising, to put over a positive image of the non-smoker, thus encouraging children to choose health.

With regard to availability of cigarettes to children, Parents Against Tobacco, a forceful association of parents organized by Mr Des Wilson, has achieved tougher legislation with regard to preventing sales of cigarettes to children.

Campaigns are at present attempting to ban, or at least restrict, advertising of tobacco. The voluntary agreement between the tobacco industry and the government has gone some way towards protecting children from tobacco advertising. For example, magazines with a readership of 200 000 or more, one third of whom are young women aged 16 to 24 years, do not advertise cigarettes. Young people are not portrayed on cigarette advertisements and posters advertising cigarettes should not be placed near schools. These are a few of the protections but a great deal more is needed. Some countries have banned tobacco advertising entirely. Action on Smoking and Health plays an active role in campaigning against smoking.

The Cancer Research Campaign funds a major programme of research into the prevention of smoking in children. The Chest, Heart and Stroke Association, the Coronary Prevention Group and numerous other charities and organizations have programmes or some other contribution to the important aim of preventing children from smoking.

What can the paediatrician do?

- Be aware of the role of parental and children's own smoking in the risks, cause and exacerbation of so many childhood health problems.
- Always ask the parent and the child, probably from the age of about 9 years upwards, if they smoke when the child is first seen for any health, growth or behaviour problems.

- Discuss with the parent or child, together or separately, the factors which lie behind their decision to smoke.
- Provide advice and help on stopping smoking for parents and children appropriate to their reasons for smoking.
- Remember to take into account the family nature of smoking at this stage in a child's life and to work with the family to achieve a smoke-free status.
- Advise mothers who are unable to stop smoking not to smoke in the house.
- Urge and help pregnant and nursing mothers to be non-smokers.
- Initiate or support actively any action against the promotion of cigarettes and tobacco.

A comprehensive review of smoking in relation to young people has been published which provides useful information for paediatricians.[75]

References

1. US Department of Health and Human Services, US Public Health Services, Office of Medical Applications of Research. Health applications of smokeless tobacco use. *J Am Med Assoc* 1986; **255**: 1045–1048.
2. World Health Organization. *Smokeless Tobacco Control.* WHO Technical Report Series 773. Geneva: WHO, 1988.
3. Thomas, M., Goddard, E., Hickman, M., Hunter, P. *General Household Survey 1992. Series GHS no. 23* (OPCS). London: HMSO, 1994.
4. Thomas, M., Holroyd, S., Goddard, E. *Smoking among Secondary School Children in 1992. An enquiry carried out by the Social Survey Division of OPCS on behalf of the Department of Health, the Welsh Office and the Scottish Home and Health Departments.* London: HMSO, 1993.
5. Doll, R., Peto, R. *The Causes of Cancer.* Oxford: Oxford University Press, 1981.
6. World Health Organization. *Prevention of Coronary Heart Disease.* WHO Technical Report Series 678. Geneva: WHO, 1982.
7. US Department of Health and Human Services. *The Health Consequences of Smoking: a Report by the Surgeon General.* Rockville, Maryland: US Department of Health and Human Services, 1982.
8. Adams, L., Lonsdale, D., Robinson, M., *et al.* Respiratory impairment induced by smoking in children in secondary schools. *Br Med J* 1984; **288**: 891–895.
9. Bewley, B.R., Bland, J.M. Smoking and respiratory symptoms in two groups of schoolchildren. *Prev Med* 1976; **5**: 63–69.
10. Benatar, S.R. Smoking and chronic respiratory symptoms in 11 to 15-year-old children. *S Afr Med J* 1979; **56**: 301–304.
11. Peat, J.K., Woolcock, A.J., Leeder, S.R., *et al.* Asthma and bronchitis in Sydney schoolchildren. *Am J Epidemiol* 1980; **111**: 728–735.
12. Charlton, A., Blair, V. Absence from school related to children's and parental smoking habits. *Br Med J* 1989; **298**: 90–92.

13   Flay, B.R., d'Avernas, J.R., Best, J.A. *et al*. Cigarette smoking: why do young people do it and ways of preventing it. In: McGrath, P., Firestone, P., eds. *Pediatric and Adolescent Behavioral Medicine*. New York: Springer-Verlag, 1983: 132–182.

14   Charlton, A. Children's opinions on smoking. *J Roy Coll Gen Practit* 1984; **34:** 483–487.

15   McNeil, A.D., West, R. Subjective effects of cigarette smoking in adolescents. *Psychopharmacology* 1987; **92:** 115–117.

16   Marsh, A., Matheson, J. *Smoking Attitudes and Behaviour: an Enquiry carried out on behalf of the Department of Health and Social Security by the Office of Population Censuses and Surveys*. London: HMSO, 1983.

17   Murray, M., Kiryluk, S., Swan, A.V. Relation between parents' and children's smoking behaviour and attitudes. *J Epidemiol Comm Hlth* 1985; **39:** 169–174.

18   Green, G., Macintyre, S., West, P. *et al*. Do children of lone parents smoke more because their mothers do? *Br J Addict* 1990; **85:** 1497–1500.

19   Charlton, A. Smoking in one parent families. *Prog in Public Educ about Cancer* 1991; **2:** 13–19.

20   Aaro, L.E., Hauknes, A., Berglund, E.-L. Smoking among Norwegian schoolchildren 1975–1980: the influence of the social environment. *Scand J Psychol* 1981; **22:** 297–309.

21   Charlton, A. The Brigantia Smoking Survey: a general review. *Public Educ about Cancer* 1984; **77:** 92–102.

22   Bewley, B.R., Bland, J.M. Academic performance and social factors related to cigarette smoking by schoolchildren. *Br J Prev Soc Med* 1977; **31:** 18–24.

23   Bewley, B.R., Bland, J.M., Harris, R. Factors associated with the starting of cigarette smoking by primary school children. *Br J Prev Soc Med* 1974; **28:** 37–44.

24   Glynn, T.J. From family to peer: a review of transitions of influence among drug-using youth. *J Youth Adolesc* 1981; **10:** 363–383.

25   Cooreman, J., Burghard, G., Perdrizet, S. L'adolescent et le tabagisme. *J Med Strasbourg* 1978; **9:** 483–486.

26   Porter, A. Disciplinary attitudes and cigarette smoking: a comparison of two schools. *Br Med J* 1982; **286:** 1725–1726.

27   Charlton, A., Blair, V. Predicting the onset of smoking in boys and girls. *Soc Sci Med* 1989; **29:** 813–818.

28   Bland, J.M., Bewley, B.R., Banks, M.H., *et al*. Schoolchildren's beliefs about smoking and disease. *Hlth Educ J* 1975; **34:** 71–78.

29   Townsend, J. Cigarette tax, economic welfare and social class patterns of smoking. *Appl Econ* 1987; **19:** 335–365.

30   Lewit, E.M., Coate, D., Grossman, M. The effects of government regulations on teenage smoking. *J Law Econ* 1981; **14:** 545–569.

31   Aitken, P.P., Leathar, D.S., O'Hagan, F.J., *et al*. Children's awareness of cigarette advertisements and brand imagery. *Br J Addict* 1987; **82:** 615–622.

32   Charlton, A. Children's advertisement awareness related to their views on smoking. *Hlth Educ J* 1986; **45:** 75–78.

33   Ledwith, F. A study of smoking in primary and secondary schools in Scotland. In: Fontana, F., ed. *Tobacco e Giovani*. Genoa: Lego Italiana per la Lotto contro i Tumori, 1981.

34   Stewart, L., Livson, N. Smoking and rebelliousness: a longitudinal study from childhood to maturity. *J Consult Psychiatr* 1966; **30:** 225–229.

35   Wills, T.A. Stress and coping in early adolescence: relationship to substance use in urban and school samples. *Hlth Psychol* 1986; **5:** 503–529.

36   DeVries, H., Dijkstra, M., Kuhlman, P. Self-efficacy: the third factor besides attitude and subjective norm as a predictor of behavioural intentions. *Hlth Educ Res* 1988; **3:** 273–282.

37   Lowe, C.R. Effect of mothers' smoking habits on the birthweight of their children. *Br Med J* 1959; **2:** 673–676.

38   Butler, N.R., Goldstein, H., Ross, E.M. Cigarette smoking in pregnancy: its influence on birthweight and perinatal mortality. *Br Med J* 1972; **2:** 127–130.

39   Haddow, J.E., Knight, G.J., Palomaki, G.F., *et al*. Cigarette consumption and serum cotinine in relation to birthweight. *Br J Obstet Gynaecol* 1987; **94:** 295–300.

40   Cnattingius, S., Haglund, B., Meirik, O. Cigarette smoking as a risk factor for late foetal and early neonatal death. *Br Med J* 1988; **297:** 258–261.

41   Bakketeig, L.S., Hoffman, H.J., Oakley, A.R. Perinatal mortality. In: Bracken, M.B., ed. *Perinatal Mortality*. Oxford: Oxford University Press, 1984: 99–151.

42   Kristjansson, E.A., Fried, P.A., Watkinson, B. Maternal smoking during pregnancy affects children's vigilance performance. *Drug Alcohol Dependence* 1989; **24:** 11–19.

43   Naeye, R.L., Peters, E.C. Mental development of children whose mothers smoked during pregnancy. *Obstet Gynaecol* 1984; **64:** 601–607.

44   Butler, N.R., Goldstein, H. Smoking in pregnancy and subsequent child development. *Br Med J* 1973; **4:** 573–575.

45   Fox, N.L., Sexton, M., Hebel, J.R. Prenatal exposure to tobacco: I effects on physical growth at age three. *Int J Epidemiol* 1990; **19:** 66–71.

46   Bulterys, M.G., Greenland, S., Kraus, J.F. Chronic fetal hypoxia and sudden infant death syndrome: interaction between maternal smoking and low haematocrit during pregnancy. *Pediatrics* 1990; **86:** 535–540.

47   Rubin, D.H., Krasilnikoff, P.A., Leventhal, J.M., *et al*. Effect of passive smoking on birthweight. *Lancet* 1986; ii: 415–417.

48   Woodward, A., Grgurinovich, N., Ryan, P. Breast-feeding and smoking hygiene: major influences on cotinine in urine of smokers' infants. *J Epidemiol Comm Hlth* 1986; **40:** 309–315.

49   Harlap, S., Davies, A. Infant admissions to hospital and maternal smoking. *Lancet* 1974; i: 529–532.

50   Colley, J.R.T., Holland, W.W., Corkhill, R.C. Influence of passive smoking and parental phlegm on pneumonia and bronchitis in early childhood. *Lancet* 1974; ii: 1031–1034.

51   Fergusson, D.M., Horwood, L.F., Shannon, F.T., *et al*. Parental smoking and lower respiratory illness in the first three years of life. *J Epidemiol Comm Hlth* 1981; **35:** 180–184.

52   Ferris, B.G.I., Ware, J.H., Berkey, C.S., *et al*. Effects of passive smoking on the health of children. *Environ Hlth Perspect* 1985; **62:** 289–295.

53   Weiss, S.T., Tager, I.B., Speizer, F.E., *et al*. Persistent wheeze: its relation to respiratory illness, cigarette

smoking and level of pulmonary function in a population sample of children. *Am Rev Resp Dis* 1980; **122**: 697–707.

54 Neuspiel, D.R., Rush, D., Butler, N.R., *et al*. Parental smoking and post-infancy wheezing in children: a prospective cohort study. *Am J Pub Hlth* 1989; **79**: 168–171.

55 Murray, A.B., Morrison, B.J. The effect of cigarette smoke from the mother on the bronchial responsiveness and severity of symptoms in children with asthma. *J Allerg Clin Immunol* 1986; **77**: 575–581.

56 Murray, A.B., Morrison, B.J. Passive smoking by asthmatics: its greater effect on boys than on girls and on older rather than younger children. *Pediatrics* 1989; **84**: 451–459.

57 Bland, M., Bewley, B.R., Pollard, V. Effect of children's and parents' smoking on respiratory symptoms. *Arch Dis Child* 1978; **53**: 100–105.

58 Charlton, A. Children's coughs related to parental smoking. *Br Med J* 1984; **288**: 1647–1649.

59 Kasuga, H., Hasebe, A., Osaka, F., *et al*. Respiratory symptoms in school children and the role of passive smoking. *Tokai J Clin Med* 1979; **4**: 101–104.

60 Luck, W., Nau, H. Nicotine and cotinine concentrations in serum and urine of infants exposed via passive smoking or milk from smoking mothers. *J Pediatr* 1985; **107**: 816–820.

61 Jarvis, M.J., Russell, M.A., Feyerabend, C., *et al*. Passive exposure to tobacco smoke: saliva cotinine concentrations in a representative sample of nonsmoking schoolchildren. *Br Med J* 1985; **291**: 927–929.

62 Willers, S., Schutz, A., Attewell, R., *et al*. Relation between lead and cadmium in blood and the involuntary smoking of children. *Scand J Work Environ Hlth* 1988; **14**: 385–389.

63 Sexton, M., Fox, N.L., Hebel, J.R. Prenatal exposure to tobacco: II effects on cognitive functioning at age three. *Int J Epidemiol* 1990; **19**: 72–77.

64 Rona, R.J., Chinn, S., Florey, C.D. Exposure to cigarette smoking and children's growth. *Int J Epidemiol* 1985; **14**: 402–409.

65 Berkey, C.S., Ware, J.H., Dockery, D.W., *et al*. Indoor air pollution and pulmonary function growth in preadolescent children. *Am J Epidemiol* 1986; **123**: 250–260.

66 Haglund, B., Cnattingius, S. Cigarette smoking as a risk factor for sudden infant death syndrome: a population-based study. *Am J Pub Hlth* 1990: **80**: 29–32.

67 Willatt, D.J. Children's sore throats related to parental smoking. *Clin Otolaryngol* 1986; **11**: 317–321.

68 Strachan, D.P., Jarvis, M.J., Feyerabend, C. Passive smoking, saliva cotinine concentrations and middle ear effusion in 7 year old children. *Br Med J* 1989: **298**: 1549–1552.

69 Corbo, G.M., Fuciarelli, F., Foresi, A., *et al*. Snoring in children: association with respiratory symptoms and passive smoking. *Br Med J* 1989; **299**: 1491–1494.

70 Ogston, S.A., Florey, C.D., Walker, C.H. Association of infant alimentary and respiratory illness with parental smoking and other environmental factors. *J Epidemiol Comm Hlth* 1987; **41**: 21–25.

71 Haneberg, B., Tonjum, T., Rodahl, K., *et al*. Factors preceding the onset of meningococcal disease, with special emphasis on passive smoking, symptoms of ill health. *Ann Norweg Inst Pub Hlth* 1983; **6**: 169–173.

72 Rubin, B.K. Exposure of children with cystic fibrosis to environmental tobacco smoke. *New Engl J Med* 1990; **323**: 782–788.

73 Janerich, D.T., Thompson, W.D., Varela, L.R., *et al*. Lung cancer and exposure to tobacco smoke in the household. *New Engl J Med* 1990; **323**: 632–636.

74 Poswillo, D., Alberman, E. *The Effects of Smoking on the Fetus, Neonate and Child*. Oxford: Oxford University Press, 1992.

75 Royal College of Physicians of London. *Smoking and the Young*. London: RCP, 1992.

7.10 Sexual counselling of teenagers

Hazel Curtis

Sexuality is part of adolescent development but some of its consequences, including sexual intercourse, pregnancy and sexually transmitted diseases, have emerged as major health concerns for paediatricians. During adolescence, the desire and need to discover and exercise one's sexuality become important. Teenagers may experience a sexual relationship with another person and they must come to understand its significance and their responsibilities. Not all are having sexual intercourse, but many are petting, masturbating or being sexual in other ways. Although some adolescents will lie about being sexually active – through guilt or lack of trust – more often they will be honest, but only if they know that their admission will be confidential.

Relationships

If counselling and support of teenagers is to be effective, the teenagers' view of what they perceive as normal behaviour needs to be explored. In a study on 761 teenagers (15–17 years) 50% of both sexes had had a relationship which they regarded as steady or more serious; one-quarter had had a less serious relationship; and just under one-fifth had never had a girl or

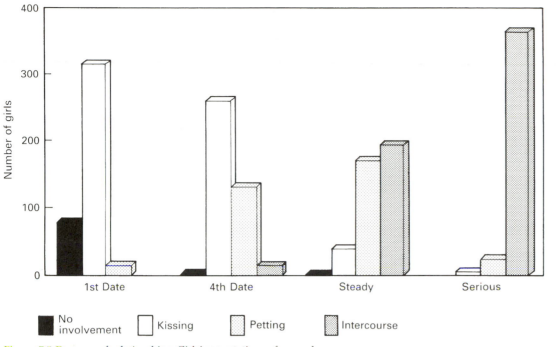

Figure 7.9 Progress of relationships. Girls' expectations of normal.

boyfriend.[1] The perception of their friends' relationships was used to explore the development of teenage relationships and the prevalence of full sexual activity. Figure 7.9 shows how the girls expected a relationship among their friends to progress, with one-fifth expecting no physical involvement on their first date, although most expected to be kissing. By the fourth date virtually all expected to be kissing and one third petting. By the time the relationship was regarded as steady, half expected their friends to be having intercourse. The pattern for the boys was not significantly different.

A steady friendship was defined by the majority as being exclusive and, in terms of the number of weeks it continued, boys defined a steady relationship as lasting one week to one year, with a median of 8 weeks, and girls one week to 18 months with a median of 11 weeks.

In becoming sexually experienced, young people often believe they are simply conforming to the norm. In the above study, although 40% who were involved in a steady or more serious relationship were sexually experienced, only one quarter of the total teenage population were experienced. The rates of sexual activity did not increase significantly with age for the girls (Table 7.21) although the rate for boys increased from 16% at 15 years to 25% at 17 years. This was regarded as a minimum estimate since the survey did not include those who were 16 years or 17 years and who had left school. Follow up of this study in 1990–91 suggests it is still the minority of under 16

Table 7.21 Sexual activity and relationships (%) in school children by age (years)

	Boys			Girls		
	15	16	17	15	16	17
Having a steady relationship	45	56	55	48	52	56
Sexually active among steady	31	49	46	40	49	41
Sexually active in whole group	16	23	25	19	25	23
$n =$	139	96	82	188	146	49

year olds who are sexually experienced.[2] The rates of intercourse were apparently not related to social class, as judged by father's occupation, or to academic achievement or activities, with the exception that the more academic 15-year-old girls were less likely to be sexually active. The girls who started their periods early were more likely to be sexually active, as has been reported in previous studies.[3,4] This might be explained by the fact that the psychological maturation of a girl is unlikely to match her physical development and she will be attractive to older boys while still at an age where she is unable to resist personal and peer pressure.

Peer pressure and peer influence is of considerable importance; people of all ages are often unwilling to admit to themselves how much they want to or need to conform to the behaviour of their friends. In the study by Curtis *et al.*, there was significant clustering of sexual activity among both boys and girls with an individual being much more likely to be sexually active when they perceived this was the norm for their friends.[1] Rates also varied considerably between comprehensive schools (and could not be accounted for by a difference in social class distribution) suggesting that the ambience and education in schools may be an important variable in the determination of sexual activity rates. For both sexes, first intercourse often occurred by default rather than as a planned progression of a relationship. Once having experienced a relationship with intercourse, even though first intercourse was often not reported as enjoyable, both sexes were likely to continue their sexual activity.[4,5]

It is common in boy/girl relationships for the boy to be older than his girlfriend. In one study on pregnant teenagers and their partners half the boys had been out with girls who were sexually experienced and often also older. These boys were likely to establish a relationship involving intercourse earlier than those who were going out with girls who were the same age, or younger, and not experienced. Within the average relationship, that is where the boy is older, it is also apparent that girls going out with sexually experienced boys are likely to indulge in sexual intercourse earlier.[6] Sexually experienced teenagers are more likely to initiate subsequent boyfriends or girlfriends into sexual intercourse.

Teenagers who start having intercourse under 16 years are more likely to have several partners over a period of time than those who start over 16 years, the boys tending to have more partners than the girls. This is important when considering risk factors for sexually transmitted diseases (STD) and cervical cancer. Most are not promiscuous, but have sex in the context of a relationship with a single person while the relationship lasts – serial monogamy. Serial monogamy exposes each partner indirectly to previous partners.

Many girls and boys regret the age at which they first had intercourse, realizing in retrospect that they had been too young.[6] A significant number of teenagers are sexually active while still at school. Society, while recognizing this fact, must do more to reinforce the normality of teenage relationships *without* intercourse. Teenagers want more discussion at school on pressures, emotions, relationships and the difference between the sexes.[7] An important aspect of counselling of teenagers, whether involved in relationships or not, is the building up of self-esteem and, alongside this, respect and responsibility towards oneself and others.

When pregnancy has been confirmed in a teenager, counselling is imperative for the girl and, if possible, for her partner and the family. Lack of counselling is reflected in the number of girls who return within a short period of time with a further pregnancy. Many girls will have decided on the outcome of the pregnancy before going to the doctor but it must be the responsibility of the doctor or a colleague to explore the three possibilities: abortion; adoption; or keeping the child. With each option it is important to ensure that the girl understands the benefit or otherwise of each possibility. An accepting, unhurried environment, in which the adolescent feels sufficiently secure to explore her own feelings about pregnancy and its consequences, is essential. Both premature parenthood and abortion may have serious long-term consequences. It is important to ensure continuing help and support irrespective of the decision made by the patient concerning her pregnancy.[7,8]

Homosexual adolescent

The homosexual adolescent may have begun to feel different from his or her peers during childhood and then, in early adolescence, to become aware of homosexual impulses or the absence of heterosexual arousal. Eventually, homosexual experimentation, a first relationship and, ultimately, a feeling of commitment to a homosexual orientation might follow during middle or late adolescence.[9]

Acceptance of homosexual orientation may be complicated by family conflict, school phobias, substance abuse, juvenile prostitution, depression and suicide. The homosexual male adolescent is at increased risk for a range of specific medical problems that warrant screening – for example, STD.

One cannot accurately guess a patient's sexual orientation based on stereotypes. If an adolescent indicates that he or she has a sexual relationship one should try to ascertain the number of sexual partners and whether the partners have been boys or girls or both sexes. It is important that the counsellor discusses the adolescent's acceptance of his/her orientation, the impact it has had on relationships at home, at school and with peers and any specific medical concerns or symptoms he or she may have.

Contraception

'Teenagers participate in sexual relations for a number of physical, psychological and social reasons that have little, if anything, to do with the availability of contraceptive services.'[10] The gap between becoming sexually active and seeking contraception results in high risk of pregnancy for teenagers. Many teenagers are at risk because intercourse is unplanned and sporadic.[4,11] Teenagers are often inexperienced at arranging their own health care. They find it difficult to communicate and negotiate in intimate relationships, they worry about being seen obtaining contraceptives. Many are self-conscious about their bodies and are, therefore, reluctant to have a medical examination or to touch themselves in the course of using certain contraceptive devices.[12]

The problems of obtaining and using contraceptives are, for many teenagers, more overwhelming than what they regard as the remote possibility of pregnancy. Ryde Blomquist suggested that those under 16 years were poor contraceptive users, because the methods available were too complicated for their psychosexual and personal development.[13] If they are too immature to use contraception, it may be they are too immature to realize the risks and responsibilities that accompany a sexual relationship.

Those over 16 years are more likely to be both initial and continuing users of contraception, suggesting that later first intercourse is associated with increased personal responsibilities. Acceptance of one's sexuality is one of the most important factors affecting whether or not a girl will use contraception. 'An irony of contraceptive usage at any age is that the more unstable the relationship the less likely contraception will be used. The younger teenagers, especially those who have not talked very much about sexual matters, may not be psychologically mature enough to anticipate their need for contraception. The younger the girl at first intercourse, the less likely that contraception will be used.'[3]

In the study from the Guttmacher Institute confidentiality was found to be an important issue, even where attitudes about sex were open – as in Sweden or the Netherlands.[14] Contraception for teenagers in the 1980s was synonymous with the pill. This resulted in many men abdicating their responsibilities, assuming that their partner was protected.[15]

In the area of contraception and relationship, attention has tended to focus on the girl and encouragement of male responsibility has been hampered by lack of information on the attitude of the adolescent male. In a study from the USA over half of the adolescent boys agreed it was important to use contraceptives wherever possible but they saw 'peers as willing to have sex and trusting to luck if contraception was not available.'[16] Fox suggested that men have a double standard, giving more support and taking more responsibility when the relationship is close and little support when it is only a casual acquaintance.

The equal responsibility of both partners in a relationship has to be clearly taught. Family planning clinics are staffed predominantly by women and are seen as 'women's clinics' reinforcing an abdication of male responsibility. In larger cities, family planning sessions for teenagers are helping to overcome this by encouraging both partners to come for counselling and advice. Once intercourse has started, the majority of teenagers will continue to have sex. It is important that contraceptive advice is given and that the most reliable form of contraception is used. It is important, however, that the implications of early intercourse –

the risk of pregnancy, sexually transmitted diseases and cervical cancer – are discussed. Those who have intercourse under 16 years are poor contraceptive users and there must be strong encouragement to delay the onset of intercourse. Female teenagers often say, when asked, that their first experiences of sexual intercourse are not always satisfactory and are not enjoyed. Male teenagers often state that it is not everything that they thought it would be. Further counselling may be needed to determine whether the teenager wishes to continue having intercourse.[5]

Confidential advice is available at family planning clinics but the teenager may not be aware that if advice is sought from a teacher the head of the school may be informed and the information subsequently passed to the parent.

Sexually transmitted diseases

In the UK, chlamydial urethritis or cervicitis is the commonest sexually transmitted disease.[17] While women infected with *Chlamydia trachomatis* may have classical symptoms of genital infection, up to two-thirds are asymptomatic.[18] Factors associated with *Chlamydia trachomatis* infection have been shown to include: a new sexual partner within the preceding 2 months; use of no contraception or a non-barrier method; and age of 24 years or less.[19] Sexually transmitted infections have special significance in the female adolescent. She is more likely to develop pelvic inflammatory disease, with its long-term sequelae of infertility, ectopic pregnancy and chronic pelvic pain, than older women.[20] It has been estimated that a sexually-active 15-year-old girl has a one in eight chance of acquiring acute pelvic inflammatory disease compared with a one in 80 risk for a sexually active 24 year old.[21]

Teenagers are often unable to appreciate the significance of the potential sequelae of pelvic inflammatory disease, although they have most to lose from it. An organism such as *Chlamydia trachomatis* that can cause devastating sequelae without causing readily apparent or easily recognizable symptomatology and is isolated from one in five asymptomatic adolescents deserves active and specific screening in all such girls.[20]

In the USA, two-thirds of reported cases of gonorrhoea occurred in persons younger than 25 years, and one in every four cases occurred among adolescents.[21]

A major sexually transmitted agent to be considered is the human immunodeficiency virus (HIV) which produces the acquired immune deficiency syndrome (AIDS). HIV infection spread over much of the world during the decade 1976–1986, mirroring, on a larger scale, the earlier spread of syphilis in Europe in the 1940s. It has become clear that AIDS is the most important and dangerous infectious disease pandemic in the developed countries since influenza at the end of World War 1.[22]

Dr Michael Merson, Director of the World Health Organization's Global Programme on AIDS, has stated: 'Geographically, AIDS is everywhere. Women are infected as much as men. It is spreading from the high risk groups to the general population world-wide. From 2 million cases now the epidemic will grow to at least 12 million by the year 2000.'[22] Dr Kouri at the eighth international AIDS conference in Amsterdam predicted that by the year 2000 90% of HIV infection will be acquired through heterosexual sex.[22]

The majority of infection will be in the developing world. Mann reinforced the facts that AIDS exploits societal weakness: 'Belonging to a marginalised or stigmatised group creates an increased risk of HIV infection and increases the risk of receiving inadequate care and support.'[22]

While much emphasis is placed, in public discussion, on the need for the development of vaccines, it is clear that, pending a vaccine with proven safety and efficacy, we must rely on the opportunities to control the pandemic offered by public education and individual risk reduction.

The government AIDS campaign has informed teenagers about transmission and the majority now have an understanding of what AIDS is. Despite this knowledge, two-thirds of teenagers in one survey did not think AIDS would personally affect them and were not particularly concerned.[1] These findings were similar to those found with adults.[23] If the spread of HIV is to be minimized, then education must be such as to create and maintain changes in behaviour.

Although the majority of young people in the study were not sexually active, only one-fifth of the population surveyed anticipated or planned to have a single monogamous relationship. What had been learned from the campaigns was the emphasis on condoms. The sheath has never been regarded as a reliable form of contraception among young people and it is unlikely, therefore, to be an effective way of preventing the spread of the HIV epidemic. AIDS programmes through schools and the media need to underline the importance of this infection and the implications for the *whole* community. The effectiveness of monogamy in preventing the spread of the virus should be proposed more forcefully.

If education is to be effective in reducing the AIDS epidemic, it must be sufficiently relevant to create and maintain changes in behaviour. It is important that education programmes are aimed at young people who are potentially the generation most at risk before they have established patterns of behaviour.

Sex and the physically and mentally handicapped

Sexuality and handicap are difficult issues for parents, professionals and for the handicapped people themselves, many of whom have poor self-image and little confidence in their ability to make and maintain relationships.[24] Disabled persons tend to be more sexually isolated than their able-bodied peers and they miss out on the opportunities to learn about sex from friends. This isolation may lead to withdrawal, immaturity and low self-esteem which are obstacles to meeting people and, ultimately, to the development of a sexual relationship.[25]

Parents find it difficult to talk about relationships and sex with their children; when the child has a disability the task is more daunting. Disabled children do need sex education; they also have to cope with the physical and emotional changes of puberty.

Sex education of mentally handicapped children needs to be simple, repetitive and innovative. A carefully planned programme can give these children a basic knowledge of sexual matters.[26] The reluctance of adults to discuss sexual matters is of more significance to the physically and mentally handicapped, for they are unable to go elsewhere and ask. Natural urges and exploration, which are part of adolescence, are suppressed and discouraged.

It would be negligent to omit a paragraph on sensory disability. For those with hearing impairment, the basic biology of reproduction can be taught but the abstract side of sex education is difficult. The idea of responsibility within relationships and the emotional aspects of friendships are difficult concepts to teach and discuss. Teenagers with hearing impairment often have language development which is delayed, compared with their peers. Related to this, they may be emotionally immature when compared with their physical maturity. Young people with visual impairment are able to discuss and learn about the non-biological aspects of relationships but teaching the biological side is difficult, because so much of this is visual – models may be used as an aid to understanding.

Many disabled teenagers are worried that they will never have a girl or boyfriend – they are surprised that this anxiety is also expressed by their able-bodied peers. Many adolescents want to get married and have children, but are anxious lest their children are disabled. Some wonder if they will be able to have children.

Sex education for the disabled needs to include the practical problems arising from the physical disabilities in a sexual relationship, the genetics of the disability, and means to help the teenager come to terms with the impairment and develop a positive self-image.[27] It is important for teenagers to be able to explore their attitudes and feelings towards sexuality in its widest sense. Organizations such as SPOD (Association to aid the sexual and personal relationships of people with a disability) and ASBAH (Association for Spina bifida and hydrocephalus) provide good material for young people, parents and professionals on all aspects of relationships.

All teenagers need people with whom they can share their anxieties and concerns regarding their sexuality and relationships. For teenagers with a disability, a parent, a trusted professional or friend who is a good listener, can be invaluable as a counsellor. The disabled adolescent has feelings which are unique to him and it is important to explore behind the outward appearance to the personality beneath. It must be remembered that sexual feelings are common to all and that these are not qualitatively affected by the disability itself. It behoves those working alongside teenagers with physical disabilities to gather information so that they can be informed and able to answer questions as they arise or know where to obtain further help.

Over recent years, great emphasis has been placed upon sexual intercourse as the ultimate within a relationship. It is essential that, for those who are unable to have intercourse, and for those who do not have a partner, the importance of other aspects of caring relationships are stressed and explored.

References

1   Curtis, H. Teenage sexuality: implications for controlling AIDS. *Arch Dis Child* 1989; **64:** 1240–1245.
2   Tripp, J.H., Mellanby, A., Phelps, F. Department of Child Health, Royal Devon and Exeter Hospital (unpublished data).
3   Bury, J. *Teenage Pregnancy in Britain.* London: Birth Control Trust, 1984.
4   Curtis, H.A., Lawrence, C.J., Tripp, J.H. Sexual intercourse and pregnancy. *Arch Dis Child* 1988; **63:** 373–379.
5   Strasburger, V.S. Sex, drugs, rock and roll. Understanding teenage sexuality. *Pediatrics* 1985; **75:** 659–663.
6   Curtis, H., Tripp, J.H., Lawrence, L., Clarke, W. Teenage relationships and sex education. *Arch Dis Child* 1988; **63:** 935–941.
7   Allen, I. *Education in Sex and Personal Relationships.* London: Policy Studies Institute, 1978.
8   Committee on Adolescence. *Pediatrics* 1989; **83:** 135-137.
9   Marks, A., Fisher, M. Health assessment and screening during adolescence. *Pediatrics* 1987; **58:** suppl 80, part 2, 131.
10 Chilman, C. Teenage pregnancy: a research review. *Social Work in Health Care* 1979; 492–498.
11 Schofield, M. *Sexual Behaviour of Young People.* London: Pelican, 1968.
12 McGee, E. *Too Little Too Late: Services for Teenage Parents.* New York: Ford Foundation, 1992.
13 Ryde Blomquist, E. Contraception in adolescence: a review of the literature. *J Biosoc Sci* suppl 5: 129–158.
14 Jones, E., Forrest, J. Teenage pregnancy in developed countries: determinants and policy implications. *Fam Plan Perspect* 1985; **17:** 53–62.
15 McAnarney, E. Adolescent pregnancy and childbearing: new data, new challenges. *Pediatrics* 1985; **75:** 973–975.
16 Fox, L.S. Adolescent male reproductive responsibility. *Social Work in Education* 1983; **6:** 32–43.
17 Communicable Diseases Surveillance Centre. STD 9 Surveillance in Great Britain 1984–1986. *Br Med J* 1986; **293:** 942–943.
18 Aryo, O., Mallinson, M., Goddard, R. Epidemiological and clinical correlates of chlamydial infections of the cervix. *Br J Venereal Dis* 1981; **57:** 118–124.
19 Hare, M., Taylor-Robinson, D., Cooper, P. Evidence for an association between *Chlamydia trachomatis* and intra-epithelial neoplasia. *Br J Obstet Gynaecol* 1982; **89:** 489–494.
20 Bump, R.C., Sachs, L.A., Buesching, W.J. Sexual transmissible infectious agents in sexually active and virginal asymptomatic girls. *Pediatrics* 1986; **77:** 488–544.
21 Oill, P.A. Venereal disease in adolescents. *West J Med* 1980; **132:** 39–48.
22 Tanne, J.H. Aids epidemic grows but response slows. *Br Med J* 1992; **305:** 209.
23 Mills, S., Campbell, M., Waters, E. Public knowledge of AIDS and the DHSS advertisement campaign. *Br Med J* 1986; **293:** 1089–1090.
24 Baker, P.A. The denial of adolescence for people with mental handicaps: an unwitting conspiracy. *Mental Handicap* 1991; **19:** 61–65.
25 Stewart, W. *The Sexual Side of Handicap.* Cambridge: Woodhead Faulkner, 1979.
26 Stevens, S., Evered, C., O'Brien, R., Wallace, E. Sex education: who needs it? *Mental Handicap* 1988; **16:** 166–170.
27 Davies, M. *Sex Education for Young People with Physical Handicap.* London: Association to Aid the Sexual and Personal Relationships of People with a Disability, 1985.

Useful addresses

ASBAH (Association for spina bifida and hydrocephalus) 42 Park Road, Peterborough, Cambridgeshire PE1 2UQ. Tel: 0733 555988.
SPOD (Association to aid the sexual and personal relationships of people with a disability) 286 Camden Road, London N7. Tel: 071 607 8851.

7.11 Genetic counselling

Elizabeth Thompson

Aims of genetic counselling

The main goal of genetic counselling is to provide information to individuals, couples and families, so that they may make informed choices in their reproductive decisions. A secondary outcome may be the prevention of the birth of handicapped children and a reduction of the burden of genetic disease on society; but it is important not to regard genetic counselling in a eugenic sense and thereby demean the status of handicapped people.

Community genetics services

This century has seen, in the western world at least, vast improvements in the treatment of environmentally caused illnesses, especially infections, so that genetic disorders are becoming relatively more important. In addition, the advent of DNA technology and rapid advances in obstetric techniques have meant that carrier detection and prenatal diagnosis are possible for an increasing number of disorders.

Traditionally, genetic counselling is provided mainly by specialist clinical geneticists in hospital centres, giving counselling to individuals in families with an established risk. Frequently, this is retrospective counselling. For example, in the absence of a positive family history, a couple only find out that they carry the gene for phenylketonuria after the birth of an affected child. This type of counselling will not provide parental choice with respect to the majority of at risk pregnancies, because first affected family members and sporadic cases are not detected before birth. A well coordinated system of population screening would allow parental choice in many more (but not all) cases.

The concept of *community genetics services* is only just beginning to be recognized. A recent report of the Royal College of Physicians (RCP)[1] pointed out the existence of a range of preventive genetics services based on population screening that are delivered by paediatricians, obstetricians, general practitioners and others, rather than by clinical geneticists. These include:

1 Neonatal screening for phenylketonuria, congenital hypothyroidism and other disorders
2 Screening during pregnancy for rhesus blood group and rubella immunity, maternal serum alpha-fetoprotein (AFP) screening for neural tube defects and Down syndrome, the offer of fetal karyotyping for older women, and second trimester ultrasound scanning for fetal anomalies
3 Population screening for carriers of haemoglobin disorders and Tay-Sachs disease.

The RCP report noted many deficiencies in these services and recommended improvements through better funding, better organization and coordination at all levels of the health service, better education of all health professionals and of the public in genetic issues, and monitoring of the services.

The recent characterization of the cystic fibrosis gene and its common mutation (ΔF508) means that soon it will be feasible to offer population carrier screening for this, the commonest autosomal recessive disorder in the European population. This is further pressure to improve services, which will involve both community child health doctors and clinical geneticists.[2] The community paediatrician therefore requires a working knowledge of genetics and an understanding of issues raised by genetic counselling and population screening.

Patterns of inheritance

It is estimated that, in humans, there are some 50 000 to 100 000 pairs of functional genes which are carried on 46 chromosomes. In somatic cells, these are arranged in a standard manner in 22 autosomal pairs, plus a pair of sex chromosomes. The basic haploid set (23) is present in gametes. After fertilization, the zygote contains a diploid set of chromosomes (46); one of each pair is maternal in origin and the other is paternal. Chromosomes (from the Greek *chromos* meaning coloured and *soma* meaning body) can be identified under the light microscope using staining techniques which give a characteristic pattern of dark and light bands (Fig. 7.10). The number, size, shape and arrangement of the chromosomes of a somatic cell of an individual is known as the karyotype.

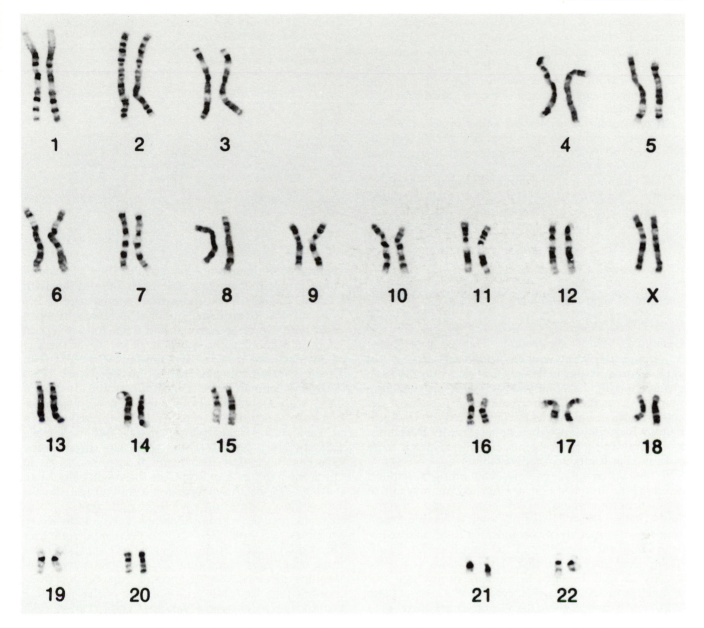

Figure 7.10 A normal female karyotype. (From the Greenwood Genetic Center, One Gregor Mendel Circle, Greenwood, South Carolina 29646, USA, by permission.)

Some genetic disorders are attributable to a visible abnormality of the chromosomes (the chromosomal disorders). Others result from a defect in a single gene as first described by Gregor Mendel (the monogenic or mendelian disorders). Many congenital malformations and common diseases have a genetic component in their aetiology and are referred to as multifactorial or polygenic disorders. The appearance of an individual (physical, biochemical and physiological) is known as the phenotype and results from the interaction of the environment and the genotype. The latter reflects the genetic constitution of an individual.

1   Chromosomal disorders

These may be numerical or structural. Numerical disorders are either polyploidy or aneuploidy. In polyploidy, the number of chromosomes is a multiple of the haploid set, exceeding the diploid number. For example, one complete extra set gives 69 chromosomes. This is triploidy (three times the haploid set). Aneuploidy refers to a chromosome number which is not a multiple of the haploid number. Examples are trisomy 21 (Down syndrome) in which there are three chromosomes 21, giving a total of 47 chromosomes, and monosomy X (Turner syndrome) in which there are only 45 chromosomes in somatic cells. Examples of structural defects include deletions, inversions, duplications, ring chromosomes and translocations. All of these result from chromosome breakage with rejoining of the wrong ends. Fragile sites are also structural abnormalities.

Chromosomal disorders are found in about 50% of spontaneous abortions and about 5% of stillbirths. In liveborns, the incidence of chromosomal aberrations is about 6.5 per 1000 births.

Most chromosomal abnormalities cause mental retardation and multiple congenital malformations. Any child with two or more congenital malformations, especially if also mentally retarded, should have the karyotype checked.

Common chromosomal disorders

A AUTOSOMAL TRISOMIES

Trisomy 21 (Down syndrome)   This is the commonest autosomal trisomy with an incidence of around 1 in 650 liveborns. Individuals with Down syndrome have a characteristic facial appearance and are mentally retarded. Congenital malformations such as heart defects and duodenal atresia are common and other problems which may arise include respiratory infections, ocular and auditory problems, hypothyroidism, acute leukaemia and atlanto-axial instability.

In normal meiosis, gametes containing a haploid chromosome number (23) are formed, as a result of disjunction or separation of homologous chromosomes. About 94% of cases of Down syndrome result from non-disjunction of chromosome 21 during meiosis in either the egg (90%) or the sperm (10%), resulting in free trisomy 21 (Fig. 7.11). Babies with free trisomy 21 may be born to mothers of any age, but advancing maternal age increases the risk (Table 7.22). For reasons which are not clear, there is a

Table 7.22 Risk of liveborn child with Down syndrome compared to maternal age

Maternal age at delivery (years)	Risk
Overall	1 in 650
20	1 in 1500
25	1 in 1350
30	1 in 900
35	1 in 400
37	1 in 250
40	1 in 100
45	1 in 30
50	1 in 7

After Table 4.5 in Harper[3]

small risk of recurrence of a child with a chromosome problem following the birth of a child with trisomy 21. This risk (under the maternal age of 35) is about 1%, comprising about 0.5% for a liveborn child with Down syndrome and 0.5% for a liveborn child with another chromosome defect. Over the age of 35 years, the risk of a woman having a child with Down syndrome begins to rise, as shown in Table 7.22. If a woman over 35 years has already had a child with Down syndrome, the risk of recurrence of Down syndrome is roughly twice the risk shown in Table 7.22 for her particular age and the chance that she may have a child with *any* chromosome defect is twice that risk again. It is unnecessary to check the parents' karyotypes as these will be normal.

About 5% of Down syndrome individuals have a translocation of a chromosome 21 onto another chromosome, usually chromosome 14, occasionally chromosomes 15 or 22, or rarely, onto another chromosome 21. Such individuals therefore have three doses of chromosome 21, comprising two freestanding chromosomes 21 and one translocation chromosome (Fig. 7.12a). In less than half of these cases, a healthy parent carries a balanced translocation (Fig. 7.12b) and is at increased risk of recurrence. Empirical data for the risk of occurrence of Down syndrome in offspring are 10% if the mother carries the translocation and 2.5% if the father is the carrier. These observed risks are less than the theoretical risks, probably because of selection of gametes and early spontaneous abortion of embryos with an unbalanced karyotype. If neither parent carries the translocation, the risk of recurrence is low (less than 1%). If a parent carries a 21:21 translocation, the risk of recurrence is essentially 100%, since normal gametes cannot be produced.

Thus in cases of translocation Down syndrome, it is important to check parental karyotypes. In addition, if a parent is a carrier, other family members should be offered counselling and testing. A further 1% of Down syndrome individuals have mosaicism.

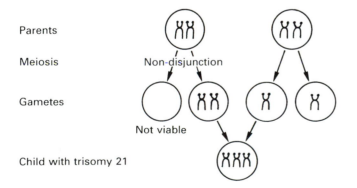

Parents

Meiosis   Non-disjunction

Gametes

Not viable

Child with trisomy 21

Figure 7.11 A diagram to show non-disjunction in trisomy 21.

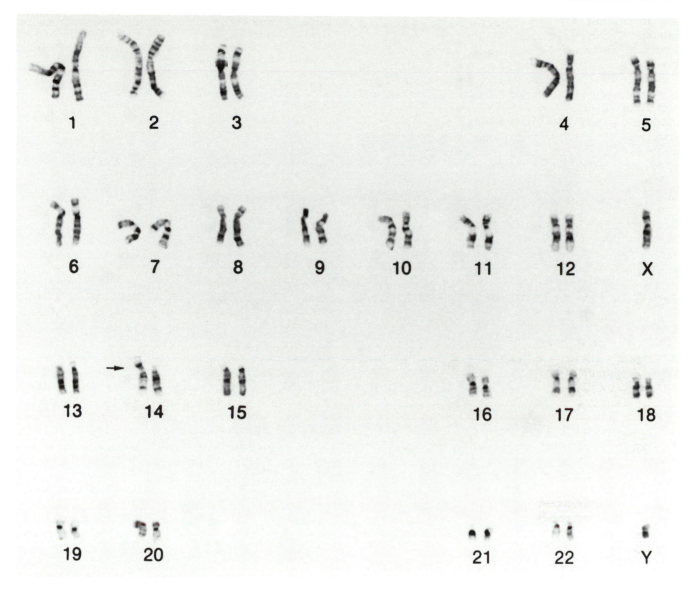

Figure 7.12 (a) Karyotype of an individual with Down syndrome with a 14/21 translocation. Note that there are two free chromosomes 21, and another chromosome 21 is attached to a chromosome 14 (arrow). There are therefore three copies of chromosome 21. (From the Greenwood Genetic Center, One Gregor Mendel Circle, Greenwood, South Carolina 29646, USA, by permission.)

Trisomy 18 (Edwards syndrome) The birth incidence is variously quoted from about 1 in 3500 to 1 in 8000, i.e. 0.29/1000 to 0.13/1000. About one-third of affected babies die within the first month, and only 10% survive the first year and are severely mentally retarded. Characteristic facial features include a small chin, short palpebral fissures, and malformed ears. The occiput is prominent, the hands are clenched in a characteristic posture, and rocker-bottom feet and a short sternum are common. Malformations of the brain, heart, kidneys and gut are frequent.

Most cases arise from parental non-disjunction, and, as with Down syndrome, there is an increased risk of non-disjunction with advancing maternal age. The risk

of recurrence of a liveborn child with this or another major chromosomal defect is about 1%. Occasionally, a parent carries a balanced translocation and is at higher risk of recurrence.

Trisomy 13 (Patau syndrome) The birth incidence quoted varies from 1 in 4000 to less than 1 in 10,000, i.e. 0.25–0.1/1000. Abnormalities include microcephaly, brain malformations especially holoprosencephaly, cleft lip and palate, scalp defects and post-axial polydactyly (extra digit(s) on the little finger side of the hand). Eye, heart and kidney malformations are common. As in trisomies 21 and 18, there is a maternal age effect. Most cases arise from non-disjunction, with a

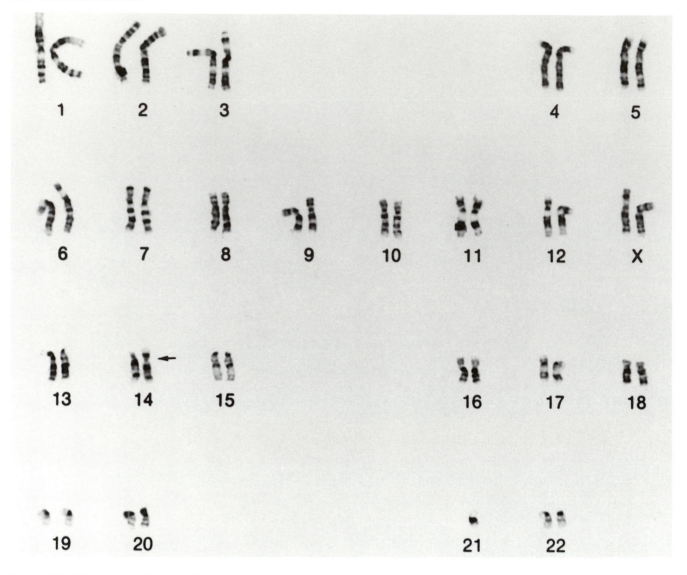

Figure 7.12 (b) Karyotype of a clinically normal 14/21 translocation carrier. Note that there appear to be only 45 chromosomes but one chromosome 21 is attached to a chromosome 14 (arrow) and the other is free. (From the Greenwood Genetic Center, One Gregor Mendel Circle, Greenwood, South Carolina 29646, USA, by permission).

low (less than 1%) recurrence risk. In about 20% of cases, however, a parent carries a balanced translocation and is at higher risk of recurrence.

B SEX CHROMOSOME DEFECTS

These generally cause less severe malformations and mental retardation than autosomal abnormalities. The phenotype becomes more abnormal, however, with a greater number of extra sex chromosomes.

Monosomy X (Turner syndrome) The incidence in female livebirths is about 1 in 2500, i.e. 0.4 per 1000. At conception, however, the frequency is considerably higher but over 95% abort spontaneously.

At birth, the only clinical feature may be lymphoedema of the hands and feet. Subsequently, short stature, lack of secondary sexual characteristics, amenorrhoea and infertility are the rule. Dysmorphic features include neck webbing, a broad chest with widely-spaced nipples and cubitus valgus. Coarctation of the aorta may be found. Intelligence is normal but some may have educational difficulties. Some growth stimulation can be achieved by the use of androgens and growth hormone. Oestrogen replacement is necessary for the development of secondary sexual characteristics.

Most cases of monosomy X arise from parental nondisjunction. In 75%, it is the maternal X chromosome which is present. Overall, 57% of individuals with

Turner syndrome have 45,X, 17% have an isochromosome of the long arm of the X chromosome (i.e. one X chromosome consists of two long arms, rather than one long and one short arm), 16% are mosaics and 10% have a short arm deletion of an X. Risks of recurrence are negligible.

Triple X syndrome   The incidence of this disorder is about 0.65 per 1000 liveborn females, i.e. 1 in 1500. Affected females may be taller than average, but usually have no or few physical abnormalities. Educational difficulties are common, and mild mental retardation is present in 15–25%. Parental non-disjunction is the cause and recurrence risks to sibs are negligible. About three-quarters are fertile and although about half of their offspring would be predicted to be chromosomally abnormal, in practice they are usually normal.

47, XXY (Klinefelter syndrome)   The incidence is about 2 per 1000 liveborn males. Affected individuals are most commonly detected as adults attending infertility clinics, since Klinefelter syndrome is the commonest cause of male infertility. Other clinical features include tall stature, small testes, poorly developed male sexual characteristics and gynaecomastia. Intelligence is usually normal, but educational and behavioural difficulties are common. Parental non-disjunction is the cause with a maternal age effect; the extra X chromosome is maternal in 60% of cases and paternal in 40%. Recurrence risks are low.

XYY syndrome   The incidence is about 1.5 per 1000 male livebirths. Many affected males probably remain undetected, but the syndrome may be associated with aggressive behaviour and mild mental retardation.

Fragile X syndrome   Also known as the Martin-Bell syndrome, this disorder occurs in about 1 per 1250 males. It is the second commonest cause of mental retardation after Down syndrome. Under certain culture conditions, the defect becomes visible as a gap (fragile site) in the long (q) arm of the X chromosome, at band Xq27.9, in a proportion of cells.

Affected males are moderately to severely mentally retarded. The phenotype includes macrocephaly and post-pubertal macro-orchidism. Older children and adults often have a long face with prominent ears and jaw.

The disorder is transmitted in a similar manner to that seen in X-linked recessive inheritance. Only about one-half of female carriers manifest the fragile X marker cytogenetically, which has made carrier detection in families difficult previously. Unusually for an X-linked recessive disorder, as many as one-third of female carriers with the fragile X marker are mentally retarded, albeit usually mildly. As many as 1 in 2500 females are affected. Even more unusual is the phenomenon of the normal transmitting male, a clinically and cytogenetically normal male whose daughters' sons may be affected. This poses genetic counselling difficulties, which have been partly resolved since the fragile X gene was discovered (see later section on DNA analysis). Carrier detection and prenatal diagnosis using a combination of pedigree analysis, cytogenetic and DNA markers can be carried out, preferably by clinical geneticists, since interpretation of results may be difficult.

C MOSAICISM

Mosaicism refers to the presence of two different cell lines derived from one zygote. About 1% of individuals with Down syndrome are mosaics with normal and trisomic cell lines. This arises after fertilization, usually in a zygote with trisomy 21 in which a normal cell line is produced at a subsequent mitosis, by non-disjunction. Less commonly, a mitotic non-disjunction produces a trisomy 21 cell line in a normal zygote. The proportion of the various cell lines varies in different tissues. Clinically, the phenotype is usually milder than in non-mosaic trisomy 21.

Occasionally, an individual with chromosomal mosaicism may have normal cell lines in peripheral lymphocytes, but a skin biopsy and culture of fibroblasts for karyotyping may reveal a chromosome defect. If the phenotype suggests a chromosomal abnormality (for example, mental retardation with congenital malformations) and lymphocyte chromosomes are normal, then a skin biopsy should be considered. In addition, unusual skin pigmentation defects and joint contractures are found in chromosomal mosaicism.

Mosaicism detected at amniocentesis and chorion villous sampling can be difficult to interpret. It is necessary to distinguish whether the mosaicism is in the fetus or the placenta, or whether it has arisen as an *in vitro* artefact. Fetal blood sampling may be needed to clarify these possibilities.

D RECIPROCAL TRANSLOCATIONS

A balanced reciprocal translocation involves exchange of chromosome material but no change in chromosome number. About 1 in 500 liveborns has a balanced reciprocal translocation and 1 in 2000 has an unbalanced translocation. In the former, the phenotype is normal but the latter is usually associated with mental retardation and physical abnormalities. A carrier of a balanced rearrangement may come to light during investigation of recurrent miscarriage or infertility, or if their child is found to have an unbalanced karyotype. In all cases of reciprocal translocation, family members should be offered specialist counselling and karyotyping. Prenatal tests can be offered to carriers.

E DELETIONS

These involve visible loss of part of a chromosome. Some are associated with a particular phenotype, for example, 4p- (Wolf-Hirschhorn syndrome) and 5p- (cri-du-chat syndrome).

The parents must be checked for a balanced reciprocal translocation, as mentioned above. With improving cytogenetic techniques, a number of syndromes have been found to be associated with small deletions (Table 7.23).

Table 7.23 Disorders associated with small chromosomal deletions

Syndrome	Chromosome
Angelman syndrome	15q
Di George syndrome	22q
Langer-Giedion syndrome	8q
Miller-Dieker syndrome	17p
Prader-Willi syndrome	15q
Retinoblastoma	13q
Wilms' tumour/aniridia syndrome	11p

q   long arm of chromosome
p   short arm of chromosome

2 Mendelian disorders

Disorders attributable to abnormalities in a single gene follow recognizable patterns of inheritance, described as follows. Some of the symbols used to draw pedigrees are shown in Figure 7.13.

A Autosomal dominant inheritance

The abnormal gene is found on an autosome (chromosomes 1–22) and so the sexes are equally affected. An individual possessing the abnormal gene (a heterozygote) has a 50% (1 in 2) chance of passing it on to each child (Fig. 7.14). In some autosomal dominant disorders, there is variable expression of the gene, even between affected members of the same family. An example is tuberous sclerosis in which one affected individual may have depigmented skin patches only, while an affected relative may have, in addition, severe mental retardation and epilepsy. Other autosomal dominant disorders, such as achondroplasia, vary little in expression and all affected individuals have a very similar clinical picture. Environmental factors may alter the expression of some dominant disorders, for example, the diet in familial hypercholesterolaemia.

Achondroplasia is an example of an autosomal dominant disorder with complete penetrance, that is all individuals possessing the abnormal gene manifest clinically. Non-penetrance refers to the absence of any clinical expression in an individual who must possess the abnormal gene. An example is shown in Figure

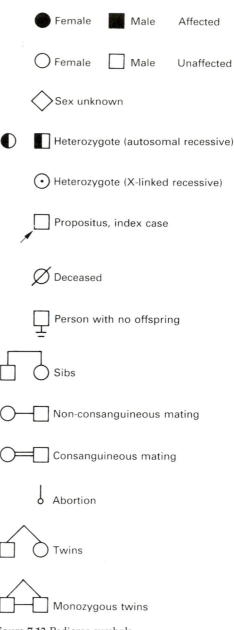

Figure 7.13 Pedigree symbols.

7.15. Non-penetrance can make genetic counselling difficult.

A pedigree of a family with an autosomal dominant disorder is shown in Figure 7.16. Sometimes a child with an autosomal dominant disorder is born to healthy parents. There are a number of reasons for this:

1 The most likely explanation is that the child represents a fresh mutation which occurred in the egg or sperm leading to the child's conception. The risk of recurrence in sibs is negligible, but the child has a

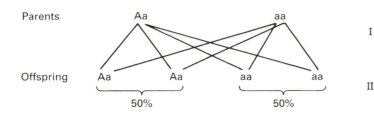

Aa is a heterozygous affected individual, aa is an unaffected individual.

Figure 7.14 Autosomal dominant inheritance.

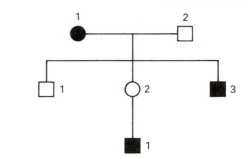

Figure 7.15 Non-penetrance. Individual II2 must have inherited the gene (as she has an affected parent and child) but is not deaf. The gene is non-penetrant in this individual. ● ■ Affected with otosclerosis.

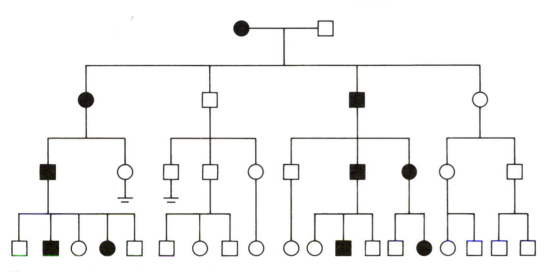

Figure 7.16 A pedigree to show autosomal dominant inheritance. Note that there are affected individuals in several generations, males and females are equally likely to be affected and male to male transmission occurs.

50% chance of passing on the gene to offspring. In some disorders, the mutation rate is high, for example in tuberous sclerosis, about 80% of cases are fresh mutations. In other conditions, such as Huntington's disease, fresh mutations are rare.

2 A healthy parent may harbour a mutation in the gonad (gonadal mosaicism). There is then a risk of recurrence in offspring. This has been proven to occur in one form of perinatally lethal osteogenesis imperfecta in which a healthy parent had (by different partners) several children with a dominant lethal form of the disease.

3 Wrong paternity can give a false impression of an affected child being born to apparently normal parents.

There are now at least 2470 autosomal dominant disorders described.[4] Some examples are:

Achondroplasia
Adult polycystic kidney disease
Crouzon syndrome
Facioscapulohumeral dystrophy
Familial hypercholesterolaemia
Huntington's disease
Marfan syndrome
Myotonic dystrophy
Noonan syndrome
Neurofibromatosis
Osteogenesis imperfecta (some types)
Tuberous sclerosis
von Hippel-Lindau syndrome

Where an autosomal dominant disorder is common, for example familial hypercholesterolaemia, which affects 1 in 500 individuals, two heterozygotes may marry relatively often. On average, one-quarter of their children are unaffected, one-half are heterozygous affected and one-quarter are homozygous affected. The latter are more severely affected and die from myocardial infarction in late childhood. However, the extent to which heterozygotes and affected homozygotes differ clinically varies between different autosomal dominant disorders. (See also section on co-dominant inheritance.)

B   Autosomal recessive inheritance

The abnormal gene is found on an autosome, so that the sexes are equally affected. Individuals carrying one copy of the gene (heterozygotes) are usually healthy. If two individuals carry the same recessive gene, there is a 25% (1 in 4) chance that each child will inherit the abnormal gene from both parents (a homozygote) and be affected (Fig. 7.17).

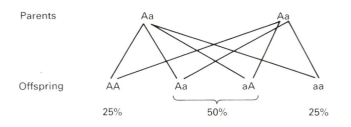

Aa is a heterzygous (unaffected carrier) individual, aa is a homozygous affected individual, AA is a homozygous normal (unaffected) individual.

Figure 7.17 Autosomal recessive inheritance.

Figure 7.18 shows a pedigree in an autosomal recessive disorder. Although carriers may have been present in both sides of the family for many generations, affected individuals are usually found only in one sibship. If heterozygotes are common in the population, as in cystic fibrosis, in which about 1 in 25 caucasians are carriers, then, occasionally, affected individuals may be seen in cousins or other family members.

A special situation arises in consanguineous matings, since there is then the chance that the couple both may have inherited the same recessive gene from a common ancestor. Based on the assumption that we each carry one abnormal recessive gene, it can be calculated that the risk of first cousins producing a child with a recessive disorder is about 3%. It is important to take a detailed pedigree and to offer the couple tests for any recessive disorders relevant to their ethnic group.

At least 647 autosomal recessive disorders have been described.[4]

Some examples are:

Congenital adrenal hyperplasia
Cystic fibrosis
Friedreich's ataxia
Fanconi syndrome
Galactosaemia
Haemochromatosis
Homocystinuria
Hurler syndrome
Oculocutaneous albinism
Phenylketonuria
Sickle cell disease
Tay-Sachs disease
Thalassaemia

C   Co-dominant inheritance

In autosomal dominant inheritance, the heterozygous affected and homozygous affected states are similar, and in autosomal recessive inheritance, the homozygous normal and heterozygous states are indistinguishable. By contrast, in co-dominant inheritance, the heterozygous, homozygous normal and homozygous abnormal states are distinguishable. Strictly speaking, the β-thalassaemia gene is an example of a co-dominantly inherited gene, rather than an autosomal recessive one. Homozygous affected individuals have β-thalassaemia major with severe anaemia. Homozygous normal individuals are completely unaffected. Heterozygous individuals may have mild anaemia, which is referred to as β-thalassaemia minor or thalassaemia trait. Sickle cell disease is also an example of a co-dominantly inherited disorder, since heterozygotes may develop sickling in situations with a low

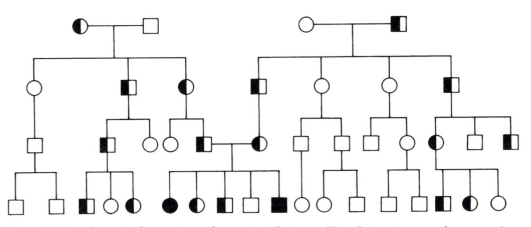

Figure 7.18 A pedigree to show autosomal recessive inheritance. Note that carriers may be present in several generations but affected individuals are usually seen only in one sibship.

oxygen tension, such as at high altitudes. However, because in both β-thalassaemia and sickle cell disease, the heterozygous states are so mild clinically, by common usage they are usually referred to as autosomal recessive disorders. As more diseases become detectable at a molecular and biochemical level, heterozygotes will be identifiable and mild clinical abnormalities in them may become apparent so that they too could be described as co-dominantly inherited disorders. However, so far as the family's perception of a normal healthy child is concerned, heterozygotes will continue to be regarded as unaffected.

D   X-linked disorders

The abnormal gene is carried on an X chromosome. A male possessing the gene (hemizygote) is affected but female carriers are usually healthy, because they also have a normal X chromosome. In fact, in any one female cell, only one X is active and the other is inactivated; this process is known as lyonization, after Mary Lyon who first described it. Whether the maternally or paternally derived X chromosome is inactivated is random in each cell. The result is that, on average, about half of a female carrier's cells have the normal X inactivated and half have the X carrying the abnormal gene inactivated. Female carriers may occasionally manifest clinical features of an X-linked disorder, for a variety of reasons. One reason is if a female carrier also has Turner syndrome (monosomy X), but this would be a rare event. Another reason is that if, by chance, relatively more cells have the normal rather than the abnormal X inactivated, then the female carrier may manifest some symptoms or signs of the disorder, but usually not to the degree seen in affected males. For example, most female carriers of X-linked anhydrotic ectodermal dysplasia show some clinical abnormality of the hair or teeth. In other X-linked disorders, such as Duchenne musclar dystrophy, it is rare for female carriers to develop clinical features such as muscular weakness, but some may have abnormally high plasma creatine kinase levels. For these examples, together with most other X-linked disorders in which female carriers usually manifest few clinical features, the term X-linked recessive is sometimes used. There are a few X-linked disorders in which female carriers usually manifest significant clinical signs and symptoms, such as incontinentia pigmenti, for which the term X-linked dominant inheritance may be used.

In each pregnancy, a female carrier has a 50% (1 in 2) risk of producing affected sons and a 50% risk that each daughter will be a carrier (Fig. 7.19). Affected males, if they reproduce, will pass on their Y chromosome to sons, who will be normal. The pedigree of an X-linked disorder therefore never shows male-to-male transmission (Fig. 7.20), whereas one in an autosomal

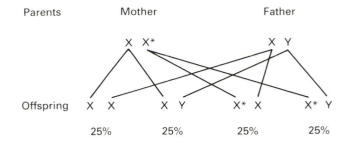

X is the normal X chromosome, X* is the X chromosome carrying the abnormal gene, Y is the Y chromosome. X X is a non-carrier female, X* X is a carrier female, X Y is a normal male, X* Y is an affected male.

Figure 7.19 X-linked recessive inheritance.

dominant disorder may. All daughters of affected males must be carriers and are referred to as obligate carriers.

As with autosomal dominant disorders, cases may arise as a result of fresh mutation. An example is Duchenne muscular dystrophy; a mother of one affected boy (with no other family history of the disease) is a carrier in two-thirds of cases but in one-third the affected boy represents a fresh mutation. Identification of female carriers in the family requires interpretation of the pedigree, creatine kinase levels in females at risk and DNA studies.

There are now about 190 X-linked disorders described.[4]

Some examples are:

Anhydrotic ectodermal dysplasia
Becker and Duchenne muscular dystrophy
Colour blindness (some forms)
Fabry's disease
Glucose-6-phosphate dehydrogenase deficiency
Haemophilia A and B
Hunter syndrome
Lesch-Nyhan syndrome
Menke syndrome
Norrie disease
Ocular albinism

E   Y-linked inheritance

An example of Y-linked inheritance is the testis-determining factor (TDF). Males transmit the gene on their Y chromosome to all of their sons and none of their daughters. To date, no examples of human Y-linked diseases have been described other than XY infertile females with mutations of the TDF gene. There is a very good reason why there are few genes on the Y chromosome other than TDF – only half of the human race has a Y.

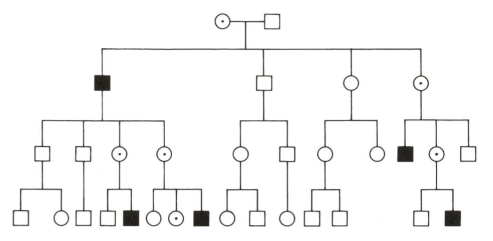

Figure 7.20 A pedigree to show X-linked recessive inheritance. Note that affected individuals are present in several generations, but they are all males and are related to each other through females. There is no male to male transmission.

F   Mitochondrial or cytoplasmic inheritance[5]

Although not described by Mendel, mitochondrial inheritance deserves to be mentioned because it is now known to be important in human disease. The human egg, unlike sperm, contains cytoplasm in which are found mitochondria, which have their own chromosomes. These cytoplasmic mitochondria are therefore transmitted from a mother to all of her children (maternal inheritance). Mutations in mitochondrial DNA have been described in Leber's optic atrophy and in some mitochondrial myopathies. There is a high risk that offspring of affected females will be affected, but a very low risk to the offspring of affected males.

G   Imprinting[6]

Until recently, it has been assumed that expression of a gene is the same whether it is inherited from the mother or father. Evidence is now accumulating in humans and mice showing that, in some disorders, a different phenotype is manifest depending on the parental origin of the gene or chromosome. For example, about half of patients with the Angelman and Prader-Willi syndromes have a small visible *de novo* deletion on the long arm of a chromosome 15, at q11–13. If the deleted chromosome is maternal in origin (that is, arose during egg formation), the child's phenotype is Angelman syndrome; if it is paternal, the child has Prader-Willi syndrome.

3   Multifactorial and polygenic inheritance

Many normal characteristics such as height and weight are determined by the combined effects of several genes and environmental factors, so that the term multifactorial inheritance may be used to describe this type of inheritance. If the environmental component is minimal, the term polygenic inheritance

can be used. The two terms are often used interchangeably. Many congenital malformations and common disorders of adult life are multifactorially determined. Examples are shown in Table 7.24. It is important to note that some multifactorial disorders such as coronary heart disease are in fact heterogeneous in aetiology; some forms are mendelian, some environmental and others are due to the interaction of genetic and environmental factors.

Normal characteristics such as height show a gaussian distribution in the general population (Fig. 7.21). For multifactorial disorders such as neural tube defect, there is a liability which has a gaussian distribution in the general population. Most people are unaffected. If a certain threshold of liability is exceeded, the individual will be affected. Relatives of an affected individual will have a shift in liability because of the genes which they share in common and a greater proportion may exceed the threshold (Fig. 7.22). Familial cases therefore occur.

Table 7.24 Common congenital malformations

Cleft lip with or without cleft palate
Cleft palate alone
Club foot
Congenital dislocated hip
Congenital heart disease
Hypospadias
Inguinal hernia
Neural tube defects, including anencephaly
Pyloric stenosis
Scoliosis

Common disorders of adult life
Diabetes mellitus
Epilepsy
Manic depression*
Schizophrenia*

*Monogenic models have also been used to explain the aetiology of these disorders

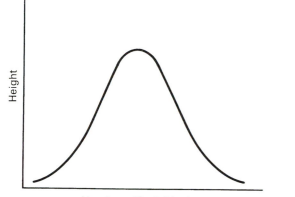

Figure 7.21 The distribution of height in the general population follows a gaussian curve.

General population

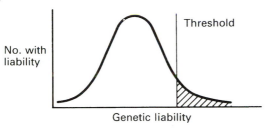

Relatives of an affected individual

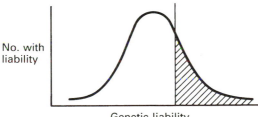

Figure 7.22 The hypothetical genetic liability for a polygenic disorder in the general population and in relatives of an affected individual. Note that the second curve is shifted to the right. Relatives of an affected individual are more likely to have an increased genetic liability and to cross the threshold (and be affected) than in the general population. □ Unaffected individuals; ▓ affected individuals.

Risks to relatives are generally much lower than those seen in mendelian inheritance. They are empirical or observed risks, derived from family studies. Certain observations have been made about this type of inheritance which reflect increased liability in a family:

1 Risks are greater to relatives closest to the proband. For example, in cleft lip and palate, the overall empirical risk to sibs is 4%, whereas the risk to second-degree relatives (nieces and nephews) is 0.6%.

2 Risks are greater if the proband has a more severe form of the disorder. For example, in cleft lip and palate, if the proband has a unilateral cleft lip only, the risk of recurrence in sibs is 2.5%, whereas the risk is 5.7% if the proband has bilateral cleft lip with cleft palate.

3 Risks are greater to relatives if the proband is of the less commonly affected sex, given that there is unequal sex incidence. For example, pyloric stenosis is more common in boys. The risk for brothers of a male proband is 3.8%; but for brothers of a female proband, the risk is 9.2%. Girls require a greater genetic liability to develop the disorder and so relatives of an affected girl will also have a greater genetic liability, than when the proband is a boy.

4 The risk is greater when several family members are affected. For example, if one child has a common congenital heart defect (CHD), the risk to sibs is usually around 3%. If two sibs have a common CHD, the risk to other sibs is 10%.

5 The recurrence risk depends on the incidence of the disorder. The risk to sibs is roughly the square root of the incidence.

6 Sib and offspring risks are similar.

It can be seen that these rules contrast markedly with those in mendelian inheritance, in which recurrence risks are not altered by the severity of the disorder, sex of the proband (in autosomal disorders), number of affected relatives and incidence of the disorder.

Genetic counselling

The process of genetic counselling involves giving information to individuals, couples and families at risk of developing or transmitting a hereditary disorder, so that they may make informed choices about their reproductive options. The term counselling is often misinterpreted to mean that genetic counsellors advise their clients whether or not to have more children or to have them at all. This is far from true. Ideally, genetic counselling should inform without being directive. In reality, it is often difficult to be completely non-directive. For example, to say that the recurrence risk is one in four sounds more pessimistic and off-putting than to say that the chance of an unaffected child is three in four. Genetic counsellors must be aware of this bias and of their own beliefs and feelings which may colour the way in which they give information. The term genetic counselling is also misleading in that the process does not usually involve an in-depth psychological and social evaluation in the sense that counselling may. These factors must however be borne in mind and the genetic counsellor must be prepared to help the occasional individual or couple who find it difficult to decide upon the best course of action. Most people who come for genetic advice, perhaps surprisingly, have little difficulty in evaluating the information and deciding what is best for them.

Effective genetic counselling occurs through a series of logical steps:

1 Establishing the correct diagnosis

Every effort must be made to verify the diagnosis, so that appropriate recurrence risks and advice may be given. A referral may mention muscular dystrophy in a relative. This may involve one of several specific entities each with its particular mode of inheritance. Hospital and other records may need to be obtained and other family members may need to be examined.

Syndrome diagnosis

Clinical geneticists are often called upon to diagnose dysmorphic syndromes. If a syndrome is recognized, costly investigations may be avoided and recurrence risk information may be available. There are at least 1800 syndromes described and most clinical geneticists have access to a computerized database of dysmorphic syndromes, such as the London Dysmorphology Database or POSSUM. The database is also in book form.[7] A short list of dysmorphic features is typed in and the computer produces a list of possible syndromes, with features and references. The successful use of such a system requires experience of dysmorphic syndromes. A manageable list of possible syndromes is produced only if searches are made using features which are considered to be *good handles*. For example, to search on frequently occurring and non-specific features such as low set ears will produce a long heterogeneous list. Good handles are usually relatively uncommon and are easily recognizable as being abnormal and do not merge with normal variation. Polydactyly and anal atresia are good handles. Even experienced users of such a system do not always make a diagnosis, but at least they should be able to give the paediatrician a list of possibilities which might lead to a diagnosis after careful evaluation of the literature.

Perinatal deaths

Another area in which diagnosis is especially important, and often neglected, is perinatal deaths. It is imperative to obtain as much information as possible so that a useful diagnostic evaluation can be made later and accurate genetic counselling given to the parents. Investigations to be considered in all perinatal deaths include chromosomes, autopsy, radiology and photography (producing the mnemonic CARP, as suggested by Dr Ian Young). For example, a baby with thanatophoric dwarfism looks clinically similar to one with camptomelic dysplasia. The former is usually sporadic (assumed to result from fresh dominant mutations) with a negligible recurrence risk, and the latter is autosomal recessively inherited, with a 25% recurrence risk. Only a radiograph can distinguish the correct diagnosis (Fig. 7.23a,b) and will allow accurate genetic advice to be given to the parents.

2 Drawing the family tree

A three generation pedigree is the minimal requirement. Specific questions must be asked about consanguinity, miscarriages, stillbirths and children who have died. The symbols used are shown in Figure 7.13.

3 Calculating the risks

Risks can be quoted as odds (one in four) or as percentages (25%). It must be remembered that many people do not have a clear understanding of either of these.

There is a variety of types of risk.

A Empiric risks

These are based on observed data and are used for chromosomal and multifactorial disorders and for heterogeneous disorders such as severe osteogenesis imperfecta in which the same phenotype may have different underlying genetic mechanisms.

B Mendelian risks

These were given above in the section on mendelian inheritance.

C Modified risks

These involve using conditional information to alter a prior risk. An example is shown in Figure 7.24.

D Risk estimates from independent evidence

These include results of investigations. An example is given in Figure 7.25.

E Communicating the risks to the patient

Risks must be put into perspective. Since about 2% of babies are born with some serious handicap, 2% can be considered as a low risk. Mendelian risks of 25% and 50% are high risks. A risk of around 10% is a moderate risk. Perception of magnitude of risk is, however, a personal matter because, strictly speaking, risk combines the probability of occurrence and the degree of damage, the latter often being a highly subjective evaluation.

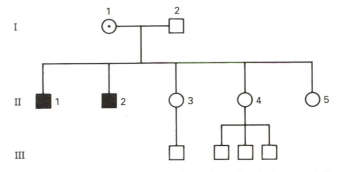

Figure 7.24 An example of a modified risk. Individuals II1 and II2 have Duchenne muscular dystrophy. Their mother (I1) is an obligate carrier. Her daughters (II3, II4 and II5) each have a 1 in 2 chance of being a carrier. This risk is modified in II3 and II4 by the fact that they have normal sons. Their modified risks are 1 in 3 (for II3) and 1 in 9 (for II4), derived using Bayes theorem.

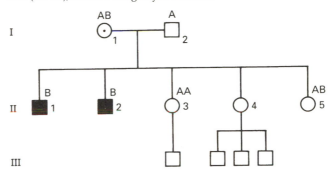

Figure 7.25 Risks from independent evidence. Continuing the example from Figure 7.24, if II3 has three normal plasma creatine kinase levels, her risk of being a carrier falls from 1 in 3 to 1 in 9 (using a standardized table). Using linked DNA markers, the maternal X chromosomes can be differentiated and may be labelled A and B. The paternal X chromosome is labelled A. Individual II3 has inherited the maternal A chromosome, whereas her affected brothers have inherited the maternal B chromosome. In this family, the Duchenne muscular dystrophy gene is tracking with the B allele. The result lowers II3's carrier risk from 1 in 9 to 1 in 160. (This figure takes into account a 5% risk of recombination between the mutation and the DNA marker.) Her risk of having a son with the disease is 1 in 320, a low risk. Conversely, individual II5 has a high (95%) risk of being a carrier. She could be offered a prenatal test (see Figure 7.26).

It is important not only to try to give risk information in a non-directive manner but also actively to seek out and correct common misapprehensions. For example, many people believe that the lack of a positive family history indicates that a disorder is unlikely to be genetic. This is untrue, since what seems a sporadic case may represent an autosomal recessive disorder, a fresh mutation for an X-linked or autosomal dominant disorder, a multifactorial condition or a chromosomal abnormality. A pitfall encountered in the understanding of mendelian risks is that the risk applies to each pregnancy; parents may wrongly assume that in autosomal recessive inheritance, for example, if they have one affected child, then the next three will be healthy. In multifactorial inheritance, however, the risks are reassessed as being higher if a second affected child is born.

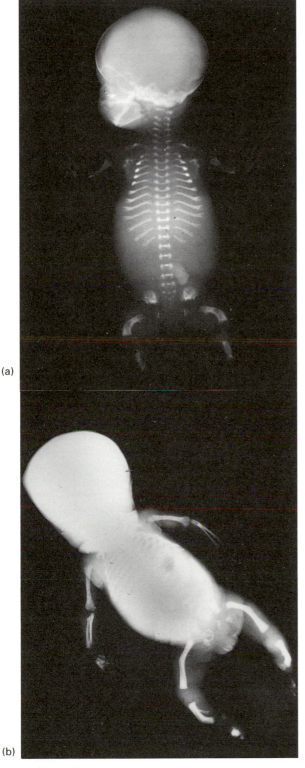

(a)

(b)

Figure 7.23 (a) A radiograph of a baby with thanatophoric dysplasia. Note the H-shaped vertebral bodies, the short horizontal ribs and the telephone-receiver-shaped femora in the anteroposterior view. (b) A radiograph of a baby with camptomelic dysplasia. Note the characteristic congenital bowing and angulation of the long bones in the legs. Reproduced from Baraitser and Winter[8] with permission.

4 Discussing the options

The options range from ignoring the risk, to deciding not to have any or more children. In between are other possibilities, such as adoption, insemination by donor and ovum donation. Prenatal diagnosis and termination of affected fetuses is another alternative which is becoming available for an increasing number of disorders. Preimplantation diagnosis may also become available in the future, as may gene therapy, that is, treatment of a genetic disorder by replacing the defective gene with a normally functioning one. Although a number of trials are taking place, it is likely that it will be some time before gene therapy is widely available.

One of the few examples of preconceptional prevention of an abnormal fetus concerns neural tube defects. There is evidence that the risk of recurrence for a woman with one affected child is reduced if she takes periconceptual folate supplements. It is unknown whether this can be applied to the general population.

The decision as to which option to take depends upon a number of factors, such as magnitude of the risk, severity of the disorder, availability of treatment, the individual's personal experience of the disorder, the mother's age, family size, ethical and moral considerations about abortion and the ability of the family to cope with another affected child.

5 Support, follow-up and genetic registers

The impact of genetic disorders on families is considerable and frequently involves guilt, anger, anxiety and sadness. Appropriate support should be arranged to be carried out by the counsellor or by colleagues such as specialist health visitors who are often members of genetic centres. Referral to appropriate lay support groups should also be offered.

Follow-up is needed to ensure that the information has been understood and remembered correctly and to update the family on any important advances in research which may have practical implications for them.

Genetic registers, compiled mainly on a regional basis, are becoming increasingly important means of fulfilling the functions of ensuring adequate support and follow up and of calling up family members at appropriate times. For example, predictive testing for Huntington's disease using DNA probes is not offered to children. At the age of 18 years, an individual at risk should be offered the opportunity to discuss the risk, with appropriate consent. A register provides a means of prompting the appropriate referral.

DNA analysis for genetic counselling

DNA analysis can be used to:

1 Clarify carrier risks of female relatives of a male with certain X-linked disorders, such as Duchenne and Becker muscular dystrophy and haemophilia A and B.

2 Detect carriers of some autosomal recessive disorders, such as cystic fibrosis, the thalassaemias and sickle cell disease.

3 Perform pre-symptomatic tests for individuals at risk of some autosomal dominant disorders, such as Huntington's disease, myotonic dystrophy, adult polycystic kidney disease, osteogenesis imperfecta and neurofibromatosis.

4 Perform prenatal tests (also see section on prenatal diagnosis).

Broadly speaking, there are two main ways in which the DNA tests are done:

1 DNA markers

DNA markers (restriction fragment length polymorphisms or RFLPs) are used to 'track' the disease gene through a family. The DNA marker might be within the gene in question (intragenic), or just outside it but very close to it (a linked marker). At meiosis, there is the chance that the disease mutation and the marker might become separated because of the process of recombination. There is therefore a small risk of an inaccurate result, which is usually no more than 5% if the marker is to be used for diagnosis. This applies more to linked rather than intragenic markers for which the risk of recombination is usually virtually zero. If, however, the disease gene is very large, as is the dystrophin (Duchenne) gene, there is a chance of recombination between an intragenic DNA marker and the actual mutation in the gene, of about 5%. Examples of the use of DNA analysis for carrier detection and prenatal diagnosis of Duchenne muscular dystrophy are given in Figures 7.25 and 7.26.

2 Actual mutation detection

The actual mutation can be detected by various methods. This means that the result of the test is very accurate. Figure 7.27 shows an example of prenatal diagnosis for cystic fibrosis, detecting the most common cystic fibrosis mutation, ΔF508. Recently, the mutation which causes the fragile X syndrome was identified,[9] which allows more accurate carrier detection and prenatal diagnosis in affected families. It consists of a highly repeated DNA sequence (a CGG trinucleotide) whose copy number varies, even in normal individuals. Carrier females and 'normal transmitting males' show an unusually increased number of copies of the sequence, which is evident on DNA testing as a small fragment of DNA inserted in the gene. Affected males and some carrier females show a large insert in the gene which represents an even greater number of copies of the sequence. It has also been noted that the size of the insert may become greater

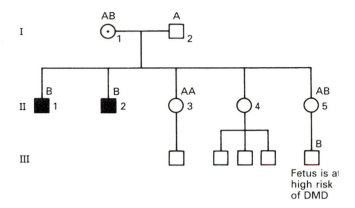

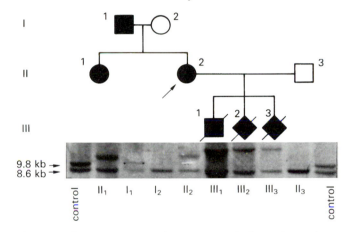

as the mutation is transmitted from one generation to the next. Similarly, the mutation which causes myotonic dystrophy has recently been discovered and involves unstable DNA. It is well recognized that this autosomal dominant disorder demonstrates 'anticipation', i.e. the clinical severity in affected individuals can increase in successive generations of a family. The mutation is a highly repeated DNA sequence (a CTG trinucleotide).[10] The number of copies of the sequence may increase as the gene is transmitted to offspring and an increased number of copies of the sequence is associated with worse clinical effects, thus providing an explanation for the phenomenon of anticipation (Fig. 7.28). These 'unstable trinucleotide – repeat expansion' mutations have emerged as a new class of human mutation, and occur not only in fragile X and myotonic dystrophy, but also Huntington's disease[11] and others.

No attempt is made in this section to describe the technical details of DNA analysis; an excellent account

Figure 7.26 Prenatal diagnosis of Duchenne muscular dystrophy (DMD) using intragenic DNA markers. Individual II5 has a high (95%) risk of being a carrier (see Fig. 7.25). Her two X chromosomes are identifiable using the DNA markers, therefore she can be offered a prenatal test, by chorion villous sampling. If a male fetus has inherited the maternal A allele, there is a low (5%) risk of DMD. Conversely, if a male fetus has inherited the maternal B allele, there is a high (90%) risk of DMD. (These figures take into account the 5% possibility of recombination at meiosis between the mutation and the DNA marker.)

Figure 7.28 Direct mutation analysis in myotonic dystrophy, to show that the clinical phenomenon of 'anticipation' correlates with increase copy number of a CTG trinucleotide sequence in the gene. The upper part of the diagram shows the pedigree, the lower part the results of DNA analysis. (Each individual's DNA result lies directly below the pedigree symbol). The DNA has been digested with the enzyme ECORI and probed with the p5B1.4 probe. In the first and last lanes are control DNA from normal individuals who are heterozygous, showing a lower 8.6 kb band and an upper 9.8 kb band. The former indicates no amplification of the CTG trinucleotide sequence, the latter shows that there are less than 30 repeats of the CTG sequence, which is in the normal range.

Individual I1 has only mild symptoms of myotonic dystrophy. His DNA shows the normal lower 8.6 kb band and an amplified upper band, indicating 260 repeats of the CTG sequence. His daughters, II1 and II2 have classical myotonic dystrophy. They both have the normal 8.6 kb lower band and amplified upper bands indicating 530 and 660 repeats of the CTG sequence, respectively. The child of II2, namely III3, died from congenital myotonic dystrophy. He had a normal lower 8.6 kb band and a greatly enlarged upper band, indicating more than 1100 copies of the CTG sequence. Fetuses III2 and III3 were similarly affected.

This diagram illustrates how the clinical severity of myotonic dystrophy can increase down the generations ('anticipation'). The number of copies of the CTG sequence in the gene can increase with transmission to offspring, and increased copy numbers are associated with greater clinical severity. Courtesy Dr Keith Johnson.

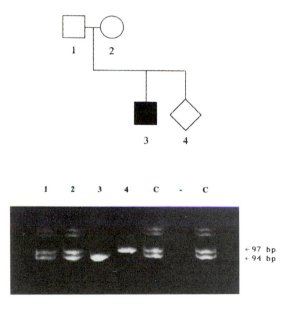

Figure 7.27 Use of direct mutation analysis in the prenatal diagnosis of cystic fibrosis. The upper part of the diagram shows a family with a son with cystic fibrosis (3) and a fetus (4). The lower part of the diagram shows the results of DNA analysis. DNA flanking the common 3 base-pair (bp) deletion (ΔF508) has been amplified by a process known as the polymerase chain reaction (PCR) and the fragments resolved on a 12% polyacrylamide gel. The normal allele is 97 bp and the mutant allele is 94 bp. The family can be offered a prenatal diagnosis as the parents (lanes 1 and 2) are heterozygous for the 97 and 94 bp fragments and the affected son (lane 3) is homozygous for the mutant (94 bp) allele. The chorion villus sample (the fetus, lane 4) is homozygous for the normal (97 bp) allele, so is predicted to be unaffected. Clearly it is important to investigate the family before a pregnancy. (The lanes labelled 'C' are control samples from known heterozygotes and the lane labelled '-' contains no DNA. The two bands above the 97 and 94 bp bands in the carriers are called heteroduplexes which arise as a result of the PCR.) (Courtesy of Dr Carolyn Williams.)

of these and their clinical application is given by Weatherall.[12]

It is important to mention that, at the present time, there is a move away from performing presymptomatic and carrier tests in children, unless there would be a direct clinical benefit to the child. This is to enable each individual to be able to take such a test with informed consent (which a child cannot give) and to avoid any unnecessary stigmatization of a child.

Prenatal diagnosis

1 General comments

Prenatal diagnosis may allow therapy to be undertaken *in utero* (for example, fetal blood transfusion in rhesus allo-immunization) or soon after birth (for example, if a fetus is found to have a treatable malformation on ultrasound scans). More often, the aim of prenatal diagnosis of an abnormal fetus is to allow the parents the option of terminating the pregnancy. Conversely, a negative diagnosis in a fetus at risk allows the pregnancy to continue with reduced parental anxiety.

Prenatal diagnosis is performed in pregnancies at risk, identified either through a positive family history or through screening carried out either before or during pregnancy. Ideally, any risk factors should be identified before a pregnancy occurs, not only because it is difficult for couples to evaluate objectively new information once pregnancy has begun, but also because prenatal diagnosis of many mendelian disorders by DNA techniques requires a family study, which may take considerable time. Certain important factors must be considered before prenatal diagnosis is contemplated:

1 Severity of the disorder. Prenatal diagnosis is presently mainly carried out if there is a risk of a severe disorder, i.e. one which causes early death or multiple physical handicaps or mental handicap.
2 Degree of genetic risk. Invasive prenatal tests are mainly reserved for pregnancies at high risk. However, due consideration must be given to the fact that a prenatal test in a low-risk pregnancy generally reduces parental anxiety.
3 Lack of availability of satisfactory treatment.
4 Availability of a reliable prenatal test.

From the counselling aspect, it is very important to discuss with the couple requesting prenatal diagnosis the following points, again preferably before a pregnancy:

1 When in the pregnancy the particular test can be done.
2 How the test is done.
3 What the risks are to mother and baby arising from the test.

4 When the results can be expected to be available.
5 The accuracy of the test. For many mendelian disorders, linked DNA markers are used to make the diagnosis and there is a small (usually no more than 5%) error rate in the result.
6 Acceptability of termination of pregnancy. This issue must be discussed specifically. Some couples requesting prenatal diagnosis, on specific questioning, would not in fact terminate an affected pregnancy, for religious or moral reasons. Many of these couples have not considered that there may be risks to the pregnancy arising from the test. In the past, prenatal tests were sometimes denied to couples who would not terminate a pregnancy, on the grounds that it was unreasonable to put a potentially normal fetus at risk of miscarriage following the test if an abnormal fetus were not to be aborted. Presently, however, it is often considered reasonable to carry out a prenatal test in this situation to allow the parents to be prepared for the birth of an affected child. Sometimes couples who had intended to abort an affected fetus change their minds when given a positive prenatal test result.

2 Types of prenatal test

The main methods of prenatal diagnosis which are currently available are shown in Table 7.25, along with the timing and risks.

A Amniocentesis

The main indications are measurement of α-fetoprotein (AFP) concentration and acetylcholinesterase activity in pregnancies at risk of neural tube defects (but see ultrasonography below) and chromosomal analysis of cultured amniotic cells in pregnancies at risk of chromosomal defects. The latter include women of advanced maternal age, women with a raised risk of having a child with Down syndrome based on serum

Table 7.25 Methods of prenatal diagnosis, usual post-menstrual age when carried out and approximate risks of miscarriage

Method	Post-menstrual age (weeks)	Risk (%)*
Amniocentesis	14–17	0.5–1
Chorion villus sampling (CVS)	>9	2–4
Fetal blood sampling	>18	1–7
Ultrasonography	18–19**	–

*Depends upon the experience of the operator.
**Detailed 'anomaly' scans are usually done at this time but level 1 scans are done in the first trimester (see text).
After Table 7, Royal College of Physicians Report.[1]

AFP (and other) levels, couples who have had a child with a chromosome defect and couples in whom one partner carries a balanced chromosome defect. In specific cases, biochemical analysis of amniotic fluid or cultured cells may be required to diagnose inborn errors of metabolism. Results may take up to 10 days for tests on amniotic fluid and up to 4 weeks for tests on cultured cells.

B Chorion villous sampling

This is used for diagnosing chromosomal abnormalities, and an increasing number of inborn errors of metabolism and disorders in which DNA analysis is possible. Common examples of the latter include:

adult polycystic kidney disease
cystic fibrosis
Duchenne and Becker muscular dystrophy
haemoglobinopathies
haemophilia A and B
Huntington's disease
myotonic dystrophy

DNA analysis may involve the use of linked or intragenic DNA markers (see Fig. 7.26), or the actual mutation may be detectable. If, for example, both parents are known carriers of the ΔF508 cystic fibrosis mutation, then this can be looked for in the chorion villous sample, and an accurate result given (see Fig. 7.27).

C Fetal blood sampling

This involves aspiration of fetal blood from the umbilical cord (cordocentesis) under ultrasound guidance. Chromosome analysis of a fetal blood sample may be required in order to clarify an ambiguous chromosome result from amniocentesis. Examination for fragile X was mainly carried out on fetal blood samples but since the discovery of the fragile X gene chorion villous samples are now being used.

D Ultrasonography

Most pregnant women in the UK have a basic (level 1) scan in the first or second trimester. This is primarily to determine gestational age together with fetal viability and number. This type of routine scan will not detect fetal malformations, unless they are gross, as in anencephaly. In some hospitals, level 2 (anomaly) scans are offered routinely at around 18–19 weeks' gestation. These are usually carried out by consultants and can detect a wide range of malformations, including congenital heart defects, clefts of the lip and palate, and microphthalmia. Level 3 scans are carried out in a few specialist centres by experts who can not only detect malformations but also carry out procedures such as fetal blood sampling. Observations of the first trimester

fetus are also becoming possible. Any woman at risk of having a child with a malformation should be referred for a good level 2 or level 3 anomaly scan, at the appropriate time.

It is argued that an expert anomaly scan alone is sufficient to diagnose neural tube defects.

To date, there is no evidence that diagnostic ultrasonography is associated with any risk to the fetus, with the exception that a normal pregnancy may be terminated after a false-positive diagnosis of a serious structural abnormality by an inexperienced operator.

E Preimplantation and oocyte diagnosis

These methods are being developed. Preimplantation diagnosis involves biochemical or DNA analysis on a single cell (blastomere) from an eight-cell embryo *in vitro*. The unaffected embryo is then replaced into the mother.[13] In oocyte diagnosis, the first polar body is subjected to DNA analysis, to allow identification of oocytes which are not carrying a particular autosomal recessive gene, so that these may be used for fertilization by the partner's sperm.[14] These procedures have been made possible by a new technique called polymerase chain reaction (PCR) which amplifies small amounts of DNA.

Population screening for genetic and congenital disorders

A simple screening process which is underused in primary care is the taking of a detailed family history before pregnancy. This is an important means of identifying some couples at genetic risk. At present, the family history is often not taken until a pregnancy occurs or its value is limited by the lack of knowledge of genetics in primary health care workers. Improved genetic education for doctors and other primary health care professionals is greatly needed.

Many genetic disorders occur in the absence of a positive family history. Some are amenable to detection through population screening programmes, described as follows.

1 Carrier detection for autosomal recessive disorders

Carrier couples should be identified by screening of populations known to be at risk, preferably before a pregnancy, so that those at high risk may choose from the available options. Examples include haemoglobin disorders in people of Mediterranean or Asian origin, sickle-cell disorders in people of African or Afro-Caribbean origin, and Tay-Sachs disease in people of Ashkenazi Jewish descent. Table 7.26 shows the various carrier frequencies. In southern Europe,

Table 7.26 Screening for carriers in ethnic groups: carrier frequencies

Disease	Ethnic origin	Carrier frequency (%)
Thalassaemias	Mediterranean or Asian	3–17
Sickle-cell disorders	African or Afro-Caribbean	8–25
Tay-Sachs	Ashkenazi Jewish	3–5
Cystic fibrosis	Northern European	4

comprehensive thalassaemia control programmes have been organized which have almost eradicated this common, severe inherited disease. In north-west Europe, including the UK, there has been a much smaller reduction in the birth incidence of thalassaemia because of the difficulties in establishing a comprehensive programme for diverse ethnic minorities.

In 1989 the gene which causes cystic fibrosis and its most common mutation, ΔF508, were identified. The latter is found in about three-quarters of British CF carriers. Now, many more mutations in the CF gene have been discovered, and at least 85% of carriers can be detected by direct gene mutation analysis. This means that soon it will be possible to offer population screening for cystic fibrosis, and it is important to consider the implications of such screening. For example, when should tests be carried out? The possibilities are at birth, in secondary school, at the family planning clinic, or in the antenatal clinic. Pilot studies are being carried out to determine public attitudes to such testing.

2   Congenital malformations and chromosomal disorders

At present, most babies with congenital malformations and chromosomal disorders in the UK are born to healthy young women with no previously identifiable risk factors. As it is not possible at present to prevent such conceptions, the only means of detecting these disorders is by population screening during pregnancy. The main disorders which can be screened for are:

Neural tube defects

A raised maternal serum α-fetoprotein (AFP) level at 16–18 weeks' gestation indicates a risk of a neural tube defect (and other fetal abnormalities such as anterior abdominal wall defect, bowel atresias and skin defects), and should lead to an expert (level 3) scan. Amniocentesis for measurement of amniotic AFP and acetylcholinesterase (which shows an extra specific band in open neural tube defects) may also be considered. About 80% of cases of open neural tube defect and over 98% of cases of anencephaly can be detected

by maternal AFP screening, but in as many as 50% of pregnancies with a raised serum AFP level, no cause is found, either prenatally or postnatally.

Down syndrome

If all mothers aged 36 years or more had amniocentesis, 30% of all Down syndrome pregnancies would be detected. In practice, less than 15% are detected, because fewer than half of the older mothers actually have an amniocentesis. A lowered maternal serum AFP at around 16 weeks' gestation indicates a risk of Down syndrome. It has been suggested that if a combination of maternal age, serum levels of AFP, human chorionic gonadotrophin and unconjugated oestriol were used, it might be possible to detect over 60% of Down syndrome pregnancies.[15] At present, this is available as a screening programme in some centres.

Other malformations

Level 2 and 3 ultrasound scans are offered in only some hospitals routinely. Under optimal conditions, it has been shown that systematic level 2 scans carried out by trained and supervised midwives, radiographers or technicians, can detect about 80% of major structural anomalies. Since over 90% of congenital malformations occur in pregnancies not at a recognizable risk, the only way to detect these is to offer skilled level 2 scanning to every pregnant woman. This carries significant resource implications.

3   Requirements for screening programmes

There are a number of requirements for effective screening programmes:

1 The tests should be safe, simple and cheap.
2 The tests should be able to give a clear result, with a minimum of false positives and negatives.
3 Adequate counselling by trained personnel should be available at all stages of testing, i.e. before the test to ensure that the individual gives informed consent to having the test and after the test, so that the individual understands the implication of both a negative and a positive result. Additional support will be required in the event of a positive test result.
4 The tests should be widely and routinely available, and those for whom the tests are intended should be aware of them through community education programmes.
5 The benefits of the tests should outweigh the costs, in material and human terms.
6 The disorder being screened for should be clearly identifiable and serious.

At present, population screening has great potential but is underused. In the future, it is to be hoped that well-coordinated community screening programmes will be developed, involving professionals in primary health care, paediatricians, obstetricians, and clinical geneticists.

References

1 Royal College of Physicians. *Prenatal Diagnosis and Genetic Screening: Community and Service Implications.* London: RCP, 1989.

2 Modell, B. Cystic fibrosis screening and community genetics. *J Med Genet* 1990; **27:** 475–479.

3 Harper, P.S. *Practical Genetic Counselling.* 3rd edn. London: Wright, 1988.

4 McKusick, V.A. *Mendelian Inheritance in Man: Catalogs of Autosomal Dominant, Autosomal Recessive and X-linked Phenotypes.* 9th edn. Baltimore: Johns Hopkins University Press, 1990.

5 Harding, A.E. The mitochondrial genome: breaking the magic circle. *New Engl J Med* 1989; **320:** 1341–1343.

6 Hall, J.G. Imprinting: review and relevance to human disease. *Am J Hum Genet* 1990; **46:** 857–873.

7 Winter, R.M., Baraitser, M. *Multiple Congenital Anomalies: a Diagnostic Compendium.* London: Chapman and Hall Medical, 1990.

8 Baraitser, M., Winter, R. *A Colour Atlas of Clinical Genetics.* London: Wolfe Medical Publications, 1983.

9 Yu, S., Pritchard, M., Kremer, E. *et al.* Fragile X genotype characterized by an unstable region of DNA. *Science* 1991; **252:** 1179–1181.

10 Harley, H.G., Brook, J.D., Rundle, S.A. *et al.* Expansion of an unstable DNA region and phenotypic variation in myotonic dystrophy. *Nature* 1992; **335:** 545–546.

11 Huntington's Disease Collaborative Research Group. A novel gene containing a trinucleotide repeat that is expanded and unstable on Huntington's disease chromosomes. *Cell* 1993; **72:** 971–983.

12 Weatherall, D.J. *The New Genetics and Clinical Practice,* 3rd edn. Oxford: Oxford Medical Publications, 1991.

13 Handyside, A.H., Kontogianni, E.H., Hardy, K., Winston, R.M.L. Pregnancies from biopsied human preimplantation embryos sexed by Y-specific DNA amplification. *Nature* 1990; **334:** 768–770.

14 Monk, M., Holding, C. Amplification of a B-haemoglobin sequence in individual human oocytes and polar bodies. *Lancet* 1990; i: 985–988.

15 Wald, N.J., Cuckle, H.S., Densem, J.W., *et al.* Maternal serum screening for Down's syndrome in early pregnancy. *Br Med J* 1988; **297:** 883–887.

Acknowledgement

The author wishes to thank Professor Marcus Pembrey for reading the manuscript and for helpful comments.

7.12 The environment and child health

Jean Golding

Introduction

A dictionary definition of environment is 'the condition or influences under which any person or thing lives or is developed'. Much epidemiology is concerned with trying to identify those features of the environment that influence health, yet the measures used are largely indirect. There are strong associations between various childhood conditions and social class, maternal age, family size, paternal unemployment, area of the country or type of housing, yet identification of such associations is merely a clue as to possible mechanisms. It is all too easy to describe a low social class association as the adverse effect of social deprivation; the causal factor in the association may merely be some identifiable substance to which those social classes are more likely to be exposed such as a particular hair dye or the method of brewing tea. Consequently, although the known associations with indirect markers such as social class are interesting, they will not be considered further in this section. Rather, I shall concentrate on specific environmental features and their (mainly intrauterine) effects.

An unknown, but probably large, proportion of childhood mortality, morbidity and disability has antecedents in the prenatal period or earlier. The major natural causes of childhood mortality include the consequences of preterm delivery, sudden infant death syndrome, congenital defects, and childhood cancer. All are strongly associated with prenatal factors, most of which may be described as environmental.

Congenital defects and childhood cancer may have similar aetiologies. With the rapid advances in genetics, many of our ideas concerning mutation and teratogenesis have been discarded. The mechanisms involved concern either an effect on the DNA such that a gene mutation (deletion) occurs and is then replicated, or an effect on the DNA which is repaired after a short period of time, but not before the development of a particular system of the developing embryo has been knocked off course, or a direct effect on particular enzymes or proteins. The potential for damaging effects has logically to be greatest during the time of maximum embryonic growth and this occurs at different gestations for different systems. It seems likely that very low doses of toxins reaching the fetus may be far more harmful than the same doses reaching the young child.

Ionizing radiation

Ionizing radiation may result in damage to a chromosome, including gene deletion or mutation; death of a cell (when this cell is in an early embryo it may be in a crucial phase of development); or activation or release of an endogenous virus.

Estimates of possible adverse effects of ionizing radiation until very recently have concerned: animal experiments with high doses over short periods of time, usually involving rodents; observational studies of atomic bomb survivors; studies of exposed groups such as thorotrast patients, radium dial painters and uranium miners occupationally exposed to radon; studies of people exposed to X-rays; or investigation of clustering of leukaemia around nuclear power stations. The focus of these studies has been cancer and other possible outcomes have been largely ignored.

Radiation can reach the human in the following ways: as natural radiation including radon, and as man-made radiation including X-rays, atomic bomb fall out, power stations and nuclear waste discharge. In general the dose received from natural sources far exceeds that from man-made ones.

Children in utero in Nagasaki and Hiroshima at the time the atomic bombs were dropped and who received a high dose of radiation had an increased risk of infant mortality compared with children receiving low doses.[1] More recently, a study in West Germany examined the secular trends in infant mortality over time and showed an upward swing in 1986. This may have been related to the increased levels of radiation due to the Chernobyl accident since the increase was greater in areas with higher levels of fall out.[2]

Animal experiments have shown that radiation may cause malformations of the heart by temporarily affecting the genetic make-up. For example Ikeda[3] showed that immediately after an acute dose of radiation to the embryonic heart, the lactic dehydrogenase (LDH) isoenzyme pattern was altered, but that this had returned to normal within 6 days. He suggested that temporal effects of normal gene expression consequent upon radiation damage may be responsible for the resulting malformation. Parental pre-pregnancy X-rays have also been shown to relate to congenital defects in animals.[4]

In humans, mothers of children with Down syndrome have been shown to have had, on average, higher doses of X-rays involving the gonads prior to conception than controls.[5,6] Three studies have tried to assess whether high *natural* radiation doses may be associated with increased rates of congenital defects.[7–9] Major problems were: unwarranted assumptions were made concerning the calculation of gonad dose; no account was taken of the dose from radon; and there was probably differential under-reporting. Consequently the inconsistent results are difficult to interpret. In the one study which had a reasonably believable rate for Down syndrome (over 1 per 1000), a positive relationship was found with background gamma radiation.[9]

Animal experiments have also indicated that irradiation in utero results in fetal growth retardation.[10] No epidemiological studies have been carried out to assess effects of natural radiation on humans. A study of women treated in childhood for Wilms' tumour found that of their subsequent pregnancies almost one-third ended in perinatal death or low birthweight if treatment had involved radiation, but no such adverse effect was present in mothers who had only had chemotherapy.[11] Animal experiments have shown an effect on postnatal growth when low level X-rays were given in pregnancy.[12] No assessment has been carried out of postnatal growth in humans exposed to natural radiation, but there was certainly a marked reduction in growth among survivors of prenatal exposure to the atomic bombs.[13]

Animal experiments have shown that low-level radiation at different developmental periods results in specific lesions in the brain resulting in structural and functional abnormality.[14] Animal experiments have also shown marked changes in both maternal and infant behaviour after exposure to radiation.[15,16] No behaviour studies exist to assess whether humans exposed to high levels of natural radiation behave abnormally. An increase in severe mental retardation rates was identified following the atomic bombs dropped on Hiroshima and Nagasaki. Infants who were in utero and at gestations between 9 and 25 weeks were most at risk. A recent review found no evidence for any threshold effect and indicated that there was a linear association between radiation dose and risk of mental retardation.[17]

Much energy has been devoted to showing that cases of childhood leukaemia cluster together in space and that some of these clusters occur near nuclear power stations.[18] There are, however, higher than expected rates of childhood leukaemia in areas where power stations were planned but not built,[19] and in isolated but rapidly growing towns.[20] There is a cluster of childhood leukaemia cases near the nuclear reprocessing plant at Sellafield, which has clearly been shown to relate to children born in the area but not to children moving to the area later in childhood,[21] and a strong relationship to paternal occupational exposure.[22]

The seminal work of Alice Stewart showed increased rates of childhood cancer after maternal X-ray in pregnancy.[23] The atomic bomb data had, however, shown no increase in rates of subsequent childhood cancer among those in utero at the time of the explosion.[1] This has been thought to relate to the increased mortality in the first year in children who would otherwise have developed cancer.

Various studies have confirmed the association between subsequent childhood cancer and fetal X-rays. Only two have assessed whether high levels of natural radiation are associated with an increased risk: one showed a cluster of T-cell leukaemia in an area of high natural radiation near Vesuvius,[24] and a study which related the incidence of childhood cancer in 12 countries to average radon levels found a strong positive correlation ($r = 0.78$, $p < 0.01$).[25]

Electromagnetic radiation

The possibility that electromagnetic radiation may have adverse effects on human health has only been raised in the past decade. There are electromagnetic fields wherever there is electric power. The major focus of attention, especially in the USA, has been the fields underneath overhead power transmission cables. Nevertheless, other types of exposure are likely to result in higher electromagnetic field exposure to the bulk of the human population. The most important of these is likely to be the electric blanket. This results in a surface electric field that is higher than that found in any house near a 500Kv power line.[26] Although electromagnetic radiation is referred to as though it is one form of radiation, it is actually composed of two separate radiations: electric radiation which is less able to pass through solid objects; thus residents of a house situated near a power line will only receive 10% of the electric radiation that they would receive if they were to stand outside the house; and magnetic radiation which is not stopped by solid objects, so that the magnetic radiation within a house due to an overhead power cable will be almost identical to that outside. Since very few people live or work near transmission lines, the major sources of electric and magnetic radiation are electric blankets and other household appliances.[26]

The field of childhood cancer has received most attention in respect of electromagnetic fields. Studies have varied in the reliability of the data and the suitability of controls. In general they have been related to the electric wiring configurations in the home. Wertheimer and Leeper[27] in Colorado first showed a positive association with high current configuration and a dose response gradient. This was not confirmed on Rhode Island[28] or in Yorkshire.[29] A study in Stockholm, however, showed more electrical constructions within 150 metres of index homes.[30] A much more recent and more thorough study has been carried out by Savitz and colleagues in Denver.[31] Although they were unable to show any association with electric blanket or heated water bed use during pregnancy, there was a dose responsive relationship between the small number of soft tissue tumours in childhood and the number of different electrical appliances used by the mother during pregnancy.[32] It should be noted, however, that this was not statistically significant. Among children, electric blanket use was associated with increased risk of all cancers.

A further study by Wertheimer and Leeper[33] examined more immediate adverse effects of electric blanket and heated water bed use during pregnancy. By comparing a group of women who used such appliances with those who did not, they have shown evidence of elevated preterm delivery rates in mothers using the electric appliances. For the mothers who used such appliances the effects varied with the season of the year, peaking during the winter months; for the non-users there were no such seasonal effects.

Noise

Although largely ignored, noise can be a health hazard in several ways: it can damage hearing permanently; animal experiments have suggested that specific genes may make one animal more susceptible to noise-induced hearing loss than another; it can mask a child's cries or attempts at communication, which may have long-term psychological consequences or even be disastrous in the short-term such as when a child is calling for help; it can affect a child indirectly through distress caused to the parents by external noise.

In both animals and humans it has been shown that high noise levels result in increased cortisol production which leads to increased blood glucose and altered immune reactions. Short-term exposure to noise results in an increase in blood pressure, as well as anxiety.[34] One study of children whose mothers were employed in noisy occupations during pregnancy showed a strong relationship with increasing risk of hearing loss the more noisy the work situation.[35] No studies of possible adverse effects of noise on the young child have yet been carried out other than those which concerned the effect of incubator noise on very preterm infants. Nevertheless, with massive hi-fi systems and the ubiquitous Walkman, children are becoming more and more exposed to very high noise levels. The long-term physical and psychological consequences should be assessed.

Toxic metals

Lead

Lead is the trace element most widely studied in relation to health and development. Lead is toxic; it accumulates in the body and is preferentially stored in bone. It derives in particular from water pipes, household dust, traffic exhaust,[36] diet, alcohol and cigarettes.[37] In Britain, Asian mothers from the Indian subcontinent are particularly prone to high levels of lead due to its presence in *surma*, the cosmetic applied to the eyelids.[38]

Basic biological effects of lead include its competition with calcium for binding sites. This is clearly demonstrated in bone where lead accumulates, but it may be even more important metabolically in the mitochondria[39] which are very sensitive to changes in calcium flux. Other elements which are replaced by lead include zinc, magnesium, copper, iron and iodine – deficiencies of all of which have possible adverse effects.

The placenta has been shown to act only as a slight barrier for the transfer of lead to the fetus.[40] The metal crosses this barrier as early as the twelfth week of gestation.[41] Studies of women occupationally exposed to lead have shown high miscarriage rates.[41] One study of women residing in a high lead exposure area found high rates of premature rupture of the membranes (17%) and high rates of preterm delivery (13%) compared with controls in the rest of the region.[42]

Perinatal deaths have, on average, higher levels of lead in the placenta and this might relate to increased exposure.[43] In stillbirths, Bryce-Smith reports lead levels in ribs and vertebrae some 5–10 times that of controls,[39] but the controls were totally inappropriate. More satisfactory data, however, concern preterm delivery: in France, maternal hair lead[44] and in Glasgow maternal blood[45] were negatively related to the duration of gestation.

Once the child is born, he is still at risk of exposure. Although breast milk only has one-tenth the lead concentration of maternal blood, this can nevertheless result in ingestion of considerable amounts.[45]

Other ways in which the infant or child may be exposed to lead vary with age. At 6 months in Cincinnati, for example, exposure relates to the diet.[46] At 18 months half the variance in blood lead was accounted for by characteristics of the housing – public housing being associated with the lowest levels. At 2 years the most significant predictor of blood lead in Boston was the level of lead in the house dust, the season and the amount of specific home improvements that had taken place such as sanding, scraping, painting.[47,48]

In New York, children with high blood levels were compared with controls to see whence the excess lead derived – the major differences were in levels of lead in house dust and the amount of lead on the hands.[49]

Another American study showed that the daily amount of lead in children's diets varied from 15 to 234 μg, the biggest contributors being canned fruit, vegetables and fruit juices.[50]

Much controversy has surrounded the possibility that high blood lead levels in childhood may be responsible for behaviour disorders and reduction in IQ. Cross-sectional studies that showed positive correlations were often unable to distinguish cause from effect – children with behaviour problems or mental retardation often exhibit pica and hence may ingest high doses of lead. Nevertheless, animal evidence is worrying. A study of rabbit pups fed various doses of lead showed a marked increase in brain lesions with high doses, lesions of the cerebellum with moderate doses and hyperactivity with mild doses.[51]

The British cross-sectional human data include four major studies. One from Edinburgh showed linear negative associations between the blood lead levels of children aged 6 to 9 years and IQ (BAS score), reading ability, number skills and matrices score. The authors found no evidence of a threshold effect.[52] Tooth lead in a study in Southampton showed a negative relationship with IQ in boys but not in girls.[53] One study of a population living adjacent to a lead smelter found no association between IQ and blood lead, but numbers with high lead levels were small.[54] Yule examined 166 children aged between 6 and 12 years living near a lead works. There were negative associations with reading, spelling and IQ scores but not with mathematics.[55] These differences remained after allowing for social class.

A comparison in New York of children with mild or borderline mental retardation and controls showed that for those children with known aetiology there was no difference in blood lead but those children with mental retardation of unknown aetiology had elevated blood lead.[56] A study comparing 26 children with dyslexia with sex and age matched controls showed marked differences in trace element status including elevated lead in both the sytems tested (sweat and hair).[57]

Prospective studies also confirm these effects. One from Boston identified three groups of children with low (<10th centile), medium (10th–90th centile) and high (>90th centile) cord blood levels. At 6 months, after allowing for various factors, there was a strong negative association with mental development[58] using the Bayley scale. Further follow-up examinations at ages 12, 18 and 24 months showed that the mental development index related best to the cord blood lead rather than the later blood lead levels.[59] There was some suggestion from the data of different effects within the upper and lower social classes.

A longitudinal study (Port Pirie, Australia) of 537 children born 1979–1982 to mothers living around a lead smelter compared the IQ assessed at 4 years with lead levels of the mother antenatally and at delivery, cord blood, and the child's blood at 6 months, 15 months, 24 months and 36 months. Of all seven measures of lead exposure, the strongest associations with IQ were found for 24–36 months' levels. Nevertheless, the best fit was found with an integrated birth to 4 year measure implying a cumulative effect. The authors conclude that there may be no clear threshold below which an adverse effect on mental development does not occur.[60]

An Italian study compared blood lead, hair lead and tooth lead with the IQ measure of 8-year-old children living in an area of high pollution.[61] There was a strong negative relationship with tooth lead but not with hair or blood lead. This supports the hypothesis that the early period of life is when lead has an adverse effect on IQ, and explains why some cross-sectional studies have failed to show any effect.

The evidence for an association between lead levels and behaviour problems is far less secure and has changed little since being summarized by Rutter in 1980.[62]

The burden of childhood lead exposure is not trivial. In the USA, using 1978 prices, it was estimated that the annual cost of lead causing learning difficulties[63] was between US $281 800 000 and US $713 200 000. Since then a large American screening programme identifies children with high lead levels and instigates a programme of treatment. Although widely implemented, there is no evidence that such a programme results in an increase in IQ levels. If, as seems likely, the lead had already succeeded in damaging the brain irreversibly, this is hardly surprising. However, it is possible that prevention of high lead levels during pregnancy and early childhood may be of more use, but more knowledge of the natural history of the process and identification of protective factors are needed before such interventions can be intelligently planned.

Cadmium

Animal experiments clearly show a teratogenic effect of cadmium; cleft palate and limb defects are the most common resulting malformations. Zinc and lead levels in the mother have been shown to have protective and augmentive features respectively.[64] Studies in animals have produced data that suggest that the teratogenic effects of cadmium may be related to the inhibition of DNA synthesis.[65] Much cadmium in a smoking mother's circulation derives from the cigarette smoke she inhales, but diet may also contribute a substantial amount.[40] Although it has been reported that cadmium does not cross the placenta,[66] it has been reliably shown that cord blood levels are about two-thirds of maternal levels.[40]

Although inverse relationships between birthweight and cadmium have been demonstrated,[67,68] studies have been weak and no strong evidence for causality

yet exists. No studies appear to have assessed whether there are long-term effects on the fetus.

Aluminium

Animal studies have shown that aluminium is a teratogen[61] and can cause fetal death and neonatal death.[69] There are only two reports showing the possibility of an association in humans. In South Wales higher levels of aluminium were found in the water supply of homes where there were children with central nervous system defects than in homes of controls.[70] In Cornwall mothers exposed accidentally to high levels of aluminium sulphate in drinking water were significantly more likely to bear a child with positional talipes.[71]

Apart from chronic toxicity in dialysis patients, little attention has been paid to the element as regards childhood disorder. Animal experiments have shown impaired neuromotor development after fetal exposure.[69] One study in 69 children showed that hair aluminium was associated with impaired visual-motor performance.[72]

Mercury

Mercury accumulates in the body and is highly toxic, especially in its organic form. Until 1973 it was widely used in cosmetics. In animals all of the mercury compounds are teratogenic and have been shown to give rise to growth retardation, postnatal behaviour aberrations and stillbirth.[41]

The potential neurotoxic effect on the fetus was demonstrated by the Minamata disaster in Japan. Women who ingested contaminated shellfish while 6–8 months pregnant gave birth to infants with major neurological problems,[73] including irritability, microcephaly, cerebral palsy and epilepsy. Many of the adults and children exposed also developed cerebral palsy.[41]

Deficiencies of essential trace elements

Although learned committees have, at various times, produced recommended dietary intakes of various elements for different age groups these have largely been derived by guesswork rather than hard scientific evidence. In addition, they do not take account of the interactions with other substances in the diet that may interfere with absorption or metabolism. Examples include: phytate interfering with absorption of zinc; or tea interfering with absorption of iron. The major deficiencies that are of concern in children are of zinc, iodine, iron and fluoride.

Zinc deficiency may arise from: a diet that is zinc deficient; a diet that although zinc sufficient includes items that impair its availability such as fibre, phytate, and alcohol; competition with iron, lead or cadmium. There is no adequate non-intrusive method of determining zinc body status other than by observing the effect of supplementation.

Zinc deficiency in childhood is, in severe cases, associated with dwarfism and hypogonadism.[74] This is particularly common in the Middle East. In the UK, severe neonatal deficiency results in acrodermatitis enteropathica.[75] Other claims of adverse effects include neonatal jaundice,[76] diarrhoea, anorexia, jitteriness, atopic dermatitis and depression.[77] Whether such associations are direct results of zinc deficiency remains to be demonstrated.

Iodine deficiency was rife in many parts of Britain until comparatively recently when the iodine content of cow's milk rose dramatically after the introduction of iodine-enriched cattle fodder.[78] Consequently in the UK, it is likely to be only small groups of vegans who have low dietary iodine.

Maternal iodine deficiency in pregnancy results in high risk of motor and mental retardation.[79] The causal nature of the association in humans was dramatically demonstrated in Papua/New Guinea using randomized injections of iodized oil pre-pregnancy.[80] The question remains as to whether there is a continuum of effect with suboptimal mental development in children exposed to mild iodine deficiency.

Iron is important for brain development. Animal experiments have shown that iron levels are more seriously affected by iron deficiency in very young animals than in older ones.[81] In humans, anaemia in early childhood has been shown in a number of studies to be associated with reduction in measures of ability[82] which do not appear to be wholly reversible with supplementation in young infants.

It is important to recognize that when zinc stores are barely adequate iron supplements can result in zinc deficiency. Clinical interventions for increasing iron status should monitor for potential adverse effects via interactions with the role of other trace elements.

Fluoride deficiency has long been shown to increase the risk of caries in childhood. Classic epidemiological studies have shown that supplementation of water supplies results in decreased caries incidence.[83] Such low levels of supplementation appear to result in no adverse effects, but nevertheless there are still areas where fluoridation of the water supply is resisted.

Housing

In England and Wales, indirect evidence has been obtained for an association between child mortality and housing. Areas with a high ratio of persons per room, and those without basic amenities such as a bath, hot water or an indoor lavatory, have higher mortality rates for ages 0–4 years but not for ages 5–14 years.[84]

Direct measures have been less clear. In the 1946 National Survey of Health and Development (NSHD) cohort, there was an association between bronchitis and pneumonia and an index of overcrowding,[85] but in the 1958 National Child Development Study (NCDS) no association was found with any measure of morbidity,[86] although the children from overcrowded homes performed less well on educational tests.[87]

It is often thought that moving from old, inadequate homes, into modern centrally-heated houses can only benefit families. Yet there are two studies which cast doubt on this. A survey of black Americans living in an inner-city area found a higher rate of illness among the children residing in newer public housing compared with those in older private housing.[88] The authors pointed out that there were many other factors which distinguished the two groups, but that most would actually predict the opposite association to the one found. For example, residents of the older private housing were exposed to higher levels of carbon monoxide and lead, and the parents smoked more.

In South Wales, a population study of respiratory illness was undertaken among children from three areas, distinguished from one another by their housing: new centrally-heated council housing; council housing with open coal fires; and traditional older housing with open fires. In comparison with the rest of the sample, children living in new centrally-heated houses had a higher incidence of colds and reduced lung function. The group living in the traditional older houses had the least number of sore throats and colds, and better lung function.[89]

There are now circumstantial data to suggest that damp and mould are related to wheezing in childhood. Martin et al.[90] in Edinburgh showed that independent assessments of damp and mould were related to reported respiratory symptoms in 101 children. Andrae et al.[91] in Sweden administered a questionnaire to parents of 5301 children and showed strong relationships between dampness and both bronchial hyperactivity and allergic asthma. Strachan[92] questioned 873 parents in Edinburgh and found a relationship between reported wheezing in the past year and fungal mould in the home. Nevertheless, he had evidence to suggest that his associations may have been due to reporting bias.

Air pollution

Air pollution is derived mainly from combustion of fuels for domestic heating or cooking, for heating or power in industry or for transport. Industrial processes may also contribute pollutants in some areas.

Two pollutant mixtures most commonly occurring are: a chemically reducing mixture associated with smoke and sulphur dioxide from burning of coal or higher molecular weight oil fractions (e.g. London fog, now controlled by the Clean Air Act which brought an end to coal fires in most urban areas); an oxidizing mixture derived via photochemical oxidation of incomplete combustion products of petrol in motor vehicles and emissions from industry (including: nitrogen dioxide, aldehydes, peroxyacetyl nitrate (PAN), nitric acid and ozone (e.g. Los Angeles smog)).

The data for the 1946 (NSHD) national birth cohort showed that upper respiratory tract infections were not related to the amount of air pollution in the child's area of residence, but that lower respiratory infections were positively correlated. Both the frequency and severity of lower respiratory tract infections increased with the amount of air pollution. The effect was found in both boys and girls and in children in middle and working class families.[93]

In reviewing the relationship between air pollution and human disease, Martin and Waller[94] pointed out that there are a number of different pollutants all of which might have different effects. These include carbon monoxide, carbon dioxide, formaldehyde, the sulphur oxides, the nitrogen oxides, and ozone.

Carbon monoxide is potentially the most dangerous indoor pollutant when released from incomplete combustion of fuels in unflued appliances or from faulty flues. Extreme exposures to carbon monoxide cause death. It is likely that less severe exposure causes some morbidity. The symptoms are ill-defined (lethargy and headache) and therefore difficult to investigate.

Formaldehyde arises from urea-formaldehyde foam used for insulation in cavity walls, from binding materials and adhesives used in chipboard furniture and other materials in the home, and from tobacco smoke.[95] Animal experiments have shown it to be a potent carcinogen and mutagen. Although it has been suggested that it may be responsible for respiratory problems in school children,[96] evidence for this is lacking. Tuthill[97] interpreted an association between new furniture or new construction and increased respiratory illness as being a result of exposure to formaldehyde, but he had no direct evidence for this.

As well as formaldehyde, isocyanates, solvents and volatile synthetic organic compounds can emanate from materials present in modern buildings. High levels can be reached and certainly cause ocular and nasal irritation. Whether there are more sinister adverse effects remains to be investigated.

In the UK, the sulphur dioxide and smoke concentrations in the external atmosphere have continued to fall over the last 20 years.[98] However, paraffin heaters in homes result in sulphur dioxide levels which increase directly in proportion to the number of hours the heater is in use.[99]

Areas of New York have been divided according to sulphur dioxide levels. There was a trend in prevalence of respiratory disease in school children in the areas with increasing levels. This persisted after allowing for passive smoking, gas cooking and other factors, although the authors were unable to distinguish the sulphur dioxide from smoke particle concentrations.[100] No similar study has been carried out in the UK.

Atmospheric nitrogen oxide and dioxide are mainly secondary pollutants formed in photochemical reactions and have been increasing over the past few years.[101] Contributions come from the nitrogenous components of fuels including the burning of tobacco. Nitrogen oxide is capable of combining with haem in blood but there is no apparent adverse health effect. Nitrogen oxide is gradually oxidized to nitrogen dioxide which is the main concern in human health. In general the concentration of nitrogen oxides is much higher in urban than rural areas, and in winter rather than summer. In general, indoor levels are lower than outdoor levels except in the presence of gas cookers without extractor hoods, paraffin heaters or to a marginal extent smoking members of the household.[102] Indoors, any unflued combustion sources can lead to concentrations of nitrogen dioxide that are often substantially higher than in streets.

A sudden increase in asthma admissions has been related to the atmospheric oxides of nitrogen in Barcelona,[103] although this was later discounted.[104] Animal experiments have certainly shown an increased susceptibility to respiratory infections after exposure to nitrogen dioxide.[99] An elaborate study in Tennessee measured the mean range of daily nitrogen dioxide concentration over a 6-month period. High levels were associated with a high incidence of acute bronchitis among infants and school children.[105] In Middlesborough,[102] the household concentration of nitrogen dioxide was influenced by gas fires, paraffin heaters and the use of the cooker for drying clothes. Bedroom concentrations were positively correlated with those of the living room. Children in bedrooms with high nitrogen dioxide concentrations were more likely to have respiratory problems.[106]

Ozone is an unstable gas with strong oxidizing ability. At one time it was thought beneficial for respiratory diseases because of its bactericidal action. Now it is recognized as one of the most dangerous irritants to eyes, throat and lungs. At times ozone constituted as much as 90% of oxidants in smog, its formation being initiated by the nitrogen dioxide–sunlight reaction.

Animal studies have shown that response to ozone is aggravated by the synergistic effect of exercise, the presence of infection and early age. The most significant transient ozone health effects observed in human clinical and field studies with exposure similar to those typically found in the atmosphere have been associated with exercising individuals and populations.[107,108]

The nature of ozone production and transport is such that ozone will accummulate to levels that may be in excess of the NAAQS (US National Ambient Air Quality Standard) or at least in excess of 100 parts per billion (ppb) for many hours during the day.[109] In some cases the concentrations will be above 100 ppb for at least 8 hours. The effects on children have been monitored using children at a summer camp.[109,110] There were four consecutive days where ozone concentrations were above 100 ppb for at least 8 hours/day. Such exposures resulted in a baseline shift in pulmonary function of children for one week after the episode. These exercising children were affected not only by the peak exposure each day but also by their total exposure to ozone.

Social drugs

Cigarettes

Tobacco smoke ties together many of the topics discussed already. It is responsible for the inhalation of higher levels of radon and its radioactive daughters, it contains cadmium and lead, and is responsible for air pollutants of various sorts. Although passive smoking in early childhood has received much attention, the balance of evidence implicates intrauterine exposure as of paramount importance in regard to child health.

Growth retardation is the topic that has received most attention in the study of maternal smoking during pregnancy with universal findings of reduced birthweight for a given week of gestation accompanied by reduced crown-heel length.[111] It has also been shown that maternal smoking is associated with increased risks of preterm delivery[112] and of premature rupture of the membranes.[113] In most studies there are usually too few perinatal deaths for valid analysis of mortality, but there was a strong association in the 1958 British Perinatal Mortality Survey between maternal smoking and both stillbirth and neonatal death which were unexplained by socioeconomic factors.[114] That other more subtle changes are taking place in utero to the infants of smoking mothers is demonstrated by narrowing of the coronary arteries,[115] an increased haemoglobin level[116] and deficiencies in serum levels of various immunoglobulins together with some evidence for reduced risk of various signs in the neonatal period such as respiratory distress syndrome,[117] irritability[111] and hyperbilirubinaemia.[118]

It has been calculated that in the USA in 1983 alone, maternal smoking during pregnancy was responsible for 35 816 low birthweight babies and 14 978 admissions to neonatal intensive care.[119] The authors calculated that the cost of maternal smoking in pregnancy relating to intensive care was $175 000 000. They suggested that the cost per infant of every smoking mother in the USA was $189 more than that of a non-smoking mother for this component alone. Elsewhere it has been suggested that reduction in smoking levels holds great promise for narrowing the socio-economic gaps in the incidence of low birthweight.[120]

During infancy there have been reported reductions in sleeping problems, but increased incidence of central apnoea,[121] and the sudden infant death syndrome.[122] Among infants whose mothers smoked during pregnancy there is reduced growth with lower triceps skin-fold thickness and weight for length compared with infants whose mothers did not smoke in pregnancy.[123] As discussed by Rantakallio,[124] longitudinal population studies have shown in Finland, the UK and the USA that the children whose mothers smoked in pregnancy continue to be disadvantaged with reduced height, reduced ability at school,[116] and increased risk of childhood cancer.[125,126]

Of particular concern in discussing the postnatal findings for maternal smoking in pregnancy is the fact that few authors have distinguished between inter-pregnancy smoking and postnatal smoking. That passive smoking is associated with lower respiratory tract infections in children is well substantiated, but there is now evidence that bronchitis in infancy is independently associated with both maternal smoking during pregnancy and passive smoking in infancy.[127]

Studies of smoking in pregnancy are confounded, however, by the social and psychological associations. For example, Newton and colleagues[128] showed in a prospective study that stressful life events during the third trimester of pregnancy were associated with preterm delivery and low birthweight. They pointed out, however, that the women who had had such life events were more likely to be heavy smokers and that there was possibly an additive or even synergistic effect. In the UK it is certainly true that mothers who smoke are more likely to be from socially-deprived groups, though less likely to be from the ethnic minority groups. The personalities of smokers have been shown to be substantially different from those of the non-smokers, and one of the most dramatic findings of Rantakallio[124] was that if the mother had smoked during pregnancy, 14 years later she was more likely to have either died, to have left home or for the family to have broken up. Measuring the smoking of the mother in isolation is therefore invalid unless one takes account of her psychosocial background.

Recent analyses from the 1970 national cohort have used the prospective design of the study to attempt to unravel the differences between maternal smoking in the first months only, smoking throughout pregnancy, and passive exposure in the first years of life. By taking account of the psychosocial background variables the following associations have become clear.[129,130]

1 *Low birthweight*: maternal smoking in last trimester.
2 *Squint and vision problems*: maternal smoking in early pregnancy.
3 *Bronchitis in early childhood*: maternal smoking in early pregnancy.

4 *Reduced growth in early childhood*: maternal smoking in early pregnancy.

5 *Behaviour problems*, especially hyperactivity by 10 years of age: maternal smoking in early pregnancy.

6 *Measles*: maternal smoking in late pregnancy.

7 *Specific components of IQ*: low *verbal* with smoking in early pregnancy, low *non-verbal* with postnatal passive exposure.

8 *Poor educational performance*: parental smoking during child's life.

9 *Childhood cancer*: maternal smoking in pregnancy[125] (numbers not large enough to detect which trimester was important).

Alcohol

Parental alcohol abuse may have profound physical and psychological effects on the child, with increased child abuse and neglect.[131] Nevertheless, most research interest has been devoted to intrauterine exposure of the developing fetus. Alcohol ingested by the mother readily crosses the placenta, and fetal blood levels are similar to those of the mother.[132]

Experiments with rats have shown increased incidence of microcephaly, developmental retardation, delayed ossification and subsequent hyperactivity as well as a variety of congenital malformations.[133] In discussing the different results obtained with different mouse strains, Chernoff[134] showed greatest alcohol effects in fetuses of mothers with low alcohol dehydrogenase activity who are thus low metabolizers of alcohol. Among humans the perfectly designed study has yet to take place. Such studies that have occurred have produced conflicting results.

It is well recognized that a number of alcoholic mothers give birth to children with distinctive facies (short palpebral fissures, hypoplastic philtrum, thinned upper lips, retrognathia, short upturned nose, hypoplastic maxilla) and associated malformations with growth retardation and mental retardation, the so-called fetal alcohol syndrome.[135,136] Of particular interest, however, is whether moderate or mild alcohol consumption of non-alcoholics is associated with congenital defects.

The evidence is far from convincing. There is one case-control study of isolated limb reduction defects from Finland which shows an adjusted odds-ratio of 1.6 (CI 1.1–2.4) for any alcohol consumption during pregnancy, but it is not clear whether or not the information was recorded prospectively during pregnancy.[137] One study of obscure methodology claims to show a dose response effect for craniofacial anomalies among 359 neonates.[138] Most studies, however, show no association between alcohol consumption and congenital defects. This includes studies of 12 440 deliveries in Boston,[139] 9236 prospectively studied pregnancies in France,[140] 7525 prospectively studied in West Germany[141] and 32 870 prospectively studied in California.[142] Although there was no overall association with malformations, the latter study did, however, show an increased rate of genitourinary defects with moderate alcohol consumption. In Japan, a pathological study of 3474 induced abortions found fewer malformations among fetuses of mothers who had drunk alcohol during pregnancy.[143]

Children of alcoholic mothers are likely to have major behaviour problems,[144] with hyperactivity, increased distractability and short attention spans.[145,146] Neonates of heavy drinkers have been reported to have abnormal sleep-awake states with longer periods awake and greater restlessness.[147] In contrast, neonates of light drinkers are reported to be more placid.[148] A major longitudinal study in Seattle has shown effects with moderate maternal consumption levels. Not only do they demonstrate dose response relationships with neonatal habituation and low arousal,[149] at 8 months there are similar relationships with feeding problems[150] and at 4 years with attention span and reaction time.[151] Nevertheless, for clinically defined behaviour abnormalities there was not a trend, but rather a threshold effect at maternal consumption of two or more drinks a day.

As already noted, children of recognized alcoholics tend to have low IQs.[152] A Swedish study comparing children fostered with those left with their biological mothers has shown equal reductions in IQ, implying a fetal rather than a postnatal effect.[144] For non-alcoholics, the Seattle study has shown a quadratic dose effect on the Bayley mental ability scale at 8 months, with children born to mothers who had had occasional drinks having higher ability than abstainers. For the Bayley motor scores, however, there was a linear effect – the more alcohol the mother had consumed the lower the scores.[150]

In conclusion, although it is difficult to compare studies because of the different ways in which information on alcohol consumption is collected, it seems possible (but by no means proven) that moderate consumption of alcohol can result in adverse outcome. If further studies show that adverse outcomes do result, it is important to assess if this is conditional on other factors, whether genetic or environmental. One of the possible defects in many of the studies quoted above is the failure to distinguish between different types of alcoholic drink. Yet studies in both France[140] and Dundee[153] have shown that beer appeared to have a more deleterious effect than wine.

Drug abuse

Heroin and methadone

Heroin users presenting at addiction clinics are usually put onto methadone, another opiate alkaloid. Both heroin and methadone have been shown to induce

CNS defects in hamster fetuses, decrease fetal body weight and inhibit pulmonary maturation in rabbits when injected late in gestation.[136]

In a comparative study in the hamster, injection during pregnancy of either heroin or methadone resulted in reduction in postnatal weight which increased with the length of survival. This study also demonstrated that a subgroup of affected infants exhibited abnormal behaviour.[154] Offspring of rats given methadone during pregnancy have postnatal hyperactivity, delayed motor development and other behavioural changes.[155]

Withdrawal symptoms are common in neonates whose mothers are addicted to opiates. Interestingly, infants addicted to methadone may not have withdrawal symptoms until several weeks after delivery, but then the irritability and other symptoms can continue for up to 6 months.[156]

One study from America[157] compared 25 children born to methadone maintained mothers with 42 mothers on multiple types of drugs and 44 controls. In all the parameters considered, methadone infants did worse than the other two groups. The infants were born at significantly shorter gestations, they were significantly lower in birthweight, 25% were small-for-gestational age compared with 5% of controls; they had significantly smaller head circumferences; 42% of the methadone group were considered abnormal neurologically at neonatal examination compared with 8% of controls, and 38% had a prolonged stay in hospital. Follow up of those infants delivered at term and not seriously ill in the neonatal period, showed the effects were still apparent. In particular, the head circumference remained small at 12 months. By the age of 12 months, 42% of the methadone group were considered suspect or abnormal neurologically compared with 6% of the multidrug group and 4% of controls. The neurological abnormalities were of tone, coordination, irritability and delayed milestones.[157]

One further adverse postnatal association of opiate dependence is the sudden infant death syndrome (SIDS). A review of five studies where infants were followed up identified 21 cases of SIDS out of 1024 infants giving an incidence of 21 per 1000, ten times the recognized rate of SIDS in North America.[158]

One long-term study followed up 22 children born to heroin dependent mothers and compared them with three control groups matched on social and environmental factors. The heroin group were shorter when examined at ages between 3 and 6 years, they weighed less, more had a head circumference below the 3rd centile, they were less well emotionally adjusted and had lower scores on psycho-linguistic ability subscales.[159]

Cocaine

Cocaine abuse is reaching epidemic proportions in the USA and, by extrapolating from various screening programmes, in some areas up to 10% of mothers have urinary test results indicating recent contact with cocaine. For example, among 3000 births in 1987–88 in San Francisco,[160] a screening programme was instigated when there was suspicion that the mother might have been exposed to drugs. Of the 601 infants screened 46% were positive for cocaine. If the index of suspicion was 100% successful in identifying those women who were using cocaine, then 10% of the total population of births were associated with cocaine use.

In Philadelphia,[161] 50 pregnancies to women on both cocaine and heroin/methadone were compared with 50 on heroin/methadone but no cocaine and 50 who took no hard drugs. The group with cocaine had the worst outcome in all parameters (birthweight, birth length, head circumference, Apgar score). In all, of the 50 on heroin/methadone and cocaine, there was one spontaneous abortion and four stillbirths. On follow up of the remaining 45 livebirths, two cases of SIDS occurred. In comparison, of the 50 on heroin/methadone, only two stillbirths and no other deaths occurred, and among the 50 controls there were no deaths.

Follow up of behaviour or intellectual ability of children whose mothers were specifically taking cocaine in pregnancy has rarely taken place. There is one report that, at 18 months of age, toddlers exposed to cocaine in pregnancy were very passive, showing no strong feelings of anger, pleasure or even distress on separation from parents.[162]

In Amsterdam, a study compared 35 infants of drug abusers on either heroin, cocaine or methadone with 37 term controls. In the neonatal period, the drug exposed group had significantly poorer neurological responses and more suspect or abnormal EEGs.[163] At one month of age, the drug exposed group were significantly more active but had worse behaviour scores.[164] When followed up at the age of 3 months, the drug exposed group were still more active and at 9 months, they were slightly better at 'duration of orienting'. In respect of their Bayley scores and their EEGs, there were no significant differences by 12 months of age.[164] Such a study is reassuring but the numbers are small and it is not possible to distinguish between the different drugs.

Follow up of exposed children should certainly take place into much later ages to look at specific learning defects and other problems. That these might well be found is indicated by a pathological examination of 10 neonatal deaths of infants born to drug-dependent mothers. The authors[165] stated that several aspects of the neuropathological findings suggest that there are primary and specific effects on the development of the nervous system.

Cannabis

Although a number of studies have questioned mothers concerning cannabis use, only one has been a truly prospective study. In this,[166] 7301 pregnancies were studied with 5% of mothers claiming to have smoked cannabis during pregnancy. Cannabis users were significantly more likely to deliver preterm, even after controlling for other factors such as parity, maternal age, alcohol consumption and tobacco smoking. There was no associaton with growth retardation, low Apgar score, congenital malformations or perinatal mortality.

Three studies have assessed the impact of maternal cannabis consumption on neonatal neuro-behavioural functioning, and all showed deleterious effects. In Canada, Fried examined 291 infants two to three days after delivery and noted an increase in tremors and startles, decreased visual responses, and poor self-quieting among babies born to regular marijuana users.[167] He noted halfway through the study that babies born to these mothers had a distinct shrill cat-like cry. A careful study in Jamaica of 20 infants born to Rastafarian cannabis smokers compared with 20 control infants born to Rastafarian non-cannabis smokers also showed significantly altered cries among the infants of cannabis smokers.[168] A study of 936 full-term infants in Boston showed a positive association between maternal marijuana use and jitteriness within the first three days of life.[169]

There appear to have been no studies that have followed up children of cannabis smokers beyond early infancy. This clearly is important at a time when cannabis smoking is not uncommon. Information showing minimal adverse effects of cannabis some years ago may not necessarily be extrapolated to today. Sexton writing in 1986 pointed out that the marijuana available then was five times more potent than that available 5 years previously.[170]

Polychlorinated biphenyls (PCBs)

This group of substances can be viewed as a paradigm for the dangers of progress. They were first manufactured in 1929 and by 1977 when their manufacture was banned, 800 million tons had been produced,[171,172] with wide application in numerous products including paints, printing inks and adhesives. The substances were, by this time, becoming widely disseminated in the environment. They are very stable and are not biodegradable. They get into the food chain and are consumed and stored in human fat. If it exists, excretion is very slow, except for the lactating mother who can excrete PCBs in her breast milk. Consequently the young infant may receive high levels.

Accidents resulting in exposure to high levels of PCBs during pregnancy have shown that it is highly teratogenic with a characteristic set of features: pigmentation of skin, gingival hyperplasia, exophthalmic oedematous eyes, intrauterine growth retardation and abnormal calcification of the skull.[171] Children exposed in utero have also been shown to have subsequent intellectual deficit,[173] but there is less evidence of long-term adverse effects related to exposure via breast milk.[174]

The burden of PCBs and similar substances is likely to remain for the foreseeable future. Adverse effects of exposure in utero have been well documented. Whether long-term exposure during childhood is of importance to health and development has still to be fully assessed.

Summary

The potential effects of the environment on the health and development of children is an enormous topic. This chapter has concentrated on specific elements in the early environment which are likely to have an effect on the long-term health of the child. For reasons of space there has been no mention of the possibility of contamination by factors such as the occupational exposure of the mother to chemicals at work or indeed in the home. The number of potentially toxic chemicals about which there is little safety information is extraordinarily broad.

The environmental features that have been discussed fall into two main groups. The features of housing and air pollution largely appear to have their effects on child health, if indeed there be adverse effects, by means of direct effect on the child after it is born. The reason for such a conclusion may well be that few have studied the possible effects of these contaminants during pregnancy. Secondly, there is definite evidence for major adverse effects on the fetus of certain environmental factors occurring during pregnancy. Hampered though we are by lack of good data, the balance of evidence at the moment is that maternal smoking in pregnancy has a pervasive and marked deleterious effect on almost all aspects of adverse outcome in the child. Other environmental features which show an equally pronounced effect on humans include hard drugs (particularly cocaine) and ionizing radiation. In addition, alcohol, especially regular alcohol use, appears to carry adverse effects, but the potential damage done by moderate alcohol consumption on the child is still a matter for debate. Of debate, too, is whether the natural radiation to which the fetus may be exposed can be of such a level as to induce adverse outcomes. The balance of the evidence is that there is no threshold for radiation effects, and that there is an increasing effect with increasing radiation levels. Current radiation levels in many homes in the UK are quite high. A study is urgently needed to assess whether there is a range of adverse outcomes at these high levels.

Although lead has been studied extensively, few prospective studies have been undertaken. Nevertheless the balance of evidence is that high levels can induce many adverse effects. There are still some important questions to be answered. In particular, what is the effect of high lead consumption during pregnancy on the later behaviour of the child. Prospective studies which take into account all other environmental features that may be affecting the child are important. Far less information is available on other toxic metals and there is some evidence that specific deficiencies may be of importance in the later outcome of the fetus.

There are clear messages from this literature review. Evidence concerning maternal smoking is devastating enough to recommend that no woman should smoke while she is pregnant. A similar message is obvious for the hard drugs. Contamination by lead should continue to be avoided, as should exposure of the pregnant mother to forms of ionizing radiation. Meanwhile there are many contaminants in our environment which need urgent investigation to assess whether or not they too should be avoided.

References

1 Kato, H. Mortality in children exposed to the A-bombs while in utero, 1945–1969. *Am J Epidemiol* 1971; **93:** 435–442.

2 Luning, G., Scheer, J., Schmidt, M., Ziggel, H. Early infant mortality in West Germany before and after Chernobyl. *Lancet* 1989, ii: 1081–1083.

3 Ikeda, T. Effects of radiation on genetically programmed development of the heart. In: Inouy, E., Nishimura, H. eds. Nagasaki: Nagasaki School of Medicine, 1978.

4 Nomura, T. Parental exposure to X-rays and chemicals induces heritable tumours and anomalies in mice. *Nature* 1982; **296:** 575–577.

5 Cohen, B.H., Lilienfeld, A.M. The epidemiological study of mongolism in Baltimore. *Ann NY Acad Sci* 1969, **164:** 320–327.

6 Alberman, E., Polani, P.E., Fraser Roberts, J.A. *et al.* Parental exposure to X-irradiation and Down's syndrome. *Ann Hum Genet* 1972; **36:** 195–207.

7 Vjeno, Y. Epidemiological studies on disturbances of human fetal development in areas with various doses of background radiation I. *Arch Environ Hlth* 1985; **40:** 177–181.

8 Gentry, J.T., Parkhurst, E., Bulin, G.V. An epidemiologic study of congenital malformations in New York State. *Am J Pub Hlth* 1959; **49:** 497–513.

9 Schuman, L.M., Gullen, W.H. Background radiation and Down's syndrome. *Ann NY Acad Sci* 1970; **171:** 441–453.

10 International Commission on Radiological Protection. *Developmental Effects of Irradiation on the Brain of the Embryo and Fetus.* Oxford: Pergamon Press, 1986.

11 Li, F.P., Gimbrere, K., Gelber, R.D., *et al.* Outcome of pregnancy in survivors of Wilms' tumour. *J Am Med Assoc* 1987; **257:** 216–219.

12 Jensh, R.P., Brent, R.L. The effects of low level prenatal X-irradiation on postnatal growth in the wistar rat. *Growth, Dev Aging* 1988; **52:** 53–62.

13 Wood, J.W., Keehn, R.J., Kawamoto, S. *et al.* The growth and development of children exposed in utero to the atomic bombs in Hiroshima and Nagasaki. *Am J Pub Hlth* 1967; **57:** 1374–1380.

14 Oster-Granite, M.L. The development of the brain and teratogenesis. In: Scarpelli, D.G., Migaki, G., eds. *Transplacental Effects on Fetal Health.* New York: Alan R. Liss, 1988: 203–226.

15 Ader, R., Deitchman, R. Prenatal maternal X-irradiation: maternal and offspring effects. *J Comp Physiol Psychol* 1972; **78:** 202–207.

16 Bayer, S.A., Brunner, R.L., Hine, R., Altman, J. Behavioural effects of interference with postnatal acquisition of hippocampal granule cells. *Nature* 1973; **242:** 222–223.

17 Pochin, E.E. Radiation and mental retardation. *Br Med J* 1988; **297:** 153.

18 Gardner, M.J. Review of reported increases of childhood cancer rates in the vicinity of nuclear installations in the UK. *J Roy Statistical Soc* 1989; **152:** 1–19.

19 Cook-Mozaffari, P., Darby, S., Doll, R. Cancer near potential sites of nuclear installations. *Lancet* 1989; ii: 1145–1147.

20 Kinlen, L. Evidence for an infective cause of childhood leukaemia: comparison of a Scottish new town with nuclear reprocessing sites in Britain. *Lancet* 1988; ii: 1323–1327.

21 Gardner, M.J., Hall, A.J., Downes, S. *et al.* Follow-up study of children born elsewhere but attending schools in Seascale, West Cumbria (schools cohort). *Br Med J* 1987; **295:** 819–822.

22 Gardner, M.J., Snee, M.P., Hall, A.J., *et al.* Results of a case-control study of leukaemia and lymphoma among young people near Sellafield nuclear plant in West Cumbria. *Br Med J* 1990; **300:** 423–429.

23 Kneale, G.W., Stewart, A.M. Mantel-Haenzel analysis of Oxford data. I. Independent effects of several birth factors including fetal irradiation. *J Natl Cancer Inst* 1976; **56:** 879–883.

24 Faiella, A., Russo, F., Fusco, F., *et al.* T-cell leukaemia in children from the province of Naples. *Lancet* 1983; i: 1333.

25 Henshaw, D.L., Eatough, J.P., Richardson, R.B. Radon: a causative factor in the induction of myeloid leukaemia and other cancers in adults and children. *Lancet* 1990; i: 1008–1012.

26 US Congress, Office of Technology Assessment. Biological effects of power frequency electric and magnetic fields – background paper, OTA-BP-E-53. Washington DC: US Government Printing Office, May 1989.

27 Wertheimer, N., Leeper, E. Electrical wiring configurations and childhood cancer. *Int J Epidemiol* 1982; **11:** 345–355.

28 Fulton, J.P., Cobb, S., Preble, L., Leone, L., Forman, E. Electrical wiring configurations and childhood

leukemia in Rhode Island. *Am J Epidemiol* 1980; **111:** 292–296.

29 Myers, A., Cartwright, R.A., Bonnell, J.A., Male, J.C., Cartwright, S.C. Overhead power lines and childhood cancer. In: *Proceedings of the International Conference on Electric and Magnetic Fields in Medicine and Biology* 1985; I.E.E.- Conference Publication 257: 126–131.

30 Tomenius, L. 50-Hz Electromagnetic environments and the incidence of childhood tumours in Stockholm County. *Bioelectromagnetics* 1986; **7:** 191–207.

31 Savitz, D.A., Wachtel, H.A., Barnes, F., John, E.M., Tvrdik, J.G. Case-control study of childhood cancer and exposure to 60-Hertz magnetic fields. *Am J Epidemiol* 1988; **128:** 21–38.

32 Savitz, D. A. Case-control study of childhood cancer and residential exposure to electric and magnetic fields. *Final report to New York State Power Lines Project, Contract #218217.* Albany, NY: New York State Power Lines Project, 1987.

33 Wertheimer, N., Leeper, E. Possible effects of electric blankets and heated waterbeds on fetal development. *Bioelectromagnetics* 1986; **7:** 13–22.

34 Moller, A.R. Noise as a health hazard. In: Last, J.M., ed. *Maxcy-Rosenau Public Health and Preventive Medicine*, 12th edn. Norwalk, Connecticut: Appleton, Century-Croft 1986: 750–763.

35 Lalande, N.M., Hetu, R., Lambert, J. Is occupational noise exposure during pregnancy a risk factor of damage to the audiotory system of the fetus? *Am J Ind Med* 1986; **10:** 427–435.

36 Annest, J.L., Pirkle, J.L., Makuc, D., Neese, J.W., Bayse, D.D., Kovar, M.G. Chronological trend in blood lead levels between 1976 and 1980. *N Engl J Med* 1983; **308:** 1373–1377.

37 Shaper, A.G., Pocock, S.J., Walker, M., *et al.* Effects of alcohol and smoking on blood lead in middle aged British men. *Br Med J* 1982; **284:** 299–302.

38 Green, S.D.R., Lealman, G.T., Aslam, M., Davies, S.S. Surma and blood lead concentrations. *Public Health* 1979; **93:** 371–376.

39 Bryce-Smith, D., Stephens, R. Sources and effects of environmental lead. In: Rose, J. ed. *Trace Elements in Health: a Review of Current Issues*. London: Butterworths, 1988: 83–131.

40 Lauwerys, R., Buchet, J.P., Roels, H., Hubermont, G. Placental transfer of lead, mercury, cadmium and carbon monoxide in women: I. Comparison of the frequency distributions of the biological indices in maternal and umbilical cord blood. *Environ Res* 1978; **15:** 278–289.

41 Schardein, J.L. Metals. In: Schardein, J.L., ed. *Chemically Induced Birth Defects*. New York: Marcel Dekker, 1985: 618–644.

42 Dilts, P.V., Ahokas, R.A. Effects of dietary lead and zinc on fetal organ growth. *Am J Obstet Gynecol* 1980; **136:** 889–896.

43 Wibberley, D.G., Khere, A.K., Edwards, J.H., Rushton, D.I. Lead levels in human placentae from normal and malformed births. *J Med Genet* 1977; **14:** 339–345.

44 Roels, H., Hubermont, G., Buchet, J.P., Lauwerys, R. Placental transfer of lead, mercury, cadmium and carbon monoxide in women. III. Factors influencing the accumulation of heavy metals in the placenta and the relationship between metal concentration in the placenta and in maternal cord blood. *Environ Res* 1978; **16:** 236–247.

45 Moore, M.R., Goldberg, A., Pocock, S.J., *et al.* Some studies of maternal and infant lead exposure in Glasgow. *Scot Med J* 1982; **27:** 113–122.

46 Clark, C.S., Bornschein, R.L., Succop, P., Que Hee, S.S., Hammond, P.B., Peace, B. Condition and type of housing as an indicator of potential environmental lead exposure and pediatric blood lead levels. *Environ Res* 1985; **38:** 46–53.

47 Rabinowitz, M., Leviton, A., Needleman, H., Bellinger, D., Waternaux, C. Environmental correlates of infant blood lead levels in Boston. *Environ Res* 1985; **38:** 96–107.

48 Bellinger, D., Leviton, A., Rabinowitz, M., Needleman, H., Waternaux, C. Correlates of low-level lead exposure in urban children at 2 years of age. *Pediatrics* 1986; **77:** 826–833.

49 Charney, E., Sayre, J., Coulter, M. Increased lead absorption in inner city children: where does the lead come from? *Pediatrics* 1980; **65:** 226–231.

50 Bander, L.K., Morgan, K.J., Zabik, M.E. Dietary lead intake of preschool children. *Am J Pub Hlth* 1983; **73:** 789–794.

51 Lorenzo, A.V., Gewirtz, M., Averill, D., Mauer, M. CNS lead toxicity in rabbit offspring. *Environ Res* 1978; **17:** 131–150.

52 Fulton, M., Raab, G., Thomson, G., Laxen, D., Hunter, R., Hepburn, W. Influence of blood lead on the ability and attainment of children in Edinburgh. *Lancet* 1987; i: 1221–1226.

53 Pocock, S.J., Ashby, D., Smith, M.A. Lead exposure and children's intellectual performance. *Int J Epidemiol* 1987; **16:** 57–67.

54 Lansdown, R.G., Shepherd, J., Clayton, B.E., Delves, H.T., Graham, P.J., Turner, W.C. Blood-lead levels, behaviour, and intelligence: a population study. *Lancet* 1974; i: 538–541.

55 Yule, W., Lansdown, R., Millar, I.B., Urbanowicz, M.A. The relationship between blood lead concentrations, intelligence and attainment in a school population: a pilot study. *Dev Med Child Neurol* 1981; **23:** 567–576.

56 David, O., Hoffman, S., McGann, B., Sverd, J., Clark, J. Low lead levels and mental retardation. *Lancet* 1976; ii: 1376–1379.

57 Grant, E.C.G., Howard, J.M., Davies, S., Chasty, H., Hornsby, B., Galbraith, J. Zinc deficiency in children with dyslexia: concentrations of zinc and other minerals in sweat and hair. *Br Med J* 1988; **296:** 607–609.

58 Bellinger, D., Leviton, A., Waternaux, C., Allred, E. Methodological issues in modeling the relationship between low-level lead exposure and infant development: examples from the Boston Lead Study. *Environ Res* 1985; **38:** 119–129.

59 Bellinger, D., Leviton, A., Waternaux, C., Needleman, H., Rabinowitz, M. Low level lead exposure, social class and infant development. *Neurotoxicol Teratol* 1989; **10:** 497–503.

60 McMichael, A.J., Baghurst, P.A., Wigg, N.R., Vimpani, G.V., Robertson, E.F., Roberts, R.J. Port Pirie Cohort Study: environmental exposure to lead and children's abilities at the age of four years. *New Engl J Med* 1988;

319: 468–475.

61 Bergomi, M., Borella, P., Fantuzzi, G., *et al.* Relationship between lead exposure indicators and neuropsychological performance in children. *Dev Med Child Neurol* 1989; **31:** 181–190.

62 Rutter, M. Raised blood lead levels and impaired cognitive/behavioural functioning. *Dev Med Child Neurol* 1980; **42:** suppl, 1–26.

63 Needleman, H.L., Bellinger, D.C. The epidemiology of low-level lead exposure in childhood. *J Am Acad Child Psychiatr* 1981; **20:** 496–512.

64 Lappe, M. Trace elements and the unborn: review and preliminary implications for policy. In: Rose, J., ed. *Trace Elements in Health: a Review of Current Issues.* London: Butterworths, 1988: 231–249.

65 Samarawickrama, G. Cadmium in animal and human health. In: Rose, J., ed. *Trace Elements in Health: a Review of Current Issues.* London: Butterworths, 1988: 21–43.

66 Ireland, M.P. Genetic aspects and trace element tolerance in man and animals. In: Rose, J. ed. *Trace Elements in Health: a Review of Current Issues.* London: Butterworths, 1988: 209–230.

67 Huel, G., Boudene, C. Cadmium and lead content of maternal and newborn hair: relationship to parity, birth weight and hypertension. *Arch Environ Hlth* 1981; **36:** 221–227.

68 Zielhuis, R.L., Stijkel, A., Verberk, M.M., van de Poel-Bot, M. Cadmium. In: *Health Risks to Female Workers in Occupational Exposure to Chemical Agents.* Berlin: Springer-Verlag, 1984: 67–73.

69 Bernuzzi, V., Desor, D., Lehr, P.R. Developmental alterations in offspring of female rats orally intoxicated by aluminium chloride or lactate during gestation. *Teratology* 1989; **40:** 21–27.

70 Morton, M.S., Elwood, P.C., Abernethy, M. Trace elements in water and congenital malformations of the central nervous system in South Wales. *Br J Prev Soc Med* 1976; **30:** 36–39.

71 Golding, J., Rowland, A., Greenwood, R., Lunt, P., Aluminium sulphate overdose: were there adverse effects on the fetus? *Br Med J* 1991; **302:** 1175–1177.

72 Marlowe, M., Stellern, J., Errera, J., Moon, C. Main and interaction effects of metal pollutants on visual-motor performance. *Arch Environ Hlth* 1985; **40:** 221–225.

73 Matsumoto, H., Koya, G., Takeuchi, T. Fetal minamata disease. *J Neuropathol Exp Neurol* 1965; **24:** 563–574.

74 Prasad, A.S., Miale, A., Farid, Z., Sandstead, H.H., Schulert, A.R. Zinc metabolism in patients with the syndrome of iron deficiency anemia, hepatosplenomegaly, dwarfism and hypogonadism. *J Lab Clin Med* 1963; **61:** 537–549.

75 Seelig, M.S. Prenatal and neonatal mineral deficiencies: magnesium, zinc and chromium. In: Lifschitz, K., ed. *Clinical Disorders in Paediatric Nutrition.* New York: Marcel Dekker, 1982; 167–196.

76 Misra, P.K., Kapoor, R.K., Dixit, S., Seth, T.D. Trace metals in neonatal hyperbilirubinemia. *Indian Pediatr* 1988; **25:** 761–764.

77 Aggett, P.J., Harries, J.T. Current status of zinc in health and disease states. *Arch Dis Child* 1979; **54:** 909–917.

78 Barker, D.J.P. Rise and fall of western diseases. *Nature* 1989; **338:** 371–372.

79 Pharoah, P.O.D., Buttfield, I.H., Hetzel, B.S. Neurological damage to the fetus resulting from severe iodine deficiency during pregnancy. *Lancet* 1971; i: 308–310.

80 Pharoah, P.O.D., Connolly, K.J. A controlled trial of iodinated oil for the prevention of endemic cretinism: a long-term follow up. *Int J Epidemiol* 1987; **16:** 68–73.

81 Lozoff, B. Iron and learning potential in childhood. *Bull NY Acad Med* 1989; **65:** 1050–1066.

82 Aukett, M.A., Parks, Y.A., Scott, P.H., Wharton, B.A. Treatment with iron increases weight gain and psychomotor development. *Arch Dis Child* 1986; **61:** 849–858.

83 Editorial. The fluoride story. *Paediatr Perinatal Epidemiol* 1987; **1:** 127–129.

84 Brennan, M.E., Lancashire, R. Association of childhood mortality with housing status and unemployment. *J Epidemiol Commun Hlth* 1978; **32:** 28–33.

85 Douglas, J.W.B. The health and survival of infants in different social classes: a national survey. *Lancet* 1951; ii: 440–446.

86 Essen, J., Fogelman, K., Head, J. Children's housing and their health and physical development. *Child Care Health Dev* 1978; **4:** 357–369.

87 Essen, J., Fogelman, K., Head, J. Childhood housing experiences and school attainment. *Child Care Health Dev* 1978; **4:** 41–58.

88 Spivey, G.H., Radford, E.P. Inner-city housing and respiratory disease in children: a pilot study. *Arch Environ Hlth* 1979; **34:** 23–30.

89 Yarnell, J.W.G., St Leger, A.S. Housing conditions, respiratory illness, and lung function in children in South Wales. *Br J Prev Soc Med* 1977; **31:** 183–188.

90 Martin, C.J., Platt, S.D., Hunt, S.M. Housing conditions and ill-health. *Br Med J* 1987; **294:** 1125–1127.

91 Andrae, S., Axelson, O., Bjorksten, B., Fredriksson, M., Kjellman, N.I.M. Symptoms of bronchial hyperreactivity and asthma in relation to environmental factors. *Arch Dis Child* 1988; **63:** 473–478.

92 Strachan, D.P. Damp housing and childhood asthma: validation of reporting of symptoms. *Br Med J* 1988; **297:** 1223–1226.

93 Douglas, J.W.B., Waller, R.E. Air pollution and respiratory infections in children. *Br J Prev Soc Med* 1966; **20:** 1–8.

94 Martin, A.E., Waller, R.E. Air pollution in relation to human disease. In: Melvyn Howe, G., Lorraine, J.A. eds. *Environmental Medicine* 2nd edn. London: Heinemann Medical Books, 1980: 104–117.

95 Higgins, I. Air pollution. In: Last, J.M., ed. *Maxcy-Rosenau Public Health and Preventive Medicine.* Norfolk, Connecticut: Appleton, Century-Croft, 1986: 576–586.

96 Pierson, W.E., Koenig, J.Q. Other environmental factors. In: Bierman, C.W., Pearlman, D.S., eds. *Allergic Diseases from Infancy to Adulthood* 2nd edn. Philadelphia: WB Saunders, 1988: 178–190.

97 Tuthill, R.W. Woodstoves, formaldehyde and respiratory disease. *Am J Epidemiol* 1984; **120:** 952–955.

98 McDowall, M. Long term trends in seasonal mortality. *Population Trends* 1981; **26:** 16–19.

99 Leaderer, B.P., Zagraniski, R.T., Berwick, M., *et al.* Assessment of exposure to indoor air contaminants from combustion sources: methodology and application. *Am J Epidemiol* 1986; **124:** 275–289.

100 Love, G.J., Shu-Ping, L., Shy, C.M., Struba, R.J. The incidence and severity of acute respiratory illness in families exposed to different levels of air pollution,

New York Metropolitan area, 1971–1972. *Arch Environ Hlth* 1981; **36**: 66–74.

101 Lindvall, T. Health effects of nitrogen dioxide and oxidants. *Scand J Work Environ Hlth* 1985; **11**: 10–28.

102 Melia, R.J.W., du V Florey, C., Morris, R.E., *et al*. Childhood respiratory illness and the home environment. I. Relations between nitrogen dioxide, temperature and relative humidity. *Int J Epidemiol* 1982; **11**: 155–163.

103 Ussetti, P., Roca, J., Augusti, A.G.N. *et al*. Another asthma outbreak in Barcelona; role of oxides in nitrogen. *Lancet* 1984; i: 156.

104 Anto, J.M., Sunyer, J., Plasencia, A. Nitrogen dioxide and asthma outbreaks. *Lancet* 1986; ii: 1096–1097.

105 Shy, C.M., Creason, J.P., Pearlman, M.E., *et al*. The Chattanooga school children study: effects of community exposure to nitrogen dioxide I and II, *J Air Pollution Control Assoc* 1970; **20**: 539–545, 582–588.

106 Melia, R.J.W., du V Florey, C., Chinn, S., *et al*. Indoor air pollution and its effects on health. *Roy Soc Hlth* 1981; **101**: 29–32.

107 Folinsbee, L.J., McDonnell, W.F., Horstman, D.H. Pulmonary function and symptom responses after 6.6 hour exposure to 0.12 ppm ozone with moderate exercise. *J Air Pollution Control Assoc* 1988; **38**: 28–35.

108 Spektor, D.M., Lippmann, M., Lioy, P.J., *et al*. Effects of ambient ozone on respiratory function in active normal children. *Am Rev Respir Dis* 1988; **137**: 313–30.

109 Lioy, P.J., Dyba, R.V. Tropospheric ozone: the dynamics of human exposure. *Toxicol Indust Hlth* 1989; **5**: 493–504.

110 Lioy, P.J., Vollmuth, T.A., Lippmann, M. Persistence of peak flow decrement in children following ozone exposures exceeding the NAAQS. *J Air Pollution Control Assoc* 1985; **35**: 1068–1071.

111 Jacobson, S.W., Fein, G.G., Jacobson, J.L., *et al*. Neonatal correlates of prenatal exposure to smoking, caffeine and alcohol. *Infant Behaviour Dev* 1984; **7**: 253–265.

112 Guzick, D.S., Daikoku, N.H., Kaltreider, D.F. Predictability of pregnancy outcome in preterm delivery. *Obstet Gynecol* 1984: **63**: 645–650.

113 Flood, B., Naeye, R.L. Factors that predispose to premature rupture of the fetal membranes. *J Obstet Gynecol Neonatal Nurs* 1984; **13**: 119–122.

114 Butler, N.R., Alberman, E.D. *Perinatal Problems: the Second Report of the 1958 British Perinatal Mortality Survey*. Edinburgh: E and S Livingstone, 1969.

115 Lehtovirta, P., Pesonen, E., Sarna, S. Effect of smoking on the fetal coronary arteries. *Acta Pathol Microbiol Immunol Scand*. (C) Section A Pathology 1984; **92**: 189–193.

116 Naeye, R.L., Peters, E.C. Mental development of children whose mothers smoked during pregnancy. *Obstet Gynecol* 1984; **64**: 601–607.

117 White, E., Shy, K.K., Daling, J.R., *et al*. Maternal smoking and infant respiratory distress syndrome. *Obstet Gynecol* 1986; **67**: 365–370.

118 Linn, S., Schoenbaum, S.C., Monson, R.R., *et al*. Epidemiology of neonatal hyperbilirubinemia. *Pediatrics* 1985; **75**: 770–774.

119 Oster, G., Delea, T.E., Colditz, G.A. The effects of cigarette smoking during pregnancy on the incidence of low birthweight and the costs of neonatal care. *Harvard University Discussion Paper Series S-86-01*, Cambridge, Massachusetts: Harvard University Press, 1986.

120 Kleinman, J.C., Madans, J.H. The effects of maternal smoking, physical stature and educational attainment on the incidence of low birthweight. *Am J Epidemiol* 1985; **121**: 843–855.

121 Toubas, P.L., Duke, J.C., McCaffree, M.A., *el al*. Effects of maternal smoking and caffeine habits on infantile apnea: a retrospective study. *Pediatrics* 1985; **78**: 159–163.

122 Golding, J., Limerick, S., Macfarlane, A. *Sudden Infant Death Syndrome: Patterns, Puzzles and Problems*. Shepton Mallet: Open Books, 1985.

123 Taper, L.J., Hayes, M., Rogers, C.S., *et al*. Influence of maternal weight, smoking and socioeconomic status on infant triceps skinfold thickness and growth during the first year. *Birth* 1984; **11**: 97–101.

124 Rantakallio, P. The longitudinal study of the northern Finland birth cohort of 1966. *Paediatr Perinatal Epidemiol* 1988; **2**: 59–88.

125 Golding, J., Paterson, M., Kinlen, L.J. Factors associated with childhood cancer in a national study. *Br J Cancer* 1990; **62**: 304–308.

126 Neutel, C.I., Buck, C. Effect of smoking during pregnancy on the risk of cancer in children. *J Nat Cancer Inst* 1971; **47**: 59–63.

127 Taylor, B., Wadsworth, J. Maternal smoking during pregnancy and lower respiratory tract illness in early life. *Arch Dis Child* 1987; **62**: 786–791.

128 Newton, R.W., Hunt, L.P. Psychological stress in pregnancy and its relation to low birthweight. *Br Med J* 1984; **288**: 1191–1194.

129 Evans, J.-A., Pollock, J.P. Parental smoking and child health and development. *Report to the Health Promotion Research Trust*, 1989.

130 Evans, J.-A., Golding, J. Parental smoking and respiratory problems in the child. In: Poswillo, D., Alberman, E., eds. *Effects of Smoking on the Fetus, Neonate and Child*. Oxford: Oxford University Press, 1992.

131 Mayer, J., Black, R. The relationship between alcoholism and child abuse/neglect. In: Seixas, F.A., ed, *Currents in Alcoholism*, vol. 2. New York: Grune & Stratton, 1977: 429–444.

132 Stein, Z., Kline, J., Smoking, alcohol and reproduction (editorial). *Am J Public Hlth* 1983; **73**: 1154–1156.

133 Streissguth, A.P., Landesman-Dwyer, S., Martin, J.C., *et al*. Teratogenic effects of alcohol in humans and laboratory animals. *Science* 1980; **209**: 353–361.

134 Chernoff, G.F. The fetal alcohol syndrome in mice: maternal variables. *Teratology* 1980; **22**: 71–75.

135 Jones, K.L., Smith, D.W., Ulleland, C., Pattern of malformation in offspring of chronic alcoholic mothers. *Lancet* 1973; i: 1267–1271.

136 Schardein, J.L. Personal and social chemicals. In: Schardein, J.L. ed. *Chemically Induced Birth Defects*. New York: Marcel Dekker, 1985: 763–800.

137 Aro, T., Haapakoski, J., Heinonen, O. A multivariate analysis of the risk indicators of reduction limb defects. *Int J Epidemiol* 1984; **13**: 459–464.

138 Ernhart, C.B., Sokol, R.J., Martier, S. *et al*. Alcohol tetratogenicity in the human: a detailed assessment of specificity, critical period, and threshold. *Am J Obstet Gynecol* 1987: **156**: 33–39.

139 Marbury, M.C., Linn, S., Monson, R. The association of alcohol consumption with outcome of pregnancy. *Am J*

Public Hlth 1983; **73**: 1165–1169.

140 Kaminski, M., Rumeau, C., Schwartz, D. Alcohol consumption in pregnant women and the outcome of pregnancy. *Alcoholism: Clin Exp Res* 1978; **2**: 155–163.

141 Mau, G. Moderate alcohol consumption during pregnancy and child development *Eur J Pediatr* 1980; **133**: 233–237.

142 Mills, J.L., Graubard, B.I. Is moderate drinking during pregnancy associated with an increased risk for malformations? *Pediatrics* 1987; **80**: 309–314.

143 Mutsunaga, E.I., Shiota, K. Search for maternal factors associated with malformed human embryos: A prospective study. *Teratology* 1980; **21**: 323–331.

144 Larsson, G., Bohlin, A.B., Tunell, R. Prospective study of children exposed to variable amounts of alcohol in utero. *Arch Dis Child* 1985; **60**: 316–321.

145 Aronsor, M., Kyllerman, M., Sabel, K.G., *et al.* Children of alcoholic mothers – developmental, perceptual and behaviour characteristics as compared to matched controls. *Acta Paediatr Scand* 1985; **74**: 27–35.

146 Spohr, H.-L., Steinhausen, H.-Chr. Follow-up studies of children with fetal alcohol syndrome. *Neuropediatrics* 1987; **18**: 13–17.

147 Rosett, H.L., Snyder, P., Sander, L.W., *et al.* Effects of maternal drinking on neonatal state regulation. *Dev Med Child Neurol* 1979; **21**: 464–473.

148 Jacobson, S.W., Fein, G.G., Jacobson, J.L., Schwartz, P.M., Dowler J.K. Neonatal correlates of prenatal exposure to smoking, caffeine and alcohol. *Infant Behav Dev* 1984; **7**: 253–265.

149 Streissguth, A.P., Barr, H.M., Martin, D.C. Maternal alcohol use and neonatal habituation assessed with the Brazelton scale. *Child Dev* 1983; **54**: 1109–1118.

150 Streissguth, A.P., Barr, H.M., Martin, D.C. *et al.* Effects of maternal alcohol, nicotine and caffeine use during pregnancy on infant mental and motor development at eight months. *Alcoholism: Clin Exp Res* 1980; **4**: 152–163.

151 Streissguth, A.P., Barr, H.M., Martin, D.C. Alcohol exposure in utero and functional deficits in children during the first 4 years of life. In: *Mechanisms of Alcohol Damage in Utero.* Ciba Foundation Symposium 105. London: Pitman Press, 1984; 176–196.

152 Naeye, R.L., Peters, E.C. Antepartum events and cerebral handicap. In: Kubli, F., Patel, N., Schmidt, W., Linderkamp, O., eds. *Perinatal Events and Brain Damage in Surviving Children.* Berlin: Springer-Verlag, 1988: 83–91.

153 Sulaiman, N.D., Florey, C. du V., Taylor, D.J., *et al.* Alcohol consumption in Dundee primigravidae and its effect on outcome of pregnancy. *Br Med J* 1988; **296**: 1500–1503.

154 Geber, W.F., Schramm, L.C. Postpartum weight alteration in hamster offspring from females injected during pregnancy with either heroin, methadone, a composite drug mixture or mescaline. *Am J Obstet Gynecol* 1974; **120**: 1105–1111.

155 Zuckerman, B.S., Parker, S.J., Hingson, R., Alpert, J.J., Mitchell, J. Maternal psychoactive substance use and its effect on the neonate. In: Milunsky, A., Friedman, E.A., Gluck, L., eds. *Advances in Perinatal Medicine Vol 5.* New York: Plenum, 1986: 125–179.

156 Caviston, P. Pregnancy and opiate addiction. *Br Med J*

157 Rosen, T.S., Johnson, H.L. Drug-addicted mothers, their infants and SIDS. In: Schwartz, P.J., Southall, D.P., Valdes-Dapena, M., eds. *The Sudden Infant Death Syndrome: Cardiac and Respiratory Mechanisms and Interventions.* New York: Ann NY Acad Sci 1988; **533**: 89–95.

158 Finnegan, L.P., O'Brien Fehr, K. The effects of opiates, sedative-hypnotics, amphetamines, cannabis and other psychoactive drugs on the fetus and newborn. *Gen Pharmacol* 1976; **119**: 653–723.

159 Wilson, G.S., McCreary, R., Kean, J., Baxter, J.C. The development of preschool children of heroin-addicted mothers: a controlled study. *Pediatrics* 1979; **63**: 135–141.

160 Osterloh, J.D., Lee, B.L. Urine drug screening in mothers and newborns. *Am J Dis Child* 1989; **143**: 791–793.

161 Ryan, L., Ehrlich, S., Finnegan, L. Cocaine abuse in pregnancy: effects on the fetus and newborn. *Neurotoxicol Teratol* 1987; **9**: 295–299.

162 Howard, J. Cocaine and its effects on the newborn. *Dev Med Child Neurol* 1989; **31**: 255–263.

163 van Baar, A.L., Fleury, P., Soepatmi, S., Ultee, V.A., Wesselman, P.J.M. Neonatal behaviour after drug dependent pregnancy. *Arch Dis Child* 1989; **64**: 235–240.

164 van Baar, A.L., Fleury, P., Ultee, C.A. Behaviour in first year after drug dependent pregnancy. *Arch Dis Child* 1989; **64**: 241–245.

165 Balian Rorke, L., Reeser, D.S. Brain defects in infants born to opiate-dependent mothers. *Pediatr Res* 1977; **11**: 1–15.

166 Gibson, G.T., Bayhurst, P.A., Colley, D.P. Maternal alcohol, tobacco and cannabis consumption and the outcome of pregnancy. *Aust NZ J Obstet Gynecol* 1983; **23**: 15–19.

167 Fried, P.A. Marijuana use by pregnant women: neurobehavioural effects in neonates. *Drugs Alcohol Depend* 1980; **6**: 415–424.

168 Fried, P.A., Makin, J.E. Neonatal behavioural correlates of prenatal exposure to marihuana, cigarettes and alcohol in a low risk population. *Neurotoxicol Teratol* 1987; **9**: 1–7.

169 Parker, S., Zuckerman, B., Bauchner, H. *et al.* Jitteriness in full-term neonates: prevalence and correlates. *Pediatrics* 1990; **85**: 17–23.

170 Sexton, M. Smoking: In: Chamberlain, G., Lumley, J., eds. *Prepregnancy Care: A Manual for Practice.* Chichester: John Wiley, 1986: 141–164.

171 Jones, G.R.N. Polychlorinated biphenyls: where do we stand now? *Lancet* 1989; ii: 791–794.

172 Rogan, W.J., Gladen, B.C., Wilcox, A.J. Potential reproductive and postnatal morbidity from exposure to polychlorinated biphenyls: epidemiologic considerations. *Environ Hlth Perspect* 1985; **60**: 233–239.

173 Jacobson, S.W., Fein, G.G., Jacobson, J.L., Schwartz, P.M., Dowler, J.K. The effect of intrauterine PCB exposure on visual recognition memory. *Child Devel* 1985; **56**: 853–860.

174 Rogan, W.J., Gladen, B.C., McKinney, J.D., *et al.* Polychlorinated biphenyls (PCBs) and dichlorodiphenyl dichloroethene (DDE) in human milk: effects on growth, morbidity and duration of lactation. *Am J Pub Hlth* 1987; **77**: 1294–1297.

Chapter 8

Health services for school-aged children

8.1 School health service

Simon Lenton

Introduction

This section reviews the development of the school health service, examines present practice, discusses current issues and provides a framework for the future evolution of services for school-age children. At the time of writing the Joint Working Party on Health Services for School Aged Children is meeting and due to report at the end of 1993. Like the Joint Working Party on Child Health Surveillance it is hoped that their report will be endorsed as national policy.[1]

An international comparison of school health programmes is excluded but the reader is referred to a recent article[2] which reviewed the major health problems and examined the school health programmes in a number of countries. It is interesting to note the wide variations in service offered to children in a school setting and that the dilemmas facing the school health service in the UK are similar elsewhere.

The needs of school-aged children and the school health service have been extensively reviewed[3-8] and most commentators agree that there have been substantial changes to the health needs of children, to the services providing for those needs and to the legislative framework in the last few decades. These issues are not new to the health service in general, but, due to reorganization, lack of national direction and the absence of a clear research and evaluation programme, it is now unclear what should be provided, by whom or where.

Historical review

Church groups first pressured the government to build schools. Their first grant was received in 1833; at the same time the first education committee was formed. In 1870, the Elementary Education Act enabled the government to set up schools where no voluntary church provision was available.

The Education Acts 1870 and 1880 introduced compulsory education and, for the first time, the poor health of children was revealed. This, together with the recognition of the poor health of men enlisting for the Boer War, led to the recommendations of the Interdepartment Committee on Physical Deterioration in 1904. This committee started a programme of social and public health legislation which included free school meals, regular medical inspections, physical training and programmes to stop juvenile smoking.

The 1907 Education (Administrative Provision) Act enabled treatment in primary schools to compensate for the lack of general practitioner or hospital-based treatment services for children. Treatment in secondary schools followed in 1918 and this combined service became the basis for the school medical service. The routine inspection of all children identified those whose abilities were limited by defects of special senses, learning difficulties and epilepsy and as a consequence local authorities started to provide special education for those so disabled. Children with behaviour problems were also recognized and by 1935 child guidance clinics, with a core team of a psychiatrist, social worker and psychologist, were part of the school medical service.

The Education Act of 1944 renamed the school medical service as the school health service and required all children in state schools to have medical inspections on entry to the primary and secondary schools and again at school leaving. Local authorities at the time provided a comprehensive service which included child guidance, orthopaedics, audiology, chiropody, orthoptics, dentistry and special investigation for asthma, enuresis and rheumatism. Provision was also made for disabilities and chronic disorders including children who were educationally subnormal, blind or partially sighted, deaf or partially deaf, speech defective, maladjusted, delicate and those with epilepsy and diabetes. In parallel to this local-authority-led service the 1946 NHS Act provided both a general practitioner and a hospital service free at the point of contact for the patient. However, the administration of these two health systems remained separate from one another and from the local-authority-led health services. A further parallel development was the Children Act 1948 which gave the local authority the responsibility of looking after children deprived of a normal home life. With time there was a growing realization that many children living at home were also deprived of physical and emotional care and that this, too, had health consequences. In 1963 and 1969 local authorities gained further powers to provide preventive, assessment and rehabilitatory services for children who appeared before the courts. These services were later delivered by social services departments.[9]

The next major transition was the NHS Reorganization Act (1974). Inspired by the need to reduce duplication of treatment services between the local authority, hospitals and general practitioners, the intention was to merge hospital and local authority services into an integrated health service. The reality was that the services were transferred from the local authority but remained intact and separately administered from community units within area health authorities.

Despite the abolition of area health authorities in 1983 and their replacement with smaller district health authorities the ideas of integration expounded in Fit for the Future[3] failed to materialize and hospital and community services continued to operate largely independently both of each other and of family practitioner services.

The NHS reorganization undertaken in 1989 separated assessment of health needs and strategic planning to meet those needs from the provision of services designed to overcome unnecessary duplication or omission from the total package of health care offered to a population. In a move towards a market economy in health care, large primary health care teams are becoming budget holders thus enabling them to buy secondary health care services for the population they serve. It remains to be seen which services they buy on behalf of school-aged children and whether this package is different from that bought by purchasers acting for the district health authority.

The Warnock Committee[10] made recommendations in 1978 which were implemented in the Education Act 1981 to ensure that children with special needs were identified, assessed and provided for, wherever possible, in an ordinary rather than a special school.

The Children Act 1989[11] provided a fundamental review of child care law particularly relevant to the social services departments of local authorities. The principles laid down are equally important to other agencies[12] and should enable children who are in need to be identified, assessed and supported, at an early stage, in a manner which involves and supports adults in their roles as parents.[13]

Health of the Nation, published in 1992,[14] outlined five key areas where health gains are sought for the targets of the WHO Health for All by the year 2000.[15] Included are a decrease in coronary heart disease and stroke, cancers, mental illness, HIV infection and accidents. Many of the determinants of these problems start in childhood and it is likely that implementation will involve a health education and promotion programme for children.

Practice today

Today, the health service offered in schools is no longer the comprehensive, largely self-sufficient system that routinely saw children at 5, 10 and 15 years and offered treatment within the same service. With the development of primary care services and their associated referral pattern to hospital-based services the demand for school-based services has diminished.

Table 8.1 gives examples of the shift of care from the school health service in 1962 to other health practitioners and agencies in 1992.

Despite this, the school health service is still seen as a service which exists to:

1　Identify children with problems that may interfere with their learning in school.
2　Assess children with learning difficulties to exclude health problems as causal or contributing factors.
3　Manage health problems and give advice to teachers and parents.
4　Offer health promotion through health education.
5　Collect health information for epidemiological or planning reasons.

The service varies considerably between different areas and the following is a description of activities though these are neither comprehensive nor universal.

The school entry review

The purpose of the school entry review is to ensure the identification of any health concerns that may affect the child's performance at school and that suitable advice is given to the school staff about the implications of those problems. Depending on the local pre-school child health surveillance programme, this may be done in school or pre-school. It may involve either the school doctor or the general practitioner and either the health visitor or school

Table 8.1 Transfer of activity from the school health service

1962	1992
School entry medical	Undertaken by family practitioner
10 year medical	Health care interview by school nurse
School-leaving medical	Discontinued
Immunization	General practitioner
Acute illness	General practitioner
Behaviour problems	Child and family psychiatry department
Disability services	Child health department
Audiology services	Undertaken largely during pre-school period
Dental services	General dental practitioners
Child protection services	Social services and child health departments
Public health	Health promotion unit
Orthopaedics	Hospital department
Medical problems	Paediatric department
Teacher training medicals	General practitioner

nurse. It will usually include a review of past records, take account of parent concerns and possibly involve a physical examination. Some areas select children to be seen by the use of parent questionnaires, others on information already known from, for example, special needs registers and others on the results of school entry screening tests or the concern of teachers.

Screening tests

The validity of screening[1] for conditions in school-aged children has been questioned, so where screening is offered a systematic evaluation should accompany practice. Screening tests in use are shown in Table 8.2.

Immunization

Immunizations for school-aged children include rubella between 10 and 13 years for girls, BCG around 13 years and tetanus and polio for school leavers. Some areas have discontinued routine BCG vaccination and substituted a protection of 'high risk' groups policy. Immunizations may be offered in a school setting but, in some areas, have become the responsibility of the general practitioner.

Consultation service

Individual children with or without their parents (depending on consent) are seen at the request of the individual, the parent or teaching staff. These referrals

Table 8.2 Screening tests in use for school-age children

Condition	Screening test	Timing
Hearing impairment	Audiometry	School entry
Visual impairment	Visual acuity	3-yearly during school period
Colour vision impairment	Screening test	Boys 9–13 years
Growth failure	Height/height velocity	School entry
Scoliosis	Scoliometer	Adolescents
Hypertension	Blood pressure	Adolescents
Cardiac defects	Physical examination	School entry
Testicular maldescent	Physical examination	School entry

Adolescent review

Few areas now offer a 10 or 15 year medical examination though some offer a selective examination for 10 year olds based on parental or school staff concerns. Instead many are moving towards a health care interview performed by a school nurse in a school setting. Health care interviews are sometimes offered at other ages often linked to the times of vision testing.

cover a wide range of problems that have usually been causing concern in the school setting. Generally the consultation is with a school doctor but increasingly school nurses are offering school-based clinics for self-referral, particularly by adolescents.

Special needs

Children with special needs require assessment so that either guidance or resources may be given to school staff to enable the child to benefit from education. The assessment process is initiated by the identification of the child and is completed when effective provision is supplied. The health service contributes reports from the school nurse and doctor, therapy services, child and family guidance and other specialists where they are involved. Health services may be provided either in or out of the school setting depending on the needs of the child and local practice.

Health promotion – health education

Health education programmes vary considerably from advice given on an individual basis at school entry review or a health care interview, to school nurses undertaking classroom teaching on health related matters or advising teachers on the contents of the curriculum.

Health promotion programmes may be initiated and coordinated by health promotion officers working within education departments. Usually these programmes are topic focused, but sometimes the whole school is the focus to ensure a health promoting environment.

Child protection

When a concern or an unexplained injury is discovered in school, school health service personnel may be asked to provide an initial assessment of the child and decide whether further investigation is required under the local child protection procedures.

Specific programmes

Specific services unavailable from a primary care or hospital setting are sometimes offered through school. These include advice concerning enuresis, encopresis, obesity and contraception. Counselling may also be available.

Career advice

The health authority has a duty to inform the careers department of the local authority on the implications of any significant health problem that may limit employment prospects.

Dental health

The roles of the community dental service are set out in HC(89)2 and guidance notes PL/CDO(89)2.

1 Dental epidemiology: to monitor the dental health of the whole population.
2 Dental health promotion: the provision of preventive programmes.
3 Provision of dental treatment for children who have difficulty obtaining dental care, for example children with complex disability.
4 Dental screening for all children in state-funded schools. At present the required ages for this are 5, 11 and 15 years, but some areas screen more frequently in populations where there is a high prevalence of dental problems.

Current issues

What are the health problems today?

It is difficult to disentangle the impact of advances in health care from changes in the physical or social environment; often data are collected in different ways over a period of time making trends difficult to establish. However, few people would disagree that there have been substantial changes since the beginning of the school health service[16] when 50% of children did not survive to 5 years of age, malnutrition was rife and infectious disease rampant causing both mortality and morbidity in school-aged children.[17,18]

Mortality rates, hospital admission rates and GP consultation rates for school-aged children are at their lowest levels but changing use of services should not be the sole criterion for judging the well-being of children. More children today with congenital malformations, organ failure and chronic disease now survive longer due to advances in medical treatment.

Few positive health status measures are collected so an estimate of the health needs of school children is notoriously difficult but must take into account the physical and social environment.[19–21]

Leading causes of death in this age group are accidents, respiratory diseases and malignancy. Self-reported long-standing illness has increased in the 5–15-year age group[22] and unfortunately there is no routinely collected data from which to ascertain a pattern of morbidity in school-aged children.[23,24]

Much of the morbidity described is worse in areas where there are high levels of deprivation. High unemployment, low levels of income, poor parent support, housing, recreational opportunities and unemployment prospects all contribute to the imbalance of morbidity across the social spectrum.[20]

Accidents are the leading cause of mortality in the 5–15 year-old age group. Morbidity is difficult to ascertain, but some estimate of the cost to the NHS has recently been surveyed.[25] While the majority of deaths are related to motor vehicle accidents, substantial numbers of children are injured in a school setting.

Infectious disease causes 10% of the deaths of all children 0–15 years. Morbidity has been reviewed[26] and there is a decreasing trend in infectious disease for which immunization is available. There has been an increase in food-related infection due to changes in food preparation methods, and an increase in infection in children undergoing increasingly intense chemotherapy for malignancy and infants who are immuno-compromised through HIV infection. Respiratory disease causes 5–10% of deaths in children and asthma is the leading cause for school absence on medical grounds.[27]

Disabilities cause considerable morbidity for school-aged children. Warnock[10] estimated 2% of all children would have a continuing need throughout childhood for special educational support, but in addition there would be a further 18% who would require support for a period of time. Bone[28] found between 3.5 and 3.8% of children had disabilities severe enough to limit their everyday activities and more than half had more than one problem. Other surveys put the figure at around 5%.[29]

Paediatricians now see fewer children with organic pathology and more children with symptoms related to social, behavioural and developmental causes. Many interfere with learning in a pre-school or school setting and the management of these difficulties has been called educational medicine[3] and recognized as the new paediatric morbidity.[30] Although these symptoms may appear to be minor in comparison with organic disease they have a marked effect on educational achievement, self-esteem, peer relationships and subsequent adult functioning.[31,32]

The prevalence of psychological difficulties is difficult to determine but eating disorders,[33,34] depression and suicide appear to be increasing particularly in urban environments.[35–38] It is presumed that these conditions are related to stress experienced by the child through separation, divorce, anxiety about their future and lack of extended family support. Sexual abuse during childhood continues to be identified but not the levels reported by adults.[31] Divorce,[39,40] bullying,[41,42] racial harassment,[43] and criminality[44] add to the stresses children experience in the course of their everyday lives.

The health behaviours of children and young people give cause for concern. Seventeen per cent of boys and 22% of girls aged 15–16 smoke regularly.[45] Alcohol is consumed in greater quantities and at an earlier age[46] and conceptions to teenagers are increasing.[47] Balding provides a full description of health behaviour in young people.[48,49]

Who and where are the children?

A database of school-aged children either resident or receiving education within the district health authority (DHA) boundaries is essential for any screening, surveillance or immunization service. Children privately educated should have access to the same service as children in state schools and a decision on whether children attending boarding schools are counted as resident or non-resident in the district needs to be made.

Having ascertained the numbers of children, health status measures need to be collected in a standardized form so that resources can be allocated appropriately.[50,51] This information may need to be collected from a number of different sources which include education departments, social services, accident and emergency departments and hospital or primary health care staff.

Information about professional activity relating to school-aged children is useful to ascertain the level of resources utilized, but gives little information about the quality or effectiveness of the service. Where information about effectiveness of interventions is not available, research or clinical audit should be initiated to answer the question whether the activity should be continued.

Communication – is information being shared?

Teachers know little about the health services available to school children,[52,53] the role of the services in health surveillance[54] or health conditions of children, for example asthma.[55] Parents are no better informed[56] than teachers and their requests for simple written information, advance notice of visits by the school doctor and nurse to the school, the name and telephone number of the school nurse, and the results of examinations seem very reasonable. Writing clear information for parents is more difficult,[57] but has been endorsed as good practice by recent reports.[4]

The school health service has been described as the invisible service due to lack of data available,[58] but it is equally invisible to primary health care teams and hospital-based teams through lack of written information after consultation in school. In the days when the service was comprehensive the school medical record functioned as a single case note for all the services involved with the child. Now, when many departments may be involved, the information after a school-based consultation needs to be shared and as school-based services become increasingly oriented towards secondary care it will be important to write to parents, with a copy to the GP and other agencies involved. Primary care contact can be recorded by adopting the national parent-held record or the education based record of achievement.[59]

Where the health problem has direct implications for the classroom teacher this should be communicated verbally and in writing to the teacher concerned as the present practice of communicating via the school-based health record is not always effective.

The development of a combined child health service should enable the development of a single secondary care record for a child and also a computerized database where information such as personal details, demographic data and essential health status measures can be stored and retrieved for audit or planning reasons.

Special needs – are services coordinated?

Children with problems which involve several different services need access to a multidisciplinary team rather than a multidisciplinary series of professionals. Key members should meet the family to review goals, set priorities and decide on an action programme which is then written down. The frequency of review depends on the child's condition and the written plan should form the basis of the review.

The team should operate in a clearly defined area (both clinical and geographical) and also meet to review local needs, revise practice-based audit and plan local development. Voluntary groups and parent representatives should be involved.

School entry examinations – routine or selective?

School entry examinations need to be seen in the context of pre-school child health surveillance and any further health or education assessments that may take place during the school years.

The purpose of entry examinations is roughly parallel to the purpose of the school health service. There are no comprehensive studies that compare the outcome of all the components of the school entry review and debate has focused purely on the medical component.

In 1986, 95% of responding health districts offered routine school entry examinations[58] and the 1986 British Paediatric Association (BPA) report[6] endorsed this practice. Studies supporting routine medicals have been written,[60–67] but papers describing a more selective practice[68–72] argue that significant defects that require medical examination are too rare to justify routine examinations of all children.

There are two key issues here: first, should a health assessment identify developmental disorders that have educational implications or is this an educational responsibility? Second, can pre-school child health surveillance adequately identify all significant physcial health problems by school entry? The first requires discussion with the education department and the second an evaluation of pre-school surveillance. Smith[71] suggests that screening all school entrants for disorders of growth, vision and hearing by a school nurse aided by parental questionnaires and review of pre-school records was satisfactory and enabled selective medical examinations to be offered in the second term, where there were concerns.

Richman and Miles[73] report similar findings. The use of a health care interview between school nurses and parents facilitated consultation with parents and allowed health education advice to be offered. Similar practice using health visitors rather than school nurses has also been described.

There appears to be agreement that there should be a school entry review when growth and special senses are screened, pre-school records and immunization status are reviewed and the concerns of parents or teachers are heard. Whether specific screening tests for other disorders of development should be routinely included is not yet clear. Where these tests are offered the results should be published as soon as possible. Children could then be selected for medical examination where there is no evidence of previous medical assessment, there is a screening test requiring medical skills, there are medical problems requiring advice to education staff or on request from parents, teachers[74] or nursing staff.

Adolescents – a health care challenge?

Adolescence is a time of enormous physical, emotional and social change and these changes are reflected in teenage behaviours which the adult world sees as challenging and can put the individual's health[75] at risk of harm either in the short or longer term.

Adolescent medicine is poorly developed in the UK compared to the USA,[76] Australia or the Nordic countries and there have been very few systematic reviews.[3,4,77–79] There are even fewer published examples of good practice[80–83] relating to the school health service.

There is little doubt that adolescents do have health concerns based on their own report and survey findings both here and abroad.[36,48,84–87] The difficulty is knowing how to meet their needs effectively either working from within the health service[88] or with other agencies.[89] The role of health promotion within the national curriculum is important, together with specific programmes to reduce morbidity. However, these interventions will not meet the needs of adolescents who have problems but find the general practitioner system difficult to use.[90]

The practice of drop-in clinics is supported in the national reviews and recently a proposal has been developed, based on the US experience, for a similar practice for this country.[91] While this may be achievable in urban areas, alternatives need to be sought as an option in smaller towns or rural areas that can build on the experience and good practice developed in such centres.

Specific advice and treatment of sexual problems, pregnancy, sexually transmitted diseases, termination of pregnancy, sexual abuse and contraception need to be provided in a coordinated manner that rarely exists in most districts. It is hoped that purchasing authorities given a mandate by *The Health of the Nation*[14] will promote better coordination of services to adolescents.

Health care interviews

Health care interviews (HCIs) are replacing the traditional periodic school medical inspection. Their development originated in the observation that fewer significant physical health problems were being detected by doctors and therefore school nurses could undertake the consultation and health education roles that normally accompanied physical examination. They would then refer the problems which they could not manage themselves. HCI practice has been described[92,93] and is established practice in 62% of areas,[94] but there have been very few attempts at evaluation.[95–97]

While this trend is sure to continue and may be very cost-effective in comparison to employing a medical person for the same activity, the tasks within the HCI must be part of a child health strategy rather than continue a process for reasons of tradition.

Immunization

BCG

BCG vaccination offers good protection against tuberculosis and is a safe procedure when given by trained staff.[98] Since the introduction of routine BCG vaccination the incidence of TB has fallen,[99,100] treatment programmes have improved and contact tracing with chemoprophylaxis has prevented the development of the disease in people at risk.

Vaccination at 13 years cannot protect the population most at risk of disseminated tuberculosis – namely infants and young children where TB meningitis has a high mortality and morbidity.[101] In view of these observations it has been suggested that routine immunization should be discontinued and a policy of immunizing high risk groups should be introduced.[102] A survey reported in 1992 indicates that 15 of the 186 districts have already discontinued routine immunization to adolescents and 148 districts have a newborn immunization policy.[103]

National policy[104] recommends continuing the routine programme because the declining incidence reported in the 1970s and 1980s has not continued into the 1990s possibly due to increased travel abroad, increasing poverty in urban areas[105] and the spread of HIV infection. Providing the present incidence of tuberculosis does not increase, it is likely that the policy of routine immunization will shift to immunization of high-risk groups starting in the newborn period. An effective policy for early investigation and contact tracing needs to be maintained and each district should have a clear policy indication who is responsible for each component of the anti-tuberculosis programme for both adults and children.

Rubella

The importance of rubella infection on the unborn child has been extensively reviewed.[106] Rubella vaccine is generally effective at preventing the disease when seroconversion takes place, although there are case reports of fetal infection in seropositive women. The policy of immunizing teenage girls has not been effective in eradicating the congenital rubella syndrome because uptake rates have been poor and this policy has not substantially altered the transmission of the disease in younger children. The recent change to measles, mumps and rubella (MMR) immunization between 12 and 18 months is proving to be both acceptable and effective at reducing the notifications for measles. Its effect on notification of congenital rubella syndrome is awaited.

There are concerns that the policy of immunization in infancy may lead to a susceptible elderly population, if immunity diminishes with age.[107,108] In Scandinavia[109] MMR vaccination is repeated in later childhood to reduce this risk, a policy predicted to eliminate the natural disease in 10 years. Depending on further epidemiological surveys, rubella immunization for adolescents will either be discontinued or a booster for MMR added. It would be convenient to combine this with school-leaving tetanus and polio immunization at 14 years of age.

Health promotion

The interdependence of health and education is self-evident but there is a limit to how individual health education can overcome environmental factors that mediate in the opposite direction, for example, anti-smoking campaigns versus tobacco advertising or good nutrition versus inadequate disposable income. *The Health of the Nation* and subsequent publications[110] highlight the key targets for the UK and as many adult behaviours have their origins in childhood[111] it will be essential to start early in life. Fundamental to changing behaviours is an understanding of their development and influences. The health field concept which underpins the Canadian health promotion strategy is a useful framework[112] for examining health issues.

Health education is part of the National Curriculum,[113] not as a separate subject but integrated across the curriculum so that year on year children build on their knowledge, alter their attitudes and eventually change their behaviour. Laudable as this approach is, evidence from the USA suggests that health education needs to be widely delivered and involve parents,[114,115] families and the local community at the planning, interaction and evaluation stages.[116,117] Teaching staff need support from health professionals to widen their approaches to health education by better information. Margaret Whitehead provides good examples of this approach.[118]

Health education items included in the National Curriculum:

- Substance abuse and misuse
- Food and nutrition
- Health related exercise

- Sex education
- Environmental aspects of health education
- Safety
- Psychological aspects of health education
- Family life education

Health of the Nation targets – reduction in:

- Coronary heart disease and stroke
- Cancer
- HIV/AIDS, sexual health
- Accidents
- Mental illness

Fundamental to the success of all these programmes is the development of positive self-esteem, an ability to value people and to adapt to change. The traditional Protestant work ethic is less applicable to a society where 10% of people are unemployed[119] and maybe the educational curriculum should reflect this reality and move towards producing individuals with a wider range of life skills.

Management and professional accountability

Health service staff working in a school setting may be managed from different units, trusts or agencies and professional lines of accountability may not always be to an individual who has previously worked in a school setting or the same professional background.

In the absence of clear national guidelines, lack of commitment over many years to research and evaluation, poor training programmes for school nurses and doctors and continuing reduction of resources, individual professionals and managers have taken decisions often in isolation from one another, which have left an inequitable service in many parts of the country. Future health services need to be based on the health care needs of the school-aged population using interventions which are known to be helpful. Staff working with children of school age require supervision, professional support and involvement on relevant clinical audit programmes.

Accommodation in school – a limiting factor

Education (school premises) regulations 1981 suggest that every school should have a medical room with a wash basin reasonably close to a toilet. A recent local survey[120] showed only 24% of schools had a medical room (almost always in a secondary school), medicals often being performed in the staff room (21%) or head teacher's office (12%). Only 18% had a couch, 34% had no wash basin and privacy was inadequate in 27%.

It seems unlikely that this situation will improve, particularly in small primary schools, and alternative accommodation needs to be found either in school or nearby if traditional hospital outpatient consultations are to devolve to a community setting. More use of health care premises is one possibility that would strengthen links with the primary health care team but good communication with the schools would have to be maintained.

New regulations (Building Bulletin BB77) recognize the need for bases for therapists and other visiting specialists in special schools but similar concepts need to be extended into mainstream schools if the policy of integrating children with special needs into these is to continue.

A framework for the future

In the past the school health service provided the majority of health care for school-aged children, but today, family practitioners, paediatric services, therapy agencies and many others contribute. It is therefore better to consider the health needs of and services to school-aged children than the school health service and plan to work with all these professional groups. This requires the responsibilities of each to be clearly defined so that there is no unnecessary duplication or omission of services provided.

Principles

Before planning services it is worthwhile establishing a number of general principles of good practice[121] that apply wherever a service (including a school health service) is offered. They include:

1 Children have rights that should be respected and promoted: for example
   to a safe and healthy environment
   to good nutrition
   to a secure and loving family life
2 Children should be seen as children first, recognizing their changing needs and abilities as they become older rather than as diseases or problems.
3 Parents and children should be actively involved in their health care.
4 Each child is a unique individual and racial, linguistic, religious and cultural backgrounds should be respected.
5 Services should be accessible and child-friendly.
6 Services should be evaluated regularly to ensure that they are meeting the evolving needs of the population.
7 Services should be both coordinated at one time and have continuity over a period.
8 Agencies should share common objectives and work together within the resources available.

Goals and aims

The goal of all professional activities with school-aged children should be to enable each child to reach the maximum potential. To do this the work of individual services should contribute towards a series of aims:

1 To promote optimal development and lifestyle of all children, for example,
   nutrition and exercise
   adequate pre-school provision
   improved physical environment

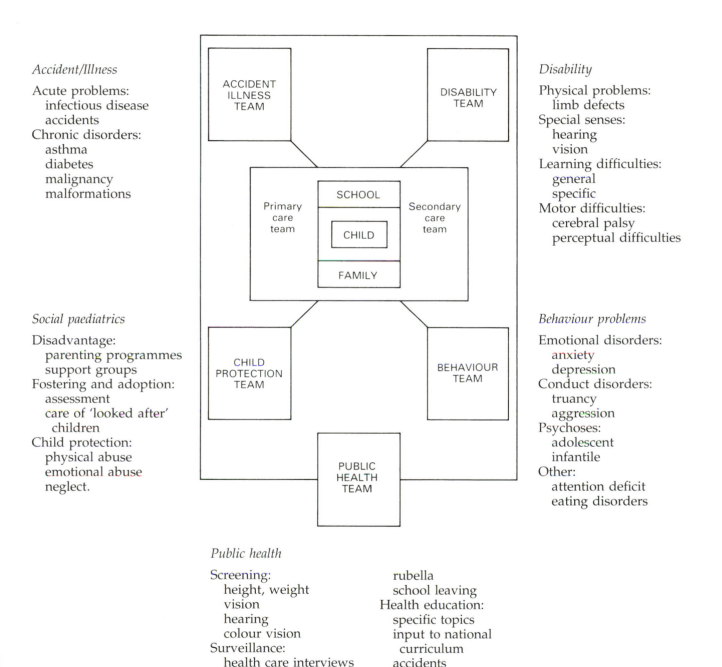

Accident/Illness

Acute problems:
   infectious disease
   accidents
Chronic disorders:
   asthma
   diabetes
   malignancy
   malformations

Social paediatrics

Disadvantage:
   parenting programmes
   support groups
Fostering and adoption:
   assessment
   care of 'looked after'
   children
Child protection:
   physical abuse
   emotional abuse
   neglect.

Disability

Physical problems:
   limb defects
Special senses:
   hearing
   vision
Learning difficulties:
   general
   specific
Motor difficulties:
   cerebral palsy
   perceptual difficulties

Behaviour problems

Emotional disorders:
   anxiety
   depression
Conduct disorders:
   truancy
   aggression
Psychoses:
   adolescent
   infantile
Other:
   attention deficit
   eating disorders

Public health

Screening:
   height, weight
   vision
   hearing
   colour vision
Surveillance:
   health care interviews
   dental health
Immunization:
   school entry

rubella
school leaving
Health education:
   specific topics
   input to national
   curriculum
   accidents
Health promotion:
   smoking
   school environment

Figure 8.1 Health education extends across all services.

2 To reduce social inequalities of health, for example,
   by targeting resources on the determinants of
   health
   improving access to health services for groups to
   whom available resources are less accessible
   improving parenting skills
3 To reduce acute events such as illness and accidents
   and their consequences, for example,
   by immunization
   accident prevention programmes
   provision of good primary and secondary care
   services
4 To reduce emotional and psychological disturbance,
   for example,
   by counselling following divorce or bereavement
   positive parenting programmes
5 To reduce disability and its consequences, for
   example,
   by prompt effective curative care
   early recognition of physical and sensory impairment
   therapy and education

Each of these five broad aims partially coincide with
the work of existing teams of individuals that already
span primary, secondary and tertiary care (see Fig.
8.2). However, the work of the members of the team
rarely relate to the explicitly stated goals or aims of the
purchaser of a service such as that of the district health
authority, local authority or family health services
authority.

A description of the needs of children relating to
each team is the starting point for the contracting process to meet those needs (Fig. 8.1).

From this broad description of needs, specific services can be developed together with monitoring
programmes, research and development ideas, and
training programmes.

These functional teams span trusts, directly managed units, fundholding practices, and they clearly
need to work cooperatively to ensure the best outcome and value for money. How this is achieved
will depend on local arrangements but a multidisciplinary professional group to develop clear policies
that span the management structures seems an obvious solution.

Public health and health promotion represent
population based interventions that may be specific
such as screening, or more general activities such as
action to ensure school is a health promoting environment. The health education elements should be consistent across all services, hence the diagram
encompassing all services by the public health team
who are responsible for monitoring the overall health
of the childhood population (Fig. 8.1).

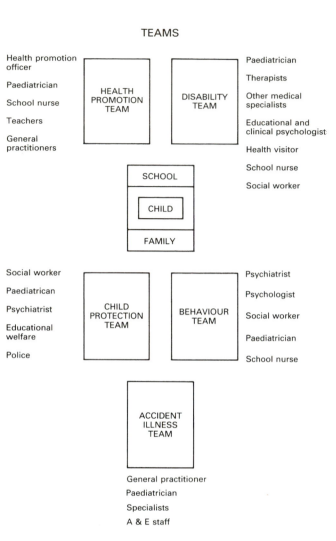

Figure 8.2 Multidisciplinary teams that span primary, secondary and
tertiary care.

The disability team – a general example

The aim of the service would be to identify, assess and
manage children with disability. The process of identification could be through a screening programme
operated by the primary health care team, for example hearing or vision, or through parent or teacher
concern depending on the condition involved. Once
a problem had been identified the child would be
referred for further assessment. This may be school,
clinic or hospital based and any problem managed
according to need. The principles outlined earlier
would apply, for example the child and parent would
be actively involved and services would be provided
in a child-friendly environment taking account of the
child's cultural background, language and ethnic
needs.

Hearing impairment – a specific example

Identification	Assessment	Management
Child health surveillance		Observation, reassessment
School entry audiogram	Hearing assessment clinic	ENT/grommets Hearing aids fitted
Parents' or teachers' concerns		Teacher for hearing impaired Speech therapist

In this example pre-school child health surveillance might be performed by the GP or health visitor, the school entry audiogram by an audiometrician or school nurse, the hearing assessment clinic staffed by community doctors or audiological physicians, ENT services provided privately or by the NHS, and hearing aids and speech therapy provided by either health or education. The source of provision in this context is unimportant. What matters is that provision is available, of good quality and the role of each component acknowledged in the whole process of identification, assessment and management of hearing impaired children.

Similar models would need to be developed for all types of disability and the agreed components included in service agreements with the commissioning bodies or fundholding GP contracts.

Implications for the school health service

The concept of a school doctor or a school nurse as someone who works only in a school setting is outdated and limits the creative provision of services for school-aged children. School-aged children require a spectrum of services provided by overlapping teams of individuals, the members of which should be clear about their role within that team. An individual doctor or nurse is likely to be a member of a number of different teams and when working within that team will work to the clinical standards that best meet the needs of the child. The physical site of provision may be within the school, if suitable accommodation is available, but it may be provided in a local clinic, health centre, home or hospital, depending on local arrangements. Whatever the physical setting of the consultation, communication with the primary health care team, educational professionals or other secondary services which may be involved is essential.

School doctors and some school nurses already work outside a school setting for some of their working time. Although working in a school environment, they are functionally part of a number of different teams including child protection or disability, and their clinical work is linked to each team.

Increasingly school doctors are providing a secondary care service, largely assessment and first-line management of problems identified by the primary health care team. School nurses increasingly undertake primary surveillance roles previously performed by school doctors and it has been advocated that these roles are the responsibility of the primary health care team. However, nurses also contribute to the secondary care of children with identified problems and so they need to link with the secondary health care teams described.

By disaggregating the purpose of the school health service into a number of aims for all children it is possible to clarify the practice that needs to develop. Subsequently an active research programme can be defined so that children of school age and particularly adolescents can fulfil their potential.

References

1 Hall, D.M.B. *Health for All Children*. Oxford: Oxford Medical Publications, 1991.

2 Stone, E.J., Perry, C.L. An international perspective and comparison of school health programmes. *School Health*, 1990; **60**: 291–382.

3 Court, S.D.M. (Chairman). Fit for the future. *Report of the Committee of Child Health Services*. London: HMSO, 1976.

4 National Children's Bureau. *Investing in the Future: Child Health Ten Years After the Court Report*. London: NCB, 1987.

5 Kings Fund Centre for Health Services Development Primary Care Group. *Changing School Health Services*. London: The King's Fund, 1988.

6 British Paediatric Association. *The School Health Services*. London: BPA, 1986.

7 Roche, K., Stacey, M. *Overview of Research on the Provision and Utilisation of Child Health Services in the Community Update IV*. Coventry: University of Warwick, Department of Sociology, 1991.

8 Watt, J, Faulkner, A, Farrow, S. *Effectiveness of the School Health Service: Review of the Background Literature*. University of Bristol: Health Care Evaluation Unit, Dept. of Epidemiology and Public Health Medicine, 1991.

9 Nash, W. *Health at School – Caring for the Whole Child*. London: Heinemann Medical Books, 1985.

10 Warnock, H.M. Special educational needs. *Report of the Committee of Enquiry into the Education of Handicapped Children and Young People*. London: Her Majesty's Stationery Office, Dept. of Education and Science, 1978.

11 The Children Act 1989. HMSO London: HMSO, 1989.

12 Working Together 1991. *A Guide to Arrangements for Interagency Cooperation for the Protection of Children from Abuse*. London: Her Majesty's Stationery Office, 1991.

13 Sheperd, S. Aspects of the Children Act – a medical perspective. *Health Trends* 1991; **23**: 51–53.

14 Department of Health. *The Health of the Nation: A*

Strategy for Health in England. London: Her Majesty's Stationery Office, 1992.

15   World Health Organization. *Health for All 2000: Targets for Health for All*. Coppenhagen: WHO, 1985.

16   Chief Medical Officer. *The Health of the School Child – Annual Report of the CMO*. London: HMSO, 1925.

17   Forfar, F., ed. *Child Health in a Changing Society*. Oxford: Oxford University Press, 1989.

18   Whitmore, K. *Health Services in Schools – a New Look*. London: Spastics International Medical Publications, 1985.

19   National Children's Homes. *Children in Britain 1992: the NCH Factfile*. London: NCH, 1992.

20   Bradshaw, J. *Child Poverty and Deprivation in the UK*. London: National Children's Bureau, 1990.

21   Kurtz, Z. Investing in the future: what is happening to children's health in the UK? *Child Soc* 1988; **4**: 335–341.

22   Office of Population and Censuses Studies. Social Survey Division. *General Household Survey*. London: Her Majesty's Stationery Office, 1989.

23   Bewley, B.R. The inadequacy of adolescent health statistics. *Comm Med* 1982; **2**: 97–98.

24   MacFaul, R. Much data but limited information in the National Health Service. *Arch Dis Child* 1988; **63**: 1276–80.

25   Child Accident Prevention Trust. *National Health Service Costs of Childhood Accidents*. London: CAPT, 1992.

26   Hall, S. Current epidemiology of childhood infections. In: Alberman, E.D., Rechman, C.S., eds. Childhood epidemiology. *Br Med Bull* 1986; **42**: 119–126.

27   Anderson, H.R., Baily, P.A., Cooper, J.S., Palmer, J.C., West, S. Morbidity and school absence caused by asthma and wheezing illness. *Arch Dis Child* 1983; **58**: 777–784.

28   Bone, M. The prevalence of disability among children. *OPCS Surveys of Disability in Great Britain, report 3*. London: Her Majesty's Stationery Office, 1989.

29   Butler, J.A. Ensuring access to health care for children with disabilities. *New Eng J Med* 1987; **317**: 162–5.

30   Haggerty, R.J., Roghmann, K.J., Pless, I.B. *Child Health in the Community*. New York: John Wiley and Sons, 1975.

31   Baker, A.W., Duncan, S.P. Child sexual abuse: a study of prevalence in Great Britain. *Child Abuse Neglect* 1985; **9**: 457–467.

32   Oberklaid, F. Children with school problems – an expanding role for the paediatrician. *Aust Paediatr* 1984; **20**: 271–275.

33   Rona, R.J., Chinn, S. The national study of health and growth: nutritional surveillance of primary school children from 1972–1981 with special reference to unemployment and social class. *Ann Hum Biol* 1985; **11**: 17–28.

34   Jobling, M. *Anorexia Nervosa: a Review of the Research*. Highlight No 63. London: National Children's Bureau, 1985.

35   Hawton, K. By their own hand. *Br Med J* 1992; **304**: 1000.

36   Rutter, M. Attainment and adjustment in two geographical areas: prevalence of psychiatric disorder. *Br J Psychiatr* 1975; **126**: 563–579.

37   Kurtz, Z. *With Health in Mind*. London: London Action for Sick Children, 1992.

38   Black, D. Mental health services for children. *Br Med J* 1992; **305**: 971–972.

39   Elliot, B.J., Richards, M.P.M. Effects of parental divorce on children. *Arch Dis Child* 1991; **66**: 915–916.

40   De'Ath, E. *Focus on Families. Divorce and its Effects on Children*. London: Children's Society, 1988.

41   Calouste Gulbenkian Foundation. *Bullying: the Child's View*. London: Calouste Gulbenkian Foundation, 1992.

42   Tatum, D., Herbert, G. *Bullying: a Positive Response*. Cardiff: South Glamorgan Institute of Higher Education, 1992.

43   Troyna, B., Hatcher, R. *Racial Harassment in School*. Highlight No 92. London: National Children's Bureau, 1990.

44   National Association for the Care and Resettlement of Offenders: *Preventing Youth Crime*. London: NACRO, 1991.

45   Goddard, E. *Smoking among Secondary School Children in England in 1988*. London: Her Majesty's Stationery Office, 1988.

46   British Medical Association. *Young People and Alcohol*. London: BMA Board of Science and Education, 1986.

47   Office of Population and Censuses Studies. *Birth Statistics 1988 for England and Wales*. Series FM1 No 17. London: Her Majesty's Stationery Office, 1990.

48   Balding, J. *Young People in 1988*. Exeter: Health Education Authority Schools Health Education Unit, University of Exeter, 1989.

49   Balding, J., Foot., G., Regis, D. *The Assessment of Health Needs at the Community Level*. Exeter; Schools Health Education Unit, University of Exeter, 1991.

50   Winn, E. *Making Use of Community Health Services Information*. London: King's Fund Institute, 1986.

51   Rigby, M. Computing school health information. *Hlth Soc Serv J* 1985; April 18th: 486–487.

52   Fox, T.K., Rankin, M.G., Salmon, S.S., Steward, M.S. How schools perceive the school health service. *Pub Hlth* 1991; **105**: 399–403.

53   Jones, C., Gordon, N. The school entry medical examination: what do teachers think? *Child Care Hlth Dev* 1991, **19**: 173–185.

54   Fitzherbert, K. Communication with teachers in the health surveillance of school children. *Mat Child Hlth* 1982; **7**: 100-103.

55   Bevis, M., Taylor, B. What do school teachers know about asthma? *Arch Dis Child* 1990; **65**: 622–625.

56   Perkins, E.R. The school health service through parents eyes. *Arch Dis Child* 1989; **64**: 1088–1091.

57   Nicholl, A. Written material concerning health for parents and children. In: MacFarlane, J.A., ed, *Progress for Child Health*. Edinburgh: Churchill Livingstone, 1985.

58   Harrison, A., Gretton, J. School health: the invisible service. *Health Care UK: an Economic, Social and Policy Audit*. London: CIPFA, 1986.

59   Lloyd Jones, G. Records of pupil achievement. *Child Soc* 1988; **2**: 178–181.

60   Whitmore, K., Bax, M. Checking the health of school entrants. *Arch Dis Child* 1990; **65**: 320–326.

61   Bax, M., Whitmore, K. The medical examination of children on entry to school: the results and use of neurodevelopmental assessment. *Dev Med Child Neurol* 1987; **29**: 40–55.

62   Jones, C., Batchelor, L., Gordon, N., West, M. The

pre-school medical: an evaluation of this examination and its role in child health surveillance. *Child Care Hlth Dev* 1989; **15**: 425–434.

63 Broomfield, D.M. Selective medicals at school entry. *Public Hlth* 1992; **106**: 149–154.

64 Rona, R.J., Allsop, M. Referral patterns after school medical examinations. *Arch Dis Child* 1989; **64**: 829–833.

65 Varley, Y. Health of school entrants in a West Yorkshire health district in 1989. *Pub Hlth* 1990; **104**: 473–477.

66 Whitmore, K., Bax, M. The school medical examination. *Arch Dis Child* 1986; **61**: 807–817.

67 Leff, S. A survey of parental concerns as children reach school entry age. *Pub Hlth* 1991; **105**: 127–132.

68 Oberklaid, F. The ritual school health examination; an idea whose time has past. *Aust Paed J* 1985; **21**: 155–157.

69 Oberklaid, F. Selective examinations on starting school. *Arch Dis Child* 1988; **63**: 225.

70 Kennedy, F.D. Have school entry medicals had their day? *Arch Dis Child* 1988; **63**: 1261–1263.

71 Smith, G.C., Powell, A., Reynolds, K. The five year school medical: time for change. *Arch Dis Child* 1990; **65**: 225–227.

72 O'Callaghan, E.M., Colver, A.F. Selective medical examination on starting school. *Arch Dis Child* 1987; **62**: 1041–1043.

73 Richman, S., Miles, M. Selective medical examinations for school entrants – the way forward. *Arch Dis Child* 1990; **65**: 1177–1181.

74 Newby, M., Nichol, A. Selection of children for school medicals by a pastoral care system in an inner city junior school. *Pub Hlth* 1985; **99**: 331–337.

75 MacFarlane, A., McPherson, A., McPherson, K., Ahmed, L. Teenagers and their health. *Arch Dis Child* 1987; **62**: 1125–1129.

76 Malus, M. Towards a separate adolescent medicine. *Br Med J* 1992; **305**: 789.

77 Bennet, D. Adolescent health in Australia: an overview of needs and approaches to care. Health education and promotion monograph. Australian Medical Association, 1984.

78 National Health Service Health Advisory Service. *Bridges over Troubled Waters: a Report on Services for Disturbed Adolescents*. London: HMSO, 1986.

79 Marks, A., Fisher, M. Health assessment and screening during adolescence. *Pediatrics* 1987; **80**: 135–158.

80 Whiting, K. Towards a school health service for adolescents the teacher–health worker team. *Child Soc* 1990; **4**: 225.

81 Crouchman, M. The role of school medical officer in secondary schools. *J Roy Coll Gen Practit* 1986; **36**: 322–324.

82 Curtis, H. Teenage relationships and sex education. *Arch Dis Child* 1988; **63**: 935–941.

83 Cherry, N. Occupational health and the school leaver. *Comm Med* 1983; **5**: 3–10.

84 Kazdin, A.E. Self-report and interview measures of child and adolescent depression. *J Psychol Psychiatr* 1982; **23**; 437–457.

85 Linday, W.R. A self report questionnaire about social difficulty for adolescents. *Adolescence* 1982; **5**: 63–69.

86 Cockett, M., Kuh, D., Tripp, J. The needs of disturbed adolescents. *Child Soc* 1987; **2**: 93–113.

87 Challener, J. Health education in secondary schools: is it working? *Pub Hlth* 1990; **104**: 195–205.

88 British Paediatrics Association. *Report of the Working Party on the Needs and Care of Adolescents*. London: BPA, 1985.

89 World Health Organization. *Young People's Health: a Challenge for Society*. Technical Report Series 731. Geneva: WHO, 1986.

90 Epstein, R., Rice, P., Wallace, P. Teenagers health concern: implications for primary health care professionals. *J Roy Coll Gen Practit* 1989; **39**: 247–249.

91 Daniel, S. *Teenage Health: a Positive Alternative for Nottingham Youth*. Nottingham: Teenage Health Care Project, 1989.

92 Mattock, C. Stepping off the medical treadmill. *Health Visitor* 1991; **64**: 154–156.

93 Waldron, S. Involving parents in school age checks. *Nursing Standard* 1992; **6**: 37–40.

94 Fletcher, K. *School Nurses do it in Schools: Trends in School Nursing Practice*. London: Amalgamated School Nurses Association, 1992.

95 Williamson, T. Health care interviews by school nurses. *Health Visitor* 1992; **65**: 402–404.

96 Holt, H. Southampton's health appraisal pilot study. *Nursing Standard* 1990; **4**: 30–31.

97 Holt, H. Southampton's health appraisal pilot study. *Nursing Standard* 1990; **4**: 26–27.

98 Fine, P.E., Rodriguez, L.C. Mycobacterial diseases. *Lancet* 1990; i: 1016–1020.

99 Silverman, M. Childhood tuberculosis in Britain: going but not gone. *Br Med J* 1988; **296**: 1147–1148.

100 Medical Research Council Tuberculosis and Chest Diseases Unit. Tuberculosis in children: a national survey of notifications in England and Wales in 1983. *Arch Dis Child* 1988; **63**: 266–276.

101 Clarke, A., Rudd, P.T.R. Neonatal BCG immunisation. *Arch Dis Child* 1992; **67**: 473–474.

102 Conway, S.P. BCG vaccination in children: routine vaccination of school children is not cost effective and could be stopped. *Br Med J* 1990; **301**: 1059–1060.

103 Joseph, C.A., Watson, J., Fern, K. BCG immunisation in England and Wales: a survey of policy and practice in school aged children and neonates. *Br Med J* 1992; **305**: 495–496.

104 Royal College of General Practitioners, OPCS, Department of Health and Social Security morbidity statistics from general practice – third national study 1981–2: London: Her Majesty's Stationery Office, 1986.

105 Cundall, D. Inner city tuberculosis and immunisation policy. *Arch Dis Child* 1988; **63**: 964–966.

106 Sidle, N. *Rubella in Pregnancy – a review of rubella as an infection in pregnancy its consequences and prevention sense*. London: The National Deaf, Blind and Rubella Association, 1985.

107 Knox, E.G. Strategy for rubella vaccination. *Int J Epidemiol* 1980; **9**: 13–23.

108 Anderson, R.M., Grenfell, B.T. Quantitative investigations of different vaccination policies for the control of congenital rubella syndrome in the UK. *J Hyg* 1986; **96**: 305–333.

109 Rabo, E., Taranger, J. Scandinavian model for eliminating measles, mumps and rubella. *Br Med J* 1984; **289**: 1402–1404.

110 Smith, A. *The Nation's Health – a Strategy for the 1990s.* London: King's Fund, 1988.

111 Barker, D.J.P., Winter, P.D., Osmond, C., Margetts, B., Simmonds, S.J. Weight in infancy and death from ischaemic heart disease. *Lancet* 1989; ii: 577–580.

112 Lalonde, M. *A New Perspective on the Health of Canadians.* Ontario: Government of Canada, 1974.

113 National Curriculum Council. *Curriculum Guidance in Health Education.* York: NCC, 1990.

114 Topping, K.J., Lindsay, G.A. Parental involvement in reading the influence of socio-economic status and supportive home visiting. *Child Soc* 1991; **5**, 306–316.

115 Elliot, H. Developing a parental survival kit: 14+. *Educ Hlth* 1992; **10**: 73–78.

116 Comer, J.P. *School Power: Implications of an Intervention Project.* London: The Free Press, Collier Macmillan, 1980.

117 Currie, L. Developing a community perspective in a primary school. *Child Soc* 1989; **3**: 226–236.

118 Whitehead, M. *Swimming Upstream – Trends and Prospects in Education for Health.* London: King's Fund Institute, 1989.

119 Smith, R. Without work all life goes rotten. *Br Med J* 1992; **305**: 972.

120 Bristol and Weston Health Authority. *School Health 1991.* Bristol: BWHA, Dept Public Health Medicine, 1991.

121 United Nations. Convention on the rights of the child. *Treaty Series 44.* London: Her Majesty's Stationery Office, 1992.

8.2 Advice to teachers, parents and children

Elizabeth Pryce-Jones

Children are at school for a large part of their lives, and it is a vital time in their emotional and physical development. They are away from caring parents, and are exposed to peer groups and a wide variety of adults. It is a bewildering time with many problems which they will find difficult. The parents of most children are beset by recurring anxieties.

The Court Report[1] in 1976 was instrumental in surveying the primary objective of the school health service. Since that time there has been some progress in carrying out the recommendations. Primary care is available to all children through their general practitioner. In the past the tendency was for parents to consult the general practitioner only when their child was ill, or when they were seen for routine immunization. It is expected that more group practices will have at least one doctor who has been specially trained in community child health, including educational medicine. They will know their local area and will have met the children and their parents before they begin school.

School doctors have a wide range of community child health duties. They have had special training, and are clinically accountable to the local consultant community paediatrician. In the non-maintained private school sector, medical care varies considerably in both day and boarding schools: the school doctor is usually appointed by the governing body and may be a local general practitioner. At a boarding school the doctor will provide both day-to-day surveillance as well as treatment. Medical examinations should be arranged where possible to permit the least possible loss of school time.

All schools should have a named school doctor and nurse[2] who, in addition to undertaking surveillance, can promote the importance of general hygiene and a healthy environment. They must be known to the parents, the school teachers and the family doctors of the children. There should be information about the school health service in the local clinics and in the GPs' surgeries. Team work is essential with the parents playing an important part. The combined intent of parents, teachers, doctors and nurses is to ensure that the child is happy and healthy at school, and is able to reach his or her full potential.

Parents much accept the responsibility of choosing the schools for their children. Each local education authority or non-maintained school will have criteria about the selection of children for their particular school. Factors considered include catchment area, social need, the attendance of siblings and, for older children, ability, when teaching programmes vary accordingly. The school has, by law, to provide education appropriate to the child's needs.

On admission to school, having obtained parental consent, the physical well-being, growth, vision and hearing of all children are screened. In some schools all children are medically examined but, increasingly, a more selective approach is being adopted whereby the doctor sees the children about whom a parent, teacher or school nurse is concerned. Thereafter routine screening continues with full access to the school doctor when it is requested or indicated. The child's pre-school health surveillance record forms the basis of continuing surveillance through the school years.

Nowhere is information sharing more important than in the planning needed for children with special educational needs. A regular meeting of parents and professionals is required. These meetings should include the children if appropriate. For older children there is a need to involve other agencies, such as the careers advisory service and adult health services who will be involved in the care of the young person. Careful records must be kept of these meetings and the parents should receive a copy of the reports.

New school doctors or nurses should be introduced to the school by the relevant clinical manager before formal work in the school.

The school nurse has a key role for parents, school staff and the doctor. She is responsible for coordinating the records and pre-school health information, and must keep written records about every child for whom there is concern. These records must be preserved in total confidence, and information only passed on with parental/carer agreement. The nurse should find out what facilities are available for medical examination and negotiate for appropriate ones. A light, warm room and a convenient waiting area is the ideal. A small storeroom is unsuitable in place of a medical room; nor should it be next to the music room, where screening of hearing will be interrupted.

The parents should have visited the school before the child starts. They can then receive an impression of the school's atmosphere. An agreeable environment is of paramount importance for children to learn in, or where they can move about with order and interest. Ideally, this should include children's pictures on the walls and play areas with grass and agreeable buildings.

The school doctor should have access to a child's teacher when necessary. The parents should have been told that the child will always be seen by the school nurse and the school doctor if necessary, and the doctor and nurse will advise the teaching staff on any health problems. A knowledge of the home background is essential for the care of a child.

General observations of children at school can be very revealing. Short sightedness and hearing difficulties affect learning. The teacher on playground duty should be aware of those who lead and those who follow. Are those who follow isolated on account of their inadequacies? Teachers are well placed to observe a child's abilities and difficulties at work and at play and feedback should be encouraged to health professionals.

Before the child enters school, and certainly before he sees the school nurse or doctor, the parents complete a questionnaire. This is designed to cover the principal features of the child's medical history. It is also advisable for the teacher to complete a form giving an impression of the child in the first two terms. This should be available to the school health team and where appropriate should be followed by an informal discussion with the head teacher or class teacher about findings related to the child's school progress. Details of previous illnesses and immunization records should also be made available to the staff. Any condition which may compromise the child's education should be explained to the teacher; these include asthma, diabetes, eczema, hay fever, seizures and recurrent ear infections. Details of other illnesses, operations or hospital admissions with dates should be included in the health record. Allergies and drug sensitivities are important especially when dealing with the child at boarding school. It is essential to know whether or not a child has any problems either with bladder or bowel control.

The number of children from ethnic minority backgrounds who live in the UK has increased. There are children who board and return abroad for holidays. Consequently, it is important to know if they need prophylactic treatment for infections such as malaria.

The Warnock Report[3] recommended that, where appropriate and practical, children with special needs should be integrated into normal schools. This may involve provision of additional teacher support or special facilities within those schools. Most parents agree with this concept. The care of these children requires careful team work and how this is provided may need discussion within the school. If a child has a specific medical condition such as diabetes, specially trained paediatric nuses can visit the school to explain to staff how best to support that child and encourage learning. This nurse is a member of the community paediatric team, and will have leaflets available to explain how the disease affects a child. However, the school doctor and nurse are the primary sources of contact with the teachers and they should always be involved in specific medical advice to the school.

Common problems

Acne vulgaris[4]

This is the most common skin condition in adolescence and its causes considerable distress. It is amenable to treatment but requires patience and understanding. Pustules will respond to antibiotics. Their therapeutic response may take 2–3 months to have an effect, although resistant cases may take a year or more. Topical agents may also be useful; benzyl peroxide is probably the most effective.

In the case of girls, oral contraceptives which contain $5\,\mu g$ of ethinyloestradiol may be combined with the anti-androgen cyproterone acetate in a single tablet, but this should be used in difficult cases only.

Allergic conditions

The most common are:

1 Hayfever
2 Allergic rhinitis
3 Asthma.

Hayfever

Hayfever causes particular concern at examination time. Pollen counts are higher in the summer. The principal remedy is, therefore, to reduce contact with pollen, but this is difficult with the child playing sport on grass. The teachers should be reassured that often the excitement of the game will produce an outpouring of adrenaline with beneficial pharmacological effects. Antihistamines afford relief when taken as a slow-release tablet. The majority of children do not suffer drowsiness as a side effect with the newer antihistamines.

Allergic rhinitis

Eye or nose irritation respond to local treatment.

Asthma

The life of an asthmatic child has become easier during the last decade due to the better range of treatments. The principal aim of management should be to enable the child to lead a normal life. Each child should be properly instructed how to use a selective bronchodilator via a pressurized aerosol inhaler or rotahaler, usually in a measured dose. In cases of exertional asthma, or wheezing exacerbated by cold air, these attacks may be prevented by using the inhaler before games. Children with severe asthma may require a combination of drugs. Severe breathing difficulties encountered during a school day should be regarded as a medical emergency and the child seen urgently by the GP or the local hospital. As with all chronic childhood disease there is a wealth of leaflets written for the lay person with basic information about the disease. Children and families may find the national asthma helpline useful.

Diabetes mellitus

Teachers must be aware of how insulin works and the place of diet. Exertion may require additional sugar, or if swimming a few dextrose tablets given beforehand. The school doctor should explain to the teacher some symptoms of a child becoming hypoglycaemic.

Some adolescents rebel against the discipline of injections and diet and an authoritarian approach may be counterproductive.

Enuresis and soiling

Ninety per cent of children are dry at night by the age of five and 95% by the age of eight. A small proportion continue to have problems into their teens and early adult life. Late development of bladder control tends to occur in families. Physical causes such as urinary infections must be excluded. Emotional factors may exist. Active management of enuresis need not be started until the age of 8 years when the school nurse can be usefully involved.

Faecal soiling may be due to chronic constipation with overflow, and children with chronic constipation need referral. Soiling may occur with symptoms of serious emotional upset. The school staff must be advised that a punitive attitude is harmful in all cases of enuresis and faecal soiling.

Epilepsy

The aim of treatment is to control seizures without side effects. Teachers should be aware that drugs only rarely adversely affect learning abilities. Few restrictions are necessary, but teachers should be advised that the child should not swim alone, climb high wall bars, go mountain climbing or take part in other dangerous activities such as cycling unaccompanied on busy roads. There should always be a well informed adult available if the child should have a seizure.

Menstrual problems

A few girls are incapacitated with their periods. The child may have severe spasmodic pain and pallor on the first day. Rest at home or in a sickroom with a simple analgesic such as paracetamol provided by a parent or carer is all that is required.

Warts

These are viral infections which may occur on any part of the body and spread by direct contact through a breach of the skin surface. Warts which often cause concern to the school staff are those found on the under surface of the foot at the sites of greatest pressure. These plantar warts characteristically appear as deep seated nodules and can be very painful. As with all viral infections the incubation period is prolonged. The consensus view is that spread is by contact with surfaces recently contaminated by the virus such as the warm moist perimeters of swimming pools. Painful warts need treatment, but most will disappear spontaneously. When treatment is necessary it may consist of application of an appropriate keratolytic paint with regular paring of the wart; curettage under local anaesthetic is rarely necessary. It is best to keep the wart covered and there is no need to exclude the child from swimming.

Conjuctivitis

Children may arrive at school with sticky eyes and a purulent discharge. Antibiotic eye drops may be useful. Personal hygiene will help to reduce transmission.

Food poisoning

When groups of children succumb to sudden gastro-intestinal symptoms, often occurring within a few hours of eating or drinking, stool culture is indicated, kitchen hygiene must be inspected and remnants of meals that may have been contaminated analysed. This is the responsibility of the Department of Environmental Health.

Athletes foot or tinea pedis

This is characterized by an itchy rash between the toe clefts. As with warts the warm steamy atmosphere of swimming baths enhances the spread of infection and early treatment with one of the topical fungicides is advisable.

Nits or Pediculosis capitis

Pediculosis is an infestation by *Pediculosis capitis* (the head louse), *Pediculosis corporis* (the body louse) and *Pediculosis pubis* (the crab louse) of the hairy parts of the body or clothing by blood sucking lice. By far the most common problem in schools are head lice who recognize no social boundaries. They exist in three forms: the egg or nits, the nymphs and the adult louse. The eggs are characteristically yellowish white, less than 1 millimetre long and are attached closely to the hair near the scalp. They are particularly seen on the hair behind the ears and along the hair partings, and are distinguishable from dandruff which readily shakes off. If nits are not treated they will become lice when the principal symptom is an itchy head. Nits are laid on the hair near the scalp and those found more than one centimetre away will probably be dead. Head lice are spread by direct contact. Lotions are effective against them when they are properly used. Children should be encouraged to brush their hair regularly and vigorously. Current schemes recommend changing the chemical used in the lotion from time to time so that resistant strains do not prevail. The school nurse should be the principal health education advisor to school children and their parents. Routine inspection of heads is not the best use of nursing time since it does not reduce infestation. The current practice of the open classroom, the sharing of tables rather than individual desks and the encouragement of constructive talk between children about their work, and closer physical contact may make the spread of lice easier.

Scabies

This is a contagious skin disease caused by the penetration of a mite, *Sarcoptes scabiei*. Characteristically the child will have an itchy rash and burrows may be found on the front of the wrist and in the webs of the fingers. Transmission of scabies is generally by close and prolonged contact. Symptoms tend to be worse when the child is warm in bed. The siblings should be examined as well as the parents. Treatment with insecticide to all members of the household simultaneously is effective.

Safety at school[5]

A safe environment in schools is essential. Schools are subject to the Health and Safety at Work Act, 1974. There is a statutory requirement that schools should have a written safety policy. Staff should have first aid certificates. Accidents resulting in death or major injury must be reported to the Health and Safety Executive. The responsibility for notification lies with the immediate local authorities. Major injury covers most fractures, the amputation of hand or foot, the loss of an eye and any other injury which results in the person being admitted to hospital as an inpatient for more than 24 hours, unless that person should be detained only for observation. Further details are available from:

The Health and Safety Executive
Room 158
Baynards House
1 Chepstow Place
London W2 4TF

In recent years greater awareness has arisen of the risks of spinal injury, particularly cervical, in diving accidents and in rugby. A code of practice has been agreed by a number of interested national organizations and physical education staff should be aware of recommended practices to avoid such injury.

In the same way, adventure training exposes many children to environmental hazards such as hypothermia. Water sports and caving pursuits increase the risk of leptospiral infection which is transmitted through skin abrasions exposed to the urine of infected rats. Wet suits should be worn appropriately and any jaundiced child exposed to the risk should be referred to hospital for investigation.

Changing views on quarantine

Quarantine was the name used for the method of preventing the spread of infectious disease from ships whereby they were kept out of port for 40 days. Advice is still given that some children should be excluded from school to prevent the spread of infection. Advice about management of cases of infectious diseases can be obtained from the appropriate medical officer to the local authority on board.

Table 8.3 gives guidance about the period of exclusion.

Table 8.3 Incubation and exclusion period for the commoner communicable diseases

Disease	Normal incubation period	Period of communicability	Minimum period of exclusion	
			Cases	Contacts*
Bacillary dysentry (shigellosis)**	1–7 days	While organism is present in stool. Faecal–oral spread	Symptom free for 48 hours unless otherwise advised by MOEH e.g. food handler etc.	Except in food handlers allow to work or attend school if symptom free
Campylobacter	(if associated with contaminated food) Variable	Person to person spread rare	Symptom free for 48 hours	Usually none
Chickenpox	11–21 days	From 1 day before to 6 days after appearance of rash	6 days from onset of rash	None
Diphtheria**	2–5 days	While the organism is present in the nose or throat	As advised by MOEH	As advised by MOEH
Food poisoning** excluding Salmonellosis	2–48 hours depending on cause	Variable depending	Formed stools	None unless symptoms
Gastroenteritis**	Variable	While organism present in stools. Faecal–oral spread	Symptom free for 48 hours	None if symptom free
Giardiasis**	6–22 days	While organism is present in stools. Faecal–oral spread	Symptom free for 48 hours	None is symptom free
German measles** (rubella)	14–21 days	From a few days before, until 4 days after onset of rash	4 days from onset of rash	None for children. Pregnant teachers unless immune should seek medical advice
Infective hepatitis (hepatitis A)**	15–50 days (commonly 28)	From 1–2 weeks before, until 7 days after onset of illness	At least 7 days from onset of jaundice	None if symptom free. Protection with human immunoglobulin may be offered
Measles**	10–15 days (commonly 10 to onset of illness and 14 to appearance of rash)	From a few days before, until 7 days after appearance of rash	7 days from onset of rash	None
Meningococcal infection** (acute meningitis)	2–10 days (commonly 2–5)	While organism is present in nasopharynx	As advised by MOEH	As advised by MOEH
Mumps**	12–26 days (commonly 18–21)	From a few days before onset of symptoms until subsidence of swelling	Swelling has subsided (7 days min.)	None
Poliomyelitis**	3–21 days	While virus is present in stools	As advised by MOEH	As advised by MOEH
Salmonellosis**	2–48 hours	While organism is present in stools	Formed stools	None

Table 8.3 Incubation and exclusion period for the commoner communicable diseases (contd.)

Disease	Normal incubation period	Period of communicability	Minimum period of exclusion	
			Cases	Contacts*
Scarlet fever** streptococcal	2–5 days	While organism is present in nasopharynx	Appropriate treatment has been given by GP	None
Thread worms	3–6 weeks	Person to person and reinfection by faecal–oral route	No exclusion. Appropriate treatment should be given by GP	None, but advise treatment of household
Tuberculosis**	4–6 weeks	While organism is present in sputum	As advised by MOEH	As advised by MOEH
Typhoid and paratyphoid fevers**	7–28 days (T) (commonly 14) 1–10 days (P)	While organism is present in stools	As advised by MOEH	Usually none unless symptoms develop
Whooping cough** pertussis	7–10 days	From 7 days after exposure, to 21 days after onset of paroxysmal cough	21 days from onset of paroxysmal cough, or earlier if adequately treated (erythromycin for 7 days)	None

* Contacts   This usually means household contacts though if a case occurs in a food handler or care staff, contacts may also include their work mates and possibly clients.
** Statutory notifiable by doctor. Early informal notification to Medical Officer of Environmental Health (MOEH) (England and Wales) or Chief Administrative Medical Officer (Wales) by staff of institutions would be very much appreciated.

References

1 Committee on child health services. *Fit for the Future.* Chairman: Court, S.D.M. London: HMSO, 1976.
2 British Paediatric Association. *The School Health Services.* London: British Paediatric Association, 1987.
3 Committee of enquiry into the education of handi-capped children and young people. *Special Educational Needs (Warnock Report).* Chairwoman: Warnock, A.M., Cmnd 7212. London, HMSO 1988.
4 Medical Officers of Schools Association. *Handbook of School Health,* 16th edn. London: MOSA, 1984.
5 Department of Education and Science. *Safety at School: General Advice,* 2nd edn. DES safety series number 6. London: HMSO, 1979.

8.3 Children with special needs

Harry Daniels

The legislative framework

The legislation governing special educational practice has a long and convoluted history.[1] It reflects the ideology of deficiency and difference within the child population and may be viewed as an expression of power relations within and between professional groupings. The most significant recent forum for the readjustment of these tensions was the Warnock Committee[2] which was set up in 1974.

The Warnock Report was commissioned by the then Secretary of State for Education, Margaret Thatcher, to:

1 Review educational provision in England, Scotland and Wales for children and young people handi-capped by disabilities of mind and body, taking account of the medical aspects of their needs together with arrangements to prepare them for entering into employment.
2 Consider the most effective use of resources for these purposes.
3 Make recommendations.

Some, but by no means all, of the recommendations of the Warnock Report formed the basis of the Educa-tion Act 1981[3] which came into force in April 1983. The

Act itself was welcomed by Mary Warnock,[4] the Chair of the Committee.

The Warnock Report may be viewed as an expression of dissatisfaction with the then legislation; with the shifting balance of power from medicine to education through psychology, with respect to the definition of children's needs; and the growing political commitment to an equal opportunities perspective in education as expressed in the 'comprehensive education for all' movement.

While the Education Act of 1981 did reflect many of these concerns it attempted to legislate for a new vision of practice without any commitment to the allocation of extra money.

The Education Act 1981

Goacher, et al.[5] in their report of research commissioned by the Department of Education and Science into procedures for assessing and making provision for children's special educational needs, identified three main groupings of principles underlying the 1981 Act. They were those concerned with:

1 The *nature* of special educational needs
2 The *rights* of those with special educational needs (and their parents)
3 The *effectiveness* of identifying, assessing and meeting special educational needs.

These principles underpin the legislation and yet are in themselves laid open to actions designed to avoid their implementation. The clearest example of these somewhat ironic legislative quirks is the intention that special educational provision should be made available in ordinary schools. Local education authorities (LEAs) were urged to make such provision but were also furnished with conditions which have been interpreted as allowing them simply to maintain the status quo:

The conditions are that account has been taken, in accordance with section 1, of the views of the child's parent and that educating the child in an ordinary school is compatible with:

a his/her receiving the special educational provision he/she requires
b the provision of efficient education for the children with whom he will be educated
c the efficient use of resources.[3]

On inspection the legislation of 1981 reveals a set of intentions, derived largely from the Warnock Report, with sets of conditions which permit the rhetoric of progress and allow for the practice of entrenchment.

Needs

The key concept within the legislation was that of special educational needs as it was this that marked the significant change if only in the rhetoric. The 1981 Education Act definition of special educational need reflects contemporary views of the causes of educational difficulty.

Section 1 of the Act relates a relativistic view of learning difficulty to the need for special provision. In this way it embodies an interactive, if not transactional view of causation.[6] Need is conceptualized in terms of provision that must be made if a child is to make educational progress:

a child has special educational needs if he has a learning difficulty which calls for special educational provision to be made for him.[3]

In the 1981 Education Act, the concept of learning difficulty replaced the 1944 Education Act's system of classifying children according to categories of handicap:

A child has a learning difficulty if:

a he or she has a significantly greater difficulty in learning than the majority of children of his age;
b he or she has a disability which either prevents or hinders him from making use of educational facilities of a kind generally provided in schools within the area of the local authority concerned, for children of his age; or
c he or she is under the age of five years and is, or would be if special educational provision were not made for him, likely to fall within paragraph a) or b) when over that age.[3]

Special educational provision is now defined in terms of resources that are required by the child and which can be clearly described in the form of a legal statement:

a in relation to a child who has attained the age of two years, educational provision which is additional to, or otherwise different from the educational provision made generally for children of his age in schools maintained by the LEA concerned;
b in relation to any child under that age, educational provision of any kind.[3]

A legal statement of a child's special educational needs should therefore outline the resources required for that child to make educational progress. The protection of the child by a statement was envisaged as a way of avoiding the practice of categorization which was not seen as necessarily guaranteeing the provision required. Critics have commented on the extent to which this new formulation of need allowed LEAs to continue to match needs with existing provision,[7] teachers to express their own needs[1] and existing practices to remain unchanged or even expand.[1,7,8]

The significant underlying feature of the concept of special educational need is the emphasis placed on the interaction between factors within the child and within the environment.[6] This move away from the restricted view of the within child categories concerning disability of mind and body was intended to allow for a continuum of educational needs. This continuum breached what were increasingly seen to be the artificial educationally and socially disadvantaging boundaries between the 1944 Act categories of handicap.

The 1944 Education Act, whatever else it did, extended the four categories of children for whom special provision was made under the 1921 Act. It also invoked the notion that associated with these new categories of disability of mind and body were appropriate forms of provision. Children were to be diagnosed, principally by medical authorities, as being members of particular disability groups with which particular forms of curriculum and, in most cases, schools were associated. The most significant of these boundaries was that between the educable and the supposedly ineducable. This particular boundary had been breached in 1970 when all children were declared educable.[9] Understanding developed that the needs of children with disabilities and difficulties are not different in nature from those of other children. It was also recognized that special educational needs may vary over time and that the handicapping effects of disabilities and difficulties defy systems of categorization.[10]

In this way the logic of defining needs in terms of provision has acquired a logic and legitimacy. The huge degree of variation in mainstream and special educational provision by LEAs has made the practice of assigning children to immutable categories appear irrelevant and unhelpful.

The concept of special educational need embodies a relativistic view of difficulty. It defines individual needs in terms of actions required in particular contexts and tacitly announces the urgency of improving that provision, which counts as 'mainstream' or 'ordinary' in order to minimize the amount of perceived difficulty and consequent special need. The legal statement of special provision represents a mechanism for ensuring the rights of children to have access to their educational entitlement.

The 1981 Act lays down the procedures which are used when it is thought that a child's special needs require extra provision. That is after the teacher in the classroom and the school as a unit have made initial attempts which have not met the criteria held for expected progress. Parents may be the first to be concerned about their child's progress and they may request assessment. If other agencies act as initiators of the process they are required to make every possible effort to contact the parents. Assessment should take place in surroundings that are familiar to the child and is undertaken by professionals from health and education. An input from social services and other sources is requested when it is considered appropriate by the LEA. Advice following assessment of needs must be given in written form. When writing this advice, professionals should have access to any advice submitted by, or on behalf of, the parents.

The current suggestion is that the whole process from initial notification of parents to the production of a draft statement should take no longer than 6 months. During this period of time educational advice should be sought from the headteachers of all the schools the pupil has attended in the preceding 18 months. They in turn should seek advice from any specialist teachers who have worked with the pupil in that time. Medical advice that is relevant to the child's educational needs should be sought from the medical officer designated by the district health authority (DHA) who may have to collate information from several doctors. All other support service advice provided by the DHA may be appended to the statement. This implies that a very wide range of DHA services may be called upon to give advice. A case conference may be called by the LEA in order to bring together the professionals offering advice and to gain a complete understanding of the child's needs. While the final responsibility for producing an assessment of the child's needs rests with the LEA there is a high demand for interprofessional collaboration and cooperation if the process is to be effective. All written professional advice is shared with the parents.

Rights of parents

The parents of children with special educational needs have an obvious duty to ensure that their children's needs are properly met with appropriate forms of provision. The notion of parental partnership in decision making as part of the identification of need and the formulation of provision was reaffirmed by the 1981 Act. Sadly, suggestions in Circular 1/83 that parents should be fully involved with frankness and openness on all sides have not always been implemented.[11]

Goacher et al. report Roger's analysis of responses to the requirement that LEAs provide parents with carefully worded letters and clear concise information booklets.[5] He found that many were misleading and difficult to use. As a consequence of this and the lack of a named person as suggested in the Warnock Report, many parents found themselves isolated and unsupported. They often appeared to feel manipulated or ignored and debarred from any genuine active involvement in the decision making process.

Goacher et al. concluded that the 1981 Act did not represent the optimal legal support for the model of parental participation encouraged in Circular 1/83: 'It may appear that the majority of parents whom we interviewed felt that they were not able to influence the outcomes of procedures in any substantial way and raised many negative issues. Certainly the structures within the LEA and the District Health Authority (DHA) and the longstanding relationships between professionals and administrators in both services, put parents at a disadvantage.'[5]

The notion of partnership is at best struggling to survive in practice. It is clear from the research that if children's needs are to be fully and properly met, then those most concerned for their care and development must attempt to share the responsibility of planning the provision required.

Provision

This new interactive concept of need also raised a number of questions concerning intervention. Rather than arrange provision in different schools to deliver different curricula to diagnosed disabilities, the community school was to provide the modifications required to enable all children to make progress and to have equal opportunity of access to common experiences in the curriculum.

David Galloway insists that one of the major obstacles to effecting an integration policy is the individualizing of children's problems.[12] His argument is that children's difficulties should be seen as the products of their schools and that it is these that need changing if children's needs are to be catered for successfully.

The principle of individualization was one often cited as a hallmark of special education. Many mainstream teachers have in the past justified referral of children to special education on the basis of the child's need for more individual attention.[12,13] Yet the very term 'individualization' is arguably the cause of considerable confusion in educational circles. Brennan distinguishes between individualized teaching and an individualized curriculum, where: 'individualized teaching means that at any given time pupils will be in a teaching or learning situation most appropriate to individual learning needs. Individual curriculum means that from all the curriculum resources of the school a selection is made of the objectives, curriculum content and learning experiences most calculated to meet the identified curricular needs of individual pupils.'[14]

Attention is drawn to the mode of pupil organization and thus pupil teacher organization on the one hand and instructional organization on the other.

Brennan failed to distinguish between individualization that allows children to develop in their own personalized ways and individualization that seeks to encourage all children to similar ends by a variety of paths. The distinction is that of the principle of control, with implications for pupil relationships. Clearly if all pupils follow different individual projects they are unlikely to be taught as even small groups, whereas some communality may be drawn across groups of children all following similar paths but at different speeds and possibly in different sequences.

In many ways, the objectives-based version of individualization diverts attention away from the context and focuses it within the child: 'The effect has been to individualise problems, locating causes in the child and the child's family, and evaluating the outcome of treatment programmes in terms of the child's adjustment to the school. Children with special needs have become the unfortunate victims of what David Hargreaves (1980) in a related context has called the "cult of the individual". I suggest that this cult is the greatest single obstacle to progress in meeting special educational needs in the mainstream.'[15]

The implication is that the system of curriculum employed can fundamentally affect the social context of learning. The tacit downgrading of the importance of contextual analysis through exclusive concentration on individual outcomes, whether these are negotiated or not, is a continuing cause of concern.

Shapiro concentrates his analysis on the way 'individualization' has been applied to exceptional children whether they be gifted or talented on the one hand or handicapped on the other. His claim is that for the gifted child 'individualization' (that which has been defined here as practices which personalize) affirms the self to a far greater extent than it does with the handicapped, where the need to engage in learning through a particular approach becomes an emblem of inadequacy.[16]

While Shaprio argues that all forms of individualizing of instruction encourage the internalization of 'already-prescribed norms', he emphasizes the extent to which special individual needs are matched to 'precisely formulated goals'.[16] For the child with learning difficulties in the USA individualization does not emphasize flexibility, instead, 'the focus is on rigidly prescribed procedures; relative latitude and opportunity for discretion is replaced by a controlled and regulated schedule.'[16]

Clearly Shapiro is arguing that the predominant form of individualization for children with learning difficulties is in fact a highly controlled process. By defining individualization in the way he does, Brennan[14] confirms this proposition as the advised form of practice in England.

This sentiment is echoed by paragraph 2.7.10 of the Fish Report: 'Schools tend to regard the identification of children with special educational needs as tantamount to referring them for special educational provision, rather than seeing identification as the first stage of a process of experimental intervention in the school which is carefully monitored.'[17]

Systems approaches

Galloway[12] also considers the case for intervening at the school and classroom system level as the first step in providing for children's special educational needs. His approach is based on assumptions which many practitioners in special schools would certainly wish to dispute, in that they represent a fundamental challenge to aspects of segregated special educational provision which embody an individualized analysis of educational difficulty.

These assumptions are:

1 Children are seen as having special educational needs when their teachers are disturbed by their progress or by their behaviour. Hence, it makes no sense to see children's needs in isolation from those of their teachers.

2 Teachers in ordinary schools can, and do, cater successfully for children with a wide range of needs. This is not, however, so likely when the children are taught in remedial or separate special classes.

3 Schools are also able to aggravate, if not create, the problems which are taken as evidence of special needs.

4 The fact that a child has special needs does not necessarily imply that the child, as an individual, needs help. The most effective way to help the child may be to review aspects of school organization, or teaching methods and resources.

5 A child's special needs are more likely to be met, with a consequent feeling of satisfaction for the teacher, if the child is seen primarily as a teaching problem, rather than as having a learning or behavioural problem.[12]

Here there is a formulation of special educational need as a function of a variety of factors. The school organization and the teachers that work within it assume a high profile in this multidimensional model. Influential in Galloway's thesis is the 'schools make a difference' group of studies.[18,19] These studies all argue that a valid analysis of difficulty in school must treat aspects of the organization of the school as independent variables. Within this framework schools may be viewed as social systems which define both competence and failure in terms of context specific criteria.

In the general discussion of special education that is the main theme of this section a description of the special schools as they exist at present forms an important component.

Special schools

Tomlinson[13] showed in her study of decision making within selected special schools that many aspects of special education were not accountable for their quality of provision.

Jones[20] has drawn attention to the comparative infrequency with which advisers and advisory teachers with responsibilities for subjects and areas of study have worked regularly with special schools. Responsibility for new teachers who specialize in areas of learning difficulty either in or out of special schools has also been the subject of concern and will continue to be during the process of integration.[20]

These, however, are relatively minor issues; the major influence on special school organization, ethos, and style has been the headteacher. This influence, to which Tomlinson[13] drew attention in her study, is so marked that any attempt at establishing links between schools will have to focus on the levels of effective control of those schools.

Ford, Mongon and Whelan[21] advanced the case for seeing special education as a form of social control. Commensurate with this position is the notion that provided special schools are not too noticeably disrupted they will be allowed to follow whatever form of practice they choose. The lack of external pressure on special schools from the demands of public examinations and, until very recently, the low level of return by pupils to mainstream settings has allowed special schools' curricula to drift in whatever direction the school and, in particular, the head choose.[13]

Tomlinson observed headteachers, in special schools, with strong charismatic personalities who had 'freedom to create a school which reflects their own views and style'.[13] Thus given the relative autonomy of headteachers in the post 1944 Act education system, special school headteachers appear to enjoy a position of extreme freedom of action. 'Headteachers, in this study, appeared to be much more idiosyncratic in using their powers to determine the goals, organisation and curriculum of their school in accordance with their own personal style than Headteachers in ordinary schools.'[13]

This research suggests that referral to a special school did not imply that any particular form of special provision was to be made. The variation between schools was, if anything, greater in the case of special schools than in mainstream schools. It was also clear that remarkably little was known about what actually went on in special schools and units, particularly in terms of curriculum provision.

This situation has now changed. Her Majesty's Inspector of Schools (HMI) has provided major reports of surveys focusing on the quality of provision in both mainstream and special settings. It is clear there is much to be done.

Schools and units making special provision for children with emotional and behavioural difficulties were criticized for the narrowness of the curriculum, the lack of planning and policy for meeting personal and social needs on a systematic and developmental basis and the lack of staff professional development with its consequences in terms of quality of work.

Their overall suggestion was that small special schools and units as they were between 1982 and 1988 were not the ideal forms of provision for meeting the needs of children with emotional and behavioural difficulties.[22]

Similarly when HMI focused attention on the services which were intended to support children in ordinary schools there were many causes for concern.[23] There was a lack of explicit policy making with clear and coordinated leadership, the lack of time, resources and financial support made available and the very wide range in provision across LEAs. This report was by no means as critical as that on emotional and behavioural difficulty schools and units and it concluded that the better support services were indeed helping schools across a broad front to make effective provision for all pupils. The survey of pupils with special educational needs in mainstream schools made the case that schools do need support. Again the inspectors found some signs of encouraging development but still noted that 75% of schools used withdrawal of pupils with special educational needs in which the work was often unrelated to the classroom and less interesting and relevant than the missed classroom activity.[24] This resulted in pupils losing continuity with classroom work in both secondary and primary classes.

The years that have elapsed since the 1944 Act was implemented have witnessed a remarkable transition. Whereas children with special educational needs (SEN) went to a special school with a special curriculum, there is now much more official emphasis on admission to a mainstream school where the curriculum is modified to meet their needs. A most emphatic endorsement of an integration policy was published in the Inner London Education Authority report of the committee reviewing the provision to meet special educational needs: 'All those responsible for providing services to children and young people, whether or not they have specific responsibilities for those with disabilities and significant difficulties, should accept the aim of integration for all.'[17]

Historically, the system of categories of disability has in turn lead to the construction of a disability focused system of provision. Fish illustrated the difficulties in making provision by the traditional approach according to disability categories. His resolution of these difficulties, particularly those of multiple disability, was that the kind of curriculum to be offered should be the major determinant of provision, with specialist teaching skills regrouped in different combinations.[17]

Also, as professionals were seen as constituent parts of provision, concerns were raised as to whose needs were being expressed.[13] Galloway[15] argued that teachers' statements concerning children's special needs may reflect their own needs or the needs of other children rather than the educational needs of the individual concerned. While the new terminology avoided sole recourse to factors within the child it also allowed for the expression of system needs at the expense of the child.

The development of, or general concept of, a continuum of needs has been associated with a variety of attempts to conceptualize a continuum of provision. Deno,[25] writing from an American perspective, promoted the notion of 'cascade' of provision which has in turn been influential on British writers.[10,26] The range of such a cascade was characterized by a decrease in incidence and increase in the complexity of learning difficulties.[10]

Fish summarized the range of special provision under the following headings:

1 Provision wholly within the ordinary class or group
   a Interpretative and social assistance
   b Consultancy
   c Co-teaching
2 Provision additional to education within the ordinary class
   a Additional special teaching
   b Therapies
   c Attendance at classes, centres and special schools outside the ordinary school
3 Special classes and units in ordinary schools
4 Separate special units
5 Day special schools
6 Boarding special schools
7 Education in other institutions
8 Education at home

Fish added to this continuum the following aspects of provision:

1 Pre-school provision
   a Home visiting teaching
   b Other peripatetic teaching services in day nurseries and playgroups
   c Nursery schools and units including nursery units in special schools and special nursery units in ordinary schools
2 Post compulsory school provision
   a Staying on in ordinary schools
   b Staying on in special schools
   c Special and ordinary provision in colleges of further education
   d Provision in special colleges
3 Post-18 provision including special access arrangements for higher education and special adult education services

The general principle underlying the notion of a continuum of provision such as this was that children would be placed in the least restrictive environment capable of meeting their needs and returned to a mainstream environment as quickly as possible. Provision organized in this way provided professionals working in the system with the problem of how to make that which counted as mainstream accessible to those who were seen as having special needs.

Professional commentators on special education were in the process of recommending changes which had implications for mainstream and special education. While the call for a more truly comprehensive system was being made from those who focused their energies on the edges of the system, similar pleas were being made from those at the centre.

Notable among these influences are two that came from the Inner London Education Authority (ILEA) in the form of the Thomas and Hargreaves Reports.[27,28] Both these reports argue that traditional schooling has an unduly limited conception of academic achievement. They both seek to incorporate aspects of personal and social development into an integrated curriculum. The Hargreaves Report for example states: 'personal and social education at its best is an important bridge between the pastoral and academic aspects of the school's work and should serve to integrate a wide range of the school's aims and practices.'[28] The argument being that this will allow more children to participate as persons in mainstream education.[28] Dessent promoted the model of a continuum of provision matching the continuum of needs and argued forcefully that there should be no breaks in either.[29] However, in practice the implementation of the 1981 Act resulted in a wide range of provision across different LEAs. In that special needs were defined in the 1981 Act in terms which were relative to the educational context of mainstream provision, then arrangements for special provision also varied as a function of existing local provision and philosophy. The Spastics Society survey[30] revealed the dearth of response at a policy level to be found in many authorities. Although this is in part attributable to the lack of funding for implementation it also attests to the reluctance of authorities to dismantle the separate systems of provision, personnel and management as advocated by Dessent. As he notes, the power relations within the system seek to maintain the position of a range of system components which are of questionable value in the context of a fully implemented 1981 Act.

The variations in response to the 1981 Act have not been uniform across all possible impairments and difficulties. Swan noted that there had been magnificent falls in numbers of pupils with sensory disabilities in special schools and, although numbers in special schools of those with physical disabilities were static, it was clear that many of these children spent much of their time in mainstream schools. Swann[8] claims that while there was a trend towards integration of children with difficulties having an organic basis there was an increase in the numbers of children in special schools for learning and behaviour difficulties, during the period 1978–83.

Goacher *et al.*[5] provide a detailed analysis of changes in the pattern of provision for special educational needs after the implementation of the 1981 Act. They noted significant differences between authorities. For all types of provision they found some LEAs electing to direct children to the sort of provision that most other LEAs were choosing to run down. There appeared to be least consensus about provision for children identified as emotionally and behaviourally disturbed.[5] Significant variations were found in the extent to which statements were made as a proportion of the local population.

The picture that emerges from the literature is that of highly localized responses to legislation which lends itself to a range of interpretations and consequent forms of implementation. Indeed in all apsects of the Act, from the formal obligation to provide special education in ordinary schools to providing parents with explicit rights to participate in decision making, there has been a continuum of local responses.

The Education Reform Act

The question of to what extent any particular authority has implemented the Act does not, of course, preclude the question of quality of provision. This question is, perhaps, best explored in the context of the 1988 Education Reform Act.[31]

Wedell[32] has recently summarized the main principles about the education of children with special educational needs. He argues that analyses of the implementation of the 1988 Education Reform Act should question whether this new legislation is informed by these principles and whether it is likely to promote the good practice that has developed during the implementation of the 1981 Act.

The main principles about education for children with special educational needs can be summarized as follows:

- Special educational needs are no longer seen as due only to factors *within* the child. It is recognized that special educational needs are the outcome of the interaction between the strengths and weaknesses of the child, and the resources and deficiencies of the child's environment.
- It is therefore not meaningful or even possible to draw a clear dividing line which separates the 'handicapped' from the 'non-handicapped'. Special educational needs occur across a continuum of degree.
- All children are entitled to be educated. The aims of education are the same for all children, but the means by which the aims can be attained differ, as does the extent to which they may be achieved.
- All schools have a responsibility to identify and meet children's special educational needs, and all children should be educated with their peers as

long as their needs can be met, and it is practicable to do so.[32]

Many of the practices which have developed in response to the 1981 Act are based upon an assumption of cooperation. The introduction of the understanding that as many as 20% of the school population may have special needs at some time during their schooling carried with it implications for cooperation between teachers. It was always assumed that the majority of educational needs would be met by classroom teachers. The slogan became 'every teacher a teacher of special needs'. The focus of intervention for the specialist teacher shifted from being exclusively the child to being some combination of the child and the teacher. Where previously the remedial teacher had withdrawn children from ordinary lessons, now the support teacher worked alongside the classroom teacher in ordinary classrooms or offered advice outside teaching time.

Arguments in favour of this change were couched in terms of difficulties in transfer of training from withdrawal settings to mainstream settings and also restricted expectations of teachers and pupils in such settings. In the case of full-time special or remedial classes concerns were raised about the narrowness of the curriculum just as they had been about separate special school classes.

The move from patterns of full-time and part-time permanent or temporary withdrawal from mainstream classes towards greater support within the classroom was only successful when teachers collaborated in teaching, planning and reviewing lessons.[33,34] In turn, these acts of cooperation were invariably most successful in schools which had developed and maintained whole school policies on special educational needs.

The term *support* became widely used and also developed many meanings. Support for teachers; support for schools; support for systems and support for children were all developed and often confused with one another. Swann[35] notes that although support teachers have begun to see themselves as agents of curriculum change they have often been frustrated in their efforts. 'In some cases they have found themselves acting mainly as teaching aides with no control or influence on lesson content and methods and able to do little more than supervise and interpret for some pupils.'[35]

Subsumed in the notion of support is the understanding that it is worthwhile enabling children to have access to whatever experiences are being provided within the school. In terms of the 1988 Act, where support was offered from outside the school, either by specialist services or other schools, the question has now become one of who will pay for these forms of cooperation in the era of local financial management of schools.

The 1988 Act introduced what was designed to be a demand led, consumer-orientated system with a built-in financial incentives scheme. Money is to be made available to schools under the Local Management of Schools (LMS) Scheme primarily on the basis of numbers of children enrolled at a school. Schools are being encouraged to market themselves in order to attract the highest number of pupils possible and thereby ensure economic security. Perhaps the most powerful indicator of school effectiveness available to these marketing exercises will be aggregated subject attainment scores. These indicators will, of course, have to be balanced against the promotion of the school on non-academic criteria.

Paragraph 81 of the report of the Elton Committee[36] provides a timely reminder that 'a school in which academic achievement is the only source of positive encouragement is likely to experience more difficulties with low achieving pupils.'[36]

It is, as yet, unclear how these influences will impinge upon the development of provision. There are, however, a number of regulations worthy of consideration at this point in terms of their likely effect on the integration or segregation of children with special needs. Paragraph 36 of circular 6/89 allows children to be taught outside their key stage.

The outcome of research concerned to identify necessary conditions for successful integration suggests that children should never be placed in classes more than 2 years below their chronological age. If children are to be taught outside their expected key stage they would, in many cases, have to be placed in classes with children more than 2 years older than themselves. In recognition of the social difficulties this would engender, schools may be tempted to recreate separate special classes for children taught outside their expected key stage. Informal arrangements such as this may be made without reference to outside agencies whereas formal disapplication or modification of the national curriculum involves elaborate procedures and possible appeals.

Four sections of the Act[31] define the possibilities for formal exemption. Sections 16 and 17 are concerned with the regulations for groups, and sections 18 and 19 are concerned with the regulations for individuals.

Section 16 allows for exemption for experimental purposes. The exact scope of the term experimental is as yet unclear. It may be that this section will be employed by some special schools as a way of maintaining a position within the education system and also meeting the needs of their pupils. Section 17 in the draft of the Bill referred to categories of children; the Act now refers to cases or circumstances. The National Curriculum Council has repeatedly suggested that there is *no* need to invoke this regulation. This, of course, does not mean that it will not be used. There is already evidence that there are differences in orientation between the Department of Education and

Science (DES), the National Curriculum Council (NCC) and the Schools Examination and Assessment Council. Suggestions made by one of these agencies are not always supported by the others. If section 17 were to be used with children with severe difficulties they could easily be placed outside education.

Section 18 is concerned with procedures for making individual legal statements of need. DES Circular 22/89 (Assessments and statements of special educational needs: Procedures within the education, health, and social services) announced that these should detail needs irrespective of the authorities' ability to make provision although they would only be expected in special schools. Statements may be written in terms of aspects of the national curriculum which should not apply, and where appropriate should include details of required extra resources. The practice of making statements since 1983 has been subject to a number of social and economic pressures and there is no reason to suppose that this should not continue.[37] Statements can be written to support children or authorities. The majority of parental appeals against what is perceived as unfair practice are not successful.[37] The future of statement writing and the specification of needs will be highly dependent on local policies and professional practice. This in turn will be reflected in the proportion of children with special needs placed in segregated provision. Section 19 allows for temporary exemption from national curriculum requirements. It is argued by the NCC and the DES that this regulation should be used sensitively and sparingly. It may be argued that this regulation could be used to hide low attainment from the gaze of school aggregated subject scores and allow second-rate provision to be made within the school. LEAs could use the 1981 Act to inspect schools which were abusing this regulation and in that way ensure that proper provision was made. This action would be conditioned by local policy regarding children with special needs. It is well established that this varies between authorities.

If analysis of causation is pursued then just as deficiency on the part of the child may have been seen as a factor so may inadequacy on the part of the curriculum. In the context of the national curriculum, the question becomes one of whether it is valuable to fund support teachers whose role is one of enabling to have access to the curriculum if the content and method is not commensurate with their needs.

This is, of course, not a new problem. Brennan[38] provided an early and very clear analysis of the issue at stake: 'The real curricular problem is that of accepting the content limitations required to achieve quality of learning in the basic subjects whilst avoiding an educational programme which is sterile, unexciting and inadequate for both personal richness and social competence.'[38]

The regulations of the 1988 Act overlay a new level of decision making and analysis on this question of curriculum adequacy. This question is intertwined with one of entitlement. The 1988 Act enshrines a child's entitlement to a broad and balanced curriculum which aims to:

a promote the spiritual, moral, cultural, mental and physical development of pupils at the school and of society; and
b prepare such pupils for the opportunities, responsibilities and experiences of adult life.[31]

While it is made clear that the national curriculum does not constitute the whole curriculum, it is questionable whether the elements of national curriculum represent an entitlement or a restraint for pupil's special educational needs. In terms of policy making this issue is of great importance for children with severe and complex learning difficulties. This group of children who, before 1970, were considered ineducable and were catered for by health authorities, could be in danger of being returned to their former educational status. If the national curriculum is not to be seen as a restraint and these children exempted from its requirements, then they may be returned to non-educational provision. However, if they are retained in education, ways and means of achieving the Education Reform Act aims will have to be sought. This will involve seeking forms of curriculum provision which bridge the gap between national curriculum demands and individual special needs.

As mentioned above, one of the features of the implementation of the 1981 Act has been the growth of cooperation between schools in planning, policy making and provision of resources. In its most highly developed form this has led to clusters of schools envisaged in the Fish report.

The development of systems for taking corporate responsibility for the changing needs of a local community was envisaged within these groups of primary, secondary and special schools.

It has been argued that the organization of provision into clusters enables mainstream schools to observe their obligations under the 1981 Act to identify and meet the special educational needs of their pupils. They could become the organizational unit within which policy making and planning can proceed across the age phases. Together with resource provision this activity may achieve particular significance in the context of local financial management and real cost charging for services, as will be discussed below. Certainly at present cluster based planning provides a context for cross service links and cooperation between the major statutory services of education, health and social services. This would help to alleviate many of the problems highlighted in DES funded research projects which focused on decision making.[39]

Interservice cooperation

Evans *et al.* noted that a great deal of time and energy has been expended in attempting to coordinate unwieldy and unresponsive networks of provision and that there have been difficulties in establishing a common approach both within and between health, social services and education authorities. The research conducted by this team concluded there had been very little joint planning between these authorities for the implementation of the 1981 Act. This in turn resulted in a lack of consultation and only allowed collaboration and cooperation to take place in unofficial and ad hoc initiatives.

They cited the difficulties created for therapists from the health service with the increased placement of children with special educational needs in mainstream schools. Lack of consultation had led to inadequate joint planning and resourcing. As a consequence while therapists supported moves towards integration they often felt frustrated by the actual practices that emerged particularly with respect to the diminution of their own effectiveness. Evans *et al.* also found that health authorities tended to have difficulty in coordinating the advice sent to LEAs for the preparation of individual statements.

To ease communication difficulties such as those sketched above, the team suggested a number of strategies:

1 Health and education authorities need to discuss, and clarify the meaning of terms such as special educational need.
2 Agreement should be sought on measurement of the effectiveness of therapies in terms of educational progress.
3 Joint financial mechanisms should be arranged for support services.
4 Services should be reorganized to ensure support of attaining normalization rather than inadvertently thwart it. (The case of retaining clinic-based assessment rather than school or home-based assessment was used as an illustration.)
5 Guidelines of responsibility for payment for aids and equipment should be established including boundary criteria, to avoid inappropriate shifting of responsibility.
6 Definition of a health service officer well briefed about children with special needs to liaise between the services.
7 The establishment of a within service system of collation and clarification of reports and advice to facilitate communication with other services.
8 Child needs should act as the reference point for advice rather than the ability of a service to provide.
9 The process of resource allocation within health services should be informed by greater knowledge of decision making processes and by monitoring of demand for services.
10 Confidentiality should be regarded as a cross service matter rather than allowing important information to be withheld within one service.
11 Parents require more systematic support in obtaining involvement of voluntary organizations.
12 Regular reviews of policy and provision should involve all three statutory services.[39]

The team made many other suggestions with respect to the organization of social and education services. The research made it very clear that there was much to be done within all three major statutory services before collaboration between them would successfully support the full implementation of the 1981 Act.

Just as between service cooperation would be facilitated within clusters, so could cooperation between schools, voluntary and community services. Clusters represent a very high level of cooperation within the education service. They may be seen as intermediaries between LEA and school levels of resource organization and as such may assume a significant role in attempts to provide community based provision in the future. This sort of cooperation between schools is seen by the NCC as a necessary part of the implementation of the Education Reform Act for children with special needs.

Ironically the 1988 Act has introduced the ideology of competition into the public provision of education. The market forces argument, that through competition quality is assured, has been applied to schooling and so schools are the units of competition. It is difficult, at present, to reconcile the need for cooperation with this new system of competition.

The role of the support services has also changed with the implementation of the 1988 Act. Educational support services will be constrained by the amount of money left in local authority control after LMS has been implemented. The amount was a maximum of 10%; it decreases to 7% within 3 years and may possibly continue to decrease thereafter. This financial arrangement places considerable strain on authorities wishing to maintain support services which work across schools. Similarly the ability of authorities to pay for real cost charged medical and therapeutic services will be limited. These funding considerations could well influence the process by which children's needs are defined.

Conclusion

Children with special educational needs are a problem, or at least they should be! The process by which their needs are identified and provision is specified should be seen as one of problem solving. Through the adoption of procedures and protocols that acknowledge that there are no simple formulae for the solution of problems, then services and school systems have the opportunity of effectively meeting needs rather than compounding existing needs or even creating new ones.

If teachers are to solve the teaching problems presented by children they must work together. Learning difficulty arises through interaction in specific contexts. The process of changing contexts so that difficulty does not arise or is minimized is complex and involves intervention at a variety of system levels. Individuals have great difficulty in effecting change when operating as isolated agents. Teachers can bring about system change within schools for the good of children with special educational needs when they plan, teach, and evaluate together. This sharing of responsibility in the problem-solving process should also extend across professional boundaries within education (across age phases and sectors) and also across the statutory services of education, health and social services.

The present legislation does not appear to encourage such sophisticated levels of cooperation. The situation demands that professionals who are concerned with children with special educational needs should seek ways of working which avoid the dangers presented by uncaring analyses of cost effectiveness, marketing and competition. The effects of the new Code of Practice introduced in 1993 are awaited.[40]

References

1 Galloway, D., Goodwin, C. *The Education of Disturbing Children: Pupils with Learning and Adjustment Difficulties*. London: Longman, 1987.

2 Department of Education and Science. *Special Educational Needs (The Warnock Report)*. London: HMSO, 1978.

3 Department of Education and Science. *The Education Act 1981*. London: HMSO, 1981.

4 Warnock, M. Introduction. In: Welton, J., Wedell, K., Vorhaus, G., eds. *Meeting Special Educational Needs: the 1981 Education Act and its Implications*. London: University of London Institute of Education, Bedford Way Papers 12, 1982.

5 Goacher, B., Evans, J., Welton, J., Wedell, K. *Policy and Provision for Special Educational Need Implementing the 1981 Act*. London: Cassell, 1988.

6 Wedell, K. Concepts of special educational need. *Education Today* 1981; **31**: 3–9.

7 Tomlinson, S. The expansion of special education. *Oxford Rev Educ* 1985; **12**: 157–165.

8 Swann, W. Is the integration of children with special needs happening? An analysis of recent statistics of pupils in special schools. *Oxford Rev Educ* 1985; **11**: 3–18.

9 Department of Education and Science. Education (Handicapped Children) Act 1970. London: HMSO, 1970.

10 Fish, J. *Special Education: the Way Ahead*. Milton Keynes: Open University Press, 1985.

11 Department of Education and Science. *Assessments and Statements of Special Educational Needs*. London: HMSO, 1983.

12 Galloway, D. *Schools, Pupils and Special Educational Needs*. London: Croom Helm, 1985.

13 Tomlinson, S. *Educational Subnormality: a Study in Decision-Making*. London: Routledge and Kegan Paul, 1981.

14 Brennan, W. *Curriculum for Special Needs*. Milton Keynes: Open University Press, 1985.

15 Galloway, D. Meeting special educational needs in the ordinary school? Or creating them? *Maladjustment and Therapeutic Education* 1985; **3**: 3–10.

16 Shapiro, S. Ideology, hegemony, and the individualizing of instruction: the incorporation of 'progressive education'. *J Curriculum Studies* 1984; **16**: 367–378.

17 Inner London Education Authority. *Equal Opportunities for All? The Fish Report*. London: ILEA, 1985.

18 Rutter, M., Maughan, B., Mortimore, P., Ouston, J., Smith, A. *Fifteen Thousand Hours: Secondary Schools and their Efforts on Pupils*. London: Open Books, 1979.

19 Reynolds, D., Jones, S., St Leger, S., Murgatroyd, S. School factors and truancy. In: Hersor, L., Berg, I., eds. *Out of School, Modern Perspectives in Truancy and School Refusal*. Chichester: Wiley, 1980.

20 Jones, N. The management of integration: the Oxfordshire experience. In: Booth, T., Potts, P. eds. *Integrating Special Education*. Oxford: Blackwell, 1983.

21 Ford, J., Mongon, D., Whelan, M. *Special Education and Social Control: Invisible Disasters*. London: Routledge and Kegan Paul, 1982.

22 Her Majesty's Inspectorate of Schools. *A Survey of EBD Provision in Schools and Units (ref 62/89)*. London: HMSO, 1989.

23 Her Majesty's Inspectorate of Schools. *A Survey of Pupils with Special Educational Needs in Ordinary Schools*. London: HMSO, 1989.

24 Her Majesty's Inspectorate of Schools. *A Survey of Support Services for Special Educational Needs*. London: HMSO, 1989.

25 Deno, E. Special education as development capital. *Exceptional Children* 1970; **37**: 229–237.

26 Topping, K. *Educational Systems for Disruptive Adolescents*. London: Croom Helm, 1983.

27 Inner London Education Authority. *Improving Primary Schools (the Thomas Report)*. London: ILEA, 1985.

28 Inner London Education Authority. *Improving Secondary Schools (the Hargreaves Report)*. London: ILEA, 1984.

29 Dessent, T. *Making the Ordinary School Special*. London: Falmer Press, 1987.

30 Rogers, R. *Caught in the Act*. London: CSIE/Spastics Society, 1986.

31 Department of Education and Science. *Education Reform Act 1988*. London: HMSO, 1988.

32 Wedell, K. The 1988 Act and current principles of special needs education: an overview. In: Daniels, H., Ware, J. eds. *The Implications of the National Curriculum for Children with Special Educational Needs*. London: Kogan Page, 1990.

33 Thomas, G. Room management in mainstream education. *Educ Res* 1985; **27**: 186–194.

34   Thomas, G. Extra people in the primary classroom. *Educ Res* 1987; **29**: 3.

35   Swann, W. Learning difficulties and curriculum reform: integration or differentiation. In: Thomas, G., Feiler, A., eds. *Planning for Special Needs: a Whole School Approach.* Oxford: Blackwell, 1988.

36   Department of Education and Science. *Discipline in Schools (the Elton Report).* London: HMSO, 1989.

37   Wedell, K., Evans, J., Goacher, B., Welton, J. The 1981 Education Act: policy and provision for special educational needs. *Br J Spec Educ* 1987; **14**: 50–53.

38   Brennan, W. *Shaping the Education of Slow Learners.* London: Routledge and Kegan Paul, 1974.

39   Evans, J., Everard, B., Friend, J. *et al. Children with Special Educational Needs: a Source Book of Information, Ideas and Discussion Points. The 1981 Education Act. Research Dissemination and Management Development Project.* Leicester: Tecmedia, 1989.

40   Education Act 1993: Draft Code of Practice on the Identification and Assessment of Special Educational Needs, DFE.

8.4 Absenteeism and school refusal

Alan Cooklin and Neil Dawson

Introduction

Doctors are at their most effective when there is a lesion, it is identifiable, and is relatively easy to treat within the resources of time, place, and equipment available in a consultation room. Absenteeism and school refusal do not fulfil any of these criteria. They do not occur in the consulting room, the cause is usually unclear, and there is no specific treatment available. This augurs badly for the doctor's success in alleviating the problem, and many doctors have been highly frustrated in their attempts to return children to school if they have tried to achieve this from within so limited a viewpoint. A wider framework of treatment is called for, one which recognizes and responds to the complex social, cultural, and relationship contexts in which the problem occurs. For some doctors this may also require a change in the role they play when responding to the complaints of parents or school about a child's non-attendance at school, or about its implied causes. This section focuses on a framework for thinking about non-attendance at school, considers the concept of cause rather than a list of causes, and the most relevant role for the doctor to play (whether as paediatrician, community paediatrician, or general practitioner) in ensuring the most effective management of the problem.

Definitions

Even at the level of definitions there are problems, so we will start with the simple question:

Why do children not go to school?

Illness

The majority of absences from school are recorded as illness.[1] If a child is too ill to return to school or has to be admitted to hospital, the local education authority has a duty to make alternative educational provision. If it is illness that is preventing the child from going to school, and there is no suggestion of avoidance of school, the only problem is to ensure the child receives adequate education.

Fear of persecution

Children will sometimes stay away from school if they are frightened of being bullied. There are many situations in schools where this is a realistic fear and the child's absence from school is an understandable avoidance of being physically assaulted by other children. Both overt and covert racism can also result in children not going to school. If children are consistently subject to racist taunts, abuse and physical attacks, they are likely to find school a frightening place and to take opportunities to stay away whenever possible.

Demoralization and academic failure

Children who do not succeed academically at school can decide to reject the activity and the institution in which they have experienced failure. In the UK, this phenomenon is particularly associated with 14–16 year olds who choose not to go to school during their last two years of school. This phase of school life, where public examinations are often the main focus of attention, highlights the distinction between those children who have succeeded and those who have failed. For members of the latter group, absence from school can be seen as an attempt to avoid being labelled as failures.

Lack of cultural or subcultural support

In some families and cultural groupings, attendance at school is not valued and absence is consequently not of significant concern to the family. Children from such families may be sent to school in accordance with the legal imperative to do so, but will be encouraged to leave school as soon as the pressure to attend is removed. Discrepancies between the social, moral or religious beliefs of the schools and those of the family or cultural grouping are likely to be at the base of the conflict. Some ethnic minority groups may find it particularly difficult to support certain school practices which are insensitive to their cultural, social or religious beliefs. For the child in these situations to be happily engaged with school activities may be a sign of disloyalty to the family's behaviours and beliefs. Absence with the tacit agreement of the family is one way the child has of avoiding an untenable situation.

A proper resolution can only be achieved by adapting the educational provision to ensure it is more congruent to the needs of the relevant group, as has been tried in a small number of community education experiments.

Not wanted

Children who go to school and are *perceived* as behaving so badly that they are eventually expelled sometimes end up with nowhere to go. How each teacher experiences a child's behaviour depends on many factors including his or her own response to the child. Some schools will ensure that there are opportunities to compare and learn from different perceptions of a particular child. However, if transfer to a second school is arranged, and this does not lead to an automatic change in behaviour and the child is asked to leave once again, a protracted period of absence from school can ensue. During this phase the education service will attempt to make decisions about an appropriate future placement for the child. Some individual tuition may be provided by the education authority but will usually be minimal. A situation can develop where the child is seen as not behaving well enough to be acceptable to any school, and therefore not welcome in any school. More or less permanent absence from school is then often covertly agreed to by all parties.

Apparently irrational fears or avoidant behaviour

Some children show extreme anxiety about going to school or into situations in school which do not appear to be anxiety provoking for most children. Such children may develop physical symptoms when attempts are made to get them to go to school and will often be absent from school for protracted periods of time. Symptoms commonly include gastrointestinal, upper respiratory (allergic and infective), and musculoskeletal complaints, or exacerbation of these or any other on-going complaint. We will discuss this group in more detail under the heading of school phobia or school refusal.

Truancy and school refusal or school phobia: traditional distinctions and definitions

Children who do not go to school provide crucial information for education researchers. Because there is a legal requirement for schools to keep an accurate record of attendance, a child's absences are recorded consistently and reliably. From the day when they first start school until the official leaving date, approximately 11 years' data for each child can be available for research. This ability to count and record absences has resulted in children who do not go to school being studied in great detail.[2,3] One of the main outcomes has been to distinguish two distinct types of absentees from school. Children whose parents apparently do not know or do not give consent for absences from school have been labelled *truants*. Conversely, children whose parents know about their child's absences from school have been labelled *school phobics* or *school-refusers*. These latter terms have been used for different purposes by previous authors but appear to refer to the same grouping and will be used synonymously in this chapter.

Truancy

Truants have been defined as those children who decide not to go to school.[4] They do not usually tell their parents and are likely to leave the house and spend their time either alone or with others keeping themselves amused in one way or another. Truancy is often associated with delinquent behaviour patterns such as stealing, lying, drug taking and other antisocial behaviour. As well as actively choosing to do other things than go to school, truants are often also actively choosing not to go to school because they consider that it does not meet their needs. They are likely to have poor relations with teachers, to feel unsuccessful and to describe school as 'boring' and say that it 'gets on their nerves'. In educational literature,[5] truants have often been described as disaffected. This has been an attempt to represent the *interactional* nature of the relationship between the child and the school. Rather than lay all the blame on the child for not liking school or even the family for not actively supporting school, educationalists have also highlighted the responsibility of the school to ensure that the curriculum and conditions at school are inviting for different kinds of children. The ability to achieve this may be limited by the introduction of external constraints, such as the national curriculum currently being introduced in the UK.

School phobia or school refusal

Children who refuse to go to school have been particularly distinguished as a group by the manifest extreme anxiety shown by the child when faced with the prospect of going to school. In contrast to truants, these children who refuse to go to school stay at home with their parents' knowledge.

School refusers have been studied more widely in child guidance and psychiatric clinics, largely because they are more likely to agree to and to attend more regularly for treatment than truants. While truants will frequently hear from teachers, welfare officers, doctors, and others that their persistent absenteeism from school is a problem, this view will often have little meaning for them. They will see psychiatric interventions as being as irrelevant and unhelpful to them as was their perception of attendance at school in the first place.

Much of the research that has been carried out on absenteeism has focused on differences between the populations of truants and school refusers. Truants are more likely to be influenced by peers than other absentees. This term was used by Galloway[2] in a way which is virtually synonymous with school refusal as used here. He also showed that other absentees were likely to have had a significantly greater history of anxiety about leaving home than truants, and that they were more likely to have expressed fear of harm befalling a parent or to have shown anxiety about a parent's health. Truants were more likely to have had a history of stealing, lying and of wandering from home in the evenings and weekends. By contrast, other absentees were more likely to stay at home in the evenings and weekends to a degree which may itself have become of concern to those outside the family.

In the traditional child psychiatric approach to school refusal, the focus of treatment was the unresolved mutual dependency relationship between mother and child.[6] Skynner[7] has stressed the importance of a family approach to school phobia, because the previous emphasis on defects in the mother–child relationship neglected a 'crucial failure of the father to help loosen the originally exclusive mutual attachment between mother and child'. Huffington and Sevitt's study[8] suggested similar characteristic patterns of family interaction in adolescent school phobia. Hersov[9] provides a detailed review of the literature on school phobia.

Absenteeism: the doctor's dilemma

By definition, a child who is ill should not go to school and should not return until he or she is well. A paediatrician or general practitioner faced with a child complaining of physical symptoms which are difficult to substantiate, or which would normally be considered routine and trivial can face a difficult dilemma, particularly if these are part of a pattern of significant absences from school. If the child's parent confirms the belief that the child is ill and therefore needs to stay away from school for protracted periods, the situation becomes even more problematic.

If a child is in pain or physically upset and the parents are worried, or believe there is some cause which needs to be identified, the doctor also has to take the symptoms seriously. If the symptoms are lightly dismissed, the doctor firstly cannot be sure, and secondly his or her professional competence can be brought into question in a way which is unhelpful to the child, while the family seeks what they imagine is more skilled advice elsewhere. On the other hand, if the symptoms are only taken at face value and treated with medication, the doctor faces the possibility of colluding with a behavioural pattern between child, family, and perhaps others, which may be encouraging a pattern of response to all life's problems in terms of increased morbidity. As well as providing treatment that would be difficult to justify, the practitioner will be aware that the treatment is likely to support the child continuing not to go to school.

This treatment/no-treatment dilemma is often central when a doctor is consulted about a child's health in a situation where non-attendance at school is a related feature. To treat the child is not satisfactory where there is no apparent physiological need. To refuse to treat the child is also unacceptable because that would be likely to leave the child experiencing symptoms and not going to school. The situation is made more complex because the symptom of not going to school is enacted in a context predominantly outside the medical world and is subject to a set of procedures administered by a complex network of professionals associated with education and schools.

The non-attendance is possibly of secondary concern to medical practitioners in relation to health considerations, whereas the absences from school are likely to be of primary concern to teachers and other education professionals. Of course it is only a dilemma when the doctor defines his or her role in so restricted a way as in the caricature introducing this section; a view which would not now be accepted as adequate by most paediatricians and general practitioners.

Clearly, to resolve the dilemma and avoid following either unacceptable course, the doctor has to introduce more choices into the situation. The introduction of more choices is an effective way of challenging debates or conflicts about causes which can develop. This conflict over cause and effect is often seen in families where children do not go to school. 'My child has a stomach ache, he is ill; because he is ill he can't go to school.'

A systemic approach

A systemic approach offers a different framework for thinking about the formulation and management of school absenteeism problems. It is essentially a way of understanding behaviour by focusing on the interconnection between behaviours, context and beliefs. Behaviours derive meaning from the context in which they are occurring. 'Stephen hit John' offers little meaning about the behaviour when compared with a similar statement, 'Tyson hit Bruno', where the context is a world heavyweight boxing match. Systemic thinking also holds that there is an interplay between a person's beliefs and their behaviour. People behave in ways that are consistent with their beliefs. The family is a self-defined system which is likely to be the most important context for the development of attachments between people. Within the family, one person's perception of another's behaviour and that other's perception of the behaviour create mutual feedback processes. Over time, this feedback modifies the family members' behaviours and interactions until an identifiable predictability and pattern emerges. This idea of pattern is connected to the individual family members' beliefs, but also to more encompassing family beliefs. A family belief is not in a steady state as it is constantly changing in relation to those beliefs handed down from the past and is always being influenced by current behaviours and events in the family and culture. The family is always in a state of tension between stability and predictability versus flexibility, or recognizable patterns versus change, often provoked by inevitable events such as births, deaths, marriages and all the associated complexities involved with living.

A systemic perspective assumes that there is no simple cause or effect. Rather it is based on the assumption that the child will be responding more or less appropriately to environmental pressures, such as concern for a father's drinking in an unhappy marriage, while the child's behaviour will itself form a pressure on the behaviour of the couple. Thus if the child, for example, befriends the mother, this may diminish her distress but also remove some of the impetus for the parents to find a real solution for their problems with each other. Furthermore, it may increase the alienation of the father. The resultant lowering of tension may be an additional incentive for the child to stay at home. To change any one of these features will necessitate and result in a change in how aspects of all these relationships fit with each other as well as with others such as the school staff. The systemic perspective provides the underpinning to the various treatment approaches under the heading of family therapy, but also to a much broader range of interventions which take into account the whole social context of child, family, school, and others.[10,11]

A systemic approach to absenteeism and school refusal

Within a systemic approach, a child who does not go to school is no longer thought of as having a symptom for which he or she is solely responsible. The child's behaviour of not going to school is conceptualized as one part that he or she plays in relation to both his or her own individual behaviour and belief interplay, but also in relation to the family's behaviour and belief framework. This is not to shift responsibility from the child and transfer blame to other family members for the child's non-attendance at school. A systemic investigation looks for connections between individual and family beliefs and behaviours, as well as to what degree these seem to fit with the beliefs and practices of the school, in such a way that the unacceptable behaviour of not going to school starts to make sense for the system. Despite the upset, discomfort, frustration, or guilt for the parents, teachers and others when a child develops any symptom and particularly panic about going to school, a systemic understanding may demonstrate why it might be preferable for the child to continue not to go to school. This apparent benefit of the continuation of the problem may be to the parents' or others' advantage as much or even more so than to the child. As well as an investigation, a systemic understanding of the child's dilemmas and the family's predicaments in relation to the non-attendance should reveal the beliefs and behaviours that need to change if the child is to be released from the need to stay away from school.

The treatment/no treatment dilemma is replaced by an attempt to challenge the family's over-simplified cause and effect framework by starting on a systemic investigation:

Mother: 'I don't know what it is, but he can't face the school. He becomes physically sick; I can't bear to watch it. He puts it all on the one teacher who seems to blame him for anything that goes wrong.'
Doctor: 'Is this something the teacher agrees with; that Ian is always in trouble?'
Mother: 'No. All the staff say he's fine in school, and in fact he's well liked.'
Doctor: 'So Ian, do you worry about Mum as much as she does about you in the mornings?'
Ian: ''Spose I do.'
Doctor: 'Did she know that?'
Ian: 'Dunno. 'Spose she did.'
Doctor (to mother): 'And when did the tummy aches start?'
Mother: 'About three weeks ago.'
Doctor: 'Are they common knowledge or is it only you who knows?'
Mother: 'No, his father knows, but blames me for worrying too much over him.'
Doctor: 'Who else worries about Ian's tummy aches?'
Mother: 'My mother.'
Doctor: 'So, who is more worried about them, you or your mother?'
Mother: 'I suppose my mother really.'

Doctor: 'What effect does your mother's concern for Ian's health have on your relationship with his father?'
Mother: 'It always leads to arguments.'

This transcript illustrates the process of using feedback from family members to connect the child's symptom to other significant relationships in the family. One can begin to see that the child's avoidance of school is playing some important part in the mother's mediation of the relationships between her husband and her own mother.

Absenteeism: an interactional event between the child, the family, the school system, the legal system, medical services, social services and education welfare services

As well as investigating the pattern of relationships in the family when a child consistently stays away from school, a systemic approach necessitates an inquiry into how the absence has activated professionals from any of the groupings mentioned above. It is difficult to identify what is an effective intervention to reduce absenteeism; it is easier to identify ineffective interventions, or those where action has been blocked by poor interprofessional coordination.

Hargreaves[5] reported that schools with very similar intakes vary in their attendance rates and that this constitutes prima facie evidence that school policies can influence attendance. He listed examples of good practice that had been observed in schools which encouraged improved attendance rates:

1 A senior teacher is charged with specific responsibility for pupil attendance.
2 Each day a list of absentees is produced quickly, ideally by morning break by the office.
3 The school devises a sensitive scheme for the immediate follow up of absentees, e.g. by telephoning home or sending out letters to parents or guardians.
4 Form tutors take care to ensure that records of attendance are accurate and that explanations for absence are produced when pupils return to school.
5 The head of year or house monitors the work of form tutors.
6 The heads of year and the teacher with responsibility for pupil attendance have regular meetings (say once a month) with the education welfare officers.
7 There are regular spot checks for lesson truancy and for pupils leaving school before the end of the school day.
8 There are rewards (in the form of praise or prizes) for individual pupils or classes with an excellent attendance record.
9 There are penalties for pupils who are persistently late.
10 Pupils with a record of truancy who return to school are quietly welcomed back and efforts are made to reintegrate them socially and academically.

Effective action may be blocked where the authority to act in relation to a child's school absence appears to have been taken away from the school and its associated educational welfare officers. This can happen if medical practitioners seem to be maintaining the problem by defining a child as ill and therefore the normal regimen cannot be used. In the face of unclear communication about a child's health, schools often do not feel empowered to take firm action in relation to persistent absence. Furthermore, legal action in relation to persistent non-attendance is rarely contemplated by educational professionals if there is a suggestion of medical professionals supporting a medical opinion in a potentially adversarial position.

A preliminary study of factors which increase the likelihood of a child successfully re-entering school[12] demonstrated that if one staff member was given full responsibility for the return of a group of children into school, and providing that this person was not at odds with the community paediatrician or general practitioner, this constituted the single most important factor in ensuring the success of a child's return to school.

The part played by doctors in the management of school refusal and absenteeism will therefore be most effective when they relate their action to these factors as well as to a formulation of the processes within the child and family. This inevitably implies some change in doctors' exclusive relationship with the patients, and requires that they form a more collaborative relationship with people, both personal and professional, in the child's world of family and educational system.

Success will be most likely if the doctor can form a positive alliance with the family, so that they perceive themselves as becoming effective rather than encouraging the notion that the child's difficulties represent a mysterious disorder (an idea which has sometimes incorrectly been seen to emanate from some child guidance clinics) from the treatment of which the parents are excluded, and which by definition implies their failure.

A case example will illustrate the complex nature of family and professional systems that can be created in relation to a child's absence from school.

Case example

Mark was 13 years old when he was referred to the Marlborough Family Service (MFS). He should have been in the third year of the local comprehensive school, but had only attended for two days in all of his secondary school career. He was referred to the MFS by the school's education welfare officer (EWO) because of her concerns about his long-term non-attendance.

MARK AND HIS GRANDPARENTS

His grandparents were in their late seventies and had brought Mark up since he was 3 months old. They had taken over Mark's care at the time when their son had separated from Mark's mother. Mark was said to see his father approximately once a month, but had not been allowed to see his mother. His grandparents were both quite frail and talked a lot about concerns for their own health and also about Mark's problems with asthma and a ganglion on his wrist. The whole of his hand and lower arm were wrapped in a bulky bandage. They said that he was awaiting an operation to remove the ganglion but that this could not take place until he had fully recovered from a recent chest infection. They said they had been advised by a consultant at the local hospital that he should not go to school until after the operation on his wrist, because if it were knocked he would suffer permanent damage. Mark behaved in a very sulky and petulant manner towards both his grandparents and refused to comply with any of their requests. His responses to questions were equally petulant and showed his development to be at a very immature level.

COMMENT

The grandparents seemed preoccupied with their own frailty and their incapacity to manage an adolescent boy. Mark's health problems appeared to give them something to concentrate on and thus deflect some attention from their own declining powers. His petulant and demanding behaviour could be said in one sense to have developed a function in keeping them from having time to worry about themselves, but was having the unfortunate effect of also wearing them out and not allowing them to enjoy the later stages of their lives in a more settled way.

THE FAMILY AND THE SCHOOL

The grandfather had been on the school's parent-teacher association. The teachers did not feel that they knew Mark, but were very concerned about his failure to get to school successfully. They said that they did not fully trust the grandfather but were not able to given any concrete evidence to support their feelings. They felt that Mark's illnesses were not as serious as his grandfather suggested and that every effort should be made to support him to behave normally and go to school.

COMMENT

Mark's non-attendance had the effect that his grandfather was better known at his school than he was.

THE FAMILY AND THE EDUCATION WELFARE SERVICE

The EWO was convinced that Mark's illnesses were not serious or adequate to prevent him from attending school. She had been trying to support the grandparents in helping Mark to go to school for the past two years but felt completely frustrated by the lack of success. She was considering implementing legal action, but felt threatened by the grandfather's reports from the local hospital.

COMMENT

The EWO was being prevented from taking potentially effective action by an unclear definition of Mark's medical condition.

THE FAMILY AND MEDICAL PRACTITIONERS

In collaboration with the EWO, a case conference was called at the local hospital where Mark had been a regular inpatient in relation to his asthma. The consultant described Mark's symptoms as very mild and said that he shared worries about the degree to which health problems seemed to be being used as a means to avoid going to school. He also gave information from the medical records that Mark had been treated at two other hospitals in the vicinity. It was agreed to share information with these other hospitals and to write to all the hospitals in the London area within reach of the family home.

COMMENT

Before this case conference neither the grandparents nor Mark had mentioned the other two hospitals. They had also reported the consultant's opinion incorrectly. The suspicion aroused caused the EWO to start a more extensive investigation of Mark's involvement with other hospitals.

OUTCOME OF HOSPITAL INVESTIGATIONS

Nine hospitals responded saying that at various times they had treated Mark for a wide range of somatic complaints. None of them knew of each other's involvement with Mark and his grandparents. Each hospital representative reported colleagues' misgivings about the need for Mark to be treated medically. Several commented that they thought Mark's behaviour towards his grandfather was worryingly aggressive, but had been unable to persuade them to take up any offers of psychiatric intervention. Mark had been operated on several times and on each occasion the surgeon was said to have been dubious about the need for the operation.

COMMENT

The alarming evidence being gathered about the extent of Mark's involvement with hospitals and the dubious nature of his need for treatment strengthened the EWO and all the other professionals involved in their resolve to challenge damaging family patterns.

THE FAMILY AND THE LAW

The grandfather had originally been quite bullying in his response to the EWO's information that she might have to resort to court action if Mark did not go to school. Once the EWO decided to pursue juvenile court proceedings, the grandfather changed his attitude dramatically and started to be much more open about the difficulties that he and his wife had had managing Mark's aggressive and disruptive behaviour and about his wish for some help so that Mark could be cared for more effectively.

COMMENT

The sharing of information between professionals and the depowering of the myths about Mark's medical condition resulted in appropriate action being carried through by the education professionals. This meant that the destructive family patterns could be firmly challenged via the medium of legal action. This seemed to be a necessary intervention in the face of a persistent pattern of secrecy in the family and lack of ability to change through persuasion alone.

In an adult this presentation might have attracted the diagnosis of Munchausen syndrome. This is a less useful term in child psychiatry, partly because the presentation of a wide range of apparently disconnected symptoms as a reason for avoiding school is both more common and more easily identified. Furthermore the child alone generally has less power to make operations happen.*

OUTCOME FOR MARK AND HIS GRANDPARENTS

The grandparents were supported in making arrangements for Mark to go to live with his aunt's family in Dorset. They continued to visit him regularly but were under much less physical and emotional strain than when they had sole responsibility for his care. Mark started to attend the local comprehensive school regularly and was reported to be doing well academically and to be captain of the school's rowing team. This information was reliable as it was received direct from the school.

* This needs to be distinguished from Munchausen syndrome by proxy[13] in which there is overt parental falsification of a child's medical history, sometimes in situations of abuse, and often including non-accidental poisoning.

What can the doctor do?

A reasonable rule is to do the least possible but to take care in identifying what that realistically is.

Three grades of intervention are possible:

Minimal

The easiest situation for the doctor is when the problem has developed suddenly, in a child who has previously done well in school, and there is a reasonable mutual understanding between parents and child about the nature of the problem. The doctor may only need to encourage the parents to take more definitive action on their own behalf, such as by enlisting the school staff's help in reviewing factors at school. If the nature of the problem is not apparent, talking to the family, as in the first example, about the significant relationships, may clarify the more appropriate issues for the family to resolve so that they themselves can then get the child back to school.

The doctor may observe a particular relationship pattern which is in part maintaining the problem, an example of which was included in the first case transcript. If the doctor asks both parents to come together with the child, it may be possible to observe the relationship pattern and to invite them to participate in a simple intervention; such as the father taking the child to school for one or two weeks. This may have the effect of removing the child from the arena of the disputes between for example the mother and the grandmother.

In all cases, the overriding principle is that it is rarely helpful to children to agree that they remain away from school as a solution. A successful return to school will often make clear the nature of the underlying problem.

Intermediate

When simple interventions fail, the doctor faces the choice of doing more of the same or of widening the arena of observation and intervention. Either or both may be necessary.

Doing *more* may include convening a number of meetings with the family until one can observe the pattern which maintains the problem, and then working out a plan with the family which returns the child to school. Other professionals such as the Education Welfare Officer may need to be recruited to make such a plan work. This is also an example of *widening* the arena. In order to understand why the child's world is not working (and to change it) the doctor may need to engage other players. Examples may include one or more grandparents, siblings, special uncles or aunts, the year head or other teachers in the school, and perhaps other medical colleagues to avoid working at cross purposes. This last point is illustrated in the last example.

Major intervention

Major intervention *may* be something some doctors will want to undertake or at least to initiate themselves, or it may be the point at which they will want to refer to specialist services or to encourage other agencies such as social service departments to take action. It takes two main forms:

1 Engaging the child and family in a major therapeutic process aimed at changing the organization of the family relationships and the way the child and family perceive relationships (including those in school).
2 Changing the educational or care context of the child. This can include an alternative type of school near home, a boarding school, or in some circumstances an alternative care provision (particularly when the opinion is formed that the overt aims of the family are actually in conflict with the developmental needs of the child – as in the last example).

These interventions have deliberately been arranged in this hierarchy to stress the importance of utilizing the family's natural resources and doing the minimum whenever possible. Even if there is a need to implement one of the major interventions, the principles used in the lesser grades should direct the doctor's approach.

References

1 Mortimore, P., Coulter, A. *Non-attendance at School: Some Research Findings.* London: ILEA Research and Statistics report 860/82, 1982.
2 Galloway, D. Research note: truants and other absentees. *J Child Psychol Psychiatr* 1983; **24**: 607–611.
3 Berg, I. The management of truancy [annotation]. *J Child Psychol Psychiatr* 1985; **26**: 325–331.
4 Kahn, J.H., Nursten, J.P., Carroll, H.C.M. *Unwillingly to School: School Phobia or School Refusal: a Psychosocial Problem,* 3rd edn. Oxford: Pergamon Press, 1981.
5 Inner London Education Authority. *Improving Secondary Schools: Report of the Committee on the Curriculum and Organisation of Secondary Schools* (Chairman, Hargreaves, D.). London: ILEA, 1984.
6 Johnson, A.M., Falstein, E.L., Szurek, S., Svendsen, M. School phobia. *Am J Orthopsychiatr* 1941; **11**: 702–11.
7 Skynner, A.C.R. School refusal: a reappraisal. *Br J Med Psychol* 1974; **47**: 1.
8 Huffington, C.M., Sevitt, M.A. Family interaction in adolescent school phobia. *J Fam Ther* 1989; **11**: 353–375.
9 Hersov, L. School refusal. In: Rutter, M., Hersov, L., eds. *Child and Adolescent Psychiatry: Modern Approaches.* Oxford: Blackwell, 1985.
10 Cooklin, A.I. Therapy, the family and others. In: Maxwell, H. ed. *An outline of psychotherapy for medical students and practitioners.* Bristol: Wright, 1986.
11 Dawson, N., McHugh, B. Families as partners. *Pastoral Care in Education* 1986; **4**: 102–109.
12 Miller, A., Cooklin, A. *Interventions in School Attendance Problems* [Report of a working group]. London: Marlborough Family Service, 1983.
13 Mrazek, D., Mrazek, P. Child maltreatment. In: Rutter, M., Hersov, L., eds. *Child and Adolescent Psychiatry; Modern Approaches.* Oxford: Blackwell, 1985.

Chapter 9

Child care and protection

9.1 Ethical issues in community paediatrics

Raanan Gillon

This section adopts a framework of ethical analysis based on the proposals of Beauchamp and Childress[1] according to which concern for four prima facie moral principles and their scope of application can be shared by all, regardless of their religious, political or philosophical backgrounds and preferences. The principles are:

1 Respect for people and for their autonomy (essentially, deliberated choices for themselves) so far as is consistent with respect for the autonomy of all concerned.
2 A requirement to help others (beneficence).
3 A requirement not to harm others (non-maleficence).
4 An obligation to behave justly or fairly to others (justice). Justice can be considered in the context of just distribution of scarce resources, justice in respect for people's rights and justice in respect for (morally acceptable) laws.

Questions of scope ask: to whom or to what do we owe these obligations? I have discussed these principles and their scope more fully elsewhere.[2]

We can accept that the central moral objective of health care is an attempt to provide net health care benefit rather than harm for the patient in the contexts of respect for the patient's autonomy and justice. So then it soon becomes clear that one of the first ethical issues that needs to be confronted is one of scope – particularly the principle of respect for autonomy. Some children are not autonomous at all (think of a newborn baby: since to be autonomous one must be able to reason or deliberate, clearly babies cannot be autonomous); while other children, though they may be to some extent autonomous in being able to deliberate about their choices and actions, are nonetheless insufficiently autonomous for their decisions to be

respected if such decisions conflict with their best interests. This issue – when does a child become sufficiently autonomous for his or her decisions to be respected in the same way as an adult's decisions should be respected, even when others believe that such decisions are not in their interests – is an inevitable theme of ethics in paediatric health care. It does also arise in various contexts of adult health care. Whenever it arises it produces problems for the central moral objective of health care for it immediately suggests the patient's autonomy is either absent or inadequately developed to be a reliably acceptable guide.

Responsibilities and rights of parents and proxy consent

What to do? I shall begin with an empirical claim. In our society, and so far as I am aware in most societies, what is done is to endow the parents of the child with the responsibility of looking after the interests of their child. In pursuit of this objective parents are granted certain rights, including the right to make certain decisions on behalf of their child; these include decisions about whether or not to consent to proposed health care treatments. In different terminology, parents are accepted as proxy decision-makers for their children until such time as they become socially recognized and respected as competent to make their own decisions. This parental responsibility and associated rights apply unless there is good moral reason for them to be withdrawn. Such a reason could be failure or threat of failure of the parents to carry out their responsibility of looking after the interests of the children, whatever the cause of that failure. Thus if parents demonstrate that they are sufficiently neglecting or damaging their children, whether because of mental disorder, alcohol, drugs, incompetence or any other cause, the child can, in our society, be made a ward of court and responsibility for the child's care, and the correlated rights of proxy decision making for the child are taken away from the parents and given to others deemed more likely to be responsible for the child's interests. Similar provisions apply in other societies. Taken to its conclusion, this process means that in an irresolvable disagreement between health care workers and the parents about what is best for the child, the parents' views should, prima facie prevail. There are of course social mechanisms for withdrawing parental rights of proxy decision making for their children and it is open to all, including health care professionals, to apply to the courts to withdraw such rights whenever they believe that the parents are sufficiently neglecting or harming their children. In the UK, this is usually done by referral to the social services department, but it can be done directly by application to the appropriate court. In emergencies, action to protect the child can be taken without prior application, though the action may have to be defended in court.

However, as indicated above, it remains open to discussion that parents ought not to be the normal proxy decision-makers for their children, or at least not in certain contexts. It might be argued for example that when parents disagree with health care workers the latter's judgements should automatically prevail. I have the impression that such a norm would be greatly preferred by some health care workers who would argue vigorously that the interests of children in general would thereby be far better protected than is currently the case. But given that such arrangements are not those pertaining in our society, that many would vigorously oppose such arrangements on the grounds that they would be more harmful overall than beneficial, and that it is morally necessary for people who wish to institute such arrangements to go through justified processes for changing our social norms (notably the processes of political argument and democratic change), then until and unless such change is democratically instituted, health care workers may not impose their decisions unilaterally on parents with whose decisions they disagree.

I must immediately qualify this unequivocal assertion for there are rare emergencies in which great harm is likely to befall the child if health care staff delay action until the normal legal processes are complete. For example if a child is likely to die in the absence of an emergency blood transfusion or, say, cardiopulmonary resuscitation, and the parents refuse permission to intervene, yet there is a reasonable expectation that with the treatment the child will not only survive but will recover to have an ordinarily acceptable quality of life, then, in the UK at least, doctors can go ahead and impose the treatment on the child where there is no time to seek advice from the court. Indeed, in the case of emergency resuscitation it is likely that any suitably qualified health care worker is entitled to intervene despite the objections of parents. If, for ex-

ample, a child seemed to have drowned and a life saver or first aider were told without explanation by bystanders claiming to be the child's parents that on no account was resuscitation to be attempted there is little doubt that the life saver would be morally (and probably legally, though that is a matter of expert legal opinion) entitled to ignore this refusal and attempt resuscitation. However, even in life-threatening circumstances, the dangers of too simplistically assuming that health care workers can impose action against the request of close relatives is vividly demonstrated by Iserson[3] who described a case where ambulance staff insisted on carrying out full life-support measures for an unconscious patient whose husband vainly explained that she was dying of incurable metastatic cancer and had explicitly rejected life support.

Thus, in summary, despite the general moral norm to the contrary, rare justified exceptions do exist which permit health care workers to override parental refusal of permission to treat their children. However, treatment should not be imposed unilaterally and where such a course of action is believed to be in the child's interests the matter should, except in emergency, be referred to a court for adjudication.

If the social norm of parental responsibility as proxy decision-makers on behalf of their children is accepted by doctors and other health care workers it is clearly in the interests of all to avoid hostile confrontation with the child's parents. The approach most likely to influence the parents to take good health care decisions on behalf of the child seems to be one of soundly reasoned and explained advice given to parents as part of the mutual objective or promoting the health of the child. By and large, health care workers are most likely to persuade parents if they behave in a supportive and non-confrontational way, acknowledging the parents' prime responsibility to take decisions on behalf of their children and the health care worker's own subsidiary role as expert adviser. If that approach fails, and if, in the health care worker's opinion, the child is sufficiently endangered, then an appeal to a court – society's referee between the two opposing sides – is usually possible. In real emergency the health care worker can act unilaterally to protect the child, and be ready to defend his or her action in court subsequently.

Autonomy and the child

What however is a child? Put differently, when should a health care worker accept that the parent is the proper decision-maker for the child or young person and when should the child or young person's own decisions, if these conflict with the parent's, be accepted? A simple answer is to offer a certain age and say that above that age the young person's decisions prevail, below it the parent's decisions prevail. To some extent such answers are supported by legislation – but only to some extent. Thus below the age of 16 years a parent is presumed in English law to be the proper person to give or withhold consent to medical treatment of the child, while at 16 years and above a young person is presumed under the Family Law Reform Act to be competent to make such decisions.[4] But as the House of Lords decision in the Gillick case makes clear this presumption may be overturned if the child under 16 years is sufficiently mature to make his or her own treatment decisions competently[4,5] (see Section 9.3). Conversely if a person older than 16 years is sufficiently mentally disabled others may be permitted to make medical treatment decisions on behalf of that person and at times against his or her wishes or apparent wishes, though this remains a muddy area so far as British law is concerned.[4,6,7]

Autonomy – literally self-rule – is, as already stated, the capacity to make deliberated choices, and in the context of action the capacity to act on those choices. Empirical aspects of autonomy have not been worked out very thoroughly. It seems reasonable to claim that to be autonomous one must have (at least) the following capacities: some ability to think or deliberate; some ability to assimilate and organize adequate information upon which to deliberate; some ability to imagine hypothetical consequences of hypothetical events and actions (what would happen if?); some ability to decide to do things and not do things (intention); some ability to overcome obstacles to one's intentions (will power); and some ability to translate decisions into mental or physical action. I have reiterated 'some ability' in each of these categories because in my view it is vital to realize that no one is *fully* autonomous and a concern with *full* autonomy is inappropriate and potentially undermining of the moral value of respect for autonomy. Rather we are required to respect the autonomy of those who are *adequately* autonomous, and thus the question of when should we accept and respect the autonomous decisions of children turns on the answer to the question when do children become adequately autonomous not when do they become fully autonomous.

Some rough guidelines exist for the degree of autonomy that a person needs for it to be respected even when others believe that such respect is against that person's interests. These are the legal guidelines provided by the House of Lords in the Gillick case.[5] Briefly, doctors were advised by Lord Scarman that if they intended to prescribe the contraceptive pill for girls under 16 years they should ensure not only that the patient understood the advice being given but also that she had sufficient maturity to understand what was involved. This includes an awareness of related moral and family questions, especially the girl's relationship with her parents, long-term problems associated with the emotional impact of pregnancy and its termination, and the risks of sexual intercourse at a young age, with and without contraception. 'It follows that a doctor will have to satisfy himself that she is able to appraise these factors before he can safely proceed upon the basis that she has at law capacity to consent to contraceptive treatment.'[5]

Thus in cases of minors below the age of 16 years, while they may be considered in English law to be adequately autonomous to make decisions about their own medical examination and treatment, the presumption must be they are not unless thorough discussion has proved otherwise. The converse is true of adults, i.e. people over the age of 18 years. They are presumed in law to be adequately autonomous for their decisions to be respected even when these decisions are against their interests. For example they can make legally valid contracts that are detrimental to their interests, whereas if an under 18 year old signs a similar contract in many contexts it is legally invalid.[8]

Beneficence and non-maleficence

Just as parents are normally the socially recognized proxies in respect of their child's autonomy so they are in the context of harms and benefits. It is prima facie for parents to decide on behalf of their children what will count as harms and benefits and how these should be balanced. Once again the role of health care workers is to offer advice about what they believe to be in the child's health interests; and it is for the parents to decide on behalf of the child whether or not to accept that advice. Once again a legal safety mechanism exists whereby parents can be legally deprived of their role as guardians if there is evidence that they are neglecting or actively harming their child. Thus again the approach most likely to be effective in promoting health care of children is for health professionals to encourage trust and confidence from parents, to avoid confrontation and hostility, to offer reasoned advice on that considered to be in the child's health care interests and to respond understandingly and sympathetically to the parents' views. Nor need disagreement about what is in the child's health care interests entail that either side is wrong.

There are many different ways of being healthy and of flourishing, and often disagreements are matters of lifestyle perceptions and preferences, or of what counts as the good life. Moreover questions of harm and benefit are always complicated by questions of probability – passive smoking almost certainly does produce some risk of harm to those who inhale other people's exhaled smoke, but the probability of this occurring is quite low. We allow each other to inflict a certain degree of risk of harm on others, including our children. For example we allow parents to take their children out for car drives. In ordinary life we accept that the risks of imposing harm on others have to be balanced by their probability and we legislate to prohibit risk on others only where there is probability of sufficient harm. If these points are ignored in the context of health care there is a real danger that health risks will be disproportionately singled out as more important than other risks that produce similar probabilities of similar degrees of harm. Such a trend would bode ill not only for health care (for the result of over-zealous concern about health risks is likely to be a backlash rejection of sensible health care) it would also bode ill for social life as a whole if health care workers became the new puritans.[9]

Nonetheless there is no doubt that in many cases parents choose unhealthy options for their children, whether by not teaching them to clean their teeth, by allowing them to smoke, drink alcohol or to take addictive drugs, by smoking themselves, by failing to have their infants immunized or by failing to give them much in the way of interpersonal stimulus such as reading and talking to them. Other parents refuse to have anything to do with orthodox health care professionals, whether for religious or other reasons, thus totally or largely denying their children the benefits of contemporary health care. And then some parents may positively abuse their children, physically, sexually or psychologically. In all such cases health care professionals may be faced with major moral dilemmas, for the more they try to impose their views on such parents the more likely are the parents to avoid having anything to do with them. Where the child is not seriously endangered a policy of continuing, patient and reasoned advice from the health care worker still seems, at least to me, to be more likely to secure the child's best interests than hostility and lecturing. However, the child's safety must be protected and at some significant level of probability of danger to the child the health care professional has to explain to the parents that he or she too has a duty of care to the child, including a legal duty under the crucially important Children Act 1989, and that this requires outside consultation with a view to protecting the child (see Section 9.3). Referral to a third party agency – social services or even in extreme cases directly to the police – needs to be seen and presented as a referral to a sort of umpire or referee to decide what is in the interests of the health and safety of the child. If this can be done then some sort of bond of shared concern may be maintainable rather than the complete breakdown of relationships that is likely to arise if a punitive or hostile approach is taken, however understandable such an approach may be in cases of severe neglect and or abuse.

Another aspect of beneficence and non-maleficence in the context of child care arises in the context of research on children. This is probably carried out more in hospital paediatrics than in community child care and I do not have space to consider it much further here. However, elsewhere[10] I have argued that if the research is therapeutic, i.e. carried out for the intended benefit of the child, then the issues of acceptable risk and of the appropriate approach to obtaining consent from the child's proxy (usually parent) can be examined in the same way as for therapy. Where the research is non-therapeutic, i.e. carried out for the intended benefit of others but not the child, then only research involving minimal risk is morally permissible. Consent from the parent or other proper proxy has to be obtained after providing adequate information concerning the non-therapeutic nature of the research, its purpose, and that the child may be withdrawn at any stage without detriment to his or her care. Much research lies on the spectrum between these two poles, the therapeutic and non-therapeutic, and a combination of moral approaches is thus required, skewed to the appropriate end of the spectrum.

Justice

Even where health care workers and parents and children are agreed about the need or desirability of some health care intervention there may still be ethical problems related to the fourth of the Beauchamp and Childress principles – justice. This is most obviously a potential problem in the context of scarce resources. The availability of growth hormone for example is restricted by its very high cost. While it is available under the National Health Service for extremely short children it has not been available for treatment of somewhat shorter than average children. Most people may well find it easy to accept that the limited resources of the National Health Service should not be used in this way, but the example raises very profound issues of distributive justice. Is height properly a concern of health care workers or is the problem just a social one, suffered by people of short stature as a result of unreasonable prejudice on the part of others? And, if the latter, does that take the issue out of health care or does it remain within its province insofar as health is partly a matter of social well-being? Also, in order to distribute health care resources according to health care needs we must know what we mean by health, and by needs. But do we? If one needs something then something undesirable will occur if one does not get it. But can we really be said to need whatever we desire? And cannot we need what we do not desire? This is an area that requires far more work, medical and philosophical, to be done, and I do not pretend to be able to give good answers to my own questions. They nonetheless demand good answers, and good reasoning because fair distribution of scarce health care resources becomes ever more important as the cost of providing health care grows exponentially. It is an area that needs urgent public and professional analysis, as much in the context of child health as elsewhere in health care. Meanwhile practitioners must go on in the realization that a conflict of moral interests arises whenever priority is given to recipients of care which is at the potential expense (or opportunity cost as the economists call it) of others who will obtain less care and less resources as a result. One morally desirable response is obvious: we must not waste the scarce resources at our disposal. But the conflict remains even if we eliminate all waste, even if governments put more resources into health care, for there will always be more demand than supply. Somehow we have to seek a balance between the interests of our patients but also of others with a proper claim on those resources, not only other actual or potential patients but also the providers of those resources, notably in our context the tax payers as represented by the government. Alas I do not have a blue print for a just system for allocation of scarce medical resources; but it is inescapable that we need to develop such a system, capable of addressing in an open and principled way this ever growing problem of health care ethics.

Finally, justice in respect of children's rights and for morally acceptable laws is of direct ethical relevance in community child care, most obviously in the context of child abuse, considered at length in Sections 9.4, 9.5 and 9.6.

References

1 Beauchamp, T., Childress, J.F. *Principles of Biomedical Ethics.* Oxford: Oxford University Press, 1989.

2 Gillon, R. *Philosophical Medical Ethics.* Chichester: Wiley, 1986.

3 Iserson, K.V. Forgoing pre-hospital care; should ambulance staff always resuscitate? *J Med Ethics* 1991; **17**: 19–24.

4 Kennedy, I., Grubb, A. *Medical Law: Text and Materials.* London: Butterworths, 1989: 182, 3–33, 290–367.

5 Gillick v West Norfolk and Wisbech Area Health Authority. The legal references to this case are: [1984] QB 581, [1984] 1 All ER 365, [1986] AC 112, [1985] 1 All ER 533 revised [1986] AC 112, [1985] 3 All ER 402 HL.

6 The Law Society. Mental Health Subcommittee's report: *Decision Making and Mental Incapacity: a Discussion Document.* London: The Law Society, 1989.

7 The Law Commission (Consultation Paper No. 129) *Mentally Incapacitated Adults and Decision-making: Medical Treatment and Research.* London: HMSO, 1993.

8 Newton, C.R. *General Principles of Law.* London: Sweet and Maxwell, 1983: 259–263.

9 Kurtz, I. Health educators: the new puritans. *J Med Ethics* 1987; **13**: 30–41, 48.

10 Gillon, R. Research on the vulnerable: an ethical overview. In: Brazier, M., Lobjoit, M., eds. *Protecting the Vulnerable: Autonomy and Consent in Health Care.* London: Routledge, 1991: 52–76.

9.2 Child protection

Murray Davies

The second half of the 20th century has seen a growing awareness, recognition and respect for the rights of children, not only in the UK but throughout the world.

On 20 November 1959 the Declaration of the Rights of the Child was adopted by the General Assembly of the United Nations; this recognized that, 'the child, by reason of his physical and mental immaturity, needs special safeguards and care, including appropriate legal protection, before as well as after birth.' This declaration only stated general principles accepted by governments, and carried no legally binding obligations. This changed on 20 November 1989 with the adoption by the General Assembly of the United Nations of the Convention on the Rights of the Child – a universal and binding policy statement on children's rights, under which nations were required to report on implementation.

The main underlying principle of the Convention is that the best interests of the child shall always be the major consideration. It states clearly that the child's own opinion shall be given due regard. The new Convention thus recognizes the child as an individual, with needs which evolve with age and maturity. It seeks to balance the rights of the child with the rights and duties of parents or others who have responsibility for the child's survival, development and protection by giving the child the right to participate in decisions which affect his or her future.

The state's obligation to protect children from all forms of maltreatment perpetrated by parents or others responsible for their care, and to undertake preventive and treatment programmes in this regard, is highlighted in Article 19 of the Convention.

In the UK the principles of the Convention are reflected in the Children Act 1989, which brought together into a single legislative framework the private and public law relating to children. The Act seeks to balance the rights of children to express their views on decisions made about their lives, the rights of parents to exercise their responsibilities towards the child, and the duty of the state to intervene where the child's welfare requires it. In all proceedings under the Act, the court must treat the welfare of the child as the paramount consideration, and this principle applies equally to care proceedings as it does to disputes between parents.

These principles had been emphasized a year earlier in the Report of the Inquiry into Child Abuse in Cleveland, 'There is a danger that, in looking to the welfare of children believed to be victims of sexual abuse, the children themselves may be overlooked. The child is a person, and not an object of concern. Professionals should always listen carefully to what the child has to say, and to take seriously what is said.'[1]

Towards the end of the 20th century, there is now a growing awareness of the need to respect the rights of children. Less than 50 years ago, the picture was very different. During the Second World War, public attention was focused on the case of Dennis O'Neal, a little boy who was boarded with foster parents and treated so brutally that he died. Concern about this case was heightened because of the widespread evacuation of children from danger areas, and the loss of parents and homes. This resulted in the appointment of a parliamentary committee, 'To enquire into existing methods of providing for children who from loss of parents or from any other cause whatever are deprived of a normal home life with their own parents or relatives.'[2]

The report demonstrated the inadequate care, and the lack of respect shown to disadvantaged and disabled children and adults, and gives the following example:

> One century-old poor law institution provided accommodation for 170 adults, including ordinary workhouse accommodation, an infirmary for senile old people and a few men and women certified as either mentally defective or mentally disordered. In this institution there were 27 children, aged six months to 15 years. Twelve infants up to the age of 18 months were the children of women in the institution, about half of them still being nursed by their mothers. In the same room in which these children were being cared for was a Mongol idiot, aged four of gross appearance, for whom there was apparently no accommodation elsewhere. A family of five normal children aged about 6 to 15, who had been admitted on a relieving officer's order, had been in the institution for ten weeks. This family, including a boy of ten and a girl of 15, were sleeping in the same room as a three year old hydrocephalic idiot, of very unsightly type whose bed was screened off in a corner.[2]

Such serious concerns, following a war fought to ensure freedom, helped to promote the view that social distress of all kinds must be a state responsibility. Freedom was described by Sir William Beveridge as something positive: freedom from want, from disease, from ignorance, from squalor, and from idleness. A policy to achieve this state of freedom was outlined by him in a report on social insurance and allied services published in 1942.[3]

The immediate post-war period saw the establishment of the welfare state. The National Health Service was established;[4] the National Insurance Act,[5] and the National Assistance Act,[6] the forerunners of social security, were introduced. Children's departments[7] were established and later developed into social services departments. Thus the foundations were set for a more comprehensive welfare service, led and provided by the state.

Historically acknowledgement of the maltreatment of children as a social ill has only come about following social change, and Gregg[8] describes some of the early abuses of children.

In the first phase of the industrial revolution, in the late 18th century, cheap child labour was used to mind machines. Child paupers were transported from London and the south of England to the cotton mills in the north. If a mill closed, the unwanted children were simply tipped out onto the roads and left alone to make their way as best they could. To the cotton master, they were as much his property as the machines they tended. The children suffered constant flogging to keep them awake, and many died of fever and ill treatment.

Initially the mills relied on water power, and were built in the country. When steam superseded water power, and factories moved to the coal field towns, work for whole families became abundant. Children were employed in factories, sometimes beginning at 3 and 4 years of age. They worked from 12 to 19 hours a day, often being whipped and beaten to keep them awake. Some, from sheer fatigue, fell into moving machinery to be killed and maimed. Parents were known to beat their own children to save them from a worse fate at the hands of the overseers. Children had to clean machinery while taking food, often while it was moving, with a result that their lungs were filled with dust and fumes, while they faced the danger of mutilation. In this factory system of slavery, a rigid discipline was enforced on adults and children alike. Factory reforms were resisted by the manufacturers on the grounds that it would increase their costs, and that it was an interference with private property. William Cobbett commented in the House of Commons,

> We have been told that our navy was the glory of the country, and that our maritime commerce and extensive manufacturers were the mainstays of the realm. We have also been told that the land had its share in our greatness, and should justly be considered as the pride and glory of England. The bank, also, has put in its claim to share in this praise, and has stated that public credit is due to it; but now, a most surprising discovery has been made, namely, that all our greatness and prosperity, that our superiority over other nations is owing to 300 000 little girls in Lancashire. We have made the notable discovery, that if these little girls worked two hours less in a day than they now do, it would occasion the ruin of the country; that it would enable other nations to compete with us; and thus make an end to our boasted wealth, and bring us to beggary.[9]

Children were employed in a variety of industries; lace, hosiery, metal, earthenware, glass, paper and tobacco. In 1843, the Children's Employment Commission reported on the conditions in many trades.[10] Children suffered hardship and abuse and frequently received only food and clothing of variable quantity and quality. Among these children were the chimney sweeps, little boys and girls who, even in the middle of the 19th century, were compelled to climb into the flues of chimneys in order to sweep them. Sometimes the children were bought, sometimes kidnapped. They were still bought and sold as late as the 1860s, and the smaller the boy the bigger the price. They formed one of the most neglected classes of the community, and often began work at about 6 years of age. When the boys first started climbing their knees and elbows were rubbed with a strong brine close by a hot fire to harden them. At first they came back from their work 'with their arms and knees streaming with blood, and the knees looking as if the caps had been pulled off.'[11] Then more brine was applied. Sheer terror of their masters drove them up the chimneys, and they were kept up by threats, sticks, pins stuck in their bare feet, or even by lighting straw below them.

The Children's Employment Commission[12] also reported on child labour in mines, where children began work as early as 4 years of age and worked for over 12 hours a day underground. The youngest children were employed as trappers, who sat in one place all day alone and often in darkness to open ventilators. Most children never saw the daylight for months at a stretch. Other children were harnessed to carts, and had to crawl on all fours to pull them. The miners wore leather straps with which they would beat the children. One child describes being beaten by the man he called, 'the corporal', who 'kicked him when he was down, pulled his ears and hair, and threw coals at him; he dared not tell his masters then, or he believes the corporal would have killed him. His brothers, one 10 the other 13 years old, are beaten until they can hardly get home, and dare not tell for fear of worse usage, and they and their father losing their work.'[8]

No authority in the 18th century had the duty of providing care and protection for children in moral danger, who often begged and roamed the streets in a neglected condition. In the new towns, the social and moral controls of the small agricultural parishes were absent, and the number of illegitimate children increased. Many babies were abandoned, murdered or sold indiscriminately. Children of destitute parents found their way with the illegitimate into the workhouse where they were often reared in groups.

Legislation to improve conditions for children, particularly in factories, mines and chimneys, appeared only after a long struggle against the resistance of interested parties. The Factory Act of 1833 limited the working hours of children in textile mills and the Mines Act of 1842 prohibited the underground employment of women and children under 10 years. Legislation in 1875 finally ended the employment of little boys as chimney sweeps.

For those children, in the 19th century, who were destitute, orphaned or deserted, it remained the duty of the Poor Law authorities to provide care for them.

Children who lived in their own homes, and with their families, whatever the extent of their neglect or exposure to moral danger were the responsibility of no one except their parents. There was no duty on the Poor Law to seek out homeless children, exposed to degradation and moral danger, and provide for them. Rescue work among children became the field of the great voluntary societies in the last half of the 19th century. The terrible conditions to which thousands of children were exposed, described by Victorian writers, roused philanthropists to action, to rescue children from neglect and cruelty. Dr Barnardo was one such pioneer; he opened his first Home for Destitute Boys in 1870. The National Children's Home opened its first home in London in 1869. By 1878 there were 50 philanthropic societies for children in London alone. Heywood[13] has provided a comprehensive picture of child care developments during the 19th and 20th centuries.

Legislation for the better protection of infant life was passed in 1872; it aimed to end the abuses of baby farming. Many mothers, unable to gain Poor Law relief, placed their children with foster mothers or nurses in the day time, or by the week, so that they could carry on with their employment. Some placed them with the knowledge, or intention, that they would die. The mortality among infants under a year put out to nurse in this way was estimated to be between 70 and 90% in the large towns.

The concern for family violence gained expression with the foundation of the Society for the Protection of Women and Children from Aggravated Assaults in 1857. While most of the Society's work was concerned with women, it also pressed for legal changes, and tried to publicize the problem of violence to children.

Gradually during the last decades of the 19th century the problem of child cruelty gained explicit expression. Official London records reveal that of 3926 children under 5 years who died by accident or violence in 1870, 202 deaths were attributed to manslaughter, 95 to neglect, and 18 to exposure to cold – all effectively due to child abuse.

It was the establishment of the National Society for the Prevention of Cruelty to Children (NSPCC) which provided the focus for recognizing the problem of child cruelty and introducing legislation. As Heywood describes, 'There was no effective method of discovering and repressing cruelty under the formation of voluntary societies for this purpose.'[13]

The founding of the NSPCC in England[14] followed the scandal of Mary Ellen which occurred in 1874. She lived in a New York tenement with her adoptive parents, and neighbours were concerned that she was being ill treated and neglected. They contacted an organization providing voluntary help to immigrants, and a visit was made to the apartment. She was found in a terrible state – neglected, beaten and cut with scissors – but the parents refused to change their treatment of her and insisted that they could do as they wished. There were laws against ill treatment of animals, but no laws to protect children; so it was decided to argue in court that Mary Ellen was a member of the animal kingdom for this purpose. The case was found proved and she was granted protection. The scandal resulted in the formation of the New York Society for the Prevention of Cruelty to Children which was the inspiration for the founding of the NSPCC in Britain which received its Royal Charter in 1895.[14] Nevertheless it was still possible in 1892 for a defence barrister in England to argue, albeit unsuccessfully, that a mother should not be convicted of the killing of her child who had suffocated when locked in a cupboard as a punishment, because parents had absolute rights over their children.

The establishment of the NSPCC and the work of others in identifying cases of cruelty led to the Prevention of Cruelty Act 1889. The Act created an offence if anyone over 16 years who had custody, control, or charge of a boy under 14 years or a girl under 16 years wilfully ill-treated, neglected or abandoned the child in a manner likely to cause unnecessary suffering or injury to health. On conviction the court could also commit the child to the charge of a relative or anyone else willing to have the care of the child. In a 5-year period 47 000 complaints were investigated by the NSPCC; 5792 people were prosecuted and 5400 convicted.

Legislation was consolidated by the Children Act 1908 which introduced juvenile courts and established the principle that young offenders under 14 years should be treated separately from adults. Although the Act was concerned with cases of cruelty and neglect, its main concern was with delinquency.

A closer link between the work for neglected and delinquent children and the work of the local education authorities, was provided by the Children and Young Persons Act 1933 which also further separated the care of neglected children from the Poor Law. The Act defined the criminal offence of wilful cruelty and wilful neglect committed against a child.

The Children Act 1948 attempted to locate responsibility for the care of children in a single government department, as recommended by the Curtis Committee. The Home Office was regarded as the most appropriate. The Act gave local authorities the duty to receive into voluntary care children whose parents were unable to care for them; to carry out child protection responsibilities; and to be responsible for children committed to their care by the courts. The old Poor Law provisions were finally replaced.

Another important concept in the Children Act was the emphasis on the status of the natural family, with the duty on local authorities to restore those received into care to their own natural home. This duty emphasized the casework aspect of the new service. As Heywood[13] described, 'Children too often remained in the care of the public assistance authorities because no casework service existed to treat the actual problem which had precipitated the reception into care.'

Medical developments, particularly in radiology, after the 1940s increased the ability to diagnose violence to children. It became possible to date fractures according to the stage of healing, and so identify repeated violence and healing fractures not previously presented for treatment. In 1946, a radiologist, Caffey,[15] described a pattern of multiple fractures and subdural haematomas in small children. The origin of the injuries was then unclear, although there was speculation they could be the result of injury rather than disease. The paper attracted little attention and no real public interest. In 1953, Silverman[16] suggested that the injuries might result from parental carelessness and in 1955 Woolley and Evans[17] first suggested the possibility of deliberate acts of injury by parents or care givers.

While there was a growing awareness of the existence of violence to children at home, the numbers were felt to be small, and the problems of neglect, delinquency and multi-problem families were much more widespread. In 1950, the government saw the need for the coordination of services to problem families and recommended the establishment of local coordinating committees for this purpose. The authorities were recommended, 'to arrange for significant cases of child neglect, and all cases of ill-treatment coming to the notice of any statutory or voluntary service in the area, to be reported to a designated officer, who would arrange for such cases to be brought before the meeting, so that after considering the needs of the family as a whole, agreement might be reached as to how the local services could "best be applied" to meet those needs.'[18]

In 1954, the American Humane Association's Children's Division began the first nationwide survey of neglected, abused and exploited children. The Children's Bureau in the USA also continued support for child abuse research, and supported Henry Kempe and his colleagues in his exploration of the physical abuse of children. He first reported his findings at a meeting of the American Academy of Paediatrics in 1961 in a paper entitled, 'The Battered Child Syndrome'.[19] Kempe argued that the syndrome was often misdiagnosed and should be considered in any child showing evidence of trauma or neglect, or where there was a marked discrepancy between the clinical findings and the story presented by the parents. His work has continued to be of central importance in the whole area of child abuse and neglect. He recommended the reporting of incidents to law enforcement or child protection agencies, and within 5 years 40 states of the USA had instituted some form of reporting law for child abuse cases.

In the UK, recognition developed more slowly but was highlighted by Griffiths and Moynihan in 1963,[20] who were concerned that cases were being incorrectly diagnosed. The British Paediatric Association (BPA) published a memorandum in 1966 which discussed the recognition and management of the problem.[21]

After outlining the clinical symptoms of the syndrome and the importance of hospital casualty officers in its recognition, the BPA recommended that, when the diagnosis was suspected, the child should be admitted to hospital while the history was investigated, and the possibility of physical disease excluded. The memorandum stressed that a purely punitive attitude to the person inflicting the injury was ill advised, and that the management of the problem was the responsibility of the medical and social welfare agencies.

Before 1968, awareness of the problem outside the medical profession was minimal. In 1968, the NSPCC established a Battered Child Research Unit which later published numerous papers disseminating knowledge and arousing professional interest in the problem.[22] In the early 1970s, a small group of doctors, lawyers, social workers and others met to study the battered child syndrome and promote public and professional awareness. The group was known as the Tunbridge Wells Study Group.[23] Sir Keith Joseph, then Secretary of State for Health and Social Services, participated because of his concern about multi-problem families, and the concept of the cycle of deprivation. The increasing knowledge about child abuse was clearly related to these concerns.

Maria Colwell was killed in 1973 by her stepfather shortly after having been returned to the care of her mother from foster parents, with whom she had lived for 5 years. This provided further impetus, particularly after the public inquiry.[24] Maria was 8 years old when she died, thus emphasizing that violence to children was not confined to battered babies.

In 1970, the government had issued a circular *Battered Babies*[25] giving guidance on the management of cases; in 1972, a second circular emphasized the need for coordination of services through case conferences.[26]

The publication of the Colwell report in 1974 was preceded by a third circular, *Non-Accidental Injury to Children*[27] which laid the foundation for the current structure of individual case coordination in the UK. It was an advisory document with no legal force but had a very significant impact on the pattern of services of statutory agencies, especially social services' departments. The circular recommended that, 'a case conference for every case involving suspected non-accidental injury to a child' should meet as soon as possible, and advised that urgent consideration be given to setting up an adequate central record of information in each area.

Concern about child abuse has not developed in a vacuum and considerable attention has been focused on the importance of using a multidisciplinary approach. The Court Report on child health services argued that, 'just as doctors, nurses and therapists must work together as a team in the health services, so the health services must work in partnership with the education and social services . . . . The planning and development of an integrated health service must therefore be done in such a way as to facilitate at every level the closest possible working relationships with those other services.'[28]

Dale and Davies[29] have discussed the dangerous aspects of inter-agency function, stressing that the ways in which agencies relate to one another can reflect the same patterns of behaviour as normal and abnormal families. 'There are healthy conflicts and rivalry; clear and blurred boundaries; alliances and scapegoats; overt and covert communication patterns and the operation of supportive, provocative and even destructive patterns of behaviour.' Difficulty in professional relationships between disciplines can seriously interfere with care of individual children.

The initial focus of interest was on battered babies and subsequently on injuries inflicted on children of all ages. As a result attention was diverted from families with other problems including neglect. The importance of neglect, which can result in retarded physical and emotional development, was highlighted by public inquiries into several fatal cases. The inquiries into the deaths of Paul Brown 1978,[30] Lester Chapman 1979,[31] and Malcolm Page 1981[32] demonstrated the consequences of neglect and the overlap between neglect and physical injury. In 1980, in a revised circular, the Department of Health and Social Security recommended the inclusion of neglect within the same procedural system as injury.[33]

A further revision of government guidance in 1986[34] led to the acceptance of child sexual abuse as a significant abuse of children. With greater publicity of this abuse, stressing the importance of believing children and emphasizing that they are not to blame, more and more adults have reported sexual abuse in their own childhood. Thus the long-standing nature of the abuse and the failure and difficulty that society has had in its recognition has been emphasized. The inquiry into child abuse in Cleveland in 1987 confirmed the existence of child sexual abuse in the UK, 'We have learned during the enquiry that sexual abuse occurs in children of all ages, including the very young, to boys as well as girls, in all classes of society and frequently within the privacy of the family. The sexual abuse can be very serious, and on occasions includes vaginal, anal and oral intercourse. The problems of child sexual abuse have been recognised to an increasing extent over the past few years by professionals in different disciplines. This presents new and particularly difficult problems for the agencies concerned in child protection.'[1]

As early as 1978, Kempe[35] reported seeing increasingly younger children who were suffering sexual abuse. He commented, 'doctors routinely ascribe specific complaints of incest, and even incestuous pregnancy, to adolescent fantasy. Often paediatricians will simply not think of incest in making assessment of an emotionally disturbed child or adolescent of either sex. Still a history of incest is so commonly found among adults who, 10 or 15 years after the event, come to the attention of psychiatrists, marriage counsellors, mental health clinics, the police and the courts and the failure to consider the diagnosis early on is somewhat surprising.'

With the acceptance that child sexual abuse exists, concerns about juvenile sex offending have emerged, demonstrating that the perpetrators of abuse are not always adult. There has been a growing awareness from victims of sexual abuse of the traumatic effects of assaults by adolescent perpetrators on children and young people. There has also been evidence from the courts of the origins in adolescence of adult, sex-offending behaviour. A number of adolescent offenders will have been abused themselves earlier in childhood, and so present as both a victim and a perpetrator.

This growing awareness of the complexity of the problem of child abuse underlines the careful arrangements required to handle cases as they come to light.

Working Together, which gave guidance on the arrangements for inter-agency cooperation for the protection of children from abuse was revised with the implementation of the Children Act.[36] *Working Together* deals with the need for professionals to have a clear understanding of child care law and its implications for them in their practice. Local authorities are given a lead role, and also a responsibility to engage other agencies to advise and assist them in their child protection and child care duties. The document continues to provide guidance on the administrative and organizational requirements for inter-agency cooperation.

The Department of Health also published *Working with Child Sexual Abuse* in 1991 to provide overall guidance on the content of child sexual abuse training;[37] 'Child sexual abuse work continues in the 1990s to be one of the most stressful for social services' staff and foster parents. The comprehensive strategy for training suggested is needed both to give the children and families the quality of service they deserve, and to recognise the considerable knowledge and skills that are required of those undertaking this very demanding and difficult work.' *Working Together* also recognized more complicated forms of abuse as evidence of the multiple abuse of numbers of children by groups of adult abusers. Organized abuse is defined in *Working Together* as 'abuse which may involve a number of abusers, and a number of abused children and young people, and often encompasses different forms of abuse. It involves to a greater or lesser extent an element of organisation.' This is not a new category of abuse, but describes the social organization and context in which the abuse, which may be physical, psychological or sexual, occurs. The abuse may take the form of a child sex ring, involve the use of a ritual to increase children's vulnerability or to frighten them, or be for the purpose of producing pornographic material. These matters were considered and commented on at the Orkney Inquiry.[38]

The inclusion of organized abuse within the guidance given in *Working Together* is to emphasize the importance of close inter-agency cooperation and agreed arrangements for agencies working together.

Recent years have seen a series of reports of abuse of children in residential care, which culminated in the Utting Report.[39] Helen Westcott has summarized the nature of institutional abuse.[40] 'Institutional abuse comprises physical, sexual, emotional abuse and neglect perpetrated by individual members of staff, in addition to system generated violations of children's rights to a healthy physical and psychological development. No systematic survey has established the incidence and prevalence of institutional abuse in the UK (or the USA) but literature from the National Association of Young People in Care and from the US suggests such abuse is widespread, and may occur at rates higher than reported rates of familial abuse. Certain similarities between familial and institutional abuse have been observed but several important differences arising from the institutional context are noted to facilitate maltreatment. Key aspects of institutional abuse include denial that abuse occurs, especially by society and institutional management, powerlessness experienced by children in care, and the role of staff at all levels in the institutional setting.'

The government made special reference to investigations in residential settings in *Working Together*, 'Children in residential settings, particularly those with disabilities, may become isolated and have very little opportunity to communicate with people outside the home or school. This renders such children particularly vulnerable to abuse. Good child-care practice should of course militate against such isolation, but even in the best settings some children find it very difficult to make their problems known.'[36]

Working Together requires well-publicized procedures on how to deal with suspected abuse; the procedures must be available to both children and staff. Recent years have seen concern that child abuse extends beyond intra-familial abuse, to a recognition that children are abused outside the family in residential settings, and in forms of organized abuse involving numbers of perpetrators.

Child abuse, in whatever form, represents a failure to respect the needs and rights of children. All children whatever their race, sex, beliefs and physical and mental abilities have the right to grow up unharmed, to have the opportunity to develop fully, and to have their basic needs met. Children and young people should be respected in body and mind, their safety and well-being ensured, and their personal dignity guaranteed. These values reflect the statements made in the UN Convention on the Rights of the Child 1989. Child protection is concerned with promoting and protecting these needs and rights.

In the UK, a comprehensive approach to child welfare and child protection has been made possible by the willingness of the government to provide a framework and guidance.

In the rest of Europe the picture is different; the different countries are at different stages of development in the recognition of and response to child abuse. All countries have definitions of behaviour that go beyond the bounds of acceptable conduct, and each country recognizes that its society should take some action and intervene when there is suspected abuse or neglect. There is also a recognition that there are times when the state should intervene to protect children, and all countries try to balance the child's safety with that of the family's privacy and security from state intervention. There are also a range of legal sanctions for the protection of children from abuse; Sale and Davies have drawn together information about child protection practices in over 20 countries in Europe and Scandinavia.[41]

In some European countries mandatory reporting exists but there is no indication that this is linked to any training or understanding about child abuse, or respect for children and young people. In France, anyone who knows that a child is being abused in a family, foster family or an institution must inform the child welfare service, and may be prosecuted if they do not. Similar requirements exist in Sweden, and were incorporated in the welfare legislation in Denmark in 1976. In Belgium, those who witness or have knowledge of criminal offences are compelled to report them; there are similar requirements in the Czech Republic and Slovakia, Turkey, Portugal and Norway.

Probably more important than mandatory reporting is the role of the public health nurse, district nurse or health visitor in providing domiciliary services to babies, young children and their parents. In many European countries this service is seen as having an important role in supporting families with young children, and in identifying abuse or neglect at an early stage. Services exist in Ireland and Norway, and in Finland, where 99% of families with children under one year of age use the network of baby clinics. In Belgium, there is a free network of nurses for children under 3 years, where the easy access which nurses have to the homes of families creates an optimal situation for the early detection of child abuse. Services exist in France, Switzerland, and in Hungary. District nurses have an important role in the Czech Republic and Slovakia as well.

These community nursing services play a key role in promoting the welfare of children; experience in the UK is mirrored in many European countries where specialist nursing staff have the knowledge and skills to assess the development of individual children, and the nature of the parenting provided for them.

Across Europe, the coordination of services and the cooperation of different disciplines are starting to grow. There is a recognition of the benefits to children and families when practitioners with different expertise work together. As in the UK, systems led and promoted by the government are more likely to have a far-reaching impact, and can provide a framework for training to take place because a national standard has been set. In Greece, for example, one of the biggest problems is acknowledged to be the lack of coordination and organization; this results in overlapping of some agency services, and also the needs of children and families being unmet. In Spain, the need for services to be better coordinated has been highlighted.

Cooperation and coordination have been demonstrated as important by two pilot schemes in Milan which began in the 1980s: the Aid Centre for the Abused Child and Family in Crisis, and the Abused Child and Family Crisis Treatment Centre. They were significant for both cooperation with the local social services and the courts which had been neglected locally. As a result, other cities adopted the same approach, and a National Council for Juvenile Problems, an inter-ministerial organization aiming to promote a unitary policy for children, was established.

A mandatory reporting system and a legally based system for intervention, do not by themselves promote an understanding of the problem of child abuse, or provide a base from which to influence professional practice and attitudes. Of greater importance are the principles and philosophies on which the activities are based. In the UK a guide was recently published[42] to assist practitioners in relating the law to good child care practice.

Statements of principles provide guidance to practice and approaches, but there are variations across Europe which influence service provision. In Switzerland, for example, almost all cantons no longer take penal action, on the understanding that measures will be taken to protect the child. Civil measures are increasingly restrictive of parents who do not voluntarily accept help which will protect the child. Help instead of punishment is thus increasingly accepted in Switzerland.

In Germany, the development of the Kinderschutzzentrum has affected public opinion regarding child abuse and how it is dealt with. Before the mid 1970s, services available to high-risk families provided practical and educational advice, and social workers had a more controlling role. Today, an important principle is that child abuse is not viewed as a criminal offence, but as a symptom of family problems that can be treated. It is argued that, with this shift, families which tended to hide are now enabled to seek help. Punishment and the penal law are used less frequently in dealing with child abuse. The safety of the child is the priority, and the criminal process is not relied upon. The basis of help is confidentiality, and help is provided on a voluntary basis.

In Sweden, the principle of voluntary participation by parent and family is enshrined in the Social Services Act of 1982. Any intervention should be planned in consultation with the parent or parents and child and designed so as to allow free play to the individual's own resources. An important principle within the country is that services are based on cooperation and mutual respect.

In the Netherlands, the government initiated an experiment in 1972 in four regions whereby a confidential doctor was appointed with social work assistance for consultations about child abuse. The philosophy underpinning the system was to operate in a non-judgmental climate. The principle of the system is not to accuse the maltreating parent but to organize help and protection for the abused child and family. Offers of help depend on motivation of the family in question to accept assistance. The confidential doctor would gain more information from doctors' and schools' records, and could make an evaluation. Confidential doctors were not involved in therapeutic programmes, but initiated action through other agencies. Thus they had an important instructional role. Since 1978, ten confidential doctor services have been established in major towns and they are now being set up nationally.

In Belgium, the principle employed by the confidential doctor service is that it is essential to the approach that child abuse and neglect is interpreted as a signal, a symptom of a serious family dysfunction. Consequently, abusers should be helped instead of punished. Again this is an important principle which will inform attitudes and responses throughout the country.

In Europe, there are different principles underpinning the approach to child abuse. There is the established view that child abuse is a signal, a symptom of family distress and must be responded to therapeutically. In the UK, we have tended to emphasize the investigation, procedures and the coordination of services, rather than beginning from a therapeutic base. In Belgium, it is argued that therapeutic programmes should be separated from the judicial system to enable a trustful relationship between therapist and family to be established. It is seen as essential that the family participates on a voluntary basis and not through submission on the threat of court action. Marneffe has written, 'Judicial and therapeutic models cannot be mixed. The role of justice being one of authoritative decisions to protect the child when parents have failed, refused or are unable to fulfil their nurturing responsibilities towards a child.'[41]

In Austria, Child Protection Centres distance themselves from pronouncements about guilt but, at the same time, ensure that families recognize their responsibilities. In Germany, in the Kinderschutzentrum, the emphasis is on voluntary help with a focus on family conflict and therapeutic provision.

In Norway, the investigation of methods for working with child abuse demonstrated the need for a family approach. Similarly, Poland considers family therapy extremely important and recognizes the importance of trying to change attitudes within the family so that behaviour patterns become more favourable.

Future judgements concerning particular approaches about the effectiveness of different methods of intervention in cases of child abuse, and more general child welfare concerns, are likely to be heavily influenced by the views of children and young people themselves. Already in the UK legislation and principles of good practice encourage professionals to work in partnership with children and parents, and to take into account the views and wishes of children. The Irish Society for the Prevention of Cruelty to Children sums up this position;[41] it believes that it is only by listening to the children themselves talking of their problems that there will be any real appreciation of the problem of child abuse. They describe the willingness of most children to suffer continued abuse and neglect in silence, rather than seek help from services which are designed from a purely adult perspective. This is an indictment of services, and a major challenge and opportunity for change. The ethos in service design must be to empower children and challenge our whole adult perspective on childhood.

In Finland over the last two decades, the status of the child has changed a great deal; the child's own wishes and views are given more weight than before. The media have been alerted to the rights of all children and one media campaign was *Don't hit a child*. The purpose of the child welfare acts was to secure the rights of a child, who should be entitled to a secure and stimulating growing environment and to harmonious and well-balanced development. A child has a special right to protection.

In Denmark, parental rights to chastise children physically continued until 1985, when the parliament changed the parental code and abolished physical punishment by parents. This shift in empowering children is noticeable throughout Europe. In Sweden, in 1950, the code of parenthood stated that parents and teachers not only had the right but also the duty to use corporal punishment in the upbringing of children. Attitudes changed in the late 1950s, so in 1958 the right to beat children at school was removed, and in 1966 the right was taken away from parents. These changes have been supported by information from the government to all Swedish households with the result that there is increased awareness that there are methods other than physical punishment which are used in the education and control of children.

Portugal is witnessing considerable public awareness of the defence of children's rights and a recognition of the need to develop suitable provisions, especially when the child's right to life, or physical and emotional welfare, is in danger.

Norway has had a Children's Ombudsman since 1981, when the Children Act at the same time protected children's rights in relation to their parents, prohibiting them from striking a child or subjecting the child to other degrading treatment. In Greece, it is recognized that there is a need to produce changes in residential care provision, and a need for the service to become more child-centred rather than staff and institution-oriented.

Increasingly children and young people will be able to influence matters affecting their rights and interests, as their position is properly respected and enhanced. In this process, they will have the support of the UN Convention with which governments will be expected to conform. The UN Convention states that governments 'shall assume that the child who is capable of forming his or her own views, the right to express those views freely in all matters affecting the child, the views of the child being given due weight in accordance with the age and maturity of the child.' This today is a very different environment to that which existed some 200 years ago, when children were transported from the south of England to cotton mills in the north, and could find themselves tipped out onto roads when they were no longer wanted. Only slowly has a proper respect for and empowerment of children begun to emerge.

Present knowledge of child abuse and neglect is based almost entirely on research and experience in western nations, and does not take into account child-rearing practices in other cultures. As Korbin has pointed out, 'in accommodating cultural variation, regardless of how painful or how harmless a practice might be . . . . It is important to remember that no culture sanctions the extreme harm that befalls children, first described by Kempe and his colleagues as the "battered child syndrome" . . . while definitions of child abuse and neglect legitimately vary across cultural boundaries, each group maintains concepts and definitions of behaviours that are beyond the standards of acceptable conduct. Although idiosyncratic child abuse and neglect may be defined differently by these groups, and may occur with different frequencies, deviance in child care behaviour is known cross-culturally as a possibility of human behaviour.'[43]

In different cultures, conditions which are detrimental to both child and adult welfare, such as poverty, and food scarcity, must be distinguished from harm inflicted or neglect perpetrated by individual parents or caretakers. Korbin identified three areas where cultural considerations come into play in identifying child abuse and neglect. The first is where a practice is viewed as acceptable by one culture, but as abusive or neglectful by another. There are examples, from different cultures, of practices that appear abusive or neglectful to a westerner. These include extremely hot baths designed to inculcate culturally valued traits, punishment such as severe beatings to impress the child with the necessity of adherence to cultural rules, and harsh initiation rites that include genital operations, deprivation of food and sleep and induced bleeding and vomiting.

Some western child-rearing practices such as isolating infants and small children in rooms or beds of their own at night, making them wait for readily available food, or allowing them to cry without immediately attending to their needs would be at odds with the child-rearing of many other cultures. There are other examples of practices accepted in some cultures but viewed as abusive by others. Korbin stated that, 'In China as recently as 30 years ago children were considered the sole property of their parents, and as such they could be dealt with in whatever manner their parents chose.'[43] Severe beatings, infanticide, child slavery, the selling of young girls as prostitutes, child betrothal and foot binding were not uncommon, but with recent changes in Chinese society so childhood experiences have been transformed.

Sarah and Robert Levine drew attention[43] to ceremonial clitoridectomy in Africa, which conforms to local ideals, but is seen as abusive by western criteria. Corporal punishment is also described as in use in traditional Africa for disobedient children. Incest is said to be treated as a religious offence rather than a crime.

The second aspect relates to definitions of child abuse and neglect which vary between cultures, but each group has criteria for identifying behaviours that are outside the realm of acceptable child care. When behaviour represents a departure from that tolerated by the culture, the behaviour may be considered child abuse or neglect.

Korbin's third area of concern was the abuse and neglect of children by society. Conditions such as poverty, inadequate housing, poor health care, inadequate nutrition, and unemployment are described as contributing more to the incidence of child abuse and neglect in western nations than parent psychopathology. These circumstances are seen as beyond individual parental control even when recognized by parents as detrimental to their child's welfare.

In Latin America and the Caribbean, the abandonment of children stems from the extreme poverty of families with millions of children living on the streets. Unemployment has increased, and education and health care have diminished, influenced by continuing foreign debt problems. Industrialization in India has seen the splitting of large families into smaller units and the moving to large towns where children are required to work, often in dangerous settings, to supplement family income.

Cultural variations occur in child rearing and child care practices. As countries become aware of different approaches, so change becomes possible when practices are detrimental to children. For the first time, through the UN Convention on the Rights of the Child, the world has a standard against which a country's provision for its children can be tested. As has been shown some abuse and neglect of children is at a societal level, where even an individual country is powerless to take remedial action, and external help and support is required. Many of the abuses of children in the third world today were present in western societies one hundred years ago.

Today there is more understanding of child abuse, and the need for action at both an individual and a societal level, and in this the needs of the individual child must never be lost from sight.

References

1 *Report of the Inquiry into Child Abuse in Cleveland 1987.* London: HMSO, 1988. (Cmnd 413.)
2 *Care of Children Committee Report* (Curtis Report). London: HMSO, 1946. (Cmnd 6922.): 38–39.
3 *Social Insurance and Allied Services.* (Beveridge Report). London: HMSO, 1942. (Cmnd 6404.)
4 National Health Service Act 1946. 9 and 10 Geo. VI, C 81.
5 National Insurance Act 1946. 9 and 10 Geo. VI, C 81.
6 National Assistance Act 1948. 11 and 12 Geo. VI, C 29.
7 Children Act 1948. 11 and 12 Geo. VI, C 43.
8 Gregg, P. *A Social and Economic History of Britain.* London: Harrap, 1965.
9 Fielden, J. *The Curse of the Factory System 1836*: 48.
10 Second Report of Children's Employment Commission 1843. XIII.
11 Children's Employment Commission 1863. Minutes of Evidence. XVIII: 297–298.
12 First Report of Children's Employment Commission 1842. XV.
13 Heywood, J. *Children in Care.* London: Routledge & Kegan Paul, 1965.
14 Jones, D., Pickett, J., Oates, M., Barbor, P. *Understanding Child Abuse.* London: Macmillan, 1987.
15 Caffey, J. Multiple fractures in the long bones of children suffering from chronic subdural haematoma. *Am J Roentgenol* 1946;
16 Silverman, F. The roentgen manifestations of unrecognized skeletal trauma in infants. *Am J Roentgenol* 1953;
17 Woolley, P.V., Evans, W.A. The significance of skeletal lesions in infants resembling those of traumatic origin. *J Am Med Assoc* 1955;
18 Joint Circular, Home Office No. 157/50, Ministry of Health No. 78/50, and the Ministry of Education No. 225/50, 31 July 1950 to Councils of Counties and County Boroughs.
19 Kempe, H. The battered child syndrome. *J Am Med Assoc* 1962;
20 Griffiths, D.C., Moynihan, F.J. Multiple epiphyseal injuries in babies (battered baby syndrome). *Br Med J* 1963;
21 British Paediatric Association. The battered baby. *Br Med J* 1966;
22 Baher, E. *At Risk: An Account of the Work of the Battered Child Research Department.* London: Routledge & Kegan Paul, 1976.
23 Department of Health and Social Security. *Report of Tunbridge Wells Study Group.* London: HMSO, 1973.
24 *Report of a Committee of Enquiry into the Care and Supervision Provided in Relation to Maria Colwell.* London: HMSO, 1974.
25 Department of Health and Social Security. *The Battered Baby.* London: HMSO, 1970.
26 Department of Health and Social Security. *The Battered Baby Syndrome.* London: HMSO, 1972.
27 Department of Health and Social Security. *Memorandum on Non-accidental Injury to Children.* LASSL (74). London: HMSO, 1974.
28 Department of Health and Social Security. Report of the Committee on Child Health Needs. *Fit for the Future (Court Report).* London: HMSO, 1976.
29 Dale, P., Davies, M. *Dangerous Families: Assessment and Treatment of Child Abuse.* London: Routledge, 1986.
30 *The Report of the Committee of Inquiry into the Case of Paul Stephen Brown.* London: HMSO, 1980.
31 *Lester Chapman Inquiry Report.* Berkshire County Council, 1979.
32 Essex Area Health Authority. *Malcolm Page: Report of a Panel Appointed by the Essex Area Review Committee.* Essex County Council and Essex Area Health Authority, 1981.
33 Department of Health and Social Security. *Child Abuse: Central Register Systems.* London: HMSO, 1980.
34 Department of Health and Social Security. *Child Abuse: Working Together.* London: HMSO, 1986.
35 Kempe, R.S., Kempe, C.H. *Child Abuse.* London: Fontana, 1978.
36 *Working Together: A Guide to Arrangements for Inter-Agency Co-operation for the Protection of Children from Abuse.* London: HMSO, 1991.
37 Department of Health. *Working with Child Sexual Abuse.* London: HMSO, 1991.
38 *The Report of the Inquiry into the Removal of Children from Orkney in February 1991.* London: HMSO, 1992.
39 *Children in Public Care: A Review of Residential Child Care (the Utting Report).* London: HMSO, 1991.
40 Westcott, H. *Institutional Abuse of Children.* London: NSPCC, 1991.
41 Sale, A., Davies, M. *Child Protection Policies and Practice in Europe.* NSPCC Occasional Paper No. 9. London: NSPCC, 1990.
42 *The Care of Children: Principles and Practice in Regulations and Guidance.* London: HMSO, 1989.
43 Korbin, J. *Child Abuse and Neglect: Cross Cultural Perspectives.* University of California Press, 1981.

9.3 Child care law

Deborah Cullen

Introduction

This section deals with the law in the UK, but involves a summary of three different legal frameworks for England and Wales, Scotland, and Northern Ireland. Only the law governing the employment of children is nearly identical in all three jurisdictions and is dealt with at the end of this section.

In broad terms, the aims of the legislation in all three jurisdictions are similar: to reinforce the responsibility of parents for the upbringing of their children, but to provide protection by the state in cases where parental care falls below an acceptable standard. The same broad aims are found in other countries and in the UN Convention on the Rights of the Child, and in certain limited areas international agreements have been painstakingly drawn up to deal with such problems as child abduction.

The law is of course also subject to change, not only in the form of new legislation, but also as a result of judicial interpretation. A major change to child care law in England and Wales has been effected by the implementation of the Children Act 1989. Northern Ireland will soon have new legislation similar to the Children Act in England and Wales, and Scottish child care law is also under review, but the possible future changes are not covered here.

England and Wales

Parental responsibility

The Children Act 1989 replaces the term 'parental rights and duties' with the concept of 'parental responsibility', which is defined as 'all the rights, duties, powers, responsibilities and authority which by law a parent of a child has in relation to the child and his property'. Where the parents of a child are married they both have parental responsibility; otherwise the mother alone has parental responsibility unless she agrees formally to share it with the father, or a court order is made in his favour. A parent cannot be deprived of parental responsibility except by an adoption order, but other orders can be made which limit his or her right to exercise that responsibility, for example a care order in favour of the local authority. Nor may parents surrender parental responsibility, but they may arrange for some part of that responsibility to be met by another person acting on their behalf (Children Act 1989 Section 2(9)). This means, for example, that a parent may authorize someone caring for a child to consent, on the child's behalf, to medical treatment.

Parental responsibility carries with it the right to determine where a child is to live, how he or she is to be educated, and the duty to care for the child and to exercise appropriate discipline. So far as consent to medical treatment is concerned, very young children are unable to consent on their own behalf to medical treatment and it is provided by statute (s. 8 Family Law Reform Act 1969) that young people over 16 years may consent to treatment. For those children who are under 16 years but who may be able to give an informed consent the position is less certain. Following the decision in the Gillick case[1] it appears that it will be a matter for the medical practitioner concerned to determine whether the young person is mature enough to give informed consent without also requiring the consent of a person with parental responsibility. Parental consent may override the refusal to consent of a child, even of sufficient understanding.[2] The Children Act (see ss 38(6), 43(8) and 44(7)) however does not allow a court order for medical examination to override the refusal of a child of sufficient age and understanding to undergo such examinations.

Individuals other than parents may acquire parental responsibility, but the fact that one person acquires parental responsibility does not mean that others lose it. In addition to parents, therefore, there may be one or more other adults who have parental responsibility, although the court may make orders which restrict the exercise of the responsibility by an individual.

Anyone who has parental responsibility for or care of a child under 16 years may also face criminal proceedings under s. 1 Children and Young Persons Act 1933 if he or she 'wilfully assaults, ill-treats, neglects, abandons, or exposes [the child or young person] or causes or procures him to be assaulted, ill-treated, neglected, abandoned or exposed, in a manner likely to cause him unnecessary suffering or injury to health.' Neglect will be deemed to have occurred if the person responsible has failed to provide adequate food, clothing, medical aid or lodging for the child. The same Act also creates a number of other specific criminal offences against children, and in its first Schedule it lists a number of offences under this and other Acts. Conviction for an offence in the Schedule against a child or young person may have a number of consequences, including a disqualification from keeping private foster children.

Children's rights

The concept of children's rights is a relatively new one and is not specifically provided for in legislation. Nevertheless, there has been a steady shift from the 19th century position where children were effectively regarded as their parents' (or rather their fathers') chattels to the position outlined in the Children Act 1989, whereby their wishes and feelings are required to be ascertained and given due weight when decisions are made about their future. The overriding principle for the courts in reaching decisions about children is however the welfare of the child and a child's wishes will not be allowed to determine an issue if the court views some alternative course as being more conducive to the child's welfare.

The Children Act 1989 gives statutory recognition to the practical reality that the chances are slim of ensuring that a young person over 16 years of age complies with an order made against his or her will. Most orders (though not care orders) will come to an end when the young person reaches the age of 16 years, and there are provisions allowing 16 or 17 year olds to decide on their own behalf whether they wish to remain in accommodation provided by the local authority under s. 20 of the Act. Younger children are not given the same rights to determine their own future, although the Act gives them a specific right to make an application themselves (with the court's leave) for a section eight (s. 8) order.

Some children have certain specific rights in relation to the local authority. Children who are 'looked after' by local authorities (which include both those who are subject to care orders, and those who are provided with accommodation on a voluntary basis under s. 20 of the Act) have a right to be consulted by the local authority (as do their parents) before decisions are made affecting them. The local authority also has a duty to safeguard and promote their welfare, to have regard to their religion, race, culture and language, to review their cases at regular intervals and, unless it is impracticable or inconsistent with their welfare, to promote contact between them and their parents, relatives and friends.

Children in need are entitled to the provision of certain services by the local authority. A child is defined as in need if: 'he is unlikely to achieve or maintain, or to have the opportunity of achieving or maintaining, a reasonable standard of health or development without the provision for him of services by a local authority under this Part [of the Act]', or if 'his health or development is likely to be significantly impaired, or further impaired, without the provision for him of such services, or he is disabled'. Local authorities are required to keep a register of disabled children in their area and to provide services for them designed to minimize the effect of their disabilities and give them the opportunity to lead lives as normal as possible. For other children in need, local authorities have a duty to provide a range of services, including day care for pre-school children, but they are given considerable discretion to decide what services they consider appropriate.

Any child in need or any child looked after by the local authority is entitled to make representations or complaints to the local authority about the way they carry out their functions under these provisions (and this right applies also to parents, foster parents and other interested parties) and the local authority is required to set up a procedure for dealing with such representations in accordance with regulations. The procedure must include the involvement of some person independent of the local authority.

In order to safeguard children who are accommodated for 3 months or more by health authorities, private residential or nursing homes, or placed in a boarding school by a local education authority, the accommodating authority must notify the child's local authority. The local authority then have a duty to consider whether to exercise any of their powers to promote the child's welfare.

Legal procedures

Introduction

Prior to the Children Act 1989 court proceedings involving children were dealt with in many separate statutes and were not always consistent. The Children Act endeavours to draw together all the major legislation governing children, although inevitably certain provisions fall outside its scope, including education (although proceedings in respect of a child's failure to attend school are contained in the Act), criminal proceedings against children and young people, and adoption (which is also under review, but still currently set out in the Adoption Act 1976).

The Children Act does however succeed in bringing together both the main provisions for dealing with disputes between individuals on the future of children, and the procedures for intervention by the state (usually in the form of the local authority). So far as is possible the legal principles and procedures are common to both and in certain situations both types of proceedings will be heard together.

General principles

Under s. 1 of the Act a court determining any question with respect to the upbringing of a child is required to regard the child's welfare as its paramount consideration. It is also required to have regard to the general principle that delay in determining the question is likely to prejudice the welfare of the child. The court must not make any order under the Act 'unless it considers that doing so would be better for the child than making no order at all'. In addition, where there are disputes over the making of a section 8 order (see below) or in applications for care orders, the Act sets out a checklist of factors to be regarded.

Proceedings between individuals

Section 8 of the Act sets out four orders that may be made concerning children, and these are collectively referred to as 'section 8 orders'. The two most important are a *residence order* 'settling the arrangements to be made as to the person with whom a child is to live' and a *contact order* requiring the person with whom a child lives to allow the child to visit or stay or otherwise have contact with the person named in the order. A *specific issue order* gives directions to determine a particular question as to an aspect of parental responsibility (e.g. directing a parent to allow the child to have certain medical treatment) and a *prohibited steps order* prevents a person from taking some step which would otherwise be within the ambit of parental responsibility.

A residence order confers on a non-parent parental responsibility for the child so that the person in whose favour an order is made will be able to take the normal day-to-day steps a parent would take in looking after the child. The making of a residence order does not however *deprive* either parent of parental responsibility and a parent therefore can continue to exercise that responsibility unless doing so is incompatible with another order.

The Children Act enables any individual (apart from local authority foster parents in some circumstances) to apply for the court's leave to seek any s. 8 order. This includes the child. In addition, parents are automatically entitled to apply without leave for any s. 8 order, and in certain circumstances other individuals (e.g. step parents) may apply for orders without first having to obtain the court's leave. No order other than a residence order may be made when the child is subject to a *care order* (see below) and a local authority may not apply for a residence or contact order.

Proceedings involving the local authority

As well as their duty to provide services, local authorities have a statutory responsibility to investigate cases where it is suspected that a child may be in need of protection. When a local authority believes that a child is receiving inadequate care it may be able to help remedy the deficiencies by providing services under Part III of the Children Act, but where this is unsuccessful or provides insufficient protection the local authority, or the National Society for the Prevention of Cruelty to Children (NSPCC), may apply for a care or supervision order. Under s. 31 of the Children Act the court may only make a care or supervision order if it is satisfied:

'a that the child concerned is suffering, or is likely to suffer, significant harm, and
 b that the harm or likelihood of harm, is attributable to:
  (i) the care given to the child, or likely to be given to him if the order were not made, not being what it would be reasonable to expect a parent to give him; or
  (ii) the child's being beyond parental control.'

The effect of a care order will be to give the local authority parental responsibility for the child and the right to determine how far the child's parents may continue to exercise their own parental responsibility. A local authority may not give parental agreement to adoption or take steps to change a child's name or religion. A supervision order requires the supervisor (usually the local authority) to 'advise, assist and befriend' the supervised child, and gives the supervisor certain powers in support of this duty. The court may attach certain requirements to a supervision order and, with the consent of the parent or other person with whom the child is living, require that person to comply with the supervisor's directions – for instance to attend with the child at a family centre for the purpose of improving the handling of the child. In addition, a supervision order may include a requirement for the child to submit to a medical or psychiatric examination provided the child (if of sufficient understanding) consents. A supervision order lasts for a maximum of one year initially, but a care order, unless it is discharged, lasts until a child is 18.

Child protection

Investigation and collaboration

By s. 47 of the Children Act the local authority have a duty to investigate whenever they have 'reasonable cause to suspect' that a child is suffering or likely to suffer significant harm, or when a child is subject to an emergency protection order or police protection. If they have insufficient information the local authority are required to take steps to obtain access to the child and, if necessary, where this is denied, to apply for a court order. To assist their enquiries they may call on the help of other agencies including any health authority or national health service trust, and that agency is required to assist them, in particular by providing relevant information and advice, unless this would be 'unreasonable in all the circumstances'.

More detailed guidance on these investigative and collaborative duties has been issued by the Department of Health. In particular *Working Together*[3] contains much detailed advice relating to child abuse, including sexual abuse, ranging from inter-agency case conferences to the operation of child protection committees. The Department of Health's social services inspectorate and children's division constantly review the position and update guidance where necessary. Detailed procedures for inter-agency collaboration will be drawn up locally by the Area Child Protection Committee in consultation with all the relevant agencies.

Orders

EMERGENCY PROTECTION ORDERS (CHILDREN ACT S. 44)

These can be made by a court (or a single magistrate) if it is satisfied that 'there is reasonable cause to believe that the child is likely to suffer significant harm' if he is not removed to other accommodation, or if he does not remain where he is. In other words, the order may be made either to enable a child to be removed from a dangerous situation or to prevent his removal from, for example, a hospital or foster home, to a harmful situation. Any individual may apply for an order on these grounds, but in addition a local authority or the NSPCC may apply if frustrated in their enquiries into suspected abuse by an unreasonable refusal of access to the child. An order lasts for 8 days with a possible extension of 7 days. While it is in force it gives the applicant parental responsibility, but he or she may only 'take such action as is necessary to safeguard or promote the welfare of the child'. Parental responsibility includes the right to give consent on behalf of a child to a medical examination, but this right may be controlled by the court giving directions with regard to the medical or psychiatric examination of the child, including an order that there should be no such examination. Even where a direction is given this cannot override the right of a child of sufficient understanding to refuse to consent to examination. The court may also give directions as to the contact to be permitted with the child by parents and others. Not only is it intended that this order should only be used in emergencies, but it is also provided that it should not necessarily involve the removal of the child if, on further investigation, such a step turns out to be unnecessary. There is also a power for the court to direct that the applicant, in enforcing the order, may be accompanied by a medical practitioner, nurse or health visitor if he chooses. This could be used to assist the applicant in assessing whether it is in fact necessary to remove the child. The police may also take a child into police protection for up to 72 hours under s. 46 of the Act.

CHILD ASSESSMENT ORDERS (CHILDREN ACT S. 43)

Orders may be made in non-urgent cases where the local authority or NSPCC suspect that a child may be suffering, or likely to suffer, significant harm, but their investigation to establish whether this is indeed the case requires a proper assessment which is prevented by the child's parents or carers. The order requires any person who is able to do so to produce the child and to comply with the court's directions as to the child's assessment and will act as an authorization to the person carrying out the assessment. Again it cannot override any refusal by a child of sufficient understanding to submit to examination or assessment. If necessary for the assessment the order may provide for the child to be kept away from home, but in any event the period of assessment cannot exceed 7 days.

This is an entirely new provision introduced by the Children Act and it remains to be seen whether it fulfils a real need.

The law and professionals

Prevention of child abuse: collaboration versus confidentiality

The duties of health professionals towards children are essentially no different from those owed to any other patients although clearly the inability of young children to consent on their own behalf to examination or treatment adds an extra dimension and children's vulnerability imposes additional responsibilities in the area of prevention of abuse, sometimes overriding the duty of confidence.

Recognition of this has been given by the General Medical Council.[4] GMC guidance emphasizes that the paramounting of the patient's interests will usually require the doctor to disclose information about neglect or abuse of the patient to an appropriate responsible person or agency.

One forum for the exchange of information about a child who may have been subjected to abuse is the case conference, but the need for professionals to consult with each other at all stages of any investigation is emphasized in *Working Together*.[3] This publication contains guidance on the investigation of possible abuse, underlining the importance of sharing information to ensure the protection of children.

Appearing in court

Not only in child abuse, but in other cases involving children, medical professionals will be called on to provide evidence in court. Under the Children Act there is greater flexibility as to which courts may hear which cases concerning children, although generally applications for care orders will be started in magistrates (family proceedings) courts. The more complex cases will usually be heard in the county courts or even the High Court, but the use of the wardship jurisdiction in cases involving the local authority, has been reduced.

In the High Court and county courts cases are heard by judges who are all qualified lawyers; the High Court judges are referred to as Mr or Mrs Justice X, and addressed as 'My Lord' or 'My Lady'; circuit judges (His or Her Honour Judge X, addressed as 'Your Honour') sit in the county courts and some are designated to specialize in care cases. The bench in the magistrates court is made up of lay justices drawn from the local community and those sitting in the family proceedings court are drawn from a special panel. Since they are not legally qualified they are advised by a legally qualified clerk, who also administers the court. They are addressed as 'Sir' or 'Madam', or 'Your Worships'.

Although documentary evidence in the form of written statements is admissible in court proceedings under the Children Act, the makers of statements must be prepared to give oral evidence, and in particular to face cross-examination on matters which are in dispute. A witness will be asked to take the oath (or make an affirmation) and will be questioned first by the lawyer for the party who has called him or her to give evidence, and then by those representing the other party or parties, and possibly by the bench. The answers should be directed to the bench, and where the evidence concerns technical matters they should be explained clearly in non-technical terms. Before referring to notes, the witness should ask the court's permission, which will almost invariably be given in the case of a professional witness, although it is important that the notes should be as near as possible contemporaneous to the events described. The notes, or clinical record, once referred to by a witness, may themselves become evidence, and be inspected by the courts and the parties. All witnesses may give evidence of facts of which they have first hand knowledge (e.g. 'I saw the child on 1 October and he had a red swelling about one inch in diameter on his right cheek'), but suitably qualified professionals may also give expert opinion evidence in their own field, so that it would be permissible for an appropriately qualified doctor to give an opinion, for example, on whether a particular injury was consistent with the explanation given by the parent. Where a person believed to have evidence relevant to a case is unwilling to appear voluntarily in court, any of the parties may ask the court to issue a witness summons (or *subpoena*) requiring that person to come to court (and possibly requiring certain documents to be brought). Once such a summons has been served on the person, it is a contempt of court to fail to comply with it but application can be made to the court for the summons to be set aside.

Northern Ireland

The Northern Ireland legal system and law relating to children resembles more closely those in England and Wales than those in Scotland, but the recent changes brought about in England and Wales by the Children Act 1989 have not yet been echoed in Northern Ireland.

Parental rights and duties

Where parents are married both have rights and duties in respect of their children; where they are unmarried the mother alone has such rights and duties, although the father may be required to contribute to the child's maintenance, and has a right to apply for custody or access under the Guardianship of Infants Act 1886 s. 5A.

Children's rights

Just as local authorities in England and Wales have duties to provide certain services for children in need, and specific duties towards children whom they are looking after, the Northern Ireland Health and Social Services Boards have similar responsibilities. In particular they are required by s. 164 Children and Young Persons Act (Northern Ireland) 1968 to make available such advice, guidance and assistance as may promote the welfare of children by diminishing the need to receive children into or keep them in care or bring them before a court. Where children are unable to be cared for by their parents, and their welfare demands it, the boards must receive them into care. This process does not however involve a transfer of parental rights, and the boards may not keep children in care under this provision against parental wishes. The ways in which parents may exercise their rights with respect to their children are similar to those which may be exercised in England and Wales by people with parental responsibility. If, however, a *fit person* order or *parental rights* order is made in respect of a child then the parents' parental rights are effectively transferred to the relevant health and social services board, subject to certain limited statutory exceptions, such as the right to consent to adoption. Criminal sanctions against ill-treatment and other forms of abuse of children are contained in Part II of the Children and Young Persons Act (Northern Ireland) 1968. When children are in care, whether under these provisions or under a fit person order, regulations similar to the parallel provisions in England and Wales make detailed provision for the way in which the boards are to exercise their responsibilities. There is however no statutory complaints procedure similar to that instituted by the Children Act 1989.

Legal procedures

General principles

The paramountcy principle applies to proceedings involving children, but there is no provision equivalent to that in the Children Act 1989 requiring the court to make an order only if that is better than making no order.

Proceedings between individuals

An order for custody of or access to a child may be made in the magistrates court under article 10 of the Domestic Proceedings Order (N.I.) 1980, when an application has been made for financial support. Under article 12 of the same order the court may make an order placing the child in the care of the social services department. Appeals from magistrates court orders are heard by the county court, which also deals with divorce proceedings. No divorce decree can be granted until the judge has found that the arrangements for the children are satisfactory, and a welfare report is required in each case to enable the judge to reach a decision. Disputed custody and access cases are heard in the High Court (Matrimonial Causes (Northern Ireland) Order 1978).

Proceedings involving the health and social services boards

Under Part V of the Children and Young Persons Act (Northern Ireland) 1968, a child or young person may be brought before a juvenile court as being in need of care, protection or control. The relevant health and social services board has a *duty* to investigate cases where information suggests that a child or young person may be in need of care, protection or control, and to bring proceedings if the grounds appear to be met, unless someone else is pursuing the matter or such a step would be contrary to his or her best interests. A police constable or the NSPCC may also institute proceedings. If the court before whom the child or young person is brought is satisfied that parental control is less than might reasonably be expected of a good parent, it may make one of a number of orders. A *supervision order* will give the child support while remaining at home, a *fit person order* removes him or her from the care and control of parents and confers most parental rights and powers on the fit person, often the health and social services board; a *training school order* will involve the child or young person's committal to a training school for a maximum period of usually 3 years.

Wardship

Any person may apply to the High Court for a child to be made a ward of court and the child then effectively comes under the custody of the court, which may make a variety of orders to promote the child's welfare. This procedure is used both by individuals and, increasingly, by the health and social services boards. It is likely, however, that when proposed new legislation comes into force, bringing the law relating to children very close to that applying in England and Wales, the use of wardship will sharply decline, as it did in England after implementation of the Children Act.

Child protection

Where a child is in need of immediate protection, a court or a justice of the peace may make an order authorizing the applicant to remove the child to a place of safety (e.g. a hospital, police station or board home) and keep him there for up to 5 weeks. The order can be extended twice for further periods of up to 5 weeks. A police constable may detain a child for up to 8 days in a place of safety without an order.

The law and professionals

Appearing in court

The court structure in Northern Ireland is similar to that in England, but in practice the High Court is used much more extensively than the county court in family matters. Magistrates (resident magistrates) are legally qualified professionals, although lay members sit alongside the resident magistrate in the juvenile court which hears applications in relation to children in need of care and protection, as well as dealing with juvenile offenders.

Scotland

Scottish child care law, like the whole Scottish legal system and court structure, differs in many ways from that in England, Wales and Northern Ireland. This section is, therefore, not set out in the same order as the previous ones.

Parents' and children's rights

Since 1991 Scots law has recognized the right of young people of or over the age of 16 to make decisions about their own financial and personal affairs. Young people who have attained 16 do not require to consult their parents or any other adult before giving consent to medical treatment. Children under the age of 16 are not usually regarded as capable of making decisions or giving any consent which has legal effect. Transactions or consents on behalf of a child are dealt with by the child's guardian, who is usually the child's parent. There is an important exception in the case of medical treatment, which is to be found in section 2(4) of the Age of Legal Capacity (Scotland) Act 1991. Under this section a person under the age of 16 has legal capacity to consent on his own behalf to any surgical, medical or dental procedure or treatment where, in the opinion of a qualified medical practitioner attending him he is capable of understanding the nature and possible consequences of the procedure or treatment. This is slightly different from the test in England, in that the emphasis is laid upon the opinion of the medical practitioner responsible for the treatment. A young child may be able to understand and consent to relatively simple procedures, but may be incapable of comprehending more complex treatment. The consent of the guardian is only required if the child cannot understand and consent to the procedure or treatment. It is not clear whether a parent may overrule the refusal to receive treatment of a child who is capable of consenting.

Guardianship is usually a parental right. Under normal circumstances a mother has such rights. A father only has parental rights if he is married to the child's mother at the time of the child's conception or subsequently. Either parent may exercise their parental rights independently of the other. The court may make an order relating to parental rights under s. 3 of the Law Reform (Parent and Child) (Scotland) Act 1986. Under this Act, the court may terminate or suspend parental rights. Such an order could relate to consent to medical examination or treatment, if the welfare of the child demanded and the order was in the child's interests.

It is an offence under s. 12 of the Children and Young Persons (Scotland) Act 1937 for anyone over 16 with custody, charge or care of any child or young person under that age wilfully to assault, ill-treat, neglect, abandon or expose them in a manner likely to cause unnecessary suffering or injury to health. A parent or other person legally liable to maintain a child will be deemed to have so neglected them, if he has failed to provide or secure, among other things, adequate medical aid.

Proceedings between individuals

The sheriff court or the Court of Session may make orders relating to parental rights in actions for divorce, judicial separation or nullity. In addition, any person claiming interest may make an application to the court for an order relating to parental rights. Parental rights are defined in s. 8 of the Law Reform (Parent and Child) (Scotland) Act 1986 to mean not only guardianship and curatory, but also custody and access and any right or authority relating to the welfare or upbringing of a child conferred on a parent by any rule of law. There is therefore considerable flexibility in Scotland as to who may apply to the sheriff or the Court of Sessions to resolve a dispute relating to a child, and the issues which may be dealt with by any court order. The court must regard the welfare of the child involved as the paramount consideration and must not make any order relating to parental rights unless it is satisfied that to do so will be in the interests of the child.

Action by the local authority

Under the Social Work (Scotland) Act 1968, children and their families are entitled to certain assistance from local authorities since s. 12 of the Act places a duty on the local authority to promote social welfare by making available advice, guidance and assistance on such a scale as may be appropriate for their local area. Local authorities also have a duty under s. 15 of the Act to receive into care children whose parents are not able to provide for them, although this does not enable authorities to receive children into care whose parents wish to look after them themselves. Such care does not of itself transfer parental rights to the local authority. The child's parent remains his or her guardian and retains the power to consent to medical treatment in so far as the child cannot consent, but the parent may delegate the exercise of his rights to the local authority. Section 16 of the Social Work (Scotland) Act 1968 does contain a procedure for the local authority to acquire parental rights in relation to children in their care, in which case the local authority is responsible as guardian of the child. An order freeing a child for adoption has a similar effect as it vests parental rights in the local authority. A full adoption order will make the adoptive parents the child's guardians, with all parental rights, and eliminate the rights of natural parents and any previous rights held by the local authority.

When parental rights are assumed under s. 16 of the Social Work (Scotland) Act 1968 this initially involves the local authority in passing a resolution which is usually dealt with by the social work committee. The child's parents will be given notice of the resolution and if they object they must notify the local authority within one month. The resolution will then lapse unless the local authority applies to the sheriff who will consider whether there are grounds under the Act for resolution, and that it is in the interests of the child for parental rights to remain with the local authority.

Child protection

Children in need of care and protection and children who commit offences are assisted through the children's hearing. Provided the child is under 16 (or under 18 if already subject to a supervision requirement) and provided one or more of the specific conditions set out in s. 32(2) of the Social Work (Scotland) Act 1968 applies, the child may be in need of compulsory measures of care. The conditions cover children who are likely to be caused unnecessary suffering or impairment to health or development due to a lack of parental care, child victims of offences, children who are members of a household where there is such a victim or a perpetrator of such an offence and children who are beyond parental control, exposed to moral danger or who abuse volatile substances, as well as child offenders and children who truant from school. Anyone, including a medical practitioner, may refer such a child to the reporter to the children's hearing, who is responsible for deciding what, if any, action is required in relation to such a child. In approximately half the cases referred to the reporter no further action is taken. A small proportion are referred to the local authority for advice, guidance and assistance. When, however, it appears to the reporter that a child is in need of compulsory measures of care he arranges a children's hearing. He must request a report for the hearing from the local authority, and they, or the reporter, may request information from other persons, including, by implication, medical practitioners. The hearing consists of three members drawn from a local panel. They are responsible for considering the child's case, together with the child, his parents and anyone else whose presence is necessary. They will decide on what course of action is in the best interests of the child. The hearing may make a supervision requirement necessitating that the child submit to supervision by the local authority. The requirement may impose conditions, including a condition of residence with particular foster parents, or in a named residential establishment. The children's hearing will review the supervision requirement at the request of the local authority, or parent (subject to certain limitations) and a requirement cannot continue without review for longer than a year. Where the grounds for referral are challenged, the case will first be heard in the sheriff court.

Emergency procedures

When children need to be removed from home as a matter of urgency a constable, or any person authorized by a sheriff or justice of the peace (JP), may detain them in a place of safety. Authority may be sought if the child is the victim of an offence, a member of the household of a victim or the household of an offender, or lack of parental care is causing unnecessary suffering or is inclement to health. A child may also himself seek refuge in a place of safety. If there are reasonable grounds to suspect that a child has been or is being assaulted, ill-treated or neglected or is the victim of an offence and he cannot be found, or entry to find him is denied, a JP may authorize a named constable to search for the child, if necessary entering by force to find him. In all cases the reporter must be informed immediately and, if he agrees the child is in need of compulsory measures of care, he will arrange a children's hearing as soon as possible. If he does not agree he will release the child. The children's hearing may authorize the continued detention of a child in a place of safety for a limited period.

Local authorities which receive information suggesting that children may be in need of compulsory measures of care are obliged to make enquiries and give such information as they may have been able to discover to the reporter.

Appearing in court

The medical profession may be called on to give evidence in proceedings between individuals relating to parental rights in the sheriff court or the Court of Session. They may find themselves giving evidence in local authority proceedings relating to an assumption of parental rights, or freeing for adoption, in the sheriff court. Medical experts may be called to give evidence to the sheriff when there is an application by the reporter relating to the grounds upon which the child has been referred to the hearing. All these are civil proceedings and the court is required to be satisfied that each material fact in the case is more likely than not to be true. The exception is when a child is referred to a hearing on the ground that they

are alleged to have committed an offence. In this event the standard of proof applicable is that which relates to criminal proceedings. When a person is prosecuted for an offence the proceedings may be brought in the district court, the sheriff court (with or without a jury), or the High Court (with a jury). The rules of evidence in criminal procedure are tighter, they generally exclude repetition of statements made by others to prove the content of the statement (hearsay) and there is a requirement of corroboration (proof of material facts from more than one source).

Sheriffs and judges are addressed as 'My Lord'. The law relating to the giving of evidence is similar to that in England and Wales.

Employment of children

This is one area where the law in all three UK jurisdictions is virtually the same, although in practice the power of the local authorities to make bye-laws means that there is no uniformity. The major relevant legislation for England and Wales is contained in the Children and Young Persons Act 1933, for Northern Ireland in the Children and Young Persons Act (Northern Ireland) 1968 and for Scotland in the Children and Young Persons (Scotland) Act 1937. The Children and Young Persons Act 1963 also governs some aspects both in England and Wales and Scotland and its provisions regarding application for a permit for a child to perform abroad apply to Northern Ireland also.

Children under 13 are not generally allowed to be employed although local authority bye-laws may allow them to be employed by their parents in light agricultural or horticultural work, and licences may be granted to individual children permitting them to take part in performances subject to certain conditions.

Children between the age of 13 and 16 may not be employed:

- Before the close of school hours on any day in which they must attend school
- Before 7.00 a.m. or after 7.00 p.m. on any day
- For more than two hours on Sunday
- To lift, carry or move anything so heavy it is likely to injure them.

Local bye-laws may modify these prohibitions to a limited extent, the most common modifications perhaps being to permit the employment of children for up to one hour before school starts, and to require employers to notify the authority that the child is employed. Bye-laws vary widely, and some require the employed child to obtain a medical certificate from the local specialist in community medicine.

In addition there are a number of other provisions in a variety of statutes prohibiting or limiting the employment of children in dangerous or morally harmful occupations or places for example in mines or on licensed premises. There are also restrictions on the types and conditions of work for 16–18 year olds. Responsibility for enforcement is divided between different government and local authority departments and is made still more difficult by the lack of uniformity as a result of the local bye-laws. The Employment of Children Act 1973 which would have allowed regulations to be made by central government in place of the bye-laws has never been implemented.

References

1   Gillick v West Norfolk & Wisbech Area Health Authority [1985] 3 All ER 402.
2   re W (a minor) (medical treatment)([1992] 4 All ER 627.
3   Department of Health. *Working Together under the Children Act 1989*, London: HMSO, 1991.
4   General Medical Council. Professional Conduct and Discipline: Fitness to Practise. Paragraph 83 (amended May 1993).

Appendix 9.1

The UN Convention on the Rights of the Child

The Convention came into force in 1990, once it had been ratified by 20 countries known as states parties under the Convention. It has now been ratified by over 90 states parties, including the UK. The Convention recognizes that children (defined as under 18, unless they achieve majority earlier) need special protection and sets out specific steps that members agree to take in an attempt to ensure children's well-being. Important matters include:

- Respect for the responsibilities and rights of parents or, where applicable, members of the extended family or community according to local custom, to provide 'appropriate direction and guidance' for the child (Article (art.) 5).
- The child's right to life and the state's obligation to ensure the child's survival and development (art. 6).
- The child's right to name, nationality and family ties (arts 7 & 8).
- The child's right not to be separated from parents against their will, except where such separation is necessary in the interests of the child (e.g. abuse or neglect) and, where this arises, legal procedures are followed and those interested allowed to participate. The child's right to maintain contact with parents even when separated, unless this is against his or her interests (art. 9).
- Children's right to have their views taken into account in procedures affecting them (arts 12 & 13).
- Freedom of thought, conscience and religion, and of association (arts 14 & 15).
- The child's right to protection from interference with privacy or family (art. 16).

- The principle that both parents have primary responsibility for bringing up their children, with their best interests as their basic concern; the state should support them in this including taking appropriate measures to ensure that children of working parents have the right to benefit from child services for which they are eligible (art. 18).
- The state's obligation to protect children from physical or mental abuse, violence and neglect, including providing preventive services (art. 19).
- The right of children deprived of their family environment or who, in their own best interests, cannot be allowed to remain there, to special protection by the state, and suitable alternative placement, with regard to the desirability of continuity and to their ethnic, religious, cultural and linguistic background (art. 20).
- Adoption, in those countries where it is allowed, only to be carried out in the best interests of the child: inter-country adoption to be considered if the child cannot be placed in a suitable alternative home in his or her country of origin; the same standards and safeguards to apply to inter-country adoption as apply in domestic adoption (art. 21).
- Special protection of refugee children (art. 22).
- The right of disabled children to enjoy a full life in conditions which facilitate the child's active participation in the community; states to promote international cooperation in the exchange of information related to preventive health care of disabled children (art. 23).
- The right of the child to the highest attainable standard of health and to facilities for treatment of illness; in particular states to take appropriate measures:
    to diminish infant and child mortality
    to ensure provision of health care to all children with emphasis on development of primary health care
    to ensure appropriate prenatal and postnatal health care for mothers
    to promote access to education on child health
    to develop preventive health care and family planning and to promote international cooperation taking particular account of the needs of developing countries (art. 24).
- The right of a child placed by the state for care or treatment to periodic reviews of the placement (art. 25).
- The right of children to benefit from social security (art. 26).
- The right of children to a standard of living adequate for their development, their parents having the primary responsibility to ensure this with support of the state where appropriate (art. 27).
- The child's right to education directed to development of mental and physical abilities to their fullest potential (arts 28 & 29).

- The right of children of ethnic minorities to enjoy their own culture (art. 30).
- Right to leisure and participation in cultural and artistic activities (art. 31).
- Protection from exploitation of labour, exposure to drug abuse, sexual exploitation, child trafficking and other forms of exploitation (arts 32–36).

- Prohibition of torture, protection from unlawful imprisonment, and rights to contact with family if lawfully detained (art. 37).
- Promotion of rehabilitative care after any injury to children (art. 39).
- Special measures to safeguard children accused or convicted of criminal offences (art. 40).

9.4 Physical abuse

Chris Hobbs

Introduction

Physical abuse (battering, non-accidental injury) refers to violence directed toward children.

The definition used to define the criteria for registration of children as physically abused is:

'Actual or likely physical injury to a child, or failure to prevent physical injury (or suffering) to a child including deliberate poisoning, suffocation and Munchausen's Syndrome by proxy.'[1]

Within these definitions, hitting a child (corporal punishment) does not constitute physical abuse unless it results in injury. However, several countries in Europe have now passed laws against the hitting of children by parents. In the UK, corporal punishment has been prohibited in state schools but not as yet in private schools. A relationship between corporal punishment and physical abuse has been claimed. Stopping hitting of children may prove to be an effective preventive strategy in physical abuse.[2]

Physical abuse may be moderate, severe or fatal. All abuse is serious and none mild; soft tissue injuries such as bruising involve considerable force in their production.

This in turn inflicts pain and is invariably associated with some degree of emotional abuse including harsh words, threats and rejection. The dangers arising from an injury relate especially to the age of the child. A small bruise in a baby should warn us of serious or fatal abuse, while a beating in an older child may pose no threat to life.

Failure to protect or deliberately placing a child in danger is as serious as a deliberate injury. Such passive abuse may reflect a conscious or unconscious urge to be rid of a child.

Children are very vulnerable and few parents who shake, hit or slap a child intend to cause serious injury. Many injuries occur when parents lose control under stress, but some are sadistic and premeditated, for example, some burns and scalds.

Historical aspects

Over the centuries, beating children was viewed as part of normal child rearing practice in many civilizations. De Mause[3] wrote that, 'the history of childhood is a nightmare from which we have recently begun to awaken. The further back in history one goes, the lower the level of child care, and the more likely children are to be killed, abandoned, beaten, terrorised and sexually abused.' In searching through history, the earliest times in which he encountered some children who may have grown up without being beaten was from 1690–1750, but there were many examples where children commonly died from hitting and beating. In Copenhagen in 1748 death statistics revealed that of 3328 who died, 987 did so because of physical abuse and most of them were children. Some states of the USA carried the death penalty for children who disobeyed their parents in the 17th century.

In the well known story of Mary Ellen in the USA in 1871,[4] her protection from battering was achieved only through Animal Protection Laws because child protective laws in the USA did not exist at that time.

In England, there is abundant evidence of physical cruelty to children in the past and the way in which it was ignored or condoned.[4]

The physical abuse of children received little attention from physicians until the middle of this century, when American paediatricians and radiologists, including Caffey,[5] Silverman[6] and Kempe,[6] encouraged the medical profession to confront the inescapable fact that children could receive serious injury at the hands of those who were caring for them.

In 1965 a Child Abuse heading appeared in the *Quarterly Cumulative Index Medicus* for the first time.

The lead, given in the USA, was followed in other countries including England, but it was not until the inquiry into the death of a battered child named Maria Colwell, who died in 1973, that public attention focused on the issue in the UK.

Since that time understanding has increased, both in recognition and management of the child and family.

Incidence and prevalence

Officially reported cases only represent a fraction of the total number of cases in the population as a whole.

Reporting depends on awareness of the problem by the public and professionals including doctors, nurses, social workers, teachers and others in contact with children.

The annual statistics of the National Society for the Prevention of Cruelty to Children (NSPCC) based on a sample of registers covering 9% of the population of England and Wales, found an increase in registration rate from 0.63 per thousand (under 17 years) in 1983 to 0.82 per thousand in 1987. The figures suggest there were over 8000 cases of physical abuse registered in England and Wales in 1987; 0.6% were classified fatal, 9% serious and 90% moderate. Figure 9.1 shows the growth in diagnosed cases in Leeds, where cases have been recorded since 1969, over the period 1969–88.

It has been estimated[7] that between 200–230 non-accidental deaths occur per year in the UK and that 1.5–2% of all children have been physically abused by the age of 17 years. Boys outnumber girls; for example in the NSPCC's series from 1983 to 1987, 55% were boys, 45% girls. Nearly half are aged 0–4 years, with about a quarter each 5–9 and 10–14 years. One in eight are aged less than a year, but 70% of serious head injuries occurred to children less than one year.[7]

Physical abuse, however, rarely exists on its own and it is important to recognize links with other forms of abuse.[8] One in six physically abused children have also been sexually abused and others have been neglected or are failing to thrive. Emotional abuse coexists in most cases.

Physical abuse occurs to children of all ethnic groups, but possibly has different frequency between the groups.

Handicapped children seem to be at increased risk and in one study[9] 13.5% of physically abused children had handicaps. In some instances, the abuse may be the cause of the handicap.

Social background

Physical abuse is reported more often from conditions of social deprivation and poverty, although it occurs in all social classes. In the NSPCC's figures,[7] only 4% of mothers and 5% of fathers were in non-manual occupational categories, but more significantly, 67% of mothers and 52% of fathers were unemployed and only 15% of mothers and 35% of fathers reported as being in paid employment.

Fifteen per cent of mothers and 43% of fathers had criminal records, but often these were unrelated to crimes toward children. However, fathers were more likely than mothers to have a record of violence against adults.

There is a greater tendency for families in which there is a physically abused child to be larger than the national average; 25% of the families have four or more children. Very nearly half of the abused children are first born. Subsequently born children also carry a significant risk, although the percentage of injured children falls with each succeeding child after the first.

Perpetrators

Natural parents or parent figures are responsible for causing the injury in over 90% of cases. Natural

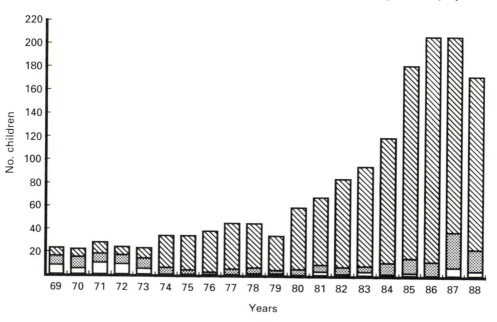

Figure 9.1 Diagnosed cases of physical abuse in Leeds 1969–88. ▨ Total; ▥ fractures; ▢ subdural, retinal haemorrhages.

mothers are responsible in one-third and natural fathers in slightly fewer.[7] If analysed according to whom the child was living with at the time, then natural mothers were implicated in 36% and natural fathers in 61% of cases where the child was living with them. While mother substitutes appear much less often in the statistics, stepfathers and father substitutes including cohabiting boyfriends of the mother, account for almost one in five cases. Stepfathers appear to be implicated relatively more often than cohabitees. Occasionally other relatives or baby-sitters are implicated.

More than half physically abused children come from families with single parents, but marital difficulties are common when both parents are in the household.

Recognition

Presentation

1 Direct report

Direct report by a child, a parent or other interested third party. Most reports are true and should, in general, be believed.

Third party reports (often anonymous telephone calls to the NSPCC or social services) should be treated seriously but sometimes are found to have no basis, or to carry malicious intent.

Worries by grandparents and other responsible family members also need careful assessment. The reasons for the reports must be identified, even if no obvious abuse is found.

2 Presentation of an injury

Following abuse, parents frequently seek help from a hospital, a health visitor or general practitioner (GP). Pointers to physical abuse include:

a Repetitive pattern of injury, but parents may use different hospitals to avoid detection.

b Injuries not consistent with the history – too many, too severe, wrong type, wrong distribution, wrong age.

c Pattern of injury which strongly suggests abuse, e.g. bruising to a young baby (there are few reasonable explanations), multiple injuries following a moderate fall, severe head injuries in babies or toddlers, rib fractures, subdural haematoma and retinal haemorrhages from violent shaking, multiple cigarette burns.

d Presence of other signs of abuse, e.g. neglect, failure to thrive, sexual abuse.

e Unusual behaviour in the parents, e.g. delay in seeking medical advice, refusal to allow proper treatment or admission to hospital, unprovoked aggression toward staff.

3 Incidental discovery of injury

Abused children are frequently allowed to go to school, to nursery or to another person's care where injuries may be found and reported. It is not unusual for parents in this situation to deny knowledge of the injury and for there to be no satisfactory explanation.

Features in the history

It is unusual for the doctor to have all the information required but the following is a checklist of important features in the history which may alert to the possibility of physical abuse.

1 Discrepant history

Does it change with telling or with who tells it? Is it vague or unclear? Exact details of time, place, person and actions are needed. For example, how did the child fall, how far, onto what. Compare your account with that of others – social worker, health visitor, policeman. Major differences need explanation. Do the father and mother give the same story?

2 Unreasonable delay

Unreasonable delay in seeking help or care for the child, especially following a fracture, serious burn or scald is a strong indicator. Denial that the child was in pain and minimization of the symptoms is common. Following a serious head injury, a baby may be left tucked up in a cot, only to be brought hours later when he refuses a feed or starts to fit. One parent of a child with a serious burn said the doctor's surgery was closed so she did not do anything for a week.

3 Family crisis

There may be a family crisis or a complicated home situation which has precipitated the injury. This could be a bereavement, loss of job or final demand for a debt. These stresses are usually revealed if parents are listened to.

4 Trigger factors

Trigger factors are behaviours in the child which precipitate the parent's violence. Inconsolable crying in the night, difficult feeding or wetting are common and in older children, stealing or lying.

5 Parents' experiences

Parents' traumatic experiences as children are important, but may be hidden or repressed. Parents may admit to being beaten themselves as children. Some may have been in care.

6 Unrealistic expectations

Unrealistic expectations coupled to a poor understanding of child development. The child is expected to love and accept the parents. When he cries or will not take his feeds, it is because he is rejecting or punishing them. An expectation that a 2-year-old will behave in model and ideal ways is likely to lead to what parents perceive as a failure on the part of the child. Obsessional and rigid patterns of child rearing may be expressed in other ways (e.g. super clean and tidy home) and can create stresses and tensions.

7 Social isolation

Social isolation from friends, extended family and professionals is a common finding in parents who abuse. Who can you turn to for help is a crucial question. As the abuse escalates, the parents find it increasingly difficult to allow anyone into their lives for fear of discovery. Abusing parents tend to attribute their problems to external factors rather than to their own difficulties.

8 Past history of child

The presence of high levels of parental anxiety, frequent admissions to hospital in the first months of life, frequent 'accidents', 'a tendency to bruise easily' are often found. The child's behaviour, growth, development and health may also be sources of difficulty. Much of this information will come from sources other than parents, who may minimize their difficulties in their search to present themselves as perfect parents.

Procedures

Key figures in the process of investigation include social workers, doctors and police officers with emphasis on inter-agency cooperation.

Vital sources of information include the general practitioner, the accident and emergency doctor or nurse, the health visitor, school nurse, midwife or paediatric nurse (if child in hospital) and other individuals, e.g. probation officer, obstetrician, adult psychiatrist and staff, and pathologist. Information may be forthcoming from other sources including other hospitals, towns, and armed forces units.

It is usual for there to be a central coordinator of information, most frequently a social worker, who will become the key worker. One task is to contact those with information and check the important facts and opinions, drawing careful distinctions between the two types of information.

The information must be collated quickly and accurately but will be discussed in more detail at the case conference.

The police may or may not know the family but certainly if a name and date of birth are available will be able to check if there is a history of violence or assault against children.

Medical examination

Medical examination is an essential step in the identification of physical abuse. Doctors undertaking this work should be experienced with children, understand growth and development and have forensic skills. They should be able to write clear and concise reports and give evidence in courts.

Examination of physically abused children requires a calm, unhurried approach with attention to detail, good note keeping and an ability to cope with distressed children and parents. The room should be appropriately equipped, including toys, soft furnishings and be quiet and private.

The following are important:

1 A full paediatric history, including note of explanations of injury, times, details etc.
2 Developmental history
3 Parent's expressed difficulties with child: behaviour, health, development
4 Detailed examination of whole child to include:
   growth: height, weight, arm circumference
   nutrition
   general demeanour and appearance
   signs of neglect, sexual abuse, emotional disturbance
   development including language, social skills
5 *Documentation of injuries*
   Diagnosis of physical abuse usually involves the assessment of lesions which are visible to the unaided eye. Accurate documentation should be by words, drawings and photographs. Each method has its own particular merits which are complementary. Such documentation permits others, including police officers, courts, social workers and other doctors providing additional opinions, the opportunity of assessing the injuries for themselves. Descriptions should be brief but detailed and include:
      probable nature of the lesion and approximate age
      site
      shape
      size (in cm)
      any unusual distinguishing features and
      where possible, an estimate of its likely causation.
   Injuries should be listed one by one and related to body outline drawings in order to demonstrate injury patterns. The size of all injuries should be recorded and all reports should be dated and signed.

Injuries in physical abuse
Classification of injuries

1 Superficial
   Bruises
   Bite marks

Other superficial injuries, lacerations, scratches, ligature marks, broken or avulsed hair or nails.

2 Fractures and bony injury
   Wrenched limbs, periosteal injury.

3 Intracranial injury (including eyes)
   Whiplash following shaking, subdural haematoma, cerebral haematoma and subarachnoid haemorrhage, contusion and oedema.

4 Abdominal injury, internal injury – stomach, gut, solid viscera, thoracic injury.

5 Burns and scalds.

6 Asphyxia, drowning and poisoning.[10]

7 Injuries arising from fabricated disorders (Munchausen by proxy).[11]

1 Superficial injury

BRUISES

Bruises are present in nine out of ten physically abused children. Bruises arise when blood is lost from the intravascular space into the skin and subcutaneous tissues. Except in rare cases of severe bleeding disorder, trauma is always implicated in their causation. Bruises do not blanch on pressure and have a characteristic colour. They can be mimicked by paint or pen marks, dye from clothes, birth marks, mongolian blue spots or café-au-lait spots. Their configuration, delineation and colour evolve with time and provide a guide to approximate age. If there is any doubt that a lesion is a bruise, serial examination will clarify the situation.

Ageing of bruises

One scheme:	Age	Colour
	0–2 days	swollen, tender
	0–5 days	red, blue, purple
	5–7 days	green
	7–10 days	yellow
	10–14 days	
	(or more)	brown
	2–4 weeks	cleared
Another scheme:	Recent (24–48 h)	reddish purple, swollen, tender
	2–3 days	brownish purple
	4–7 days	brownish green
	7 days +	yellow

These differing schemes highlight the caution which doctors should adopt when discussing the ages of bruises in court.

Sites for inflicted bruises

Buchanan[12] analysed sites for superficial injuries of all kinds in 251 abused children. The figures refer to the number of injuries and the total obviously exceeds the total number of children, denoting that injuries were present in several sites in some children:

Forehead	37
Lower jaw	18
Arms	119
Chest	23
Around eyes	49
Ears	49
Hands	7
Abdomen	16
Cheeks	114
Mastoid	11
Legs	82
Back	60
Mouth	10
Feet	4
Buttocks	52

General points about sites

Bruises on the buttocks, lower back and outer thighs are often related to punishment.

Injuries to the inner thigh and genital area suggest either sexual abuse or punishment for toileting misdemeanours. The penis may be pinched or pulled and sometimes tied with string, hairs or rubber bands.

Injury to the head and neck is common. Slap marks are found on the sides of the face and ears, extending onto the scalp. Bruises to the external ear are unusual following accidents because of the protective effect of the triangle created by the shoulder, skull and base of neck which greatly reduces injury to the ear following a fall. Bruises to the lower jaw and the mastoid are strongly associated with abuse. Other sites are the neck, suggesting choking, and the eyes and mouth. Bruising around the eye can occur in normal school children from a direct injury but it takes a very hard blow to the forehead for blood to track down around one or both eyes.

Injury to the upper lip and frenulum may follow forced feeding and an old tear of frenulum may persist.

Bruises distal to the elbow and knees generally carry less significance than those on thighs and upper arms. Bruises to the trunk (chest and abdomen) are also suspicious of abuse and lower abdominal bruises should suggest sexual abuse.

Age of injuries

Multiple bruises have often been inflicted on a number of occasions and there will be different ages as well as size and shape. This polymorphic pattern of injury is typical of abuse. After a single accident, bruises will be of the same age and few in number. Falls downstairs are not associated with multiple bruises in many sites and of different ages.

Patterns of bruises

Inflicted bruises arise in a number of different ways:

Hand marks
Marks of implements, e.g. straps, sticks, buckles
Bruises from throwing, swinging or pushing child onto hard object

Bites
Bizarre marks.

HUMAN HAND MARKS

1 Grab marks or fingertip bruises involving extremities, face, or chest wall.
2 Hand print or linear finger mark.
3 Slap mark – may be seen indistinctly as two or three finger-sized linear marks with stripe effect. Rings may leave a tell-tale mark.
4 Pinch marks – a pair of crescent-shaped bruises, facing each other.
5 Poking marks – finger nail may cut the skin.

MARKS FROM IMPLEMENTS

The Newsons[13] found among a community sample of 700 ordinary children, that by 7 years of age, 26% of boys and 18% of girls had been hit with an implement of some kind. In both use and threat, the order of preference was: first strap or belt, second cane or stick, third slipper, fourth miscellaneous objects.

Belts or straps leave parallel sided marks which tend to curve with the contours of the body, whereas stick marks are less clearly defined linear marks over prominent areas, usually thinner than strap marks. Loops of flex show circular closed-end thin lines.

Large confluent areas of bruising, commonly on buttocks, arise from slipper beatings.

Tie marks cause circumferential bands around limbs and gags cause abrasions at the corners of the mouth.

BITE MARKS[14]

Bites can be inflicted by an animal, an adult or a child. Identification of the perpetrator is possible if the mark is recent and clear.

Animal bites result in puncturing, cutting and tearing of the skin by the carnivorous dentition.

The human diet is omnivorous and the teeth similar in size, shape and prominence. The resulting bruises are crescent-shape and individual teeth marks may be identified, if the injury is recent. In a very aggressive bite, the skin may be broken. To differentiate between an adult and a young child (under 8 years) it should be remembered that the intercanine distance (third tooth on each side) is greater than 3.0 cm in the adult or older child and less than 3.0 cm in a child with primary teeth.

Arch width differences between a 5-year-old child and an adult are 4.4 mm in the maxilla and 2.5 mm in the mandible, that is the difference is not great.[15] In the same study by Moores, the cumulative widths of the six upper deciduous teeth were 10 mm smaller in the primary than in the secondary dentition. In the lower arch, the differences were approximately 7 mm.

Suspect identification can be attempted with the help of a forensic dentist or odontologist. A series of photographs as soon as the injury is identified should be taken at intervals of 24 hours with a millimetre rule incorporated. Suspected perpetrators are asked to provide a dental impression to compare with the photographs.

Saliva: ABO blood groups can be determined from saliva washings of the skin surrounding a bite. Approximately 0.3 ml of saliva are deposited and it can be difficult to obtain sufficient by swabbing.

BIZARRE MARKS

Unusual bruises may arise when a child is struck through clothes and then the pattern of the weave may appear. Puncture wounds, e.g. from nappy pin, cord burns and self-inflicted injuries all produce unusual non-accidental marks. Petechial (pin-prick) bruises are common and arise when capillaries rupture producing small haemorrhages around them. They can be seen if an arm has been held tightly, around the neck if strangulation has been attempted or between the fingers of a handslap.

ACCIDENTAL INJURIES

In non-abused children, up to 10–12 bruises may be seen at any one time. In 400 children[16] aged from 2 weeks to 11 years, some injury was found in 37% but with increasing prevalence to the end of the third year of life. The commonest site was the lower leg (21.5%), thigh and buttock (9.25%) and arms (8.5%). In contrast, bruises to the head and face were found in only 6.5% of non-abused compared with 60% of 119 non-accidentally injured children. Accidental injuries to the shins, bony prominences (e.g. foreheads) in toddlers and to the hands and feet were prominent, but bruising to the lumbar region showed a marked variation with age – unusual before the age of 3 years, but present in 15% of children between the ages of 6 and 11 years. Bruising in young babies (2 weeks to 2 months) was found in only four out of 60 and in two there was a clear history of injury. Bruising was uncommon between 3 and 9 months (only one in eight children affected) but increased as the children became more mobile and active, so that 50–65% of children aged between 12 months and 11 years had lesions, usually minor bruising. Injuries to genitalia (two children, both easily explained) and to chest and upper back (maximum 5% in all the age groups) were uncommon, as too were burns (three only) and none had fractures.

NON-TRAUMATIC CAUSES OF BRUISING

Occasionally children are encountered where non-accidental injury is suspected and a bleeding disorder is encountered.[17] Wheeler and Hobbs over 10 years found that 23 out of 50 children with lesions suspicious of non-accidental injury were referred with possible bruising. Of these, five had bleeding disorders. Of other possible causes, Mongolian blue spots, capillary haemangioma, allergic peri-orbital swelling and dye ink or paint were described.

O'Hare and Eden[18] reported that routine tests of clotting in every child with bruising suspected of being non-accidental in aetiology, resulted in abnormal initial investigations in 16%. While children with spontaneous bleeding or bleeding for trivial trauma were found, many of the other children had several features supporting a diagnosis of non-accidental injury. *The coexistence of a bleeding disorder and physical abuse does occur and the diagnoses are not mutually exclusive.* The risks to a child from abuse, who has a bleeding disorder, may well be greater so that concern for the child's well-being may increase on discovering an abnormality.

Tests to exclude a bleeding disorder in non-accidental injury include:

1 Full blood count film
2 Platelet count (size and shape)
3 Partial thromboplastin time
4 Prothrombin time
5 Thrombin time
6 Fibrinogen
7 Bleeding time.

In addition, the drug history is important since salicylates, for example, can induce a platelet disorder.

OTHER SUPERFICIAL LESIONS

Scratches are common in abused children and may result from finger nails or nappy pins. Children have also been stabbed with knives; nails can be pulled out and traumatic alopecia result if they are grabbed by the hair. The hair may spiral, following overstretching, at the broken end and the scalp may be tender with petechiae at the hair roots. Differentiation from alopecia areata, common in deprived, poorly nourished children, involves the absence of loose hair at the periphery, inflammation or scaling of the scalp. Violent traction forces on the scalp, e.g. lifting the child by his hair, can lead to the diffuse extensive boggy swelling of a subgaleal haematoma between the scalp aponeurosis and the calvarium. These lesions may present without history and then abuse should be implied.

2 Fractures and bony injury

Fractures are classified as serious physical abuse. They may occur in any bone, be single or multiple, clinically obvious or occult, and detectable only on radiograph.

It was mainly the recognition of fractures which prompted the identification of what was called in 1946 by Caffey,[6] 'the parent–infant stress syndrome' and later renamed by Kempe, 'the battered baby syndrome'.[6]

Caffey drew attention to the metaphyseal avulsions at the end of long bones which he thought resulted from indirect traction, stretching and shearing; there were acceleration and deceleration stresses on the periosteum and articular capsules rather than direct impact stresses to the bone itself.

Fractures in abuse arise in a wide variety of ways, usually involving considerable force. The presence of a fracture usually implies a high level of force and therefore violence and the potential for a fatal outcome in the child.

PREVALENCE

Four per cent of 4037 physically injured children had long bone fractures and 2% had fractures in other bones.[7] The majority of fractures occur in young children. In one study of physically abused children 58% were under 3 years old and they sustained 94% of the fractures.[19] The proportion of children presenting with fractures from abuse rises to a maximum in the first year of life, when it may be as high as a half.[20] A high index of suspicion is required at this stage.

MECHANISMS OF PRODUCTION OF FRACTURES

Fractures occur when children are struck (with a hand or implement), thrown, grabbed, swung (impacting against a hard object such as wall or floor), shaken, or squeezed or when limbs are twisted or pulled. Most accidental fractures in young children result from falls.

Helfer and colleagues[21] reviewing 246 children aged 5 years or less who fell out of bed (219 at home and 95 in hospital), found three who sustained skull fractures with no serious intracranial injury, three fractured clavicles and one fractured humerus. The height of the fall was around 90 cm (3 feet) onto carpeted or non-carpeted floors. Seventeen per cent of the children had bumps, lumps, bruises or scratches. Roberton, Barbor and Hull[16] recorded no recent fractures, although as discussed earlier, many had bruises. Fractures in young children must always be assessed carefully and correlation attempted between:

1 The type of injury observed
2 The known mechanisms required for its production
3 The proposed mechanism of its production.

If there is a lack of correlation, then abuse must be considered.

DETECTION OF FRACTURES DUE TO PHYSICAL ABUSE

Children present with pain, excessive crying, refusal to use the affected limb. An arm may lie limply by their side, or they may refuse to walk. With a baby, a swelling may be noticed, e.g. haematoma over skull fracture. With older fractures, symptoms will regress and detection will depend on history and radiology. Fractures in hidden sites, for example the chest, will only be detected by radiology.

COMMON PATTERNS

1 Single fracture where there is other evidence of abuse, e.g. multiple bruises.
2 Multiple fractures, e.g. limb bones, ribs, skull, at different ages of healing possibly with minimal or no soft tissue injuries. In these cases, questions about metabolic or genetic bone disease will arise.
3 Metaphyseal-epiphyseal injuries, often multiple, and associated with violent shaking. An associated head injury including subdural haematoma may be present.
4 Isolated rib fractures. In the absence of a specific history of direct chest trauma, which is unusual, these provide strong evidence of abuse.
5 The formation of new periosteal bone. This arises when a limb is twisted or wrenched and takes time to develop. Other possible causes, e.g. infection, Caffey's disease, may need expert radiological assistance.
6 A skull fracture associated with intracranial injury is strongly associated with abuse when a young child has been injured in the home.

SKELETAL SURVEY

It is not always necessary to undertake a full skeletal survey if one suspects physical abuse. However, consider a skeletal survey in the following circumstances:

- When a child presents with a fracture which suggests physical abuse
- All physically abused children less than 3 years old
- Older children with severe bruising
- For localized pain, limp or reluctance to use arm or leg
- A previous history of recent skeletal injury
- Children dying in unusual of suspicious circumstances.

TYPES OF FRACTURE

There are a great many different fractures which can occur in the developing skeleton and their understanding is complex. Reference to a specialized textbook is essential in difficult cases.[22]

LIMB BONE FRACTURES

Children may be grabbed, pulled, swung or shaken by arms or legs or struck by fists or implements, or kicked. A wide range of fractures reflects the multifarious nature of violence to children.

The task of the clinician (paediatrician, surgeon, radiologist, pathologist) is to construct a likely mechanism of injury and compare it to the parent's history.

Some common sense points to consider

1 Fractures are painful and lead to immediate loss of function.

2 If children are said not to cry or express pain we must ask why. Abused children are sometimes too frightened to complain and we can recognize the frozen and watchful child in the accident and emergency department.[23]
3 Children do not continue to walk or play normally with a fracture, but parents who have abused may ignore the injury.
4 Pain is at a maximum at the beginning and swelling, bleeding and bruising take a while to develop in full. As these develop, pain may lessen.
5 Many fractures show no bruising.
6 As many of the fractures in abused children involve areas of bone dislodged from the main shaft or incomplete (greenstick) breaks, all the classical signs of fracture are not always present. Loss of function is the most important sign of a recent fracture. Once healing is under way, there may be no clinical signs of fracture detectable, but radiology will reveal the old injury. In abuse, this is especially important because there may be fractures of different ages in the same child.

Types of fracture in long bones

1 Metaphyseal lesions: high specificity for abuse[24] (corner fractures, bucket handle lesions).
2 Cartilaginous epiphyseal plate injury (Salter and Harris type I and II) occur in accidents and abuse.[25]
3 Transverse or oblique fractures of the shaft. Oblique are the more usual fractures in childhood. Transverse fractures may result from direct force, i.e. a blow.
4 Spiral fractures due to torsion injury.
5 Subperiosteal new bone formation. This can be seen following trauma in abused children but is also noted following infections and metabolic causes. New bone formation usually occurs 10–14 days after the injury. In abuse, excessive traction and torsion forces which occur when a child's limb is grabbed, pulled or twisted lead to stripping of the loosely attached periosteum along the long bone shaft.

Other fractures include compound, comminuted, impacted and pathological (underlying bone disease). Thus it can be seen that the type of fracture, with the exception of the metaphyseal or epiphyseal injury help little in diagnosis, and other features are needed. The presence of metaphyseal or epiphyseal fracture(s) does however make abuse very likely.

Rib fractures

Rib fractures in infants comprise between 5 and 27% of fractures in abused children.[19,26,27] They can occur antenatally and a case is described of a woman who had attempted to abort her fetus by banging her abdomen against tables and by falling downstairs.[28] Multiple healing rib fractures were discovered radiologically.

Cardiopulmonary resuscitation rarely, if ever, causes rib fractures and can be safely disregarded as a factor.[29] Other non-abuse causes of rib fractures include motor vehicle accidents, rickets, osteoporosis, surgery and osteogenesis imperfecta. If there is no history of specific major trauma and no radiological evidence of intrinsic bone disease, unexplained rib fractures are highly specific for abuse.

Diagnosis Rib fractures are usually diagnosed radiologically. They are frequently multiple and bilateral and most often situated posteriorly near the costotransverse process articulation. Fractures can also occur further anteriorly and sometimes multiply in the same rib.

Kleinman,[30] suggests that rib fractures occur when a child is violently shaken. Anteroposterior compression occurs when the infant's chest is held with palms situated laterally, thumbs anteriorly and fingers posteriorly. In evidence of this, he quotes an abuser's confession and the findings of periosteal disruption and new bone formation on the ventral aspect of the rib surfaces. The rib cage is viewed as a single functional unit comprising a series of parallel struts; forces are distributed widely throughout the cage leading to multiple fractures of similar age.

Radiology Acute changes on X-ray may be difficult to see but callus is usually well developed within 2 weeks and the only remaining evidence at a month may be slight cortical thickening.

Skull fractures

Injury to the skull is all too common in the seriously battered child. Fracture of the skull implies an impact between a solid object and the head. When a child has been violently shaken, there may be serious intracranial injury without skull fracture unless impact against a blunt object has also occurred. Accidental skull fractures in young children usually follow falls, but it is as well to emphasize that this is an infrequent occurrence in the usual kind accidents which occur.

In two series,[21,31] with a combined total of 594 young children sustaining falls of up to 90 cm (about 3 feet) from table or worktop height, only five (1–2%) sustained a skull fracture which in all cases was single and linear. None sustained intracranial injury.

Patterns of skull fractures[32] Fractures should be accurately described and measured, on the radiograph or at autopsy. The following classification is recommended.

Single linear: this is a single fracture consisting of an unbranched line in straight, zig-zagged or angled configuration. The fracture margins are closely opposed with the maximum width between

them, usually no more than 1–2 mm and often less than 1 mm.

Multiple or complex: this term applies where there is more than one fracture or where a single fracture has multiple components including a branching pattern. There may be a stellate configuration with several branching lines converging on a central point.

Depressed: this is a fracture where the normal curvature of the skull is interrupted by the inward displacement of bone. There may be comminution of the fracture with a fragment displaced inwards.

Growing fractures:[33] these are enlarged linear fractures usually 3 mm or more at maximum width. They may continue to enlarge over time, sometimes with the formation of a leptomeningeal cyst.

Reports of skull fractures should include:

1 Site – which bone(s).
2 Whether suture lines crossed.
3 Configuration, e.g. linear, crazy paving, stellate, branching.
4 Orientation – horizontal, vertical, oblique.
5 Length (cm) of each component × maximum width (mm).
6 Other features e.g. depression, growing.
7 Presence of soft tissue swelling (use bright light source).

Comment should also be made on sutures, whether widened or not, with a measure of width.

Anatomy of skull fractures in abuse and accident[32]

	Accident (60 cases)	Abuse (29 cases)
Single linear	55	6
Multiple complex	3	23
Depressed	3	12
Maximum fracture width (3 mm or more)	4	10 (of 13 measured)
Growing	2	6

These figures are from a study of 89 children with skull fractures aged 0–2 years; 29 of the children were abused.

Site The most commonly fractured bone, in either an accident or abuse, is the parietal which is large, prominent, relatively thin and vulnerable to injury. Frontal fractures are much less commonly seen, either in abuse or accident, while occipital fractures have a special predominance in abused children. A depressed occipital fracture is virtually pathognomonic of abuse.

Fractures of the temporal bone and anterior and middle fossa are also uncommon and usually follow severe trauma.

Site and extent of cranial fractures[32]

	Accident (60)	Abuse (29)
Parietal	57	27
Occipital	3	16
Frontal	0	4
Temporal	1	5
Anterior or middle cranial fossae	1	4

Number of bones involved

1	56	7
2	3	11
3 or more	1	11

It is frequently possible to recognize, in a child with fractures involving more than one bone or non-parietal bones, that the history denotes a more severe fall. For example, one child with a fracture extending from the parietal across into the temporal bone sustained his injury when he fell from a first floor window (4 metres) onto the ground below. Such an injury would be most unlikely to arise from a fall of 1–2 metres. This child suffered from disturbed consciousness for 2–3 days but made a full recovery.

Growing skull fracture[33] Most fractures which occur innocently following falls of a few feet are narrow, hairline cracks, usually in the parietal bone. The width can be measured on a radiograph with a millimetre rule. Occasionally wider fractures are seen of 3 mm or over and rarely a fracture may exceed 5 mm in width. These latter fractures are considered to be growing and require special consideration since they are more likely to be associated with abuse.

Growing fractures are uncommon, although they are reported in small numbers in the neurosurgical literature. The essential features are:

1 A skull fracture in infancy or early childhood.
2 A dural tear at the time of injury.
3 Brain injury beneath the fracture.
4 Subsequent enlargement to form a cranial defect.

Out of 89 cases of skull fractures of all kinds in the children studied in Leeds[32] aged up to 2 years, there were three growing fractures which required surgical treatment. By the time treatment is required, the defect is obvious as a smooth pulsatile swelling over the defect and the edges of the defect are palpable. Growing fractures are linked to severe injury and abuse should be suspected if they are found.

Other fractures in child abuse
Almost any bone can be affected. The clavicle is one of the most commonly fractured bones in childhood. Injury to the lateral portion of the clavicle is less common than midshaft fracture in abuse but may be more suggestive of abuse. Scapular and sternal fractures are highly suggestive of abuse but are uncommon. Fractures of the small bones of the hand and feet are also described including metacarpal and metatarsal injury but are unusual. Fusiform swelling of the digits may mimic juvenile arthritis. Repetitive beatings of the hands or feet may induce reactions in the small tubular bones.

Spinal injury
This usually results from forced extension and flexion injuries causing damage at several levels. Defects in lucency of the anterior superior edges of the vertebral bodies, often the low thoracic and upper lumbar region with narrowed disc spaces is typical. There may be no associated spinal cord injury.[34]

DATING FRACTURES[35]

Fractures in child abuse often present late. Discrepancy between the claimed age of the injury and that ascertained from radiological assessment is strong presumptive evidence of abuse. The presence of fractures of different ages and at different stages of healing is also strong evidence of abuse. In abuse, repeated trauma to the same site may complicate the process of healing.

PROCESS OF HEALING

Stages:

I Induction. This is the interval between injury and appearance of new bone. Haemorrhage and swelling occur, pain subsides as early as one to two days after injury and the process of repair begins with ingrowth of capillaries, removal of non-viable tissue and cellular reorganization.

II Soft callus. Osteoblasts proliferate and lay down new bone, often seen first around the periosteum. This takes 10–14 days in older children but less in infants. This stage lasts 3–4 weeks until the fracture line begins to obliterate.

III Hard callus. The fracture is solidly united and lamellar bone replaces periosteal and endosteal bone. This takes 2–3 months in adults but less in children. Infant fractures may unite in a quarter of the time of older children.

IV Remodelling. The gradual restoration of the original configuration of cortex and medulla can continue for 1–2 years after the original injury. The potential for this process to achieve extreme degrees is greatest in children.

A timetable for radiographic changes in children's fractures is shown in Table 9.1.

DIFFERENTIAL DIAGNOSIS OF SKELETAL ABNORMALITY IN CHILDREN

1 Normal variant, e.g. symmetrical periosteal, new bone formation in healthy infants.
2 Pseudofracture, e.g. aberrant sutures on skull X-ray.
3 Accidental trauma including birth trauma (clavicle, humerus).
4 Osteogenesis imperfecta.[36]
5 Infection, e.g. osteomyelitis, congenital syphilis, Caffey's disease.
6 Nutritional, e.g. scurvy, rickets, vitamin A intoxication.
7 Malignancy, e.g. leukaemia, tumour.
8 Osteoporosis, copper deficiency.[37]
9 Child abuse.
10 Other, e.g. congenital indifference to pain, Menke's syndrome.

In reviewing 10 years of non-accidental injury in Leeds,[17] out of 2578 referrals there were 1912 children with suspected physical abuse. Of these, 50 children had lesions resembling abuse where another cause was found, excluding accidents. Eight of them had bony lesions as follows:

Birth injury (clavicle)	1
Calcified cephalhaematoma	1
Osteoporosis secondary to neuromuscular disorder	1
Caffey's disease	1
Congenital hydrocephalus	1
Normal skull variant	1
Scoliosis	1
Osteomyelitis	1

Table 9.1 Timetable for radiographic changes in children's fractures[35]

	Category	Early (days)	Peak (days)	Late (days)
1	Resolution of soft tissues	2–5	4–10	10–21
2	Periosteal new bone	4–10	10–14	14–21
3	Loss of fracture line definition	10-14	14–21	
4	Soft callus	10-14	14–21	
5	Hard callus	14–21	21–42	42–90
6	Remodelling	3 months	1 year	2 years to epiphyseal closure

Note that repetitive injuries may prolong categories 1, 2, 5 & 6.

3 Intracranial injury

The prognosis of a head injury relates to the intracranial component. Injury to the brain is the commonest cause of death from physical abuse; 95% of serious head injuries in the first year of life result from abuse.[38] Serious head injury following an alleged minor fall in a baby should alert one to the possibility of abuse. The pathology of head injury includes:

1 Scalp injury – bruises, traumatic subgaleal haematoma.
2 Skull fracture.
3 Subdural and subarachnoid haemorrhage.
4 Cerebral contusion, haemorrhage and oedema.

SUBARACHNOID HAEMORRHAGE

This rarely occurs spontaneously in childhood and then follows rupture of an arteriovenous malformation or aneurysm. It may also occur as part of a wider pattern of injury after trauma.

SUBDURAL HAEMORRHAGE

This gives rise to haematoma which is nearly always traumatic in origin. While birth injury or clotting disorders are possible early causes, subdural haematoma almost invariably results from violent shaking which leads to disruption of bridging veins and bleeding into the subdural space.[39,40]

A detailed history should enable birth trauma to be distinguished from abuse. The presence of retinal haemorrhages is another important sign in abuse; they usually disappear in a few days in the newborn but may persist long after abuse. They occur particularly after violent shaking, but also after a whiplash injury of the infant who has a relatively large and unsupported head. The haemorrhages are thought to follow the acute rise in intracranial and central retinal vein pressure.

CEREBRAL CONTUSION, HAEMORRHAGE AND OEDEMA

Areas of cerebral injury may be scattered throughout the brain leading to fits, raised intracranial pressure and long-term handicap. Between 3% and 11% of children in hospitals for the retarded were handicapped as a result of physical abuse in one study.[41] Clinical conditions included epilepsy, post-traumatic hydrocephalus, changes to visual pathways and cerebral infarction leading to atrophy and microcephaly.

Children presenting without a history of trauma who have unexplained hydrocephalus, raised intracranial pressure or fits may have been abused. The fundi should be carefully examined for retinal haemorrhages and a skeletal survey considered.

4 Abdominal injury[42,43]

Abdominal injuries are less commonly recognized in physical abuse than limb fractures or craniocerebral injuries. Their importance lies in the threat to life, particularly if there is delay in diagnosis. Intra-abdominal trauma usually results from a kick or punch and injury to gastrointestinal as well as solid organs may result.

DIAGNOSTIC POINTS

1 There may be no signs of external injury, e.g. bruising.
2 Delay in presentation and denial of a history of trauma make diagnosis difficult.
3 Doctor's attention may be attracted to other injuries, e.g. head and limbs.
4 Free abdominal gas is found in the minority of cases.
5 A high index of suspicion is required, especially if general condition of child poor or shock present.

TYPES OF INJURIES

Perforation of gut:	stomach
	duodenum and duodeno-jejunal flexure
	jejunum
	ileum
Haemorrhage	major vessel
Laceration, contusion, haematoma	liver, spleen, duodenum, pancreas, mesentery, kidney

MECHANICS OF INJURY

1 Compression
A punch or kick to the abdomen will squeeze the intestinal tract especially the stomach or colon. Susceptibility to injury is greatest when the organs are distended by food or gas. The result is likely to be rupture if the organ is unable to withstand the increased pressure.

2 Crush injury
This results if an organ is compressed against the spine or rib cage. An example is in blunt abdominal trauma, when the relatively fixed duodeno-jejunal flexure is crushed against the spine producing shearing forces which result in rupture or bleeding into the wall. Other susceptible organs include the pancreas, liver, spleen or kidney.

3 Sudden acceleration and deceleration injuries
When the child is swung or thrown into a solid object. This is likely to interrupt the vascular supply to the bowel without perforation.

5 Burns and scalds[44,45]

Burns and scalds occur in about 10% of physically abused children and 5% of sexually abused children and in 15% of those both physically and sexually abused.[8]

Accidental injury follows brief lapses in parent's protection, most often of toddlers who sustain scald injuries from hot drinks and hot water in the kitchen or bathroom. Burns and scalds are often associated with serious neglect and young children may die in house fires when left alone unattended.

Deliberately inflicted burn or scald injuries may be impulsive or premeditated. They include sadistic acts and those designed to punish or invoke fear.

CLASSIFICATION OF BURNS AND SCALDS

Scalds occur from contact with hot water or liquid foods; sogginess and blistering results. Patterns reflect pouring or splashing with variable depth of injury frequently modified by clothing.

Contact or dry burns are caused by conduction from hot and often metallic solid objects, e.g. irons, fires and surrounds, curling tongs. The typical pattern is sharp and demarcated with uniform depth.

In abuse, contact is enforced leading to a deeper burn than would occur following the rapid reflex withdrawal from a painful stimulus.

Flame burns are caused by fires or matches and tend to be deep with charring and burned hairs.

Cigarette burns are circular (with a tail if brushed contact), of full thickness (if inflicted) and heal leaving depressed pale thin scars. They may be multiple.

Electrical burns are small and deep with exit and entry points. Other burns include friction, chemical and radiant burns.

In assessing the depth of a scald or burn, the parameters of time and temperature are related by means of the Moritz–Henriques equation.[46] For example, at 44°C it may take several hours to produce a full thickness burn whereas at 60°C about 10 seconds. The thickness of the skin and age of the child are other factors.

IMPORTANT SITES AND PATTERNS

Scald accidents in toddlers and older infants affect the face, shoulders, upper arms and upper trunk, especially the anterior chest. Children immersed in hot baths may have extensive scalds. The patterns of such injuries should be carefully matched to the parents' account by manipulating a dolls' limbs and immersing a doll into water to see what patterns of immersion result. Forced immersion patterns have been described and include the glove and stocking distribution and the hole in doughnut effect when the child's bottom is forced onto the cooler base of the bath leaving an area of spared skin.

Contact burns may affect any area but the hands (especially dorsum),[44] soles of feet and legs are common sites. Burns around the mouth may follow forcible attempts to feed a child with excessively hot food.

THE HISTORY IN INFLICTED BURNS

The cardinal point is that the history does not match the injury. Some parents deny that the injury is a burn and other causes will then need to be excluded. The incident may be unwitnessed or the parent disclaim any knowledge of how it occurred or the child himself held responsible. Repeated and multiple burns are especially worrying.

ASSESSMENT

It may be necessary to compare the alleged source of the burn with the injury or to undertake a detailed re-enactment of the incident measuring water temperatures for example to see whether the history is consistent with the injury.

Police or forensic investigators with experience of this work will be required. Visits to the home will be essential. It is important to document the injuries and their pattern including photography. Sexual abuse should be considered.

DIFFERENTIAL DIAGNOSIS

This includes impetigo, eczema, epidermolysis bullosa, severe nappy rash, sensory deficit including congenital insensitivity to pain and unusual and unlikely accidents. Chemical burns or hypersensitivity, e.g. to nickel have been confused.

Munchausen syndrome by proxy

There is now no doubt that Munchausen syndrome by proxy is a manifestation of child abuse. In 1951 Asher described Munchausen syndrome in adults who related symptoms of illnesses which did not exist thereby encouraging physicians to investigate and treat on the basis of these fabricated diseases.

In 1977 the term Munchausen syndrome by proxy was first used by Meadow to describe the syndrome in children where the proxy was usually the mother. Munchausen syndrome by proxy arises in the context of a disturbed parent-child relationship where there is often a lack of empathy with the child. Harm results from both the actions of the carer coupled with the adverse effects of unnecessary investigations, hospitalization and medical or surgical treatment.

True Munchausen syndrome by proxy requires a partnership between the parent and physician who interact to develop themes of induced illness. Unfortunately some physicians, notably those who have difficulty recognizing abuse, are particularly vulnerable to participating in this kind of abuse.

Ironically Munchausen syndrome by proxy came into the public's consciousness following the murder

of several children by a nurse at a hospital in Grantham in Lincolnshire, UK. In fact, she did not 'suffer' from the syndrome and would have been more accurately described as a serial killer of children.

With greater understanding of the whole area of induced illness in children[47] it is now appreciated that there is a spectrum of effects.[48]

1 *excessive parental anxiety and perceived illness* Excessive concern that a child is ill may reflect other anxieties or past experiences, e.g. parents who have experienced a previous child death.
2 *doctor shopping* Repeated second opinions leading to excessive medical contacts and investigation can be potentially harmful and certainly unpleasant for the child.
3 *enforced invalidism* Exaggerating disability thereby preventing the child from experiencing normal life and activities is detrimental to the child's development.

These three aspects of illness behaviour are commonly encountered in everyday paediatric practice and are an extension of normal behaviour concerning illness in children. When the behaviour becomes extreme then it may become abusive. Much time is spent in outpatient clinics helping and encouraging parents to adopt reasonable and appropriate responses to issues of care for their children.

4 *fabricated illness* This includes more active and conscious deception. Parents may:

- lie about symptoms
- artificially create abnormal physical signs
- interfere with laboratory samples
- interfere with monitoring and treatment apparatus
- administer drugs and poisons
- alter or distort measurements and record charts
- withhold food

As a result, illnesses may be suspected or diagnosed and unnecessary investigations and treatments started. Not only are parent and doctor involved, but the child frequently becomes an active participant in these activities, sometimes adopting the illness role including playing out the symptons.

The diagnosis is usually suspected after illnesses fail to take their usual course or when conventional treatment does not have its expected effect. The behaviour usually extends into the hospital ward on admission and its absence when the parent is not present or actively excluded may provide the first clue. Common clinical presentations include:

Seizures: real, induced or fabricated
Apnoea and drowsiness: induced by drugs or suffocation
Diarrhoea or vomiting, e.g. by drugs or pharyngeal stimulation

Rashes: scratching, caustics or dyes
Failure to thrive: active withholding of food
Bleeding: fictitious history, blood added to specimens, administered anticoagulants.

Non-accidental poisoning and suffocation have links with the Munchausen by proxy syndrome.

The consequences of Munchausen syndrome by proxy can be very serious including death or chronic illness. The condition is often persistent, the average length before diagnosis is over one year. The average age at diagnosis is in the preschool age period. Older children may become adult sufferers. Mortality figures up to 10–20% have been described.[49] The psychological morbidity is extensive.

Links with other abuse, physical, sexual and emotional are well described.[50] Most if not all of the mothers (fathers are responsible in less than 5% of cases) have experienced serious abuse or neglect as children. Psychiatric disorder is quite common.

Management

Critical and informed paediatric practice must acknowledge this problem. Beware the mother who is over-attentive of you as the doctor or who thrives in the medical environment.
Share concerns and observe carefully.
Learn to question and challenge when things do not add up.
Remember to check other professionals' records and also verbally especially with the GP and colleagues in hospital. Talk to the child alone without the parent present.
Check that all charts and records are clear.

Remember this is a child protection issue and close cooperation with other agencies including social services, police and other appropriate professionals is required. Gather evidence and confront the parents, but be prepared to protect the child.

Parents will need support. A good outcome for the child and family requires a planned, comprehensive, therapeutic package over a sustained period of time. This requires a well coordinated approach by a multidisciplinary, multi-agency team working with the child and family members.[47]

Many children however who remain at home living with the abusing parent will show impaired functioning and development.

Reporting non-accidental injury

If a doctor is worried about the possibility that an injury may have been inflicted, he should discuss this with others, including senior nurses, other doctors, and contact the social services department, either in the hospital or the area where the child lives, by telephone.

It is important to emphasize that the diagnosis of physical abuse involves both a medical opinion and a social work assessment of the family. In some cases, where the doctor is worried, he may ask for the social services, NSPCC, health visitor and others to check their records.

Investigation of abuse should be conducted on an inter-agency basis, following locally agreed guidelines, since no one agency can hope to protect a child by working in isolation. Local guidelines should indicate the point at which the police become involved. In many areas early consultation between social services and the police takes place in all cases of certain or suspected physical abuse in order to agree an investigation procedure.

Medical reports

These are written for the social services department and NSPCC, who have a statutory responsibility to protect children. The child's GP and the community child health service, who may both have responsibilities toward the child and family, should be notified.

Important areas to be included (not necessarily in order)

1 The doctor's name, qualifications and appointment, the date and place of the examination.
2 The child's name, date of birth and age at examination. Siblings can be included in the same report.
3 Referral pathway and requesting agency or individual.
4 Parents' or others' statements regarding how the injuries occurred.
5 Statements by the child using the child's words, including anything said to the doctor.
6 Other medical or social information relevant to the assessment.
7 The manner, demeanour and behaviour of the child, his physical and emotional state, and indicators of poor care or neglect.
8 Height and weight, including centile ranking, and a clinical assessment of growth and nutrition.
9 A developmental assessment.
10 Injuries listed and described.
11 Examination of the child's genitalia and anus.
12 The results of X-ray examinations or blood tests.

The opinion

It is important to express an opinion about the injuries and an overall view of the child. Example: 'It is my opinion that the pattern, number and distribution of injuries indicates that this child has been non-accidentally injured. The bruising to the left side of the face is not consistent with parents' explanation of a fall downstairs, but is more likely to have resulted from a blow with an outstretched hand. The 1.0 cm circular cratered scarred lesion on the left thigh is consistent with an inflicted cigarette burn and not with the child scratching or picking himself.'

Other concerns should also be listed. Example: 'This child's weight is below the 3rd centile and he appears poorly nourished. It is my opinion that he is suffering from failure to thrive due to an inadequate intake of food. The fairly severe nappy rash, dirty fingernails and generally unkempt appearance suggest that he is being physically neglected. It is likely that the child's poor language development assessed as being about 12 months delayed at the age of three, reflects inadequate stimulation.'

Child Protection conferences in physical abuse[51]

The physically abused child may require urgent protection by means of a Child Protection Order (previously Place of Safety Order) and this should be sought from a Magistrate's Family Proceedings Court as necessary. The Child Protection conference is available to allow discussion and exchange of information after abuse has been confirmed or is suspected.

Child Protection conferences followed recommendations incorporated in the 1980 Department of Health and Social Security circular which gave advice to social services departments on a systematic approach to the management of child abuse. One of its recommendations was that an inter-agency case conference should be called where appropriate.

In cases of suspected or confirmed physical abuse, the timing of the conference is important. After an injury has been recognized, an investigation is instituted into the circumstances and an assessment made of the family situation and likely source of the abuse. The child will usually be placed in a safe location, be it a foster home, with a suitable relative or a hospital ward. Occasionally the child remains at home with the abusing parent(s) where it is judged that the risk of further injury is low and the parents are showing appropriate cooperation. However, with severe injury, a period of separation is advisable to allow assessment of the risk of returning home and to enable plans for future management of risk to be made.

It is advisable for the child to remain in a safe place until such time as the Child Protection conference has been held and decisions made. It is not always necessary to keep the child in a safe place under an order from the court as for instance when the parents are cooperative and show willingness to leave the child in hospital.

Attendance at the Child Protection conference involves:[51]

Social services. The chairman may be a senior social work manager, depending on the local arrangements. He should not have direct decision making responsibility for the case. The social worker and the team leader are always present. Other social workers who may be present include probation officers, if involved with either parent, and the education welfare officer who will liaise with school.

Police. Many areas now have trained and dedicated officers for child abuse work. The officer involved in the investigation will make a report.

Health. GP, health visitor, school nurse, nurse manager. These are all important members with information about the child and family. Paediatrician, preferably of senior grade, either consultant or SCMO or senior registrar. Other doctors such as from accident and emergency, child psychiatry are occasionally required.

Child abuse coordinator or advisor is in an important position to advise on case management and is often in a neutral position, not having had contact with the family.

Solicitor will be present to advise and guide the conference on legal matters.

Others include hospital nursing staff, housing, teachers and members of voluntary organizations.

Parents. There are new guidelines issued in *Working Together*,[1] 'while there may be exceptional occasions when it will not be right to invite one or other parent to attend a Child Protection conference in whole or in part, exclusion should be kept to a minimum and needs to be especially justified.' The decision to exclude rests with the chair of the conference.

Whether parents are invited or not to the Child Protection conference, it is essential that they are kept fully involved and informed about the basis of an investigation or intervention as well as the outcome and decisions of the conference. Parents and children (where appropriate) are asked to submit their views in writing if possible to the conference.

Decisions of the Child Protection conference[52]

The Child Protection conference should focus on the child as the primary client whose interests must transcend those of the parent where there is any conflict. The conference will develop a plan for the child.

A decision will be taken regarding registration of the child's name under the appropriate category on the child protection register. Once this is done, the child automatically becomes the subject of an inter-agency protection plan which must be reviewed at least every 6 months. The conference will also decide who the key worker should be and discuss how the information regarding decisions will be imparted to and discussed with the parents.

The Child Protection conference may wish to make recommendations regarding such matters as the institution of care proceedings and the appropriate immediate placement of the child, but the responsibility for these decisions does not lie with the case conference.

Siblings

Where a child has been identified as suffering abuse within a family, it is always necessary to consider the position of any siblings. Information should be collected, including a paediatric assessment and all siblings discussed at the case conference. Very often there will be evidence of difficulties with siblings who, even if not injured, may well have experienced violence within the family and have lived within a stressful and dysfunctional situation. A Child Protection conference may choose to register a sibling when another child has been harmed in the household.

The statutory agency may decide to accommodate the child on a voluntary basis if the parents are agreeable for his protection but, in view of the nature of child abuse, parents frequently deny that their child is at risk of harm and a decision must then be taken to institute care proceedings. The local authority, police and NSPCC all have the power to bring care proceedings.

Emergency protection can be secured by obtaining an Emergency Protection Order under the Children Act[48] which will provide protection for 8 days, renewable under exceptional circumstances for another 7 days. Interim care orders, supervision and care orders are sought in the Magistrate's Family Proceedings Court or the county court. Complex and difficult cases may be taken to the High Court.

Management of child and family

The aims of management are to secure a safe environment for the child, to provide for his future needs and prevent further abuse.

After a period of assessment, the small number of children for whom substitute or alternative care is required should be identified. The majority of children will return or remain at home with a plan of management to protect the child.

Strategies include:

1 Address the sources of stress within the family.
2 Alleviate material difficulties – housing, debt.
3 Empower parents to improve their parenting skills.
4 Provision of day care.
5 Improve community support.
6 Use of family aides, home helps.
7 Promote non-violent ways of coping with stress.
8 Facilitate improved relationships within family and extended family.
9 Inform about child development.

The plan should incorporate input from a variety of different agencies, and should be coordinated by the key worker.

Concerns about the children must be honestly expressed to the parents and the need for change spelled out clearly. Expectations and standards of care must be

explicitly stated. If there is a legal order, control is with the statutory authority within the terms of the order. Otherwise cooperation must be achieved voluntarily which is often difficult in child abuse work.

In addition to addressing the needs of the child, it is important that the parents' needs are addressed otherwise they will not be able to provide differently for their child. Sometimes a separate worker is assigned to give special attention, for example to a mother or a father, leaving the key worker to focus on the child's needs.

Part of successful management is periodically assessing the child's well-being and development. It is useful for the family and closely involved 'face workers' to have an assessment by a paediatrician who can comment on the child's progress highlighting improvements as well as areas of development which need to be addressed.

Encouraging the parents to make their own observations and assessments is also part of such programmes as the Child Development Project being used by health visitors in some areas.[53]

When satisfactory progress has been made, and the family appears to be functioning at an acceptable level, the child's name may be removed from the register and the intensity of work reduced, although contact will usually be maintained after this time.

References

1 *Working Together Under the Children Act 1989.* London: HMSO, 1991.
2 Newell, P. *Children are People Too. The Case Against Physical Punishment.* London: Bedford Square Press, 1989.
3 De Mause, L. *The History of Childhood.* London: Souvenir Press, 1974.
4 Radbill, S.X. Children in a world of violence. In: Helfer, R.E., Kempe, R.S., eds. *The Battered Child*, 4th edn. Chicago: University of Chicago Press, 1987.
5 Caffey, J. On the theory and practice of shaking infants. *Am J Dis Child* 1972; **124**: 161–169.
6 Kempe, C.H., Silverman, F.N., Steele, B.F., Droegmueller, W., Silver, H.K. The battered child syndrome. *J Am Med Assoc* 1962; **181**: 17–24.
7 Creighton, S.J., Noyes, P. *Child Abuse Trends in England and Wales. 1983–1987.* London: NSPCC, 1989.
8 Hobbs, C.J., Wynne, J.M. The sexually abused battered child. *Arch Dis Child* 1990; **65**: 423–427.
9 Smith, S.M., Hanson, R. 134 battered children: a medical and psychological study. *Br Med J* 1974; **iii**: 666–670.
10 Rogers, D., Tripp, J., Bentovim, A., Robinson, A., Berry, D., Goulding, R. Non accidental poisoning: an extended syndrome of child abuse. *Br Med J* 1976; **i**: 793–796.
11 Meadow, S.R. Munchausen syndrome by proxy. *Arch Dis Child* 1982; **57**: 92–98.

12 Buchanan, M.F.G. *Physical Abuse of Children* (video tapes and accompanying booklet). University of Leeds Audio-Visual Service, 1989.

13 Newson, J., Newson, E. *Findings on Use of Physical Punishment on 1, 4, 7 and 11 year old Children, Together with Some Sequel in Later Life*. University of Nottingham, Child Development Research Unit, 1986.

14 Bernat, J.E. Bite marks and oral manifestations of child abuse and neglect. In: Ellerstein, N.S., ed. *Child Abuse and Neglect. A Medical Reference*. New York: J. Wiley & Sons, 1981, 141–164.

15 Moores, C.F.A. *The Dentition of the Growing Child*. Massachusetts: Harvard University Press, 1959, 79–110.

16 Roberton, D.M., Barbor, P., Hull, D. Unusual injury? Recent injury in normal children and children with suspected non-accidental injury. *Br Med J* 1982; **285**: 1399–1401.

17 Wheeler, D.M., Hobbs, C.J. Mistakes in diagnosing non-accidental injury, 10 years' experience. *Br Med J* 1988; **296**: 1233-1236.

18 O'Hare, A.E., Eden, O.B. Bleeding disorders and non-accidental injury. *Arch Dis Child* 1984; **59**: 860–864.

19 Herndon, W.A. Child abuse in a military population. *J Paed Orthopaed* 1983; **3**: 73–76.

20 McClelland, C.Q., Heiple, K.G. Fractures in the first year of life. A diagnostic dilemma? *Am J Dis Child* 1982; **136**: 26–29.

21 Helfer, R.E., Slovis, T.L., Black, M. Injuries resulting when small children fall out of bed. *Pediatrics* 1977; **60**: 533–535.

22 Kleinman, P.K. *Diagnostic Imaging of Child Abuse*. Baltimore: Williams & Wilkins, 1987.

23 Ounstead, C. Gaze aversion and child abuse. *World Med* 1975; **12**: 27.

24 Silverman, F.N. Radiology and other imaging procedures. In: Helfer, R.E., Kempe, R.S. eds. *The Battered Child*. Chicago: University of Chicago Press, 1987, 214–246.

25 Salter, R.B., Harris, W.R. Injuries involving the epiphyseal plate. *J Bone Jt Surg* 1963; **45A**: 587–622.

26 Swischuk, L.E. Spine and spinal cord trauma in the battered child syndrome. *Radiology* 1969; **92**: 733.

27 Barrett, I.K., Koszlowski, K. The battered child syndrome. *Australian Radiology* 1979; **23**: 72–82.

28 Gee, D.J. Radiology in forensic pathology. *Radiology* 1975; **41**: 109–144.

29 Feldman, K.W., Brewer, D.K. Child abuse, cardiopulmonary resuscitation and rib fractures. *Pediatrics* 1984; **73**: 339–342.

30 Kleinman, P.K. ed. Bony thoracic trauma. In: *Diagnostic Imaging of Child Abuse*. Baltimore: Williams & Wilkins, 1987, 87–89.

31 Kravitz, H., Driessen, G., Gomberg, R., Korach, A. Accidental falls from elevated surfaces in infants from birth to one year of age. *Pediatrics* 1969: **44**: (suppl) 869–876.

32 Hobbs, C.J. Skull fracture and the diagnosis of abuse. *Arch Dis Child* 1984; **59**: 246–252.

33 Lende, R.A., Erickson, T.C. Growing skull fractures of childhood. *J Neurosurg* 1961; **18**: 479–489.

34 Akbarnia, B., Torg, J.S., Kirkpatrick, J., Sussman, S. Manifestations of the battered child syndrome. *J Bone Jt Surg* 1974; **56A**: 1159–1166.

35 O'Connor, J.F., Cohen, J. Dating fractures. In: Kleinman, P.K. ed. *Diagnostic Imaging in Child Abuse*. Baltimore, Williams & Wilkins, 1987, 103–113.

36 Taitz, L.S. Child abuse and osteogenesis imperfecta. *Br Med J* 1987; **295**: 1082–1083.

37 Shaw, J.C.L. Copper deficiency and non-accidental injury. *Arch Dis Child* 1988; **63**: 448–455.

38 Billmire, M.E., Myers, P.A. Serious head injury in infants: Accident or abuse? *Pediatrics* 1985; **75**: 340–342.

39 Guthkelch, A.N. Infantile subdural haematoma and its relationship to whiplash injuries. *Br Med J* 1971; **11**: 430–431.

40 Caffey, J. On the theory and practice of shaking infants. *Am J Dis Child* 1972; **124**: 161–169.

41 Buchanan, A., Oliver, J.E. Abuse and neglect as a cause of mental retardation: a study of 140 children admitted to subnormality hospitals in Wiltshire. *Br J Psychiatr* 1972; **131**: 458.

42 Cooper, A., Floyd, T., Barbour, B. Major blunt abdominal trauma due child abuse. *J Trauma* 1988; **28**: 1483–1487.

43 Touloukain, R.J. Abdominal visceral injuries in battered children. *Pediatrics* 1968; **42**: 642–646.

44 Hobbs, C.J. When are burns not accidental? *Arch Dis Child* 1986; **61**: 357–361.

45 Hight, D.W., Bakalar, H.R., Lloyd, J.R. Inflicted burns in children. Recognition and treatment. *J Am Med Assoc* 1979; **242**: 517–520.

46 Moritz, A.R., Henriques, F.C. Studies of thermal injury. The relative importance of time and temperature in the causation of cutaneous burns. *Am J Pathol* 1947; **23**: 695–720.

47 Gray, J., Bentovim, A. The management of induced illness in children. Paper presented at the 2nd BASPCAN National Congress, University of Bristol 5th–8th July 1994.

48 Meadow, S.R. Munchausen syndrome by proxy. *ABC of Child Abuse*, London: BMJ Publishing group, 1993.

49 Rosenberg, D.A. Web of deceit: a literature review of Munchausen syndrome by proxy. *Child Abuse & Neglect* 1987; **11**: 547–63.

50 Bools, C.N. Neale, B.A. Meadow, S.R. Comorbidity associated with fabricated illness (Munchausen syndrome by proxy). *Arch Dis Child* 1992; **62**: 77–9.

51 MacMurray, J. Case conferences. In: Meadow, S.R. ed. *ABC of Child Abuse*. *Br Med J* 1989; 42–44.

52 *An Introduction to the Children Act 1989*. London: HMSO, 1989.

53 Early Child Development Project Evaluation Paper No. 8. 1988, 103–105. From: University of Bristol, 22 Berkeley Square, Bristol BS8 1HP.

9.5 Neglect and emotional abuse

Kim Oates

Although neglect and emotional abuse of children occur in approximately one in 300 children, they are conditions which often leave no physical signs and which may therefore not always come to medical attention. To aid in recognizing and understanding neglect and emotional abuse of children this section looks at requirements for normal mental health, definitions and incidence of neglect and emotional abuse, types of neglect with emphasis on non-organic failure to thrive and types of emotional abuse as well as prevention and treatment strategies.

Requirements for good mental health

The foundation for good mental health is laid in infancy. Bowlby stated in 1951 that it is essential for mental health that the infant and young child should experience a warm, intimate and continuous relationship with his mother,[1] although he felt this did not exclude other caretakers as long as there was regularity and continuity.[2] Rutter believes that there are six characteristics necessary for adequate mothering or parenting, the absence of which may lead to emotional deprivation or neglect.[3] They are a loving relationship which leads to attachment, which is unbroken, which provides adequate stimulation, in which the mothering is provided by one person and which occurs in the child's own family. Children also have to have other needs met such as adequate nutrition, opportunities for conversation and play, protection from danger and discipline based mainly on teaching and role models for behaviour. Pringle[4] lists children's needs as love and security, opportunities for new experiences, praise, recognition and responsibility.

As well as having an awareness of these needs for understanding emotional abuse and neglect, it is important for these needs to be considered when making treatment programmes for abused and neglected children.

Not all children have all of these needs adequately met, but some children seem to fare far worse than others. Children have a mixture of strength and vulnerability. They influence their parents' behaviour and in turn they develop according to the way their parents behave towards them. Solnit, using an example of a crying infant, points out that the normal behaviour of one infant may be experienced by one set of parents as healthy, another as sick and by another as violent. One set of parents, aware of normal infant behaviour, will see the crying and fussiness as normal and will soothe the child. The other parents may think the crying and fussiness is due to an illness and will only be reassured once the child has been checked and declared well, while the third set of parents, whose own needs for dependency are great and who fear the demands of their infant, will see the crying baby as demanding. They may get into a vicious cycle where the infant's behaviour evokes tense responses, leading to increased crying and perhaps even leading to a situation which puts the infant at risk for abuse and neglect.[5] Why some children seem more resilient and some more vulnerable is not well understood.

Definitions and incidence

A community workshop in the USA convened by Whiting[6] produced this definition for emotional neglect: 'Emotional neglect is a result of subtle or blatant acts of omission or commission experienced by the child, which cause handicapping stress on the child and which is manifested in patterns of inappropriate behaviour.' Skuse[7] defines emotional abuse as: 'The habitual, verbal harassment of a child by disparagement, criticism, threat and ridicule, and the inversion of love; by verbal and non-verbal means rejection and withdrawal are substituted.' Garbarino prefers the term psychological maltreatment[8] where there is a pattern of psychically destructive behaviour which is a concerted attack by an adult on a child's development of self and social competence.

Neglect is somewhat different as it involves failing to meet the child's developmental needs for stimulation and a failure of physical caretaking. In infants neglect often leads to non-organic failure to thrive defined as 'a condition where growth progress fails to keep up with a previously established growth pattern and which responds to a combination of providing an adequate caloric intake and providing for the child's emotional needs.'[9] This definition while acknowledging the emotional deprivation commonly associated with the condition also emphasizes the need for an adequate caloric intake.

The current definitions in use in England and Wales are:

Emotional abuse: actual or likely severe adverse effect on the emotional and behavioural development of a child caused by the persistent or severe emotional ill-treatment or rejection. All abuse involves some emotional ill-treatment.

Neglect: the persistent or severe neglect of a child, or the failure to protect a child from exposure to any kind of danger, including cold or starvation, or extreme failure to carry out important aspects of care, resulting in the significant impairment of the child's health or development, including non-organic failure to thrive.

It is difficult to obtain figures about the incidence of these conditions although it would be reasonable to assume that incidence figures are an underestimate. A study in the USA in 26 representative communities found that 3.2 per 1000 children were victims of emotional abuse and neglect.[11]

Neglect

Neglect results from inadequate or negligent parenting. Some aspects of neglect may seem obvious. The children are not well cared for, inadequately clothed, do not receive sufficient good quality nutrition and may be delayed in their development, especially their language skills. However, overzealousness in the detection of neglect can easily lead to confusing neglect with poverty or ignorance. A family which is poor, unemployed, living in inadequate housing and generally overwhelmed by their circumstances may have children who are inadequately clothed and fed and perhaps even lacking in hygiene. To label the parents as neglectful when they are in circumstances over which they have little control is unfair. These families need help. Only if they refuse reasonable services to help their children should neglect be considered.

Infants who are neglected are more likely than other infants (but not exclusively so) to use persistent self-stimulating behaviour such as rocking or head banging. They also appear to be insecure in their play and behaviour. In contrast to abused infants whose play is likely to have a high activity level, but which is not of high quality and is sometimes destructive, neglected infants are more likely to have low levels of play behaviour, to be passive and sometimes show little interest in toys.[12] Language delay is also common in neglected children[13] and seems to be more affected than visuospatial abilities.[14]

Schmitt[15] describes five types of neglect: medical; safety; educational; physical; and emotional deprivation. The neglect of a child's medical care and safety needs are the two types of neglect which could lead to a fatal outcome. Medical practitioners are most likely to be aware of medical neglect. This can include the refusal of blood transfusions for religious reasons and refusing to sign consent forms for other necessary and perhaps life-saving conditions. Court intervention is usually necessary to solve these problems. However, undue conflict with the parents should be avoided and where possible they should be involved in careful discussion rather than argument, and be involved in the decision-making process even when this involves legal intervention.

Medical neglect can also include refusing to give regular medication for chronic conditions such as diabetes mellitus, embarking on bizarre diets which may lead to vitamin deficiency and anaemia and refusing proven medical treatment in favour of unproven, unorthodox treatments for chronic or potentially fatal diseases. This becomes particularly complex in cases of malignant disease although, when the standard treatment offers a reasonable chance of cure, legal intervention may be needed to ensure treatment. Potential problems in these areas can often be overcome if the doctor makes sure that the parents have plenty of opportunity to ask questions so as to understand the treatment, that they are materially able to comply with the treatment and that other assistance such as interpreters, relatives or trusted friends are involved if necessary to help the parents understand the treatment. This is particularly important if they have misapprehensions based on past experience, cultural beliefs or language barriers. Medical neglect can also include parents not availing themselves of some essential components of normal child health care such as immunization.

Schmitt defines safety neglect as a situation where an injury occurs because of gross lack of supervision.[15] A recent example seen at The Children's Hospital in Sydney was a mother who left her toddler at home alone with an electric radiator turned on. The toddler put a stool next to the radiator and then dropped a blanket over the stool and radiator to make a cubby house. The blanket caught fire and the child sustained extensive, disfiguring burns. Close supervision and careful monitoring of the child's environment to remove hazards and avoid dangerous situations are essential in the first 3 or 4 years of life.

Educational neglect involves keeping children away from school, perhaps to work at home or to do baby sitting. It may involve collusion with a child who has school phobia rather than seeking treatment.

Physical neglect involves not meeting the child's needs for food, shelter and clothing, recognizing the danger of confusing physical neglect with poverty.

Emotional deprivation leads to withdrawal, delay in language and gross motor development and sometimes inappropriate displays of affection to strangers. Many emotionally deprived children will have features of non-organic failure to thrive.

Non-organic failure to thrive

Failure to thrive is a description rather than a diagnosis. It is used to describe an infant who shows a decline from a previously established growth pattern and is sometimes reserved for infants whose failure to gain weight places them below the third centile for age. Linear growth may also be affected, although usually to a lesser extent, and there may be evidence of delay in psychomotor development. When investigation of these children fails to reveal an organic cause for the growth disorder, and when the history is suggestive of emotional or nutritional deprivation or both, the condition is termed non-organic failure to thrive. The implication is that the child's social, emotional or nutritional environment is disturbed to the point where it interferes with normal growth and development. Between 15% and 50% of children with failure to thrive fall into this non-organic group.[16,17]

Growth failure was first noted to be associated with emotional deprivation in children living in institutions where death rates were high. In 1915 Chapin reported that the death rate in children under 2 years living in infant asylums in the USA was 42%.[18] He called this 'the cachexia of hospitalisation' which he believed to result from a combination of poor physical environment and lack of individual care and nurturing in the institution.[19] Chapin's concern for infants in institutions did not attract a great deal of attention until Spitz[20] and Bakwin[21] again reported this condition, stressing the lack of emotional stimulation as being the main reason for growth failure. In 1957 Coleman and Provence[22] pointed out that the clinical syndrome of growth failure due to deprivation could also occur in children living in their own homes.

Clinical features of non-organic failure to thrive

A careful history from the parents and observation and examination of the infant are more useful than ordering a large battery of laboratory tests. The history and examination generally suggest which, if any, investigations should be ordered. Sills[23] reported that out of 2067 laboratory tests performed on 185 children with failure to thrive only 36 (1.4%) were of positive diagnostic assistance. No test was of positive value in the absence of a specific indication for doing that test derived from the history and physical examination.

One approach to non-organic failure to thrive is to make the diagnosis only after exhaustively excluding all possible organic causes for the child's growth failure. However, because emotional or environmental disorders are such a common cause of failure to thrive, non-organic causes should be considered in parallel with the search for a hidden organic cause.

The infant's growth pattern may assist in reaching the diagnosis although the features are not diagnostic. Previous weights from clinics, if available, should be plotted to show the curve of the child's growth pattern. The infant's weight is the parameter which deviates most from normal. If linear growth is also affected, it suggests that the condition has been present for some time. It is unusual for head circumference to be affected except in long-standing cases. The usual pattern to be found when measurements are plotted on centile charts is for the head circumference to be normal and for the weight to be reduced out of proportion to any reduction there may be in length. Physical examination shows few signs apart from the evidence of growth failure. As well as loss of fat, muscle wasting is common and is best noted in the large muscle groups. Wasting of the gluteal muscles reveals loose folds of skin at the buttocks, best demonstrated when the legs are extended at the hip. Developmental assessment usually shows that the infant is delayed in all milestones.[24] These infants have been noted to have cold hands and feet,[25] minimal smiling and decreased vocalization,[26] apathetic and withdrawn behaviour[24] and abnormal persistence of infantile posture.[27] Indiscriminate seeking of affection has been noted in toddlers, while infants have been reported as disliking being touched and held.[28]

Although deprivation dwarfism and non-organic failure to thrive are often discussed together, children with deprivation dwarfism seem to constitute a distinct group. Whereas in failure to thrive it is the marked weight loss that is the striking feature, in deprivation dwarfism it is the short stature that first brings the child to attention. Although these children are dwarfed, they do not present a picture of malnutrition.

Five published series of deprivation dwarfism (Table 9.2) show that although the children were often underweight for height, this was not reported as a striking feature. The reported ages of children with deprivation dwarfism, ranging from 2 to 16 years, encompass a quite different range from that seen in non-organic failure to thrive which usually presents in children under 2 years. The behaviour of deprivation dwarfism children is also quite different. They are reported to steal and hoard food, to gorge

Table 9.2 Documented characteristics of deprivation dwarfism

Author	No. cases	Age (years)	Growth improves as environment improves	Weight in relation to height
Silver and Finkelstein[29]	5	4–6	Yes	Low
Powell et al.[30,31]	13	3.3–11.5	Yes	Thin, not malnourished
Apley et al.[32]	9	2–15	—	Weight corresponded to height
Kreiger and Mellinger[33]	7	3.4–10.1	Yes	Low
Hopwood and Becker[34]	35	2–14	Yes	Half mildly underweight for height

themselves, to eat large amounts of unusual foods such as condiments and to eat from garbage cans.[34] The relationship of growth hormone production to deprivation dwarfism is not clear. In the much quoted study of Powell et al.,[31] six of the eight children studied had low growth hormone levels and all six had an increase in growth hormone production following improvement in their environment. Other researchers have found growth hormone to be low in a smaller proportion of children with deprivation dwarfism[32,34] and for growth hormone response to an improvement in the environment to be variable[33] or absent.[35]

Deprivation of calories or affection?

There is conflicting evidence about whether the growth failure of these infants is due to deprivation of affection and stimulation or simply due to deprivation of calories. Spitz,[20] in a study of infants separated from their mothers, and Widdowson,[36] in a study of older children from orphanages in post-war Germany, claim that the harsh environments rather than lack of food were responsible for the growth failure. However, no analysis of actual food intake was reported in these studies. Whitten et al.,[37] in a well-designed and somewhat disturbing study, kept 13 infants with non-organic failure to thrive for 2 weeks in a windowless room where they received minimal handling but an adequate diet. Despite the emotional and sensory deprivation all but three had an accelerated weight gain. Six of these infants then received a high level of mothering and sensory stimulation, but with no improvement in their diet. There was no change in the rate of weight gain in this group. These researchers concluded that if children are given enough food they will grow and that the problem of growth failure in maternal deprivation is due to inadequate caloric intake.

Non-organic failure to thrive is probably not due solely to a lack of calories or a lack of affection. There are also likely to be factors within the child and defects of the interaction between the child and parents as well as a combination of poor caloric intake and insufficient affection and stimulation which are responsible for the condition.

Characteristics of the parents

Descriptions of the characteristics of the parents of these children have a common theme noting multiple problems within the family. These include poverty, overcrowding, unemployment, illegitimacy and seriously disturbed marital relationships. The mothers are reported to be lonely and isolated and the fathers are often absent, uninvolved in family life and unsupportive.[24,38,39] Maternal depression and suicide attempts have been described[40] and, in a psychological study of the mothers,[41] there was found to be a common theme of profound emotional and physical deprivation in the mothers' own early childhood with them having little to spare from their own meagre stores of affection to pass on to their offspring. Although most of the families described have come from low socioeconomic groups, the condition can occur in stable, intact families from favourable economic circumstances.[42,17]

Three groups of authors have attempted to construct profiles of mothers whose children had non-organic failure to thrive.[43–45] The characteristics of the mothers in each group are summarized in Table 9.3. Each group of authors classified the mothers into three groups and suggested that treatment became more difficult from group one to group three. The profiles differed somewhat and it is likely that a proportion of mothers involved did not fit readily into any of these groups. The usefulness of this sort of approach is that it helps to determine which mothers are more likely to be amenable to help. It is also a reminder that parents of children with non-organic failure to thrive are not a homogeneous group and that it is essential that the individual problems of the family should be assessed before starting a treatment programme.

Hess et al.[46] compared the intelligence quotients of eight mothers of children with non-organic failure to thrive, eight mothers whose infants had failure to thrive for organic reasons and eight mothers whose children were growing normally. The groups were matched for socioeconomic status but the observer was not blinded. The mothers from the non-organic group had a lower intelligence score on the vocabulary test of the Stanford-Binet intelligence scale. It would have been interesting to have had the mothers tested on measures of intelligence other than verbal

Table 9.3 Three attempts to create profiles of mothers whose children have non-organic failure to thrive

	Kempe et al.[43]	Evans et al.[44]	Jacobs and Kent[45]
Group I	Basically capable, temporarily overwhelmed	Young, immature, depressed	Deficient in basic mothercraft skills
Group II	Immature, chronically deprived and depressed	Poor health, chaotic lifestyle, need structural support	Passive, low affect, overwhelmed
Group III	Antisocial, aggressive, sees baby as bad	Extreme anger and hostility	Significant psychological disorder

abilities because, if these mothers are like their children, it may be that the greatest discrepancy in intelligence would be found to lie in the area of verbal ability.

When Pollitt et al.[47] compared 19 pre-school infants with non-organic failure to thrive with a comparison group matched for age, sex and race, but not for socioeconomic status, no significant differences were found between the two groups in marital history, family structure, household crowding or history of psychiatric disorders. The mothers in the study group were more likely to express annoyance and to slap their children and were less likely to praise, kiss or caress them. Studies such as this should be repeated, preferably with matching social class, to determine which of the described family characteristics contribute to the system and which are more likely to be related to other factors, such as social class.

Non-organic failure to thrive should not be regarded as being solely due to maternal factors. The child may also contribute to the condition.

Characteristics of the children

It is becoming increasingly apparent that babies are born with different temperaments and that these differences can be detected at birth.[48,49] The feeding behaviour of babies with non-organic failure to thrive is often reported as being difficult from the earliest weeks of life. They have been described as refusing the nipple, falling asleep or crying during feeding, having poor appetites, posseting and vomiting frequently as well as fighting against the person who feeds them.[50,51] It is likely that an infant with this type of temperament, born to a mother with the characteristics already described and who therefore does not have the nurturing skills to overcome these feeding difficulties, will fail to thrive.

There have been several reports of distinct personality and behaviour patterns in these infants. Rosenn et al.[28] showed that they preferred distant social encounters and inanimate objects to close personal interactions such as being touched and held. Hypotonia, when they are held and cuddled, without any neurological abnormalities, and apprehensive, frightened,

apathetic and withdrawn behaviour with infrequent smiling and vocalization have been noted. These infants may show delay in the establishment of specific, strong attachment to their parents and may not show anxiety with strangers or displeasure at being left by their parents.

Non-organic failure to thrive appears not to be a condition produced either by the parent or by the child. Children with non-organic failure to thrive have been shown to have developmental idiosyncrasies which combine with social and familial factors to give the profile of non-organic failure to thrive.[52] The traditional view of the condition being exclusively parentally induced should be abandoned with emphasis on the biological and behavioural attributes of the children as well as the parents.

Subsequent development

Growth

Follow-up studies which have looked at the growth of these children are summarized in Table 9.4. Most suggest that the majority of children do have catch-up growth. A problem with these studies is that the loss to follow up is quite high. For example Mitchell et al.[59] were able to review only 12 of a group of 30 infants who had non-organic failure to thrive. Although most of this group was of normal size, much of the value of the study is lost because of the high proportion of the original group that was not reviewed.

The physical features of the parents, which have some influence on the child's size, were considered in only one of these studies.[40] This showed that from an initial group of 24, only one child of the 21 reviewed was below the tenth centile for height when corrected for mid-parent height. Prader and Tanner[58] have reported that catch-up growth following starvation or severe illness can often restore the situation to normal in pre-pubertal children. It is likely that as these children become older and less dependent on an adult to feed them, they learn to fend for themselves. A meta-analysis of eight comparable follow-up studies showed that while hospitalization significantly enhanced the probability of sustained catch-up growth,

Table 9.4 Catch-up growth following non-organic failure to thrive

Author	No. cases	Length of follow up	Weight above 3rd centile (%)	Height above 3rd centile (%)
Glaser et al.[54]	40	3 years 5 months	65	68
Elmer et al.[42]	15	3–11 years	47	47
Chase and Martin[55]	19	3 years 6 months	32	47
Hufton and Oates[40]	21	6 years 4 months	76	95
Ayoub et al.[56]	35	14 months	80	—
Mitchell et al.[53]	12	1–4 years	84	92
Oates et al.[57]	14	12 years 6 months	100	93

hospitalization had only a comparatively small effect on the psychosocial development.[59]

Intellectual development

Although severe and prolonged malnutrition in the early years may lead to a decrease in intellectual function,[60,61] it would be wrong to draw parallels between studies of this nature and those of children with non-organic failure to thrive where the degree of malnutrition is usually less severe.

Whether or not the child remains in an unstimulating environment is likely to be an equally important factor. Richardson[62] found that malnourished children with a favourable social background had an average IQ only two points lower than those who had not been malnourished, while malnourished children from an unfavourable background had an average IQ nine points lower than controls.

Most follow-up studies of children with non-organic failure to thrive show a high proportion of developmental disorders. Elmer et al.[42] found six of 15 children to be mildly retarded and four others to be moderately retarded, with slow speech development and difficulty in conceptual thinking being reported in many of the children. A study of 21 children reviewed after 6 years showed that 14 had a reading age 1 or 2 years below their chronological age and that 10 were described by their teachers as functioning below average.

A follow-up study of 14 children who had been admitted to hospital, on average, $12\frac{1}{2}$ years previously with non-organic failure to thrive showed that compared with a control group matched for social class, the study children were significantly lower on the verbal scale of the WISC-R and were significantly lower in verbal language development and in reading abilities.[57]

Emotional development

The high incidence of emotional disorders found in these children on follow up is summarized in Table

9.5. Hufton and Oates[40] looked at behaviour in the siblings of the index children and found significantly fewer behaviour disorders. When two-thirds of this group were again reviewed $12\frac{1}{2}$ years after presentation they had significantly more behaviour problems on a teacher rating scale and lower levels of social maturity than a control group.[57]

The environment in which these children remain is likely to be responsible for their adverse intellectual and emotional development. It has also been shown that these children are at risk for physical abuse[63,64] as well as intellectual and emotional disadvantage. Although the studies that have been described show problems in intellectual and personality development in approximately 15–65% of these children, this leaves a large proportion of the group who appear to develop normally. This supports Rutter's assertion[65] that many children are particularly resilient and can do well despite adverse social circumstances.

Management of non-organic failure to thrive

The approach of excluding organic disease, keeping the child in hospital until weight gain has been achieved and then discharging the child to the same situation is of short-term benefit unless the home environment can also be improved. This approach may even be counter-productive if the child is simply placed in hospital and cared for by other females who are efficient and competent. This may be a demonstration to the mother that others can succeed where she has failed, thus reinforcing her feelings of inadequacy.

While hospital admission is often necessary, both for diagnosis and treatment, it is important to work closely with the family during this period. From the outset the parents should be encouraged to become active members of the hospital team. The mother should be encouraged to live in the hospital and staff should take a warm, encouraging, non-judge-

Table 9.5 Studies of intellectual and emotional sequelae of non-organic failure to thrive

Author	No. cases	Average age at review	Mean interval to review	Emotional status	
Glaser et al.[54]	40	4 years 6 months	3 years 5 months	28%	Behaviour or psychological problems
Elmer et al.[42]	15	3 years 3 months to 11 years 7 months*	4 years 9 months	47%	Behavioural disturbance
Hufton and Oates[40]	21	7 years 10 months	6 years 4 months	48%	Abnormal on teacher rating scale
Mitchell et al.[53]	12	3–6 years*	1–4 years	3%	Behavioural problems, no different to controls
Oates[9]	14	13 years 9 months	12 years 6 months	44%	Abnormal personality profiles. No abnormalities in controls.

* Range of ages – average age not stated.

mental approach to her so as to help her recognize her baby's needs and respond to them appropriately. This warm, supportive relationship should be continued at home with home visits and use of community resources.

In making a treatment plan, an assessment of the mother's personality and capabilities is required. Fischoff et al.[66] described character disorders as being common in these mothers, claiming that while a problem-solving approach is appropriate for treating a psychoneurotic problem where the mother has the capacity for introspection, a mother with a character disorder has a limited ability to perceive and assess the environment and needs of her child. Where patterns of thought are concrete, emphasis on treatment should be on providing basic help in all phases of the mother's life with practical help in feeding, child-rearing and other general aspects of child care.

The classifications of mothers that have been described are also useful in planning treatment. Those who are immature, overwhelmed or with a chaotic lifestyle respond well to a structured programme, while those with significant psychological disorder and antisocial behaviour are much more difficult to help.

Non-organic failure to thrive is not a simple problem. It is one which is caused by a variety of factors in the parents, none of which are specific, and which may be contributed to by the child, particularly the interaction between the child and the parents. While the controversy as to whether it is due to deprivation of calories or of affection remains unresolved, the follow-up studies indicate that despite a good chance of catch-up growth, these children often do poorly in their intellectual and emotional development. Non-organic failure to thrive requires more than nutritional rehabilitation in hospital. Specific, practical help on a long-term basis should be provided for the mothers and an individual programme of stimulation and education should be provided for the child if the long-term adverse sequelae of this condition are to be avoided.

Emotional abuse

A hidden problem

Emotional abuse is a hidden form of child abuse. It often does not come to the notice of medical practitioners because there are no physical features. If it does manifest as a behaviour disorder, the underlying emotional abuse may not be recognized. These may be some of the reasons why emotional abuse is much less well documented than other forms of abuse. Yet this form of abuse may be even more damaging than physical abuse and neglect. Garbarino[8] believes that, rather than emotional abuse being part of the spectrum of child abuse and neglect, it is at the very heart of the issue in physical and sexual abuse because of the

psychological messages of worthlessness and debasement which are given to children whose parents physically and sexually abuse them.

It is not only parents who can emotionally abuse children. Emotional abuse can be caused by relatives (especially if they are living in the family home), by neighbours, by those caring for children in institutions, in detention homes, in centres for the intellectually disabled, by child care workers, in hospitals, even in child welfare departments, by school teachers – in fact by any adult who is in a position of power in relation to the child and who should have some responsibility for the child's welfare. In general terms, emotional abuse by the child's own parents is likely to be more serious, although, if the child has no parents, or is in substitute care, emotional abuse in these circumstances can be equally serious. Emotional abuse of children is always totally unacceptable. However, cultural norms have to be remembered. Behaviours which may seem abusive in some cultures may be acceptable in others, but when the behaviour towards the child conveys a culture-specific message of rejection, or when it impairs a socially relevant psychological process, such as the development of self-esteem,[67] then it should be regarded as emotional abuse, whatever the family's cultural norms.

Types of emotional abuse

Garbarino[67] has defined psychological maltreatment or emotional abuse as a concerted attack by an adult on a child's development of self and social competence. He labels it as a pattern of psychically destructive behaviour which can take five forms:

1 *Rejecting*, which involves behaviours that communicate or constitute abandonment such as a parent refusing to touch or show affection to a child.
2 *Terrorizing*, involving threatening the child with extreme or vague but sinister punishment, intentionally stimulating intense fear, creating a climate of unpredictable threat or setting unmeetable expectations and punishing the child for not meeting them.
3 *Ignoring*, referring to the parent being psychologically unavailable to the child because the parent is so preoccupied with herself that there is no ability to respond to the child's behaviours.
4 *Isolating*, involves parental behaviour which prevents the child from taking advantage of normal opportunities for social relations.
5 *Corrupting*, referring to parental behaviours that mis-socialize children and reinforce them in antisocial or deviant patterns, especially in the areas of aggression, sexuality or drug abuse.

To understand better these five forms of emotional abuse, Garbarino believes they should be looked at in each of the four major stages of development; the first 2 years, years 2 to 5, the early school years and adolescence.[67] Garbarino shows how the five types of psychological maltreatment may take different forms at different ages. For example rejection in infancy may mean refusal to respond to the child's smiles and vocalizations, while rejection in adolescence may mean subjecting the adolescent to humiliating and excessive criticism. Similarly isolation in early childhood may involve punishing the child for making social overtures to children and adults while for the school-aged child it may mean preventing the child from going to play with other children or from inviting them home.

Parental characteristics

A characteristic of these parents is that they often do not know enough about child development to cope with the normal demands resulting from the child's behaviour at different developmental stages.[68] They may also tend to isolate themselves from the community, although because of their behaviour, neighbours in the community may also isolate the family. Emotional maltreatment seems to be more common in poorer communities where there is high unemployment, poverty and a sense of powerlessness and frustration among the parents.[69] Of course, it also occurs in middle and upper-class families where there is stress, tension and aggression coupled with inadequate parenting skills and unrealistic expectations for the children. However middle and upper-class families may be better able to hide the emotional abuse of their children and the professionals treating them may be more reluctant to consider this diagnosis. Parental behaviour includes being unable to meet their children's psychological needs,[70] responding inappropriately to the child by giving them too many responsibilities and punishing them when they fail,[68] inappropriately infantalizing their children so as to prevent them from reaching their potential, lacking respect for the child's thoughts and feelings[71] and being inconsistent in parenting so that the child receives conflicting and contradictory messages and sees the parents as being unreliable.[72]

One of the few control studies in this area[73] compared seven emotionally abusing parents with a closely matched group of seven so-called problem parents in a day nursery. The emotionally abusing parents showed poorer coping skills, poorer child management techniques and more difficulty in making relationships. They also reported more deviant behaviour in their children than did the control parents. It is clear from the studies of emotionally abusing parents that emotional abuse is multi-factorial and, when a sufficient cluster of factors occurs, the parent or other caregiver may be particularly likely to inflict emotional abuse.

Characteristics and responses of the children

The way children respond to emotional abuse will depend on the type of abuse and the age of the child. Emotionally maltreated infants usually respond by being apathetic or irritable and not being able to be easily calmed by their parents. Because of their parents' lack of appropriate response to them, they do not learn to act in the way Brazelton[74] has described as 'taking turns' where the parents' and infant's movements and vocalizations are in harmony with each other. Older children come to see the world as a place hostile to them. They become distrustful and are therefore difficult to help. They tend to develop low self-esteem and to have a negative view of the world sometimes with anxiety and antisocial behaviour. These effects can be long-lasting and can interfere with the child's ability to make satisfactory relationships throughout childhood and in adult life.[75]

Intervention and treatment

The initial aspect of intervention is a careful assessment of the family. This will determine what type of intervention is needed and whether it can be made with family cooperation or whether legal backing is necessary. Because some of the problems in emotionally abusing families are stress-related, it may be important to focus at first on some of the family's concrete problems, such as family resources, as these are likely to be more acceptable to the family. Treatment aimed solely at family dynamics, which ignores some of the family's practical needs, is not likely to be successful. It is important that any interventions have realistic goals and meet the needs of the family. It is also essential that interventions have inbuilt evaluations to make sure that scarce resources are being used appropriately.

Simply making suggestions to improve family functioning may not be enough. Very practical help may be needed. Practical home-based services for neglectful families have been shown to support and improve the functioning of families who would otherwise have had their children removed from home. These programmes are also more cost-effective than placing the child in care.[76]

Other measures of intervention may include marital counselling, family therapy, neighbourhood support systems, home visiting and helping the parents to understand more accurately their children's development and behaviour so that they can come to tolerate the developing child's curiosity, exploration and failures as the child develops and tries to master the environment. Helping the parents to understand, rather than misinterpret, these normal behaviours and providing them with the resources to cope with them can be an effective method of intervention in families where there is some degree of motivation.[77]

Intervention with the child may involve play therapy, day care, the use of a therapeutic pre-school where the child can learn from alternative role models, social skills training and interventions to help the child develop and improve self-esteem. Ideally parent and child treatment should proceed simultaneously so that parental confidence and self-esteem is improved along with that of the child.[78]

In addition to looking at prevention at the individual level, Lally has suggested that prevention should be considered at the level of the social systems in our society and the fundamental and cultural beliefs our society has about children.[79] At the level of government assistance, families usually come to the attention of governments only when problems arise. Policy is generally set to react to problems rather than to ensure that systems are available to help families and children when economic factors which affect families such as inflation, recession and under-employment come into play. At a community level, larger systems, such as neighbourhood and community resources, may need to become involved in helping families cope more effectively.

Neglect and emotional abuse of children can have long-term consequences, not only for the children concerned but for their ability to make satisfactory adult relationships and to become successful parents. This is a compelling reason why prevention and effective treatment of these children and their families, while not easy, should be a priority.

Acknowledgements

Some of the material on non-organic failure to thrive has been reproduced by permission of the publishers of the *Australian Paediatric Journal*.

References

1 Bowlby, J. *Maternal Care and Mental Health*. Geneva: World Health Organization, 1951.
2 Bowlby, J. *Can I Have My Baby?* London: National Association for Mental Health, 1958.
3 Rutter, M. *Maternal Deprivation Reassessed*. Harmondsworth, Middlesex: Penguin, 1972, 15–28.
4 Pringle, M.K. *The Needs of Children*. London: Hutchinson, 1975.
5 Solnit, A.J. Theoretical and practical aspects of risks and vulnerabilities in infancy. *Child Abuse and Neglect* 1984; **8**: 133–144.
6 Whiting, L. Defining emotional neglect. *Children Today* 1976; **5**: 2–5.
7 Skuse, D.H. Emotional abuse and neglect. *Br Med J* 1989; **298**: 1692–1694.
8 Garbarino, J. The psychologically battered child: toward a definiton. *Pediatr Ann* 1989; **18**: 502–504.
9 Oates, K. ed. Failure to thrive. In: *Child Abuse, a Community Concern*. Sydney: Butterworths, 1982, 119–129.
10 Her Majesty's Stationery Office. *Working Together*. London: HMSO 1991.
11 Burgdorff, K. *Recognition and Reporting of Child Maltreatment: Findings from the National Study of the Incidence and Severity of Child Abuse and Neglect*. Washington DC: National Center on Child Abuse and Neglect, 1980.
12 Harmon, R.J., Morgan, G.A., Glicken, A.D. Continuities and discontinuities in affective and cognitive-motivational development. *Child Abuse and Neglect* 1984; **8**: 157–168.
13 Fox, L., Long, S.H., Langlois, A. Patterns of language comprehension deficit in abused and neglected children. *J Speech Hearing Dis* 1988; **53**: 239–244.
14 Haywood, C. Experiential factors in intellectual development: the concept of dynamic intelligence. In: Zubin, J., Jarvis, G.A. eds. *Psychopathology and Mental Development*. New York: Grune & Stratton, 1967.
15 Schmitt, B.D. Child neglect. In: Ellerstein, N.S. ed. *Child Abuse and Neglect, a Medical Reference*. New York: Wiley, 1981, 29–306.
16 Hannaway, P. Failure to thrive, a study of 100 infants and children. *Clin Pediatr* 1970; **9**: 96–98.
17 Shaheen, E., Alexander, C., Truskowsky, M., Barbero, G.J. *Clin Pediatr* 1968; **7**: 255–261.
18 Chapin, H.D. A plea for accurate statistics in infants' institutions. *Arch Pediatr* 1915; **32**: 724–726.
19 Chapin, H.D. Are institutions for infants necessary? *J Am Med Assoc* 1915; **64**: 1–3.
20 Spitz, R. Hospitalism, an inquiry into the genesis of psychiatric conditions in early childhood. *Psychoanalyt Study Child* 1945; **1**: 53–74.
21 Bakwin, H. Emotional deprivation in infants. *J Pediatr* 1949; **35**: 512–521.
22 Coleman, R.W., Provence, S. Environmental retardation (hospitalism) in infants living in families. *Pediatr* 1957; **19**: 285–292.
23 Sills, R.H. Failure to thrive, the role of clinical and laboratory evaluation. *Am J Dis Child* 1978; **132**: 967–969.
24 Bullard, D.M., Glaser, H.H., Heagarty, M.C., Pivchik, E.C. Failure to thrive in the neglected child. *Am J Orthopsychiatr* 1967; **37**: 680–690.
25 McCarthy, D. Deprivation dwarfism viewed as a form of child abuse. In: Franklin, A.W., ed. *The Challenge of Child Abuse*. London: Academic Press, 1977, 96–107.
26 Leonard, M.F., Rhymes, J.P., Solnit, A.J. Failure to thrive in infants, a family problem. *Am J Dis Child* 1966; **111**: 600–612.
27 Krieger, I., Sargent, D.A. A postural sign in the sensory deprivation syndrome in infants. *J Pediatr* 1967; **70**: 332–339.
28 Rosenn, D.W., Loeb, L.S., Jura, M.B. Differentiation of organic from non-organic failure to thrive syndrome in infancy. *Pediatr* 1980; **66**: 698–704.
29 Silver, H.K., Finkelstein, M. Deprivation dwarfism. *J Pediatr* 1967; **70**: 317–324.
30 Powell, G.F., Brasel, J.A., Blizzard, R.M. Emotional deprivation and growth retardation simulating idiopathic hypopituitrism I: endocrinologic evaluation of the syndrome. *New Engl J Med* 1967; **276**: 1271–1278.
31 Powell, G.F., Brasel, J.A., Blizzard, R.M. Emotional deprivation and growth retardation simulating idiopathic hypopituitrism II: endocrinologic evaluation of the syndrome. *New Engl J Med* 1967; **276**: 1279–1283.

32 Apley, J., Davies, D.R., Silk, B. Dwarfism without apparent physical cause. *Proc Roy Soc Med* 1971; **64**: 135–138.

33 Krieger, I., Mellinger, R.C. Pituitary function in the deprivation syndrome. *J Pediatr* 1971; **79**: 216–225.

34 Hopwood, N.J., Becker, D.J. Psychosocial dwarfism: detection, evaluation and management. *Child Abuse and Neglect* 1979; **3**: 439–447.

35 Castells, S., Reddy, C., Choo, S. Permanent panhypopituitrism associated with maternal deprivation. *Am J Dis Child* 1975; **129**: 128–130.

36 Widdowson, E.M. Mental contentment and physical growth. *Lancet* 1951; **i**: 1316–1318.

37 Whitten, C.F., Pettit, M.G., Fischoff, J. Evidence that growth failure from maternal deprivation is secondary to undereating. *J Am Med Assoc* 1969; **209**: 1675–1682.

38 Oates, R.K., Yu, J.S. Children with non-organic failure to thrive – a community problem. *Med J Aust* 1971; **2**: 199–203.

39 Kerr, M.A.D., Bogues, J.L., Kerr, D.S. Psychosocial functioning of mothers of malnourished children. *Pediatrics* 1978; **62**: 778–784.

40 Hufton, I.W., Oates, R.K. Non-organic failure to thrive: a long-term follow up. *Pediatrics* 1977; **57**: 73–77.

41 Togut, M.R., Allen, J.E., Lelchuck, L.A. A psychological exploration of the non-organic failure to thrive syndrome. *Dev Med Child Neurol* 1969; **11**: 601–607.

42 Elmer, E., Gregg, A., Ellison, P. Late results of the failure to thrive syndrome. *Clin Pediatr* 1969; **8**: 584–588.

43 Kempe, R.S., Cutler, C., Dean, J. The infant with failure to thrive. In: Kempe, C.H., Helfer, R.E., eds. *The Battered Child* 3rd edn. Chicago: University of Chicago Press, 1980, 163–182.

44 Evans, S.L., Reinhart, J.B., Succop, R.A. Failure to thrive. A study of 43 children and their families. *J Am Acad Child Psychiatr* 1972; **11**: 440–457.

45 Jacobs, R.A., Kent, J.T. Psychosocial profiles of families of failure to thrive infants – preliminary report. *Child Abuse and Neglect* 1977; **1**: 469–477.

46 Hess, A.K., Hess, K.A., Hard, H.E. Intellectual characteristics of mothers of failure to thrive syndrome children. *Child: Care, Health Dev* 1977; **3**: 377–387.

47 Pollitt, E., Eichler, A., Chan, C.R. Psychosocial behaviour of mothers of failure to thrive children. *Am J Orthopsychiatr* 1977; **45**: 525–537.

48 Thomas, A. *Temperamental and Behavioural Disorders in Childhood*. New York: New York University Press, 1968.

49 Brazelton, T.B. *Neonatal Behavioural Assessment Scale. Clin Develop Med No. 50*. London: William Heinemann Medical Books, 1973.

50 Freud, A. The psychoanalytic study of infantile feeding disturbances. *Psychoanalytic Study of the Child* 1946; **2**: 119–132.

51 Pollitt, E., Eichler, A. Behavioural disturbances amongst failure to thrive children. *Am J Dis Child* 1975; **130**: 24–29.

52 Bithoney, W.G., Newberger, E.H. Child and family attitudes of failure to thrive. *Dev Behav Pediatr* 1987; **8**: 32–36.

53 Mitchell, W.G., Gorrell, R.W., Greenberg, R.A. Failure to thrive: a study in primary care setting: epidemiology and follow-up. *Pediatrics* 1980; **65**: 971–977.

54 Glaser, H.H., Heagarty, M.C., Bullard, D.M., Pivchik, E.C. Physical and psychological development of children with early failure to thrive. *J Pediatr* 1968; **73**: 690–698.

55 Chase, H.P., Martin, H. Undernutrition and child development. *New Engl J Med* 1970; **282**: 933–939.

56 Ayoub, C., Pfeifer, D., Leichtman, L. Treatment of infants with non-organic failure to thrive. *Child Abuse and Neglect* 1979; **3**: 937–941.

57 Oates, R.K., Peacock, A., Forrest, D. Long-term effects of non-organic failure to thrive. *Pediatrics* 1985; **75**: 36–40.

58 Prader, A., Tanner, J.M., Von Harnack, G.A. Catch-up growth following illness or starvation. *J Pediatr* 1963; **62**: 646–659.

59 Fryer, G.E. The efficacy of hospitalisation of non-organic failure to thrive children: a meta-analysis. *Child Abuse and Neglect* 1988; **12**: 375–381.

60 Hertzig, M., Birch, H.G., Richardson, S.A., Tizard, J. Intellectual levels of school children severely malnourished during the first two years of life. *Pediatrics* 1972; **49**: 814–824.

61 Stoch, M.B., Smyth, P.M. Fifteen year developmental study of effects of severe undernutrition during infancy on subsequent physical growth and intellectual functioning. *Arch Dis Child* 1976; **51**: 327–336.

62 Richardson, S.A. The relation of severe malnutrition in infancy to the intelligence of school children with differing life histories. *Pediatr Res* 1976; **10**: 57–61.

63 Koel, B.S. Failure to thrive and fatal injury as a continuum. *Am J Dis Child* 1969; **118**: 565–567.

64 Oates, R.K., Hufton, I.W. The spectrum of failure to thrive and child abuse. *Child Abuse and Neglect* 1977; **1**: 119–124.

65 Rutter, M. The long-term effects of early experience. *Dev Med Child Neurol* 1980; **22**: 800–815.

66 Fischoff, J., Whitten, C.F., Pettit, M.G. A psychiatric study of mothers of infants with growth failure secondary to maternal deprivation. *J Pediatr* 1971; **79**: 209–215.

67 Garbarino, J., Guttman, E., Seeley, J.W. *The Psychologically Battered Child*. San Francisco: Jossey-Bass, 1986.

68 Herrenkohl, R.C., Herrenkohl, E.C., Egolf, B.P. Some antecedents and developmental consequences of child maltreatment. In: Rizley, R., Cicchetti, D., eds. *Developmental Perspectives on Child Maltreatment*. San Francisco: Jossey-Bass, 1981.

69 Brown, S.E. Social class, child maltreatment and delinquent behaviour. *Criminology* 1984; **22**: 259–278.

70 Egeland, B., Sroufe, A., Erickson, M. The developmental consequence of different patterns of maltreatment. *Child Abuse and Neglect* 1983; **7**: 459–469.

71 Patterson, G.R., Thompson, M. Emotional child abuse and neglect: an exercise in definition. In: Volpe, R., Breton, M., Mitton, J., eds. *The Maltreatment of the School-Aged Child*. Lexington, Massachusetts: Heath, 1980.

72 Fontana, V. *Somewhere a Child is Crying*. New York: Macmillan, 1973.

73 Hickox, A., Furnell, J.R.G. Psychosocial and background factors in emotional abuse of children. *Child: Care, Health and Development* 1989; **15**: 227–240.

74 Brazelton, T.B. Joint regulation of neonate–parent behaviour. In: Tronick, E.Z., ed. *Social Interchange in Infancy: Affect, Cognition and Communication*. Baltimore: University Park Press, 1982.

75 Rohner, R.P., Rohner, H.C. Antecedents and consequences of parental rejection: a theory of emotional abuse. *Child Abuse and Neglect* 1980; **4**: 189–198.

76 Van Meter, M.J. An alternative to foster care for victims of child abuse/neglect: a university-biased program. *Child Abuse and Neglect* 1986; **10**: 79–84.

77 Martin, H.P. Intervention with infants at risk for abuse and neglect. *Child Abuse and Neglect* 1984; **8**: 255–260.

78 Pawl, J. Strategies of intervention. *Child Abuse and Neglect* 1984; **8**: 261–270.

79 Lally, R. Three view of child neglect: expanding visions of preventive intervention. *Child Abuse and Neglect* 1984; **8**: 243–254.

9.6 Child sexual abuse

Harry Zeitlin and Ruby Schwartz

Introduction

With the fall of morbidity in childhood, reflecting the control of infection, the effects of more persistent problems have become increasingly evident. They include congenital disorders, oncology and abuse. Following a sequence of physical abuse, neglect and emotional abuse, sexual abuse of children has deservedly received much greater attention in recent years. Throughout this section a note of caution is struck, not to diminish the seriousness of abuse but to guide the reader to be prepared to consider the possibility under a wide range of circumstances, and then discriminate between abuse and other problems.

Definitions

Child sexual abuse is defined as the involvement of dependent developmentally immature children and adolescents in sexual activities that they do not truly comprehend, to which they are unable to give in-formed consent and that violate the social taboos of family roles.[1,2] An alternative and more succinct definition is 'the exploitation of the child for sexual gratification of an adult'.[3]

All definitions include acts that have a sexual connotation to the perpetrator and that involve a child. They also have a very wide ambit so that the nature of the acts, the frequency, intrusiveness, associated physical and psychological trauma and the significance for the child can all vary enormously.

Classifications have been made according to the nature of the abuse. Kempe and Kempe[2] gave the following categories of abuse: incest, paedophilia, exhibitionism, molestation, sexual intercourse, rape, sexual sadism, child pornography, child prostitution.

None of these except perhaps the last specifies the nature of the effect on the child. Sexual abuse is better not considered a diagnostic entity but either the cause of disturbance observed in a child or a description of the actions of an adult.[4] This approach helps in the distinction of requirements for clinical care and criminal proceeding purposes.

From an investigatory point of view the types of sexual activity involved may be divided into two basic groups (Table 9.6); the first includes those most likely to result in physical evidence.

Table 9.6 Grouping of types of abuse according to contact or no contact

A   Those involving contact between the perpetrator and their victim e.g.:

1   Inappropriate touching or fondling
2   Masturbation
3   Oral intercourse
4   Insertion of fingers or foreign objects into the vulva or anus
5   Intracrural intercourse
6   Actual or attempted vaginal or anal intercourse

B   Non-contact abuse where the child inappropriately witnesses a sexual act, but there is no contact between the perpetrator and the abused victim e.g:

1   Exhibitionism
2   Pornography
3   Masturbation by an adult in the presence of a child

Incidence/prevalence

The incidence of child sexual abuse is almost impossible to estimate accurately. It seems clear that it is common and has in the past been under-reported. Finklehor[5] gave an anonymous questionnaire to 755 undergraduates in New England and found that 19% of the females and 9% of the males reported having been sexually victimized as children. In Great Britain 2019 men and women aged 15 and over were interviewed as part of a Mori survey; 10% reported that they had been sexually abused before the age of 16.[6] The variable nature of abuse and of its effects make such statistics on prevalence difficult to interpret. There are also some high risk groups, and not surprisingly high rates have been reported among adolescents who run away from home, who abuse drugs or other substances, become sexually promiscuous or self poison.[7] The overall figures, rather than indicating that 10% of the population have been psychologically traumatized, would endorse a need for all children to receive education on self protection against inappropriate behaviour from adults.

What is normal acceptable behaviour?

Evaluation of abuse in the community needs to be against a background of some understanding of acceptable normal social behaviour, though defining that is not easy. Parents ask, 'Is it all right for my children to come into bed in the morning?' 'What if my daughter gets into the bath with me?'. 'Should we be seen naked by our children?' To a large extent what is acceptable can only be determined by knowledge of what is common behaviour, in spite of the inherent circularity of that argument. Rosenfeld et al.[8,9] investigated family bathing practices and also the frequency of children touching parents' genitals. Bathing with children of the opposite sex decreased as the children grew older, and was uncommon after the age of 8 to 9 years. They found also that genital touching was common in non-clinical families. Both behaviours they felt could be part of abuse but could not be taken as indicative of it without supporting evidence; reports of genital touching were more a reason for educating parents on child sexual development. The definitions of abuse given above relate to the motivation of the adult with regard to gaining sexual gratification and while that is often difficult to ascertain it remains an essential component to distinguishing normal behaviour. Perhaps the best advice to parents is to continue to behave as is customary in their family but to give more active thought as to how they will instruct their children in appropriate modesty and personal rights.

When does abuse occur?

Sexual abuse may occur to children of all ages, either sex and in any part of society though the circumstances which cause it are not fully understood. It is perhaps clearer for incest and intrafamilial abuse and Finklehor[10] proposed four preconditions:

1 A parent who is capable of crossing adult/child boundaries.
2 A vulnerable child.
3 The opportunity.
4 The ability to overcome external and internal inhibitions.

On a pragmatic level Bamford and Roberts[11] listed some more direct risk factors as:

1 Previous incest or sexual deviation in the family.

2 New male member of the household with a record of sexual offences.
3 Loss of inhibition due to alcohol.
4 Loss of maternal libido or sexual rejection of the father.
5 Paedophilic sexual orientation especially in relation to sex rings and pornography.

Presentation

Children who have been the victims of child sexual abuse present in three main ways: with physical signs, behavioural changes, and allegations or disclosures. Occasionally suspicion is aroused by the behaviour of the perpetrator.

Physical presentation

Not all abuse results in physical signs; when present the signs may be transient and, apart from gross injury, few signs are pathognomonic of abuse. When physical signs are the presenting manifestations they may be acute and the dramatic results of a recent episode of abuse. They include vulval abrasions and bruising, genital or perineal bleeding, bladder or bowel penetration, genital injuries or more widespread results of forcible rape. The victim may attend an accident and emergency department, a general practitioner or present at a police station.

The non-acute physical presentation may have aroused suspicion prior to medical referral but can also present as incidental findings on examination for apparently unrelated reasons. Many abuse cases start with the discovery of anatomical or physiological abnormality of the ano-genital region. Both genital[12] and anal[13] findings have been found to be common in validated cases of sexual abuse. However there is a dearth of studies showing the prevalence in the non-abused population.

Emans' study goes a little way towards this with control comparisons for vulval and vaginal findings, but the results need careful interpretation.[12] The study showed, for example, that scars on the hymen are far more likely in abused girls (9%) than non-abused girls without vaginal disorder (1%). However, if 10% of all girls have been abused the probability of a girl with hymenal scars having been abused would be 50%; a reason for great concern but with equal chance of other causes. The same applies to most other signs such as redness or increased vascularity; while each was associated with abuse the majority of children in the community with each sign probably had not been abused. Eighty-four per cent of those with vaginitis and 80% with vulvitis had no evidence of sexual abuse. Such findings in a child are nonetheless of major importance as identifying a group with a raised likelihood of abuse.

For anal findings, data are really not available to make similar comparisons. Anal dilatation and other anal pathology does occur commonly after actual or attempted anal penetration. Hobbs and Wynne[13] say that in their clinical experience the signs are otherwise uncommon but there is little evidence concerning prevalence in the whole population. A recent study by McCann[14] suggests that dilatation up to 1.0 cm occurs in about 50% of children. Dilatation over 2.0 cm was much more specific to abused children but the finding was only valid when the rectum was empty and the child relaxed. There is also no available comparison of findings in children with ano-rectal problems, including constipation, thread-worm, thrush etc. There is now agreement that examination in the knee–chest position produces a different appearance in some children from that seen in the more usual left lateral position.

A suggested principle for practice would be that sexual abuse should be considered as one of the possible causes of genital and anal pathology with the physician being aware that many investigated cases will have other causes.

A working party of the Royal College of Physicians of London has produced a recent report in which the physical signs associated with sexual abuse (Table 9.7) in children are discussed.[15]

Behavioural presentation

Most forms of behavioural disturbance have been described as resulting from abuse.[16] With any unexplained change of behaviour the possibility of abuse should be considered. Two types of behaviour are more constantly associated with abuse: evidence of sexualization and evidence of traumatization. The former would include abnormal sexual behaviour such as preoccupation with his or her own genitals, or expression of genital or sexual interest in play. There is a danger though that the interest shown by adults after an alleged abuse could begin to induce such play.

The evidence for traumatization is less clearly identifiable but includes anxiety, fearfulness, expression of guilt, panic, nightmares, sleep disturbance, withdrawal, oppositional and conduct disorder. While aggression in children is a relatively non-specific behaviour some abused children will replicate the aggression that they have experienced.

Allegations

The first presentation of abuse may be disclosure of details of the abuse to a trusted adult or an allegation may arise in the course of investigating physical or behavioural criteria. There are indications as to the characteristics of a valid allegation. The child usually shows an appropriate effect, is able to expand on the basic statement and refers to him or herself in the first person.[17] The more central an event is in the child's life the better it is remembered, and children over the age of eight can usually recollect events as accurately as an adult. The younger the child the more possible it is to distort the child's 'recollection' by pressure.

Table 9.7 Physical signs of sexual abuse[15]

	Diagnostic	Supportive but not diagnostic
Vulval and vaginal signs	a Laceration or scars in the hymen which may extend to posterior vaginal wall b Attenuation of the hymen with loss of hymenal tissue	a Enlarged hymenal opening b Notch in hymenal edge which may be associated with scarring c A bump on hymen with some disruption d Localized erythema and oedema, pouting urethra and hymen e Moulded scar in posterior fourchette

Perianal signs	a Laceration or healed scar extending beyond the anal mucosa on to the perianal skin in the absence of reasonable alternative explanation	a Anal laxity without other explanation
		b Reflex anal dilation greater than 1 cm
		c Acute changes: erythema
		        swelling
		        fissures
		        venous congestion
		        bruising
		d Chronic changes e.g: funnelling
		  i thickness of anal verge skin with reduction in anal verge skin folds
		  ii increased elasticity
		  iii reduction in power of anal sphincter
		  i–iii may occur with frequent anal intercourse

Rate of validation of suspected abuse

About 70% of allegations eventually prove to be valid,[18,19] and about 5% prove to be the result of deliberate falsification. The rate of validation falls if the allegation takes place in the context of a custody or access dispute varying between 35% and 55%.[20,21] Accusations are not the only way that abuse is identified or at least suspected and the overall rate of validation appears to be lower. Shetky gave a validation rate of under 50%[22] for anal and genital findings. In another series of 608 children thought to have been sexually abused 337 were confirmed giving a validation rate of 55%.[23]

As already noted, most criteria associated with abuse are of relatively limited specificity. The presence of several factors, even when each one is of limited specificity, dramatically increases the chances of identifying abuse as the probabilities are multiplied rather than added together. It should be remembered that if abuse is not the cause of any findings then something else is wrong for which the child and family probably need help. In all cases therefore clarification is essential and further information can be derived from several sources including:

1 Statements made by the child.
2 Observations of the child's behaviour at play.
3 Specific play.
4 Full assessment of emotional and behavioural status.
5 Physical and forensic assessment.

The purpose of investigation and action

The acute management varies according to the way in which the child presents and also the agency to which the allegation is brought. It can be easy in abuse cases to lose the perspective of the purpose of the investigation and hence the nature of appropriate action. Table 9.8 outlines some essential tasks and the relevant agencies. Some functions overlap as for example social workers carrying out supportive and reparatory work with families, but it is important to distinguish clearly between the main tasks.

Health service

Referral within the health system enables more detailed and specialist investigation and perhaps specialist knowledge in the interpretation of previous findings. Referral is most commonly to medical or psychiatric services but may be to paediatric surgery, neurology, dentistry etc. The specialist paediatric physician or psychiatrist will provide firstly more detailed investigation as to whether anything physically or emotionally is wrong, evaluation of the nature and severity of the disorder, if present, and evidence of cause. Secondly, the specialist may be able to advise on and implement a treatment or management programme to tackle the disorder. At any point in this process it may be considered that sexual abuse is sufficiently likely to indicate consultation with social services and police and initiation of joint investigation procedures.

Social services/NSPCC

The social services have special and statutory duties with regard to the care and protection of children. The most important aspect of involvement of the social services is to invoke the procedures for such protection. Confidentiality and the contract with the family concerned are changed on referral to the social services. If a community paediatrician or general practitioner has reason to suppose that a child is at risk from avoidable damage, either physically or emotionally, then rapid referral to social services is indicated. Wherever possible this should be with the knowledge of the family concerned. The social services also have a role in advising and supporting stressed and distressed families. It should not be forgotten that referral to social services is frequently for the benign reason of providing practical and constructive help.

Police

Child abuse is against the law. If any health care professional knows or believes that a crime has been committed and particularly if it is thought that a crime will be committed again against a child, then investigation and prevention of further crimes is the task of the police. The criteria for criminal investigation overlap but are not the same as those for either further medical investigation or care proceedings concerning the child. It is sometimes forgotten that the law has been broken by the perpetrator and not the child. Once abuse has been confirmed and its effect on the

Table 9.8 Basic functions of main agencies involved in abuse cases

Agency	Purposes	Special function
Health service	Investigation/ management of physical disorder Investigation/ management of psychiatric disorder Advice	Health care Same confidentiality as GP i.e. interests of the child are paramount
Social services	Support with child care Child protection Child protection register Instituting legal proceedings	Protection Statutory duties
Police	Investigation of past or potential crime	Action against perpetrator

child ascertained then great care must be taken to avoid further abuse to the child by subjection to continued enquiry as part of a criminal investigation.

The differences between each of these referrals are important, but it would be a daunting task for any primary care physician to spend several hours contacting each agency and discussing the findings and concerns. If indications for referral are present, then it is usually only necessary to refer to one agency. All Area Child Protection Committees (ACPCs) in England and Wales are responsible for the production of inter-agency guidelines which describe the procedures to be followed in individual cases. The flow chart in Figure 9.2 summarizes referral sequences.

Who should investigate abuse?

Health professionals become involved in the assessment of child sexual abuse in two main ways, either when specifically asked to advise and investigate in cases where a suspicion has already been aroused, or when a referred child is found to have a criterion that raises suspicion.

1 A paediatrician may be involved in the assessment of acute or non-acute cases:
   a Treatment of any injuries.
   b Long-term therapy for any infection or illness uncovered.
2 A divisional surgeon or forensic medical examiner undertakes collection of forensic evidence and assessment of acute abuse cases.
3 A child psychiatrist may be involved in diagnosis and acute and long-term management of victim and family.
4 Nursing staff may be involved in initial observation of the child's status and statements.

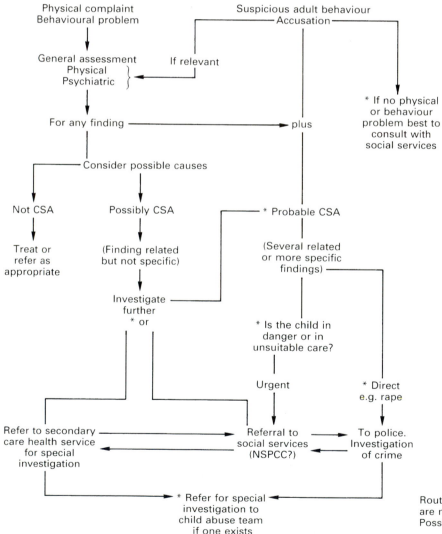

Figure 9.2 Flow chart for referral. CSA child sexual abuse.

All four groups are also actively involved in education for other health and non-health professionals, e.g. police and social services.

Management

Initial plan of action

The varied nature of abuse makes a single stereotyped plan for all cases hazardous but there are some general principles that should be adhered to. First, the interests of the child should be paramount whether or not that conflicts with the rights of adults. That also implies that the investigation and management should themselves carry the lowest possible risk of adverse effects.

The first level of action is to support and advise parents or teachers to understand the possible significance of what they have seen or heard. An essential perspective is to consider all possible causes and then how to narrow down those possibilities.

The second level of action is for the professionals first involved to consider from their own expertise what steps are necessary to clarify matters further and if abuse remains a serious possibility when to involve the other main services.

If suspicion or serious doubt remains after the initial steps then health services, social services and police should be involved in an initial strategy discussion or actual meeting. In this way, the safety of the child is checked, the plan for further investigation agreed and the roles of each agency identified. If it is felt that the likelihood of abuse requires further investigation, then arrangements are made which usually include the interview of the child and family by social services and/or the police. Dependent on the nature of the abuse, it may result in the child being assessed medically.

Practical investigation of sexual abuse

In all cases a full history and thorough physical examination are indicated though the urgency of these vary according to the nature of abuse. The relation of physical findings to the type of abuse is summarized in Table 9.9.

Physical investigations

Although it is always essential to ensure the medical well-being of a patient, diagnostic findings are often very limited and form a very small part of the diagnostic procedure.

The medical examination in the assessment of child sexual abuse involves taking a full medical history. Specific details of the events that may have occurred should be requested from the informant. If there are physical signs the child may be asked about them and

Table 9.9 Relation of type of abuse to clinical findings

Type of abuse	Findings on physical examination
1 Non-contact abuse	
i Exhibition	None
ii Pornography	None
2 Contact	
a Touching or fondling	No physical signs will be left unless this has been violent in which case bruising or bite marks may be seen soon after the event.
b Oral contact	If recent, semen, spermatozoa or saliva may be detected. Forensic swabs would be required.
c Masturbation	
i Adult in presence of child	None ⎫
ii By child of adult	None ⎬ may be forensic evidence on clothing etc.
iii By adult of child	May lead to redness but unless recent will probably not leave signs
d Insertion of fingers or object into vulva or anus	Physical signs may be present and therefore examination of value. If very recent (previous 48 hours) forensic evidence must be sought. If occurred a long time before and not ongoing will be of minimum value as healing occurs usually without significant scar formation. In these cases, examination only indicated if patient symptomatic.
e Vaginal, anal or oral intercourse. Intracrural intercourse	Physical findings may be present if recent. Also forensic evidence maybe available.
f Genital contact with parts of body	Unlikely to leave any signs

told that it is 'OK' to say whatever they like. It is important then to listen and record whatever is said without putting the child under pressure. If the child has already been questioned as part of a child protection investigation then relevant factors may be provided by social services and/or the police. The height and weight of the child are always measured. A full physical examination follows. In this procedure the following signs are looked for:

1 Physical disorder.
2 Neglect or deprivation.
3 Physical injury or accidents.
4 Emotional disturbance.
5 Sexual abuse.

In the majority of cases ano-genital examination involves the inspection of the genitalia with a bright light and a magnifying lens. Internal examinations are generally not indicated in prepubertal children but may be necessary in sexually active adolescents. The genitalia are inspected with a bright light, and a magnifying lens or a colposcope may be used. A colposcope allows accurate measurement of the hymenal orifice and facilitates photography but is not recommended for general use. The child is examined in a comfortable position, usually with the legs drawn up in the frog position but the knee/elbow position may be used. The anus is usually examined with the child lying in the left lateral position. However, if the child is young and very frightened, a full assessment can be done with the child sitting on a trusted adult's knee.

Swabs may be taken from the child and these may be sent for bacteriological assessment or for forensic analysis. If the latter is necessary, a doctor trained in the collection of forensic evidence must be present at the time of the assessment and the swabs appropriately handled and labelled in order to preserve the chain of evidence required in a court of law.

An internal examination may be required if there has been acute trauma. In this case heavy sedation or an anaesthetic is usually needed particularly in the prepubertal child. If sedation is used care is needed when determining the degree of opening of the anus or hymenal orifice because of effects of relaxation.

Prior to a medical examination, consent is required from the child's guardian and a child who is old enough to understand the procedure. During the medical examination it is often advisable to have two doctors present; both of them should be experienced in the assessment of abnormal findings. In this way the child is spared multiple medical examinations for second or third opinions. It is also good practice to have the mother, both parents or a trusted adult present for the child. Although internal examinations are not done the child is touched in the genital region and a small, distressed child may construe this as abuse. The taking of swabs may be particularly distressing but upset can be reduced by allowing the child to hold a swab and assist in the process.

The medical examination is rarely absolutely diagnostic and the findings must be taken in conjunction with the other evidence. Strongly suggestive findings include confirmation of sexually transmitted disease (excluding the neonate where infection may occur during the passage through the birth canal) and positive forensic evidence. Pregnancy in a child or young person under the age of 16 years indicates abuse or unlawful sexual intercourse.

The medical examination should be a carefully planned non-traumatic experience and should not compound any abuse that may have occurred previously. Not all children with genital symptoms have been abused and many children who have been abused have no physical findings. The family and other professionals involved should be warned at the start that the examination may not be diagnostic.

After the examination, it is important to let all parties, including the child, know what has been found. Although, ideally, only one examination should be performed, this is not always possible if there has been trauma or infection. As in any other field of medicine, it is always important to assess whether injuries and illness have been satisfactorily cured. Hence the need for subsequent review.

Emotional and behavioural investigation

The psychological assessment of potentially abused children has several purposes: first to assess overt distress or disturbance, secondly to help the child clarify what has happened to them, thirdly to assess risk to future mental health and finally to determine immediate and long-term action.

The first task for all adults, including the initial examining physician, is to observe and listen to the child. The professionals should be interested, concerned and friendly and it is most important that the child should feel and be safe.

If, at the strategy or planning meeting, further investigation is thought to be indicated then the purpose of that investigation and its mode of execution should be planned. The developmental status of the child must be taken into account, the younger the child the more difficult the assessment from all aspects. A teenager making an allegation is usually well able to make a clear statement to a trained police officer investigating the offence. It may also be necessary to evaluate the child's mental state and to hear from him or her preferences or concerns over safety. The younger the child the more likely that the assessment should be carried out by mental health professionals with appropriate experience.

Standard assessment of the child's mental health may assist in establishing the nature and cause of any behavioural disturbance. The absence of overt or reported disturbance should act as a caution against intervention which carries its own risk unless there is very strong reason. Separation of a child from a parent is one such action that carries a risk.

During a general assessment or at any point from first suspicion it may become apparent that a child is fearful of talking or that there are secrets they are under pressure to keep. There are several actions that help. The child should be enabled to feel safe. That may require several sessions over a period of time. If the parents are not implicated or deny implication it helps to get them to endorse openly that the child may say what he or she likes.

The concept of disclosure is best avoided since it carries the assumption that abuse has occurred and implies the use of techniques that are pressing and leading. The term facilitation describes a more appropriate technique of picking up clues that the child gives and helping the child explain and feel as safe as possible in doing so. During an interview leading or circular questions are unhelpful though at times the child may need firm encouragement to go on once they have started to explain. Dolls with representation of genitalia and body orifices (anatomical dolls) can help where the child has difficulty in explaining[24] but should be used on the basis of 'show me' rather than 'is this what happened?' It has been reported that casual play with the dolls differs between abused and non-abused children with the former showing more persistent sexually orientated interest.[25] In this context finger exploration of orifices was considered to be a natural reaction of a child to a new play thing. Interpretation of such unstructured use of the dolls is hazardous particularly if little is known about the developmental status, social environment and education of the child.

At the strategy or planning meeting it should be possible to agree on how to minimize the number of interviews, who should carry them out, whether there should be observers and how to obtain and record the information that the other professionals require for their particular tasks. Closed circuit TV and video recording are useful adjuncts to accurate recording.

Confirmation of suspected abuse

The need to search for criteria of the highest specificity and the importance of identifying several criteria has been referred to above. Reliance on physical examination alone will result in both false-positive and false-negative conclusions and it is the collation of data from several sources that ensures the lowest risk. This cannot be achieved by one isolated person and a multidisciplinary approach to the assessment of children who may have been abused is vital.

Further action

Once all the information has been collated, it is discussed at a case conference following which specific action may be taken. With the changes introduced in the 1989 Children Act parents will usually be present and it is important that after this meeting the family are offered help whether or not it is thought that sexual abuse has occurred. This may be directed at other problems or the traumas of investigation.

If abuse is thought probable then a series of tasks will have to result. These will include:

1 Protecting the child
   a identifying the perpetrator
   b separation of the child from the perpetrator
   c determining whether appropriate action will be agreed with parents
   d agreeing on legal action if necessary
2 Working with the family
   a identifying key social worker
   b agreeing investigation and management goals with family
   c identifying other essential professional support
3 Treatment of the child
   a identifying safe environment
   b ascertaining need for treatment
   c identifying treatment resource
4 Dealing with perpetrator
   a clarifying with police need for criminal investigation
   b clarifying with police need for criminal prosecution
   c agreeing on methods of obtaining forensic evidence
   d considering treatment for perpetrator

The management is summarized in Figure 9.3.

Psychological treatment

The psychological treatment of abused children depends on the nature of the abuse and its impact. The more intrusive, traumatic and persistent the abuse the more likely that there will be long-term effects.

The general principles of treatment of the children include the provision of:

1 Safety to be able to relate damaging experiences.
2 Support in recognizing their own lack of guilt.
3 Education for future safety.
4 Normalization: a move from sexual interests to other values in the children.
5 Specific therapy for other effects such as depression.

Prevention

Management of sexual abuse involves dealing with the consequences and trying to protect children by prevention. The primary care physician has a principal role in prevention since he normally acts as an adviser to families on child development. Jenny et al.[26] have described a developmentally based schedule for primary care physicians teaching 'parents and children

Management

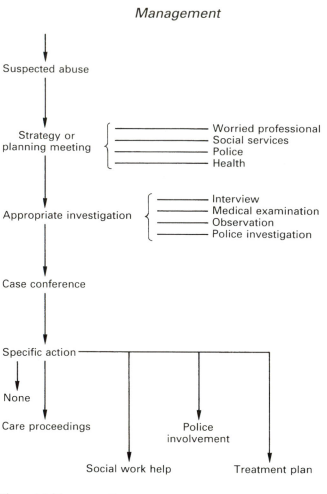

Suspected abuse

Strategy or
planning meeting
— Worried professional
— Social services
— Police
— Health

Appropriate investigation
— Interview
— Medical examination
— Observation
— Police investigation

Case conference

Specific action

None

Care proceedings

Police
involvement

Social work help

Treatment plan

Figure 9.3 Management.

reasonable protective behaviours'; a synopsis of this is given in Table 9.10.

Misunderstandings and myths

Child sexual abuse arouses strong passions with resulting misunderstanding and misinterpretation of data both by the public and professionals. Arguments have become polarized with half truths being held as dogma. Originally sexual abuse of children was ignored or denied with gross under-reporting of cases. The position has now moved to one in which there is a much greater readiness to consider abuse when any relevant criterion is present but where the presenting problem may instead be part of a far more complex case. The professional's ability to cope with anxiety and doubt is often tested to the limit and the need for clarity of thought and adherence to basic principles cannot be overemphasized.

Some of the more common confusions have already been referred to and this section is meant mainly to act as a reminder. Reliance on any single criterion for abuse is hazardous and corroborative evidence should always be sought. The physician's role is important but physical evidence is only sometimes present and rarely diagnostic in its own right. The statement that 'Children do not lie' is usually true, deliberate lying occurs in very few cases.[17] However it is probable that up to 25% of allegations may be due to genuine misunderstanding and only about 70% are eventually validated.[18]

There is a tendency to consider that if abuse has clearly occurred but with no evidence as to the identity of the perpetrator, then it is probably the father. Fathers and stepfathers are an important and major group

Table 9.10 Protocol for sex education and abuse prevention in well-child care

Age	Developmental issue	Prevention plan
Newborn	Complete dependency	Discuss choosing (reliable) day care and baby sitters
6 months	Discovery of pleasant feelings associated with genitals	Discuss normal infant self-exploratory behaviour
18 months	Beginning of language development	Encourage parents to teach acceptable, preferably 'anatomic' names for body
$2\frac{1}{4}$–4 years	Establishment of gender identity	Identify children with sex role confusion
3–5 years	Increasing independence Recognition of sexual differences	Encourage parents to give children permission to say no to advances. Reassure parents about normal sexual curiosity
5–8 years	Increasing independence Starting school	Discuss safety away from home. Encourage parents to teach safe behaviours. Encourage children to talk about frightening behaviours
8–12 years	Developing sexuality Highest incidence of abuse	Discuss parental planning for sex education
13–18 years	Developing adult identity	Discuss personal safety and risk taking behaviour, alcohol, drugs, sexually transmitted disease, birth control

Modified from Jenny *et al.*[26]

among abusers, but together constitute less than half of all abusers, except in studies only considering incestuous abuse.[23] Thus if there is no indication as to the identity of the abuser automatic separation of the father from the child is not justified without further evidence.

'Women are rarely involved in abuse' as a statement is true since direct sexual abuse is perpetrated by men in the large majority of cases. This has led to a hazardous assumption that if the male perpetrator is separated from the child all has been done to ensure safety. However, in some 40% of cases there is evidence that the mother has known of the abuse or has colluded with it.[27] This does not constitute a majority but is enough to require constant consideration. There are reports that the number of cases of direct abuse by women is being seriously underestimated[28] but if only 5% of children are directly abused by women then any unit with experience of over 100 abused children would expect to have seen some cases.

References

1 Schechter, M.D., Roberge, L. Sexual exploitation. In: Helfer, R.E., Kempe, C.H., eds. *Child Abuse and Neglect: The Family and the Community*. Cambridge, Mass: Ballinger, 1976.
2 Kempe, R.S., Kempe, C.H. *Sexual Abuse of Children and Adolescents*. New York: W.H. Freeman and Company, 1984.
3 Fraser, B.G. Stranger child abuse: the legislation and the law in the United States. In: Mrazek, P.B., Kempe, C.H., eds. *Sexually Abused Children and their Families*. Oxford: Pergamon Press, 1981.
4 Zeitlin, H. Investigation of the sexually abused child. *Lancet* 1987; ii: 842–844.
5 Finklehor, D. *Sexually Victimized Children*. New York: Free Press, 1979.
6 Baker, D., Duncan, S. Child sexual abuse: a study of prevalence in Great Britain. *Child Abuse and Neglect* 1985; 9: 457–467.
7 DeVine R.A. Sexual abuse of children: an overview of the problem. In: *Sexual Abuse of Children: Selected Readings*. Washington D.C. US Department of Health and Human Services, 1980.
8 Rosenfeld, A.A., Siegel, B., Bailey, R. Familial bathing patterns: implications for cases of alleged molestation and for pediatric practice. *Pediatrics* 1987. 79: 224–229.
9 Rosenfeld, A.A., Bailey, R., Siegel, B., Bailey, G. Determining incestuous contact between parents and child: frequency of children touching parents genitals in a non-clinical population. *J Am Acad Child Psychiatr* 1986; 25: 481–484.
10 Finklehor, D. *Child Sexual Abuse: New Theory and Research*. London: Collier Macmillan, 1984.
11 Bamford, F., Roberts, R. Child sexual abuse:. In: Meadow, R. ed., *ABC of Child Abuse*. London: British Medical Journal, 1989.
12 Emans, S.J., Woods, E.R., Flagg, N.T., Freeman, A. Genital findings in sexually abused symptomatic and asymptomatic girls. *Pediatrics* 1987; 79: 778–785.
13 Hobbs, C.J., Wynne, J.M. Buggery in childhood: a common syndrome of child abuse. *Lancet* 1986; ii: 792–796.
14 McCann, J., Voris, J., Simon, M., Wells, R. Perianal findings in prepubertal children selected for non-abuse. *Child Abuse and Neglect* 1989; 13: 179–193.
15 *Physical Signs of Sexual Abuse in Children*. London: Royal College Physicans, 1991.
16 Bentovim, A. The diagnosis of child sexual abuse. *Bull Roy Coll Psychiatr* 1987; 11: 295–299.
17 Jones, D.P.H., McQuiston, M. *Interviewing the Sexually Abused Child*, 3rd edn. Royal College of Psychiatrists Publication. London: Gaskell Press, 1988.
18 Jones, D.P.H., McGraw, J.N. Reliable and fictitious accounts of sexually abused children. *J Interpersonal Violence* 1987; 2: 27–45.
19 Herman, J., Russell, D., Trocki, K. Long term effects of incestuous abuse in childhood. *Am J Psychiatr* 1986; 143: 1293–1296.
20 Green, H. True and false allegations of abuse in child custody disputes. *J Am Acad Child Psychiatr* 1986; 25: 449–456.
21 Schetky, D.H., Benedek, E.P. *Emerging Issues in Child Psychiatry and the Law*. New York: Brunner/Mazel, 1985.
22 Schetky, D.H. Emerging issues in child sexual abuse. *J Am Acad Child Psychiatr* 1986; 25: 490–492.
23 Hobbs, C.J., Wynne, J.M. Child sexual abuse: an increasing rate of diagnosis. *Lancet* 1987; ii, 837–841.
24 Boat, B.W., Everson, M.D. *Using Anatomical Dolls: Guidelines for Interviewing Young Children in Sexual Abuse Investigations*. Chapel Hill: University of North Carolina, 1986.
25 Jampole, L., Weber, M.K. An assessment of the behaviour of sexually abused and nonsexually abused children with the anatomically correct dolls. *Child Abuse and Neglect* 1987; 11: 187–192.
26 Jenny, C., Sutherland, S.E., Sandhal, B.B. Developmental approach to preventing the sexual abuse of children. *Pediatrics* 1986; 78: 1034–1038.
27 Russell, D., Finklehor, D. Women as perpetrators: review of the evidence. In: *Child Sexual Abuse New Theory and Research*. London: Collier Macmillan, 1984.
28 Wilkins, B. Women who sexually abuse children. *Br Med J* 1990; 300: 1153–1154.

9.7 Adoption and fostering

Marion Miles

Adoption

The historical perspective

The process of adoption secures a permanent home, in a family, for a child whose parents are unable or unwilling to provide care themselves. Such provision of care by adults other than the natural parents has occurred throughout history; adoption was recorded as early as 2350 BC and Oedipus and Moses provide examples of substitute care.[1,2] Adoption was confirmed in English law by the Adoption of Children Act 1926, and in Scottish law in 1930. Thus, by means of a court order, parental rights are totally and irrevocably transferred to the adopters and the child becomes a full member of a new family.

The Adoption Act was introduced as a result of the recommendations contained in the Hopkinson Committee Report 1921, and later reports of the Tomlin Committee in 1925 and 1926.[3,4] The First World War highlighted many social problems particularly those of illegitimate children, whose numbers rose during the war years, and those of children who were orphaned or who had lost one parent. Informal adoption placements were arranged but the children lacked legal security. They were exposed to stigmatization and insecurity since they could not obtain a birth certificate in the new family name, could be removed by their birth parents, or returned to them by their adopters. The Hopkinson Committee recognized that the welfare of the child was of paramount importance, that family life was preferable to institutional life and that children would be better protected by legal provision for adoption. However, it also stressed that efforts should be made to maintain the mother–child relationship and 'to avert such severance taking place on economic grounds'.[3] These diverging views led to debate, but the Tomlin Committee concluded that legalized adoption should be introduced. With considerable foresight the committee expressed concern about the policy of complete secrecy which was practised by existing adoption agencies. Despite this reservation the adoption process, which provided a welcome solution to the twin problems of illegitimacy and infertility, continued to be invested with secrecy, which often extended to the children also.

In 1945, the Curtis Committee was convened to consider the existing provision for children who were deprived of a normal family life and to identify the measures needed to compensate for parental care.[5] The committee acknowledged that adoption was the most satisfactory method of providing children with a substitute family and its report led to the Children Act 1948. Although the Act was not directly concerned with adoption it had significant implications for adoption practice since it led to the establishment of children's departments and the involvement of local authorities in adoption work.

A further Adoption of Children Act 1949 required a probationary period of 3 months before an adoption order could be made, during which time the placement was supervised. The Act also enabled adopted children to inherit as a member of the adoptive family rather than from the birth family. In 1950, further amendments allowed an adopted child to inherit property, but not a title, from adoptive parents.

During this period, adoption became separated from the mainstream of child care although, originally, it was regarded as one option in the range available to disadvantaged children. This separation may have been fuelled by the desire for secrecy, but for whatever reason persisted until the Children Act 1975 when adoption again became part of the spectrum of services available to children who could not be cared for by their birth parents.

In 1973, Rowe and Lambert published the results of an important research study commissioned by the Association of British Adoption Agencies.[6] They estimated that approximately 7000 children with special needs awaited a family placement in a foster or adoptive home. Five per cent needed a direct adoption placement and a further 25% a foster home with a view to adoption. However, for a variety of reasons which included pressure of other duties on social workers' time, poor recording and poor decision-making, the majority of the children remained in limbo in local authority residential care, no longer in touch with their birth families. Fortunately, the Houghton Committee had been established in 1969 to consider adoption and to identify any desirable changes.[7] The committee's report reaffirmed confidence in adoption and stressed the need to give first consideration to the welfare of the child.

The Children Act 1975 was built on the work of the Houghton Committee. The main thrust of the Act was to give priority to the long-term welfare of the child even if this meant overriding the wishes of the parents. Previously, adoptions which were likely to be contested were rarely processed because adoption orders were seldom if ever granted in the absence of parental consent to adoption. The Act also required local authorities to provide an adoption service and made third party adoption arrangements (through intermediaries such as doctors, midwives, clergymen and lawyers) illegal.

The Act introduced very significant changes to adoption and was one of three influences that promoted a new approach to the placement of children with special needs. The other influences were concern about the outcome of long-term fostering and the success of the British Adoption Project in recruiting families for children with special needs. Their effects are considered later in the chapter.

Further adoption provisions of the Act were contained in the Adoption Agencies Regulations (AAR) 1983[8] and are of particular interest to doctors concerned with child health. The regulations introduced the statutory requirement to appoint a medical adviser to adoption work. Thus the contribution of what had previously been good practice was recognized and made mandatory.

The Children Act 1989 was implemented in 1991 and strikes a new balance between family autonomy and child care. With these changes and a shift in adoption practice, which now involves older children rather than babies, a review of adoption law, policy and practice is indicated. A comprehensive consultation process is currently underway in England and Wales which will formulate proposals for new legislation to reflect the developments in practice which have taken place over the past two decades.

Table 9.11 Numbers of adoption orders 1974–1990 England and Wales

Year	Children
1974	22502
1976	17621
1978	12121
1980	10609
1982	10240
1984	8648
1986	7892
1988	7390
1990	6533

OPCS Survey. London: HMSO, 1991.

The numbers involved

In 1930, 4500 adoptions were recorded and this figure included children adopted by relatives and step-parents. By 1940 the figure had doubled. During the Second World War there was an increase in the number of babies born to unmarried mothers. This together with other effects of its aftermath resulted in a further rise and in 1950 14 000 adoption orders were granted.

During the 1960s, there was a dramatic change in social and sexual activity which was reflected in the adoption figure for 1968 when 27 000 adoption orders were granted involving 9000 babies.

However, by 1972 the Houghton Committee was able to note the fall in the number of babies available for adoption and related it to improved methods of birth control, the availability of legal abortion, a more flexible approach to family life and better social support which enabled unmarried mothers to keep their babies. On the other hand the number of prospective adopters remained high.

By 1980, adoption orders had dropped to around 10 000 of which less than 25% involved babies. Currently less than 7000 children are adopted annually of which only 16% are infants.

The following trends emerge (Tables 9.11 and 9.12):

- There has been an appreciable and continuous fall in the total number of adoption orders granted.
- There has been a gradual increase in the number of older children adopted.

The adoption process

How adoptions are arranged

Adoptions can only be arranged through an adoption agency, unless the child is a close relative of the prospective adopters or the placement follows an order of the High Court.[9]

An arrangement made by an authorized agency is known as an agency placement. The child is placed with prospective adopters either at the direct request of a parent or by the local authority which is looking after the child. In most cases, the adopters are unknown to the child and his family, unless they are foster parents who apply to adopt and are already providing care.

The 1976 Adoption Act required all local authorities to ensure that an adoption service was available

Table 9.12 Age at adoption England and Wales (OPCS)

Year	Age (years)					
	Under 1 (%)	1–4 (%)	5–9 (%)	10–14 (%)	15–17 (%)	All ages
1974	5172 (23)	6148 (27)	7462 (33)	3132 (14)	588 (3)	22502
1979	2649 (24)	2183 (20)	3572 (33)	2013 (19)	453 (4)	10870
1984	1836 (21)	1935 (22)	2605 (30)	1728 (20)	526 (6)	8648
1989	1115 (16)	1875 (27)	2244 (32)	1331 (19)	458 (7)	7044

and most of these adoption agencies are based in local authority social work departments. There are also many voluntary adoption agencies which cover wider geographical areas than social services departments. The number of voluntary societies has dropped as fewer babies become available for adoption. Many of those remaining have developed specialized family finding services for needy children; some are linked to specific religious groups. Examples include Barnardo's, who operate on a country-wide basis, the National Children's Home and the Catholic Children's Society. Voluntary adoption societies are subject to approval by the Secretary of State and they are regularly inspected by social services inspectors.

The agencies provided by local authorities together with the approved voluntary societies constitute the statutory adoption service. A useful guide to all adoption agencies is regularly produced by the British Agencies for Adoption and Fostering (BAAF).

All adoption agencies assess children and prospective adopters, place children, provide post-placement support and counselling, and advise adopted people seeking access to their original birth records. However post-adoption services are variable and improvements in provision are under review.

Local authority adoption work is provided free, but most voluntary societies are charities and rely on contributions.

Non-agency applications to adopt can be made by step-parents, other relatives who care for the child and non-relatives who might be private or local authority foster parents.

The adoption order

Application for an adoption order which makes the adoption legal can be made to a magistrate's court, county court, High Court or, in Scotland, to the sheriff court or the Court of Sessions. When the child has been placed by an agency, or the adopter is a relative, an order can be made as soon as at least one of the adopters has cared for the child at home for a period of 13 consecutive weeks. In other cases there is a qualifying period of 12 months. However, because of court timetables, the interval is usually longer. When the child has special needs a longer settling-in period is usually advisable. When the adoption is contested by the birth parent(s) further delay may ensue. In baby placements, the 13 week period commences when the baby is 6 weeks old. An adoption order may be made on a young person up to the age of 18 unless he or she is married. Once the order is made, an adoption certificate is issued by the Registrar General.

The adoption order states the child's original and new name and the names of the birth parents and a copy is sent to the adoptive parents. A short adoption certificate gives the child's new name only, a full certificate has the details of the order showing the adopters as the parents. The adoption certificates have the same legal status as birth certificates.

Under the British Nationality Act 1981 a child becomes a British citizen when the adoption order is made in the UK if one of the adopters is already a British citizen. Children with British citizenship in their own right retain it when adopted by a foreign national.

Access to birth records and the contact register

The need for adopted people to know about their origins is acknowledged within section 57 of the 1976 Adoption Act which enables people who were adopted after 1975 to have automatic access to their original birth certificates on reaching the age of 18. Those adopted before 1975 are required to see a counsellor before having access. In Scotland the age limit is 17 and access has been possible since 1930. Triseliotis, in Scotland, interviewed people who had applied for their certificates and concluded that those who had good relationships with their adoptive parents were less likely to seek access to their original birth records. Following the 1976 Adoption Act, the Registrar General operated an informal register for adopted people and their birth relatives. However, the number of adopted people who sought information increased during the 1980s and reached 33 000 in l990. Privately run registers which provided reunion facilities mushroomed, using the information on the birth certificate to trace birth parents and other relatives. However, using this system there was no way of knowing whether contact by the young person would be welcome or not. The provision of an official register offered a safe, confidential way for birth parents and other relatives to indicate that contact would be welcome and to offer an address for future reference. After several years of campaigning, an official adoption contact register run by the Registrar General and covering England and Wales began operation in 1991.

The register is in two parts. Part 1 lists adopted people and Part 2 birth parents and other relatives. For both parts there is a registration fee. On request from the adopted person the Registrar General sends the name and address of any relative who has registered and notifies the relatives that this has been done. The flow of information is one way and information about the adopted person cannot be given to the birth relatives. The register will only help an adopted person to learn about his relatives who have entered the register. It does not put relatives who do not wish for contact at risk.

There are many issues around contact and both the adopted person and the birth relatives need to approach any reunion gradually. In most cases, support and sensitive counselling is needed at each stage of the newly developing relationship.

Who can adopt?

Adoption is undertaken for many different reasons. They include infertility, a desire to increase the family without adding to the population, a wish to share the advantages of a happy home with a less fortunate child and a considered decision to help a child with a specific disability. Having decided to adopt, prospective adopters approach an adoption agency and should choose one which can most closely relate their needs to the resource they are offering. Most agencies offer group sessions where adoption and the children available are discussed. If commitment is sustained, then the assessment process is commenced by agency social workers.

The assessment is comprehensive and takes place over a period of many months. Reasons for wanting to adopt are explored together with details of each applicant's personal life, interests, family lifestyle, potential for parenting, understanding of child care and the resource being offered. In addition, personal references from people who know the applicant, a check of police records, and local authority enquiries are required by law.

On satisfactory completion, a report is presented to the adoption panel so that a recommendation to approve the applicants can be made to the agency. The high quality of the assessment process is reflected by the approval rate of most panels, although approval can be deferred if more information is requested.

There are few eligibility criteria prescribed in statute in the selection of people who would like to adopt, but agencies have a relatively free hand and may impose their own restrictions. Since the issues which may influence decisions are not defined by either legislation or guidance, prospective adopters often criticize the apparent inconsistencies between the threshold criteria of different agencies. This aspect is now under review and clearer guidance may be forthcoming.

Age of applicant

Lower age limits are prescribed in legislation; an adopter must be at least 21 years old, or 18 years when a parent is adopting his or her own child jointly with a step-parent.

Agencies operate their own upper age limits. When a healthy infant is being placed, many agencies seek couples in their 20s or 30s and do not consider applicants when the wife is over 35 years of age. These limitations are imposed to take into account the fact that 2 years are likely to pass before a child can be placed because of the assessment process and the small number of babies available for adoption. They also reflect the wishes of many mothers placing their babies who express a preference for young couples. Childless couples argue against this limit pointing out that over 60 000 women a year give birth to babies when they are 35 years or over. However, this figure still accounts for less than 10% of live births. Since the number of potential adopters far exceeds the number of available infants (the National Association for the Childless estimates that each year there are approximately 35 000 adopters compared to 500 infants) these limits also serve as a rationing device and avoid raising the expectations of older couples unnecessarily. Another dilemma faces infertile couples since infertility investigations can last several years by which time the couples may be in their late 30s or early 40s before being able to commit themselves to adoption.

Greater flexibility about age limits is exercised when older children, sibling groups or those with special needs are being placed. Under these circumstances the maturity and experience of the applicants warrant special consideration since the number of such children needing families far exceeds the number of families available. Nevertheless, age can never be discounted and agencies must be satisfied that adopters can remain sufficiently healthy and vigorous to care for children until they are grown up.

Health

There are no statutory health requirements, but the Adoption Agencies Regulations (AAR) require adopters to obtain a comprehensive medical report to include personal and family health history, current state of health, details of the consumption of tobacco, alcohol and other habit-forming drugs, for consideration by the medical adviser to the agency. Health factors which give rise to debate include smoking, obesity (when the body mass index is greater than 30) and an alcohol consumption above the recommended limit. A smoking habit raises particular concern because of the effects of passive smoking and the presentation of a poor role model to the child. Many agencies exclude applicants who smoke, but will reconsider once the habit ceases. Other situations which may require sensitive consideration by the medical adviser include the presence of genetic conditions which have led adopters not to have children of their own, cardiovascular problems, treated cancer, degenerative problems and visual impairment. Many agencies will only place babies with couples with established infertility.

Marital status

A sole applicant may apply to adopt a child. If two people apply to adopt jointly they must be married thus complying with the European Adoption Convention which prohibits adoption by unmarried couples. Agencies look for stability in an adoptive partnership and some stipulate minimum periods during which the couple have been married or have lived together. The greater likelihood of divorce in the case of second or third marriages requires agencies to consider applicants appropriately.

Generally speaking, agencies prefer adoptive couples to single applicants. However, some older children, and those with disabilities, require undivided attention which can be successfully offered by a single adopter. In the case of a single applicant who is living with a partner, assessment involves both partners.

At least one of the adopters concerned has to confirm the intention to make a permanent home in the UK. The question of adoption by lesbians or male homosexuals is controversial. Some agencies consider that such applicants should not be excluded if they can provide a home which meets the child's best interests. Opinions are divided and the subject is under review in England and Wales.

The adoption panel

All agencies are required to provide a counselling service for parents, and for the children depending on their age and understanding, before a decision can be made about adoption. The counselling procedure ensures that birth parents understand the nature and implications of adoption and provides them with an opportunity to express their views and anxieties. Subject to this process every adoption agency is required to establish an adoption panel and the Adoption Agencies Regulations 1983 clearly defined the composition and functions of a panel.[8]

Panel composition

The panel is established by the management committee of an approved adoption society or by the social services committee in the case of a local authority adoption service and is accountable to that committee. The maximum number of panel members is ten, the minimum seven, and there must be at least one man and one woman. The quorum for meetings is five. The agency appoints the chair who is usually a social worker. The regulations require that two panel members be social workers employed by the agency and there has to be, in addition, a management representative, a medical adviser and at least two members who are independent of the agency. The latter are expected to make a special contribution and the regulations allow the agency to make imaginative appointments. They often include representatives of an ethnic minority group, adoptive parents, teachers, psychologists, workers from another agency and cultural advisers. A legal adviser is not required to be a member of the panel but is usually present since the agency must obtain legal advice about every case that is presented to the panel.

Appointments to the panel can be made for whatever period seems appropriate, but are usually reviewed on a 3-yearly cycle.

Panel functions

The panel considers all the cases referred to it by the agency and makes recommendations to the agency who in turn makes decisions. The panel is required to meet and cannot carry out business by correspondence. For each child being considered the panel must make a recommendation whether adoption is in the child's best interests, and, if so, whether the child should be freed for adoption. Freeing is the process whereby parental responsibility is transferred to the agency. It enables the mother to relinquish legal care of her baby at an early stage and was intended for use mainly in baby adoptions where the mother and agency are working together to secure the baby's future. It is also used to protect prospective adopters from complicated and distressing legal situations, when adoption is contested by the birth parent or parents, so that the dispute is between the parents and the local authority not the birth parents and prospective adopters. Either at the same time or subsequently the panel has to make a recommendation about a proposed placement when a child is matched to suitable adopters. Recommendations about the suitability of prospective adopters can be made by any agency panel, but only the one considering the placement can make a recommendation about matching. The agency who makes the placement assumes responsibility for follow-up procedures. All recommendations are recorded in writing.

In order to fulfil its functions the panel is presented with detailed, comprehensive reports about the child, the birth parents and prospective adopters which include personal, family, social and health information. At any stage the panel can request further information to assist in its task and the agency is required to meet such a request. At all times first consideration must be given to the child's welfare and best interests. Whenever possible his wishes and feelings must be considered, together with those of his parents, about religious upbringing.

Once the agency has made a decision, based on the panel's recommendations, the following procedures are undertaken:

- Notification of decision to parents.
- Notification of decision to free child for adoption.
- Notification to prospective adopters that they are considered suitable to adopt.
- Notification to prospective adopters that they are suitable for a particular child or children.
- The child is informed about the placement, taking account of age and understanding.
- Prospective adopters are supplied with written information (including details of history, religious and cultural background, health, developmental and educational status and any identified problems or needs) about the child *before* placement.
- Health information about the child is sent to the adopters' general practitioner *before* placement.

- Adopters' local authority is notified.
- Adopters' health authority is notified and thereby the health visitor and other relevant health services.
- Adopters' local education authority is notified if
  a the child is of compulsory school age
  b or is considered to have special educational needs.

When a baby is involved in the placement the proposed new name is used and NHS registration can be modified accordingly. With older children this is rarely appropriate or practicable especially when the child has been with prospective adopters for some time in a foster placement.

In addition to the statutory procedures listed above most medical advisers alert a colleague in the area to which the child is moving when there are or there are likely to be health or developmental problems.

At all times, the agency case records are treated as confidential and must be securely stored for at least 75 years.

Adoption allowances

In the past, some families who wished to offer children adoptive homes were unable to do so because of financial considerations. In order to overcome this obstacle a system was introduced in England and Wales in 1982 whereby adoption agencies could develop individual adoption allowance schemes subject to approval by the Secretary of State. Payment of an allowance is designed to secure an adoption placement and should not be seen as a reward for the adopters.

In 1991 new regulations came into force under the Children Act 1989 which replace the earlier schemes. Now agencies have to consider, assess and pay allowances in accordance with the regulations and do not have to submit their schemes to the Secretary of State for approval. Any agency, whether a local authority or an approved society, can pay an allowance subject to the regulations. Allowances will continue to be the exception rather than the rule. They cannot be granted retrospectively and should take account of the adopters' financial circumstances.

A recommendation to pay an allowance is made by the adoption panel. The agency then makes the final decision.

Specific circumstances for payment of an allowance are set out. They include:

- Foster parents who wish to adopt a child who has developed a strong attachment to them, but who cannot afford to lose the fostering allowance. A subsequent adoption allowance will take account of the child benefit allowance to which they become entitled as adopters.
- Facilitation of a placement with siblings or another child with whom the child has developed close ties.
- Placement of a child with special needs.

- Anticipation of the need for an allowance at some future date for a child with special needs.

Adopters in receipt of an allowance are required to notify the agency if there is a significant change in their financial affairs, which are also considered at an annual review.

The actual amount of the allowance therefore reflects the adopters' financial resources and the needs of the child. A record of the allowance is included in the adoption case records, is treated confidentially and preserved for 75 years.

Complaints

There are no statutory requirements in adoption legislation for a complaints procedure to be available to adopters. Users of the statutory agencies have access to a procedure established by local authorities under the Local Authority Social Services Act which came into effect in 1991. Voluntary societies usually provide a mechanism for review but are not required to do so by the Act.

Role of the medical adviser

The AAR recognized the importance of health information in the context of adoption and require the appointment of a named medical adviser (MA) to the adoption panel. The adviser has to be involved in every case presented to the panel because of the possible significance of health factors which should be considered in the wider context of the panel's discussion. The MA must be suitably qualified, well informed about adoption practice, and able to work closely with social workers. Local authority agencies usually approach the district health authority for advice about a suitable appointment. Voluntary agencies usually make appointments on a more personal basis.

In practice, MAs include community child health doctors, consultant paediatricians, community physicians, child psychiatrists and general practitioners. Most MAs belong to the Medical Group of BAAF which started under the guidance of Dr Hilda Lewis, a child psychiatrist, who was deeply concerned with the care of deprived children. The group has an educative role, advises on good practice by contributing to the production of BAAF Practice Notes and regularly responds to Department of Health consultation documents. The group has played an important role in the development of a child-centred adoption service and the removal of the label unadoptable from children with special needs.

The MA has to ensure a high standard of medical practice in the work of the agency and should be consulted on all policy and procedure matters related to the disclosure of health information.

Larger agencies may have more than one MA in which case it is usual for one adviser to assume a coordinating role.

The MA is involved in the following specific tasks:

1 Obtaining health information about the birth parents, the child and adopters

When medical information is sought the use of BAAF forms designed to meet these requirements has been recommended in Department of Health guidance to agencies.[8,10] The forms have been produced to facilitate the collection of information which focuses on the needs of children. When information is requested from a doctor it is usual to send the form accompanied by a letter signed by the MA which sets out the reasons for the request and emphasizes the need for background information which will assist in the placement of the child.

All reports are stored securely. In addition to panel members, access is limited under special circumstances to courts, guardians ad litem and ombudsmen.

Health information about the birth parents should be sought from a doctor who knows the parent, usually the GP. In practice, it is often difficult to locate a doctor who has adequate information so a form is available, which can be completed by the parent and social worker, to give background health details, which can be scrutinized by the MA. The MA can then highlight and pursue various items as necessary. Appropriate obstetric information is also obtained, subject to maternal consent. It is essential to explain to the parents the importance of health information to the child and future caregivers if their cooperation is to be obtained.

Accurate and up-to-date information about the physical and mental health of prospective adopters is required and usually requested from their GP. Again an explanatory letter about the purpose of the report is recommended to ensure a full exchange of information. Complementary health information may be requested by the MA from specialist services. Information is updated on a 2-yearly basis unless a new health issue arises.

Prospective adopters have no legal right to see their medical reports which are exempt from obligatory access under the Access to Personal Files Act 1987.

A recent and comprehensive report on the child's health history, health and developmental status is required under the regulations. Depending on age a neonatal report or a summary of perinatal events is also required. The results of any screening tests which the MA recommends must also be recorded. The use of the appropriate BAAF forms ensures a high standard of information collection and collation.[10] The intention is to build up a full picture of the child's health and development, including strengths and weaknesses, in order to identify any specific needs. In this way the adoption panel, prospective adopters, and future

health providers can be well informed. The MA may or may not undertake the examination personally, but in any case will need to approach other sources for supplementary information including the GP, the community child health service and the school health service.

2 Ensuring access to medical services

Children under consideration for adoption may have received less than adequate previous medical care. The variety of physical, developmental and emotional problems encountered is considerable. The MA needs to have a good understanding of these problems and to establish a wide network of colleagues able to provide information and ready advice including physicians, surgeons, psychiatrists, psychologists, and geneticists. The MA must keep abreast of new developments in child health. For example, issues around HIV infection are likely to occur more frequently and the MA needs to know where to seek specialist advice in an area complicated by the difficulties of early diagnosis and confidentiality. It is sometimes possible and desirable to place a newly born baby with prospective adopters when it is too early to pronounce with any certainty about the baby's health and development. Such a placement can only be considered when the mother has had time before the birth to reflect on her decision and when the MA has no obvious reservations about health risks or perinatal complications.

Under these circumstances the implications of an early placement have to be explained to the prospective adopters and the MA must ensure that a careful assessment is undertaken when the baby is 6–8 weeks old.

In advance of any adoptive placement a written report about the child is sent to the adopters' GP. The MA retains responsibility for maintaining an overview of the health needs of all children from the time of referral to the agency until an adoption order is granted.

3 Interpreting medical information

When making decisions about adoption, relevant medical information is considered, in conjunction with social and other reports, by social workers and members of the adoption panel. The responsibility for interpretation and assessment of this information rests with the MA. This process ensures that all health issues relating to the child are recognized and taken into account and that the physical and mental health of adopters is also carefully considered when assessing their ability to care for a child.

The MA has to advise prospective adopters about health issues and may do this personally or arrange meetings with appropriate specialist colleagues. Whether facilitating or participating in counselling sessions, the MA needs to understand the social, emotional and educational implications of disability and deprivation and to have skills in communicating such knowledge.

When applicants cannot be accepted as adoptive parents for wholly or mainly medical reasons, the MA has an important part in deciding how best to advise them in the least damaging way.

Many MAs participate in the recruitment and preparation of adoptive parents thereby describing and advising about the health issues which may arise.

4 Attending panel meetings

In addition to interpreting medical information for other panel members, the MA also has to function as a full panel member with the same voice and vote in discussions as other members. This role is often more difficult to fulfil, but can be facilitated during sessions when the panel meet and train as a group.

Telling children about adoption

During recent decades, practitioners have encouraged adopters to tell their adopted children that they were adopted, and to do so from an early age, but there is no legal obligation to do so. Adoption is a life-long process involving the birth parents, the child and the adoptive family to varying degrees and forming an adoption triangle. Children have a right to know about their past, including from whom they get their physical characteristics. It is impossible to keep adoption a secret forever and potentially disastrous for a child to learn about adoption from an outside source. Opportunities to talk about adoption occur naturally and if dealt with on this basis help the child to accept and understand the situation gradually as he grows older.[11] The process is facilitated by using a lifestory book containing photographs, mementos and written information. Depending upon age it is usual for a child to move to an adoptive home with a rudimentary or detailed lifestory book which has been compiled by the agency social worker and can be added to as further details emerge.

What children understand about adoption

Research in America shows that all children reach an understanding about adoption at about the same age regardless of whether they are in adoptive families or not.[12] Most of their understanding is gathered in a general social way rather than by information from parents. Understanding of and knowledge about the adoption process change with their own development, consequently their concern and interest are focused on different aspects at different stages.

The pre-school period

When the words adoption and adopted are used about children from the beginning there is usually no precise moment at which they are told that they are adopted. Early telling is advocated but young children may appear to understand more than they really do. They know that the word adopted applies to them and they repeat what they have heard, but do not understand the significance of not being born into the families they know.

Older children

Around the age of 6 years, most children can differentiate between birth and adoption. At this stage it is important for them to know about their birth and that they were born in the same way as most other people. Talking about the birth leads naturally into explaining why the child was placed for adoption. It recognizes that there is a history which antedates joining the family and reassures the child that he can think and talk about that period. In these discussions, the birth father should not be ignored even when information is scanty.

Children develop an understanding of blood relationships by 8–9 years and can appreciate different kinds of relationships. However, they do not understand the legal implications and may develop anxieties about being reclaimed by their natural parents. With growing awareness of adoption comes understanding about separation and they may grieve for their natural parents. This may take the adoptive parents unawares but offers an opportunity to reassure and explore other feelings.

The legal permanence of adoption is understood by 11 year olds, by which time children want to know more about the relationship between their birth parents, particularly whether or not they were married.

Difficult questions can be asked and dealt with at this stage. Indeed the answers may provoke greater anxiety in the parent than the child.

Adolescents

By 13 years, young people fully understand the adoption process and more clearly appreciate the reasons for adoption. Teenagers need to separate from their parents and to do so need to learn who they are in relation to their parents. Adopted children have to learn in relation to two sets of parents before they can fully develop their identities. Adopted teenagers are usually curious about their birth parents. Their adoptive parents may find this a very stressful period and benefit from advice and support in order to prevent discussions becoming confrontational and hurtful. Many agencies offer a post-adoption advisory service; the Post Adoption Centre is a voluntary agency which offers a specialist service.

Children with special needs

Until the 1980s, children with special needs were considered hard to place in a permanent substitute family. The children involved comprise three main groups:

1 Children with disabilities, learning difficulties or other problems whose parents have agreed to adoption, but for whom adoptive homes have been difficult to find. Most of these children spend time in a foster or residential home before being placed for adoption.
2 Children described by Rowe and Lambert as 'children who wait'.[6] Typically they have been received into the care of a local authority, have experienced several changes of care and unsuccessful attempts at rehabilitation with their birth parents. These children are usually older and include sibling groups. Many will no longer be in contact with their birth parents.
3 Children who have been in care for shorter periods of time following abuse or neglect and who are still attached to their birth families.

Children from minority ethnic groups may be included in any of these categories. However, their main needs often revolve around the importance of maintaining their racial, cultural and religious identities. Most agencies now accept that placements for these children should reflect these needs and, since recruitment of suitable families sometimes proves difficult, that they should be considered to have special needs.

Permanent substitute families offer the children security, stability and the opportunity to make lasting relationships. The benefits are well summarized by Triseliotis, 'a family for life with its network of support systems not only for them but also their future children'.[13] Attempts to meet the needs of the children defined in group 1 may be made by any agency, who may recruit specific families by advertisement. Other agencies, including Parents for Children and the Thomas Coram Foundation, specialize in finding families for children with disabilities or other problems.

There is danger that placement plans for children in group 2 may drift because of complex legal problems or the logistics of placing, for example, a sibling group of three or more children. These children are exposed to system abuse resulting from the continued impermanence of their placements. Many children from groups 2 and 3 are placed for adoption against the wishes of their birth parents. In the 1980s, Thorburn and Rowe considered 1165 placements of children with special needs and found that for 31% of the children, adoption was contested.[14]

Studies which have tried to identify the characteristics which contribute to the successful parenting of children with special needs have failed to identify many common features. Perhaps this is not surprising since the parenting of a baby with Down Syndrome requires very different skills from those needed to support a disturbed 12 year old or a group of four siblings. Some factors seem to increase the risk of breakdown, for example the presence of a natural child of the family whose age is within 3 years of the age of the newcomer. Interestingly a proportion of those who have parented successfully have been previously rejected when applying for more conventional placements.

Outcomes of placements of children with special needs

Given the vulnerability of children with special needs it is important to consider how often the placements break down. Thorburn and Rowe[14] found that up to 22% of placements terminated within 6 years. They also confirmed that the age at placement was related to disruption – the older children did less well. In Scotland, O'Hara and Hoggan found a disruption rate of only 4.6% for children aged under 10 years at placement compared to 21.7% for those who were older at placement.[15]

Other reviews by Wolkind and Kozaruk considered 108 children with medical and developmental problems aged 3 months to 11 years at placement. The least successful outcomes involved children who were over 5 years at placement, who had been in residential as opposed to foster care for over 2 years prior to placement, or who had significant learning difficulties.[16,17]

Wedge and Mantle studied sibling group placements involving 160 children. Follow up at 4 years revealed that 21% of placements had broken down.[18] Thus attempts to define a simple breakdown rate would be misleading. The outcome depends upon the age at placement, the special needs of the child, and the time at which the assessment of success is made.

Children from minority ethnic groups

Within this group there are particular issues which relate to the placement of black children. The term black is used in relation to children from the following groups: African Caribbean; Asian, including Indian, Pakistani, Indonesian, Chinese; African; Arab.

They are considered together because they have cultural needs which are different from those of white children and they are at risk of experiencing racism. It is acknowledged that some individual members of these groups may not define themselves as black but, in an attempt to meet the needs of the children, a general approach is adopted.

Background

In the 1960s, black children in care were found to be, and consequently defined as, *hard to place*. The British Adoption Project – a research project – sought and found placements for 53 black children with 51 couples, 80% of whom were white. Following the success of this project, which had not had the benefit of the opinions of black people, transracial placement was accepted and became commonplace. At the time it was seen as a liberal, tolerant approach which could assist in the formation of an integrated society. Gradually black people challenged this practice and older black children, who had been reared in white families, suggested that their placements, while loving, had not always equipped them to cope with racism. Most agencies now support the view that black children should be placed whenever possible in families of the same race, culture and religion in order to help the children develop a positive black identity and to cope with racism.[19] Tizard argues for a more flexible approach and is concerned that rigid policies lead to unacceptable delay in placement.[20]

Agencies who specifically recruit black families find that they are available. However, there are resource implications and it is essential to involve black workers who can draw upon their own valuable experience of being black in Britain and respond sensitively to the needs and fears of the black families. When a transracial placement of a black child in a white family is considered to be in the best interests of the child it is important that the family has access to appropriate advice and support and can incorporate a black role-model into the family network.

Useful guidance from the social services inspectorate was issued in 1990 in which the arguments about race and culture are well set out. Advice on the principles which should inform placements is offered to agencies and practitioners. The guiding principle is identified thus: 'other things being equal and in the great majority of cases, placement with a family of similar ethnic origin and religion is most likely to meet a child's needs as fully as possible and to safeguard his or her welfare most effectively.'[21]

Step-children and adoption

A step-family is created when a partner brings to the family a child by a previous relationship. Under these circumstances the adults concerned often feel the need to make the family a legal unit and look to adoption as the way of achieving it.[22] Step-families face several problems. The newcomer suddenly has an instant family. The children may grieve for the parent and the life they have lost. There may be behaviour problems. The children may be uncomfortable having a different name from the rest of the family. The children's other parent may undermine relationships within the new unit. The advantages of adoption appear tempting since it gives all members of the family the same name, recognizes the family by law, resolves problems around inheritance and severs legal links with the previous family. There

are, however, disadvantages. The children may be confused since the adoption certificate registers both parents as adoptive parents. Children are legally separated from members of the previous family and when this involves grandparents it may cause unnecessary distress. The legal separation may emphasize the sense of loss experienced by most adopted children and obstruct the desired openness about origins which is recognized as being helpful to adopted children. There may also be practical disadvantages since the adoption severs any rights to inheritance from the other birth parent or that parent's family.

The Houghton Committee recognized that 'the legal extinguishment by adoption of a child's links with one half of his family was inappropriate and could be damaging'.[7] The Children Act 1989 introduced the strongly supported concept of parental responsibility which is shared by married birth parents, but lost to one through adoption into the new family. This loss is contrary to the philosophy of the Act and the courts are unlikely to grant an adoption order which would conflict with the principle of continued involvement.

Under the Act, the courts are able to make a different, possibly more appropriate order – a residence order. Under this order, which defines the arrangements about the person with whom a child is to live, that person also acquires parental responsibility. However, under a residence order the step-parent cannot agree to adoption nor can the child's name be changed. At the same time a contact order can be made in favour of the other birth parent and grandparents. In granting an adoption order under these circumstances, the court will consider the relationship between the child and the step-parent. If there is still meaningful contact with the birth parent and relatives, the court is less likely to agree to adoption. In any case, the court will wish to know the child's views and feelings and take them into account. When the application to adopt is made the local authority is required to investigate and report to the court. All those involved will be interviewed by a social worker. Useful information about the process is produced and regularly updated by BAAF and can also be obtained from the National Stepfamily Association.

The numbers of children adopted by their own parent or parents increased in the 1960s from 4369 in 1962 to 10 751 in 1971. Changes in practice resulted in a reduction in the 1980s to 2872 (31.8% of adoptions) which reflects the move from secrecy.

Developments in adoption practice

Open adoption

The closed model of adoption, which severs relationships with the child's birth parents, seemed entirely appropriate when legislation was introduced in 1926. Unmarried parents and the children escaped the contemporary stigma of illegitimacy and adopters gained the children they desperately wanted in an atmosphere of secrecy. Doubts about the closed model grew and were strengthened as more and more older children, with a well-developed history and considerable information about their birth families, were adopted. The problems associated with breaking parental contact for older children have been well documented.[23] Open adoption has been the subject of debate for several years. It is differently interpreted by adoption workers and might be better described as openness in adoption. At one end of the spectrum it is adoption with contact where information about a child's progress, sometimes including photographs, is passed to the birth parents directly or through the adoption agency. At the other end of the spectrum is open adoption where the birth parent is actively involved in the selection of adopters and meets them. Open adoption is more commonly practised when babies are placed and is popular with voluntary agencies. New Zealand has successfully promoted open adoption for a decade where the majority of birth parents help to choose adopters. Over 60% meet the adopters and post-placement contact in varying degrees is the norm.[24]

The impetus for change has come in different ways. First, studies in the 1960s by McWhinnie[1] and 1970s by Triseliotis[25] revealed the effect of secrecy about adoption on adopted people. The reluctance of some adoptive parents to tell children they were adopted and to share background information with them led to mistrust. Those adopted felt inferior and incomplete. The study by Triseliotis contributed to the legal changes which made it possible for adopted people to gain access to their birth records. Adopted people repeatedly ask for more openness in adoption and adoptive parents are now both better informed about birth parents and better prepared to tell children about adoption. A recent study by Craig confirms the benefits of openness for parents and children alike.[26]

Secondly, other studies have identified the long-term adverse effects on birth mothers required to relinquish their children.[27] The mothers felt continued anxiety about their children's past and present well-being and some entered a state of perpetual mourning. The expectation is that open adoption will make relinquishment easier for mothers and reduce the psychological impact. Follow up in New Zealand suggests that these expectations are realistic.[28]

When discussing open adoption it is useful to consider the possible advantages and disadvantages for the people involved.

The children

If open adoption enhances feelings of well-being and promotes a sense of identity and positive self-image, the behavioural and emotional difficulties which culminate around adolescence should be reduced. Open adoption avoids sudden revelations and the child will grow with an understanding that he has a biological and a psychological family. Long-term studies are awaited. Short-term ones are reassuring.[29]

The argument against open adoption proposes that attachment to the adoptive family is impeded by continued links with the birth family and that the child becomes confused. However, there is evidence that children can relate appropriately when the adults concerned behave harmoniously.[28] With older children, the maintenance of meaningful links helps them to settle into their new families.[30]

Birth parents

The adverse effects on birth mothers have been described above. Pannor and Barran report that open adoption helps birth parents to cope with loss and mourning.[31] The expectations of birth parents vary. The New Zealand study suggests that birth mothers do not seek lasting relationships with the adoptive families.[28]

Adoptive parents

The advantages for adoptive parents are less obvious. Open adoption should help adopters to acknowledge the difference between biological and adoptive parenthood. However, they are likely to be fearful and question whether they can be successful parents if not in full control. Being legally secure should minimize these fears. When older children are involved adopters largely reject continuing contact.[32]

Open adoption provides a challenge but its development seems inevitable. On balance the evidence to date supports greater openness in adoption. Further research will serve to advise about different types of contact and decisions should be made on a case-by-case basis to ensure that the child's best interests are met.

Inter-country adoption

Inter-country adoption (ICA) usually involves inter-cultural or transracial placement of a child. Until recently it occurred infrequently in Britain but, as the number of babies available for adoption became smaller, potential adopters have looked more often to ICA as a solution to their problems. ICA has been more widely practised in America (especially after the Second World War and the Korean conflict), Scandinavia and Holland and it is from these countries that most of the outcome studies emanate.[33]

Concern about the process centres on the removal of children from their own society and culture to be reared elsewhere. This concern is heightened when the motivating forces are the needs of childless couples in the west. When placements are made, without careful selection of the adopters or counselling for the natural parents, which may involve the exchange of money it is difficult to see that the interests of the child are being served. Debate therefore revolves around moral and practice issues.

Ngabonziza has recently provided a comprehensive overview of the subject by considering the three main types of ICA:[34]

1 Priority given to the needs of the child. In this situation there is identification of appropriate adoptive parents by a recognized agency with preparation of the child and family and supervision and monitoring of the placement.
2 Adoption undertaken by a relative in another country. In this situation the child remains connected to its own family even if the ties are tenuous.
3 Adopters seek children from abroad because children are not available in their own country. In this situation the children often come from deprived areas. Both they and their families are vulnerable to exploitation. In some cases the adopters look abroad because they have not been approved by a panel in Britain.

Ngabonziza acknowledges that in exceptional circumstances ICA may be in the child's best interests. However, Article 3 of the 1986 UN Declaration on Social and Legal Principles states that the first priority is for a child to be cared for by its own parents. The prime responsibility for individual states is to enable parents to do so. The resource implications are considerable but so are the amounts of money spent on ICA by adopters. Selman[35] and Tizard[36] rehearse the arguments for and against ICA and summarize the research on outcomes.

Hoksbergen makes the important point that while adoption has largely moved from being a service for childless couples to a service for children needing families, the move in ICA has been in the other direction.[33]

In Britain adopters engaged in ICA tend to be older and to have higher incomes than other adopters. Nearly 50% of adopters meet at least one birth parent and most of the adoptions are arranged through agencies.[37]

ICA process

There is no comprehensive record of the number of children brought into the UK for adoption. An application for entry clearance is made and processed by the local high commission, embassy or consulate. The application is considered by the Home Office and referred to the Department of Health for advice on adoption and welfare aspects. Until recently children could be brought into the UK without entry clearance and the Home Office identified only 50 to 75 such children annually.

Between 1984 and 1991, entry clearance was granted to 202 children. Of the 131 non-relative adoptions, 75% of the children were under 2 years of age. Over 50% of

the other 71 children were over 5 years of age and were adopted by relatives. Most of the children came from India.

Over the same period of time, 266 children entered the UK without entry clearance, all from Central and South America and 75% were less than 12 months old. The ratio of boys to girls was 3:4. The recent plight of Romanian children resulted in 278 coming to the UK with entry clearance during 1990 and 1991. A further 93 children entered without clearance. Ninety-five per cent of the children were less than 3 years old, 58% less than 12 months of age. The ratio of boys to girls was 2:3.

Outcomes

The general picture which emerges from research indicates that many of the children involved in ICA have poor or very poor health on arrival in their adoptive country. In Holland 59% were found to have a serious disease or malnutrition but by 2 years had made remarkable recoveries.[38] In Britain, more recently, nearly 50% of the children were in good health on arrival.[37]

Overall around 80% of the children progress satisfactorily.[39] There are issues of racial, cultural and personal identity for a substantial minority and educational performance is likely to be lower than that of other adopted and non-adopted children.[40]

The knowledge base about the outcomes of ICA is still limited. Experience to date suggests that, as with all adoptions, each child should be considered individually with careful pre-placement assessment and appropriate support during the placement and post-placement stages. Some children will have continuing health, emotional and educational problems.

In the UK there are no agencies who deal specifically with ICA. In America, where specialist agencies have evolved, there is concern that they lose their focus on the welfare of children and become agencies for finding families for childless couples.

Outcomes of adoption

Most adoption studies have considered the placement of babies, although some have looked at children with special needs. Overall it appears that less than 3% of placements break down before adoption becomes legal. Adoption remains popular and the outcomes are generally positive.

Many of the studies on adoption have looked at the characteristics of adoptive families and sought to define how natural and adoptive parenthood and the children differ. In 1964, Kirk concluded that adoption is most successful when the differences between being a natural and adoptive family are openly acknowledged thus allowing origins to be freely discussed.[41] This was a valuable study but did not give information about success rates since it did not include placements from which children were removed.

In Sweden, 168 children, who had been placed for adoption as babies, were followed and compared with children who were returned to their birth parents, children in foster homes and a sample from the general population. Success was based on school performance and the satisfaction of parents at the ages of 11, 15, 18 and 23 years. Overall the boys showed more maladjustment than the girls. The boys who were fostered or returned home fared less well than the adopted and control groups.[42] In Britain, Raynor and Kornitzer considered the satisfaction of adoptive parents and their children. Raynor found that 80% of 160 adopters and 85% of adoptees expressed satisfaction with their experiences.[43] Kornitzer studied 164 families covering adopted children and adults and reported that 75% were successful.[44]

The outcome of baby placements was studied by Lambert and Streather in 1980 as part of the longitudinal National Child Development Study conducted by the National Children's Bureau.[45] There were 145 adopted children and a control group. At 7 years they were doing well and 70% of placements were judged to be satisfactory and a further 20% as fairly satisfactory. At 11 years they were reported to be progressing well at school, but when corrections were made for social disadvantage their social adjustment was less good than children living with their birth parents.

Reassuringly, Kadushin reported in America that 78% of 91 placements of older children, aged 5 to 11 years, who had experienced multiple changes of care, neglect and ill-treatment, were judged by their adoptive families to be successful 6–10 years after placement.[46] In Britain, Triseliotis and Russell found that 82% of the 44 young adult adoptees, who were placed between the ages of 2 and 10 years, were enthusiastic about their placements. Objective measurements including alcohol abuse, criminal records and adjustment in later life confirmed an 80% success rate.[47]

Howe and Hinings found that adopted children were over-represented in a child guidance clinic.[48] Other studies suggest that adopted children display more problems in their middle and teenage years compared to children in matched control groups.[49] Evidence from adopted adults confirms that a small group have problems of identity.[13]

Other researchers have concentrated on the placement of black children. In America, Grow and Shapiro reported on the transracial placements of 125 black children.[50] Assessments were made of the children's attitude to race and parents and their teachers were interviewed. They concluded that 77% had adjusted successfully. Also in America, Zastrow found no difference in outcome, in terms of parental satisfaction, between 44 black children placed in white families and 44 same race placements of black children.[51] Of greater concern were the findings of Simon and Alstein that 20% of the adoptive families of 133 children, placed transracially and reviewed at 11 years, identified problems related to racial difference.[52]

Shireman and Johnson began a longitudinal study of 118 black children placed for adoption under the age of 3 years with single parents, black parents and white parents. Follow up at 4 and 8 years, on the basis of reports, observations and standardized tests, showed that for 79% adjustment was rated good or excellent. Further data will be collected.[53] The children in transracial placements were reported to have a good sense of racial identity at 8 years, but that it had not progressed to the same extent as it had for those children in same race families.

Some studies have specifically considered adoptive placements which have disrupted – though less than 3% disrupt before being legalized. Kadushin found a significant relationship between the age at placement and the outcome.[54] Over 10% of children in successful placements were aged 6 years or more. In failed placements this figure rose to 30%. Sibling placements are also more likely to disrupt and 28% of sibling placements failed compared with 1.2% when the children were placed singly. Since more children placed in sibling groups are also older at placement these factors appear to operate together.

Foster and other care

The phrase *in care* under the Children Act 1989 only refers to children who are subject to care orders. Previously the term included children who were *received* into care on a voluntary basis and others who had been *taken* into care on a court order. Now children are *looked after* by a local authority when they are provided with *accommodation* for more than 24 hours on a voluntary basis, namely by agreement with the parents or children themselves when they are aged 16 years or more, or as the result of a court order.

In the process of being looked after children may be placed with foster carers or in residential settings such as children's homes. Residential placements are used less frequently now, usually for young people rather than children, and may be made for a specific reason or when other arrangements have broken down. The duty of the local authority is to promote the safety and welfare of all children who are being looked after, working with their parents in a constructive way and taking account of the wishes of the children as well as their ethnic, cultural and religious needs.

The children involved

Many children enter the public care system with health, developmental, behavioural and educational problems resulting from material and emotional deprivation.

In a study by Bebbington and Miles of 2500 children admitted to care, deprivation was identified as a common factor among all the children.[55] Only 25% of the children were living with their parents, nearly 75% of the families received income support, over 50% lived in disadvantaged neighbourhoods and only one in five lived in owner-occupied housing. Other associated factors included overcrowding, young mothers, and parents who were of different racial origins. A further disturbing finding was that the association between deprivation and the need for local authority care was greater than that shown in an earlier study in the 1960s. A similar study by Wedge and Phelan found that contributory factors included disrupted family relationships, which occurred in over half of all admissions to care, and parental deprivation or ill health.[56] A recent study in Newcastle revealed that 60% of children placed with foster parents had experienced abuse or neglect at some time.[57]

Overall there has been a lack of emphasis on the health needs of these children, but some important information has emerged from various studies. The National Child Development Study (NCDS), a longitudinal study of a group of children born in 1958, showed a greater prevalence of developmental difficulties in children in care and that, at the age of 16 years, they were more likely to be clumsy and to have speech problems than their peers. The same study also showed that children who had been in care were more likely to be shorter and lighter at 7 years and enuretic at 11 years than their peers who had never been looked after by local authorities. Disability is common among those children who are looked after because their parents cannot or will not care for them or because they have been abused or neglected.

In papers commissioned to consider the physical and mental health needs of children in care, Wolkind concludes that the children are among the most vulnerable in terms of psychological disturbance[58] and Bamford deplores the lack of information about their physical health.[59] They suggest various reasons why these needs have been inadequately addressed to date.

The reasons include:

- The loss of a health advocate who is intimately familiar with the child's history or alert to symptoms which an ordinary parent would notice.
- The low priority given to history taking and medical examination coupled with a frequent absence of health information.
- The poor use of growth charts.
- The poor use of data from health records.

The requirements of the Children Act should ensure some remedies to these issues since there will be better collection of health information and thereby more efficient identification of needs so that appropriate treatment and support can be offered (Table 9.13).

The figures shown in Table 9.13 reflect changes in practice over the past decade which, by providing greater support to families, have reduced the total number of children admitted to care and increased the number of placements in foster homes. Information as it is currently collected does not, unfortunately, indicate the turnover of children nor the number of placements they experience.

With regard to black children, Rowe found that they were over-represented, accounting for 19% of admissions to care. Asian children were under-represented in all age groups, while African and Afro-Caribbean children were over-represented particularly in the preschool children and those aged 5–10 years (Table 9.14).[60]

Bebbington and Miles calculated that children of mixed racial parentage were 2.5 times as likely to be looked after as white children especially in the preschool age group.[55] As a group they also experienced multiple re-admissions to care.

The low figures for Asian children possibly reflects the support of the extended family, but may suggest that child care services are not acceptable to their parents.

Table 9.13 Number of children in care (England and Wales) DOH

	1980	1990
Total	100158	63810
Percentage		
a) By age		
under one year	1.4	2.7
1–4 years	9.2	14.8
5–9 years	19.0	20.1
10–15 years	46.3	39.1
16 years and over	24.2	23.2
b) By sex		
boys	58.9	53.7
girls	41.1	46.3
Manner of accommodation (%)		
	1979	1989
Foster home	36.0	55.0
With relative or friend	18.4	14.2
Community home	30.8	17.7
Other	14.8	13.1

A further breakdown of a representative sample revealed that foster homes provided the following percentage of placements:

0–4 years	77
5–10 years	65
11 years or more	15

Table 9.14 Percentage of admissions to care

White	81%
Mixed parentage	8%
Afro-Caribbean	6%
African	2%
Asian	1%
Other	2%
Total number of children	3748

From Rowe[60]

The fostering service

Since, overall, 55% of the children who are looked after by local authorities are placed with foster parents it is important to consider the fostering service.

Foster care is the preferred way of providing care and nurture in a family setting for children who cannot be cared for by their own families and who are not placed for adoption. Fostering is a skilled task and foster parents are important members of the professional team concerned with child care.

Foster parents do not automatically acquire parental responsibility for the children in their care. When children are accommodated it is retained by the parents; when children are subject to court orders it is shared by the parents and the local authority. However, under section 3(5) of the Children Act, foster parents may do 'what is reasonable to promote the child's welfare'.

The fostering task

Children may be placed in a foster home for a variety of reasons and for each child the nature and purpose of the placement has to be defined. Thus foster care may be provided on a short-term or long-term basis. The usual limit to the number of foster children in a family is three. This does not apply to larger sibling groups; it may also be in the best interests of a child to limit the number to one.

Examples of short-term placements include care given during a family crisis or that provided for a baby before an adoption placement is identified. Respite care is a specialized short-term service provided for families and other carers. By offering short breaks for families with disabled or chronically ill children, admission to residential care may be avoided. Some short-term placements address a specific task and help to prepare disadvantaged or disturbed children for a move to a more permanent home. These placements offer a specialist bridging service whereby children can experience, often for the first time, stability in a family setting. In this way the risk of disruption of adoptive placements is reduced.

Long-term fostering more frequently involves older children who do not want to be adopted or for whom adoption is not viable because of the extent of their disturbance or emotional damage. The regulations require that the placement plan agreed between parents, the agency and the foster parents states the expected duration of the placement. In this way placements do not drift and decisions about rehabilitation with the birth family or placement in a permanent substitute family are kept to the fore.

Recruitment of foster carers

Foster parents may be recruited during local campaigns for general or specialized schemes or for a child with specific needs. Precisely focused campaigns may be used to attract carers from particular racial, cultural or religious groups.

Assessment and approval of foster parents

Potential foster parents are assessed by social workers who are required to explore attitudes, family lifestyles, relationships and accommodation. Specific items for discussion include the applicants' understanding of racial, cultural and religious issues and they have to undertake not to use any form of physical punishment. The upper age limit applied to foster parents is more flexible than that usually applied to adopters but the general health and mental health status of all applicants are scrutinized and police records are consulted. Foster carers have access to any medical reports supplied about them under the Access to Medical Reports Act 1988. The applicants are required to name two referees both of whom have to be interviewed by a social worker. Once the assessment process has been satisfactorily completed a report is considered for approval by a fostering or combined fostering and adoption panel. Approval is confirmed in writing and the nature of the service being offered clearly defined. This is important since the demands of the various types of fostering are very different. Family members may be assessed and approved as foster carers of children related to them.

The Foster Placement (Children) Regulations 1991 replace the Boarding-out of Children (Foster Placement) Regulations 1988. The emphasis of the new regulations is on approval of foster parents rather than a household as previously. Better regulation of foster homes has been achieved by the new arrangements which allow foster parents to be approved by only one local authority or voluntary organization responsible for child placement. Having been approved, the foster parents can be used by other agencies subject to the consent of the approving agency or organization. The assessment process includes preparation for the fostering task but continuing support and training is essential. The former is supplied by social workers and other experienced foster parents who form local networks. Training may be arranged at local level with participation of health professionals. The National Foster Care Association (NFCA) serves to promote good foster care. It has developed valuable training programmes and a counselling and advisory service for foster carers.

Foster parents are paid allowances which vary between agencies. Enhanced payments may reflect the age and special needs of each child.

Private foster care

Private fostering describes an arrangement made by a parent for the care of a child within a family for more than 28 days by a person who is not a relative. The proposal to foster has to be notified to the local authority who has to visit the home and be satisfied that the arrangements are satisfactory and that the child's health, developmental, emotional, educational and social needs are met. Medical reports on the children are recommended but not required. However, when medical advice is sought, general practitioners may be the first to learn of privately fostered children since all arrangements are not regularly reported.

Private foster carers are not assessed and approved in the same way as other foster parents and they do not have to be registered. The usual upper limit of three children applies unless the placement involves a larger sibling group. Financial arrangements are agreed between the foster carers and the parents.

Other family care situations

Children on care orders may be placed back with their parents most commonly during the period leading up to the discharge of the order. Under these circumstances the local authority has to review the accommodation, consider other members of the household, review contact with other family members, identify the child's health and educational needs and define the support services that are required. A check on police records is made and medical advice about the carers' health status is sought.

Childminding

Childminders provide day care in a family setting for children up to the age of 8 years. They are required to keep records of the children in their care. The local authority maintains a register of childminders and inspects accommodation, equipment and arrangements for play out of doors. Fitness to care for children is carefully considered and takes account of the minder's physical and mental health. Prospective childminders are required to supply references and police checks are undertaken. The recommended childminder : child ratios are:

- 1:3 for children aged less than 5 years
- 1:6 for children aged between 5 and 7 years
- 1:6 for children aged less than 8 years of whom no more than three are under 5 years.

In all cases the ratios include the childminder's own children.

Childminders are recommended to agree a contract with parents to cover fees, times for leaving and collecting the children, diet, behaviour management and other matters. A model contract has been prepared by the National Childminding Association.

Health care for children who are looked after by local authorities or voluntary organizations

The relevant responsible authority or organization is required to act as a caring parent and to adopt a positive approach to health surveillance as well as the treatment of illness and accidents. Many of the children concerned have received irregular or inadequate health care and some may have complex conditions such as multiple disabilities, learning difficulties, emotional and behavioural disturbances and poor growth. Problems may emerge after some time, so continuing review is essential. A child may come from a dysfunctional family, apparently in satisfactory health, only to disclose previously unsuspected abuse at a much later date, when feeling secure enough to share the pain with the carers. Under these circumstances foster parents need easy access to support and advice in order to respond in a sensitive, constructive way to assist the child's recovery.

A child in foster care must be registered with a general practitioner and receive dental care. Under the Arrangements for Placement of Children (General) Regulations 1991, a medical examination and written health assessment are required before placement, if possible, or as soon as is practicable afterwards if not. In either case a comprehensive health and developmental assessment is recommended using an appropriate BAAF form.[61]

When an urgent placement is arranged a preliminary medical report is compiled to provide basic information for the carers. A comprehensive examination can be undertaken within the following weeks. In this way a baseline is provided from which to monitor the child's health and development while in foster care. Under the Review of Children's Cases Regulations 1991, further health and developmental assessments are required at 6-monthly intervals for children under 2 years of age and at yearly intervals thereafter. Further examinations are recommended before each change of school or as indicated by the child's needs.

Medical and developmental examinations may be undertaken by a general practitioner, community child health doctor, paediatrician or other specialist. Arrangements vary depending upon local preferences and resources. Unlike the Adoption Agencies Regulations, there is no provision under the Children Act for a named medical adviser to agencies who look after children. However, in all cases, specialist advice must be available to the responsible authority to interpret the reports and advise on health care. Frequently the specialist advice is provided by the medical adviser to the adoption panel or a child health colleague.

A copy of the medical report is sent to the child's general practitioner and other relevant health professionals. The foster parents must have comprehensive, written information about any child in their care and this includes details of the child's health and health needs. It is common practice to provide a foster parent with a copy of the medical report. To avoid fragmentation of health information contacts with health professionals can be recorded in a parent- (or carer-) held child health record. Older children can be encouraged to contribute to a health record and usually enjoy doing so. A suitable booklet, *My Health Passport*, has been published by BAAF and has been used enthusiastically by children aged 8 years and over.

Consent to examination or treatment

Issues around consent have been identified in Section 9.3 and are usefully discussed in a BAAF practice note.[62]

Arrangements for consent must be clearly defined for children who are fostered and will vary according to whether or not the local authority has parental responsibility. A parent, or the local authority, can delegate authority to give consent to examination or treatment to a foster parent. A suitable card has been designed for this purpose by NFCA. Whenever possible, major procedures should be discussed with parents and they should be kept informed of health matters. Young people of 16 and over can give or withhold consent to examination and treatment. Younger children, if judged by the doctor to understand the implications of the situation, have the same rights. However, it is the responsibility of the agency, while informing children of their rights, to encourage them to understand the importance of health care and treatment.

Although the proportion of children being looked after by agencies in foster homes continues to increase, 15–18% of the group as a whole are placed in community homes. For them the health care requirements are the same as those outlined above for foster children. A health record for each child is kept in the community home in addition to separate records which are maintained by general practitioners, the community child health service and others.

Outcomes

In 1991, the Department of Health published an important review of the outcomes of children placed in foster homes, residential units and for adoption.[63] The document emphasizes the need to rehabilitate the family quickly if lengthy separations are to be avoided. Most children who remain separate from their families after 6 weeks continue to do so for a very long time. Only one child in three ceases to be looked after by a local authority in less than one month. By 6 months only 50% have returned home. After 6 months one child in three continues to be looked after for more than one year. When separation is unavoidable the need for permanence of placement is stressed. The lack of security implicit in many fostering arrangements of the 1960s and 1970s contributed to the high breakdown rate of around 50% within 5 years of placement reported by George and others.[64]

Rowe and her colleagues studied a group of children who had been in foster homes for more than 5 years; most had been placed when under 5 years of age. Emotional disturbance was reported in 30% of the children and was thought to reflect the sense of insecurity identified by parents and children.[65]

With regard to the breakdown of foster placements, Berridge and Cleaver found that up to 40% of children placed with strangers experienced disruption. Breakdown appeared to be related to the higher ages of children at placement and the presence of a natural child of the foster family whose age was similar to or younger than the foster child.[66] Other factors include previous placement breakdown, unsuccessful attempts to return home, ambivalence or opposition on the part of the child to the placement, unrealistic expectations of the care giver, severe behaviour problems and loss of contact with relatives and friends.

In 1984, Triseliotis and Russell reviewed 40 adults who had grown up in foster homes. In 60% of the sample, satisfaction was expressed by the parents and those fostered and a further 15% were satisfied but had experienced difficulties.[47]

More recently, Rowe and colleagues undertook a large-scale survey of foster care placements. Success rates varied between authorities from 56% to 69%.[60] It is now recognized that when trying to assess the level of success it is helpful to differentiate between various placement arrangements. Not surprisingly, placements made with a view to adoption are among the most successful. Foster placements with relatives are also stable.

Most short-term placements are thought by parents and children to have achieved what was intended, usually support during a family emergency.[67]

Medium-term placements are frequently made to achieve a specific purpose or to effect a change in behaviour or relationships and are less successful.[60]

Long-term placements usually involve older children and are more frequently associated with problems of rehabilitation.[68]

Few young people leave care with academic qualifications and this reflects the low expectations of achievement that frequently operate. Research has shown that being in care is not the cause of educational failure. Children bring their problems with them into a system which fails to remedy their deficiencies. It has been shown that children with below average attainments fare no worse in foster homes than similar children receiving support in their own homes.[69] The reason why they do not do better is perhaps because they lack a sense of permanence in their placements.[70] This theory is supported by Garnett's finding that children who have grown up in care in settled placements have higher educational achievements than children who enter the care system, at a later date, from dysfunctional families.[71]

Leaving the system

Young people cease to be looked after by an agency at the age of 18 years, but still need support as much as ever. Many foster parents continue to maintain contact after the official age of providing care. One young person summed up his situation, 'It's not being in care. What matters is when you've got to leave it. Where are you gonna be? Where are you gonna go? What's gonna happen?'[72] Research shows that many young people become homeless and that the proportion of those leaving care who are unemployed is higher than the local average.[73] Garnett found that one in seven of the girls leaving care was already pregnant.[71] Young men who have been looked after are over-represented among male prostitutes and many start adult life with a prison sentence.[73,74]

It is therefore important to note the recommendations given in the guidance on the Children Act in relation to preparation for leaving care.[75] Three broad aspects to preparation are identified:

- Enabling young people to build and maintain relationships with others (general and sexual relationships).
- Enabling young people to develop their self-esteem.
- Teaching practical and financial skills and knowledge.

Among the latter are listed health education, sex education and registration with a doctor and dentist.

Practice and policy issues surrounding adoption and fostering are still evolving and varying degrees of change are inevitable. However, what is undertaken to serve the best interests of the children concerned will also, hopefully, serve their best interests as adults.

Useful addresses in the UK

British Agencies for Adoption and Fostering (BAAF)
11 Southwark Street
London SE1 1RQ

National Foster Care Association
Francis House
Francis Street
London SW1P 1DE

Parents for Children
41 Southgate Road
London N1 3JP

Thomas Coram Foundation for Children
40 Brunswick Square
London WC1N 1AZ

Post-adoption Centre
8 Torriano Mews
Torriano Avenue
London NW5 2RZ

Independent Adoption Service
121-123 Camberwell Road
London SE5 0HB

National Stepfamily Association
72 Willesden Lane
London NW6 7TA

National Childminding Association
8 Masons Hill
Bromley
Kent BR2 9EY

Parent to Parent Information on Adoption Services
Lower Boddington
Daventry
Northants NN11 6YB

References

1 McWhinnie, A. *Adopted Children, How They Grow Up.* London : Routledge and Kegan Paul, 1966.
2 Triseliotis, J. *Evaluation of Adoption Policy and Practice.* Edinburgh: University of Edinburgh, 1970.
3 *Committee on Child Adoption* (Hopkinson, A., chairman). London: HMSO, 1921. (Cmnd 1254.)
4 *Child Adoption Committee* (Tomlin, J., chairman). London: HMSO, 1925. (Cmnd 2401.)
5 *Committee on the Care of Children* (Curtis, J., chairman). London: HMSO, 1946. (Cmnd 6922.)
6 Row, J., Lambert, L. *Children Who Wait.* London: Association of British Adoption Agencies, 1973.
7 *Committee on the Adoption of Children* (Houghton, D., chairman). London: HMSO, 1972. (Cmnd 5107.)
8 Department of Health and Social Security. *Adoption Agencies Regulations 1983.* London: HMSO, 1984. (LAC(84)3, HC(84)1).
9 Adoption of Children Act 1976.
10 British Agencies for Adoption and Fostering. *Using the BAAF Medical Forms: Practice Note 27.* London: BAAF, 1991.
11 Chennells, P. *Explaining Adoption to your Adopted Child.* London: BAAF, 1987.
12 Brodzinsky, D. New perspectives on adoption revelation. *Adoption Fostering* 1984; **2**: 27–32.
13 Triseliotis, J.P. Identity and security in adoption and long term fostering. *Adoption Fostering* 1983; **1**: 22–31.
14 Thorburn, J., Rowe, J. A snapshot of permanent family placement. *Adoption Fostering* 1988; **3**: 29–34.
15 O'Hara, J., Hoggan, P. Permanent substitute family care in Lothian: placement outcomes. *Adoption Fostering* 1988; **3**: 35–38.
16 Wolkind, S., Kozaruk, A. The adoption of children with medical handicap. *Adoption Fostering* 1983; **1**: 32–40.

17 Wolkind, S., Kozaruk, A. 'Hard-to-place' children with medical and developmental problems. In: Wedge, P., Thorburn, J. eds. *Finding Families for 'Hard-to-Place' Children*. London: BAAF, 1986.

18 Wedge, P., Mantle, G. The placement of sibling groups with permanent substitute families. Norwich: University of East Anglia, 1990.

19 British Agencies for Adoption and Fostering. *The Placement of Black Children. Practice Note 13*. London: BAAF, 1987.

20 Tizard, B., Pheonix, A. Black identity and transracial adoption. *New Community* 1989; **15**: 427–437.

21 Department of Health, Social Services Inspectorate. *Issues of Race and Culture in the Family Placement of Children*. London: HMSO, 1990. (C1(90)2.)

22 Masson, J., Nobury, D., Chatterton, S.G. *Mine, Yours or Ours? A Study of Step-parent Adoption*. London: HMSO, 1983.

23 Triseliotis, J. Adoption with contact. *Adoption Fostering* 1985; **4**: 19–24.

24 Mullender, A. The spread of openness in New Zealand: the two ends of the process meeting in the middle. In: Mullender, A., ed. *Open Adoption BAAF Practice Series 19*. London: BAAF, 1991.

25 Triseliotis, J. *In Search of Origins*. London: Routledge and Kegan Paul, 1973.

26 Craig, M. *Adoption: Not a Big Deal*. Edinburgh: Department of Social Policy and Social Work, Edinburgh University, 1990.

27 Bouchier, P., Lambert, L., Triseliotis, J. *Parting with a Child for Adoption*. London: BAAF, 1991.

28 Dominick, C. Early contact in adoption: contact between birth mothers and adoptive parent at the time of and after adoption. Research Series 10. Wellington: Department of Social Work, 1988.

29 Fox, N. Attachment of Kibbutz infants to mother and metapelet. *Child Dev* 1977; **48**: 1228–1239.

30 Fratter, J. *Family Placement and Access*. London: Barnar, 1989.

31 Pannor, R., Barran, A. Open adoption as standard practice. *Child Welfare* 1984; **3**: 245–250.

32 Lambert, L., Buist, M., Triseliotis, J., Hill, M. Freeing children for adoption. *Adoption Fostering* 1990; **1**: 36–41.

33 Hoksbergen, R.A.C. *Adoption in Worldwide Perspective*. Lisse: Swets and Zertlinger, 1986.

34 Ngabonziza, D. Inter-country adoption. *Adoption Fostering* 1988; **1**: 35–40.

35 Selman, P. *Inter-country Adoption: What can Britain Learn from European Countries?* Newcastle: Newcastle University, 1990.

36 Tizard, B. Inter-country adoption. A review of the evidence. *J Child Psychol Psychiatr* 1991; **5**: 743–756.

37 International Bar Association. *The Inter-country Adoption Process from the UK: the Adoptive Parents' Perspective*. London: IBA, 1991.

38 Hoksbergen, R.A.C. Inter-country adoption. Coming of age in Netherlands: basic issues, trends and developments. In: Alstein, H., Simon, R.J., eds. *Inter-country Adoption*. New York: Praeger, 1991.

39 Thorburn, J. *A Review of Research which is Relevant to Adoption*. London: Department of Health, 1990.

40 Dalen, M., Saetersdal, B. Transracial adoption in Norway. *Adoption Fostering* 1987; **4**: 41–46.

41 Kirk, D. *Shared Fate*. London: Collier-Macmillan, 1964.

42 Bohman, M., Siguardsson, S. Negative social heritage. *Adoption Fostering* 1980; **3**: 25–32.

43 Raynor, L. *The Adopted Child Comes of Age*. London: Allen and Unwin, 1980.

44 Kornitzer, M. *Adoption and Family Life*. London: Collier-Macmillan, 1980.

45 Lambert, L., Streather, J. *Children in Changing Families*. London: Macmillan, 1980.

46 Kadushin, A. *Adopting Older Children*. New York: Columbia University Press, 1970.

47 Triseliotis, J.P., Russell, J. *Hard to Place: the Outcome of Adoption and Residential Care*. Aldershot: Gower, 1984.

48 Howe, D., Hinings, D. Adopted children referred to a child and family centre. *Adoption Fostering* 1987; **3**: 44–47.

49 Humphrey, M., Humphrey, H. *Families with a Difference*. London: Routledge, 1988.

50 Grow, L.J., Shapiro, D. *Black Children–White Parents: a Study of Transracial Adoption*. New York: Child Welfare League of America, 1974.

51 Zastrow, C.H. *Outcomes of Black Children – White Parents Transracial Adoptions*. San Francisco: R and E Research Associates, 1977.

52 Simon, R.J., Alstein, H. *Transracial Adoption*. New York: Wiley, 1977.

53 Shireman, J., Johnson, P. A longitudinal study of black adoptions. *Social Work* 1986; **31**: 172–176.

54 Kadushin, A., Seidl, F.W. Adoption failure: a social work post-mortem. *Social Work* 1971; **16**: 37.

55 Bebbington, A., Miles, J. The background of children who enter local authority care. *Br J Social Work* 1989; **19**: 349–368.

56 Wedge, P., Phelan, J. The impossible demands of child care. *Social Work Today* 1988; **19**.

57 Stone, J. *Children in Care: the Role of Short Term Fostering*. Newcastle-upon-Tyne: Social Services Department, 1990.

58 Wolkind, S. *The Mental Health of Children in Care: Research Needs*. London: Economic and Social Research Council, 1988.

59 Bamford, F. *The Physical Health of Children in Care: Research Needs*. London: Economic and Social Research Council, 1988.

60 Rowe, J., Hundleby, M., Garnett, L. *Child Care Now: A Survey of Placement Patterns*. London: BAAF, 1989.

61 British Agencies for Adoption and Fostering. *Using the BAAF Medical Forms. Practice Note 27*. London: BAAF, 1991.

62 British Agencies for Adoption and Fostering. *Consent to Medical Treatment for Children. Practice Note 23*. London: BAAF, 1991.

63 Department of Health. *Patterns and Outcomes of Child Placement*. London: HMSO, 1991.

64 George, V. *Fostercare*. London: Routledge and Kegan Paul, 1970.

65 Rowe, J., Cain, H., Hundleby, M., Keane, A. *Long-term Foster Care*. London: Batsford, 1984.

66 Berridge, D., Cleaver, H. *Foster Home Breakdown*. Oxford: Blackwell, 1987.

67 Packman, J., Randall, J., Jaques, N. *Who Needs Care?* Oxford: Blackwell, 1986.

68 Farmer, E., Parker, R. *Trials and Tribulations: Returning Children from Care to their Families*. London: HMSO, 1991.

69 Heath, A., Colton, M., Aldgate, J. Educational progress of children in and out of care. *Br J Social Work* 1989; **19**: 447–460.

70 Aldgate, J. Foster children at school: success or failure? *Adoption Fostering* 1990; **14**: 38–49.

71 Garnett, L. *Leaving Care for Independence: a Follow-up Study to the Placement Outcome Project*. London: HMSO, 1990.

72 Stein, M., Carey, K. *Leaving Care*. Oxford: Blackwell, 1986.

73 Stein, M. *Leaving Care and the 1989 Children Act*. Oxford: First Key, 1991.

74 Minty, B. *Child Care and Adult Crime*. Manchester: Manchester University Press, 1988.

75 Department of Health. *The Children Act 1989, Guidance and Regulations for Residential Care*. London: HMSO, 1991.

Chapter 10

Neurological problems

10.1 Development of the central nervous system

Bert Touwen

There are two main aspects to the development of the central nervous system: morphological and functional. Much is known about each separately but less about how they interrelate. This section will discuss both aspects.

Structural development

About the third week after conception the neural plate is formed by a thickening of the ectodermal cells on the dorsal aspect of the embryo. This event marks the onset of a process called neurulation in which the first phase of neural tube formation occurs with development of the neural folds and neural groove, and closure of the anterior and posterior neuropores. In the second phase of neural tube formation (less precise than neurulation) there is significant differentiation of the neural axis with neuronal proliferation occurring in the germinal matrix around the central canal and ventricles, and then migration of these cells to their definitive locations. This process reaches its peak around 12 weeks after conception and is practically complete by 24 weeks after conception (Fig. 10.1).[1] This process is followed by outgrowth of axons and dendrites from the cells and the formation of synapses. The latter processes continue during postnatal life, and result in the network production which is so characteristic of the central nervous system.

While axonal, dentritic and synapse formation is occurring, physiological neuronal cell death is also taking place in many areas particularly in the spinal cord.[2,3]

Myelination and transmitter production take place in parallel to the axonal growth and synapse formation, and all these processes continue postnatally with qualitative and quantitative differences. Around birth, muscle fibres are multiply innervated but soon after, retraction of axons occurs and the muscle fibres then display mononeuronal innervation.[4]

In the cortex, where structural layering is completed during the last months of pregnancy and the first postnatal months, network formation and synapse production are especially impressive during the first years of life. At the end of the first year synapse density reaches its maximum, but thereafter it decreases until adult densities are reached at the age of about 7 years.[5,6] Synapse elimination seems to be an active, genetically steered process, although competition between neurones cannot be excluded, which takes place in various cortical areas at the same time.[6]

Glial cell proliferation, which also starts very early in pregnancy, continues during the postnatal years. Glial cells play a role in metabolic processes, and furnish a frame for the neuronal networks.

When all these processes are taken together it appears that most of the morphological changes take place after mid-pregnancy. It is then necessary to question how they relate to the development of brain function.

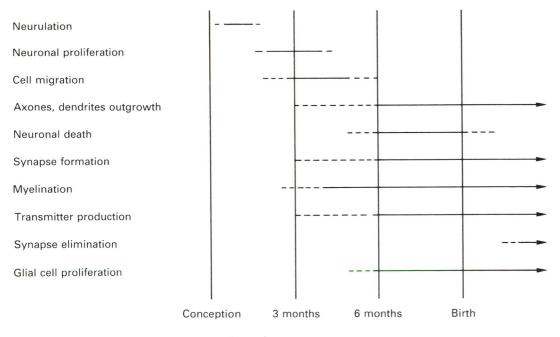

Neurulation

Neuronal proliferation

Cell migration

Axones, dendrites outgrowth

Neuronal death

Synapse formation

Myelination

Transmitter production

Synapse elimination

Glial cell proliferation

Conception   3 months   6 months   Birth

Figure 10.1 Neural developmental processes during human ontogeny.

Timing of possible insults

The central nervous system is most vulnerable to damage during periods of rapid change which is when the constituents of the neural networks are being formed. Teratogenic substances, such as drugs, are especially damaging in the early weeks of pregnancy. For example, the anticonvulsant drug sodium valproate can cause neural tube defects if taken in the third week after conception during neurulation.[7] Irradiation, rubella and hepatitis B viruses have their main damaging effects in the first trimester of pregnancy during neuronal proliferation. Maternal alcoholism appears to have a teratogenic effect at and following the second and the third month of gestation.[7]

Infections with organisms such as cytomegalovirus or *Toxoplasma gondii* can damage the neural developmental processes over a much longer period – throughout pregnancy. Cytomegalovirus transmission through the placenta seems to be particularly clinically significant when occurring during the first two trimesters of pregnancy.[8] Toxoplasmosis is similarly most devastating in early pregnancy, although the protection against materno–fetal transmission is also greatest at that stage. Late third trimester infections may be asymptomatic, but this does not preclude a poor prognosis. In contrast to cytomegaloviral infections which can be both teratogenic and inflammatory, toxoplasma infection is mainly inflammatory.[7]

Damage to the developing nervous system from maternal or fetal metabolic disease will depend in part on the protective or compensatory effect of the placenta. In some instances neural damage may occur after birth when this protective mechanism is removed. While myelination occurs from mid-pregnancy onwards, it becomes particularly important postnatally when absent or disordered myelination will be evident by slow developmental progress. Migration failures, which are said to be responsible for some types of epilepsy and dyslexia, come about during the second trimester. Circulation disturbances have different effects according to the timing of their occurrence. All conditions able to cause reduced blood flow to the uterus may lead to an impairment of fetal oxygenation. Maternal hypotension from any cause, even anxiety, occurring at any point in pregnancy or labour can do this, especially if the fetus is already at risk, for example from intrauterine growth retardation.[9] From the developmental angle, the parts of the nervous system which are metabolically most active need intensive vascularization. These areas are notably the germinal matrix around the central canal and ventricles during the phase of cell proliferation and initial migration and, at later fetal ages, those areas to which the cells have migrated where axonal ramification and synapse formation are taking place, e.g. the cortex and basal ganglia. As a result, watershed zones arise, due to topographical organization of the vascularization of the brain. Thus hypoxic and ischaemic attacks have different effects depending on the stage of neural development resulting in periventricular leucomalacia and haemorrhage in young preterm babies and cortical and basal ganglia involvement in term infants. Primary haemorrhages are subependymal with or without rupture into the ventricular system. Their prognosis is relatively good. They are usually due to hyperperfusion followed by a breakdown of the capillary bed. The haemodynamic background is hypoxia. Rupture into cerebral parenchyma may occur, leading to cyst formation or (asymmetrical) ventricular dilatation.

When ischaemia is present, periventricular leucomalacia (PVL) or subcortical leucomalacia may occur, often followed by secondary haemorrhagic infarction; porencephalic cysts may arise, and the prognosis depends largely on their occurrence, size and location. PVL with cystic degeneration may develop *in utero* or show itself up to at least a month postnatally. Neurological sequelae can postpone their appearance until the destroyed areas reach the time when they would normally display their specific function.

Functional development

Ultrasound studies have shown that in normal fetuses the first signs of movement can be discerned at about 7–8 weeks post-conceptional age, and that the movement repertoire of the fetus expands astonishingly fast. At 20 weeks' gestation, all the types of movements are present which are found in the normal term fetus; they consist of well organized and complex patterns (Table 10.1). Remarkably, there is no distinct cranio-cerebral or proximodistal sequence in the development of these types of subcortically mediated movements, which are thought to be important for a proper development of joints, musculature, skin, lungs and intestine; in general they reflect their postnatal counterparts by which time gravity is impinging on the infant.[10,11]

When the temporal patterns of morphological and functional development are compared, there seems only a weak relationship. Direct contact between motor neurones and muscle fibres, and between afferent and efferent cells in the spinal cord coincide with the first discernible fetal movements,[12] but the large range of movement types develops in the period in which the major morphological processes are as yet in their very beginning, i.e. in the first trimester of pregnancy. It seems that a very low level of structural development is sufficient for the primary types of movements described. That movement occurs to this degree at this stage is proof of the capacity of the very immature fetal brain to generate active motor patterns (besides the reactions and reflexes which were shown by Hooker and Humphrey in the 1930s and 1940s).[13,14]

So far as our knowledge goes, it seems that an enormous expansion of brain architecture is needed for adequate and adaptive use of the motor capacities which become so evident postnatally. The recognition that the central nervous system is not required merely for movement, but rather for the quality of movement, for example, through its ability to use movements for various functions or to perform seemingly similar movements in various ways is important in the early detection of abnormal movement patterns and developmental deviations. For instance, although movement patterns of term and even more of preterm newborn infants are limited compared with those of older infants or a young child, they have a highly variable character compared with those of a neurologically deviant newborn who moves in a monotonous and stereotyped way.[15–17] This is also seen in prenatal life: growth-retarded fetuses show less variable movements than normal fetuses.[18]

Postnatal development

Normal sensorimotor function displays much variability. Conversely, stereotypic functional patterns (those showing a lack of variability) suggest developmental disturbance. It should be remembered that the maturational phase of the neonatal brain does not permit specifically localized function and that the very young brain has only a limited number of ways, syndromes or constellations of signs, in which to express its dysfunction (Table 10.2).

During infancy, variability increases in order to respond to environmental influences and limitation of variability is an early sign of developmental disturbance.[19] An infant who is consistently late with three or four sensorimotor items has a high risk of abnormal development.[20] A list of stereotypes which can be considered as alarm symptoms for deviant development is given in Table 10.3.

After infancy

A toddler shows increasingly adaptive variability in contrast to the indiscriminate variations of the infant. It is as if the toddler is beginning to select strategies for specific purposes. Sensorimotor functions become child specific rather than age specific.

Table 10.1 Characteristics of fetal motor patterns[11]

Character	Type of movement
Slow	Generalized, head, hand to face, stretches
Fast	Startles, hiccups
Slow and fast	Arm, leg and jaw
Steady increase	Breathing, rotation of the head, jaw opening, sucking and swallowing
Increase until plateau	Generalized, arm
Increase followed by decrease	Extension of the head, startles, hiccups, hand to face
Neither increase nor decrease	Leg, forward flexion of the head, yawns, stretches

Table 10.2 Neonatal neurological syndromes

Syndrome	Presentation
Abnormal excitability	Seizures
	Hyperexcitability: hyperkinesis, irritability, tremulousness, hyperreflexia
	Apathy: floppy and poorly responsive, hypotonia, hyporeflexia, reduced movement
	Coma
Abnormal muscle tone	Hypertonia
	Hypotonia
Abnormal movement patterns	Jittery, hyperkinesis, hypokinesis, later involuntary movements
Asymmetry of movement	
Central hemisyndrome	Asymmetric posture and movements
Peripheral hemisyndrome	Interruption of reflex arc, e.g. brachial plexus lesion
Brainstem syndromes	Deviation of eyes
	Abnormal eye movements
	Hyperreflexic brainstem responses e.g. snout reflex, glabella reflex (both of these are often accompanied by retrojection of the head), vestibulo-ocular response (doll's eye phenomenon) and Moro response
	Dissociated responses between head/trunk and limbs i.e. absent brainstem responses and eye movements combined with generalized hypertonia and hyperreflexia (serious) or vice versa (often less serious, and more frequent)
Structural defects	Spina bifida cystica
	Hydrocephalus
Combinations	

Table 10.3 Alarm symptoms in infancy

1 Poverty of movement
2 Stereotyped postures, e.g. fisting, arm flexion, clawing of toes, equinovarus. May be unilateral or bilateral
3 Neglect of limbs
4 Infant slips through hands in vertical suspension
5 Head lag during traction or sitting
6 Tremor during voluntary movements when not crying
7 Restless, awkward and fidgety movements of trunk, face and tongue. Rapid jerky movements of the limbs
8 Extended posture at hip, knees and feet in vertical suspension
9 Extension of the legs in vertical suspension with the baby swaying to and fro and side to side. This is abnormal in a baby over 5 months corrected age
10 Persisting asymmetric tonic neck reflex
11 Opisthotonic posture with extension of head, neck and spine
12 Sitting posture on lumbosacral spine not upright on buttocks
13 Poorly reactive to sound
14 Poor following movements of the eyes. Visual lack of interest
15 Persisting strabismus
16 Abnormal rate of change in growth of head circumference
17 Setting sun phenomenon, vomiting, wide sutures, tense fontanelle
18 Delayed functional development

Table 10.4 Alarm symptoms in a toddler

1	General	Global delay, any stereotyped movement or posture, fidgety, toddling* still apparent after age $2\frac{1}{2}$–3 years, strabismus, impaired eye movements and ability to localize sound, poorly alert
2	Sitting	Rounded back with legs extended, sitting between knees when kneeling, impaired rotation
3	Stance	Clawing of toes, asymmetrical balance on instep, scissoring or marked adduction of legs, impaired balance, inability to pick up object from floor (after 2 years), Gower's sign positive – climbing up the legs with the arms when rising from the floor
4	Gait	Toe walking, clawing of toes, impaired balance, circumduction of one leg, scissoring or marked adduction of legs, broad based and no rotation of trunk (after 3 years)
5	Hand function	Excessive laterality, tremulous, over grasp, difficulty handling more than one small object at a time, mirror movements

* Toddling: this describes the characteristic stiff legged gait of toddlers or very young children seen between 1 and $2\frac{1}{2}$ years, in contrast to the supple and harmoniously flowing movements thereafter.

A morphological counterpart of this change can possibly be seen in the process of synapse elimination coincidentally taking place in the cortex, and which reaches its peak at this age.[6] It is thought to lead to a shaping of cortical connectivity. Central conduction velocities also increase in this period, promoting the possibility of sending complex messages through cortico-spinal pathways.[21] If indiscriminate variability persists, hyperkinetic, dyskinetic or clumsy motor behaviour could be the result. Table 10.4 gives symptoms based on lack of development of adaptive variability. They can be considered as alarm symptoms for deviant development in a toddler.

In conclusion, the relationship between morphological and functional brain development in terms of sensorimotor activity is still poorly understood. But variability as a characteristic of normal development and a lack of it at appropriate ages as seen in abnormal development, are valuable concepts in the understanding and early detection of neurological impairment during infancy and childhood.

References

1 Dobbing, J. The later development of the brain and its vulnerability. In: Davis, J.A., Dobbing, J., eds. *Scientific Foundation of Paediatrics*, 2nd edn. London: Heinemann, 1981: 744–759.

2 Purves, D., Lichtman, J.W. *Principles of Neural Development*. Sunderland, Massachusetts: Sinauer, 1985: 131–154.

3 Forger, N.G., Breedlove, S.M. Motoneural death during human fetal development. *J Comp Neurol* 1987; **264**: 118–122.

4 Thompson, W.J. Changes in the innervation of mammalian skeletal muscle fibers during postnatal development. *Trends Neurosci* 1986; **9**: 25–28.

5 Huttlenlocher, P.R., de Courten, C., Garey, L.J., v d Loos, H. Synaptogenesis in human visual cortex – evidence for synapse elimination during normal development. *Neurosci Lett* 1982; **33**: 247–252.

6 Rakic, P., Bourgeois, J.P., Eckenhoff, M.F., Zecevic, N., Goldman-Rakic, P.S. Concurrent overproduction of synapses in diverse regions of the primate cerebral cortex. *Science* 1986; **232**: 232–235.

7 Volpe, J.J. *Neurology of the Newborn*. Philadelphia: Saunders, 1987: 672.

8 Zaia, J.A., Lang, D.J. Cytomegalovirus infection of the fetus and neonate. *Neurol Clin* 1984; **2**: 387.

9 Myers, R.E., de Courten-Myers, G.M., Wagner, K.R. Physiotherapy and biochemistry of perinatal asphyctic brain injury. In: Yabuuchi, H., Watanaba, K., Okada, S.,

eds. *Neonatal Brain and Behaviour*. Nagoy: University of Nagoy Press, 1987: 1–14.

10 De Vries, J.I.P., Visser, G.H.A., Prechtl, H.F.R. The emergence of fetal behaviour. I: Qualitative aspects. *Early Hum Dev* 1982; **7**: 301–322.

11 De Vries, J.I.P., Visser, G.H.A., Prechtl, H.F.R. In: Prechtl, H.F.R., ed. *Continuity of Neural Functions from Prenatal to Postnatal Life*. Oxford: Blackwell Scientific Publications Ltd, 1984: 46–64.

12 Okado, N., Kojima, T. Ontogeny of the central nervous system: neurogenesis, fibre connection, synaptogenesis and myelination in the spinal cord. In: Prechtl, H.F.R., ed. *Continuity of Neural Functions*. Clinics in Developmental Medicine No. 94. Oxford: Spastics International Medical Publications with Blackwell, 1984: 31–45.

13 Hooker, D. *The Prenatal Origin of Behaviour*. Lawrence: University of Kansas Press, 1952.

14 Humphrey, T. Function of the nervous system during prenatal life. In: Stave, U., ed. *Perinatal Physiology*. New York: Plenum, 1978: 651–683.

15 Touwen, B.C.L. Variability and stereotypy of spontaneous motility as a predictor of the neurological development in preterm infants. *Dev Med Child Neurol* 1990; **32**: 501–508.

16 Cioni, G., Prechtl, H.F.R. Preterm and early post-term motor behaviour in low-risk premature infants. *Early Hum Dev* 1990; **23**: 159–191.

17 Ferrari, F., Cioni, G., Prechtl, H.F.R. Qualitative changes of general movements in preterm infants with brain lesions. *Early Hum Dev* 1990; **23**: 193–231.

18 Bekedam, D.J., Visser, G.H.A., De Vries, J.J., Prechtl, H.F.R. Motor behaviour in the growth retarded fetus. *Early Hum Dev* 1985; **12**: 155–165.

19 Touwen, B.C.L. Neurological development in infancy. Clinics in Developmental Medicine No. 58, 150. London: Heinemann, 1976.

20 Neligan, G., Prudham, D. Potential value of four early developmental milestones in screening children for increased risk of later retardation. *Dev Med Child Neurol* 1969; **11**: 423–431.

21 Eyre, J.A., Koh, T.H.H.G Maturation of descending pathways in man from birth to adulthood. *J Physiol* 1988; **296**: 58.

10.2 Central motor deficit (including cerebral palsy)

Carlos de Sousa and Christine Bungay

The term *central motor deficit* encompasses all non-progressive abnormalities of motor control, function and development in childhood which are not due to lesions of muscle, peripheral nerve or spinal cord. This wide definition includes all those disorders often grouped together under the heading of *cerebral palsy*, as well as all other non-progressive motor disorders, and includes some which in the past have not fitted easily or consistently into a single category. Central motor deficits arise prenatally, perinatally or postnatally because of abnormal brain development, deranged metabolism, cerebrovascular disease, cerebral hypoxia, neurological infection, trauma or exposure to toxic agents. Central motor deficits can occur alone or together with other abnormalities, when they may be a feature of a syndrome (sporadic or genetic, sometimes due to a chromosomal abnormality) which will include other recognizable features.

Although there are occasions when the terms *central motor deficit* and *cerebral palsy* can be used interchangeably, the former is preferred in this section. The use of the term *central motor deficit* is likely to enjoy even wider currency in the future.

Studies of prevalence rates are made difficult by methodological issues. The reported prevalence of children with stable motor handicaps who are alive at the age of school entry is about 2 per 1000 live births in industrialized nations.[1] Studies of the prevalence of cerebral palsy have used different case definitions which make comparisons between studies hazardous. Some definitions exclude known congenital malformations or postnatally acquired abnormalities. Others use a much wider definition of cerebral palsy which becomes almost synonymous with the term central motor deficit as used here.

Childhood central motor deficits are prevalent in all communities. In some poorer countries, such as Nigeria, there is a higher proportion of children with identifiable and potentially preventable causes.[2] A study from Saudi Arabia has shown prenatal causes to be present to a similar degree as in industrialized countries.[3] Social class differences in the prevalence of some motor disorders suggest the likely part that environmental factors play in their aetiology. In particular, socioeconomic disadvantage increases the prevalence of spastic hemiplegia and diplegia.[4]

Types of central motor deficit

The child has an abnormal motor pattern in which spasticity, dyskinesia, ataxia or hypotonia may predominate. These are descriptions of clinically detectable abnormalities and they are not diagnostic entities. More than one abnormal pattern can coexist at a given age (for instance spasticity plus dyskinesia, or hypotonia plus ataxia). Most children with central motor deficits pass through stages in which different patterns may predominate – for instance, early hypotonia and later spasticity. By using the predominant pattern of involvement as a denominator, some broad but clinically useful categories can be delineated.

Spastic disorders

Spastic disorders are characterized by exaggerated stretch reflexes in the muscles of affected limbs (giving rise to hypertonicity), hyperreflexia and an upgoing plantar response (positive Babinski sign).

Spastic hemiplegia

Spastic hemiplegia is the commonest type in many series and accounts for between one-third and one-half of children with predominantly spastic disorders. Spastic hemiplegia is of prenatal origin in over two-thirds of affected children, and more commonly affects the right side. An abnormality is seldom recognized at birth, and most congenital hemiplegias become apparent between 6 months and 1 year of age. Initially there may be only reduced movements in the affected arm, and the hand on that side may be held closed for more time than not. The Moro reflex may be asymmetric and from 6–9 months, so also may be the forward parachute response. The baby may reach out for toys less on the affected side. The older child often maintains the arm in a typical posture, flexed at the elbow, wrist and fingers, with an adducted thumb; spasticity and hyperreflexia become more evident with increasing age. Usually the leg is less severely affected than the arm, and a leg abnormality may not be noted until the child is walking, which is often delayed. Asymmetric toe walking may be a presenting feature of a hemiplegia. The limbs of the affected side tend to be smaller in hemiplegias of prenatal origin. There may be mild facial weakness. Intellectual deficits (usually in the mild to moderate range) occur in 15–40% of affected children.[5] Approximately one half of children with spastic hemiplegia will have seizures, which may have their onset at any age.[6] A hemianopia occurs in 25% of patients and may be undetected in the younger child.[7] Perceptual defects may occur on the involved side. There may be associated hemisensory loss.

Spastic diplegia

In spastic diplegia there is functional disability of both legs secondary to increase of tone and deep tendon reflexes in the lower limbs. The upper limbs show few neurological signs though some functional disability is usually evident, most easily demonstrable in the older child. Its relative frequency in different population based studies of spastic disorders varies from over 50% to less than that of spastic hemiplegia. Some studies have shown a decrease in the incidence of spastic diplegia which began with the introduction of good basic neonatal care, although in recent years this trend has been reversed, possibly due to the increased survival of very low birthweight infants.[8] Spastic diplegia is rarely postnatally acquired.[9] Between one-half and two-thirds of the children are born prematurely. Spastic diplegia associated with preterm birth has some distinguishing features such as an often normal intellect, a low incidence of seizures and the frequent association of periventricular leucomalacia identified by imaging or neuropathological studies.[10] Spastic diplegia in children born at term is more likely to be associated with developmental brain anomalies. The typical postural abnormalities of spastic diplegia begin to evolve in the first year. The lower limbs are flexed, internally rotated and adducted at the hips because of spasm and contracture, with knee flexion and equino-valgus of the ankle and foot (Fig. 10.2).

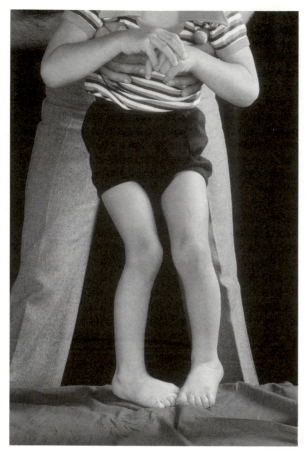

Figure 10.2 Child with spastic diplegia.

Most children will achieve independent walking by 48 months; many show mild incoordination with bimanual tasks; signs may be asymmetric down the body.[11] Most have good intelligence, with 70% having an IQ above 70.[7]

Spastic quadriplegia

Children with a spastic disorder involving all four limbs are described as having spastic quadriplegia, although the terms tetraplegia, double hemiplegia and total body involvement have also been applied. This is the smallest group of children with spastic disorders, less than 25% of the total in many series, but they have the greatest degree of motor, as well as other, impairments. Intelligence is rarely within the normal range and epilepsy is common. Visual impairments, feeding difficulties often secondary to pseudobulbar palsy, and severe communication problems occur in the majority.[12] A number of different neuropathological abnormalities may be associated with spastic quadriplegia: including multicystic changes sparing infratentorial structures; neuronal migration defects; other cerebral malformations; and defects of myelin formation.[13] Quadriplegia is postnatally

acquired in about 15% of cases.[14] Among children with central motor deficits acquired after the perinatal period, spastic quadriplegia is the commonest type. Most affected children have severe spasticity, affecting the muscles of the upper limbs rather more than the lower limbs. There is often some asymmetry of involvement between the two sides, and this can be important in the evolution of skeletal abnormalities such as hip dislocation and scoliosis.

Dyskinetic disorders

Some children with central motor deficits have a striking excess of involuntary movements as their principal abnormality. Such movements may be fleeting or sustained, they may predominate in one group of muscles or move from one group to another and they will vary in the rapidity with which they recur. Sustained, mobile spasms of agonist and antagonist muscles, recurring without great rapidity are termed *athetosis*. Fleeting localized movements recurring unpredictably and rapidly are described as *chorea*. *Dystonic* spasms are sustained abnormal postures of limbs, which can be maintained for a considerable time. Many of these movements are exacerbated by attempts at voluntary control.

In some children with dyskinetic disorders there will be a history of kernicterus or hypoxic ischaemic encephalopathy as an antecedent event. In early infancy such children are usually markedly hypotonic, the movement disorder often evolves over several years and athetoid movements may become particularly prominent. Other children have a peculiar delay in the onset of dystonia, which may follow an antecedent perinatal cerebral insult by many years.[15] Less commonly, non-progressive movement disorders (with dystonia prominent) can be acquired in childhood, following neurological infection, hypoxia or trauma.

Many children with a pure dyskinetic disorder have low muscle tone and do not have exaggerated tendon jerks. In others there may be a mixed pattern of involvement, with varying degrees of spasticity and sometimes ataxia as well. Cognitive development is more likely to be normal (especially when a dyskinetic disorder is of prenatal or perinatal onset) than in many other types of central motor deficit.[7] In the past, deafness frequently occurred in those children with a dyskinetic disorder which followed kernicterus.

Ataxic disorders

A small number of children have a central motor deficit presenting predominantly with ataxia. Some children with spastic diplegia have a marked ataxia, and are then separately classified as having an ataxic diplegia. The majority of ataxic disorders are of prenatal origin. There is a higher familial occurrence with this type of motor deficit than with most others. Some rare progressive ataxic syndromes may initially manifest themselves in this way. Imaging of the brain may show developmental abnormalities, particularly affecting the vermis. The dysequilibrium syndrome is a subtype in which there is markedly defective postural function affecting the trunk and legs with sparing of the upper limbs.[16] Many children with congenital ataxic motor deficits are markedly hypotonic in early infancy, and sitting is often not achieved until 15–18 months of age. Ataxia becomes more apparent towards the end of the first year of life and sometimes only later. Prognosis for intelligence is worse than in children with hemiplegia or diplegia; half have an IQ less than 70.[7]

Hypotonic disorders

Many children with central motor deficits are hypotonic in early infancy. In most this evolves into a predominantly spastic, dyskinetic or ataxic pattern. A few retain hypotonia as a predominant motor abnormality. This group includes a high proportion with significant mental handicap. Chromosome disorders (such as Down syndrome) and cerebral malformations (such as lissencephaly) may be associated with this pattern of motor development. In some children with hypotonic motor deficits there may be a delay in the rate of normal myelination within the central nervous system, and this can be demonstrated by magnetic resonance imaging.[17] A combination of central hypotonia and metal retardation often contributes to a marked delay in acquisition of motor milestones. Hypotonia usually becomes less pronounced in the older child.

Transient central motor deficits

Not every child identified as having a non-progressive central motor deficit in their first year will retain abnormal motor development into later life. There are some who exhibit motor patterns which are transient variants from the norm. These may include hypotonia, mild generalized hypertonus, or a delayed acquisition of motor milestones without a significant abnormality of tone or movements. Such variants rightly give rise to concern, and these infants need careful examination and re-examination. There is often a family history in parents or in a sibling of a similar pattern of early motor development, with later development being normal. In some, a combination of factors conspire to slow early motor development, for instance a family pattern of late walking combined with excessive ligamentous laxity.

Nelson and Ellenberg[18] drew attention to the frequent normalization of motor abnormalities in children sufficiently abnormal to be diagnosed as having cerebral palsy at one year of age. Caution needs to be exercised in attaching undue prognostic significance to some motor abnormalities in early infancy, especially if these are not severe. On the other hand, there is not likely to be later normalization in the one-year-old infant who has clear evidence of a spastic hemiplegia or a mixed spastic and dyskinetic quadriplegia.

Origins of central motor deficits

Many different processes can give rise to central motor deficits. Certain patterns are more commonly associated with particular antecedents such as spastic diplegia with preterm delivery and dyskinetic disorders with kernicterus. In other cases events such as hypoxic ischaemic encephalopathy in the newborn may be followed by outcomes as varied as complete normality, a dyskinetic disorder with normal intellect or spastic quadriplegia with mental handicap and epilepsy. Such a range of outcomes is likely to be a result of the variable combination of several different processes.

Individual factors which underlie central motor deficits can be grouped into those beginning to operate prenatally, perinatally or postnatally.

Prenatal factors

Cerebral malformations

Cerebral malformations which result in central motor deficits include migrational disorders (schizencephaly, lissencephaly, neuronal heterotopias and microgyria) which occur because of failure of neurones to migrate normally from the periventricular germinal layer out to the cortex, in the first 25 weeks of gestation.[19] Some migrational disorders may be the result of congenital infection or metabolic disorders (including peroxisomal disorders), whereas others may comprise part of a syndrome (such as Aicardi syndrome with optic colobomata, callosal dysgenesis and infantile spasms). Hydrocephalus is often associated with central motor deficits, hypotonia and ataxia. A number of developmental abnormalities of the cerebellum occur, including Dandy-Walker malformation (vermian agenesis and fourth ventricular cyst), and ataxia as well as other motor deficits may result.

Destructive brain lesions

Destructive brain lesions may also arise prenatally and go on to cause motor deficits. Fetal parenchymal or subdural haemorrhage may occur, sometimes due to a coagulopathy.[20] Prenatal ultrasound has also demonstrated the onset of periventricular leucomalacia and porencephalic cysts before birth in preterm infants who may go on to exhibit a motor deficit.[21]

Minor congenital malformations

There is an increased incidence of minor congenital malformations in children with central motor deficit.[22,23] Their occurrence is an indicator of abnormal embryogenesis extending beyond the nervous system.

Recognizable genetic disorders

Recognizable genetic disorders are also a cause of some central motor deficits.[24] They are most frequently linked with congenital ataxia, which is due to a genetic disorder (usually autosomal recessive, sometimes dominant or X-linked) in up to half of affected children. An example is Joubert syndrome, which is autosomal recessive, and also includes dysgenesis of the cerebellar vermis, episodic tachypnoea and abnormal eye movements. Spastic disorders are less likely to be genetic, although there are significant recurrence risks (around 10%) in siblings of children with spastic diplegia or quadriplegia in which no other causative factors exist.[25] Segawa's syndrome, in which there is progressive limb dystonia with diurnal variation, is rare but important to recognize. Children with this probably dominantly inherited disorder usually show good response to treatment with dopa.[26] Dyskinetic disorders may be caused by inborn errors of metabolism including Lesch-Nyhan syndrome (X-linked) and glutaric aciduria type 1 (autosomal recessive).

Congenital infection

Congenital infection, with for instance cytomegalovirus or *Toxoplasma gondii*, may result in a central motor deficit in combination with other neurological abnormalities. Prenatal exposure to a variety of *toxins* may lead to later motor deficits. These include alcohol, causing fetal alcohol syndrome, mercury, causing fetal Minamata disease and *crack* cocaine.[27] Many of these prenatal factors also cause poor fetal growth. Even in the absence of other factors, fetal growth retardation is significantly associated with spastic disorders.[28]

Perinatal factors

Perinatal asphyxia

Although there is no doubt that some infants who suffer from perinatal asphyxia go on to develop central motor deficits, asphyxia is not the major cause of such deficits. Permanent motor deficits occur in less than 2% of infants who have been asphyxiated at birth. Among infants with spastic, dyskinetic or mixed disorders, the occurrence of perinatal asphyxia is between 6% and 12%.[29,30] Prenatal factors, including growth retardation and minor malformations, often coexist as antecedents in this group of asphyxiated newborns who later show motor deficits.

Low birthweight

Infants of very low birthweight (< 1500 g) have a much increased risk of developing central motor deficits, as much as 35 times that of other newborns,[31] and this incidence has shown little change with time. Neurological infection and metabolic disorders, especially hypoglycaemia and hyperbilirubinaemia in the postnatal period, add significantly to the risk of developing a motor abnormality.

Bilirubin encephalopathy

Bilirubin encephalopathy in the newborn period is considerably rarer now. This has been due to the improved obstetric and neonatal management of rhesus allo-immunization and the other causes of neonatal hyperbilirubinaemia. There has also been a fall in the number of children who develop a dyskinetic disorder with deafness, which can be attributed to bilirubin encephalopathy. This has been accompanied by an increase in the proportion of children with dyskinetic disorders due to other causes.[32]

Postnatal factors

Postnatally acquired central motor deficits are about five times less common than prenatally or perinatally acquired deficits.[9] Sometimes these are termed postnatally acquired cerebral palsy, but this term has more than one definition with a variable age limit for its onset and different interpretations as to which non-progressive motor deficits should or should not be included.

Infection

Infection of the central nervous system is the major cause of postnatally acquired motor deficits.[33,34] Infectious causes include bacterial meningitis, tuberculous meningitis, cerebral abscess, cerebral malaria and viral encephalitis. The human immunodeficiency virus (HIV) is a neurotropic virus which can cause a progressive or static encephalopathy following congenital infection. This frequently includes a central motor deficit, often presenting as a progressively worsening diplegia, although acute hemiplegia may occur,[35] and extrapyramidal involvement may also be a feature.[36]

Trauma

Trauma is an important cause of acquired motor deficits, especially in older children. About 20% of children who survive severe head injuries show motor impairments as a result.[37] Many of these survivors also have cognitive impairments. They include a high proportion of children from socially deprived backgrounds, and their rehabilitation benefits from involvement of their local multidisciplinary community-based team.[38] Another important cause is cerebral infarction, which can be the result of infections such as mycoplasma and chicken pox; inborn errors of metabolism such as homocystinuria, ornithine carbamyl transferase deficiency and mitochondrial cytopathy; and vascular anomalies such as moya-moya disease. Cerebral hypoxia following drowning, suffocation, electrocution, cardiac arrest or status epilepticus may cause a motor deficit and children with cerebral tumours with progressive symptoms at the time of presentation, may have a non-progressive motor deficit after successful surgical resection.

Spastic quadriplegia is relatively more common among those acquired postnatally compared to prenatal or perinatal cases, accounting for 30–50% of the total. Cerebral infarction often results in hemiplegia. Hypotonic, dyskinetic and ataxic disorders are uncommon, although a dyskinetic disorder may follow basal ganglia infarction from carbon monoxide poisoning.

Pathophysiology of central motor deficits

The central motor deficits of childhood arise as a result of processes which interfere with cerebral function at a time when the nervous system is still developing. The impact of such processes may depend upon their timing.[39] If they occur early in development there may be considerable scope for remodelling; but, conversely, early lesions may interfere more profoundly with later integration of neural function. Some direct evidence for the remodelling that can take place is provided by studies using transcortical magnetic stimulation. Stimulation of the motor cortex in patients with congenital hemiplegia shows there to be bilateral corticospinal tract representation in the intact cerebral hemisphere at different sites.[40] This is not the case with postnatally acquired hemiplegias, in which the intact hemisphere only has corticospinal tract connections to the contralateral side (Evans, 1992, personal communication).

Assessment and diagnosis

Assessment and diagnosis of a child with a central motor deficit is best achieved by combining the skills of different professionals. In most cases this will include a paediatrician and a physiotherapist, and others likely to be involved include speech and occupational therapists, audiologists, psychologists, teachers, specialist nurses, and ophthalmic and orthopaedic surgeons. Families can, and frequently do, become bewildered at the multiplicity of professionals their child needs to see, and it is essential that one professional assumes a key role as coordinator and communicator. At the stage of first assessment and diagnosis this will usually be a paediatrician.

The first assessment establishes a baseline of a child's abilities and deficits, not only in motor development, but also in other areas, such as cognitive development and use of special senses. The process of assessment commences at the time of first contact with a therapist or paediatrican, and is a continuing process by which all the professionals involved identify changes in the child's condition and evaluate the effects of intervention. This information is used to plan further management and is the property not only of professionals, but also of the child and his family. Diagnosis aims to establish the neuropathological and aetiological basis for the motor deficit. It synthesizes information gained from the assessment together with the child's medical and family history and the results of special investigations. Diagnosis allows for prognosis to be more clearly established, for genetic advice to be given to the family and sometimes for specific treatments to be used.

Medical history and examination

The gathering together of information about a child's past will not always be completed satisfactorily at a single interview. It is often useful to provide parents with a questionnaire in advance to collect details of the developmental history with greater accuracy. The exact structure of an interview depends upon the circumstances but, especially at first contact, it is important to ask parents their main areas of concern. This can be followed by establishing the child's current attainments. The information gained from the questionnaire can then be developed, ensuring at the same time that doctor and parent are using terms in the same way. The family history should be recorded in detail, even if not apparently of immediate relevance. Again, parents may find it easier to recollect details by means of the questionnaire. Information about the pregnancy, delivery and postnatal period should, wherever possible, be supplemented by contemporaneous medical records or direct enquiries from professionals involved.

Sometimes parents attach undue significance to events around the time of the labour and delivery. It is never fair to expect parents to be the sole judges of whether there was perinatal asphyxia or a significant medical problem in the postnatal period. Information should therefore be gathered about possible maternal drug exposure or major illness in pregnancy; concerns about fetal growth; fetal movements in comparison to previous pregnancies; gestation, mode of delivery and duration of labour; medical problems encountered during labour and delivery; birthweight (in comparison with previous pregnancies) and birth head circumference; condition when born, including time to establishing first breath and cord blood pH if measured; type of resuscitation required, for how long and its outcome; medical problems encountered in the postnatal period, including need for ventilatory support, seizures, renal failure; duration of stay in neonatal unit; time taken to establish oral feeding and condition at the time of discharge from hospital. Information regarding early feeding difficulties, irritability, disturbed sleep pattern or excessive passivity should be sought. Other medical problems, for instance seizures, frequent vomiting, or respiratory infections should be recorded. Information about home circumstances and parents' employment is important.

Medical examination of the child aims to assist with diagnosis. It includes measurement of the child's growth – height, weight and head circumference. Unusual physical features and minor malformations, including any skin anomalies or abnormalities overlying the spine, should be sought. A general physical examination should include a search for evidence of otitis media and respiratory disease secondary to aspiration and gastro-oesophageal reflux. The eyes should be examined for their ocular movements, possible squint, cataracts, lens dislocation and pigmentary retinopathy. Refractive errors are common in children with motor deficits, and their full assessment will require the involvement of an orthoptist and ophthalmic surgeon.

In practice, particularly with very active or easily frightened young children, examination of the motor system should proceed according to opportunity, with the intention of making a full examination eventually. There are some benefits to using standardized methods of recording findings, particularly if information is to be used for research purposes, but also to maintain a consistent approach between different observers. A very useful form has been produced as *A standard recording of central motor deficit*[41] and it includes items on the nature of motor involvement, functional severity and associated problems.

The face should be examined for evidence of weakness, which is sometimes present in children with hemiplegia. Orofacial dyskinesia is not uncommon in children with dyskinetic motor deficits. Tongue thrust and dribbling are common in spastic quadriplegia when associated with pseudo-bulbar palsy. Note should be made of abnormally prolonged retention of sucking and swallowing reflexes, poorer tongue function than expected for age, an exaggerated gag reflex and dribbling.

Abnormal involuntary movements of the limbs and trunk should be described (these may only be present on extending the arms), as should the child's preferred posture. If the child is able to walk, this should be observed with particular reference to any asymmetry or generalized gait abnormality. The child should be encouraged to walk slowly, then to run, stoop, sit and rise from the floor, jump, hop and stand on one then the other foot, according to his capabilities. Balance in turning, whether from a sitting or bending posture, is a useful observation. A ball for throwing, catching and kicking is an effective way of demonstrating motor skills where appropriate and one with which most children feel comfortable. Similarly children where able enjoy pencil and paper activities and these permit observation of hand preference, pencil grasp and the type of perceptuo-motor skills possible. The child should be observed in the supine position, and more time will need to be spent with this part of the investigation in the very young child, or if motor abilities are very limited. Posture should be observed, including any tendency to asymmetry, fisting of the hands, adduction of the legs (scissoring) or abnormal extensor tone. Head turning to one side may induce an asymmetric tonic neck reflex (with extension of the arm and leg on the side to which the head is turned) at a time when this reflex should have disappeared (around 6–7 months) (Fig. 10.3). On pulling to sitting there may be excessive head lag, and when held in the sitting position head control may be poor, sometimes with a relative overactivity of neck extensors as compared to neck flexors. Sideways saving can be assessed by gently tipping the sitting child towards either side. A normal and symmetrical forward parachute response should be sought in children over 6 months of age by suspending the child in the prone position and rapidly moving the body head first and downwards. The child's normal sitting position should be observed and recorded.

In all infants it should be possible to assess limb tone in response to passive muscle stretching, which should be done slowly at first and then more rapidly. If there is an exaggerated sensitivity of muscles to stretch, which suddenly lessens, then spasticity is likely in that limb. The limb should always be examined several times, as tone is influenced by state of arousal, particularly anxiety, irritability and crying. The range of passive movements possible should be measured at different joints and the presence of fixed contractures determined. Palpation of the wrist and hand may reveal spasticity in wrist and digit flexors. Hand and foot

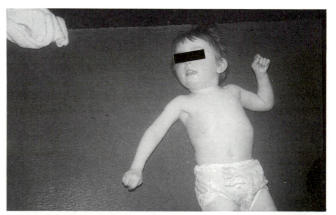

Figure 10.3 Retained asymmetric tonic neck reflex in a 2-year-old child with a spastic central motor deficit.

sizes should be compared, and leg length measured with the child supine. The range of abduction of each hip should be measured with the knees flexed, this normally being greater than about 45°. Note should also be made of any hip flexion contracture (the Thomas test, flexing one hip with the knee bent while leaving the other extended) and the amount of internal and external rotation at the hip. Restricted knee extension, due to spasticity of the hamstring muscles should be assessed. The range of dorsiflexion of the foot is measured with the foot held in varus and the knee partly flexed. The feet are inspected for positional abnormalities such as valgus, a cavus deformity (forefoot equinus with high arch) and toe deformities.

Information obtained from eliciting the tendon reflexes may complement that from the examination of posture and tone. These reflexes should be elicited with the head in a central position, to eliminate the possible effect of a retained asymmetric tonic neck reflex. It is normal for tendon reflexes to be much less brisk in the arms than the legs of children. Of particular significance in children with central motor deficits are excessively brisk tendon reflexes, especially if they can be obtained over a wider site than normal, or if there is marked and consistent asymmetry. Tendon reflexes tend to be normal in purely dyskinetic motor deficits, and may be normal or suppressed in ataxic disorders. A crossed adductor response (adduction of the opposite hip on tapping the patellar tendon) indicates severe spasticity. The plantar response is variable in normal young infants. Even in older children with spastic central motor deficits an extensor plantar response is not a consistent finding.

The spine should be regularly assessed in every child with a central motor deficit, from the side and from the back. There may be inequality in the height of shoulders, and, in the child who can stand, the appearance of a rib hump on trunk flexion denotes a structural scoliosis. The level of the curve, whether thoracic or lumbar, the type of curve, whether C or S shaped, and the direction of its convexity should be noted.

A complete medical examination of a child with a motor deficit is time consuming, but likely to be rewarding in terms of the amount of information that can be derived, and the practical use to which this information can be put.

Young children are less able to cooperate with examination and more easily alarmed by intervention. The value of observation at rest and then in play, both when moving around or sitting, cannot be underestimated. It is always a good way to begin examination, and the use of a ball, crayons, bricks and tiny objects to pick up, give considerable information on motor function and indirectly on motor signs. Gaining a child's confidence in this way may make the difference between achieving full examination or not, and maximizes the chance of getting at least some useful information from examination.

Investigations in diagnosis and assessment

There is no such thing as a routine series of investigations for central motor deficit. The choice of tests is determined by the type of motor deficit, its apparent time of onset, any associated features and the presence or absence of plausible aetiological factors. The results of investigations may assist in making a diagnosis, which could have genetic implications; they may facilitate understanding of the processes underlying the deficit; and they may reveal the presence of complications of associated conditions. Investigations should not be done if there is a likelihood of their causing harm or unnecessary distress, or if they have no direct relevance to the child's condition. In circumstances where the central motor deficits are non-progressive, it may be appropriate to wait until a child is old enough to understand and to cooperate with investigations. However, most investigations (and this includes brain scanning with X-rays or magnetic resonance) can be satisfactorily achieved in very young infants, and definitive early results may aid the family in the process of adjustment to their child's condition, and may be necessary for genetic counselling.

It is important to ensure that neonatal screening for *phenylketonuria* and *hypothyroidism* has been completed. This will almost certainly be the case with current practice in the UK, but may not necessarily have happened with some children who were born in other countries. Both of these conditions can give rise to motor deficits.[42,43]

Chromosomal analysis should be undertaken in the majority of children with motor deficits. Most children with major chromosomal abnormalities have central motor deficits, usually with generalized hypotonia and delayed motor development being most prominent, but sometimes also giving rise to spasticity or ataxia. Detectable chromosomal abnormalities are more likely if there is growth retardation of prenatal origin, microcephaly or macrocephaly, other congenital malformations or dysmorphic features.

Computed tomography (CT) is abnormal in over 75% of children with non-progressive central motor deficits. A range of abnormalities may be demonstrated, including maldevelopments of early prenatal origin, periventricular leucomalacia, cortical and subcortical atrophy.[44,45] Many of the changes demonstrated may be slight. There is often little correlation between the clinical severity and the extent of the radiological abnormality. Occasionally very extensive malformations may occur in children with only a moderate deficit (Fig. 10.4). *Magnetic resonance* (MR) imaging provides better anatomical delineation and is also particularly good at demonstrating lesions in the periventricular white matter, and abnormal or delayed myelination.[46] There may be some correlation between white matter loss and clinical severity. Proton magnetic resonance spectroscopy is a research tool which can be

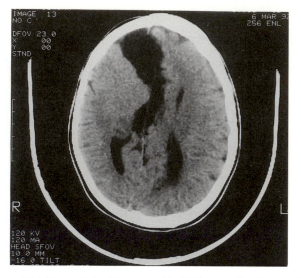

Figure 10.4 Computerized tomographic (CT) scan of a 12 year old with a left hemiplegia, epilepsy and mild learning difficulties. There is an extensive congenital malformation of the brain with agenesis of the corpus callosum, an interhemispheric 3rd ventricular cyst and a migrational abnormality involving the right frontal lobe.

used to estimate neuronal loss within a localized region of interest in the brain. Single photon emission computerized tomography has demonstrated cerebral blood flow abnormalities in children with motor deficits who have no CT-scan abnormality, but this is also a research tool, and there is poor concordance between the clinical findings and the alterations in blood flow.[47]

Brain imaging should be performed in all children with central motor deficits which are either postnatally acquired or apparently progressive. In those children with a static motor deficit of prenatal or perinatal origin imaging may provide much important information about aetiology. MR appearances in particular are often an indicator of the severity of the disorder and may be a guide to later outcome. Brain imaging, and especially MR, will be done with increasing frequency in children with central motor deficits in the future.

Evidence of *congenital infection* with rubella, cytomegalovirus and toxoplasmosis should be sought in all children with motor deficits of prenatal origin. Investigations are more informative when done soon after birth. Investigation for a possible congenital infection may also require testing of maternal blood samples, including a sample obtained at the time of booking in early pregnancy.

Some *inborn errors of metabolism* cause abnormal motor development. In most cases it will be apparent that there is an acquired and progressive motor deficit. In some, however, the period of normality prior to presentation in early infancy may be so brief, or the rate of progression so slow, that these children appear to have non-progressive central motor deficits. Progressive neurological disorders are discussed in more

detail in Section 10.4. These disorders are individually rare, and their diagnosis relies upon the appropriate use of specialized laboratory investigations in selected cases. Some children with organic acidurias have hypotonia, spasticity or dyskinesias.[48] Children with glutaric aciduria type I, and less commonly those with propionic acidaemia and methylmalonic aciduria may have an onset of a dyskinetic disorder following an episode of metabolic decompensation.[49] Chromatography of urine for organic acids will enable the diagnosis to be made. Arginase deficiency, a rare urea cycle defect, can give rise to progressive spasticity, with features resembling a spastic diplegia.[50] There will be hyperammonaemia and abnormal plasma and urinary amino acids. Some female carriers for ornithine carbamyl transferase (OCT) deficiency, another urea cycle defect, may experience stroke-like episodes, and the diagnosis may only be apparent with a protein or other loading test.[51] Other metabolic causes of cerebral infarction in children are homocystinuria (including some heterozygotes), which is detectable on plasma and urinary amino acid analysis; and mitochondrial respiratory chain defects (mitochondrial encephalopathy, lactic acidosis and stroke-like episodes or MELAS) in which plasma and CSF lactate levels are elevated, and muscle biopsy shows characteristic abnormalities.[52] Mitochondrial defects can give rise to a variety of motor deficits, either central or due to neuropathies and myopathies. Plasma lactate measurements on their own are frequently misleading, and if a mitochondrial disorder is suspected, CSF lactate should be measured and muscle biopsy considered. Lesch-Nyhan syndrome, an X-linked disorder of purine metabolism in which there is hyperuricaemia, is characterized by early hypotonia and later dyskinesia and compulsive self-injurious behaviour in affected males. Confirmation of the diagnosis is by assay of the enzyme hypoxanthine guanine phosphoribosyl transferase (HGPRT).

Children with those leucodystrophies which present in infancy usually have a major central motor abnormality at an early stage. Metachromatic leucodystrophy (due to arylsulphatase deficiency) is the commonest type, and in the form presenting in infancy there is progressive spasticity, with loss of motor abilities and later loss of other abilities also. Krabbe's disease (due to galactocerebrosidase deficiency), Canavan's disease (due to aspartoacylase deficiency) and Alexander's disease have these same features in common. Macrocephaly (in Krabbe's and Alexander's diseases) and peripheral neuropathies (in metachromatic and Krabbe's leucodystrophies) are distinguishing features. Pelizaeus-Merzbacher disease is a leucodystrophy, often of onset in very early infancy, in which there are markedly abnormal eye movements (horizontal and rotatory nystagmus) present at an early stage, optic atrophy, a progressive motor disorder with spasticity and dystonia and sometimes congenital stridor. The inheritance is most often X-linked, and in those with very early onset there may be confusion with a non-progressive motor deficit. Abnormal brainstem auditory evoked responses are frequently present as a distinguishing feature. The diagnosis of these disorders will be assisted by abnormalities on brain imaging, and can be confirmed (except in the cases of Alexander's and Pelizaeus-Merzbacher diseases) by enzymology. Leucodystrophies which present in later childhood, including adrenoleucodystrophy (an X-linked peroxisomal disorder) often have cognitive decline as a prominent early feature, with motor abnormalities becoming more apparent later.

Specialist metabolic investigations for these and other inborn errors of metabolism should be reserved for those children with familial disorders, with probably progressive or unexplained postnatally acquired disorders, when special features referred to above are present or where there are specific indicators from the results of other investigations.

Physiotherapy

The child with a central motor deficit is disadvantaged in the acquisition of movement skills. Given the best treatment available motor skills will be acquired at the cost of considerable effort on the part of the child and family, and an investment in time and expertise from the therapist. Therapeutic aims will vary according to the degree of motor dysfunction, learning deficit and any associated conditions. It is essential that energy and resources should be directed to the needs of the individual child with respect to his pathology, personality and circumstances. The primary aims can be grouped as:

- Reducing discomfort
- Minimizing the risk of deformity
- Enhancing functional skills
- Increasing mobility
- Maximizing independence
- Teaching parents and carers techniques of handling.

The child is an integral part of a family. He is dependent on the family for his daily needs. The family of a child diagnosed as having a central motor deficit inevitably need to make some adaptation to their child's particular needs. Many authors and parents describe this process as a grief response.[53] The selection of treatment approach must respect and take into account the point the family have reached in this process of adaptation. Asking a family to learn and execute a complex programme six times daily when they are numb with shock is a recipe for disaster. That same family may well become active partners in a vigorous therapeutic programme when they have moved towards reorganization and adaptation. It is,

however, worth noting that adaptation is not a linear progression and families move back and forth between phases over many years as their child matures and new events occur. Therapeutic expectations must move with them and adapt to their changing needs as well as those of the child.

For over half a century orthopaedic surgeons, physicians and therapists have developed techniques to aid the habilitation of children suffering from motor deficits. Each approach has a following and claims for unique success. On close scrutiny these approaches appear to derive from wide ranging, often conflicting, theory and practice. There remains a paucity of scientific evaluation of the effect of treatments. Most therapists synthesize a model of practice based on standard techniques supplemented by their own experience and that which seems most suited to the circumstances.

Most syntheses take root in the work of Karel and Berta Bobath[54] and Andras Peto.[55] Specific techniques from Rood and Vojta[56] may be used. A significant influence on current practice has been the service delivery model of the Portage service.[57] A number of centres exist to promote the controversial work of Doman and Delacato.[58]

Neurodevelopmental treatment

The Bobath approach

Philosophy: based on the belief that the disability associated with central motor deficit arises from 'an interference with the development of normal postural control against gravity.'[54] Abnormal patterns of coordination arise in association with disorders of postural tone and reciprocal innervation.

Techniques: treatment is executed by *handling* the child in such a way as to elicit reactions that are as *normal* as possible. Through this experience and by constant repetition new and more normal sensorimotor patterns are established.

Treatment does not correct or teach movements. Nor does it follow absolute developmental sequences or perfect one skill before moving on to another. It aims to facilitate new skills that are relevant to preparing the child for future functional skills. Parent training is emphasized. The parent is responsible for the home management of the child. The gains made during therapy sessions must be carried over into the child's daily life and activities. Parents are present during treatment sessions. They are not given lists of exercises but learn and practise techniques to continue at home.

Example: a therapist will show a parent ways of positioning a young child during carrying, such as astride the hip, so that spasticity is inhibited and active control of head and trunk is facilitated.

This approach requires commitment and consistency between carers. It works well with children in their early stages of development and when the approach is shared by all individuals involved with the child including family, school staff and respite carers.

Key words: handling; facilitation; postural control.

Conductive education

The Peto approach

Philosophy: the motto above the door of the Institute for the Motor Disabled in Budapest reads: 'Not because of, but in order to'. A dysfunction is not perceived as the *property* of the child but of the interaction between *the way the child is* and the environment.

Education is orchestrated by a *conductor* who has been trained for 4 years in aspects of medicine, psychology, physiotherapy and education that relate to the physically handicapped child. The child actively engages in his own learning throughout his waking day in an environment that generates positive expectations of the child.

Techniques: the institute *facilitates learning* rather than *offers treatment*. The programme aims to develop a sense of personal responsibility in the child to work actively towards specific goals in locomotion, self-care and communication. Work is carried out in groups selected according to salient similar characteristics. The programme uses minimal apparatus (slatted plinths, ladderback chairs, quoits, simple walking poles and sticks) in a wide variety of ways to achieve functional independence.

Example: a small group of children and parents (or educators) work with a conductor towards a specific target, such as functional grasp. Work centres around repetitive activities reinforced with simple rhymes to assist *rhythmic intention* (enabling the child to use language to cue himself in preparation for an activity). The child may lie on a slatted plinth and learn to grasp the rungs in order to assist rolling over or sitting up.

This approach has much to offer children who are alert, motivated and aware of their peers. Some internal language is required to participate fully in what is a very interactive programme. Children who enjoy friendly competition blossom in the fun of a well structured group.

Key words: conductor; orthofunction; rhythmic intention.

Home-based early intervention

The Portage model

Philosophy: the Portage project explored the possibility of developing a model for an 'early education programme for handicapped children' that could be replicated by others. The underlying premise is that parents are the most powerful educators of their children regardless of their own education, economic status or intellectual capacity. The home is the natural environment for effective work with the young child and family. Each child has a unique profile of strengths and weaknesses which need to be addressed in a task focused, developmentally sequenced approach.

Techniques: the programme takes place at home, supported by a home teacher through a weekly visit. An individual curriculum is prepared from a base line established using a checklist-centred assessment of the child's abilities. Goals are set with the family. These are broken down into steps that the child can aim to reach over the following week. Parents or principal care givers work with the child each day using an individual programme of instructions. Response is charted in order to give feedback to the parent and teacher.

Example: the family may indicate that they want to work with their child to improve sitting balance. The Portage worker (with the advice of a physiotherapist if necessary) will define a target that should be achievable within one week. A detailed activity chart will be written. This will define when, where, how, how often, under what conditions and for how long the child will practise achieving that target. This will include a correction procedure for when the activity deviates and a reward for a successful practice.

This model offers families a reliable structure in which they can work with their child, sets clear attainable targets and gives parents very tangible rewards in documenting the effects of their work with their child. It requires considerable skill to adapt the model to children who have major physical impairment. However, the importance of focusing on the development of the whole child is particularly important for this group and Portage can provide a balanced counterpoint to more therapeutically focused intervention.

Key words: home teacher; activity chart; goals; partnership.

Patterning treatment

The Doman-Delacato approach

Philosophy: this approach to habilitation is based on the premise that mental handicap, learning problems, movement disorders and behavioural difficulties are caused by poor neurological organization and all of these problems lie somewhere along a single continuum of brain injury. The view is held that the only effective treatment is that advocated by this approach and that its effectiveness is in direct relationship to the frequency, intensity and duration of treatment. Children are constantly exposed to a rigid developmental sequence and are discouraged (at times actively prohibited) from participating in activities that are not stage appropriate, for instance walking before a child can crawl.

Techniques: an assessment is made of the child against certain developmental criteria used with this technique. Following this a profile is drawn up and a programme established. This programme will deliver a number of motor and sensory experiences in order to facilitate neurological organization. The experiences are intended to improve: visual competence; auditory competence; tactile competence; mobility; language and manual competence. Treatments are delivered at regular intervals, occupying up to 18 hours a day. Commonly four helpers take the child through the prescribed programme. The child is largely the passive recipient of the programme and given only limited opportunities to generate ideas or activities.

Many workers in this field of disability have serious concerns about the claims made by the institute, the relentless stress put upon families and the deprivation of normal experience some children incur.[58–60] However, many families continue to seek the clear, firm, structured approach of what they perceive as a positive thinking movement. The methods used and results claimed may be questionable, but there are lessons to be drawn from this perception.

Key words: patterning; amphibian creeping; reptilian crawling; hanging and brachiation.

The eclectic approach

As has been stated earlier most therapists synthesize a repertoire of treatment skills derived from the standard techniques and applied to their and their client's situation. Despite the diversity in techniques, strands of similarity emerge. A recurring theme is that of activity being goal directed, carried over into the child's day-to-day activities and involving the active support of parents, carers and educators.[61] Recent interest in the practice of implementing individual family service plans may serve as a future framework for engaging parents and carers in working towards realistic objectives relevant to the child's daily life.[62] An appropriate programme, put into effect by a therapist and a dedicated and committed family, will encourage and enable the child to develop independence as far as is possible.

Positioning, splinting and mobility aids

The selective use of positioning, splinting and mobility aids can help to maintain and supplement a therapeutic programme.

Positioning

Positioning may be achieved through the use of side lying cushions or boards, prone standers, standing frames and corrective seating (Fig. 10.5). The object of these devices is to enable the child to experience a wide variety of positions and play situations while maintaining or improving posture and function.

Splinting

Splinting may be used either to maintain or improve the range of movement at targeted joints, or to stabilize one joint in order to facilitate function. Dynamic splinting may be used to control the range or quality of movement and sometimes to re-educate systematically a pattern of movement.

When embarking on the use of splints it is important to consider:

- Why is this joint to be splinted?
- What can be achieved by this?
- What effect will it have on other joints?
- How long should splinting be applied to be effective?
- When and how will the effect be apparent?
- What effect will using this aid have on the quality of life of the child and family?

Splinting to maintain or increase range of movement can be applied to a number of target joints either singly or as a group. Most commonly it will be used for the ankles, knees, hips, wrists and elbows. Splints are designed to oppose any deforming forces, such as a pull of the foot into equinus, flexion of the wrists or adduction of the hips. The splint can be made of plaster of Paris, mouldable plastic materials or metal and leather. The splint will be made at the position of maximum tolerable correction. As the range of movement improves re-splinting will be necessary for maximum benefit.

Many therapists use the technique of serial casting in which a light cast is applied at weekly intervals for a period of 6 weeks. At each cast change a little more correction is gained. After casting a plastic orthosis may be necessary to sustain the improvement. This method can delay or avoid the need for surgery, such as elongation of the tendo Achilles. During growth spurts, serial casting may need repeating at 6–9 monthly intervals

Splinting to stabilize may be applied to a single joint or a group of joints. It is used in order to break tasks down into smaller components, for instance splinting the feet in a plantigrade position and the knees in extension in order to enable a child to develop control of his pelvis in standing. All the child's conscious effort can be directed at working on head, trunk and pelvic balance. As skill increases, the support from the splints can be reduced – first at the knees and then at the ankles. *Dynamic splinting* often involves sophisticated splints with joints in multiple planes to limit, guide and correct movement simultaneously. In the simplest form, this may be an ankle foot orthosis with a hinged ankle joint allowing dorsiflexion but preventing plantar

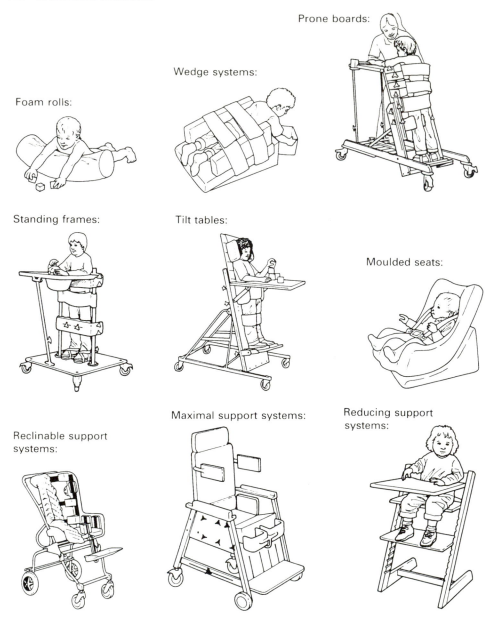

Figure 10.5 Seating and positioning aids for children with central motor deficits.

flexion. Other systems exist which modify and assist the use of hip movement, such as hip guidance orthoses.

Mobility

Mobility may be assisted in a number of ways given regard to the child's physical stage and level of maturation (Fig. 10.6). Early mobility characteristically emerges from the prone position and may be assisted by the use of tummy trolleys or scooter boards. Mobility may be achieved in the sitting position using a variety of go-carts and wheeled chairs. These may be hand or power controlled. Mobility on feet may be achieved by the use of prone leaning walkers (Cheyne style), walking devices that incorporate caliper type devices (Leeds walker, David Hart walker) or custom selected walking frames, crutches and sticks.

Medical problems and their management

Treatments for spasticity

Children with spasticity have increased stretch reflexes and impaired voluntary movements. Some muscle groups are affected more than others, and can contribute to the abnormal postures seen. There are situations in which a reduction in spasticity is desirable, allowing for a fuller range of unrestricted movements

Trundle toys:

Walking frames:

Forward support: Rear support: Maximal support:

Wheeled chairs:

Go-carts: Wheelchairs (manual):   Wheelchairs (power assisted):

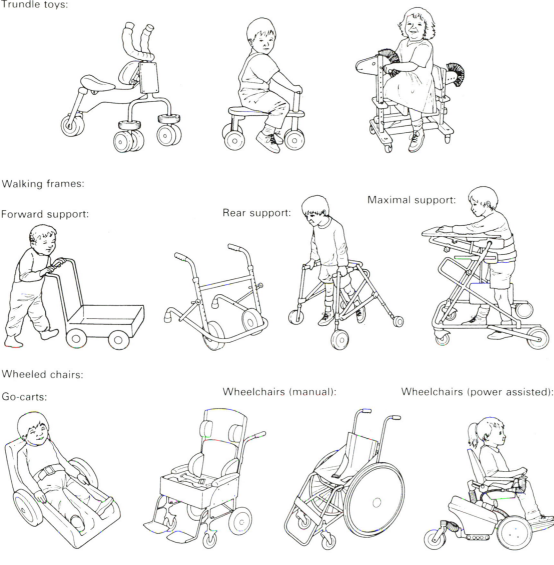

NB Power assisted wheelchairs may be designed for indoor or outdoor use. In the UK there is no agency with a statutory responsibility to provide outdoor, user driven power assisted mobility.

Figure 10.6 Aids to mobility for children with central motor deficits.

at particular joints and permitting better positioning of children. However, most treatments are not selective in their reduction of tone, and whereas there may be benefit from reducing tone in spastic muscles it may be outweighed by the effects of the reduction in tone in non-spastic muscles. Some children who are able to stand or walk need a degree of rigidity in order to maintain a standing posture. The benefit of any treatment to reduce spasticity should be evaluated following a trial period in an individual patient.

Drugs

Baclofen is the drug most widely used to reduce spasticity in childhood central motor deficits. It acts as an agonist at gamma aminobutyric acid ($GABA_B$) presynaptic receptors, resulting in the inhibition of spinal cord polysynaptic reflexes, as well as antagonizing the actions of excitatory neurotransmitters at post synaptic receptors. When given orally it reduces muscle spasm and pain, and may improve mobility.[63] Effective doses can also increase weakness, and the sedative side effects of treatment may be considerable. *Intrathecal baclofen* treatment was introduced for the treatment of spinal spasticity in adults, but it has also been used with some success to treat spasticity of cerebral origin in children.[64] A continuous dose of intrathecal baclofen is administered by a programmable pump with a catheter going into the lumbar subcutaneous space. This treatment has far fewer of the side effects of oral baclofen, but the benefit to patients with spasticity of cerebral origin is less than that seen in patients with spinal spasticity.[65] The decrease in spasticity is usually most marked in the lower limbs.

Other drugs used for the treatment of spasticity include *diazepam*, which also has GABA-agonist actions, and *dantrolene*, which produces its effects directly on muscle. *Vigabatrin*, which is an anticonvulsant which acts by enhancing GABA levels, may also have some antispasticity effects.

Surgery

The surgical treatment for spasticity which has commanded the most attention is *dorsal root rhizotomy*. The procedure involves an L2 to L5 laminectomy, followed by selective division of chosen lumbosacral dorsal spinal nerve rootlets, based on their electromyographic responses to peroperative electrical stimulation.[66] The intention is to identify and destroy those rootlets, thereby modulating abnormally processed afferent input. Selective division avoids the problems of sensory loss which occur with complete division of the dorsal roots. This technique has considerable claims for its efficacy following the careful follow up of groups of patients.[67,68] The greatest benefits are seen in intelligent children with spastic diplegia who can walk, have good strength and are aged 3–8 years, and also if the technique is coupled with a programme of intensive physiotherapy. Unfortunately there has never been a controlled study of this technique, and there are theoretical and practical criticisms of applying a costly, time consuming and invasive form of treatment which at present is of unproven efficacy.[69]

Stereotactic brain surgery has been used in a few centres for children with motor deficits since the 1960s. The greatest benefit has been in children with dystonia or tremor, and to a lesser extent in those with spasticity, particularly spastic diplegia.[70] Techniques used include ablation of the globus pallidus, the thalamus or the cerebellar dentate nucleus. Although there are encouraging results from these techniques, there have never been controlled studies of their use.

Preventing and treating structural deformity

The most common structural deformity in children with central motor deficits is *hip dislocation*. In the majority this is an acquired deformity and estimates of overall prevalence vary from 5% to 10%.[71,72] A combination of factors gives rise to dislocation in children with spastic motor disorders.[11] Of particular importance are the overactivity of the iliopsoas muscle, the principal hip flexor and medial rotator, together with overactivity of the hip adductor muscles. The femoral head subluxes laterally and eventually dislocates to the posterolateral surface of the ilium. Subluxation of the femoral head is accompanied by acetabular dysplasia, as normal modelling of the acetabulum in the first few years of life is dependent upon contact with the femoral head. Deformities in the shape of the femoral head develop and there is degeneration of its articular cartilage. The result is a joint which allows only a restricted range of movements, which may be painful.

Hip dislocation is particularly common in children with spastic quadriplegia, affecting between 16% and 50% of this group,[72,73] although some children with spastic diplegia and, less commonly, hemiplegia are also affected. Hip dislocation is uncommon in those children who acquire the ability to stand and walk. Scoliosis and hip dislocation often occur in the same child, but the evidence points to both of these deformities occurring as a result of the severity of the motor disorder, rather than one deformity predisposing to the development of the other. Hip dislocation is considerably rarer in postnatally acquired central motor deficits.

A dislocated hip may be suspected when there is flexion and internal rotation of the leg at rest or with adduction, or if there is limitation of abduction and external rotation with the hip extended and the knee flexed. The only certain method of diagnosis is to X-ray the hip. The important measurement is the percentage of the femoral head uncovered by the acetabulum, the migration percentage (Fig. 10.7).[71] Subluxation has been defined as a migration percentage of 33; when it is above 50, rapid dislocation often follows. In those children particularly at risk, pelvic radiographs should be repeated annually.

Although improved positioning, correct seating and the promotion of standing are advocated for motor disorders, there is no evidence that these measures prevent subluxation or dislocation of the hip.[11,73] A number of orthopaedic procedures are available to help prevent hip subluxation progressing to dislocation. These include soft-tissue procedures such as tenotomies and myotomies, intended to weaken the adductor muscles. These procedures can be combined with anterior branch obturator nerve neurectomy or transfer of the origin of the adductor. The effectiveness of a soft-tissue procedure alone is controversial in preventing dislocation or in treatment of established hip dislocation.[74] The likelihood of success following surgery is much greater in independent walkers. Another approach is to weaken the iliopsoas

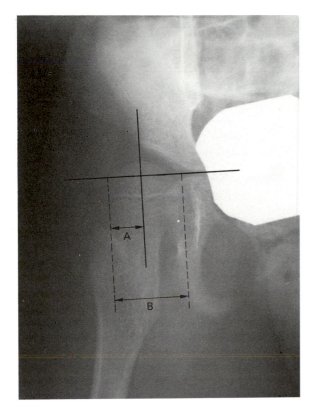

Figure 10.7 Percentage migration of femoral heads (X-ray) (migration percentage = A/B × 100).

patients who had undergone surgical procedures to the hip were compared with 50 who had received no treatment.[76] There were no differences between the groups in their level of pain, sitting ability, pelvic obliquity, scoliosis, nursing care difficulties, decubitus ulceration or fractures.

Scoliosis, like hip dislocation, is more prevalent in non-ambulant children with central motor deficits than those who are ambulant. A significant scoliosis is one in which there is lateral curvature of the spine which does not fully correct on forward flexion. The extent of curvature is best assessed from anterioposterior radiographs of the spine taken with the patient sitting, and the essential measurement is the Cobb angle, measured as the angle subtended by the upper surfaces of the first and last vertebrae in the primary curve (Fig. 10.8). The curve may be C-shaped or S-shaped, with the former being more common in children with severe motor deficits; most curves are thoracolumbar or lumbar. The reasons why some children with motor deficits develop scoliosis are not clear, but one factor must be asymmetrical truncal muscle tone, particularly where motor signs are seen more on one side of the body than the other.

Once a structural scoliosis is present the amount of curvature is likely to increase with age, and there may be particularly rapid progression around the time of the adolescent growth spurt. The rate of progression

by tenotomy, or carry out an iliopsoas transfer to elongate the muscle. By combining such a procedure with adductor tenotomy and obturator neurectomy, there is a much greater likelihood of preventing dislocation in the non-ambulant child with spastic quadriplegia.[11] However, such unilateral soft-tissue procedures need to be used with caution, as there may be deleterious effects on the opposite hip joint.[73] In non-ambulant children, the likelihood of success may be significantly influenced by postoperative management of posture.

In older children with subluxation, or if there is established hip dislocation, an open reduction procedure, combined with femoral or pelvic osteotomy, is likely to be necessary. If hip dislocation has been long-standing there may well be degeneration of the articular cartilage and a very dysplastic acetabulum. If the hip is a cause of pain, then a resection of the femoral head, possibly combined with an arthroplasty or other procedure, is often advocated.[75]

Despite the numerous reports of benefit to individual children or small groups, there is a lack of controlled studies of the orthopaedic management of hip dislocation in children with central motor deficits. That caution should be used when advocating surgery for non-ambulant children with already dislocated hips is illustrated by a retrospective study from the Arizona Children's Hospital, in which 50

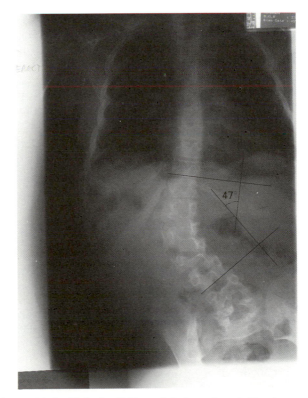

Figure 10.8 Scoliosis: the Cobb angle is that subtended by the upper surfaces of the first and last vertebrae in the primary curve.

slows considerably after growth is completed. Scoliosis may lead to increased problems with seating and there may be restrictive lung disease with the more severe thoracic curves. It is the prevention and management of these complications which leads to intervention; a severe degree of curvature on its own is not an indication for treatment, in particular surgery.

For curves of up to 20%, observation together with radiographs at annual intervals are sufficient in many cases. If a curve of up to 40% is present then orthotic bracing may be used.[77] A variety of different devices are available, with moulded polypropylene braces which fit under the arms being among the most acceptable. The intention is to prevent progression of the curve, and therefore to delay or possibly abolish the need for surgical treatment.

Surgical treatment is best reserved for those curves of over 40%. Orthoses are unlikely to be helpful in this situation. A number of different procedures are available to the orthopaedic surgeon, and there have been considerable technical advances in recent years.[11,78] If surgery is contemplated, it is important not to postpone it so long that progressive curvature causes severe restrictive lung disease and makes the risk of anaesthesia unacceptably high. Most surgical techniques rely upon a combination of fusion of the vertebrae, together with distraction and correction of the curvature using a rod device. The orthopaedic surgeon may use posterior fusion of the spine only, or a combined anterior and posterior approach. Among the most widely used fixation devices are Harrington rods and the Luque device. The latter consists of two steel rods, one on either side of the spine, held in place by wire loops.

Scoliosis surgery is time consuming and success requires preoperative preparation and skilled operative and postoperative management. Apart from the expected hazards of such major surgery, there is a risk of permanent spinal cord injury. Intraoperative monitoring using cortical evoked potentials is usually carried out in an attempt to monitor spinal cord function. In selected patients scoliosis surgery can produce excellent correction and a comfortable sitting posture.

A rare but important acquired spinal abnormality occurs in some patients with central motor deficits. *Cervical spine instability* can occur in some children with dyskinetic motor deficits, in whom it is usually ascribed to frequent abnormal movements and postures.[79] Cervical myelopathy may occur and deterioration may be sudden, or may not be appreciated in the face of other motor abnormalities. Less commonly, cervical myelopathy may develop in patients with spastic motor deficits without an associated movement disorder.[80]

Surgical treatment is useful for a small number of children where the central motor deficits cause *upper limb deformities*.[11,81] Although splints are often used to prevent deformity, it is uncertain whether these are of benefit. Splints worn during the daytime may interfere more with hand function than benefit it. Surgery has as its primary goal the improvement of upper limb function especially of the hand in activities of daily living. Appearance may also be improved. The best candidates for this type of surgery are children with spastic hemiplegia, without a significant dyskinetic element, who retain some good voluntary control of hand movement and are able and old enough to be well motivated.

Shoulder deformities do not often give rise to significant impairment in hand function. Typically in children with spastic hemiplegia there is adduction and internal rotation at the shoulder. Occasionally surgery may be undertaken to reduce the effects of contracture of the subscapularis or pectoralis major muscle. Elbow flexion deformities of greater than about 60° may interfere with function, and may be helped by procedures to lengthen the biceps tendon. Forearm pronation deformities may be improved by pronator teres tenotomy.

Wrist flexion deformities are common in children with spastic hemiplegia, often in combination with ulnar deviation. The orthopaedic surgeon can help to restore active wrist extension by tendon transfers of the flexor carpi ulnaris to a selected site on the extensor side. Such a procedure will only improve hand function if voluntary release is not impaired.[82] Finger flexion deformities may be improved by lengthening of the individual flexor tendons.

The adducted thumb deformity seriously impairs useful hand function. The aim of surgery is to enable effective grasp to be attained between thumb and fingers. A number of surgical techniques are used, most of which involve release of the adductor policis muscle. In older children, arthrodesis of the metacarpal–phalangeal joint may be done. Finger deformities which interfere with function include swan-neck deformity due to hyperextension at the proximal interphalangeal joint. They often improve if surgery is carried out to correct wrist flexion contracture, but a persistent severe deformity can be overcome by surgery to the digital flexor tendons.

The range of orthopaedic surgical treatments for *deformity and functional abnormality of the lower limbs* of children with central motor deficits is very great indeed.[11,83] The capacity for bringing about significant functional improvement is great, as is the possibility of at best obtaining no net benefit or at worst causing significant new impairment. In an effort to refine decision making, sophisticated systems of gait analysis have been employed.[84,85] At their most complex these combine video filming with electromyographic (EMG) recording and data recorded from strain gauges attached to force plates on the floor. Reflective markers located at standard points on the patient's limbs are used to generate signals which are

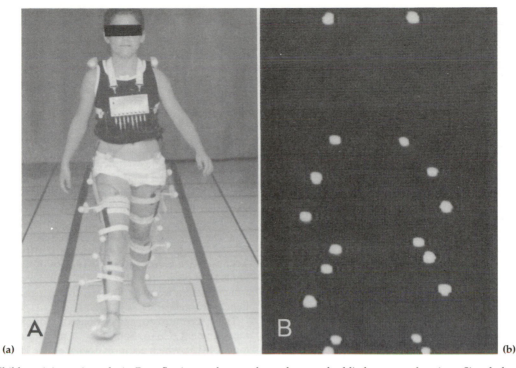

Figure 10.9 (a) Child receiving gait analysis. Retroflective markers are located at standard limb segment locations. Signals from each marker are recorded by three cameras, one anterior and two lateral. (b) Limb segment marker positions are tracked by the computer and used to form kinematic graphs. The child is wearing a telemetry unit that transmits data from both surface and fine wire elecromyographic electrodes. She is shown as her feet strike pressure-sensitive force plates. (Reproduced form Deluca[84] by kind permission of the authors and publishers).

processed by a computer attached to recording cameras (Fig. 10.9). By using such a system the different functional pathologies underlying similarly abnormal gait patterns can be appreciated. Proponents argue that such systems can be used to evaluate patients preoperatively, to plan surgery and to assess the effects of treatment.[86] It remains to be seen whether the full panoply of sophisticated methods of analysis is required to improve clinical decision making. The methods themselves may be so invasive as to bring about gait abnormalities during recording; this may happen with the placement of EMG electrodes.[87] It may be that methods of analysing energy expenditure can provide complementary information about the effects of abnormal gait in children with central motor deficits.[88] Technically very simple methods, which may require only the measurement of heart rate and walking velocity, can be used to derive a physiological cost index which can be used to evaluate the effects of intervention.[89]

Flexion deformity of the knee is common in children with spastic central motor deficits. Spasticity of the hamstrings is a major contributor to this, but co-spasticity of the quadriceps contributes to a stiff-legged gait.[90] A variety of different surgical procedures can be used to reduce the effects of hamstring spasticity, and these may be combined with transfer of the rectus femoris tendon to overcome stiffness.[91] A few children have a hyperextended knee gait, probably caused by a predominance of quadriceps spasticity, and they may be helped by tenotomy or tendon lengthening to that muscle.

Equinus foot deformity (excessive plantar flexion) is another very common abnormality in children with spastic disorders. In the majority of children there is a dynamic deformity due to altered muscle tone without evidence of contracture. Equinus may be perceived to be unsightly, and in the child with spastic hemiplegia it often contributes to the asymmetry of gait. However, in other children, particularly those with spastic diplegia, a degree of dynamic equinus usefully counteracts the effects of hamstring spasticity and knee flexion. Lengthening of the tendo Achilles should be reserved for those children with increasing deformity with clear functional deterioration.[92] Surgical treatment may also be necessary to help overcome the effects of valgus deformity of the foot, which is not uncommon in children with spastic diplegia.

Epilepsy and its management

Epilepsy occurs with a greater frequency in children with central motor deficits than in the rest of the population. It is particularly common in children with spastic quadriplegia, 90% of whom experience epileptic seizures.[14]

Epilepsy in children with motor deficits often has an onset in early infancy, with infantile spasms a not uncommon presentation.[93] Any type of seizure may occur, with generalized tonic-clonic seizures the most common. Partial seizures, either simple partial motor seizures or complex partial seizures with psychomotor features, occur particularly in children with hemiparetic disorders, about 50% of whom experience seizures. These partial seizures may become secondarily generalized. EEG abnormalities occur in far more children with spastic hemiplegia than actually experience seizures.[15] Childhood absence epilepsy (classical petit mal) is *not* observed with increased frequency in children with motor deficits.

Epilepsy in children with motor deficits has a poorer prognosis than in children who are otherwise neurologically normal. They are less likely to respond to monotherapy, less likely to be able to discontinue anti-epileptic drug treatment and more likely to relapse if treatment is discontinued.[93] The principles underlying the treatment of seizures are detailed in Section 10.7. The same principles apply to children with central motor deficits as to other children. A firm *clinical* diagnosis of epilepsy must be made, backed up as necessary by EEG findings. In some children with dyskinetic motor deficits or with severe spastic quadriplegia there may be confusion between what are seizures and what are fluctuating or sustained motor abnormalities. Patient and repeated observations, video recording and the appropriate use of EEGs during abnormal episodes can help to distinguish epileptic from non-epileptic abnormalities. The aim of treatment with anti-epileptic drugs is to render the child free of seizures, which are inconvenient and potentially hazardous because of their capacity to disrupt daily activities, cause physical harm during episodes and result in status epilepticus. The treatment must be free of side effects such as unacceptable sedation or behavioural changes.

Carbamazepine is likely to be the drug of first choice for both generalized and partial seizures in children with central motor deficits. *Sodium valproate*, which is particularly useful for generalized seizures, may very rarely cause serious hepatoxicity, most often in younger infants on a combination of treatments. *Phenytoin* remains a useful anti-epileptic drug for generalized and partial seizures, although drug monitoring is necessary because of the narrow target range of drug levels and its zero order kinetics. The benzodiazepines, particularly *clobazam* and *clonazepam* are useful either as monotherapy or in combination with other agents, although tolerance often develops; rectal *diazepam* may be administered to halt seizures. *Vigabatrin* is used in the treatment of partial and generalized seizures, and may also be effective in infantile spasms. *Lamotrigine* is another newer anti-epileptic drug which is finding a place alongside the more established drugs in the treatment of partial and generalized seizures.

Vision and hearing deficits; communication disorders

Defects of the special senses may have an enormous impact on the child with a central motor deficit, who is already restricted in the ways in which he can interact with his environment. Such defects may be difficult to recognize or to quantify in the face of multiple handicaps, and their optimum management is a part of a coordinated multidisciplinary approach to treating the child.

The principles employed in diagnosing and treating visual and hearing deficits are detailed elsewhere in this book. Some particular aspects only will be highlighted here.

Decreased visual acuity occurs in as many as 70% of children with central motor deficits.[94] The majority of those children have a *cerebral visual disturbance*. This term encompasses a group of abnormalities due to damage or dysfunction of the optic tracts, the visual cortex and other cortical areas subserving higher visual function. In addition to decreased acuity, these children may have defects of visual attention, of voluntary eye movements and perceptual difficulties.[95] Squint is a common problem, with a significant risk of developing amblyopia. Cerebral visual disturbance may become less pronounced with age, a process described as delayed visual maturation.[96]

Hearing impairments also occur with increased frequency in children with central motor deficits. The prevalence has been estimated at 12.5%,[97] but is likely to be less today than in the past because of a decrease in the incidence of neonatal bilirubin encephalopathy. Other high risk groups include children with intrauterine infections, survivors of meningitis, children with head injuries and those with craniofacial abnormalities. Hearing impairments often occur in those children with the most severe motor deficits, along with visual and cognitive deficits. Diagnosis and management are likely to be most difficult in this group.

A combination of factors can make *communication* difficult for children with central motor deficits. There are the effects of disordered motor control on language production. Poor postural control and difficulty in maintaining visual contact are sometimes a problem. Hearing impairment and cognitive deficits may contribute significantly. Alternative systems of communication have to be appropriate to the child's developmental attainments and they have to be suited to the child's motor deficits. Aids to communication include signing systems (such as Makaton), symbol systems (such as Blissymbols) and synthesized speech systems (such as a touch talker).[98]

Mental retardation and behavioural disorders

Around 35% of children with central motor deficits have *severe mental retardation* (an IQ of less than 50).[99] An increasing proportion of children with severe mental retardation have motor deficits. The reasons for this increase are several, but include the increased survival of babies of very low birthweight. Children with postnatally acquired motor deficits[9] and those with spastic quadriplegia have the greatest likelihood of having severe mental retardation.

These pupils pose a great challenge to teachers of children with special needs, especially when it comes to meeting the requirements of the Education Reform Act 1988 which included a nationally prescribed curriculum and the requirement to quantify progress in designated areas.[100] Some children have specific learning difficulties which may only become evident with time, including visual perception disorders and visual motor disorders. Other children with central motor deficits have above-average intelligence, with approximately 5% having IQs above 110 and 1% having IQs above 130.[101] If the accompanying motor, sensory or communication difficulties are severe, particular problems may arise in these children of at least average attainment. This has been the case in the past with a few children with dyskinetic motor deficits. Social and emotional adjustment may at times be more difficult than educational progress.

Behavioural difficulties occur with increased frequency among children with central motor deficits. Often these undermine the confidence of parents or other carers. Disturbed sleep patterns and misbehaviour around mealtimes are particularly challenging in the young child. Self-injurious behaviour, occurring in boys with Lesch-Nyhan syndrome, as well as in other children with central motor deficits and severe mental retardation, can be difficult to modify.[103] Approaches to management which include behaviour modification techniques enjoy mixed success when dealing with these problems. Occasionally when confronted with very difficult behaviours there may be a temptation to resort to methods of management which deprive a person of their dignity. It is of paramount importance that any treatment respects the human rights of the patient, whatever his combination of emotional, cognitive and physical problems.

Feeding, growth and gastrointestinal problems

Feeding difficulties are common in children with motor deficits, especially in early childhood. A number of possible mechanisms, sometimes operating in combination, can underlie these difficulties:

- Excessive oral sensitivity, which may result in foods or utensils inducing tongue thrusting, gagging and other abnormal responses.
- Persistence of primitive reflexes, such as rooting and sucking, which may interfere with the establishment of more mature feeding patterns.
- Cognitive delay, decreasing the ability to learn new skills.
- Oropharyngeal muscular incoordination.
- Inappropriate positioning, with the child's posture contributing to the difficulties around the time of feeding.
- Emotional factors are very important. A great deal of social interaction takes place around feeding. A tired, angry or depressed parent or carer is likely to communicate these emotions while feeding a child. A child with a limited ability to communicate may seize upon the opportunity to disrupt the feeding process.
- Learnt abnormal patterns, stemming from any of the above, may persist long after the reason for their appearance, and may contribute to making the experience of feeding a frightening or unhappy one for a child.

Feeding difficulties are among the greatest practical problems that parents and carers of very young children with motor deficits face.[103] Many of these problems can be reduced by a programme of early intervention and home support by professionals with the appropriate skills, such as speech therapists, physiotherapists and dietitians. Examples of practical measures that can be taken include the provision of special feeding aids or utensils (Fig. 10.10); correct positioning with adapted or special seating; the teaching of feeding techniques which modify the rate of feeding, the amount of each mouthful or its direction of presentation; and dietary planning to ensure that foods with the most acceptable texture and taste can be provided in a nutritionally complete form.[104] Specific help may need to be directed towards behaviour modification, and periods of respite care may be helpful.

Drooling is a considerable problem in children and adults with motor deficits. The principal mechanism is an overflow of saliva from the mouth due to dysfunctional voluntary oral motor activity and swallowing.[105] In very young children drooling is socially acceptable. In older children and adults it may cause skin irritation and may cause an offensive smell. Its principal drawback is its social unacceptability. In a very few children there is a risk of aspiration. Several different approaches are available for the management of drooling:

- Behavioural modification techniques include electronically controlled prompts to swallowing.

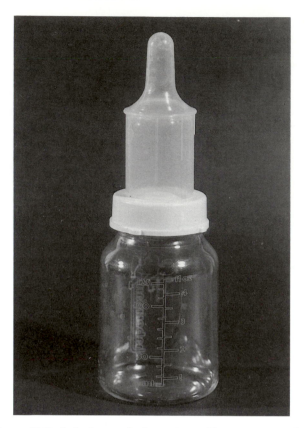

Figure 10.10 A feeder employing a teat with a one-way valve. (Haberman Feeders, 44 Watford Road, Herts, WD7 8LR.)

- Drug treatments include the use of anticholinergics such as benzhexol chloride or transdermal scopolamine,[106] which are tolerated for periods of as long as 2 years without significant side effects in many children.[107]
- Surgical techniques include transposition of the parotid or submandibular ducts to the tonsillar fossa.[108]

In most children drooling becomes less noticeable with age, and this knowledge should also be used to guide the choice of treatment.

The need for good *dental hygiene* should not be overlooked. Tooth cleaning may present difficulties to a carer or to the child who has learnt to use a brush. This may be helped by using toothbrushes with adaptable handles or electric toothbrushes. Orthodontic abnormalities including malocclusion are more common among children with motor deficits, and will require expert surveillance until a decision is made about intervention.[109]

Gastro-oesophageal reflux occurs with a much greater frequency in children with central motor deficits than in their peers and can continue to be a problem even in the older child. There may be a history of vomiting or of regurgitation of stomach contents. Recurrent respiratory infections, probably due to aspiration, suggest

the problem. Reflux may cause oesophagitis, resulting in anaemia and pain. The vomiting may be so frequent or so severe as to interfere with nutrition, but symptoms characteristically vary in severity with time and some children with reflux do not vomit much. The mechanism for reflux is probably centrally mediated incoordinate action of oesophageal motor activity, the cardiac sphincter and gastric emptying. The occurrence of reflux can be suggested by the features listed above, but, especially if surgical intervention is being considered, additional investigations should be done. A barium cine swallow is helpful if abnormal, but this investigation has an appreciable false-negative rate. A chest X-ray and blood count may be abnormal. Oesophageal pH monitoring is a more sensitive indicator of reflux than radiography.

A variety of measures can be used to treat reflux, depending upon the age of the child and the severity of the problem:

- Changing the consistency of feeds with agents such as Carobel or Nestagel is sometimes helpful, especially in very young infants.
- Drug treatments include: antacids, such as Gaviscon; cimetidine as an H_2-receptor antagonist to reduce gastric acid secretion; and domperidone or cisapride as agents to increase gastric motility.[110]
- Surgical treatments include fundal plication, a major operation which will limit the ability to vomit under any circumstances. It should only be carried out if it has been demonstrated that reflux is causing major ill health, and that medical treatment has failed to control the problem.

Constipation is another common gastrointestinal problem in children with central motor deficits. There may be a combination of reasons for its occurrence, including insufficient fluid intake (as a result of feeding difficulties or reflux); insufficient dietary fibre; defective centrally mediated control of colonic and anorectal muscle activity; and poor posture or inadequate abdominal and pelvic floor muscle activity. The child who learns that defecation is a painful process is more likely to postpone it, setting up a cycle of increasing problems. Useful measures include increasing dietary fluid and fibre; judicious use of laxatives; and promoting a good position for defecation.

Growth is frequently impaired in children with central motor deficits. In some there is poor intrauterine growth, and continued poor growth is yet another indicator that central motor deficits are but single features of multi-system disorders. It is likely that abnormal muscle tone and activity contribute directly to impaired growth, possibly by disrupting a trophic influence from the brain[111] and this may be another reason why children with the most severe motor deficits tend to have the poorest growth. In some children, sub-optimal nutritional intake, because of feeding difficulties, gastro-oesophageal reflux or increased metabolic requirements, may contribute to reduced growth.

It is important to distinguish those children who are nutritionally compromised from those who are small, but healthy and with a normal growth velocity. Accurate serial measurements of weight are necessary. Assessment of linear growth may be made difficult because of fixed joint contractures, in which case alternative measurements, such as upper-arm and lower-leg length, can be used and compared with normal standards.[112] It is also useful to look for other indicators of poor nutritional status, such as the results of haematological or biochemical tests.

Complementary routes of feeding should be considered if there is disproportionately poor weight gain for linear length, and if adequate nutritional intake cannot be maintained in spite of employing some of the measures outlined above. The methods most often used are nasogastric tube feeding and gastrostomy feeding. The former is likely to be the method of first choice in most children.[113] If catch-up growth can be demonstrated using a nasogastric tube, and if there are also other clear benefits to the child, then a gastrostomy can be used.[114] So-called button gastrostomies can be placed endoscopically, and are well tolerated (Fig. 10.11). However, as with any treatment for children with motor deficits, clear goals need to be established before deciding on such intervention.

Outcome

Measuring outcome and the effects of intervention

Accurate assessment of the benefits, if any, of specific treatment for individuals with central motor deficits requires validated and responsive measures of change in overall motor function. Indices which are to be used to evaluate change in function should comprise items which are clinically relevant and capable of detecting change.[115] Such items should give consistent responses, and the inferences drawn from the results must be truthful. At present there are insufficient indices which are designed specifically to detect change in motor function with time and which have

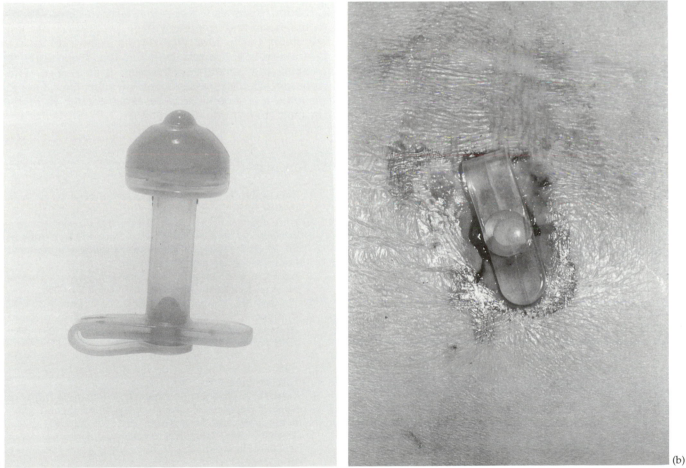

(a) (b)

Figure 10.11 Button gastrostomy: (a) before and (b) immediately after placement.

been validated when used to measure the effects of intervention. In addition to measuring technical outcome, studies of intervention should include data on functional outcome – whether the therapy for the child meets functional needs in adulthood – and also data on patient satisfaction.[116]

The proliferation in therapies for children with motor deficits, the claims made for them and the investments in them (principally in time and energy from the family) dictate that the outcome of such therapies must be assessed objectively.[117] There have been a number of studies of the effects of physiotherapy on motor disorders in the last 20 years.[61,118,119] Many studies appear flawed in their design. Few fulfil the majority of the criteria suggested by Tirosh for the design of an adequate study: randomization of subjects to treatment groups; representative study groups; detailed description of intervention; avoidance of additional therapies; blind assessment of outcome; detailed description of measures; accounting for all patients entered; ascertainment of compliance; assessment of all relevant outcomes (technical, functional, patient satisfaction); consideration of clinical and statistical significance.[118] The study which has come closest to fulfilling these criteria is that of 48 children with spastic diplegia from Baltimore, USA, treated with physiotherapy or an infant stimulation programme.[119] Neither this nor any other well designed study has demonstrated the technical or functional benefits of physiotherapy. What is certain, however, is that families very frequently describe satisfaction not only with outcome but also with the way in which care is provided by physiotherapists. The role of the physiotherapist is much more than just a provider of therapy, but is that of an expert case manager, advising on a range of functional problems, recommending specific treatments, managing complications, monitoring progress and caring for the individual.[116] Other forms of intervention (orthopaedic, pharmacological and neurosurgical) are in need of the same type of rigorous assessment as physiotherapy.

Survival and mortality

Children with central motor deficits have an increased mortality compared with the remainder of the population. Approximately 10% will have died before reaching adulthood. Mortality is greatest among those children with spastic quadriplegia and dyskinetic disorders.[120] Other factors which are associated with a significantly increased mortality are mental retardation, immobility and seizures. Children with central motor deficits who are neither immobile nor severely intellectually subnormal have a 99% chance of reaching adulthood.

Determining the cause of death in children with central motor deficits is made difficult for many reasons, including the lack of good data on death certificates.[121] Deaths are attributed to respiratory causes in almost 30% of cases. Post-mortem examination is performed in less than one-third of cases, and even in these the information provided may not be very illuminating. Status epilepticus is a cause of death in some children with motor deficits and epilepsy. Asphyxial episodes may occur in some children and young adults due to their positioning in bed at night.[122] Most frequently this is due to obstruction of the airway because of flexion of the neck, or some other abnormal posture. It is likely that impaired mobility in bed contributes to the danger of such episodes. There may be preventable factors in some of these deaths.

Conclusion

This section has dealt in the main with the medical and physical therapy aspects of central motor deficits. These are among the most prevalent neurological handicaps of childhood. Our knowledge of these disorders has increased enormously in recent years, and so have the number of ways in which these patients can be cared for. At times it seems that technical innovations in diagnosis and treatment have progressed beyond our ability to consider what is truly in the individual's best interest. The future provides the opportunity to combine the benefits of the new technologies with rigorous scientific assessment of outcome, and to maintain a compassionate advocacy for the rights of the child and young adult.

References

1   Paneth, N., Kiely, J. The frequency of cerebral palsy: a review of population studies in industrialised nations since 1950. In: Stanley, F., Alberman, E., eds. *The Epidemiology of the Cerebral Palsies*. Clinics in Developmental Medicine No. 87. London: Spastics International Medical Publications 1984: 46–56.
2   Nottidge, V.A., Okogbo, M.E. Cerebral palsy in Ibadan, Nigeria. *Dev Med Child Neurol* 1991; **33**: 241–245.
3   Al-Rajeh, S., Bademosi, O., Awada, A., Ismail, H., al-shammasi, S., Dowodu, A. Cerebral palsy in Saudi Arabia: a case control study of risk factors. *Dev Med Child Neurol* 1991; **33**: 1048–1052.
4   Dowding, V.M., Barry, C. Cerebral palsy: social class differences and severity or disability. *J Epidemiol Comm Hlth* 1990; **44**: 191–195.
5   Sussova, J., Zdenek, S., Faber, J. Hemiparetic forms of cerebral palsy in relation to epilepsy and mental retardation. *Dev Med Child Neurol* 1990; **32**: 792–795.
6   Tizard, J.P.M., Paine, R.S., Crothers, B. Disturbances of sensation in children with hemiplegia. *J Am Med Assoc* 1954; **155**: 628–632.
7   Olow, I. Children with cerebral palsy. In: Gordon, N., McKinlay, I., eds. *Neurologically Handicapped Children:*

Treatment and Management. Oxford: Blackwell Scientific Publications, 1986, 60–81.

8 Hagberg, B., Hagberg, G. The changing panorama of infantile hydrocephalus and cerebral palsy over forty years: a Swedish survey. *Brain Dev* 1989; **11**: 368–373.

9 Pharoah, P.O.D., Cooke, T., Rosenbloom, L. Acquired cerebral palsy. *Arch Dis Child* 1989; **64**: 1013–1016.

10 Koeda, T., Suganuma, I., Kohno, Y., Takamatsum, T., Takeshita, K. MR imaging of spastic diplegia: comparative study between preterm and term infants. *Neuroradiology* 1990; **32**: 187–190.

11 Bleck, E. *Orthopaedic Management in Cerebral Palsy*. Clinics in Developmental Medicine No 99/100. London: MacKeith Press, 1987.

12 Edebol-Tysk, K. Epidemiology of spastic tetraplegic cerebral palsy in Sweden: I, Impairments and disabilities. *Neuropediatrics* 1989; **20**: 41–45.

13 Krägeloh-Mann, I., Hagberg, B., Petersen, D., Riethmuller, J., Gut, E., Michaelis, R. Bilateral spastic cerebral palsy – pathogenetic aspects from MRI. *Neuropediatrics* 1992; **23**: 46–48.

14 Edebol-Tysk, K. Epidemiology of spastic tetraplegic cerebral palsy in Sweden: II, Prevalence, birth data and origin. *Neuropediatrics* 1989; **20**: 46–52.

15 Burke, R.E., Fahn, S., Gold, A.P. Delayed-onset dystonia in patients with 'static' encephalopathy. *J Neurol, Neurosurg Psychiatr* 1980; **43**: 789–797.

16 Hagberg, B., Sanner, G., Steen, M. The dysequilibrium syndrome in cerebral palsy. *Acta Pediatr Scand* 1972; **61**: Suppl 226.

17 van der Knaap, M.S., Volk, K., Bakker, C.J. *et al.* Myelination as an expression of the functional maturity of the brain. *Dev Med Child Neurol* 1991; **33**: 849–857.

18 Nelson, K.B., Ellenberg, J.H. Children who 'outgrew' cerebral palsy. *Pediatrics* 1982; **69**: 529–536.

19 Barth, P.G. Disorders of neuronal migration. *Can J Neurol Sci* 1987; **14**: 1–16.

20 de Sousa, C., Clark, T., Bradshaw, A. Antenatally diagnosed subdural haemorrhage in congenital Factor X deficiency. *Arch Dis Child* 1988; **63**: 1168–1170.

21 Skolnick, A. New ultrasound evidence appears to link prenatal brain damage, cerebral palsy (medical news and perspectives). *J Am Med Assoc* 1991; **265**: 948–949.

22 Miller, G. Minor congenital anomalies and ataxic cerebral palsy. *Arch Dis Child* 1989; **64**: 557–562.

23 Coorssen, E.A., Msall, M.E., Duffy, L.C. Multiple minor malformations as a marker for prenatal etiology of cerebral palsy. *Dev Med Child Neurol* 1991; **33**: 730–736.

24 Hughes, I., Newton, R. Genetic aspects of cerebral palsy. *Dev Med Child Neurol* 1992; **34**: 80–86.

25 Bundey, S., Griffiths, M.I. Recurrence risks in families of children with symmetrical spasticity. *Dev Med Child Neurol* 1977; **19**: 179–191.

26 Boyd, K., Patterson, V. Dopa-responsive dystonia: a treatable condition misdiagnosed as cerebral palsy. *Br Med J* 1989; **298**: 1019–1020.

27 Singer, L.T., Garber, R., Kliegman, R. Neurobehavioural sequelae of fetal cocaine exposure. *J Pediatr* 1991; **119**: 667–672.

28 Blair, E., Stanley, F. Intrauterine growth and spastic cerebral palsy. *Am J Obstet Gynecol* 1990; **162**: 229–237.

29 Torfs, C.P., van den Berg, B.J., Oechsli, F.W., Cummins, S. Prenatal and perinatal factors in the etiology of cerebral palsy. *J Pediatr* 1990; **116**: 615–619.

30 Naeye, R.L., Peters, E.C., Bartholomew, M., Landis, J.R. Origins of cerebral palsy. *Am J Dis Child* 1989; **143**: 1154–1161.

31 Escobar, G.J., Littenberg, B., Petitti, D.B. Outcome among surviving very low birthweight infants: a meta-analysis. *Arch Dis Child* 1991; **66**: 204–211.

32 Kyllerman, M. Dyskinetic cerebral palsy. II: pathogenetic risk factors and intrauterine growth. *Acta Paediatr Scand* 1982; **71**: 551–558.

33 Stanley, F., Blair, E. Postnatal risk factors among the cerebral palsies. In: Stanley, F., Alberman, E., eds. *The Epidemiology of the Cerebral Palsies*. Clinics in Developmental Medicine No. 87. London: Spastics International Medical Publications, 1984: 135–149.

34 Arens, L.J., Molteno, C.D. A comparative study of postnatally acquired cerebral palsy in Cape Town. *Dev Med Child Neurol* 1989; **31**: 245–246.

35 Schmitt, B., Seeger, J., Kreuz, W., Inenkel, S., Jacobi, G. Central nervous system involvement of children with HIV infection. *Dev Med Child Neurol* 1991; **33**: 535–540.

36 Belman, A.L., Diamond, G., Dickson, D.W., Llena, J., Lantos, G., Rubinstein, A. Pediatric acquired immunodeficiency syndrome: neurological syndromes. *Am J Dis Child* 1988; **142**: 29–35.

37 Mahoney, W.J., D'Souza, B.J., Haller, J.A., Rogers, M.C., Epstein, M.H., Freeman, J.M. Long term outcome of children with severe head trauma and prolonged coma. *Pediatrics* 1983; **71**: 756–762.

38 Crouchman, M. Head injury: how community paediatricians can help. *Arch Dis Child* 1990; **65**: 1286–1287.

39 Wigglesworth, J. Brain development and its modification by adverse influences. In: Stanley, F., Alberman, E., eds. *The Epidemiology of the Cerebral Palsies*. Clinics in Developmental Medicine No. 87. London: Spastics International Medical Publishers, 1984, 12–26.

40 Cohen, L.G., Zeffiro, T., Bookheimer, S. *et al.* Reorganisation in motor pathways following a large congenital hemispheric lesion in man: different ipsilateral motor representation areas for ipsi- and contralateral muscles. *J Physiol* 1991; **438**: 33P.

41 Evans, P., Johnson, A., Mutch, L., Alberman, E. A standard form for recording clinical findings in children with a motor deficit of central origin. *Dev Med Child Neurol* 1989; **31**: 119–127.

42 Raine, R.S. The variability and manifestations of untreated patients with phenylketonuria (phenylpyruvic aciduria). *Pediatrics* 1957; **20**: 290–302.

43 Smith, D.W., Klein, A.M., Henderson, J.R., Myrianthopoulos, N.C. Congenital hypothyroidism: signs and symptoms in the newborn period. *J Pediatr* 1975; **87**: 958–962.

44 Wiklund, L.M., Uvebrant, P., Flodmark, O. Computed tomography as an adjunct in etiological analysis of hemiplegic cerebral palsy. I: children born preterm. *Neuropediatrics* 1991; **22**: 50–56.

45 Koch, B., Braillier, D., Eng, G., Binder, H. Computerized tomography in cerebral-palsied children. *Dev Med Child Neurol* 1980; **22**: 595–607.

46 Yokochi, K., Aiba, K., Horie, M. *et al*. Magnetic resonance imaging in children with spastic diplegia: correlation with the severity of their motor and mental abnormality. *Dev Med Child Neurol* 1991; **33**: 18–25.

47 Taudorg, K., Vorstrup, P. Cerebral blood flow abnormalities in cerebral palsied children with a normal CT scan. *Neuropediatrics* 1989; **20**: 33–40.

48 Brandt, N.J. Symptoms and signs in organic acidurias. *J Inherited Metab Dis* 1984; **7**: suppl 1, 23–27.

49 de Sousa, C., Piesowicz, A.T., Brett, E.M., Leonard, J.V. Focal changes in the globi pallidi associated with neurological dysfunction in methylmalonic acidaemia. *Neuropediatrics* 1989; **21**: 199–201.

50 Terheggen, H.G., Lowenthal, A., Lavinha, F., Colombo, J.P. Familial hyperargininaemia. *Arch Dis Child* 1975; **50**: 57–61.

51 de Grauw, T.J., Smit, L.M.E., Brockstedt, M., Meijer, Y., Moorsel, J.K., Jacobs, C. Acute hemiparesis as the presenting sign in a heterozygote for ornithine transcarbymalase deficiency. *Neuropediatrics* 1990; **21**: 133–135.

52 Pavlakis, S.G., Philipps, P.C., di Mauro, S., de Vito, D.C., Rowland, L.P. Mitochondrial myopathy, encephalopathy, lactic acidosis and stroke-like episodes: a distinctive clinical syndrome. *Ann Neurol* 1984; **16**: 481–488.

53 Mitchell, D., Brown, R., eds. *Early Intervention Studies for Children with Special Needs*. London: Chapman and Hall, 1991.

54 Bobath, K. *A Neurophysiological Basis for the Treatment of Cerebral Palsy*: 2nd edn. Clinics in Developmental Medicine No. 75. London: Spastics International Medical Publications, 1980.

55 Cottam, P.J., Sutton, A. *Conductive Education: a System for Overcoming Motor Disorder*. London: Croom Helm, 1986.

56 Scrutton, D. *Management of the Motor Disorders in Cerebral Palsy*. Clinics in Developmental Medicine No. 90. London: Spastics International Medical Publishers, 1984.

57 Jesien, G. Home-based early intervention: a description of the Portage project model. In: Scrutton, D., ed. *Management of Motor Disorders of Children with Cerebral Palsy*. Clinics in Developmental Medicine No. 90. London: Spastics International Medical Publications, 1984: 36–48.

58 Cummins, R.A. *The Neurologically Impaired Child: Doman Delacato Techniques Reappraised*. Melbourne: Croom Helm, 1988.

59 American Academy of Pediatrics. *Policy Statement: the Doman-Delacato Treatment of Neurologically Handicapped Children*. *Pediatrics* 1982; **70**: 810–812.

60 Sparrow, S., Zigler, E. Evaluation of patterning treatment for retarded children. *Pediatrics* 1978; **62**: 137–150.

61 Bower, E., McLellan, D.L. Effect of increased exposure to physiotherapy on skill acquisition of children with cerebral palsy. *Dev Med Child Neurol* 1992; **34**: 25–39.

62 Meisels, S., Shonkiff, J., eds. *Handbook of Early Childhood Intervention*. Cambridge: Cambridge University Press, 1990: 702.

63 Milla, P.J. A controlled trial of baclofen in cerebral palsied children. In: Jukes, A.M., ed. *Baclofen: Spasticity and Cerebral Pathology*. Cambridge: Cambridge Medical Publications, 1978: 16–22.

64 Albright, A.L., Cervi, A., Singletary, J. Intrathecal baclofen for spasticity in cerebral palsy. *J Am Med Assoc* 1991; **265**: 1418–1422.

65 Armstrong, R.W. Intrathecal baclofen and spasticity: what do we know and what do we need to know. *Dev Med Child Neurol* 1992; **34**: 739–745.

66 Abbott, R., Forem, S.L., Johann, M. Selective posterior rhizotomy for the treatment of spasticity: a review. *Child's Nervous System* 1989; **5**: 337–346.

67 Peacock, W.J., Staudt, L.A. Spasticity in cerebral palsy and the selective posterior rhizotomy procedure. *J Child Neurol* 1990; **5**: 179–185.

68 Vaughan, C.L., Berman, B., Peacock, W.J. Cerebral palsy and rhizotomy: a 3-year follow-up evaluation with gait analysis. *J Neurosurg* 1991; **74**: 178–184.

69 Landau, W.M., Hunt, C.C. Dorsal rhizotomy, a treatment of unproven efficacy. *J Child Neurol* 1990; **5**: 174–178.

70 Trejos, H., Araya, R. Stereotactic surgery for cerebral palsy. *Stereotactic Functional Neurosurg* 1990; **54** and **55**: 130–135.

71 Scrutton, D. The early management of hips in cerebral palsy. *Dev Med Child Neurol* 1989; **31**: 108–116.

72 Cooke, P.H., Cole, W.G., Carey, R.P.L. Dislocation of the hip in cerebral palsy: natural history and predictability. *J Bone Joint Surg* 1989; **71B**: 441–446.

73 Gamble, J.G., Rinsky, L.A., Bleck, E.E. Established hip dislocations in children with cerebral palsy. *Clin Orthopaed Rel Res* 1990; **253**: 90–99.

74 Sherk, H.H., Pasquariello, P.D., Doherty, J. Hip dislocation in cerebral palsy: selection for treatment. *Dev Med Child Neurol* 1983; **25**: 738–745.

75 McHale, K.A., Bagg, M., Nason, S.S. Treatment of chronically dislocated hip in adolescents with cerebral palsy with femoral head resection and subtrochanteric valgus osteotomy. *J Paediatr Orthopaed* 1990; **10**: 504–509.

76 Pritchett, J.W. Treated and untreated unstable hips in severe cerebral palsy. *Dev Med Child Neurol* 1990; **32**: 3–6.

77 Zimbler, S., Craig, C., Harris, J., Soh, R., Rosenberg, G. Orthotic management of severe scoliosis in spastic neuromuscular disease: results of treatment. *Orthopaed Trans* 1985; **9**: 78–82.

78 Rinsky, L.A. Surgery of spinal deformity in cerebral palsy. *Clin Orthopaed Rel Res* 1990; **253**: 100–109.

79 Ebara, S., Harada, T., Yamazaki, Y., et al. Unstable cervical spine in athetoid cerebral palsy. *Spine* 1989; **14**: 1154–1159.

80 Reese, M.E., Msall, M.E., Owen, S., Pictor, S.P., Paroski, M.W. Acquired cervical spine impairment in young adults with cerebral palsy. *Dev Med Child Neurol* 1991; **33**: 153–158.

81 Koman, L.A., Gelberman, R.H., Toby, E.B., Poehling, G.G. Cerebral palsy: management of the upper extremity. *Clin Orthopaed Rel Res* 1990; **253**: 62–74.

82 Hoffer, M.M., Lehman, M., Mitani, M. Long-term follow-up on tendon transfers to the extensors of the wrist and fingers in patients with cerebral palsy. *J Hand Surg* 1986; **11A**: 836–841.

83 Bleck, E.E. Management of the lower extremities in children who have cerebral palsy. *J Bone Joint Surg* 1990; **72A**: 140–144.

84 Deluca, P.A. Gait analysis in the treatment of the ambulatory child with cerebral palsy. *Clin Orthopaed Rel Res* 1991; **264**: 65–75.

85 Patrick, J.H. Use of movement analysis in understanding abnormalities of gait in cerebral palsy. *Arch Dis Child* 1991; **66**: 900–903.

86 Shapiro, A., Susak, Z. Malkin, C., Mizrahi, J. Preoperative and postoperative gait analysis in cerebral palsy. *Arch Phys Med Rehabil* 1990; **71**: 236–240.

87 Young, C.C., Rose, S.E., Biden, E.N., Wyatt, M.P., Sutherland, D.H. The effects of surface and internal electrodes on the gait of children with cerebral palsy, spastic diplegic type. *J Orthopaed Res* 1989; **7**: 732–737.

88 Rose, J., Gamble, J.G., Burgos, A., Medeiros, J., Haskell, W.L. Energy expenditure index of walking for normal children and for children with cerebral palsy. *Dev Med Child Neurol* 1990; **32**: 333–340.

89 Mossberg, K.A., Linton, K.A., Friske, K. Ankle-foot orthoses: effect on energy expenditure of gait in spastic diplegic children. *Arch Phys Med Rehabil* 1990; **71**: 490–494.

90 Gage, J.R. Surgical treatment of knee dysfunction in cerebral palsy. *Clin Orthopaed Rel Res* 1990; **253**: 45–54.

91 Sutherland, D.H., Santi, M., Abel, M.F. Treatment of stiff-knee gait in cerebral palsy: a comparison by gait analysis of distal rectus femoris transfer versus proximal rectus release. *J Paediatr Orthopaed* 1990; **10**: 433–441.

92 Fulford, G.E. Surgical management of ankle and foot deformities in cerebral palsy. *Clin Orthopaed Rel Res* 1989; **253**: 55–61.

93 Aksu, F. Nature and prognosis of seizures in patients with cerebral palsy. *Dev Med Child Neurol* 1990; **32**: 661–668.

94 Schenk-Rootlieb, A.J.F., Nieuwehuizan, O.V., van der Graaf, Y., Wittebol-Post, D., Willemse, J. The prevalence of cerebral visual disturbance in children with cerebral palsy. *Dev Med Child Neurol* 1992; **34**: 473–480.

95 Foley, J. Central visual disturbances. *Dev Med Child Neurol* 1987; **29**: 116–120.

96 Tresidder, J., Fielder, A.R., Nicholson, J. Delayed visual maturation: ophthalmic and neurodevelopmental aspects. *Dev Med Child Neurol* 1990; **32**: 872–881.

97 Robinson, R.O. The frequency of other handicaps in children with cerebral palsy. *Dev Med Child Neurol* 1973; **15**: 305–308.

98 Enderby, P., ed. *Assistive Communication Aids for the Speech Impaired*. Edinburgh: Churchill Livingstone, 1987.

99 Nicholson, A., Alberman, E. Cerebral palsy: an increasing contributor to severe mental retardation. *Arch Dis Child* 1992; **67**: 1050–1055.

100 National Curriculum Council. *Curriculum Guidance: 2. A Curriculum for All: Special Needs in the National Curriculum*. York: NCC, 1989.

101 Bowley, A.H., Gardner, L. *The Handicapped Child: Educational and Psychological Guidance for the Organically Handicapped*: 4th edn. Edinburgh: Churchill Livingstone, 1980.

102 Murphy, G., Wilson, B., eds. *Self Injurious Behaviour*. Kidderminster: British Institute of Mental Handicap Publications, 1985.

103 Reilly, S., Skuse, D. Characteristics and management of feeding problems of young children with cerebral palsy. *Dev Med Child Neurol* 1992; **34**: 379–388.

104 Croft, R.D. What consistency of food is best for children with cerebral palsy who cannot chew? *Arch Dis Child* 1992; **67**: 269–271.

105 Sochaniwskyj, A., Koheil, R.M., Bablieh, K., Milner, M., Kenny, D.J. Oral motor functioning, frequency of swallowing and drooling in normal children and in children with cerebral palsy. *Arch Phys Med Rehab* 1986; **67**: 866–874.

106 Siegel, L.K., Klingbeil, M.A. Control of drooling with transdermal scopolamine in a child with cerebral palsy. *Dev Med Child Neurol* 1991; **22**: 1010–1014.

107 Reddihough, D., Johnson, H., Staples, M., Hudson, I., Exarchos, H. Use of benzhexol chloride to control drooling of children with cerebral palsy. *Dev Med Child Neurol* 1990; **32**: 985–989.

108 Burton, M.J. The surgical management of drooling. *Dev Med Child Neurol* 1991; **33**: 1110–1116.

109 Koster, S., Rosenstein, S.N. Orthodontics in cerebral palsy. In: Rosenstein, S.N., ed. *Dentistry in Cerebral Palsy and Relating Handicapped Conditions*. Springfield: CC Thomas, 1978: 95–110.

110 Brueton, M.J., Clarke, G.S., Sandhu, B.K. The effects of cisapride on gastro-oesophageal reflux in children with and without neurological disorders. *Dev Med Child Neurol* 1990; **32**: 629–633.

111 Growth and nutrition of children with cerebral palsy [editorial]. *Lancet* 1990; **i**: 1253–1254.

112 Spender, Q.W., Cronk, C.E., Charney, E.B., Stallings, V.A. Assessment of linear growth of children with cerebral palsy: alternative measures to height or length. *Dev Med Child Neurol* 1989; **31**: 206–214.

113 Sanders, K.D., Cox, K., Cannon, R., *et al*. Growth response to enteral feeding by children with cerebral palsy. *J Parenter Enteral Nutr* 1990; **14**: 23–26.

114 Remple, G.R., Colwell, S.O., Nelson, R.P. Growth in children with cerebral palsy fed via gastrostomy. *Pediatrics* 1988; **82**: 857–862.

115 Rosenbaum, P.L., Russell, D.J., Cadman, D.T., Gowland, C., Jarvis, S., Hardy, S. Issues in measuring change in motor function in children with cerebral palsy: a special communication. *Phys Ther* 1990; **70**: 125–131.

116 Goldberg, M.J. Measuring outcomes in cerebral palsy. *J Orthopaed* 1991; **11**: 682–685.

117 Harris, S.R., Atwater, S.W., Crowe, T.K. Accepted and controversial neuromotor therapies for infants at high risk of cerebral palsy. *J Perinatol* 1988; **8**: 5–13.

118 Tirosh, E., Rabino, S. Physiotherapy for children with cerebral palsy: evidence for its efficacy. *Am J Dis Child* 1989; **143**: 552–555.

119 Palmer, F.B., Shapiro, B.K., Wachtel, R.C. *et al*. The effects of physical therapy on cerebral palsy. *New Eng J Med* 1988; **318**: 803–808.

120 Evans, P.M., Evans, S.J.W., Alberman, E. Cerebral palsy: why we must plan for survival. *Arch Dis Child* 1990; **65**: 1329–1333.

121 Evans, P.M., Alberman, E. Certified cause of death in children and young adults with cerebral palsy. *Arch Dis Child* 1990; **65**: 325–329.

122 Brogan, T., Fligner, C., McLaughlin, J.F., Feldman, K.W., Kiesel, E.L. Positional asphyxia in individuals with severe cerebral palsy. *Dev Med Child Neurol* 1992; **34**: 169–173.

10.3 Neuromuscular diseases

Adnan Manzur and John Heckmatt

Introduction

In a survey of world literature, Emery estimated the overall prevalence of common neuromuscular disease in both sexes to be around 286×10^{-6} – 1 in 3500 of the population as a whole.[1] If rare neuromuscular disorders and the severe ones manifesting in infancy are included, the overall prevalence could possibly exceed 1 in 3000.

Clinical diagnosis

A comprehensive description of these disorders is available elsewhere.[2,3] We intend to highlight those problems which should alert a community paediatrician to the presence of neuromuscular disease, and those aspects of management likely to be of specific relevance.

Neuromuscular disease may present as a floppy infant, later with delay in motor milestones, as weakness in early childhood with difficulty walking and more extreme activities, or in the school age child as difficulty with school sports. A child may first be referred to an orthopaedic surgeon because of lower limb deformities.

In the floppy infant it is important to differentiate floppiness with weakness from floppiness without weakness. The most significant pointer to the presence of neuromuscular disorder is muscle weakness in association with hypotonia.[4] The infant with good antigravity limb movements is more likely to have a central, chromosomal, metabolic or a benign aetiology. A history of poor or absent fetal movements and of polyhydramnios is suggestive of an in utero onset, but is not specific to muscle disease.[5] Fixed talipes, abnormal respiratory muscle activity, ophthalmoplegia, facial weakness, sucking and swallowing difficulties are strongly suggestive of a neuromuscular problem.

Disproportionate delay in motor development occurs in ligamentous laxity, which is characterized by hypermobile joints, normal muscle strength, and a good prognosis. Motor delay with muscle weakness (with or without lax joints) is neuromuscular in origin. Isolated motor delay occurs in intermediate spinal muscular atrophy as affected children are very intelligent. In Duchenne muscular dystrophy the pattern may be of global delay.[6]

The strong toddler with delayed motor milestones, for example with mental retardation, can often pull himself to stand and cruise around furniture. The weak child is frequently unable to pull to stand, but when put into standing position, may be able to stand and cruise.

The pre-school child with Duchenne muscular dystrophy (DMD) may present with frequent falls without a waddling gait. Diagnosis is often missed by failure to recognize the early phase of the Gower's sign[7] or to observe the child running which exaggerates the waddling gait. Despite overt disability the diagnosis may be delayed until school age when the child is noted to have calf hypertrophy and is physically and maybe intellectually slow compared to his peers.

In the school-age child, foot deformity is suggestive of hereditary motor sensory neuropathy (HMSN). Detailed muscle strength testing to find the distribution of weakness and testing of sensation is possible at this age. In the congenital myopathies and in facioscapulohumeral muscular dystrophy, for example, the mild facial weakness can be picked up by inability to bury the eye lashes completely on closing the eyes tightly or to show the teeth fully.

A detailed family tree going back three generations is essential. Examination of parents and siblings can be revealing. For example, calf hypertrophy is present in manifesting carriers of DMD, foot deformity in mildly affected relatives with HMSN, and mild muscle weakness and facial weakness in congenital myopathy. There is a typical denial of symptoms in families with myotonic dystrophy, but careful examination reveals facial weakness and myotonia.

Special investigations

Serum creatine kinase (CK)

The methodology is not standardized and the laboratory should always report its own normal range. Serum CK is elevated into the thousands in Duchenne and Becker muscular dystrophies, even before development of clinical signs. Serum CK is raised in only 50% of patients with congenital muscular dystrophy and acute juvenile dermatomyositis, and is almost always normal in the chronic neuropathies.[8]

Electrophysiological studies

a *Motor nerve conduction velocity*

This can be measured easily with surface electrodes. Velocity is markedly reduced in the demyelinating peripheral neuropathies (for instance HMSN type 1), but is normal in the axonal neuropathies (such as HMSN type 2) in which case the amplitude of the motor action potential is markedly reduced.

b *Electromyography (EMG)*

This is performed by insertion of a fine needle electrode into the muscle. Three common patterns may be noted:

1 Denervation (neuropathic) with spontaneous fibrillation at rest, lack of full interference pattern and presence of high amplitude fasciculation potentials. These changes are characteristically seen in anterior horn cell disease.
2 Myopathic with low amplitude polyphasic potentials seen in dystrophies and congenital myopathies.
3 Myotonic with spontaneous bursts of trains of potential with waxing and gradual waning, is seen in myotonic dystrophy and myotonia congenita.

Muscle ultrasound

This recent development is more acceptable as it is non-invasive and may, where available, obviate the need for routine EMG. It is a good screening investigation for muscle disorders in general and is important for choosing an appropriate muscle for needle biopsy in patients who have selective muscle involvement.[9,10] Specific patterns of involvement have been described in dystrophy, spinal muscular atrophy (SMA) and dermatomyositis.[11]

Muscle biospy

This is performed with a Bergstrom needle under sedation and local anaesthesia on a day-case basis[12] and should only be carried out at specialized centres where facilities for histochemistry, immunocytochemistry and dystrophin assay are available. The biopsy must be interpreted in conjunction with the history and the clinical picture to get a satisfactory diagnosis.[13]

Management

It is important to realize that severe neuromuscular disease may cause intense psychological, social and financial stress on the family. With help in all these areas and appropriate modification in housing, transport, schooling and lifestyle, there may be a successful adaptation to a devastating and long illness.

Definitive curative treatment is available for only a minority of neuromuscular disorders. The aim of management in the majority of cases is to maintain and prolong functional mobility and to prevent and control contractures and bony deformities.

Joint contractures put limbs at a mechanical disadvantage, limit walking and cause discomfort. Regular passive stretching is essential to prevent progression. Specific exercises as a part of physiotherapy regimen may strengthen various muscle groups and promote motor milestones. Children with neuromuscular disease show a rapid deterioration in strength and function if they are confined to bed for any reason. It is important to give physiotherapy to maintain muscle strength and to mobilize the child back to walking as quickly as possible. Parents of children with intermediate severity spinal muscular atrophy should be taught the techniques of chest physiotherapy.

A skilled orthotist capable of working with polypropylene and aluminium alloy is invaluable as heavy and poorly fitting orthoses are seldom tolerated and quite useless. Ankle-foot orthoses may be used as night splints to prevent equinus deformity of the feet or, during the day, to stabilize joint laxity or to correct the drop foot gait in HMSN. Light-weight, ischial weight-bearing, long-length calipers (knee-ankle-foot-orthoses), can be worn under trousers and are used to promote standing and walking. A moulded thoracolumbar spinal orthosis (spinal brace) may slow the progression of scoliosis and enable the child with severe trunk weakness to adopt the sitting posture for the first time.

Surgical correction of deformities needs to be carefully timed in the context of a particular child's age, muscle power and natural history of disease. In a mobile child, correction of lower limb deformities should be aimed at improving ambulation rather than anatomical correction for its own sake. Scoliosis needs careful monitoring for progression. The risk of respiratory complications in spinal stabilization surgery is high in patients with a forced vital capacity below 30% of expected. In the non-ambulant child a balance has to be struck between the need to allow adequate spinal growth and the need to perform the operation early to prevent progression and the associated deterioration in respiratory function.

Physical handicap may dictate major alteration to the house or rehousing to ground floor adapted accommodation. This needs to be coordinated with the occupational therapist, employed by the local authority, who can assess the patient at home in the light of the disability and prognosis. A detailed guide of specialized aids is available.[14] The Muscular Dystrophy Group of Great Britain employs several family care officers who are based at the neuromuscular centres. They liaise with the statutory and voluntary organizations in the community and facilitate the provision of services to the affected families.

Respiratory failure in neuromuscular disease

Respiratory muscle weakness may lead to sleep hypoventilation[15] predisposing the patient to develop chronic respiratory failure. Sleep hypoventilation may present with severe symptoms, including disturbed sleep, morning drowsiness, nausea and headaches. In some disorders such as the relatively nonprogressive congenital myopathies, this occurs at a stage when the patient is ambulant. The patient with sleep hypoventilation may remain stable, may slip gradually into chronic respiratory failure or may present with acute-on-chronic failure during an otherwise trivial respiratory infection.

Chest shape and breathing movements should be assessed for evidence of diaphragmatic and intercostal muscle weakness.[16] Respiratory reserve is frequently diminished in neuromuscular disease and we recommend routine measurement in the clinic of forced vital capacity with a portable spirometer such as that made by Micromedical. Sleep hypoventilation can be easily detected by overnight oxygen saturation monitoring with an oximeter.

Treatment of sleep hypoventilation can dramatically improve the patient's quality of life. It has been attempted in the past with the iron lung, rocking bed, or negative pressure ventilation via cuirass pump and jacket.[16] The equipment involved was often unwieldy and noisy and not very effective. Positive pressure ventilation via tracheostomy has been used but is invasive.

The management of chronic respiratory failure has been revolutionized with the advent of nocturnal nasal mask ventilation.[17,18] The patient's breathing at night is augmented with breaths delivered by a compact portable ventilator with a snugly fitting mask on the nose. This corrects sleep hypoventilation without noise or encroachment on living space or restriction of travel. Reliable portable ventilators are available such as the Ventimate (Thomas Respiratory Systems, London) and the BIPAP/ST (Medic Aid, Sussex, UK) at a present cost of £3–4000. Ventilation in DMD poses more difficult ethical issues and is discussed later.

Genetic counselling

A firm and precise diagnosis is an essential prerequisite. Members of the family who may be affected or are potential carriers should, when possible, be identified and counselled. Gene location for many of the disorders is now known. Of the common severe diseases, antenatal diagnosis is available for DMD and is being established for severe SMA (Werdnig-Hoffmann disease). Genetic counselling using DNA analysis requires a sample of blood from the patient. If the disorder is severe or progressive, blood should be taken and stored.

The muscular dystrophies

The term muscular dystrophy is used for a group of genetic disorders with primary, progressive degeneration of the skeletal muscle. Various subtypes are defined on the basis of clinical distribution, severity of muscle weakness and pattern of inheritance. With advances in medical genetics, it is likely that gene localization to particular chromosomes and presence of gene deletion will also become part of the criteria for subclassification of dystrophies.

Duchenne muscular dystrophy

This is a well-defined, X-linked recessive disorder; the gene is carried and transmitted by females and manifests itself in males. The incidence of DMD is about 1 in 3500 male births.[1] The prevalence in the population as a whole is about 3 per 100 000.[19] The biochemical defect is the almost complete absence of the large molecular weight protein dystrophin.

Clinical features

The onset of symptoms is usually before the age of 5 years; loss of ambulation occurs by the thirteenth birthday and death is in the late teens or early twenties.

Parents are usually unaware of a problem until after the boys start walking. Walking is delayed beyond 18 months in half of affected children. Once walking, there is a tendency to fall frequently and unexpectedly and to have difficulty in rising.[20] There may be a waddling gait, and there is always difficulty running and climbing stairs. Weakness of hip extensors leads to gradual development of a forward tilt of the pelvis and a compensatory lordosis to maintain the upright posture. Enlargement of calf muscles is usual but not invariable; however, the calves usually feel firm to palpation. Gower's sign is prominent in school-age boys and becomes more laborious and takes longer as the disease progresses. An affected boy is never able to hop.

The distribution of weakness is symmetrical and proximal. Weakness of the arms is not symptomatic in the early stages but can be found on clinical testing. There is no facial weakness, no bulbar weakness and no abnormality of sphincter control. Some tightness of the tendo Achilles and iliotibial bands (fascia lata) is often present by 5 years of age. With progression of these contractures and with increasing weakness, the gait becomes progressively more up on the toes and broad based.

The mean age of loss of independent walking is 9.5 years, with a range from 7 to 12 years. Confinement in the wheelchair is associated with rapid development of contractures of hip and knee flexors and ankle plantiflexors. In 90% of cases a progressive thoracolumbar scoliosis develops, the maximum progression of which occurs in conjunction with the pubertal growth spurt.

There are remarkably few data on the mode of death of these patients. Death commonly occurs suddenly and unexpectedly during a relatively trivial intercurrent infection. Respiratory insufficiency is probably the main cause, but cardiac involvement is also important.

The onset of respiratory failure is insidious with limitation and progressive decline of forced vital capacity once independent walking is lost. Nocturnal hypoxaemia is relatively asymptomatic, but occasionally patients develop severe symptoms of sleep hypoventilation.

The ECG is abnormal in almost all patients over 10 years, showing sinus tachycardia, tall R waves in right precordial leads and deep Q waves. Cardiac ultrasound scanning shows little abnormality until about the age of 14 years. Cardiac failure is rare and usually a terminal event.

There is an associated non-progressive intellectual impairment, not explained by the lack of educational opportunity or physical handicap. The mean IQ in most series is in the region of 85, compared with a mean normal population IQ of 105 using the Wechsler scale.[2] The range of IQ follows a normal distribution curve with 30% of boys with DMD below IQ 75 and a small proportion with IQ above 110.

Investigations

Serum CK activity is elevated to at least 10 times the upper limit of the normal adult range. The EMG shows a low-voltage myopathic pattern. Muscle ultrasound shows increased echogenicity with preservation of muscle bulk.

Muscle biopsy is performed for definitive diagnosis. Dystrophic change is characterized by proliferation of endomysium and perimysium, active degeneration and regeneration and progressive replacement of the muscle by adipose tissue. The degree of change on the biopsy does not correlate well with the clinical severity. Dystrophin assay on muscle tissue with immunofluorescence and immunoblotting techniques shows absence or almost complete absence of dystrophin.

Identification of a deletion in the gene by DNA studies on blood gives a precise molecular genetic diagnosis. The deletion can however be identified in only about 60% of the affected boys and is of limited value in determining disease severity.

Management

While the child is ambulant, he should have daily passive stretching of the tendo Achilles, iliotibial bands and hip flexors to prevent fixed contractures. This can usually be done by the parents with regular help and support from the physiotherapist. Night splints are required when the feet cannot be dorsiflexed to beyond the neutral position (90°), and can often be made of plaster of Paris.

Weight watching and healthy eating should be encouraged to avoid obesity which may add to the difficulty in walking. Weight loss in overweight boys is safe[21] and weight charts designed by Griffiths and Edwards may be used as a guide.[22] Constipation is another common problem amenable to diet.

At the moment of loss of independent walking, the majority of boys are suitable for prolongation of walking by rehabilitation with ischial weight bearing knee-ankle-foot orthoses.[23] This has psychological benefits, prevents contractures and postpones development of scoliosis. Regular physiotherapy assessments allow preparation of the family and selection of optimal time for intervention. Rehabilitation involves percutaneous Achilles tenotomies, intensive inpatient physiotherapy over 4 weeks and requires special expertise particularly with the orthotics. The mean period of prolongation of walking in a series of 93 patients was 21 months.[24]

Rideau and co-workers[25] have introduced early radical surgery for patients between the ages of 4 and 6 years. This innovative treatment involves release of the pelvic head of rectus femoris, complete excision of fascia lata, formal lengthening of the tendo Achilles and tenotomies of the hamstrings and other muscles. They claim to achieve a more normal gait, freedom from physiotherapy, and stabilization or improvement in function. Their results are uncontrolled, however, and a randomized controlled trial has failed to confirm any benefit.[26]

Once the child is wheelchair bound, the progression of limb and spine deformities is rapid and inevitable. Equinus deformity of the feet should be prevented with continuous wearing of ankle-foot orthoses. This is practical if the child has had previous Achilles tenotomy for rehabilitation. Use of a spinal brace is generally recommended although its benefit in slowing the progression of scoliosis is uncertain. The Luque operation involving placement of two rods alongside the spine with laminar wiring to each vertebra has revolutionized the management.[27] In our unit, the operation is carried out once the Cobb angle is about 20–30°, before puberty or in early puberty, and while the forced vital capacity is still above the critical 30% value.

Management of respiratory failure in DMD poses difficult ethical issues. Various factors have to be considered; symptoms, quality of life with and without treatment, the wishes of the patient and his family and availability of resources. Over the years, many workers have documented prolongation of life using traditional techniques of mechanical ventilation,[28–30] but at the expense of an increased burden of care on the family.[31] The advent of nasal ventilation unquestionably shifts the ground in favour of offering ventilation and this technique is dramatically effective in relieving acute symptoms.[18] There are no long-term published results yet and, in general, ventilation is only offered if and when the patient presents with symptoms. This is perhaps an unsatisfactory situation, and a controlled trial of prophylactic nasal ventilation to try to clarify its place in management is currently under way.

Genetics and carrier detection

The DMD gene locus at XP21 is the largest known human gene. The gene contains at least 65 exons distributed over 2.5 million base pairs.[32] A deletion in one or more of the exons can be demonstrated in at least 60% of the affected cases. The protein product coded for by the normal gene has been named dystrophin.[33] It is a large (400 kd), extremely low abundance protein associated with the membrane fraction from the muscle.

The gene has a high spontaneous mutation rate and one-third of all cases are fresh mutations. In the offspring of a carrier, each son has a 50% chance of being affected and each daughter has a 50% chance of being a carrier.

There have been dramatic advances in the last decade in genetic counselling. Serum CK is elevated in a majority of carriers and its estimation may detect 70–75% of carriers. There is, however, an overlap between the normal population and DMD carrier's CK levels so a normal CK does not rule out carrier status. Only a small proportion of carriers (8%) show muscle weakness and large calves – the so called manifesting carrier. Estimation of carrier risk for an individual female using CK and other data was therefore often imprecise. Calculation of risk is now much more accurate, taking into account gene deletion and linkage analysis, pedigree and serum CK levels.[34] Dystrophin estimation at biopsy also has useful application in identification of carriers and isolated manifesting carriers.[35]

Genetic counselling of the mother should be undertaken at the time or shortly after diagnosis of the index case. Potential female carriers in the family are not usually tested before the age of 16 years. Antenatal diagnosis is carried out only in women who plan to terminate the pregnancy if the fetus is found to be affected. In families where the index case has a dystrophin gene deletion, it is simple to screen the fetus for that specific deletion. These tests are carried out on tissue obtained by chorion villus sampling at 10 weeks of gestation. This procedure however carries a 1–3% risk of fetal loss and is generally considered appropriate only if the carrier's risk is more than 5%.[34]

Screening

In a population where diagnosis is made at 4–5 years of age, 30–40% of cases come from families having more than one affected boy.[36] The Muscular Dystrophy Group report that the mean age at diagnosis of boys with DMD is 5.2 years whereas the mean age at the initial presentation to a doctor is 2.7 years. Earlier diagnosis would allow early detection of carriers and prevention of secondary cases in the family.[37] Wallace and Newton studied patterns of standing and emphasized two components of the Gower manoeuvre: (1) the child adopts the prone position on all fours before attempting to stand; and (2) the child 'walks up the legs'. Adoption of the prone position is a normal developmental phase in toddlers but its persistence after 36 months suggests either central hyptonia or a neuromuscular disorder.[7]

The most effective method of early detection would be by a population based neonatal screening programme. Serum CK is elevated from birth. It can be elevated in the normal newborn, secondary to trauma of delivery, but drops rapidly over the first few days.[38] Screening for DMD can thus be performed by estimation of CK in male infants after the third day of life. Serum CK assay can be done on a drop of blood dried on a filter paper.[39] Neonatal DMD screening has not been widely adopted as it does not fulfil the traditional criteria; also early studies showed families did not act on information given and secondary cases were not prevented. As a compromise, Gardner-Medwin suggested screening all boys not walking at 18 months of age[40] on the basis that 50% of boys with DMD do not walk until after 18 months. A trial programme based on this approach was introduced in Wales for an 18 month period[41] but was not considered to be worthwhile as it would reduce the number of cases by less than 10% and was also impracticable. Nevertheless, the diagnosis should be considered in any 18-month-old boy who presents to the paediatric clinic with unexplained language delay or delay in walking. Smith[42] re-examined the attitude of mothers to a programme of neonatal screening and found most would opt for a screening programme if offered and would also choose termination to prevent severe handicap. Now that effective genetic counselling and accurate diagnosis with dystrophin assay are available, neonatal screening should be reconsidered.

Becker muscular dystrophy

Becker muscular dystrophy (BMD) is similar to DMD in muscle weakness distribution and inheritance, but it has a later onset and slower progression with better prognosis. Though the onset may be in childhood, the course is slow and mild, and affected individuals remain ambulant beyond 16 years of age. BMD is compatible with a normal life span and there is no associated mental retardation. The calves may be prominent and there may be cramps in the legs on exercise and episodes of myoglobinuria. Changes in the ECG are common, and occasionally one sees heart block and cardiomyopathy in the ambulant patient. In those patients with myoglobinuria, there is a risk of severe hyperpyrexial type reactions and myoglobinuria with certain anaesthetics such as halothane, but general anaesthesia should be safe so long as appropriate precautions are taken.

The serum CK is elevated as with DMD. Muscle biopsy shows dystrophic change and reduced quantity of dystrophin, which may also be abnormal in molecular weight.[43]

The genes for Duchenne and Becker muscular dystrophy are allelic. Though it has been shown that deletion of exons containing Hind III fragments 33 and 34 and 33 to 35 is commonly associated with BMD,[44] the differentiation between BMD and DMD should be based on the severity, course and progression of the disease.

With the identification of gene locus, some workers refer to DMD and BMD under the umbrella term XP21 muscular dystrophy. This term conveys no information about severity or prognosis. We recommend that the traditional eponyms should still be used; DMD with loss of ambulation by the 13th birthday, and BMD with walking preserved beyond 16 years. In practice, there are some boys who lose ambulation between 13 and 16 years of age; they are referred to as the intermediate severity group or Duchenne outliers.

Limb girdle muscular dystrophy

This is a disorder of variable severity with progressive muscle weakness mainly affecting the proximal muscles of the limbs. The gene locus is on chromosome 15 with autosomal recessive inheritance, affecting both boys and girls. It is comparatively rare in Europe with a prevalence less than 5×10^{-6}, but is more common in certain in-bred Arabian communities.[1]

The course is very variable, although the majority of patients probably have a milder disease than DMD. In girls, toe walking may be prominent and antedate the difficulty in walking. There may be cramps on exercise. Early cardiac involvement, such as treatable arrhythmia or cardiomyopathy, needs to be recognized.

In males, the differential diagnosis is Duchenne and Becker muscular dystrophy. In females, the differential diagnosis includes atypical cases of Duchenne and Becker muscular dystrophy affecting females (severely manifesting carriers, Turner's syndrome, XO/XX mosaics, X autosome translocation with breakpoint at XP21). It is therefore important

to perform chromosome karyotype, dystrophin gene deletion studies and dystrophin assay to rule out XP21 dystrophy. This differentiation and precision in diagnosis is crucial to accurate genetic counselling. The inheritance is autosomal recessive, while in contrast manifesting Duchenne and Becker carriers may pass the condition on and there may be asymptomatic female carriers in the family.

Facioscapulohumeral dystrophy

Weakness predominantly affects the face and the shoulder girdle muscles. Inheritance is autosomal dominant with variation in severity within the family. The gene has been localized to 4q35-qter.[45]

The common presentation is in adolescence or adult life, though childhood cases occur and can be found on examining affected families. Facial weakness may predate the weakness in the shoulder girdle. Characteristic upward rotation of scapulae and terracing of shoulders can be seen on abduction of the arms.[3] The condition is variable within individual families with some having mild non-progressive involvement and others severe progressive disability. There is no cardiac or intellectual impairment. Patients with marked difficulty in elevation of shoulders may benefit from orthopaedic fixation of scapulae to the thoracic wall.

A variety of changes are reported on muscle biopsy including small angular fibres suggestive of denervation and full-blown dystrophic changes.

Congenital muscular dystrophy

This disorder often presents in infancy with floppiness and weakness in association with dystrophic change on muscle biopsy. Contractures of varying severity may be present at birth manifesting as arthrogryposis, or may develop in early childhood. Overt facial weakness may be present. Respiratory failure in the neonatal period is an uncommon presentation. The apparent onset in some children is delayed past infancy; they present with delayed walking and contractures. Although the condition is termed muscular dystrophy, the weakness is non-progressive and there may actually be improvement in strength with age. Intellectual impairment occurs in a minority, although it is a consistent feature in the Fukuyama-type subgroup described in Japan.

The serum CK is normal to mildly elevated; muscle ultrasound is markedly echogenic and is a useful screening investigation. Muscle biopsy shows a striking dystrophic picture with marked proliferation of connective and adipose tissue.

The inheritance is probably autosomal recessive. The gene locus has not yet been identified.

Early diagnosis is important to institute a programme of passive stretching of contractures, night splints and physiotherapy. Children too weak for independent ambulation may benefit from standing or walking orthoses. Occasionally there is sufficient improvement to allow the child to progress to walking without the calipers. Unfortunately children often present too late for rehabilitation.

The congenital myopathies

Nemaline (rod body) myopathy

The common presentation is in infancy with floppiness, mild facial and generalized muscle weakness with preserved antigravity movements, but with disproportionate difficulty in swallowing and risk of recurrent aspiration. Muscle weakness is non-progressive, but there may be significant respiratory muscle weakness and nocturnal hypoventilation may develop.

Kyphoscoliosis may emerge during puberty despite ambulation. Rarely the condition may present in the newborn with respiratory failure in which case prognosis is poor. The inheritance is usually autosomal recessive. Rod-like structures are seen on the Gomori trichrome stained sections of muscle biopsy.

Myotubular (centronuclear) myopathy

Common features are muscle weakness and external ocular ophthalmoplegia. Three clinical and genetic subtypes are described:[46]

1 Severe X-linked type, presenting with ventilatory failure, skeletal muscle weakness and ophthalmoplegia; the prognosis is poor. The gene locus is at Xq 28.[47]
2 Less severe infantile type, which is probably recessively inherited.
3 Mild juvenile or adult type, which is autosomal dominant in some families.

A histological feature common to all subtypes is the presence of large central nuclei in muscle fibres.

Mitochondrial myopathies

The common features shared by this diverse group of syndromes are the presence of ragged red fibres seen on muscle biopsy sections stained with the modified Gomori stain. In-vitro studies of mitochondrial metabolism show various defects of the respiratory chain, predominantly affecting complex IV in children.[48] Presentation may be with a myopathy characterized by marked fatiguability in which the main differential diagnosis is myasthenia.

Three clinical encephalomyopathy syndromes are also described, although many cases have a combination of features.

1 Kearns-Sayre (oculo-crano-somatic) syndrome (KSS).
The main features are progressive external ophthalmoplegia, ptosis, ataxia, short stature, retinitis pigmentosa, fatiguability and muscle weakness in limbs and neck flexors.
2 Syndrome of myoclonic epilepsy and ragged red fibres (MERRF).
3 Syndrome of mitochondrial encephalopathy, lactic acidosis and stroke-like episodes (MELAS).

The majority of patients with the KSS syndrome are not familial. Maternal (mitochondrial) transmission has been described in MERRF and MELAS.[49] Autosomal recessive transmission is responsible for severe cytochrome oxidase deficiency which presents with progressive weakness in infancy.

Central core disease

Common presentation is that of mild and non-progressive weakness which is proximal or generalized and may present in early infancy or childhood. Talipes and congenital hip dislocation are frequent associations. There is an increased risk of hyperpyrexial reaction with certain anaesthetics[50] and a medic-alert necklace or bracelet is advisable. Inheritance is autosomal dominant with the gene locus at 19q12-q13.2.[51] In any child with musculoskeletal deformity it is therefore important to look for other deformities and take a careful family history. On muscle biopsy, with the oxidative enzyme reaction (NADH-TR), the cores are seen on transverse sections as holes in the centre of the fibres.

Malignant hyperthermia

Malignant hyperthermia (MH) is a dominantly inherited state of susceptibility to potentially fatal hyperpyrexial reaction (rise of temperature to 44°C, muscle rigidity, cyanosis, acidosis, convulsions and myoglobinuria) on exposure to suxamethonium, halothane and various other anaesthetics.[52] Most susceptible individuals are fit and healthy prior to anaesthesia, though about 50% have elevated CK and some may have a subclinical myopathy or musculoskeletal deformities (kyphoscoliosis, foot deformity, hip dislocation, joint contractures, recurrent dislocation of patella).

The gene locus at 19q13.1-q13.3 overlaps with the gene locus for central core disease and the two disorders may be allelic. Diagnosis is suspected by history of anaesthetic-related incidents or death in the family or in a child with unexplained musculoskeletal deformities; it is confirmed by in-vitro contracture testing. The parents and siblings should also be investigated. Surgery can be performed using anaesthetics other than those known to trigger an adverse reaction in the person.

Identification of the rare King's syndrome[53] can avert a potential disaster. These children have short stature, cryptorchidism, multiple skeletal deformities, ptosis and susceptibility to hyperpyrexial reaction and represent the severe end of the spectrum of the autosomal dominant type or possibly a separate autosomal recessive variant.

Metabolic myopathies

A specific metabolic abnormality can be identified in certain muscle disorders. Type II glycogenesis is due to acid maltase deficiency. The severe fatal form is Pompe's disease which presents in infancy with hypotonia, weakness, and hypertrophic cardiac failure. There is a milder form which presents in the second decade with proximal muscle weakness or insidious sleep hypoventilation and respiratory failure. The ECG shows large QRS complexes and a short PR interval. Excess glycogen is seen on muscle biopsy. The gene locus is at 17q and inheritance is autosomal recessive.

Type V glycogenesis (phosphorylase deficiency, McArdle's disease) is characterized by cramps on exercise. Although diagnosis is often not made until adult life, symptoms can be traced to childhood. There may be myoglobinuria after excessive exercise. Gene locus is at 11q and inheritance is autosomal recessive. Diagnosis is made histochemically on muscle biopsy.

Juvenile dermatomyositis (JDM)

This is an acute or subacute multisystem autoimmune disorder with primary involvement of skin and muscle with an underlying vasculitic pathology. It differs from adult dermatomyositis in its lack of association with underlying malignancies and the good response to treatment.

Three major presenting features are muscle weakness, misery (often the first sign) and rash, developing over a period of weeks or a few months. Muscle weakness is progressive, proximal and symmetrical. Difficulty in swallowing is common. The skin rash, which is not always present, is characteristically violaceous on the upper eyelids and rather erythematous on the knuckles, elbows and knees. There is often elbow and Achilles tendon tightness which resolves as treatment is started.

Skin and soft tissue calcification is characteristic, often developing as the disease starts to resolve. Clinically detectable vasculitic involvement of the gastrointestinal tract is rare but potentially fatal, leading to haemorrhage or perforation. Mortality has been dramatically reduced by treatment with steroids.

The diagnosis is based mainly on the clinical picture; the serum CK is elevated in only 50% but the EMG is usually myopathic and may also show fibrillation potentials at rest. Muscle ultrasound may show a characteristic alteration in echogenicity on angulating the transducer in the horizontal plane.[11] Muscle biopsy may be normal but may show perifascicular atrophy, degeneration and inflammatory cellular response.

The disorder is very steroid sensitive. High-dose prednisolone (2 mg/kg/day) or intravenous methyl prednisolone is still favoured in some centres, but there have been excellent results over the years with a low dose prednisolone regimen, starting with 1 mg/kg/day and tapering gradually over the following months but without going over to alternate day.[54] The low dose regimen avoids the serious side effects of steroid therapy (hypertension, osteoporosis, cataracts, avascular necrosis of bone) and growth suppression is temporary. Partial response to steroids or relapse may necessitate immunosuppression with azathioprine or cyclosporin A.[55] Loss of ambulation as a consequence of relapse must be avoided, as permanent contractures can develop; physiotherapy during the acute and remission phase is essential.

Myotonic syndromes

Myotonia is characterized by delayed muscle relaxation; for example, slow extension of the fingers when opening the hand after making a fist. Two of the more common myotonic conditions, myotonic dystrophy and myotonia congenita, will be discussed.

Myotonic dystrophy (Steinert's disease)

The onset is usually in adolescence or adulthood with full manifestation in the fourth and fifth decade. Prevalence rate in adults is around 50×10^{-6}. The inheritance is autosomal dominant and the gene locus is at 19q13.2-q13.3.[56]

Patients may be aware of difficulty in relaxing their grip. The full form has multisystem involvement with ptosis, facial weakness, wasting of sternomastoids, weakness with distal muscle involvement, frontal baldness in males, cataracts, cardiomyopathy with conduction defects and gonadal atrophy. The course may be progressive with marked muscle weakness, loss of ambulation and respiratory or cardiac problems. There is a very wide variation in disease expression and some patients may have only minimal facial weakness and myotonia or only pre-senile cataract. Smooth muscle involvement may cause constipation.

Myotonic dystrophy can have its onset in childhood and cases can be recognized if children of affected adults are examined. At this stage, however, the problem is usually limited to mild facial weakness and myotonia. Intellectual development may be delayed. Denial of symptoms is common.

Congenital myotonic dystrophy has an incidence of at least 1 in 3500 live births. Mildly affected infants are floppy and have facial weakness and difficulty in sucking and swallowing. Severely affected infants have respiratory failure from birth but may not have severe generalized weakness. There is usually a history of poor fetal movements and polyhydramnios.

Ventricular dilatation is present from birth and can be detected on ultrasound scanning.

Although congenital myotonic dystrophy is dominantly inherited, it is invariably the mother who is the affected parent. She is usually mildly affected and hitherto undiagnosed. The explanation is now known to relate to the basic defect which is a variable DNA sequence at 19q13.[57] Diagnosis is confirmed by examining the mother and documenting myotonic discharges on her EMG.

The prognosis varies with the initial severity. Affected neonates who require ventilation from birth for more than 4 weeks are unlikely to survive beyond 15 months even if they eventually come off the ventilator.[58] Delayed motor milestones and intellectual impairment is the rule, irrespective of initial severity.[59]

Antenatal diagnosis is now available for congenital myotonic dystrophy by linkage analysis. Having identified the index case, it is important to identify, if possible, all the other affected family members. Mildly affected adults are at risk during general anaesthetic of oversensitivity to muscle relaxants and the anaesthetist should be forewarned.

Myotonia congenita (Thomsen's disease)

This dominantly inherited condition presents with myotonia and muscle hypertrophy in childhood. Patients become aware of grip myotonia and difficulty in initiating movements after rest. Myotonia is aggravated by cold, may be brought on by sudden fright and is relieved by repetitive movement. Severity of myotonia varies in different patients and, if troublesome, may be treated with phenytoin, quinine or procainamide.

Diseases affecting lower motor neurones

Chronic hereditary disease of the lower motor neurone pertaining to childhood falls into two main groups: spinal muscular atrophy (primary anterior horn cell degeneration) and hereditary motor sensory neuropathy (primary involvement of peripheral nerves).

Spinal muscular atrophy (SMA)

The term is best reserved for a group of autosomal recessively inherited, proximal, symmetrical muscle atrophies associated with degeneration of anterior horn cells of the spinal cord. Following the original descriptions, attempts have been made by many authors to classify various subtypes of SMA on the basis of severity, age of onset, age of death. The chaos has been further compounded by introduction of the descriptive terms acute and chronic SMA. Dubowitz[60] recommended subdividing SMA into three categories as follows:

1 Severe SMA. Unable to sit unsupported.
2 Intermediate SMA. Able to sit unsupported but unable to stand.
3 Mild SMA. Able to stand unaided.

Severe spinal muscular atrophy (Werdnig-Hoffmann disease)

Onset is in the first few weeks or months of life, or may be intrauterine with reduced fetal movements. Usually the infant appears normal and then has an insidious onset of weakness. The characteristic picture is that of an infant with severe paralysis of proximal muscles but who has bright alert facies. The arms are often internally rotated at the shoulders (jug handle position). The tendon reflexes are invariably absent, and if present invalidate the diagnosis. There is no facial weakness, but fasciculation of the tongue is common. Contractures of any severity are uncommon. Bulbar weakness is uncommon unless there is a superimposed chest infection.

Severe weakness of the intercostal muscles with sparing of the diaphragm leads to gradual development of a characteristic bell-shaped appearance of the chest. Early on the breathing has a characteristic see-saw motion due to the relatively good diaphragm and weak intercostal muscles. The cry is weak and the cough absent or ineffectual. The prognosis is uniformly poor and most infants succumb to chest infection within the first year of life. Accurate prediction of exact weeks or months of survival is difficult, however, and in general should be avoided.

Intermediate spinal muscular atrophy

Onset is usually between 6 and 18 months of age when the child, having sat unaided, cannot take weight on legs and is unable to stand. Weakness is always symmetrical and affects proximal more than distal muscles. Arms are less affected than legs and there is antigravity power at the shoulder girdle while the legs are very weak. Tendon jerks are absent. There is no facial or bulbar weakness. Fasciculation and atrophy of the tongue are common. Fine tremor of the hands is frequently present.

Intercostal muscle weakness is usually not severe, there is no diaphragmatic weakness and respiratory failure is uncommon unless the child has a severe scoliosis.

The muscle weakness is not progressive and survival into adolescence or adulthood is common. Prognosis depends on the degree of involvement of the respiratory muscles; those with severe involvement have a narrow chest and poor cough, and may succumb to chest infections. Scoliosis is a frequent complication; it has an early onset and a rapid progression before puberty.[61] Those children who are wheelchair bound are predisposed to hip and knee flexor contractures and equinus deformity of the feet.

Mild spinal muscular atrophy (Kugelberg-Welander syndrome)

Motor milestones in infancy are normal, standing and walking may be on time or delayed. At this stage, parents may notice mild muscle weakness which is proximal in distribution. These children may have a waddling gait and get up from the floor with a Gower's manoeuvre. Laxity at the ankles may cause a flat-footed gait with external rotation of the feet. Hand tremor is common. Muscle strength is well maintained and there may even be some improvement. Prognosis is good and ambulation is maintained for many years though there may be deterioration in function in association with weight gain or pubertal growth spurt. There is usually no significant respiratory weakness. Scoliosis may develop but it usually only poses a serious clinical problem in a small subgroup who lose ambulation, become wheelchair bound and have not been rehabilitated.

Investigations

Muscle ultrasound shows a moderate increase in echogenicity accompanied by loss of muscle thickness with increased subcutaneous tissue depth.[62] EMG is neuropathic. In the intermediate type, the EMG shows a tremulous pattern of the baseline which reflects fasciculation of the skeletal muscle and is extremely useful diagnostically.

Muscle biopsy shows a neurogenic change with presence of atrophic fibres involving both type I and type II fibres. The atrophic fibres are clustered together, often whole bundles (group atrophy). These are interspersed with fascicles containing markedly hypertrophied fibres which are mainly type 1.

Genetics

SMA is the second most common autosomal recessive disorder in the UK, after cystic fibrosis. At the moment it seems that the mutations responsible for all cases of classical autosomal recessive, proximal symmetrical SMAs of infancy and childhood are allelic for the gene locus at 5q.[63] Intrafamilial variability in severity of SMA may occur but is uncommon.

Antenatal diagnosis by linkage analysis is now possible in informative families, if appropriate tissue specimens (preferably blood to extract DNA) from the index patient are available. It is crucial that blood for DNA extraction is taken and saved from all infants affected with severe SMA and the poor prognostic subgroup in intermediate SMA.

Management of severe SMA

Precise diagnosis and counselling are essential. An initial period of hospitalization may be needed to assess the problem and to teach parents how to suction the pharynx to clear secretions, etc. Chest infections account for the inevitable demise, and the parents must be counselled and prepared for this. Mechanical ventilation is inappropriate and not advisable unless there is need to gain time to clarify the diagnosis.

Management of intermediate SMA

There should be vigorous and early treatment of chest infections with antibiotics and physiotherapy, promotion of ambulation and management of scoliosis.

Physiotherapy should be initiated at an early stage to encourage activity and to prevent contractures. Children should be reviewed frequently to assess muscle strength. In general, in the second year of life, rehabilitation in standing calipers with a pelvic support band can be started, with a view of progressing to ischial weight-bearing knee-ankle-foot orthoses (KAFOs). Scoliosis is treated with an external spinal brace which enables better sitting posture and prevents severe fixed deformity at an early age. Ambulation in orthoses is associated with a slower rate of progression of scoliosis[61] and should be encouraged. Scoliosis may progress in spite of these measures and we recommend a Luque fusion operation in a non-ambulant child with SMA when the curvature is 40° or more and clearly progressing, almost always before puberty.

Management of mild SMA

If there is loss of ambulation, provision of KAFOs can often prolong useful walking for several years and prevent development and progression of scoliosis. Unfortunately, patients with this condition are still being referred too late for rehabilitation.

Hereditary motor sensory neuropathies (HMSN)

Early description under the umbrella terms Charcot-Marie-Tooth disease or peroneal muscular atrophy were based on clinical presentation and contained many subgroups which are now identified more precisely, based on inheritance, clinical, electrophysiological and pathological features. Reported prevalence varies widely but seems to be around 100×10^{-6}.[1] Only the commoner types will be discussed here.

HMSN type I

Presentation is in the first decade with pes cavus. Weakness is distal in distribution, starting in the peroneal group of muscles, with a slow progression to proximal muscle groups. Wasting of the affected muscles is present but not a striking feature (in contrast to HMSN II). Weakness of ankle dorsiflexion causes foot drop and a steppage gait. Clawing of the hands may occur at a later stage. Tendon reflexes are diminshed or lost. Sensory deficit may be evident on electrophysiological testing but is often not apparent clinically in childhood. Peripheral nerves may be palpably enlarged.

The underlying pathological lesion is demyelination of the peripheral nerve, resulting in slowing of motor nerve conduction velocity to less than half the normal value. Nerve biopsy, which is not necessary for diagnosis, shows evidence of demyelination and a characteristic onion bulb appearance.

Inheritance is autosomal dominant. Penetrance is variable and all family members should have a clinical examination and measurement of motor nerve conduction velocity.[64] The course is slowly progressive and ambulation is usually not lost. The gene locus has been identified at 17p[65] and 1q[66] in different families.

HMSN type II

Presentation is similar to type I, but onset is later, atrophy of affected muscles is more striking, peripheral nerves are not enlarged. The pathological lesion is axonal degeneration. Motor nerve conduction velocity is not appreciably slowed, but amplitude of the motor action potential is markedly reduced. The inheritance is autosomal dominant.

HMSN type III

This variety runs a more severe course with onset in infancy with delayed walking, gradual decline and possible loss of ambulation in adult life. Peripheral nerves are palpably enlarged. Motor nerve conduction velocity is slow and biopsy appearances are similar to type I. Inheritance, in contrast, is autosomal recessive.

Patients should be encouraged to remain active. Ankle-foot orthoses may help to counteract foot drop and keep feet in a better posture. Surgical correction of foot deformities may help to improve function in late adolescence.

Myasthenia gravis

Abnormal fatiguability after sustained muscle activity, improvement after rest and a variability in strength during the day is characteristic of myasthenia gravis. The prevalence is about 2–4 per 100 000,[67] but is much rarer in childhood. About 4% have onset of symptoms in the first decade and a further 20% in the second decade.

Juvenile myasthenia

This autoimmune disorder is the biggest subgroup and is usually associated with the presence of circulating acetyl-choline receptor antibodies. Females outnumber males 4 : 1. The onset is insidious, although may seem to be precipitated by an intercurrent febrile illness. There may be a history of diplopia on reading, increasing difficulty in chewing or swallowing during a meal, or worsening hand writing in the course of a lesson or on examination. Virtually all the patients have ptosis, with or without ophthalmoplegia. Weakness commonly involves facial muscles, chewing, swallowing, speech, neck and trunk muscles, shoulder and hip muscles. Respiratory muscle weakness and particularly diaphragm involvement may result in hypoventilation and respiratory failure. There is a steady worsening in symptoms towards the end of the day and there may be fluctuation in severity from day to day. The fatiguability can often be tested for by asking the patient to hold out the arm or to look upwards for a prolonged period.

An important diagnostic test is the use of the short-acting anticholinesterase, edrophonium (Tensilon). When injected intravenously, edrophonium produces a temporary improvement in strength effective within half to one minute. This test should only be done in hospital with full resuscitation facilities immediately available because of the possibility of a dramatic worsening following injection.

Treatment is with neostigmine or pyridostigmine, which are longer acting (about 2 and 4 hours respectively) and can be taken orally. Thymectomy is usually required to induce remission.[68] Some patients with an unresponsive and protracted course may need additional immunosuppressive treatment with prednisolone (alternate days) and azathioprine. Plasmapheresis may result in temporary improvement for 3–5 weeks and may be helpful to tide over an acute crisis or operation.

Transient neonatal myasthenia

Infants of myasthenic mothers may present usually within a few hours of birth, or at the very latest the first 72 hours, with feeding difficulty, generalized weakness, poor respiratory effort and inability to handle pharyngeal secretions. The infant is affected secondary to passive transplacental transfer of antibody. Most respond to anticholinesterase drugs.[69]

Familial infantile myasthenia

This non-autoimmune type is characterized by episodes of severe respiratory and feeding difficulties at birth or during infancy. Extra-ocular movements are normal, and patients show a good response to anticholinesterase treatment and a high remission rate. Although the disease occurs frequently in siblings it is not present in the mother, and inheritance is probably autosomal recessive.[70]

Acknowledgements

We are grateful to the Muscular Dystrophy Group of Great Britain for financial support and thank Miss Anjli Jagpal for typing the manuscript.

References

1 Emery, A.E.H. Population frequencies of inherited neuromuscular diseases: a world survey. *Neuromusc Disorders* 1991; **1**: 19–29.

2 Dubowitz, V. Muscle disorders in childhood. *Major Problems in Clinical Pediatrics*. Philadelphia: W B Saunders, 1978.

3 Dubowitz, V. *A Colour Atlas of Muscle Disorders in Childhood*. London: Wolfe Medical Publications, 1989.

4 Dubowitz, V. *The Floppy Infant*. London: Heinemann, 1969.

5 Heckmatt, J., Dubowitz, V. Neuromuscular disorders. In: Levene, M.I., Bennet, M.J., Punt, J., eds. *Fetal and Neonatal Neurology and Neurosurgery*. Edinburgh: Churchill Livingstone, 1988.

6 Smith, R.A., Sibert, J.R., Harper, P.S. Early development of boys with Duchenne muscular dystrophy. *Dev Med Child Neurol* 1990; **32**: 512–517.

7 Wallace, G.B., Newton, R.W. Gower's sign revisited. *Arch Dis Child* 1989; **64**: 1317–1318.

8 Heckmatt, J.Z., Dubowitz, V. Biochemical aspects of muscle disorders. In: Clayton, B.E., Round, J.M., eds. *Chemical Pathology and the Sick Child*. Oxford: Blackwell Scientific Publications, 1984: 463–485.

9 Heckmatt, J.Z., Dubowitz, V. Ultrasound imaging and directed needle biopsy in the diagnosis of selective involvement in neuromuscular disease. *J Child Neurol* 1987; **2**: 205–213.

10 Heckmatt, J.Z., Dubowitz, V. Diagnostic advantage of needle muscle biopsy and ultrasound imaging in the detection of focal pathology in a girl with limb-girdle dystrophy. *Muscle Nerve* 1985; **8**: 705–709.

11 Heckmatt, J.Z., Dubowitz, V. Real-time ultrasound imaging of muscles. *Muscle Nerve* 1988; **11**: 56–65.

12 Heckmatt, J.Z., Moosa, A., Hutson, C., Maunder-Sewry, C.A., Dubowitz, V. Diagnostic needle muscle biopsy, a practical and reliable alternative to open biopsy. *Arch Dis Child* 1984; **59**: 528–532.

13 Dubowitz, V. *Muscle Biopsy: a Practical Approach*. London: Bailliere Tindall, 1985.

14 Harpin, P. *With a Little Help* vol I–VIII. The Muscular Dystrophy Group of Great Britain, Natrass House, 35 Macaulay Road, London SW4 0QP. Tel 071 720 8055.

15 Bye, P.T.P., Ellis, E.R., Ossa, F.G., Donelly, P.M., Sullivan, C.E. Respiratory failure and sleep in neuromuscular disease. *Thorax* 1990; **45**: 241–247.

16 Heckmatt, J.Z., Loh, L., Dubowitz, V. Nocturnal hypoventilation in children with nonprogressive neuromuscular disease. *Pediatrics* 1989; **83**: 250–255.

17 Ellis, E.R., Bye, P.T.P., Bruderer, J.W., Sullivan, C.E. Treatment of respiratory failure during sleep in patients with neuromuscular disease: positive pressure through a nose mask. *Am Rev Respir Dis* 1987; **135**: 148–152.

18 Heckmatt, J.Z., Loh, L., Dubowitz, V. Night-time nasal ventilation in neuromuscular disease. *Lancet* 1990; i: 579–582.

19 Gardner-Medwin, D. Clinical features and classification of muscular dystrophies. *Br Med Bull* 1980; **36**: 109–115.

20 Emery, A.E.H. *Duchenne Muscular Dystrophy*: Oxford Monographs on Medical Genetics No 15. Oxford: Oxford Medical Publications, 1987.

21 Edwards, R.H.T., Round, J.M., Jackson, M.J., Griffiths, R.D., Lillburn, M.F. Weight reduction in boys with muscular dystrophy. *Dev Med Child Neurol* 1984; **26**: 384–390.

22 Griffiths, R.D., Edwards, R.H. A new chart for weight control in Duchenne muscular dystrophy. *Arch Dis Child* 1988; **63**: 1256–1258.

23 Heckmatt, J.Z., Dubowitz, V., Hyde, S.A., Florence, J., Gabain, A.C., Thompson, N. Prolongation of walking in Duchenne muscular dystrophy with lightweight orthoses: review of 51 cases. *Dev Med Child Neurol* 1985; **27**: 149–154.

24 Rodillo, E.B., Fernandez-Bermejo, E., Heckmatt, J.Z., Dubowitz, V. Prevention of rapidly progressive scoliosis in Duchenne muscular dystrophy by prolongation of walking with orthoses. *J Child Neurol* 1988; **3**: 269–274.

25 Rideau, Y., Duport, G., Marie-Agnes, Y., *et al*. Traitement des dystrophies musculaires: resultats d'une cooperation franco-italienne. *Sem Hôp Paris* 1987; **63**: 438–443.

26 Manzur, A.Y., Hyde, S.A., Rodillo, E., Heckmatt, J.Z., Bentley, G., Dubowitz, V. A randomised controlled trial of early surgery in Duchenne muscular dystrophy. *Neuromuscular Disorders* 1992; **2**: 379–387.

27 Luque, E.R. The anatomical basis and development of segmental spinal instrumentation. *Spine* 1982; **7**: 256–259.

28 Rideau, Y., Gatin, G., Bach, J., Gines, G. Prolongation of life in Duchenne muscular dystrophy. *Acta Neurol* 1983; **38**: 118–124.

29 Bach, J.R., O'Brien, J., Krotenberg, R., Alba, A.S. Management of end stage respiratory failure in Duchenne muscular dystrophy. *Muscle Nerve* 1987; **10**: 177–182.

30 Mohr, C.H., Hill, N.S. Long term follow up of nocturnal ventilatory assistance in patients with respiratory failure due to Duchenne type muscular dystrophy. *Chest* 1990; **97**: 91–96.

31 Miller, J.R., Colbert, A.P., Osberg, J.S. Ventilator dependency: decision making, daily functioning and quality of life for patients with Duchenne muscular dystrophy. *Dev Med Child Neurol* 1990; **32**: 1079–1086.

32 Koenig, M., Hoffman, E.P., Bertelson, C.J., Monaco, A.P., Feener, C., Kunkel, L.M. Complete cloning of Duchenne muscular dystrophy (DMD) cDNA and preliminary genomic organisation of the DMD gene

in normal and affected individuals. *Cell* 1987; **50**: 509–517.

33 Hoffman, E.P., Brown, R.H., Kunkel, L.M. Dystrophin: the protein product of the Duchenne muscular dystrophy focus. *Cell* 1987; **51**: 919–928.

34 Hodgson, S.V., Bobrow, M. Carrier detection and prenatal diagnosis in Duchenne and Becker muscular dystrophy. *Br Med Bull* 1989; **45**: 719–744.

35 Clerk, A., Rodillo, E., Heckmatt, J.Z., Dubowitz, V., Strong, P.N., Sewry, C.A. Characterisation of dystrophin in carriers of DMD. *J Neurol Sci* 1991; **102**: 197–205.

36 Zellweger, H., Simpson, J., Ionasescu, J. Twenty years – Iowa muscle clinic: reminiscences and prospects. *Eur J Pediatr* 1982; **138**: 17–22.

37 Gardner-Medwin, D. Recognising and preventing Duchenne muscular dystrophy. *Br Med J* 1983; **287**: 1083–1084.

38 Drummond, L.M. Creatine phosphokinase levels in newborns and their use in screening for Duchenne muscular dystrophy. *Arch Dis Child* 1979; **54**: 362–366.

39 Dellamonica, C., Collombel, C., Cotte, J., Addis, P. Screening for neonatal Duchenne muscular dystrophy by bioluminescence measurement of creatine kinase in blood sample spotted on paper. *Clin Chem* 1983; **29**: 161–163.

40 Gardner-Medwin, D., Bundey, S., Green, S. Early diagnosis of Duchenne muscular dystrophy. *Lancet* 1978; **i**: 1102.

41 Smith, R.A., Rogers, M., Bradley, D.M., Sibert, J.R., Harper, P.S. Screening for Duchenne muscular dystrophy. *Arch Dis Child* 1989; **64**: 1017–1021.

42 Smith, R.A., Williams, D.K., Sibert, J.R., Harper, P.S. Attitudes of mothers to neonatal screening for Duchenne muscular dystrophy. *Br Med J* 1990; **300**: 1112.

43 Hoffman, E.P., Fishbeck, K.H., Brown, R.H., *et al.* Dystrophin characterization in muscle biopsies from Duchenne and Becker muscular dystrophy patients. *New Engl J Med* 1988; **318**: 1363–1368.

44 Hodgson, S., Hart, D., Abbs, S., *et al.* Correlation of clinical and deletion data in Duchenne and Becker muscular dystrophy. *J Med Genet* 1989; **26**: 682–693.

45 Wilmenga, C., Frants, R., Brouwer, O., Moorer, P., Webe, J., Padberg, P. Localization of fascioscapulohumeral muscular dystrophy gene on chromosome 4. *Lancet* 1990; **ii**: 651–653.

46 Heckmatt, J.Z., Sewry, C.A., Hodes, D., Dubowitz, V. Congenital centronuclear (myotubular) myopathy. A clinical and genetic study in eight children. *Brain* 1985; **108**: 941–964.

47 Starr, J., Lamont, M., Iselius, L., Harvey, J., Heckmatt, J. A linkage study of a large pedigree with X-linked centronuclear myopathy. *J Med Genet* 1990; **27**: 281–283.

48 Harding, A.E., Holt, G.J. Mitochondrial myopathies. *Br Med Bull* 1989; **45**: 760–771.

49 Egger, J., Wilson, J. Mitochondrial inheritance in mitochondrially mediated disease. *New Engl J Med* 1983; **309**: 142–145.

50 Central core disease (editorial). *Lancet* 1988; **i**: 866.

51 Kausch, K., Lehman-Horn, F., Janka, M., Wieringa, B., Grimm, T., Muller, C. Evidence for linkage of the central core disease locus to proximal arm of human chromosome 19. *Genomics* 1991; **10**: 765–769.

52 Ellis, F.R. Malignant hyperpyrexia. *Arch Dis Child* 1984; **59**: 1013–1015.

53 Steenson, A.J., Torkelson, R.D. King's syndrome with malignant hyperthermia: potential outpatient risks. *Am J Dis Child* 1987; **141**: 271–273.

54 Miller, G., Heckmatt, J.Z., Dubowitz, V. Drug treatment of juvenile dermatomyositis. *Arch Dis Child* 1983; **58**: 445–450.

55 Heckmatt, J., Hasson, N., Saunders, C., *et al.* Cyclosporin in juvenile dermatomyositis. *Lancet* 1989; **i**: 1063–1066.

56 Shaw, D.J., Harper, P.S. Myotonic dystrophy: developments in molecular genetics. *Br Med Bull* 1989; **45**: 745–759.

57 Harley, H.G., Rundle, S.A., Rearden, W., *et al.* Unstable DNA sequence in myotonic dystrophy. *Lancet* 1992; **339**: 1125–1128.

58 Rutherford, M.A., Heckmatt, J.Z., Dubowitz, V. Congenital myotonic dystrophy: respiratory function at birth determines survival. *Arch Dis Child* 1989; **64**: 191–195.

59 Harper, P.S. Congenital myotonic dystrophy in Britain: clinical aspects. *Arch Dis Child* 1975; **50**: 503–513.

60 Dubowitz, V. Chaos in classification of the spinal muscular atrophies of childhood. *Neuromusc Disord* 1991; **1**: 77–80.

61 Rodillo, E., Marini, M.L., Heckmatt, J.Z., Dubowitz, V. Scoliosis in spinal muscular atrophy. *J Child Neurol* 1989; **4**: 118–123.

62 Heckmatt, J.Z., Pier, N., Dubowitz, V. Assessment of quadriceps femoris muscle atrophy and hypertrophy in neuromuscular disease in children. *J Clin Ultrasound* 1988; **16**: 177–181.

63 Munsat, T.L., Skerry, A.S., Korf, B., *et al.* Phenotype heterogeneity of spinal muscular atrophy mapping to chromosome 5q11.2-13.1 (SMA 5q). *Neurology* 1990; **40**: 1831–1836.

64 Vanasse, M., Dubowitz, V. Dominantly inherited peroneal muscular atrophy (hereditary motor and sensory neuropathy type I) in infancy and childhood. *Muscle Nerve* 1981; **4**: 26–30.

65 Vance, J., Nicholson, G., Yamaoka, L., Stalich, J., Stewart, C., Speer, M. Linkage of Charcot-Marie-Tooth disease neuropathy type Ia to chromosome 17. *Exp Neurol* 1989; **104**: 186–189.

66 Bird, T., Ott, J., Giblett, E. Evidence for linkage of Charcot-Marie-Tooth neuropathy to the Duffy locus on chromosome 1. *Am J Hum Genet* 1982; **32**: 99.

67 Hokkanen, E. Epidemiology of myasthenia gravis in Finland. *J Neurol Sci* 1969; **9**: 463–478.

68 Rodrigues, M., Gomez, M.R., Howard, F.M., Taylor, W.F. Myasthenia gravis in children: long-term follow up. *Ann Neurol* 1983; **13**: 504–510.

69 Namba, T., Brown, S.B., Grob, D. Neonatal myasthenia gravis: report of two cases and review of the literature. *Pediatrics* 1970; **45**: 488–504.

70 Robertson, W.C., Chun, R.W.M., Kornguth, S.E. Familial infantile myasthenia. *Arch Neurol* 1980; **37**: 117–119.

10.4 Degenerative disease

Stuart Green

Those children who degenerate or regress represent only a small percentage of children with developmental problems. Each individual degenerative disease is rare, but cumulatively they are an important group to recognize. The majority of them are genetic and probably account for between 2% and 5% of neurological disability. It is important to be aware of the broad pattern of these conditions, so as to know when they should be further referred because of the implication of future management and genetic counselling. Progressive disease is a particular problem for community paediatricians because no sooner has an assessment been made of the child and placement arranged in an appropriate school with supportive services, than the condition itself begins to change and the needs of the child also change. It is important to understand the nature of these diseases and their particular symptoms, so that appropriate planning is made for support at each stage.

History is all important. A detailed neurological examination indicates which parts of the nervous system are involved, but the history gives the time course of the disease, which is critical in making a diagnosis.

For the most part we are dealing with metabolic genetic disease. Occasionally, non-genetic diseases, e.g. subacute sclerosing panencephalitis (SSPE), hydrocephalus and very occasionally tumour may present with regression, although tumours usually have other signs and symptoms too. Only very rarely can specific treatment be offered but assessment, management, genetic advice, counselling and support should always be available.

It should be remembered, however, that there are a number of conditions which can appear to be degenerative but which are not. Sometimes this is known as pseudo-degeneration.

Pseudo-degeneration

Epilepsy

Any child especially one mentally handicapped who has severe epilepsy, may have phases when the epilepsy control is poor. This may not be obvious as the attacks can be non-convulsive, subclinical, or simply unrecognized. The child's attention will be poorer, he may become more hyperactive and appear to lose skills. When this happens a critical review of the child's epileptic status, management and drugs is required. It may be that drug therapy is inadequate, or that too many drugs are the cause of the problems. Readjustment may stabilize the child again. There are some children with very severe epilepsy who do appear to degenerate slowly and in only a few of these can a metabolic cause be elucidated, and in most cases a cause is never determined.[1]

Growth and development

Some children with neuromuscular problems or cerebral palsy (non-progressive conditions), appear to get worse when they go through the preadolescent growth spurt. One possibility is that they are getting bigger and heavier and this may cause secondary problems in gross motor skills, such as walking. Another factor is that as the children get older they may be expected to do more than before, so previous lack of skills is only then recognized. This may give a false appearance of deterioration.

Psychological factors

Children who are physically handicapped or mildly retarded as they approach teenage life occasionally become inwardly reflective, easily dissatisfied and sometimes depressed. This depression can result in apparent blunting of intelligence, and will affect both attention and learning to give the impression of loss of skills. Careful attention must be paid to children in this category and they may benefit from referral for psychological support.

False interpretation of IQs

Sometimes the child's development quotient is cited as evidence for degeneration; for example a child at the age of 5 years who has a quotient of 75, at the age of 8 or 9 years a quotient of 65 and at 13 or 14 years a quotient of 55. This gives the impression that the child is deteriorating, but quotients are not very accurate, they measure different things at different ages, and some retarded children reach a plateau at an early age.

Regression

In order to make a diagnosis of regression, a history is critical, and the use of independent reports, teachers' comments, photographs and videos is very helpful. It is surprising the number of people who have these available.

Regression in some diseases may occur very quickly such as in amino acid or organic acid disorders, and may be triggered by infection so that clinically the situation can appear to be an acute encephalopathy and the diagnosis of regressive disease be missed. On the other hand in conditions like Friedreich's ataxia, regression is slow over many years, so that it may not even be noted until a few years after the onset. In the early stages of such a disease development outstrips regression easily masking the degenerative aspect.

It is often extremely difficult to date the onset of a progressive disease like Friedreich's ataxia as the early signs are so subtle and may merge into the range of normal variation. It is often easier however, with hindsight, especially in the case of a second child in a family with the same condition, for the parent to make the diagnosis much earlier, even before the medical profession.

Some special considerations

1 Occasionally tumours may mimic and present with dementia without much in the way of other signs in the early stages, such as frontal tumours and small tumours causing hydrocephalus by aqueduct block.
2 Chronic poisoning: carbon monoxide and lead should always be thought of in a school-age child who is falling off in intellectual and behavioural skills.
3 Sensory defects: deafness or visual defects may be static and may present with apparent failure to progress at school mimicking dementia. These functional skills must be assessed.
4 Social problems and psychological factors can cause an apparent regression.
5 Some cases of profound handicap when only seen for the first time at a late stage, may appear to be static, whereas in fact there has been a degeneration earlier in life and then stasis. This particular problem can arise when earlier history is unavailable.
6 Some of the spinocerebellar degenerations and genetic spastic paraplegias are associated with extremely slow mental regression which takes many years (even decades) to manifest itself.

This chapter is mainly concerned with those diseases which show regression after a period of initial normality in infancy (first year). Diseases with regression within the first year tend to be more acute and accompanied by seizures, coma, hypotonia and other neurological signs.[2]

Regression will be dealt with under the following headings:

1 Loss of intellectual skills, language and change of behaviour.
2 Regression with seizures.
3 Language deterioration.
4 Progressive difficulty in walking or coordination.
5 Progressive visual loss.

Loss of intellectual skills, language and change of behaviour

Adrenoleukodystrophy
Metachromatic leukodystrophy
Batten's disease
San Fillipo and other mucopolysaccharidoses
Wilson's disease
SSPE
Hypothyroidism
HIV infection

Adrenoleukodystrophy (ALD)

This disease has been known for many years as a sex-linked recessive form of leukodystrophy, but only recently has it been recognized as being due to one of the peroxisomal disorders.[3] Plasma very long-chain fatty acids are elevated. It occurs in males and presents in the school-age child with attention problems, learning problems, language difficulties, dysphasia, disorientation, and eventually dementia. The diagnosis in the early stages may be very difficult and the child may be suspected of having behavioural problems. Eventually more specific signs such as hemianopia, hemiparesis and ataxia develop. At this stage it is often thought that the child has some form of tumour. It is one of the very few metabolic diseases where there may be focal unilateral signs. Focal seizures are a late phenomenon. Occasionally adrenal insufficiency presents as an acute problem. Even without this problem death usually ensues within 4 or 5 years, probably in an average of 2 years. A child may remain in a semi-comatose state requiring tube feeding for a long period of time. Recently there has been a suggestion that the administration of a diet low in long-chain fatty acids may have some therapeutic value. Trials are at the moment being pursued.[4]

It is extremely important to make the diagnosis in these children early, because mother and siblings may be asymptomatic carriers. Carrier testing and prenatal diagnosis are available.

Metachromatic leukodystrophy

Although the commoner forms of metachromatic leukodystrophy present with spasticity or walking difficulties in the first few years of life, occasionally this condition may present with a picture of regression in the school-age child, with a progressive dementia. This may occur late in the first decade or second decade of life. The mental findings may appear before the classical signs of ataxia or spasticity. Symmetrical low attenuation in the central cerebral white matter on CT scan may make one suspicious, but the diagnosis is confirmed by leucocyte enzyme assay of arylsuphatase A. Treatment is symptomatic, including diazepam for muscle spasms, and therapeutic support to aid feeding and positioning. Genetic counselling should be offered as prenatal diagnosis is available for this recessive condition. Bone marrow transplant has been attempted, but results are too few to analyse.[5]

Batten's disease

Batten's disease (neuronal ceroid lipofuscinosis) is an autosomal recessive disorder of uncertain aetiology where excessive pigment is deposited in the brain and other cells in the body. It is possibly due to some disorder of oxidative metabolism. The diagnosis is by the clinical picture and confirmation by skin or rectal biopsy. No biochemical tests at the moment exist.

Two clinical pictures are seen outside infancy.

1 The late infantile type: in this the child develops normally over the first few years of life, then language begins to fail or does not really develop; seizures, often of a myoclonic type, start and the child becomes ataxic. It is often first diagnosed as a myoclonic type epilepsy or a variant of Lennox Gastaut epilepsy. There is slow progression often with fluctuation, with gradually increasing retinal blindness and spasticity. By 5 or 6 years of age the child is severely handicapped and survives for a few more years in this stage. Additional clinical clues are that the head is small (rather than large as in the other storage diseases), and the blindness is due to a retinal, not an optic nerve problem.

2 The juvenile type: the child is usually normal until the age of 4 or 5 years when vision begins to fail. The child may attend a unit for the partially sighted, often no specific diagnosis is made at this stage and then vision fails completely. Sometimes the child is labelled as having optic atrophy or retinitis pigmentosa. By the age of 9 or 10 years the child starts to develop seizures and begins to dement. By the age of 13 or 14 years a Parkinsonian-like state ensues. Language is often reasonably good until the age of 8, 9 or 10 years. This slowly degenerates to very specific mumbling dysarthria. These children may survive until early 20s. They do not develop as much spasticity as the late infantile type and may be still walking at late teenage.

Management of the juvenile type of Batten's disease is a challenge to therapists, paediatricans, school teachers and teachers of the visually impaired. Despite the regression, these children do somehow retain their own personality until late into teenage life. They need all the help and support they can get. Most often these children will finish up in a special unit attached to a blind school or one of the specialist schools for both the blind and handicapped.

San Fillipo disease

San Fillipo disease is one of the mucopolysaccharide storage diseases. However, coarsened facial features and skeletal deformities are hardly present, and hence the diagnosis may not be suspected. The main presenting feature is very slowly progressive retardation. This starts about the age of 3 or 4 years and the child may be labelled as simply slow and may progress at first. As time passes the few skills that these children have gained over the years begin to be lost. From the age of 5 or 6 years onwards there is no improvement. The child's behaviour may be very difficult to manage in terms of hyperactivity and negativity. Even in the second decade of life there may be little or no physical findings, maybe a slight coarsening of the hair and a barrel-shaped chest. Neurological signs and seizures are rare. One of the problems of diagnosing this group of children is that they may have been labelled as severely retarded and be institutionalized for years, the assumption being made that degeneration is due to some secondary psychiatric problem.

Confirmation of diagnosis is by analysis of urinary mucopolysaccharides and prenatal diagnosis is available. There is a very active Mucopolysaccharide Society which can help support the families of these children, and those with classical Hurler's disease. There has been interest in the possibility of bone marrow transplantation for this group of children and others, but the results are still uncertain.[5]

Wilson's disease

This is a disorder of copper metabolism. Very occasionally it may present with a dementia, usually in the older child, but occasionally from 7 or 8 years onwards. However, in most cases there is a history of jaundice and other features such as dystonia are associated. Kayser Fleischer rings on the limbus of the iris are nearly always present, and specialist biochemical tests are necessary for confirmation. The importance of making this rare diagnosis is that this disease is potentially treatable, and the symptoms reversible in the early stages.[6]

Subacute sclerosing panencephalitis (SSPE)

This slowly progressive encephalitis emerges a number of years after an attack of measles. The measles has usually occurred at a relatively early age and the interval to presentation of SSPE symptoms may be 4 or 5 years after the infection. It is still not clearly understood whether it occurs due to some abnormal immunity to the measles virus by the child or by modification of the initial measles virus. It is a rare disease and becoming more so with widespread measles vaccination.

The disease may present slowly, subacutely, and rarely acutely with a wide variety of manifestations. It is usually associated with some form of learning problem, dementia, or visual attention difficulty, less commonly with an acute hemiparesis, hemichorea or raised intracranial pressure. Myoclonic jerking is an early feature. It may have very minor manifestations as simple as nodding, but the characteristic feature is that it is periodic, occurring at intervals of anything between 20 seconds and 2 or 3 minutes, when it is established. No other disease gives this classical periodicity. The time course of the disease from the initiation of symptoms to total incapacity (blindness, spasticity, gross dementia) may vary from a few months to a few years. In the early stages it may be mistaken for other causes of dementia, myoclonus or behavioural problems, but once established the picture is classical. The EEG is pathognomonic and measles antibodies are raised in the CSF and serum.

It is a condition in which there is a challenge to the management team as the patient progresses to a pre-terminal stage of spasticity, blindness, feeding difficulties and myoclonus. The child may stay at this stage for many years. A variety of treatments including arabinoside and intrathecal interferon have been tried without any success.

It appears that measles immunization very significantly diminishes the chances of developing this disease, and the figures from the USA, where measles immunization has been available for a number of years, seem to support this. It is hoped and expected that this trend will follow in the UK.

Other diseases: hypothyroidism, HIV infection

Hypothyroidism should always be considered in someone with retardation of unknown origin especially if the facial features are coarse. This is very unlikely in a young child born in this country, who will have been screened for thyroid deficiency in the newborn period, but it should be remembered in any child who has been born abroad. Very occasionally chronic lead poisoning may present with a dementia. In this case there will usually be a background history of access to old lead paint most often on toys or in old houses.

In the 1990s we can expect to see some children presenting with dementia, usually associated with other neurological signs, as part of the HIV infection complex.[7]

Regression with seizures

Lennox Gastaut syndrome
Alpers' disease
Rett's syndrome
Angelman's syndrome
Neurocutaneous disease

Lennox Gastaut syndrome

Lennox Gastaut syndrome is a term loosely applied to a group of children who have severe mixed myoclonic epilepsy, usually starting at the age of 2 or 3 years, and appear to regress clinically. Typically they have myoclonic, akinetic and generalized seizures. Sometimes this occurs in a child who had infantile spasms in early life (and who may even have tuberous sclerosis) and sometimes occurs for no obvious reason. There is often, as with infantile spasms, an apparent arrest in development when the seizures start. Very few children regain normality even with seizure control which is rarely achieved despite multiple use of drugs, and many slip back to a lower level and then stabilize, although there is great fluctuation with severity of the seizures. In a few of these children an underlying metabolic disease may be found, and sometimes Batten's disease is the cause. This is one of the very difficult areas where it is often uncertain whether a child has a true degenerative disease or not. If there is a true degenerative neurological disease, other signs such as spasticity or visual problems will ensue.

Alpers' disease

This is another not very well-defined condition in which children start to have explosive epilepsy in the first few years of life, often asymmetrical, sometimes even with epilepsy partialis continuans. They may become ataxic and then develop intellectual retardation. They often die within a year or two and finally develop fatal liver disease. It is a condition where the pattern of inheritance is unknown. It may well bear some relationship to Leigh's syndrome and possibly have a basis in some form of mitochondrial disorder.[8]

Rett's syndrome

This disease, virtually unknown in the 1980s, is now recognized as probably the second or third most common cause of mental retardation in girls. Previously described by Rett in 1956 and redescribed by Hagberg and others in the early 1980s,[9] this clinical syndrome of retardation occurring in girls still defies pathological analysis. The clinical picture seems to be fairly well defined. There is a progressive loss of skills occurring with a prevalence of 1 : 10000 to 1 : 15000 (probably only in girls). These children appear to be normal or near normal for the first year of life, (in retrospect, they were never very skilled) but sometime toward the end of the first year of life or before 18 months, there is a period of slowing down of development, followed by a period of arrested development. It is sometimes associated with a period of irritability and seizures may emerge. This period of irritability then seems to settle down. The child is left with an autistic-like picture, development of hand skills ceases as also does language, and these children may or may not stop walking. The head stops growing at a normal rate. These girls then develop a number of peculiar behavioural patterns. They have episodes of hyperpnoea and apnoea without obvious cause. They seem unable to use their hands, although there is no physical abnormality. They develop stereotypies, most particularly hand wringing, hand tapping or hand flicking. They have very minimal communication skills, although some parents believe the child's understanding is greater than the level of speech suggests. The mental deterioration stabilizes, the seizures are not usually a major problem, but there is a gradual increase in spasticity or ataxia. By late teenage or early adult life, they have often lost the typical stereotypies. It is therefore difficult to know whether some adult females with severe mental retardation and small heads have Rett's syndrome, unless the early history is very clear.

The diagnosis is essentially a clinical one. There are no pathological or neurophysiological markers. There may well be a number of children who have a *forme fruste* of Rett's syndrome, and this is discussed extensively in Hagberg's paper.[10] One theory is that this may be a sex-linked dominant condition lethal in males and manifest in females, although this has not been proved.

Children with this condition have been mistakenly diagnosed as having cerebral palsy, Batten's disease, spinocerebellar degenerations, Friedreich's ataxia and post-encephalitic syndrome.

Angelman's syndrome

Angelman's syndrome, otherwise known as the happy puppet syndrome and now known to be associated with deletion in chromosome 15, is another disease with very slow progression and deterioration.[11] The clinical features are not very obvious in early life, but there is delayed motor development with ataxia and often but not always myoclonic seizures. There slowly emerges a picture of severe retardation with superimposed language problems, ataxia, incoordination and a tendency to giggle and laugh, awkwardness and jerking movements (hence the name happy puppet) and a protruding jaw, (although the latter may not be obvious until the child is older). It is the history, the facies and the characteristic movement which should suggest the diagnosis. There are certain specific EEG findings.[1] Degeneration is slow and these children

may survive until their early twenties. No specific therapy is available but anticonvulsants may help. Recent research has suggested that this is one of the few conditions in which genetic imprinting may take place. Prenatal diagnosis is becoming available by DNA technology.

Neurocutaneous disease

It is always important in any child with epilepsy and retardation to check the skin for neurocutaneous problems.

Broadly speaking with very few exceptions, significant mental retardation does not occur in the neurocutaneous group of conditions in the absence of epilepsy. The epilepsy is not necessarily the cause of the retardation but is closely associated with it. None of the diseases briefly discussed below are truly degenerative. The epilepsy associated with them may come on suddenly. The child may appear initially to go through a phase of loss of skills, following a significant bout of seizures.

Tuberous sclerosis

Tuberous sclerosis is a dominant condition with variable expression, manifested by seizures, developmental retardation and variable neurocutaneous findings.[12] If young children, particularly below the age of 2 years, present with infantile spasms or any complex seizure disorder, particularly if there is more than one type, it is important to look meticulously for depigmented patches with a Wood's light. Although a CT scan will usually show the characteristic areas of calcification in the cerebral ventricular wall, below the age of 2 years these may not be present. Adenoma sebaceum does not usually show until a later age. Seizure onset later on in life, after the age of 5 years, is not usually associated with developmental retardation.

Sturge-Weber syndrome

Sturge-Weber syndrome is associated with a port-wine stain predominantly down one side of the face covering at least the area of the ophthalmic division of the trigeminal nerve. It is associated among other things with angiomatous malformation on the ipsilateral side of the brain.

The diagnosis is usually obvious at birth, although the port-wine stain may not be very dark until a few months of life. It is commonly (more than 80%) associated with contralateral seizures which may be difficult to control. The child may have periods of stability followed by episodes of uncontrollable seizures, following which there may be temporary hemiparesis, which may occasionally become permanent. Learning difficulties are more common in those children who have frequent seizures.

It is not a clearly inherited condition and the origin is unknown.

Hypomelanosis of Ito

Although described a number of years ago this neuro-cutaneous syndrome has only come into prominence recently. Characteristic findings include patchy depigmentation often in a linear or streaked appearance, on the trunk or on the back of the lower limbs. This may be very faint and often missed in Caucasian people. It is more obvious in Asian or black children. It is commonly associated with seizures and microcephaly and a variety of ophthalmic problems. The whole expression of the condition may be very wide and it is unlikely the whole spectrum is known. It may be that a number of children with mild epilepsy have this condition without it being diagnosed. Genetics are complicated and many of the children show chromosomal mosaicism. Again as with the other groups it is not truly degenerative, though the epilepsy may cause significant continuing problems.

Language deterioration

There are some children where the main clinical feature is a loss of language in the absence of any obvious dementia in the early stages. Occasionally this is a feature of Batten's disease, or of adrenoleukodystrophy.

In the relatively rare condition of Landau Kleffner syndrome a slow loss of language is the early presenting symptom. At first these children may be mistaken for deaf, they start to shout and appear not to understand, but then language gradually disappears. This may be ushered in by a few seizures, but these are not usually a prominent feature. These children are often labelled as hysterical. The EEG usually shows a focus on one side, but is not necessarily very abnormal. There are often no other neurological signs but the children may be left profoundly handicapped linguistically. A number of subvarieties have been described,[13] and management consists of confirming the diagnosis, treating any seizures although these are not usually a major problem, and intensive language therapy. Even with the best management, the outlook is not very good.

There are a group of disorders sometimes referred to as degenerative language problems. These are children who fail to develop language in the first few years of life and deteriorate. They appear to be separate from the Landau Kleffner group, and broadly overlap with a group of children with autistic features, sometimes referred to as having a pervasive developmental disorder. A more detailed review of this subject is given by Gillberg.[14]

Progressive difficulty in walking or coordination

Duchenne dystrophy
Mitochondrial myopathy
Other myopathies
SMA II and III
HMSN I and II
Spastic paraparesis
Friedreich's ataxia
Progressive dystonia
Ataxia telangiectasia
Arnold-Chiari malformation/hydrocephalus
Spinal cord lesion
Pelizaeus Merzbacher disease
Other metabolic diseases

Neuromuscular diseases

A number of children with progressive neurological conditions present with difficulty in walking, coordination, tremor, or any combination of these. They usually present at school age and the child appears to have progressive difficulty in walking in the presence of normal intellect. It is important to distinguish a number of different conditions. Neuromuscular diseases, particularly Duchenne and other muscular dystrophies, spinal muscular atrophies and the peripheral neuropathies should always be considered. In these, features of a low motor neurone lesion are usually obvious but the symptoms may reflect several different diagnostic possibilities. For instance children with cerebral palsy may present with a waddle rather like Duchenne dystrophy, and toe walking may be a feature of spastic paraparesis, Friedreich's ataxia and other spinocerebellar degenerations as well as muscular dystrophy. These conditions are discussed in more detail in Section 10.3.

Spastic paraparesis

There are a number of different genetic subgroups within this entity.[15] The evolution of the difficulty with walking is usually quite slow and may or may not be noticeable, but gradually over a number of years the gait becomes more stiff and awkward. Occasionally there are associated problems such as mental retardation, optic atrophy, peripheral wasting, deafness. The nosology of this disease is complex. Different forms may represent different genetic conditions. Progression may be so slow that it takes many years to realize there is an actual degenerative condition.

It is important to exclude spinal cord compression.

Friedreich's ataxia

This may present with progressive ataxia, and must be distinguished from non-progressive cerebellar ataxias. Cerebellar tumours rarely may give rise to walking difficulties, there are other signs and the deterioration is usually much faster.

Progressive ataxia in the early years may well be due to Friedreich's ataxia. There is a slow evolution of gait ataxia, incoordination of hand movements, nystagmus and slurring of speech. Reflexes gradually become depressed and plantar responses extensor. Most children develop a cardiomyopathy. The condition is recessive. The children become gradually more incapacitated towards the end of their school life, but are rarely in wheelchairs before teenage years. This condition must be distinguished from other forms of progressive cerebellar ataxia, which are rarer. These are well discussed in Harding's monograph.[16] In Friedreich's ataxia nerve conduction studies show that there is normal or slightly slow motor conduction and absent sensory conduction.

Progressive dystonia (torsion dystonia)

In this condition, which is of unknown origin but probably represents one or more genetic variants, there is a slow onset of focal dystonia over 5 to 10 years. It usually starts with an abnormal gait, and walking in a bizarre crab-like way.[17] The abnormality progresses to involve an arm or a leg until eventually all four limbs are affected. In the most severe cases the child is confined to a wheelchair within 3 or 4 years. Speech is not usually affected, but may be. The child becomes extremely handicapped. In the milder cases there may be only difficulty in walking or coordination. It is probably genetically heterogeneous. Dementia does not usually take place.

Diseases that should be excluded are Wilson's disease, Hallervorden-Spatz and juvenile Huntington's chorea.[1] These diseases are very rare.

One of the early diagnostic difficulties is that despite the marked and bizarre symptoms, examination on a couch reveals very little abnormality. Many of the children have already seen a child psychiatrist. Some of the children respond very well to several drugs including artane, carbemazepine and levo dopa. There is a well organized support group.

Ataxia telangiectasia

Ataxia telangiectasia is a rare genetic condition which presents with a slowly evolving picture rather like ataxic cerebral palsy. It may be so slow in its evolution that the child is incorrectly labelled as having cerebral palsy in the first few years of life. Often, but not always, there are recurrent sinusitis and pulmonary infections.

At the age of 6 or 7 years classical telangiectasia on the bulbar conjunctivae, the ear lobes and elbow flexural creases may be seen. Ocular motor problems become prominent although vision and intellect remain stable. By teenage life, the child is usually very severely handicapped. Bowel lymphomas may develop.

The alpha-feto protein is often low, so is immunoglobulin A. The formal diagnosis rests on the finding of specific sensitivity to chromosomes on ultraviolet radiation. Prenatal diagnosis is available.

Hydrocephalus

Although chronic hydrocephalus (of whatever cause, for example Arnold-Chiari malformation) usually presents with an enlarging head and spasticity, a mild to moderate degree of hydrocephalus may present with an ataxic syndrome often with only a slight degree of spasticity. There may also be some titubation of the head. In all children with a slowly progressive ataxia, it is important to measure the head size and consider, in the absence of any other diagnosis, a CT scan.

It is often very difficult to know in the first few years of life if the child with cerebellar disease has cerebral palsy (an ataxic diplegia) or truly progressive disease. There are a number of rare progressive cerebellar diseases.[18]

Spinal cord lesions

Spinal cord lesions may occasionally present with an ataxia. It is important in any ataxic child to check the power, tone and reflexes in the lower limbs, to look for bladder problems and to try to identify a sensory level. Syringomyelia may be very slowly progressive.

Pelizaeus Merzbacher disease

This progressive leukodystrophy, of as yet uncertain origin, may present with early nystagmus and progressive ataxia and spasticity. It has an X-linked inheritance, therefore usually occurs in males and may have a very protracted course. The diagnosis is clinical and supported by findings on magnetic resonance imaging.

Metabolic disease

Very occasionally the late onset gangliosidoses due to hexoseaminidase A and B deficiency may present with a picture rather like that of a Friedreich's ataxia. Usually a dementia supervenes. Diagnosis is by white cell enzyme analysis.

Progressive visual loss

Visual degeneration

Leber's optic atrophy
Batten's disease
Optic nerve glioma
Optic atrophy
Adrenoleukodystrophy
Subacute sclerosing panencephalitis

Most children who have progressive loss of vision over a long period of time are referred to ophthalmologists, rather than paediatricians or paediatric neurologists. In some cases the answer is fairly clear in that these children have developed some progressive retinal, optic nerve or anterior chamber disease and will be appropriately diagnosed. However, in some cases of progressive visual loss there are very few if any ophthalmic signs at all, and in certain cases although ophthalmic signs are diagnosed, they are misinterpreted. The common diseases presenting with chronic visual loss are discussed.

Leber's optic atrophy

This is a disease which usually presents subacutely, but may present acutely or chronically in which there is progressive loss of acuity. One eye may be affected first then the other. Vision diminishes dramatically without any other symptoms. It seems in the very early stages the fundi may show an inflammatory picture of the optic nerve head which may be mistaken for optic neuritis. Other cases show slow evolution of a progressive optic atrophy.

In nearly all cases the patient is a male in the second decade of life. There is sometimes a family history with an uncle or maternal grandfather being affected. The condition usually progresses to fairly significant visual loss, and then often stabilizes. If there is a family history it often appears at first to be sex linked, but closer examination sometimes shows inconsistencies such as female to female transmission. This is because the disease is not sex linked, but probably one of the manifestations of so called 'mitochondrial cytopathies'.[19]

Batten's disease

On a number of occasions children are initially diagnosed as retinitis pigmentosa of unknown origin. They subsequently deteriorate and turn out to have the Spielmeyer Vogt form of Batten's disease.[17] They may have no signs other than visual signs early on with a diminished electroretinogram, then by the age of 10 or 11 years start to show other neurological signs. It is important to be very careful in making a diagnosis of isolated retinitis pigmentosa or optic atrophy, especially if the condition appears to be worsening.[20]

Optic nerve glioma

Here is another condition which can easily be misdiagnosed. A child may be labelled as hereditary or progressive optic atrophy (there are some dominant forms),[15] yet have a slowly evolving optic nerve glioma which has been missed both clinically and on CT scan.

Any child who presents with progressive optic atrophy and loss of vision, whether or not there is a family history, must have a good CT scan looking at the area of the optic chiasm. An optic nerve glioma can occur in association with neurofibromatosis so that it is important to look for *café-au-lait* patches, as the optic atrophy may be part of a more generalized syndrome.

Optic atrophy

Optic atrophy otherwise may be truly part of a wide number of degenerative diseases of the spinocerebellar type.[16] In this case, visual loss is not the main symptom, but a secondary syndrome often found sometime after the disease is first diagnosed. These diseases include hereditary spastic paraparesis, Behr's disease, and Friedreich's ataxia.[15]

Adrenoleukodystrophy

This disease may present as indicated above with visual cortical loss, and children are apparently unable to find their way around rooms, losing their visual memory, although not obviously blind.

Subacute sclerosing panencephalitis (SSPE)

Although this disease most commonly presents with dementia and myoclonus, the earliest features may be a wide variety of neuro-ophthalmic syndromes. The condition may present with progressive visual loss due to optic atrophy, or a neuroretinitis. It may also present with a slowly progressive cortical visual loss, not unlike that described with adrenoleukodystrophy. The wide variety of visual symptoms may be thought by the ophthalmologist to be just due to ocular pathology. It is always important in these cases[21] to consider SSPE. The diagnosis is by confirming high measles antibody titre in the blood and CSF and the typical EEG.

Management

Although in the majority of these disorders there is no specific therapy, much can be done to help children with degenerative CNS disease. In those cases where there is no specific therapy, supportive therapy can be given. This may take the form of anticonvulsants for epilepsy, analgesia for pain, antispasticity agents and drugs to control movement disorders. Physiotherapy is often required to correct deformities temporarily and help with posture and balance; occupational therapy for assistance with seating, communication aids and self help skills; a speech therapist to advise on feeding and communication; special education, home support and in some cases specialized relief care. The community paediatrician will often be central in co-ordinating the management of such a child and must liaise closely with the hospital paediatrican, the general practitioner, other medical and paramedical specialists.

One of the major problems with such children is the question of assessment. An assessment which may be valid in a child with a degenerative disease at the first stage may no longer be valid 6 months or a year later, because other symptoms have evolved. Should the child be placed in a school suitable for his needs at the time, or in one more appropriate to his needs a year or so hence? The community paediatrician will have to liaise between a wide number of different therapists. Frequest visits to hospitals for epilepsy or recurrent infection pose a problem. Does the child necessarily have to be admitted for every intercurrent problem and can the local school cope? It is the role of the local community paediatrician to liaise with the school and inform on management. An identified liaison nurse is a great help. A time may come when it is of little benefit to send a child to school, at which stage it is important to reassess who benefits by school placement – the child or the parent? Home tuition may be a better alternative at that stage. This may be provided by a combination of a home teacher plus therapists and district nurses.

As a disease progresses some children are left in a semicomatose state, and problems with nutrition and feeding arise. Discussion has to be with the parents as to how this is best arranged. Should a nasogastric tube be put down – how is this supervised and organized?[22] It is important to remember that the child with progressive degenerative disease may have a number of other conditions as well which may cause distress or pain. These might include local sepsis especially dental, recurrent chest infections, gastro-oesphageal reflux, peptic ulceration, constipation (a major problem), painful deformity and dislocation. It must also be remembered that members of the family suffer socially and financially because of the problems, and younger siblings too may be very distressed because they fear they have caused the disease or because they fear they might develop it themselves. Privacy must be respected.

Genetic counselling must be followed up to make sure the family have understood the situation, especially the implications for other children.

When the preterminal phase comes, sensitive discussions have to be entered into with the family as to how the latter days of the child should be managed, whether this is more appropriate at home or in hospital, or in some specialized hospice.[23]

Addendum

A number of support groups have developed over the past few years which have contributed a great deal to the support of children, parents and families with degenerative disease. Some of them are also actively involved in information gathering, have a great deal of knowledge of the practicality of rare disease and are actively involved in research.

Some of the main organizations dealing with degenerative diseases are listed here with contact telephone numbers. An up-to-date list of all parent support groups including rare diseases, can be obtained from:

'In Touch', 10 Norman Road, Sale, Cheshire
M33 3DF
Tel: 061 905 2440

Research Trust of Metabolic Disease in Children
Tel: 0270 250221

Mucopolysaccharide Diseases Society
Tel: 0494 762789

Ataxia
Tel: 0252 702864

Dystonia Society
Tel: 071 329 0797

UK Rett's Syndrome Association
Tel: 068 4833357

Tuberous Sclerosis Association
Tel: 0527 871898

Acknowledgements

I am very grateful for the secretarial help of Mrs Gill Knutton with the manuscript and Miss Beryl Holmes, Metabolic Liaison health visitor.

References

1 Stephenson, J.B.P., King, M.D. *Handbook of Neurological Investigations in Children*. London: Wright, 1989.
2 Green, S.H. Degenerative disorders of the infant central nervous system. In: Punt, J., Levene, M., Bennett, M.J., eds. *Fetal and Neonatal Neurology and Neurosurgery*. Edinburgh: Churchill Livingstone, 1988: 469–483.
3 Naidu, S., Moser, H.W. Peroxisomal disorders. *Neurol Clin* 1990; **8**: 507–527.

4 Green, S.H. Adrenoleukodystrophy. *Arch Dis Child* 1991; **66**: 830–831.

5 Krivit, W., Shapiro, E., Kennedy, W., *et al*. Treatment of late infantile metachromatic leukodystrophy by bone marrow transplantation. *New Eng J Med* 1990; **322**: 28–32.

6 Arima, M., Takeshita, K., Yoshino, K., Kitohara, T., Suzuki, Y. Prognosis of Wilson's disease in childhood. *Eur J Paediatr* 1977; **126**: 147–154.

7 Elder, G.A., Sever, J.L. Neurological disorders associated with AIDS retroviral infection. *Rev Infect Dis* 1988; **10**: 286–302.

8 Harding, B., Egger, J., Portman, B., Erdohazi, M. Progressive neuronal degeneration of childhood with liver disease. *Brain* 1986; **109**: 181–206.

9 Hagberg, B., Aicardi, J., Dias, K., Ramos, O. A syndrome of autism, dementia and loss of purposeful hand movement in girls: Rett's syndrome, a report of 35 cases. *Ann Neurol* 1983; **14**: 471–479.

10 Hagberg, B., Goutieres, F., Hanefeld, F., Rett, A., Wilson, J. Rett syndrome: criteria for inclusion and exclusion. *Brain Dev* 1985; **7**: 372–373.

11 Robb, S.A., Pohl, K.R.E., Baraitser, M., Wilson, J., Brett, E.M. The 'happy puppet' syndrome of Angelman: review of the clinical features. *Arch Dis Child* 1989; **64**: 83–86.

12 Gomez, M.R. *Neurocutaneous Diseases: a Practical Approach*. Boston: Butterworths, 1987.

13 Deonna, T., Beaumanoir, A., Gaillard, F., Assal, G. Acquired aphasia in childhood with seizure disorder: a heterogenous syndrome. *Neuropaediatrie* 1977; **8**: 263–273.

14 Gillberg, C. Neurobiology of infantile autism. *J Child Psychol Psychiatr* 1988; **18**: 297–321.

*15 Baraitser, M. *The Genetics of Neurological Disorders*. 2nd edn. Oxford: Oxford University Press, 1990.

*16 Harding, A. *Hereditary Ataxias and Related Disorders*. Edinburgh: Churchill Livingstone, 1984.

*17 Brett, E.M. *Paediatric Neurology*, 2nd edn. Edinburgh: Churchill Livingstone, 1991.

*18 Bundey, S. *Genetics and Neurology*. Edinburgh: Churchill Livingstone, 1985.

19 Di Mauro, S., Bonilla, E., Zevioni, M., *et al*. Mitochondrial myopathies. *J Inher Metab Dis* 1987; **10** supp 1: 113–128.

20 Santavuori, P. Neuronal ceroid-lipofuscinosis in childhood. *Brain Dev* 1988; **10**: 80–83.

21 Green, S.H., Wirtschafter, J.D. Ophthalmoscopic findings in subacute sclerosing panencephalitis. *Br J Ophthalmol* 1973; **57**: 780–787.

22 Booth, I.W. Enteral nutrition in childhood. *Br J Hosp Med* 1991; **46**: 111–113.

23 Baum, J.D., Dominica, F., Woodward, R.N. *Listen: My Child Has a Lot of Living to Do*. Oxford: Oxford University Press, 1990.

* These are also general references.

10.5 Neural tube defects and hydrocephalus

Matgorzata Borzyskowski

Introduction

The term spina bifida has been in use since the 17th century,[1] although it is not known who first introduced it. Indeed it seems that congenital defects of the neural tube are at least as old as man himself. Morgagni who detected the relationship between spina bifida and hydrocephalus also described spina bifida and anencephaly as expressions of the same anomaly and deduced that the abnormalities in the lower limbs, bladder and rectum were secondary to neuronal damage in the defective spinal cord.[2]

The outcome of these children was very poor until new materials and techniques became available for the treatment of hydrocephalus. In 1956 Eugene Spitz implanted a ventriculo-atrial silastic drain into an infant boy with hydrocephalus whose father, John Holter, had designed a valve mechanism for the drain enabling control of pressure and unidirectional flow.

By the end of the 1950s reliable ventriculo-atrial and ventriculo-peritoneal systems were available and, with the development of better antibiotics, primary surgical closure of the defect for all newborns with myelomeningocele was available. This aggressive management uncovered new problems in particular of an orthopaedic and urological nature. It became apparent that multidisciplinary teams were necessary to deal with the neurosurgical, orthopaedic and urological problems of these children. We are now also aware of the learning difficulties and psychosocial problems that these children encounter.

Incidence

Spina bifida is more common in Europeans than Asians or Africans. In India, it is more common in Sikhs, and in the UK it is more common in Northern Ireland than south east England.[3] It is thought that ten times as many fetuses with neural tube defects spontaneously abort than are born with the defect.[4] It is more common in females and recurs in siblings and this together with the ethnic variation suggests that genetic factors play a part although environmental factors are also thought to be important.

The incidence has fallen in England and Wales from 4.26/1000 live births in 1972[5] to 1.26/1000 live births in 1984.[6] Prenatal diagnosis and abortion of affected fetuses in the last 12 years has influenced the birth prevalence but it may not altogether account for the drop in numbers. Indeed a decrease was seen before prenatal diagnosis was available and has also occurred in the Republic of Ireland where there is no screening programme and termination of pregnancy is not available.[7] The decline has been greatest in the areas of highest prevalence suggesting an environmental influence.

In recent years it has been thought that periconceptional supplementation with multivitamins and folic acid may prevent the occurrence of neural tube defects.[8] However, although recent publications have shown conflicting results,[9-11] a recent trial funded by the Medical Research Council has provided clear evidence of the role of folic acid in preventing neural tube defects.[12] Thus it has been recommended that all women who have had an affected pregnancy should have folic acid supplements before starting a further pregnancy.

Antenatal screening

All women who have had a child with a neural tube defect should be offered antenatal screening by means of measurement of amniotic alpha fetoprotein and high resolution ultrasonography. In some parts of the country all women are screened by measurement of venous alpha fetoprotein at around 16 weeks' gestation. However, this is not universal practice. Termination performed on the result of raised alpha fetoprotein levels is unselective. Some discrimination may be provided by ultrasonography but this needs to be validated by long-term follow up. The author has seen a few affected infants in the last 5 years who either had no antenatal care or in whom the defect was not detected by either measurement of alpha fetoprotein or ultrasonography or was picked up too late for any action to be taken.

Genetic counselling

All families who have had an affected child should be offered genetic counselling as it is known that there is an increased risk of recurrence in subsequent pregnancies. It should be remembered that open and closed spina bifida and anencephaly behave as part of the same group with a recurrence risk of 1 in 25. There is also an increased risk of isolated hydrocephalus in these families. If two children have been affected the recurrence risk rises to 1 in 10. The risk of recurrence in the offspring of an adult with spina bifida is about 3%.[13] There is also an increased risk in mothers taking sodium valproate.

The risk of recurrence of sacral agenesis (which is more common in diabetic mothers) is low in both diabetic and non-diabetic mothers.

Type of defect

Spina bifida is a developmental defect due to failure of fusion of the neural tube around the 28th day of gestation. The neural tube may be affected anywhere along its length and results in anencephaly if the forebrain does not develop.

Failure of fusion of the neural tube causes defective closure of the vertebral canal. The most common lesion is thoracolumbar, then lumbosacral, then thoracic and least common is a cervical lesion. Herniation of the medulla and cerebellar tonsils through the foramen magnum results in the Arnold-Chiari malformation obstructing the flow of cerebrospinal fluid (SF) and causing an obstructive hydrocephalus.

In a meningocele the meninges form a sac lined by arachnoid membrane and dura containing CSF and rarely a small amount of nervous tissue. The skin over the sac is usually intact, whereas in a myelomeningocele the spinal cord and all the nerve roots are outside the vertebral canal though still covered by a membrane centrally and skin peripherally. There may be associated lipomata or tethered nerve roots. If there is no sac and the spinal cord is flattened and is wide open on the surface, this is known as a rachischeisis.

The term closed spina bifida is used to describe all significant lesions with a skin covering and should not be confused with the term spina bifida occulta which occurs in at least 5% of the population and consists of a narrow defect of laminar fusion of L5 and/or S1. On its own spina bifida occulta is not regarded as significant.

Closed spina bifida is twice as common in girls and may present with asymmetric limb growth, contractures, pes cavus, sensory or reflex loss, a cutaneous lesion such as lumbosacral lipoma, a hairy patch, a sinus or dimple above the sacrum or a naevus or scarred area, bladder dysfunction or constipation. The abnormalities found include: a low conus, split spinal cord (diastematomyelia) with or without a bony or fibrous septum, lipomas with intraspinal lesions, meningoceles, dermoid cysts and dermoid sinuses and significant pure bony defects without radiological spinal cord abnormalities. All these children should have an antero-posterior and lateral X-ray of the lumbosacral spine and further investigations and management as indicated. However, attitudes to investigation and surgical treatment of closed lesions vary because of doubt that the neurological deficit progresses. It has been suggested that the progression may be caused by tethering of the lower spinal cord either by stretching and ischaemia or compression by a central septum, meningocele or dermoid cyst.

The usual indications for investigation of closed spina bifida are the presence of a vertebral defect and some evidence of progressive neurology. In addition, a significant bladder problem in a child with a vertebral defect should be investigated further. Surgical intervention is indicated for progressive neurology with a potentially treatable pathology. It is uncertain whether untethering prevents later deterioration; each case must be fully discussed with the neurosurgeons after full investigation. Even though the neurological deficit may be minor, these children have all the same problems with neuropathic bladder and bowel dysfunction as children with much more severe neurological dysfunction. Indeed, their bladder dysfunction is often very severe and dangerous in terms of renal function.[14] Associated hydrocephalus is rare.

Assessment of severity at birth

In recent years the management of spina bifida and hydrocephalus has been affected by prenatal diagnosis, the option of termination of affected pregnancies and the availability of surgical intervention after birth. The decision to operate or not should only be made after full discussion with the parents.

Poor prognostic factors at birth are: gross hydrocephalus, severe paraplegia with a voluntary motor level of L3 or less, kyphosis or scoliosis or both, thoracolumbar or thoracolumbosacral lesions, and the presence of associated major malformations.

Hunt[15] has recently published the results of follow up of 117 consecutive cases of open spina bifida born between 1963 and 1970 and treated unselectively. Forty-eight children died before the age of 16. Of the 69 survivors, 60 had had a shunt and two were blind following shunt dysfunction, 22 were mentally retarded, 35 were wheelchair dependent, 52 were incontinent, 33 were unable to live without help or supervision and only 17 were capable of open employment. Hunt found that the sensory level at birth was a good predictor of the likely degree of handicap in adult life in this group of patients. Those with sensory levels above T11 (at or above the umbilicus) if treated from birth have the greatest morbidity and mortality; those with sensory levels below L3 (below knees) have a 75% chance of survival, 80% have normal intelligence, 90% are ambulant as adults, 40% would be continent, 95% would have minimal or moderate disabilities and 85% would be totally independent.

Whether or not a selection policy is carried out, all babies born with spina bifida should be examined by a paediatrician or paediatric neurologist experienced in assessing such babies and their long-term management. In addition, the child should be seen by a neurosurgeon or paediatric surgeon. The following are assessed in particular:

1 *The skull*: the head circumference is measured and plotted, the sutures and fontanelle are palpated for evidence of distension and raised intracranial pressure, the fundi are examined and eye movements are assessed.
2 *Cranial nerves*: these are assessed by observations of the movements of the face, tongue, palate and by watching the baby suck.
3 *Spine*: the spine is palpated along its entire length as there may be other lesions. The length and width of the lesion is measured and its level noted.
4 *Limbs*: the baby is examined for talipes equinovarus and congenital dislocation of the hips. Movements of the limbs should be assessed by observation and by stimulating the legs and muscle power is assessed against gravity and with and without resistance and by testing for neonatal reflexes. The deep tendon reflexes should be tested.
5 *Sensory level*: this is important and best assessed using pin prick and ice.
6 *Bowel and bladder*: it is important to see if the bladder is palpable, to look for dribbling of urine and to assess the urinary stream. The anal reflex should be tested using an orange stick and the anal tone assessed.

The findings and their implications should be discussed with both parents. If considered appropriate, it is preferable to operate as soon as possible, but this is not mandatory and can be deferred if the parents require more time to make a decision.

Because the children will have multiple problems, a team approach involving the paediatrician, paediatric neurologist, neurosurgeon, orthopaedic surgeon, urologist and the therapists is vital. Although some of the child's problems may require assessment and management at specialist regional clinics, the local paediatrician should be in overall charge of the child's management.

Associated problems

1 Hydrocephalus

This is rare in children with closed lesions and unusual in association with a meningocele. In children with myelomeningocele, hydrocephalus occurs in a large majority and is usually associated with the Arnold-Chiari malformation which, in its mildest form, consists of downward displacement of the medulla oblongata and cerebellar tonsils through the foramen magnum, and in the severest form, herniation of the cerebellum. The malformation obstructs the free flow of CSF either directly or secondarily through arachnoiditis with adhesions and so may cause hydrocephalus.

It may also be responsible for the later development of syringomyelia.

The hydrocephalus may be evident at birth or develop after closure of the back. Thus the child should be carefully monitored by daily measurement of the head circumference, palpation of the fontanelles and sutures and by ultrasonography. In addition there may be feeding problems, vomiting, swallowing difficulties and cranial nerve palsies.

The decision to intervene is based on the rate of head growth, regular assessment of ventricular size by ultrasonography and CT scanning and the child's well-being. It is important to differentiate between arrested hydrocephalus which may need no treatment and progressive hydrocephalus which will require intervention.

The surgical procedure for the relief of hydrocephalus consists of draining CSF from the lateral ventricles via shunts into the right atrium (ventriculo-atrial), or more often peritoneal cavity (ventriculo-peritoneal). Various forms of shunts consisting of tubes and valves opening at different pressures are available. Occasionally a reservoir is inserted into the system which allows the ventricles to be tapped easily and the pressure of the CSF measured.

Medical treatment with isosorbide has been used successfully[16] and in some cases the need for a shunt may be averted. As it is an osmotic diuretic the electrolytes should be measured regularly and the drug should be avoided in those with impaired renal function.

There are many complications that may occur in children who have ventricular shunts. The main problems are infection of the shunt and blockage resulting in raised intracranial pressure. Shunt infection occurs in 12% of treated children[17] and *Staphylococcus*, usually coagulase negative, is the commonest organism. The associated low-grade bacteraemia may cause fever, anaemia, failure to thrive and splenomegaly. Very rarely shunt nephritis may occur in a child with a ventriculo-atrial shunt. Infections require antibiotics and often shunt replacement. Blockage may occur proximally from the choroid plexus growing into the proximal catheter or distally by withdrawal of the shunt from the right atrium secondary to growth. This results in raised intracranial pressure and usually requires revision of the shunt and replacement of the valve. The use of a ventriculo-peritoneal shunt may reduce the problems related to growth as surplus tubing can be left in the peritoneal cavity. The components of the shunt may separate, pressure necrosis may occur and there may be a decompression effect if the valve pressure is too high. In addition, children with ventriculo-atrial shunts may rarely develop acute pulmonary emboli and chronic pulmonary hypertension.

It is thus apparent that any child with treated hydrocephalus requires close monitoring and easy access to a neurosurgeon should problems arise.

2 Orthopaedic problems

These children have a variable degree and variety of lower limb weakness and paralysis. Deformity may occur as a result of muscle imbalance. Hip dislocation occurs early in spinal lesions at the level of L4 and above and contractures of the feet are common in sacral lesions. Sensory loss may aggravate the motor handicap because of impaired sensory feedback and pathological fractures are common because of disuse. Kyphosis and scoliosis may occur with growth. The aim of management of these children is for the child to walk. However, children with lesions of T12 and above are usually wheelchair bound; with L1–3 lesions, they are predominantly wheelchair users but can walk with long calipers; children with L4–S1 lesions usually walk using short calipers and a walking aid; and those with S2–5 lesions walk unaided.

It is important that the child is assessed orthopaedically as soon as possible after birth. Muscle charts are useful but it is important to realize that some of the observed movements may be reflex or involuntary.

Passive stretching and careful splinting are all that is required until the prognosis is clear. Orthopaedic surgery is rarely necessary until it is clear that the child will be able to stand and walk. However, sometimes a simple tenotomy of the adductors of the hip or a deforming tendon at the knee or ankle may allow more effective conservative treatment and prevent gross, progressive deformity. Major surgery is reserved for those who are going to walk usefully and to aid satisfactory positioning in a wheelchair. Dislocation, subluxation and dysplasia of the hip are very common. It is now thought that if both hips are dislocated they should be left alone unless there is a pure lower motor neurone lesion and the child is going to be an active walker, probably without any aids at all. A single dislocated hip should only be replaced if the child is going to walk well. Rarely though the hip dislocation causes pain necessitating surgical intervention.

Orthoses of some kind will be required by most patients. A wide range is available and ideally the orthopaedic surgeon, paediatrician or paediatric neurologist, orthotist and physiotherapist should work closely seeing the child in combined clinics if at all possible. Often a pelvic band is necessary to start with, progressing to long leg or short leg orthoses and appropriate surgery where indicated. If a pelvic band continues to be necessary, it is unlikely to be used as an adult as it will be too cumbersome and a wheelchair will probably be preferred. If it becomes clear that elaborate orthoses are not going to be used as an adult then further training should be directed towards providing wheelchair independence. Children who are independent in long or short leg orthoses will usually continue to use these as adults unless walking becomes too laborious and exhausting.

The aim of orthopaedic surgery is to allow the child to be as independent as possible. Regular physiotherapy by the parents under the supervision and guidance of the physiotherapist is an integral part of orthopaedic management and ensuring that the parents and children (depending on maturity) understand management and its aims is more likely to lead to compliance and success.

3   Neuropathic bladder

It is now well recognized that the majority of children with spina bifida will have neuropathic vesico-urethral dysfunction. It is very rare for this not to be the case and is only seen in the occasional child who has a meningocele with no neurological involvement. It is often the children with more minor lesions who have the most dangerous bladder dysfunction in terms of renal function.[14]

It is therefore important to monitor the micturition pattern of the infant by noting the presence of a poor or good urine stream, or any dribbling or urine, to palpate the abdomen for a large bladder and to carry out ultrasonography to look for hydronephrosis (this can be done at the same time as cranial ultrasonography is done to assess ventricular size). As soon as feasible after back surgery and treatment of hydrocephalus (if warranted), bladder and urethral function should be assessed by video-urodynamics or if not possible by a micturating cysto-urethrography to look for reflux and to assess the degree of bladder emptying. Obviously if hydronephrosis has been identified earlier these investigations should be done at that time and the hydronephrosis treated (usually by an indwelling catheter or vesicostomy).

The advent of video-urodynamic studies in the last 15 years has transformed the management of these children. It enables us to identify those most at risk from renal damage, i.e. those with high pressure bladders, vesico-ureteric reflux, detrusor sphincter dyssynergia (DSD) (failure of the distal urethral sphincter to relax when the detrusor muscle contracts and thus poor emptying and raised pressure) and to monitor them very closely. Ultrasonography by an experienced radiologist enables detection of early changes related to high pressure and poor emptying without exposing the child to X-ray irradiation and can thus be carried out very frequently (monthly if necessary in the child at risk). Management can then be suitably modified. These children are particularly prone to urinary tract infections because of poor emptying and in the presence of DSD and reflux renal damage invariably occurs unless this situation is modified.

The aims of management are preservation of renal function, continence and normality of life. Whatever management is used, preservation of renal function is the most important consideration.

In order to achieve continence there needs to be a reasonable bladder capacity, a reasonable degree of outflow obstruction, satisfactory bladder emptying and a low pressure bladder.

Management has to have realistic expectations and it is not possible to achieve complete continence in all cases. However, if a child needs only one pad a day instead of nine, this is a successful result.

The adverse factors for renal function are DSD, reflux, raised intravesical pressure, reduced bladder compliance and recurrent infections. Management is aimed at reducing these in order to preserve renal function and promote continence.

All children must have bladder and renal function assessed fully and reassessed at regular intervals. Creatinine is not a good indicator of renal function in these children because of their reduced muscle bulk. Glomerular filtration rate is a much better measure. Dysfunction changes with time and the first 5 years and teenage years are the most vulnerable in terms of both continence and renal function. Life-long supervision will be required.

Control of infection is important particularly if vesico-ureteric reflux is present; the use of prophylactic antibiotics is advocated in those who have reflux and those with frequent symptomatic infections. Infections in these two groups should of course be treated with the appropriate antibiotic. Regular urine culture is important. Asymptomatic infections do not all require treatment and some children on clean intermittent catheterization (CIC) or with an indwelling catheter nearly always harbour organisms in their urine. Adequate bladder drainage is fundamental in the prevention of urinary tract infections.

An important member of the multidisciplinary team caring for these children is a home liaison nurse who not only sees the children when they attend hospital, but visits them at home and at school, and is responsible for liaison between the hospital and community. The nurse can advise on various forms of nappies, pads and incontinence appliances. In addition, she can teach children and their carers techniques such as CIC.

The key factors in management are an understanding of the pathophysiology of bladder and urethral dysfunction, video-urodynamic assessment, and a realistic approach to management.

Three types of vesico-urethral dysfunction are recognized:[18]

a *Contractile*: incontinence occurs with high pressure contractions, but voiding is incomplete and capacity usually reduced. The bladder neck is competent in 50% of the children and the distal sphincter is dyssynergic in most of them.

b *Intermediate*: there is poor compliance due to a thick contracted bladder wall and ineffective contractions. The bladder neck is incompetent and the distal sphincter is static with incomplete voiding and leakage at a critical pressure. Often there is continuous incontinence.

c *Acontractile*: the detrusor does not contract and the bladder neck is incompetent. The distal sphincter is static with leakage occurring when a critical volume is reached.

In general, although drugs may improve bladder capacity indirectly by reducing detrusor overactivity, medical management aims to improve bladder capacity by improving bladder emptying and so increasing the interval between voids. The limiting factor for achieving continence is severe sphincter weakness. Effective bladder emptying can be achieved by:

i *Clean intermittent catheterization*: this is a means of removing residual urine and has made a tremendous difference to the management of these children. It is particularly useful in those with DSD where bladder emptying and protection of the upper tracts is achieved and this group, i.e. the contractile, have the best chance of achieving continence. If there is leakage due to high pressure contractions, anticholinergic agents are often beneficial. Mild degrees of bladder neck incompetence may respond to alpha adrenergic drugs. Children with very small capacity bladders (because of reduced compliance) or hyperreflexia (uninhibited spontaneous abnormal contractions) which does not respond to anticholinergics, or those with marked sphincter weakness, will not become dry and may require surgical intervention to do so.

ii *Bladder expression*: this is often disliked by young children and is not recommended in the presence of DSD or reflux.

iii *Bladder straining*: this may achieve bladder emptying in the older well-motivated children in whom the innervation of the abdominal wall musculature is preserved. However, they may leak because of sphincter weakness.

iv *Continuous catheterization*: this may be the only way to achieve continence in the severely handicapped wheelchair bound girl and is mandatory in those presenting with upper tract dilatation secondary to urinary outflow obstruction. It is usually disliked by the mobile child.

In addition, continence can be helped by:

a *Penile appliances*: if there is no obstruction to urinary outflow, although a good fit is difficult to achieve in young boys.

b *Pads*: a large variety to suit different needs is now available.

c *Pharmacological agents*: the most useful are:

i *anticholinergic agents*: these have proved to be the most beneficial and act by reducing detrusor hyperreflexia and indirectly increasing bladder capacity. They can be used on their own or in combination with CIC. Propantheline bromide and oxybutynin chloride have been used most commonly. The latter is effective in 75% of cases.[19]

ii *alpha adrenergic agents*: these are used to increase the tone of the bladder neck region. Ephedrine is used most commonly, but does not prevent stress incontinence if bladder neck weakness is severe.

If these two agents are used bladder emptying must be ensured. They can be used in combination in a child using CIC who has both hyperreflexia and bladder neck weakness.

iii *antibiotics*: see above.

If despite all these measures the child is unacceptably wet or renal function shows signs of deteriorating or both, then serious consideration has to be given to surgical intervention. Deterioration of renal function is usually due to outflow obstruction at the distal sphincter and may be made worse by reflux and high pressure contractions which have not responded to medical management. Detailed discussion of surgical techniques is beyond the scope of this section, but surgical techniques such as augmentation cystoplasty to increase bladder capacity and reduce intravesical pressure not responding to medical management (as seen in small, contracted, thick walled hyperreflexic bladders) or substitution cystoplasty (bladder replacement) are available. Bladder neck weakness can be dealt with by the implantation of an artificial urinary sphincter and in the child with spina bifida this nearly always means some form of bladder surgery at the same time.

The timing of surgical intervention is critical. If renal function is deteriorating, then surgical intervention will be determined by this. If, however, surgery is being considered because of incontinence which has not responded to other means, full discussion with the child and parents is vital so that the best time can be chosen, for example avoiding important school examinations. It is preferable to wait until after puberty.

Urinary diversion is rarely performed but may be the only option in a very small number. Undiversion is now being requested by some and can be performed, but this may require fairly major surgery. It is usually not just a matter of reconnecting the ureters to the bladder, but usually requires major bladder reconstruction. Artificial urinary sphincter implantation may be necessary and the patient may subsequently have to catheterize intermittently in order to empty the bladder. Thus although the patient looks more normal, they are rarely rendered normal so that careful selection is mandatory.

Close cooperation between the paediatrician and urologist ideally at a combined clinic is very important; this emphasizes once again the value of team work in the management of these children. Life-long supervision and regular reassessments are necessary and should be carried out by a team understanding the nature of the problem.

4 Neuropathic bowel

It is much more difficult to achieve bowel continence than urinary continence. In addition marked constipation may affect bladder function. The underlying problem is deficient sensation of the lower bowel, rectum and anus often in the presence of a patulous or atonic anal sphincter. It is important to achieve motions which are of normal consistency and a high fibre diet is very useful to promote this. In addition, when passing a motion, the child needs to be able to push down with the abdominal muscles and this needs to be practised regularly from an early age. Thus a regular toileting regimen, for example twice daily, is useful although there is no point expecting the child to sit and push for 30 minutes. For some children, regular manual evacuation may be the answer. Laxatives may be required although a high fibre diet together with a regular toileting regimen is preferable. Occasionally suppositories or enemas are indicated. It can be a long process to achieve the correct balance in any individual child. However, if the child and family are motivated the outcome is usually successful. Surgical intervention may be required in the occasional child when everything else has failed.

5 Vision

Many of these children have optic atrophy (secondary to hydrocephalus) or a squint and require ophthalmological follow up.

6 Trophic ulceration

This is common and difficult to manage; it requires bed rest, elevation and exposure to the air of the affected area. Antibiotic treatment may be necessary. Meticulous care of the areas with sensory loss is essential at all times and the children should be taught to check their feet every day. Prompt action must be taken as soon as there is any sign of skin trauma.

7 Intellectual development

Surveys have shown that children with hydrocephalus have lower IQs than their brothers and sisters; intelligence is particularly affected in those who have required shunts.[20] These children show a discrepancy between their verbal and performance skills with a small but statistically significant effect on the performance section of the Wechsler Intelligence Scale for Children (WISC). Motor and perceptuo-motor skills are most affected. Visual perception is often impaired and visual scanning may be affected in children with hydrocephalus. In addition, hand function may be impaired by tremor or poor coordination as a result of cerebellar involvement in the Arnold-Chiari malformation.

Most of these children given an impression of normal verbal ability and yet have an apparent lack of understanding.

It is therefore important that they should be seen from an early age by a developmental paediatrician for regular review. Thus problems can be anticipated and, if necessary, intervention with advice by a speech therapist or occupational therapist or both arranged.

In addition, the majority will require regular physiotherapy supervision. If the child is likely to have special educational needs, the education authority should be notified, so that an assessment of needs can be completed before school entry in order to ensure appropriate educational provision. This will need to be reviewed at the recommended intervals with the involvement of the multidisciplinary team.

The adult

It has been stressed throughout this section that regular surveillance by a multidisciplinary team is vital in the management of these children. The transition from the paediatric service to the adult service needs to be carefully planned. Often the orthopaedic surgeon and urologist will remain unchanged, but far too often the young adult gets lost to the system and follow up ceases until an emergency arises. This may be because the patient fails to turn up for an appointment or because no suitable provision is available. Young people should be involved in the decision as to whether they remain under paediatric care until they leave school or transfer to the adult service.

The family

It must never be forgotten that the whole family is affected by the birth of a child with spina bifida. Family life will never be as normal as it was and this must always be taken into consideration by all those involved in the management of these children. Adequate counselling of parents and siblings is essential. It is also important that the consultant, rather than junior doctors, sees the child in outpatients whenever possible and is available for consultation by the family if the need arises, to provide optimum consistency of care and to coordinate multidisciplinary care.

References

1 Skinner, H.A. *The Origin of Medical Terms*. Baltimore: Williams & Wilkins, 1961.

2 Morgagni, J.B. *De Ledibus et Causis Morborum per Anatomen Indagatis*, Libri V; Venice: Ex Typographia Remondiana: 1761.

3 Leck, I. Causation of neural tube defects; clues from epidemiology. *Br Med Bull* 1976; **30**: 158–163.

4 Creasy, M.R., Alberman, E.D. Congenital malformations of the central nervous system in spontaneous abortions. *J Med Genet* 1976; **13**: 9–16.

5 Bradshaw, J., Weale, J., Weatherall, J. *Congenital Malformations of the Central Nervous System* (Population Trends No 19). London: HMSO, 1980: 13–18.

6 Office of Population Censuses and Surveys. Congenital malformations. *OPCS Monitor*, MB3 85-2, London: HMSO, 1985.

7 Kirke, P.N., Elwood, J.H. Anencephaly in the United Kingdom and Republic of Ireland. *Br Med J* 1984; **289**: 1621.

8 Smithells, R.W., Sheppard, S., Schorah, C.J., *et al.* Apparent prevention of neural tube defects by periconceptional vitamin supplementation. *Arch Dis Child* 1981; **56**: 911–918.

9 Mullinare, J., Cordero, J.F., Erikson, J.D., Berry, R.J. Periconceptional use of multi-vitamins and the occurrence of neural tube defects. *J Am Med Assoc* 1988; **260**: 3141–3145.

10 Mills, J.L., Rhoads, G.G., Simpson, J.L., *et al.* The absence of a relation between the periconceptional use of vitamins and neural tube defects. *New Eng J Med* 1989; **321**: 430–435.

11 Milunsky, A., Jack, H., Jick, S.S., *et al.* Multivitamin/ folic acid and supplementation in early pregnancy reduces the prevalence of neural tube defects. *J Am Med Assoc* 1989; **262**: 2847–2852.

12 MRC Vitamin Study Research Group. Prevention of neural tube defects, results of the Medical Research Council vitamin study. *Lancet* 1991; **ii**: 131–137.

13 Baraitser, M. *The Genetics of Neurological Disorders*. Oxford: Oxford University Press, 1982.

14 Borzyskowski, M., Neville, B.G.R. Neuropathic bladder and spinal dysraphism. *Arch Dis Child* 1981; **56**: 176–180.

15 Hunt, G.M. Open spina bifida: outcome for a complete cohort treated unselectively and followed into adulthood. *Dev Med Child Neurol* 1990; **32**: 108–118.

16 Lorber, J. Isosorbide in the treatment of infantile hydrocephalus. *Arch Dis Child* 1975; **50**: 431–436.

17 Brett, E.M., ed. Hydrocephalus and congenital anomalies of the nervous system other than myelomeningocele. In: Brett, E.M., ed. *Paediatric Neurology*. Edinburgh: Churchill Livingstone, 1983: 404.

18 Mundy, A.R., Shah, P.J.R., Borzyskowski, M., Saxton, H.M. Sphincter behaviour in myelomeningocele. *Br J Urol* 1985; **57**: 647–651.

19 Borzyskowski, M., Mundy, A.R.M. The management of the neuropathic bladder in childhood. *Paediatr Nephrol* 1988; **2**: 56–66.

20 Halliwell, M.D., Carr, J.G., Pearson, A.M. The intellectual and educational functioning of children with neural tube defects. *Z Kinderchir* 1980; **31**: 4.

10.6 Severe mental handicap

David Taylor

The categories used to describe very low levels of intellectual functioning keep being changed in an attempt to avoid stigma. As used in the original sorting process from lowest to highest, they were idiot, imbecile and moron, all of which words have since entered the vocabulary of abuse. Mentally subnormal, mentally retarded, and mentally handicapped have officially all come and gone. In the USA the expression 'exceptional child' is a nice euphemism for an idiot on the one hand but on the other does not help much with how a child prodigy might otherwise be described in English. Recently the categories of moderate learning difficulties and severe learning difficulties have come into use. But how are we now to describe bright capable children who also have some severe learning difficulties? All this reveals 'severe mental handicap' as a social and administrative category that is strongly associated with stigma.

The parents of a handicapped child can be seen as having made a social gaffe, brought into being an unwanted sort of child. No person would choose to bring into being a child who is burdened by imperfections. Services for the mentally handicapped are those that help with the management of stigma and its attendant pain and with the various types of problems that are more liable to occur when the brain does not work very well. These problems arise from failure of cerebral function, from seizures, palsies, problems of self-care and health care management as well as a range of psychiatric disorders. Advocacy, both for appropriate citizen rights and for appropriate recognition of their health care needs, is the most urgent requirement of the handicapped.

In considering the needs of this population, it is necessary to ask first what sort of physical and structural processes are operating and what is their origin, that is, the disease, diagnosis and aetiology. Secondly, ask what sort of illness might this person be experiencing? Despite their low IQ they might be very well but there might also be symptoms in a variety of systems; for example pain which they cannot describe. Thirdly, what is the nature of this person's predicament? How are they placed in the world? Do not just consider their personal environment but give thought to the pattern of their relationships, their access to ordinary resources, their sources of joy and enrichment. Are they contained in a drab and uncongenial situation, remote from potential friends, deprived of proper clothes and unrelieved by appropriate work and recreation? Are they institutionalized in their own home, as much unrelieved as they might be in an asylum with two thousand others?

Prevalence

Since the category is purely administrative, *prevalence* of severe mental handicap can be variously defined. A social measure of severe mental handicap is those persons who will always need help with managing their lives. On the basis of a measured IQ below 50, prevalence would encompass three to four persons per thousand of the population. Nearly all persons would have evidence of organic cerebral disorder, diagnosable at the 'disease' level in about 75%. At this level of functioning the incidence of epilepsy is around 30%, and half of the population would have recognizable psychiatric disorder.

McKinlay (1988, personal communication) has tabulated some useful figures for a health district of 250 000 persons (Table 10.5).

In his figures there are at any one time 1000 people with severe learning difficulties of whom 200 are school children. McKinlay argues for the need for joint planning with other services such as education and social services, and with adult physicians at the time of school leaving for the continuing proper health care of mentally handicapped adults. However, it is extremely uncertain who has the responsibility for managing these patients' health care once they are located in the community, and it is also very problematic to provide it adequately. It is uncertain who will develop the expertise to diagnose those severely handicapped persons' physical ailments; who best will manage their seizures; and who will have the resources to treat their mental disorders when the hospitals for the mentally handicapped are finally closed.

Causes of severe mental handicap

Approximately one-third of all severe mental handicap is due to Down syndrome. This figure could be usefully reduced by programmes of surveillance and selective abortion in older mothers, but the bulk of cases still comes from sporadic chromosomal disorders in young mothers. Only some form of blood test can contribute usefully to more precise screening. Many parents consider it worthwhile to raise a child with Down syndrome and refuse abortion. There is a widespread range of ability within the syndrome and it is not certain how this occurs. Down syndrome is a multisystem disorder and apart from the brain abnormality the facies achieve a remarkable degree of similarity in configuration and development of the heart and the gut may be compromised *in utero*.

Other aetiologies of mental handicap can only be mentioned in note form in this brief section. A good schema for considering causation is given in Table 10.6.

General effect of brain damage

It is well recognized that very major changes in the ordinary configuration of the brain, for example extreme degrees of hydrocephalus or very large chronic tumours, are compatible with apparently normal levels of functioning. So is the converse true, that many persons with extremely low levels of functioning show little major structural brain disorganization. Equally these extremes must not be allowed to obscure the truth that there is an association between damage and difficulties. The disappointment for structuralists remains the very modest level of our knowledge of specific behavioural syndromes to associate with known sorts of brain disorder. However the general effects of damage are consistent and some are seen in the following ways:

Cognitive

It is axiomatic in this section that the causative disorder will have impaired the child's cognitive capacity. Usually this is global but some interesting findings are emerging such as the marked impairment in performance skills of children with Turner syndrome and the various exceptional skills seen in some children with infantile autism (Kanner's

Table 10.5 Approximate number of people per health district of 250 000

	Children	Leavers/ year	Adults
Total	50 000	4500	200 000
Severe learning difficulties	200	15–20	800
Moderate learning difficulties and special needs	400	30–40	800
Cerebral palsy	100	8–10	400
Spina bifida	50	3–5	200
Severe epilepsy	80	6–8	300
Severe autism	25	2–3	100
Blind/partially sighted	100	8–10	1300*
Deaf/hard of hearing	100	8–10	1200**

* Visual acuity <6/18 in better eye at home
** Hearing loss >50dB in better ear

Table 10.6 Cause of severe mental handicap

Preconceptual	Existing genetic traits in parents, masked or apparent. These may be recessive or dominant and of variable penetrance. The resulting syndrome may be structural or metabolic. Some are revealed by characteristic dysmorphologies. Relatives may be affected to various degrees by a similar syndrome.
Conceptual	Error may occur in the microgenesis of the sperm or ova or in their reformation at fusion. Certain chromosomal deficits and gene deletions seem to occur at this stage of development. Relatives will not be similarly affected.
Intrauterine	The environment of the child in utero can be the deleterious factor. For example: 1 Poisoning from drugs taken by the mother e.g. alcohol, 'street drugs' and also prescribed medications. 2 Exposure of the mother to X-rays. It is possible that background radiation could also be important. 3 Multiple births and other problems of placentation and intrauterine nutrition can interfere with implantation. Infection in utero can be blood borne or local. Viruses, such as cytomegalovirus, and protozoa such as toxoplasmosis and bacteria such as syphilis may be sexually transmitted to the mother and then passed vertically to the baby. Rubella damages a fetus in relation to its developmental age at the time of infection. Other viral infections may have similar effects. Migrational: the flow of neural masses can be variously disrupted. Anencephalics rarely survive birth, hydrocephalus can be associated with fusion failure (spina bifida) and heterotopias of the brain can be associated with clinical abnormalities such as in Aicardi syndrome.
Perinatal	Perinatal problems: there is a clear relationship between birthweight/gestational age and perinatal problems, which link in turn to respiratory distress syndrome, hypoxia, intracranial haemorrhage and periventricular leucomalacia. Obstetric factors play less part except for occasional disasters and it is important to recognize the maternal account of the pregnancy and delivery may reflect her concern for the child rather than 'objective' information. Seizures in the newborn unless due to hypocalcaemia are an index of potentially severe cerebral dysfunction. Infection by meningitis and encephalitis can lead to severe mental impairment.
Postnatal	Injury via domestic accident, child abuse, or road traffic accidents. Infection – meningitis or encephalitis Neoplasms Cerebral degenerative disease Metabolic disorders such as phenylketonuria and hypothyroidism The epilepsies of childhood signal a considerable proportion of those children who will have severe or moderate learning difficulties. Early diagnosis can permit genetic counselling and treatment may modify outcome.

syndrome) or Asperger syndrome against a background of cognitive impairment.

Behavioural

The interesting question is whether the behavioural anomalies which are recorded in various of the retardation syndromes, for example the self-biting of the Lesch-Nyhan syndrome can be said to constitute behavioural phenotypes. This approach is favoured for the overactive, over eager winsomeness of children with Williams syndrome, and the shallow overtalkativeness or cocktail party chatter seen in some children with hydrocephalus. There is a strong association between tuberous sclerosis (TS) and early infantile autism. This may be secondary to infantile spasms (common in tuberous sclerosis) which seem to disrupt the organizational basis of language and communication in a similar way to that seen with loss of language, following seizures in the Landau-Kleffner syndrome.

Seizures

Epilepsy occurs in at least one-third of the severely mentally handicapped and seizures will have occurred at some time in even more of them. Neonatal seizures, early onset epileptic encephalopathy, infantile spasms and the Lennox Gastaut syndrome predominate in early childhood, together with a lifelong increased propensity to sporadic grand mal.

Prolonged episodes of major generalized status epilepticus are probably directly causative of further cerebral damage. This may be limited to mesial temporal sclerosis, but the sclerosis can extend to the entire hemisphere and lead to infantile hemiplegia.

In prolonged episodes of minor status the electrical signals from the brain trigger major generalized disorganization of functioning. The individual presents as an obtunded, fatuous, vacuous form of being who nevertheless can adequately perform routine tasks and achieve some social interaction. Such episodes can last hours, days, months. They may occur electrically during sleep and not be noticed for a long time. These episodes may impair the child's best available level of functioning at other times.

Motor function

Some dysfunction is gross enough to be revealed in standard neurological examination. Much of what is important, both in fine motor functioning and gross motor performance is better assessed using more dynamic strategies such as by watching the child dress, draw, walk, run, or attempt to hop. If parents and carers are helped to understand such dysfunctions it becomes easier for them to understand some of the child's difficulties which might otherwise be attributed to wilfulness and not wanting to try.

Special senses

Special techniques and complex apparatus may be required to test the special senses since cooperation of the children with simpler tests is often absent. Optimum hearing and vision are crucial so these pathways must be carefully checked since they may have been affected by the same event as caused the mental handicap, as for instance in congenital rubella syndrome.

Modifiers of the effects of brain damage

Some of the lack of association between aetiology and severity of effect, and between those two and behaviour, are due to the influence of other variables such as:

1 Age of onset of influence of the injurious agent.
2 Sex of the child.
3 Location of the lesion within the brain. Thus there are variable effects of tuberous sclerosis with the location of the tubers such as whether they are within the limbic system or are lesions of the left or right brain.
4 Severity of insult for example of anoxia, haemorrhage, or the influence of genetic modifiers in Down syndrome.
5 Social environment created for the management of unwanted behaviours and the promotion of skills.
6 Temperament and specific genetic make-up of the child.

Psychological effect of brain damage

Apart from the direct effect on learning, mental handicapping syndromes produce psychological effects within the environment of their care through other important mechanisms which deserve to be recog-

nized since they are to some extent, modifiable. These mechanisms include:

Stigmata

Stigmata are the outward signs and behaviours which indicate 'outgroup' membership. In mental handicap the stigmata are many.

Dysmorphology

The classic stigmata described by Langdon Down enabled medical categorization and eventually revealed the chromosomal disorder. However the characteristic facies may, on the one hand, betray membership of a stigmatized group, but may alternatively indicate to the public that it should modify its expectations of such a person. Not to be possessed of such a social signal while being liable to unconventional behaviour could be a disadvantage.

Motor and communication behaviour

Unusual patterns of ambulation ('funny walks') betray deviance as do the dystonias, athetosis, and clumsiness. Dyspraxias, drooling, and disorders of voice regulation (pitch, timbre, prosody) all may betray or suggest the person is mentally handicapped.

Odour

Some metabolic disorders create unpleasant smells. Faecal or urinary incontinence create both odour and the likelihood of wearing nappies. Both of these are signs of special category membership.

Threat of sudden death

Handicapped people create anxiety in their carers who use devices to control them as if supervising younger children. Because the mentally handicapped person cannot guard against common dangers, they tend to be closely watched to the extent of intruding on their personal privacy. Their natural exploratory drives are thwarted.

Handicapped people with epilepsy are additionally at risk from sudden death in a seizure or in accidents caused by fits and this further promotes over vigilant, over cautious supervision. Consequently some lack respite or even brief periods of relaxation for themselves.

Shortened life span

The life span of severely handicapped people is reduced considerably. Down syndrome people are at great risk from early dementia but all handicapped persons have an increased risk of life-threatening disease being overlooked or misinterpreted.

Limited sensory input

Mentally handicapped children are more limited in their opportunities to explore their environment either because they lack mobility, or lack judgement, or because they have reduced sensory inputs due to compromised visual or auditory function. These restrictions are further constraints on learning for children whose cognitive capacities are already impaired.

Threatened personal identity

The administrative category, mentally handicapped, is of itself a limiting and constraining category. Within it are found further categorizations, such as Down syndrome, which in one sense argues that the children resemble others of that category rather more than they resemble members of their nuclear family, and argues against particular individuation. The child is thus more likely to be seen as 'a mongol' than as his father's son with all the potential that implies. Equal constraints can be seen in other similar diagnoses. This labelling has, properly, been criticized by social scientists advocating on the children's behalf. Plastic surgery has been resorted to in an attempt to break the strength of such categorizations by removing the stigmatizing features. But the mentally handicapped child is constrained by so many considerations, for example physique, movement, communication and social patterns as has been argued above, that these stigmata are not easily eradicated.

Thus to be mentally handicapped works directly against one of the prime tasks of development which is to achieve an individual identity. Failure to become an individual person is to become a stereotyped member of the stigmatized mentally handicapped group.

Psychosocial areas affected by mental handicap

Reward and satisfaction

The fact that breaking the news to parents about handicap in their child requires skill and delicacy is a measure of the impact that the loss of perfection will have on the parents. Part of the gratification of parenting is to see the synthesis of the two parental selves emerging and flowering in a new individual. Great work and resource is required to raise an infant and the joy and satisfaction are the rewards of this investment. Parents can come to terms and make good with different levels of achievement and satisfaction to an astonishing degree. Even so there often lurks a residual resentment, guilt and sadness at their lot.

Financial problems

Financial difficulties are usually evident. The work career of carers will be disrupted, limits placed upon their work mobility and flexibility of hours of work. The parents may be fatigued to a point where their work capacity suffers. Various consultations, alternative medicine, diets and regimens result in increases in parents' living costs if they are to contend with the handicap and 'do their best for their child'. Special transport, equipment and medicines can be necessary.

These financial burdens are met to some degree by special provisions in the form of state allowances. These represent the community's way of caring and assisting with the burden.

Life cycle crises

Birth

The crisis of birth is heightened by the ambivalence created by disappointment and concern about the new member of the family. Rejection sometimes occurs but hope usually triumphs and, having experienced shock, numbness, denial, rage, and depression, the family usually manages to cope. Physicians have the task of recognizing failure of coping and providing skilled assistance.

School

School is the first occasion in which the child is subjected to systematic evaluation and selection by the community, though the arrangements for this selection are now moved to well before the ordinary school years. The family is challenged to 'go public' with their child. They may prove very defensive and very critical of the provisions available.

Puberty

Emergent sexual development at puberty is associated with recrudescence of those original anxieties about a handicapped child. There are anxieties about exploitation and defencelessness, but also quite deep fears about reproduction and sexual behaviour in such imperfectly informed and ill-prepared persons. These amplify parents' ordinary anxieties about sexual development. Parents and other guardians sometimes, quite irrationally seek to curtail this sexuality and so inhibit the threat they see it imposing.

Masturbation may become a problem at any age. Carers become concerned and question whether it should be stopped. Giving clear directives about privacy, creating distraction rather than confrontation, and providing alternative activities offer the best chance of helping. The questions surrounding the control of fertility by the use of oral contraceptives or sterilization raise moral and ethical issues which have to be addressed on an individual basis.

Marriage

Marriage is improbable for the severely handicapped and reproduction is actually unlikely as fertility is often impaired. Perhaps it is in the disappointment of these realities that the anxiety over sexuality is projected.

Work

While parents can see clearly that *working* for a living will not occur, the issue of work is translated into questions about the degree of self-care that is likely to be achieved. These anxieties usually presuppose the parents' own death and relate to the time when their handicapped and limited child will be left entirely to the mercy of others.

Through the inability to work gainfully, two other of the goals of development fail to be realized. There is *no employment* and this implies a *failure to be independent* of parents. Work failure really entails failure of three measures: independence, work, and identity. Perhaps parents see this when, even in childhood, they look for an answer to this summarizing question, 'will he ever go out to work doctor?'

Mental disorder and severe mental handicap

Mentally handicapped people are liable to all the mental disorders that afflict more able people. The probability of disorder is higher, not only because of the factor of cerebral disease but because of the aggregation of a large number of social factors which impinge upon the handicapped person either directly, or indirectly through their relatives or carers.

Many of the vicissitudes of rearing an ordinary child, the problems of sleep, the problems of feeding, infantile tantrums, developing continence, learning the rules of social engagements, guarding against dangers will all be enhanced by maturational, cognitive, and situational problems. It is more difficult to explain, harder to train and, in addition, the actual maturational progress of the handicapped child is delayed, so stretching the processes of infancy well beyond their ordinary years. Parents may, more easily, simply give in until they find that they are being dominated by an angry, determined, aggressive youngster who is implacably demanding. The parents' problem is that they have to remain the principal advocates of their child who, in reality, is their tormentor.

Major psychosis

This can include early infantile autism (Kanner's syndrome) or atypical autism where the problems not only include disorders of communication, symbolization, and socialization inherent in that diagnosis, but are likely to include severe problems of hyperkinesis as well. Onset is usually before 30 months, can be severe in non-mentally handicapped people, but the prognosis is worse where there is also handicap. Autism is not a single entity but more a collection of features which are particularly common to a greater or lesser extent in children with mental handicap. In treatment some consideration should be given to the hyperkinesis, and special schooling and training are needed for autistic children. Handicap *due* to autism, which would remit were the autism treated, is improbable.

Affective and schizophrenic disorders can supervene though the clinical picture may be atypical, for example the depressive content may not be describable and hallucinations may only be inferred from behaviour. Referral to appropriate psychiatrists is necessary and drug treatment will follow lines used in non-handicapped people.

Hyperkinetic syndrome

Frantic, persistent, restless, joyless pursuit of transiently novel stimuli; overactivity, dysphoria and aggressiveness characterize this syndrome in brain dysfunctional children. It was best described by Ounsted in epileptic children. It tends to be severely exacerbated by barbiturates and benzodiazepines. It can be exacerbated by almost any form of sedative medicines. Drug treatment by amphetamine or methylphenidate deserves the benefit of a double-blind trial in each case using two different dosage schedules.

Self injurious behaviour

Certain forms of cerebral dysfunction seem particularly to give rise to a tendency towards self injury. These behaviours evoke rapid responses from care givers and are therefore very likely to be reinforced. Eye poking, self-biting, scratching, head banging, self-slapping, pinching and coprophagia (dung eating) are among the more prominent items. Well organized, researched and maintained behaviour modification is a treatment but it is important to ensure that no medically correctable sources of pain or distress such as toothache, constipation with painful tenesmus or oesophageal reflux are the basis of the distress.

Pica

Some severely handicapped children tend to mouth the objects they explore (like the Kluver-Bucy syndrome[1] in bilateral severe temporal lobe damage) and they ingest inedible objects that can be swallowed. This may lead to poisoning or to obstruction.

Multidisciplinary care

Community mental handicap (learning disability) teams manage the clinical needs of people with mental handicap within their own family homes and within a network of community services. The work is focused on a bio-psycho-social model, being multidisciplinary, requiring consideration and sharing of ideas between professionals.

The core disciplines are usually those of psychiatry, nursing, psychology, occupational therapy, physiotherapy, speech therapy and social work; there are frequently links with music, art and dance therapy as well as close links with the day centres, hostels, hospitals and general practitioners.

In childhood, the primary task is to diminish or prevent disability, in adulthood the management of the effects of disability take primacy. While most teams work with adults there is a great importance in life-long coordinated services for children and adults who develop disabling conditions. Good liaison between the child development services and the adult services is essential. In many districts, children with learning disability are looked after by the child development team, with care passing to the community mental handicap (learning disability) team when the child leaves school, though in the last school years both teams often work together.

The moves towards community care may place a greater responsibility on the local authority to provide services, however, there will be a continuing necessity for a multidisciplinary approach in the assessment and management of clinical problems in this group of people who have extremely complex biological, psychological and social needs.

Many districts hold mental handicap registers which list young people with significant learning disability. It is probably better to have these registers than not, as they provide information on those people with specific needs permitting more appropriate support and assisting in service planning. On the other hand, such registers represent a potential conflict of interests between privacy and record keeping.

Surveillance and screening programmes

Optimum health is promoted by specific screening programmes for some conditions: it is recognized that Down syndrome is associated with an increased incidence of congenital heart disease, duodenal atresia, imperforate anus, thyroid disorders, Hirschsprung's disease, atlanto-axial instability and leukaemia. Care

is directed at detecting these conditions early in order to treat appropriately. There are no established recommendations for frequency of thyroid function screening and there are so many features common to both Down syndrome and hypothyroidism that the latter may not be obvious clinically. A high index of suspicion with regular thyroid function tests perhaps every 2 years until the age of 30 years and annually thereafter is one suggested approach.[2] Prospective studies are also in hand to define the natural history of thyroid function test results in children with Down syndrome of all ages in order to determine optimum screening times.[3] The incidence of Hirschsprung's disease in children with Down syndrome is not known but investigation is indicated when any Down syndrome child presents with severe constipation.[4,5]

Many questions have been asked about atlanto-axial instability which is thought to be present in about 15% of children with Down syndrome. In particular, what is its natural history and how useful are cervical spine radiographs in determining the risk of dislocation? Past views have swung from seeing radiographs as unhelpful[6] to a recommendation that they be obtained between 2 and 6 years[7,8] with a repeat at 8 years;[7] justification for screening has been the potential complications of atlanto-axial dislocation, the difficulty individuals have in verbalizing specific symptoms and the possible importance of knowing the cervical spine status prior to anaesthesia when increased neck manipulations may occur. However, only about 20 cases of atlanto-axial dislocation have been reported in world literature over the last 25 years[9] so the risk appears to have been overemphasized. In 1990, Roy concluded radiological screening was inappropriate[6,10] and in 1991, Selby that it was unreliable[11] as radiological findings are partly dependent on the positioning of the patient and fluctuating muscle tone. It is also clear that when upper cervical cord compression does occur, physical signs, particularly gait disturbance are evident early though the hypotonia, flat everted feet and broad based gait of many persons with Down syndrome may mask the true clinical picture for a time.

Surveillance and special screening programmes for learning impaired people whether with Down syndrome or any other disorder have to be set against the thrust by carers to normalize the lives of their charges. Programmes that may seem medically justifiable may not meet with the realization of other important ambitions of the individuals. Doctors need to think carefully about screening programmes considered worthwhile.

Conclusion

Severe mental handicap has a prevalence of three to four per thousand. It is usually associated with diagnosable cerebral disorder and precise diagnosis may permit a programme of prevention. Physical illness deserves special consideration and epilepsy is common and requires special judgement in prescribing medication. Psychiatric disorder is seen in about half the cases. The family are sorely burdened and may require specialist help.

References

1 Klüver, H., Bucy, P.C. Preliminary analysis of the functions of the temporal lobes in monkeys. *Arch Neurol Psychiatr* 1939; **42**: 979–1000.
2 Dinani, S., Carpenter, S. Down's syndrome and thyroid disorder. *J Mental Defic Res* 1990; **34**: 187–193.
3 Cutler, A.T., Benezra-Obeiter, R., Brink, S.J. Thyroid function in young children with Down syndrome. *Am J Dis Child* 1986; **140**: 479–483.
4 Leung, A.K., Seagram, G.F. Hirschsprung's disease and mongolism (letter). *J Natl Med Assoc* 1991; **83**: 660.
5 Leung, A.K., Mui, C.Y., Lau, S.J. Hirschsprung's disease and mongolism. *J Natl Med Assoc* 1986; **78**: 443–446.
6 Davidson, R.G. Atlanto-axial instability in Down syndrome: a fresh look at the evidence. *Pediatrics* 1988; **81**: 857–865.
7 Pueschel, S.M., Scola, F.H., Pezzullo, J.C. A longitudinal study of atlanto-dens relationships in asymptomatic individuals with Down syndrome. *Pediatrics* 1992; **89**: 1194–1198.
8 Msall, M.E., Reese, M.E., Digaudio, K., Griswold, K., Granger, C.V., Cooke, R.E. Symptomatic atlanto-axial instability associated with medical and rehabilitative procedures in children with Down syndrome. *Pediatrics* 1990; **85**: 447–449.
9 Chaudry, V., Sturgeon, C., Gates, A.J., Myers, G. Symptomatic atlanto-axial dislocation in Down's syndrome. *Ann Neurol* 1986; **21**: 606–609.
10 Roy, M., Baxter, M., Roy, A. Atlanto-axial instability in Down's syndrome – guidelines for screening and detection. *J Roy Soc Med* 1990; **83**: 433–435.
11 Selby, K., Newton, R.W., Gupta, S., Hunt, L. Clinical predictors and radiological reliability in atlanto-axial in Down's syndrome. *Arch Dis Child* 1991; **66**: 876–878.

10.7 Seizure disorders in children

Fritz Dreifuss

In managing epilepsy the major strategy is the elimination of seizures. Seizures are symptoms of cerebral disturbance and the most effective treatment is aimed at the underlying cause. However, the majority of cases of epilepsy have to be treated symptomatically and the mainstay of such treatment is the administration of anticonvulsant medications.

The need to eliminate seizures is based on the assumption that they are deleterious to the person. This can be directly by causing further neuronal impairment, or possibly through mechanisms of kindling with perpetuation of seizures; or it can be indirectly by causing physical, social, psychological, vocational and recreational impairment, thereby irreversibly altering the quality of life and ability to cope.

It is recognized that the degree of disruption to the person depends on the nature, severity, frequency and predictability of the seizures. Thus isolated nocturnal seizures, reflex epilepsy in response to reading and self-limiting benign rolandic seizures have a different implication in terms of disruption to recurrent status epilepticus, atonic drop attacks and episodes associated with prolonged periods of confusion. While this probably does not alter the underlying goals of management, it tends to modify the urgency and vigour of treatment in the context of the risk/benefit analysis of any treatment choice.

The prevention of potentially epileptogenic events is a concept of paramount importance. This includes the prevention of head injury and some central nervous system infections, better antenatal care and reduction of birth trauma, early and vigorous treatment of inflammatory illnesses and improved immunization rates. It may be that some epilepsies can be prevented by prophylactic administration of anticonvulsant medication after head injury or for recurrent febrile seizures.

Seizure control can usually be accomplished by appropriate anticonvulsant therapy (pharmacological and surgical) and by avoidance of precipitating factors. These include alcohol, sleep deprivation, certain sounds and other reflex precipitating stimuli, and in some individuals photic stimulation. Severe prolonged seizures cause neuronal changes, but at present there is no reliable pathological evidence that absence seizures or isolated short tonic-clonic seizures cause histological change. In the case of severe prolonged seizures energy requirements of the brain may be greater than can be met and relative anoxia, hypotension and acidosis may contribute to neuronal dissolution.[1] Even when glucose and oxygen are administered and paralysis of peripheral musculature is accomplished, experimental seizures may result in neuronal change indicating that even in the absence of overt convulsions the metabolic requirements of actively discharging neurones may be excessive. It would seem reasonable to suppose that all seizures are to a degree stressful and potentially deleterious to the maintenance of energy homeostasis in the nervous system. Prolonged and repeated epileptic seizures may result in secondary epileptogenesis with development of foci removed from the primary epileptogenic site[2] and clinical experience suggests that long-standing epilepsy becomes more intractable with time. Early treatment is thus prophylactic.

Epilepsy has psychosocial consequences which may be as disabling as the primary condition and also eminently preventable. Social, educational and vocational handicaps should not be allowed to develop or, if they have, to continue.[3]

Whether therapy is pharmacological or surgical, the major goal should be good control with minimal cerebral damage. Many surgical procedures have been developed for the treatment of epilepsy and these have included ablation of areas of the brain including superficial and deep focal lesions, the division of commisural tracts and the removal of expanding lesions both benign and malignant. Such procedures whilst they can arrest seizures may still be associated with significant surgical morbidity. Side effects of drugs may limit satisfactory seizure control and cause sedation if large doses are required. In a few cases, the cost of medication may be economically unviable, compromising compliance and potential seizure control.

Principles of treatment

1   A diagnosis must be established regarding the type of seizure. Where possible, aetiological factors should be identified and eliminated.
2   Specific treatment should be commenced which in most instances will be based on pharmacological principles.
3   Factors which influence the patient's quality of life as a result of epilepsy will need attention.

An accurate diagnosis is the single most important factor in choosing the best approach to patient management. Sophisticated and seizure-specific antiepileptic drugs have been developed, but to some extent they are all attended by side effects. This potential for side effects makes it particularly important to analyse the risk/benefit ratio before commencing medication, and highlights the need to choose the drug that is most efficacious for the patient's particular seizure type. At the same time, it is important to select a drug that meets the patient's other needs. For example, the woman who wants to become pregnant, the teenager who needs a convenient drug regimen with single daily dosage, and the patient with intercurrent illnesses that compromise metabolic pro-

cesses all have special requirements to which an anticonvulsant management programme must be specifically tailored.

Some syndromes presenting with seizures may not require medication because the seizures are relatively benign or because the medications used are potentially more harmful than the occasional seizures. This is the case with benign febrile convulsions and with occasional isolated seizures that occur many years apart. Epilepsy that is triggered by specific circumstances such as forms of musicogenic or other reflex epilepsy, and seizures that occur in response to specific medications such as phenothiazines, may be managed by avoidance of the triggering factors, even though the predisposition to seizures remains unchanged.

There also exists a large and increasingly recognized group of non-epileptic seizures. It is essential to differentiate these from epileptic seizures for several reasons. Non-epileptic seizures may result from underlying conditions that require specific therapy and without appropriate treatment may be life threatening. Patients whose seizures are incorrectly assumed to be epileptic may receive inappropriate medication which does not improve the symptoms and also produces side effects. In an effort to improve seizure control, the dosage of these drugs is frequently increased.

Differential diagnosis of recurrent episodes

Syncope

Episodes of syncope can be associated with convulsive activity caused by prolonged cerebral ischaemia. Syncope may result from autonomic or postural changes, or emotional states that affect peripheral vascular resistance. Other possible causes include decreased cardiac output from vasovagal slowing, diminished venous return, or direct cardiac causes such as arrhythmias or outflow obstruction.

If a careful history is taken, the differential diagnosis is usually not difficult. The patient with syncope frequently experiences premonitory symptoms, and observers usually report that the patient appears pale or ashen prior to loss of consciousness. Precipitating causes are frequently present, such as emotional trauma in simple fainting, prolonged standing, or in the case of outflow obstruction, physical effort on exertion.

If syncope is suspected, the patient should have a thorough cardiac evaluation, including a prolonged electrocardiogram to evaluate rhythm changes and possible abnormalities such as prolonged Q–T intervals which predispose to potentially fatal ventricular fibrillation.

Hyperventilation

Recurrent episodes of lightheadedness, paraesthesia, a feeling of constriction in the chest, tremulousness, abnormal postures of the hands and feet, and altered consciousness may result from prolonged hyperventilation of which the individual may be unaware. The symptoms can usually be reproduced by three minutes of vigorous overbreathing. This syndrome of hyperventilation occurs particularly during stress or in teenagers.

Benign paroxysmal vertigo

Benign paroxysmal vertigo occurs during the first 3 or 4 years of life.[4] The child appears frightened, frequently turns pale, and runs to the mother. If the child is sufficiently aware and verbal he or she will complain of feeling dizzy and is frequently sick. The electroencephalogram (EEG) is normal. Benign paroxysmal vertigo may be a variant of migraine, but abnormal vestibular function has been demonstrated.

Abdominal migraine

In most instances this is actually a migraine phenomenon. Although the usual manifestations of migraine are bright scotomata and unilateral headaches, early-onset childhood migraine may be characterized by nausea, vomiting, recurrent abdominal pain and confused behaviour. The clue to the nature of these episodes is their periodicity and their frequent occurrence in children with motion sickness.

The differential diagnosis can be difficult because the EEG may show unilateral centrotemporal spike activity like rolandic epilepsy, and benign childhood partial seizures frequently coexist with migraine.

Differential diagnosis also includes basilar artery migraine and occipital epilepsy of childhood as described by Gastaut.[5] Both conditions are associated with visual disturbances, hemianopia or even blindness, and may be followed by altered consciousness, confusion and occasional unilateral or bilateral hemiparesis of limited duration. In occipital epilepsy, spike and wave discharges occur in the occipital region when the eyes are closed.

Hemiplegic migraine, mitochondrial encephalopathy with lactic acidosis and cardiovascular accidents also have to be distinguished from partial epilepsy, particularly the HHE (hemiplegia, hemiatrophy and epilepsy) syndrome.

Pseudoseizures

In any practice which manages difficult epilepsy problems, pseudoseizures figure in the differential diagnosis. A useful tool to distingish between epileptic seizures and pseudoseizures is the closed-circuit television EEG (CCTV-EEG) during episodes (Fig. 10.12).[6]

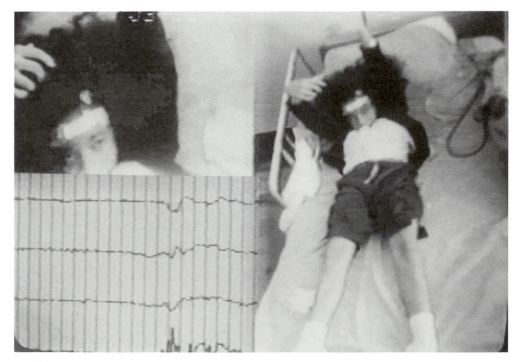

Figure 10.12 Frontal lobe tonic seizure with EEG suppression, arising during sleep; this could probably have been regarded as a pseudoseizure.

There are several important points to keep in mind in the diagnosis of pseudoseizures: a bizarre seizure is more likely to be epileptic than non-epileptic; epilepsy and pseudoseizures are not mutually exclusive and more often than not coexist in the same patient; the absence of EEG abnormalities in the scalp recording during a seizure does not necessarily exclude epilepsy because there may be no surface manifestation, or abnormalities may be obscured by artefact, and epileptic seizures may be triggered by severe emotional stress.

Other factors differentiating pseudoseizures from epilepsy are that they do not occur during sleep and usually not just before or after waking. Injuries, incontinence and postictal confusion are rare. Epileptic seizures usually respond at least partially to the administration of anticonvulsant drugs, whereas pseudoseizures do not. While bizarre seizure manifestations may occur with epilepsy, such behaviours as asynchronous independent thrashing of limbs, pelvic thrusting and forced eyelid closure usually do not.

Many pseudoseizures are mixed with true seizures in the same patient, the use of the label Munchausen's syndrome[7] reflects in this context pseudoseizures only. The practitioners of this syndrome present such plausible yet fictitious accounts of illness that even trained medical personnel may resort to heroic measures, including intubation and intravenous diazepam administration in their management.

A recent development is the recognition of Munchausen syndrome by proxy, which is a bizarre manifestation of child abuse.[8] An example is when a small child is brought to a paediatrician or neurologist for the management of what are described as intractable seizures. However, these are only ever observed by one of the parents (usually the mother) who commonly is quite solicitous and apparently well informed, and who allows the child to be subjected to extensive investigation and therapy. Over time the child is shown to have no seizure disorder.

Breathholding attacks

Recurrent episodes of breathholding may be confused with seizures. They usually begin between the ages of 6 months and 3 years and occur in response to pain or a temper tantrum. The child begins to cry, sometimes quite quietly, recurrent sobs can be detected by thoracic movement which becomes fixed in expiration, and the child may become cyanotic. At this stage there may be some convulsive movement, upward rolling of the eyes and afterwards the child may appear sleepy.

Gastro-oesophageal reflux

This condition, also known as Sandifer's syndrome, is seen in early infancy and is characterized by apnoea, frequently accompanied by laryngospasm and leading to cyanosis.[9] Gastro-oesophageal reflux in children is often associated with opisthotonus (extensor posturing) of the upper extremities. Because of its association with feeding and the frequent accompanying failure to thrive, a pH probe and swallowing studies are usually conducted. Feeding a child with this condition in the propped-up position is often beneficial.

Sleep disorders

Recurrent disturbances during sleep are important in the differential diagnosis of epilepsy. These include myoclonus, night terrors, sleep walking and narcolepsy.

Differentiating the epilepsies

Once it has been established that the patient suffers from epilepsy it is important to ascertain the type of seizure, the epileptic syndrome of which the seizure is a manifestation, and when possible the cause. Only then can the most appropriate therapeutic plan be developed.

Classification of seizure types ICES[10]

Ultimately, the decision to treat the epileptic patient with medication or surgery as well as the choice of antiepileptic drug will depend on identification of the type of seizures.

The international classification of epileptic seizures (ICES) (Table 10.7)[10] is based primarily on descriptions obtained from patients or witnesses to the seizure, together with interictal and where available ictal EEG recordings. Of all the diagnostic methods, a detailed history of the nature of the seizures is most important. Actual visualization and recording of the seizure are of such importance that special techniques have been developed, such as video (CCTV-EEG) or prolonged cassette recording in which the EEG is time-linked to clinical events.

Although in many instances the underlying mechanism of epilepsy cannot be determined, seizure types can usually be categorized as either partial or generalized.

Partial seizures

Partial seizures originate in a fairly discrete area of the brain and usually remain relatively localized for a sufficient period of time to allow identification of their focal nature. Partial seizures that subsequently involve both sides of the brain are called secondarily generalized seizures.

Partial seizures are referred to as simple when consciousness is preserved and complex when conscious-

Table 10.7 International classification of epileptic seizures (ICES)[10]

I *Partial seizures* (localization related)
A Simple partial seizures (consciousness not impaired)
  1 With motor symptoms
  2 With somatosensory or special sensory symptoms
  3 With autonomic symptoms
  4 With psychic symptoms
B Complex partial seizures (with impairment of consciousness)
  1 Beginning as simple partial seizures and progressing to impairment of consciousness
    a With no other features
    b With features as in A.1–4
    c With automatisms
  2 With impairment of consciousness at onset
    a With no other features
    b With features as in A.1–4
    c With automatisms
C Partial seizures with secondary generalization
  1 Simple partial seizures evolving to generalized
  2 Complex partial seizures evolving to generalized
  3 Simple partial seizures evolving to complex partial seizures evolving to generalized
II *Generalized seizures* (Bilaterally symmetrical and without local onset)
A 1 Absence seizures
  2 Atypical absence seizures
B Myclonic seizures
C Clonic seizures
D Tonic seizures
E Tonic-clonic seizures
F Atonic seizures
III *Unclassified epileptic seizures* (inadequate or incomplete data)

---

ness is impaired. Simple partial seizures emanate from the cerebral cortex and do not affect regions of the brain involved in the maintenance of consciousness. These regions are, however, involved in complex partial seizures, when they frequently become bilaterally disturbed.

Generalized seizures

Generalized seizures involve the brain bilaterally from the outset. The initial symptom is frequently loss of consciousness and the clinical manifestations include absence, myoclonus, tonic, clonic and tonic-clonic seizures.

Classification of epilepsies and epileptic syndromes ICE[11,12]

Seizure types are one component of an epileptic syndrome or form of epilepsy. Other factors to consider are aetiology, age of onset, precipitating factors, severity, chronicity, structural abnormalities of the brain, clinical course and frequency, and EEG phenomena.

The international classification of epileptic syndromes (ICE)[11,12] is summarized in Table 10.8. This goes further than the ICES by recognizing the clinical accompaniments of the seizure type. Thus there are localization related and generalized epilepsy syndromes reflecting the partial and generalized seizure types.

Further sub-classification taking in both seizure type and epileptic syndromes is into primary (idiopathic or genetically determined) epilepsy, secondary (symptomatic) epilepsy with a known cause and cryptogenic epilepsy (cause unknown though presumed symptomatic). The aetiology of the brain disorder causing the seizures is the most important factor influencing overall prognosis. Patients with primary epilepsy generally have a better prognosis than those with symptomatic disease.

Most of the epileptic syndromes appear during childhood.[13] Common examples include neonatal seizures, febrile seizures, infantile spasms, Lennox-Gastaut syndrome, petit mal epilepsy, juvenile myoclonic epilepsy, benign rolandic epilepsy, primary generalized epilepsy with generalized tonic-clonic seizures, temporal lobe epilepsy and progressive myoclonic epilepsy.

Using the ICE classification:

Localization-related epilepsies

These occur at any age and are mostly secondary (symptomatic) to focal brain disorders. However, they can also be primary (or idiopathic) as with benign rolandic epilepsy;[14] this usually ceases by puberty, its principal seizure type is partial, commonly beginning in the face, and the natural history and familial nature of this condition indicate that it is of primary origin. The seizures occur most often during sleep, have a simple partial onset and rarely generalize. A positive family history is often found. The EEG shows focal spike activity, classically centro-temporal.

Generalized epilepsies

These are characterized by absences, myoclonic and tonic-clonic (classic grand mal) seizures; onset is usually during childhood or adolescence, aetiology is most likely genetic and usually there is no other evidence of brain abnormality. Typical absence seizures occur in petit mal (or pyknoleptic) epilepsy; and juvenile myoclonic epilepsy; atypical absences occur in Lennox-Gastaut syndrome.

Classic petit mal or pyknolepsy[15] (now referred to as childhood absence epilepsy) and juvenile absence epilepsy are benign and usually cease in adolescence. The tendency to develop this type of epilepsy is inherited, probably as an autosomal dominant trait

Table 10.8 International classification of epilepsies, epileptic syndromes and related seizure disorders (ICE)[11,12]

---

1 Localization-related (focal, local, partial) epilepsies and epileptic syndromes
  1.1 *Idiopathic (with age-related onset) or primary*
       Benign childhood epilepsy with centrotemporal spikes (benign rolandic epilepsy BRE)
       Childhood epilepsy with occipital paroxysms
       Primary reading epilepsy
  1.2 *Symptomatic or secondary*
       Chronic progressive epilepsia partialis continua of childhood (Kojewnikow syndrome)
       Syndromes characterized by seizures with specific modes of precipitation (include:
          partial seizures following acquired lesions, usually involving tactile or proprioceptive
          stimuli; partial seizures precipitated by sudden arousal or startle epilepsy)
       Temporal lobe epilepsies
       Frontal lobe epilepsies
       Parietal lobe epilepsies
       Occipital lobe epilepsies
  1.3 *Cryptogenic* defined by seizure type, clinical features, aetiology, anatomical localization
2 Generalized epilepsies and syndromes
  2.1 *Idiopathic (with age-related onset) or primary*
       Benign neonatal familial convulsions
       Benign neonatal convulsions
       Benign myoclonic epilepsy in infancy
       Childhood absence epilepsy (pyknolepsy)
       Juvenile absence epilepsy
       Juvenile myoclonic epilepsy (impulsive petit mal[2])
       Epilepsy with grand mal seizures on waking (GTCS)
       Other generalized epilepsies (not defined above)
       Epilepsies with seizures precipitated by specific modes of activation
  2.2 *Cryptogenic or symptomatic*
       West syndrome (infantile spasms, Blitz–Nick–Salaam Krämpfe)
       Lennox–Gastaut syndrome
       Epilepsy with myoclonic-astatic seizures[3]
       Epilepsy with myoclonic absences
  2.3 *Symptomatic or secondary*
       Non-specific aetiology
          Early myoclonic encephalopathy
          Early infantile epileptic encephalopathy with suppression–burst EEG
          Other symptomatic generalized epilepsies not defined above
       Specific syndromes (including diseases in which seizures are a presenting or predominant
          feature)
3 Epilepsies and epileptic syndromes undetermined whether focal or generalized
  3.1 *With both generalized and focal seizures*
       Neonatal seizures
       Severe myoclonic epilepsy in infancy
       Epilepsy with continuous spike-waves during slow wave sleep
       Acquired epileptic aphasia (Landau–Kleffner syndrome)
       Other undetermined epilepsies not defined above
  3.2 *Without unequivocal generalized or focal features*
4 Special syndromes
       Situation-related seizures
       Febrile convulsions
       Isolated seizures or isolated status epilepticus
       Seizures occurring only when there is an acute metabolic or toxic event such as due to
          eclampsia, alcohol, drugs, non-ketotic hyperglycaemia

---

with age-dependent expression. Monozygotic twins are 85% concordant for the three-per-second EEG trait and 75% concordant for the seizures.[16]

In juvenile myoclonic epilepsy[17] both absence and tonic-clonic seizures may occur. They begin in late childhood or adolescence and absences are more prolonged than those seen in classic petit mal. Approximately one-third of patients have early morning myoclonic jerks; in some the jerks are repetitive and culminate in a clonic-tonic-clonic seizure and in others generalized clonic-tonic-clonic seizures are the chief manifestation. Treatment with sodium valproate is usually effective, but the tendency to seizures is permanent. In juvenile myoclonic epilepsy the ictal discharges may consist of polyspikes and polyspike-wave complexes with frequencies of 4 to 6 and 8 to 12 per second. Petit mal and juvenile myoclonic epilepsy overlap in both seizure type and age distribution.

Infantile spasms and Lennox-Gastaut syndrome are discussed together because they share several common features. Both are caused by diverse disorders that produce permanent brain damage, both occur in primary, secondary, and cryptogenic forms, and both previously were grouped among the myoclonic epilepsies of childhood. In some patients the disorder begins as infantile spasms that evolve to the Lennox-Gaustaut syndrome. The response to therapy and prognosis for both are better when the syndrome is cryptogenic than when secondary to a diagnosable brain disorder.

Infantile spasms can be either a seizure type or part of an epileptic syndrome. As the seizure type, they usually appear before 12 months and abate by 5 years of age. West syndrome is a combination of infantile spasms, EEG pattern of hypsarrhythmia and developmental arrest or regression.[18] Many patients with infantile spasms have other types of seizure before or concurrent with the spasms. In about half of the cases, the epilepsy persists after the spasms subside, sometimes taking the form of the Lennox-Gastaut syndrome. Early diagnosis and prompt initiation of therapy with ACTH improve the outlook.

Lennox-Gastaut syndrome is a severe form of epilepsy characterized by multiple seizure types, an EEG pattern of slow ($1\frac{1}{2}$ to $2\frac{1}{2}$ per second) spikes and waves with bursts of fast rhythms in sleep, and developmental arrest or regression. The seizure types include atonic or drop attack seizures, absence and atypical absence seizures and axial (contractions limited to the trunk) tonic seizures.[19]

Other secondary epileptic syndromes include disorders in which epilepsy is a prominent feature but which are associated with specific diseases such as lipidosis, ceroid lipofuscinosis, progressive myoclonic epilepsies of the Lafora and Baltic types and the mitochondrial encephalopathies. Also included here are the progressive epilepsies of early childhood engendered by other inborn areas of metabolism such as the amino acid disorders.

Special syndromes: febrile seizures[20]

Febrile seizures occur among children aged 3 months to 5 years who have a fever and no other aetiological evidence for a seizure disorder. These seizures occur in approximately 2 to 5% of children under 5 years in western countries, about one-third of whom have more than one. The younger the patient, the greater the chance of recurrence. A national cohort study based on nearly 15 000 children in the 1970 British birth survey showed that only 2.4% of children with febrile seizures go on to manifest epilepsy by age 7 years, and in the few who do there is little evidence that this has been caused by the febrile convulsions.[21] Two other large cohort studies in the USA reached remarkably similar conclusions.[22-24] The risk of later epilepsy may increase to 7% with follow up to age 25 years.[24] A recent study has shown an association between childhood febrile seizures and hippocampal sclerosis but is not able to clarify if this is a causal relationship[25]. While prophylactic treatment of febrile seizures with long-term anticonvulsant drugs may reduce the number of seizure recurrences, there is no evidence that anticonvulsant therapy reduces the risk of later epilepsy and there is evidence that the intermittent administration of rectal diazepam early in the course of a febrile illness may be the preferred method of seizure prophylaxis should this be deemed necessary.[26] Very prolonged seizures lasting much more than half an hour may be damaging.[27,28] Prolonged (greater than 15 minutes) convulsions should be prevented[29] and to this end parents may give rectal diazepam. Recently a joint working group of the Royal College of Physicians of London and the British Paediatric Association produced guidelines for managing febrile convulsions[30] but did not resolve whether rectal diazepam should be given as soon as a convulsion begins or only after 5 minutes.

Treatment considerations

The choice of the anticonvulsant drug will depend upon the nature of the underlying seizure (Table 10.9). In view of the fact that anti-epileptic drugs may cause neurological and other side effects the administration of multiple drugs given simultaneously increases these difficulties. In most instances monotherapy is effective in controlling seizures. Monotherapy should be used until the seizures are controlled, until adequate therapeutic anticonvulsant blood levels have been obtained or until toxicity precludes further increase in drug dosage. If single drug therapy is unsuccessful the administration of more than one drug may become necessary. Where appropriate, and possible, it is important to tailor the drug regimen to the convenience of a school day and to avoid a midday dose. Social, emotional, educational or vocational pressures may interfere with successful management. A multidisciplinary approach in a specialized epilepsy centre may be needed to achieve optimal seizure control. All changes in drugs should be made as gradually as possible with only one change at any one time. Whether to withdraw the initial drug and replace it with another drug or whether to lower the dose of the first and add a second are questions of judgement. Common errors in seizure management include inadequate determination of seizure type leading to the use of inappropriate therapy. Another

Table 10.9 Individual anticonvulsant drugs used for specific seizure types or syndromes

Neonatal seizures	The drug of choice is phenobarbitone with an initial dose of approximately 20 mg/kg and a maintenance dose of approximately 6 mg/kg with an aim to achieve blood levels at around 30 µg/ml. Depending on the nature of the underlying disease neonatal anticonvulsant drug therapy is a temporary measure
Recurrent febrile seizures	If prophylactic treatment is indicated, rectal administration of diazepam 0.25 mg/kg may be useful in a febrile illness. Long-term prophylactic anticonvulsants are rarely needed.
Infantile spasms	Cryptogenic infantile spasms (West syndrome) are treated with ACTH as soon as the diagnosis is made. Vigabatrin may be an alternative first line choice of treatment. Alternate day prednisolone has fewer side effects than ACTH. For other forms of severe infantile myoclonic encephalopathy, sodium valproate or benzodiazepines (clonazepam, clobazam) should be considered, but there is a relatively high risk of hepatic toxicity in severely ill patients in this age group with sodium valproate[31]
Lennox-Gastaut syndrome	There is no certain treatment for this condition. Recent evidence suggests lamotrigine may be very effective. Sodium valproate, benzodiazepines (clonazepam, clobazam), carbamazepine and all other anticonvulsant drugs have been used, most with little success. Occasionally, there is an increase in slow spike-wave discharges with carbamazepine. Felbamate has been used with some success in the USA.[32]
Benign simple partial seizures of childhood (Rolandic epilepsy)	Therapy can be withheld unless frequent seizures occur. Drugs of choice include carbamazepine, sodium valproate or phenytoin
Pyknoleptic (petit mal) epilepsy	Ethosuximide or sodium valproate are the drugs of choice. Ethosuximide is usually the first drug in patients who have absences alone but sodium valproate is the drug of first choice where other seizure types particularly generalized tonic-clonic seizures or myoclonic seizures complicate the clincial picture
Juvenile absence and juvenile myoclonic epilepsy	These are best treated with sodium valproate. Juvenile absence is frequently a concomitant of the juvenile myoclonic epilepsy syndrome
Epilepsies associated with simple partial seizures, complex partial seizures with or without secondarily generalized seizures of the tonic-clonic variety	The drugs of choice include carbamazepine, sodium valproate and phenytoin. Phenobarbitone is undesirable because of its effect on cognitive function. Differences in drug efficacy may be difficult to discern, but varying side effects between individuals may influence the long-term choice of anti-epileptic drug. Lamotrigine and vigabatrin and gabapentin are proving of considerable benefit though side effects with vigabatrin are sometimes unacceptable.
Reflex epilepsies in response to flashing lights, sounds, reading, warm water immersion, sudden movement	These respond well to sodium valproate, benzodiazepines, carbamazepine or phenytoin. Sodium valproate is usually preferred

area is impatience. Knowledge of pharmacokinetics indicates that an adequate steady state blood level may take several days or weeks to be obtained and frequent changes in drugs or the addition of more drugs is not required until after an adequate trial of the primary agent. Intercurrent events such as an illness may alter anticonvulsant drug metabolism and require blood level monitoring with appropriate changes in dosage.

New anti-epileptic drugs are under study and are being developed with the rationale revealed by basic research on neurotransmitter pharmacology. Recent additions are lamotrigine, vigabatrin and gabapentin. Lamotrigine is thought to stabilize neuronal membranes by inhibiting the release of glutamate, the excitatory neurotransmitter that plays a key role in the generation of epileptic seizures. Lamotrigine appears to be particularly effective where the interictal EEG shows a generalized spike and wave abnormality, and in the generalized epilepsies particularly atypical absences. The mode of action of vigabatrin is predominantly that of gamma aminobutyricacid (GABA) enhancement by blocking the GABA-degradative enzyme, GABA-transaminase. GABA is an inhibitory neurotransmitter which is thought to help limit seizure activity. Vigabatrin is particularly useful in complex partial seizures, as also is gabapentin. To date lamotrigine, vigabatrin and gabapentin have been mainly used as add-on therapy to existing anti-epileptic drugs. Other drugs under development include felbamate and various excitatory neurotransmitter antagonists and agents, such as flunarizine, which block calcium channels.

Other anti-epileptic drugs in the management of intractable disorders include bromides, ethotoin, methsuximide, chlormethiazole and paraldehyde.

The ketogenic diet may occasionally be useful in the Lennox-Gastaut syndrome.

In every individual treatment plan many factors must be considered in the patient's overall management which consists of much more than the administration of medication and the evaluation of drug levels.[33] The participation of social workers, educational consultants and vocational rehabilitation counsellors add to the quality of life and may influence the degree of seizure control. In every instance a professional in the community familiar with all professional and voluntary resources upon which the person with epilepsy can draw should be a member of the treatment team.

areas of normal activities that has in the past been a greater disadvantage to the existence of the person with epilepsy than has the epilepsy itself. The more the pity that this has to a large degree been an avoidable cause of misery.

Epilepsy education should form part of every treatment programme and should be directed at all levels with which a person with epilepsy is likely to come in contact – from family to school, to departments concerned with public safety, and the public in general. Professional education aimed at school nurses, medical students, paediatricians and family practitioners should be undertaken.

Restrictions on persons with epilepsy

There is a major temptation to shield children with epilepsy from potential harm. Protectiveness however very easily yields to over-protectiveness, to the extent that the person is deprived of those exploratory activities which are necessary for the attainment of independence and confidence. No one can ever be completely guarded against harm by being deprived of the dignity of risk. Some restrictions are necessary. These include the operation of a motor vehicle until a certain seizure-free interval has occurred in response to medical treatment. No one with a history of seizures should operate an aircraft or a commercial passenger vehicle. Persons with epilepsy should not bath in a house by themselves as drowning is not uncommon under these circumstances, particularly as immersion in warm water is sometimes a triggering factor for seizures. Supervised sports including swimming are usually not contraindicated. Common sense indicates that in the case of absence seizures precipitated by hyperventilation, the playing of wind instruments in the school band should probably be avoided in favour of percussion instruments. Sports in which head injury is a frequent consequence are not favoured. One might oppose boxing for anyone, not only for persons with epilepsy, as its very essence is an attempt to cause a head injury. The question as to whether the person should play football is not resolved. Probably most persons with epilepsy whose seizures are well controlled can play football but if the seizures are a consequence of head injury, this sport should also be restricted. Occupational restrictions include the operation of unguarded machinery and moving equipment. Some exceptions may be made if seizures are well controlled or if seizures always occur during sleep. In general, many of the restrictions placed on the employment of persons with epilepsy and participation in competitive activities have been unnecessarily broad. To some extent the situation is being redressed by provisions in legislation relative to the employment of the handicapped. It is the exclusion from large

Duration of therapy

There are no hard and fast rules as to duration of therapy after seizures are controlled. In pyknoleptic petit mal and benign rolandic epilepsy, conditions which have a natural history of going into abeyance during adolescence, discontinuation of medication after a 1–2 year seizure-free period is reasonable.[34] Seizures which have as their basis an underlying structural lesion are more likely to continue indefinitely though even here, with maturation of the brain, the tendency becomes less with age, and efforts to discontinue medication should be considered after a 4-year seizure-free interval.[35] Each patient should be individualized. For example, if the patient is a child, reduction and cessation of medication is tried with more confidence than if the patient is a teenager about to apply for a driver's licence, to start dating, or to live away from home. The patient should participate in the decision and be told the potential risks of discontinuing medication and these depend on the syndrome involved. If the patient is a woman desiring pregnancy, early discontinuation of medication before a lengthy seizure-free period has elapsed may be a smaller risk to take than that of potential teratogenicity to a fetus from an anticonvulsant drug.

Some syndromes carry a high rsk of continuation of seizures. These include epilepsies with focal neurological abnormality, mental retardation, an abnormal interictal EEG background and a strong family history of continued seizures. An example is juvenile myoclonic epilepsy which often recurs after medication is discontinued.

The situation regarding driving is confused by the autonomy of various jurisdictions around the world and even within a country, such as the USA, where driving prohibitions vary from 3 months to 2 years after the last seizure, where reporting of seizures may or may not be mandatory and where the physician may or may not be immune from actions generated after his opinion has been given in good faith. In the UK, the regulations concerning driving and epilepsy were revised in 1994. These allow persons with a history of epilepsy to apply for a driving licence if they have been seizure free for one year, or in the case of attacks occurring in sleep, if such attacks have been confined to sleep over the previous 3 or more years. There is no distinction made between different types or causes of epilepsy or between those persons on or off medication.

References

1 Meldrum, B.S. Metabolic factors during prolonged seizures and their relation to nerve cell death. In: Delgado-Escueta, A.V., Wasterlain, C.G., Treiman, D.M., Porter, R.J., eds. *Advances in Neurology*, 34. New York: Raven Press, 1983.

2 Morrell, F. Secondary epilepsy in man. *Arch Neurol* 1985; **42**: 318–335.

3 Dreifuss, F.E. *Paediatric Epileptology: Classification and Management of Seizures in the Child*. Boston: John Wright PSG Inc, 1983: 265–276.

4 Basser, L.S. Benign paroxysmal vertigo of childhood: a variety of vestibular neuronitis. *Brain* 1964; **87**: 141–152.

5 Gastaut, H. A new type of epilepsy: benign partial epilepsy of childhood with occipital spike-waves. In: Akimoto, H., Kazamatsuri, H., Seino, M., Ward, A.A., eds. *Advances in Epileptology*, Proc. of XIIIth international congress of the ILAE. New York: Raven Press, 1982: 18–25.

6 Holmes, G.L., Sackellares, J.C., McKiernan, J., *et al*. Evaluation of childhood pseudoseizures using EEG telemetry and video-tape monitoring. *J Pediatr* 1980; **97**: 554–558.

7 Asher, R. Munchausen syndrome. *Lancet* 1951; **i**: 339–341.

8 Meadow, R. Munchausen syndrome by proxy: the hinterland of child abuse. *Lancet* 1977; **ii**: 343–345.

9 Kinsbourne, M. Hiatus hernia with contortion of the neck. *Lancet* 1964; **i**: 1058.

10 Commission on Classification and Terminology of the International League against Epilepsy. Proposal for revised clinical and electroencephalographic classification of epileptic seizures. *Epilepsia* 1981; **22**: 489–501.

11 Commission on Classification and Terminology of the International League against Epilepsy. Proposal for classification of epilepsies and epileptic syndromes. *Epilepsia* 1985; **26**: 268–278.

12 Commission on Classification and Terminology of the International League against Epilepsy. Proposal for revised classification of epilepsies and epileptic syndromes. *Epilepsia* 1989; **30**: 389–399.

13 Roger, J., Dravet, C., Bureau, M., Dreifuss, F.E., Wolf, P., eds. Epileptic syndromes. In: *Infancy, Childhood and Adolescence*. London: John Libbey, Eurotext, 1985.

14 Beaussart, M. Benign epilepsy of children with rolandic (centro-temporal) paroxysmal foci. *Epilepsia* 1972; **13**: 795–811.

15 Drury, I., Dreifuss, F.E. Pyknoleptic petit mal. *Acta Neurol Scand* 1985; **72**: 353–362.

16 Metrakos, J.D., Metrakos, K. Genetics of convulsive disorders: part II, genetic and electroencephalographic studies in centrencephalic epilepsy. *Neurology* 1961; **11**: 464–483.

17 Janz, D., Christian, W. Impulsiv-petit mal. *Dtsch Z Nervenheilkd* 1957; **176**: 3246.

18 Jeavons, P.M., Bower, B.D. Infantile spasms: a review of the literature and a study of 112 cases. Clinics in Developmental Medicine No 15. London: Spastics Society and Heinemann, 1964.

19 Gastaut, H., Roger, J., Soulayrol, R., *et al*. Childhood epileptic encephalopathy with diffuse slow spike-waves (otherwise known as 'petit mal variant') or Lennox syndrome. *Epilepsia* 1966; **7**: 139–179.

20 Nelson, K.B., Ellenberg, J.H. *Febrile Seizures*. New York: Raven Press, 1981.

21 Verity, C.M., Golding, J. Risk of epilepsy after febrile convulsions: a national cohort study. *Br Med J* 1991; **303**: 1373–1376.

22 Nelson, K.B., Ellenberg, J.H. Predictors of epilepsy in children who have experienced febrile seizures. *New Eng J Med* 1976; **295**: 1029–1033.

23 Nelson, K.B., Ellenberg, J.H. Prognosis in children with febrile seizures. *Pediatrics* 1978; **61**: 720–727.

24 Annegers, J.F., Hauser, W.A., Shirts, S.B., Kurland, L.T. Factors prognostic of unprovoked seizures after febrile convulsions. *New Eng J Med* 1987; **316**: 493–498.

25 Kuks, J.B.M., Cook, M.J., Fish, D.R., Stevens, J.M., Shorvon, S.D. Hippocampal sclerosis in epilepsy and childhood febrile seizures. *Lancet* 1993; **342**: 1391–1394.

26 Knudsen, F.U. Intermittent diazepam prophylaxis in febrile convulsions. *Acta Neurol Scand* 1991; **83**: 1–24, Suppl 135.

27 Meldrum, B.S. Secondary pathology of febrile and experimental convulsions. In: Brazier, M.A.B., Coceani, F., eds. *Brain Dysfunction in Infantile Febrile Convulsions*. New York: Raven, 1976: 213–222.

28 Vannucci, R.C. Metabolic and pathological consequences of experimental febrile seizures and status epilepticus. In: Nelson, K.B., Ellenberg, J.H., eds. *Febrile Seizures*. New York: Raven, 1981: 43–57.

29 Wallace, S.J. *The Child with Febrile Seizures*. London: John Wright, 1988: 81, 126.

30 Joint Working Group of the Research Unit of the Royal College of Physicians of London and the British Paediatric Association. Guidelines for the management of convulsions with fever. *Br Med J* 1991; **303**: 634–636.

31 Dreifuss, F.E., Santilli, N., Langer, D.H., *et al*. Valproic acid hepatic fatalities: a retrospective review. *Neurology* 1987; **37**: 379–385.

32 Ritter, F. *et al*. Felbamate in the treatment of Lennox-Gastaut Syndrome. *New Eng J Med* 1993; **328**: 29–33.

33 Penry, J.K. *Epilepsy, Diagnosis, Management, Quality of Life*. New York: Raven Press, 1986.

34 Sato, S., Dreifuss, F.E., Penry, J.K. Long term follow-up of absence seizures. *Neurology* 1983; **33**: 1590–1595.

35 Dean, C.J., Penry, J.K. Discontinuation of anti-epileptic drugs. In: Levy, R.H., Dreifuss, F.E., Mattson, R.H., Meldrum, B.S., Penry, J.K., eds. *Antiepileptic Drugs* 3rd edn. New York: Raven Press, 1989: 133–142.

10.8 The transition to adulthood

Andrew Thomas

The provision of services for young people with physical disabilities in Britain has been described as being the 'worst in Europe'.[1] This is principally because there are major gaps in the support services for young people with physical disabilities that occur after the statutory school-leaving age of 16 years.[2–4]

Around this age, all young people may begin to encounter major changes that affect the delivery of a wide range of services. The organization and delivery of health care, for example, is subject to change, with a movement from paediatric to adult-orientated services. This is also a time at which changes in education are likely to occur; young people may experience a move from school to further education, employment, training, or day care. Moving away from the family home also tends to become an issue around this time, with additional options for people with disabilities ranging from independent living to sheltered accommodation and residential care. The age of 16 years also marks the point at which young people become financially independent and entitled to claim state benefits in their own right.

The need for specialist advice and help for people with disabilities is crucial at this time. However, despite the need for support during the transition to adulthood a recent review of the literature indicates that young people with physical disabilities continue to lack the necessary health and support services.[4]

This section considers the difficulties faced by young people with physical disabilities as they move from being a teenager to a young adult. The section is divided into two parts: the first considers the needs of young people with physical disabilities and the difficulties they face in meeting these needs through the statutory services; the second part discusses the role of the clinician in organizing and providing appropriate services.

The needs of people with physical disabilities

The research literature indicates that young people with physical disabilities have wide ranging needs.[3–5] These are summarized in Table 10.10.

A distinction is drawn here between three classes of needs: the need for personal autonomy, service needs, and social needs. This distinction is made because the

Table 10.10 The needs of young people with physical disabilities

Personal autonomy
Awareness
  information about entitlement to services
Choice
  advice
Accessibility
  transport
  physical access

Service needs
Health care
  general health
  specialist health, such as bowel and bladder; skeletal; sensory; epilepsy
  speech therapy
  physiotherapy
  occupational therapy
  psychological and psychiatric services
  dental care
Health education
  dealing with incontinence and pressure sores
  sex education
  contraceptive advice
  genetic counselling
Training and education
  basic education such as reading, writing, etc.
  further education such as exam-based courses
  assessment
  rehabilitation
  training for independence
Employment
  employment training
  open employment
  sheltered employment
  adaptations to the work environment and the nature of work
Housing
  independent living or sheltered housing
  adapted housing
Financial support
  benefits
  grants for aids and equipment

Social needs
Relationships
  friendships
  sexual relationships
  social skills
Recreation
  hobbies and pastimes
  outdoor pursuits

range of services currently available is often viewed as being provided by professionals who view their clients' needs from the perspective of a service provider. The effect is to view all people with physical disabilities as a homogeneous group for whom the same services are thought to apply. However, it is clear that in the same way that able-bodied people have a range of differing needs, so too do people with disabilities. To many, personal autonomy – the ability to be an individual – and choice are often seen as being denied by the services that are currently available.

Personal autonomy

In recent years there has been a considerable shift in attitude towards people with disabilities. At one time considered the passive recipients of services, people with disabilities are now steadily demanding a greater say in the way in which services are organized and delivered.[6,7] Indeed, for people with disabilities to function in society on equal terms with able-bodied people it is essential that they are allowed their independence and personal autonomy. The notion of independence is often construed (incorrectly) as meaning the ability to do things physically alone.[8] However, for some people with severe disabilities this is clearly inappropriate. The two key issues that arise are, first, that people with disabilities are able to make independent decisions for themselves, and secondly, having made a decision there need to be services available that enable those decisions to be acted upon. Yet, the majority of services continue to pay only lip-service to this issue. In order to bring about a change in emphasis and move away from treating people with disabilities as passive recipients, the organization and delivery of services must reflect three basic principles: awareness of entitlement, choice, and accessibility.

First, people should be aware of the services to which they are entitled. One of the major problems that arises is a lack of awareness of the services and facilities that are available. Cash benefits are a typical example. The DHSS[9] has estimated that in 1979 only two-thirds of those eligible were receiving the supplementary benefit (now income support) to which they were entitled. More recently Cooke et al.[10] found that of a sample of nearly 400 children with disabilities, the take up of attendance allowance* was between only one-half and two-thirds of those eligible, and one in five families were not claiming the mobility allowance* to which they were entitled.

Second, a prerequisite to independent thought and action is the need for choice. This may be a choice between a range of service options, or the choice to accept or reject any service offered. People with disabilities are rarely offered a range of choices; where

* Now subsumed with disability living allowance (DLA).

there are choices to be made these are often made by other people such as parents, key workers, or the service providers themselves.[5]

Third, there is the need for accessible services. Too often people with physical disabilities are excluded from services or facilities either because they are unable to travel to them, or because buildings have been designed without sufficient thought to their accessibility. People with mobility difficulties may wish to use certain facilities but the only way to get there for them can be by taxi – an expensive option for most people, but particularly for this group of people who are more likely to be living solely on state benefits. Equally, many people with disabilities are excluded from taking part in a range of activities – employment, training, recreation – because the buildings are inaccessible. Narrow doors, stairs, a lack of ramps and a paucity of lifts make access into, and movement around, a building particularly difficult, if not impossible, for people with restricted mobility or who use a wheelchair.[4,5,11]

The degree to which a person with disabilities is aware of, and has access to, services and facilities determines the extent to which that person can live as an independent individual in society. In the UK, the idea that people with disabilities may wish to take charge of their lives and be active members of society has been slow to gain ground. It is essential, however, that in order to enable people with disabilities to participate fully in society they must be involved in the design of their environment – living accommodation, shops, employment, recreational facilities, transport – as well as the design of services to meet their needs.

Service needs

Health care

A major problem that arises in the provision of health care for young people is the lack of coordinated health service contact after leaving school. For example, in a survey of 18–21 year olds with severe disabilities carried out by Hirst,[3] of those who had regularly seen a physiotherapist, speech therapist, psychologist, dentist or doctor at school, 81%, 79%, 92%, 50% and 70%, respectively, no longer did so. It may be argued that such levels of contact are simply a reflection of a minimal need for health care. A study by Thomas et al.[4] would appear to contradict this; 89% of a sample of 112 young adults with physical disabilities had health problems requiring regular medical attention, yet only 28% received regular hospital treatment and only 20% regularly consulted their general practitioner. In addition, young adults with multiple impairments often have the greatest health needs (particularly where there are both physical disabilities and mental impairments) yet are the least likely to have regular medical consultations after leaving school.[12]

Few studies have documented the health needs of young people with physical disabilities in any detail but recent research has shown that there are a number of areas of medical concern. For example, a clinical survey[4] in which 60% of the sample had either cerebral palsy or spina bifida, found a wide range of health-related problems requiring regular medical attention: overweight and obesity (20%; particularly for people with a diagnosis of spina bifida, 44%); cardiac problems (19%; rising to 45% for people with spina bifida); respiratory problems (17%); incontinence of bowel (54%) and bladder (56%); skeletal problems including kyphoscoliosis (18%; 44% for people with spina bifida), joint contractures of the legs (59%), foot deformation (26%) and restricted hand movements (64%); and 34% of the sample of young people had problems with skin care. The link between bowel and bladder incontinence and skin care problems was considerable, the likelihood of such problems increasing twofold in the presence of incontinence; again, this was primarily associated with the spina bifida group. Other problems identified included problems of visual acuity (26%) together with abnormal eye movements, either squints or nystagmus (18%); hearing problems (21%); communication problems, including athetosis and dysarthria (47%). Just under one-third of the sample were found to be epileptic. Most of these young people were using anticonvulsant drugs for the control of epilepsy, yet for many a specialist review of their medication had not been carried out for some years.

Such findings, reflected in other studies[13–15] indicate a wide range of health problems that are often very severe. Many of these are adequately dealt with while the person is still at school; the difficulty arises when they leave. The health care provided during the school years, in many instances, is not continued into the adult years. As a consequence many young people with physical disabilities have deteriorating health conditions that remain untreated, or are treated on an irregular or ad hoc basis.

The same problem of continuity of care arises in the provision of speech therapy, physiotherapy and dental services.[3,16] Thomas et al.[4] report that 'over four-fifths of the young people examined by the doctors had difficulties with walking. For the majority of these, regular physiotherapy would have been beneficial by ensuring greater mobility . . . only 33% saw a physiotherapist on a regular basis.' Similarly, 'the provision of speech therapy was also seen to have declined sharply after leaving school . . . the mismatch between the need for speech therapy and its provision was particularly marked . . . overall, only 26% of young people requiring speech therapy were receiving it.'

Psychological problems may also be prevalent in this client group. For example, the Ontario Child Health Study[17] found that in an epidemiological survey of 3294 4–16 year olds, chronic illness and physical disability were associated with a threefold risk of psychological disorders, compared with children and young adults with no such problems; they were also five times more likely to have problems of social adjustment, defined as isolation, low social participation and low social competence. Similarly, a study of 15–19 year olds with cerebral palsy or spina bifida also demonstrated an association between psychological adjustment and the severity of the disability, people with moderate or severe disabilities being the most likely to have psychological problems (boys 45%, girls 48%).[18] While girls in this study were found to exhibit more marked psychological problems than boys, in particular anxiety and depression, the boys were more likely to show antisocial behaviours. In this context, a study by Tew and Laurence[19] is of particular interest. They have suggested that the presence of a disabled child in a household may have a detrimental effect on the rest of the family; they recorded a fourfold increase in maladjustment among siblings of children with spina bifida. However, despite these elevated rates of psychological problems little use appears to be made of the psychological services by this client group. Thomas et al.,[4] for example, report that while 35% of their study group had behaviour problems and 70% displayed problems of a more social nature, only 2% were receiving the services of a counsellor or a psychologist to help them with these problems. In all cases this help was paid for privately rather than being provided through the National Health Service.

Health education

All young people, whether able-bodied or disabled, should have a good knowledge of their bodily functions, common illnesses and the physical changes that occur with puberty, as well as an awareness of the importance of personal hygiene, the need for regular exercise and a good diet. Equally, it is important that people with disabilities should have an understanding of the nature of their disability, together with its physical consequences and implications for the future. It is clear from the available research evidence that this is a much neglected area, yet one that is of considerable importance in the maintenance of good health. Typical areas to be addressed are the importance of maintaining an adequate and stable weight, the causes and consequences of pressure sores, the susceptibility of anaesthetic areas of the body to accidental damage in spina bifida, paraplegia etc, and the need for regular maintenance therapy through exercise routines and home physiotherapy as a way of promoting and maintaining increased physical independence.

Sex education and genetic advice tend to be handled very poorly for people with physical disabilities. While there is comparatively little known about the sexual knowledge of teenagers with physical disabilities, some research suggests that their sexual knowledge can be very poor. Dorner's study[20] of 18–19 year olds with spina bifida, for example, indicated that only 45% knew how children were conceived. In an earlier study,[21] Dorner found that, in common with able-bodied people, people with disabilities tend to worry a great deal about their sexuality. For people with physical disabilities those worries are often of a more fundamental and practical nature. Teenage girls, for example, tend to be particularly worried about their ability to conceive, boys about their potency. There are also frequent worries expressed about their ability to maintain sexual relationships as well as the practicalities of making love where there are problems of restricted mobility, paralysis, or incontinence.

The risk of passing on a disability to one's children is also a topic of great concern to many teenagers with physical disabilities.[18,20] In Thomas et al.'s study,[4] while 88% of the study sample had received some form of sex education, it was said to be geared to the needs of people with disabilities in only 10% of instances; overall two-thirds felt that their sex education had been inadequate because it had not addressed their special needs. Similarly, while many of the disabling conditions seen in this study did not have a genetic risk, over three-quarters of the sample did not know whether their disability was hereditary and expressed considerable worries to the research team about their future prospects for starting a family.

Education, training and employment

There is now considerable evidence to suggest that few people with physical disabilities will have reached their full potential by the statutory school-leaving age of 16.[11,22,23] This occurs for a variety of reasons including interruptions to schooling through ill health and admission to hospital and educational programmes whose focus has been on learning independence skills rather than the more usual range of school subjects leading to academic qualifications. This means that people with physical disabilities generally have fewer academic qualifications than their able-bodied counterparts,[24] with considerable repercussions for the educational and employment prospects of this group of young adults.

Typically, young people with physical disabilities have difficulties in obtaining education after the age of 16 years, including tertiary education.[25] They find it difficult to obtain places on further education and degree courses because their frequently interrupted schooling does not provide them with sufficient academic qualifications; very few tertiary institutes provide the physical requisites in the form of acceptable access and building adaptations for people with physical and locomotion difficulties; and careers advice to this group of people is generally felt to be

inadequate.[25] This is compounded by the lack of support available: Stowell's survey[26] of the provision for students with special needs in further and higher education found that only 38% of courses provided support for students with physical difficulties, and only 21% provided support for people with learning difficulties. Almost half had inadequate access arrangements into buildings and 60% stated that they might have to deny a place on a course to a student with a physical disability because of problems of access or because of the absence of the necessary support services.

In general, the employment prospects for school leavers with disabilities are also worse than their able-bodied counterparts. In a major study for the Warnock Committee, Walker[27] found that people with disabilities were less likely to be in paid employment and experience more periods of unemployment than able-bodied people; when in work they were also less likely to be in skilled and professional work, and experienced worse working conditions. The financial remuneration of people with disabilities also tends to be lower than the national average.[28]

The alternative to open employment for many young people with disabilities is sheltered employment: this may either be in the form of a workshop environment (e.g. Remploy or similar workshops run by local authorities or charitable bodies) or a sheltered placement with an ordinary commercial employer. While attitudes to these options are very mixed, sheltered employment opportunities are also very scarce. Head and Griffiths,[29] in their London study, considered sheltered employment to be a 'virtually non-existent option', with only one in 50 physically disabled school leavers finding such a placement.

A major difficulty in the employment of people with disabilities, particularly for those who have a physical or locomotor disability is that work environments are rarely suitable for this group of people. Narrow doors, stairs, the absence of ramps and lifts all contribute to the difficulties a person with a disability may encounter in being able to find and maintain work. Financial grants are available through the employment service to enable employers to adapt both the physical environment as well as any machinery or equipment that is used by the individual. Both employers and people with disabilities, however, tend to have little awareness of the adaptation grants that are available.

Housing

Moving away from the family often becomes a priority in the teenage years. This applies to able-bodied people and people with disabilities alike. While the cost of renting or buying a property is a universal problem for young people, in the latter case there are additional problems that need to be overcome.

These include problems of access and the need for ramps into the building; difficulties with stairs, and facilities such as kitchens and bathrooms that may be adequate for able-bodied people but pose serious problems for people with mobility problems or who use a wheelchair.

Housing adaptations play a major part in the provision of housing for people with disabilities and are often preferred to specialist housing designed for people with disabilities. Adaptations are available through local authority social services departments. However, it is apparent that very few homes have been properly adapted to meet the needs of a young adult with a physical disability:[4] many adaptations are of poor quality and in many instances quite inappropriate for the type of disability. A number of studies have now shown that housing adaptations can be extremely successful, particularly where the person with a disability is involved in the design. However, two major complaints about housing adaptations continually occur – errors in the design of the adaptation, and the length of time taken to provide them.

Financial aspects of disablement

People with disabilities and their families are likely to be financially disadvantaged as a consequence of their disability. There are two main contributory factors: increased family expenditure and reduced family income.[30,31] Increased expenditure is likely to occur through increased wear and tear on clothes and shoes, the cost of transport and incontinence aids, increased laundry, extra heating and housing adaptations. Reduced family income is likely to occur because many young people with disabilities are unable to find work; those that do find work tend to earn substantially less than able-bodied people.

It is essential, therefore, that this group of people claim the cash benefits to which they are entitled. Yet, for this group of people, the take up of benefits is often low. Hirst,[3] for example, found that only 28% of his sample of 17–21 year olds were receiving the maximum amount in benefits to which they were entitled. While there is a large range of pamphlets and information leaflets available for people with disabilities, research work with the elderly has suggested that most have never seen any of them. In general, the worst informed tend to be those seen regularly by social workers, district nurses, health visitors, home helps and general practitioners.[32] In part this may be because these professionals do not see it as their role to provide such information. Alternatively, they may feel that someone else is dealing with the problem. It is clear, however, that any agency that has regular contact with a person with a disability could play a major role in identifying an outstanding need and ensuring that this need is met by referring the individual to the relevant agency.

The social consequences of physical disability

Relationships

Adolescence is generally considered to be a time of increased social activity and rapid expansion of a teenager's social circle, yet many young people with physical disabilities grow up in a socially impoverished environment. Due to restricted access and mobility, and, in some cases, the lowered expectations of others, teenagers with physical disabilities are given little social preparation for adult life.[18,33] While adolescents with disabilities share the same desires as other young people to develop personal independence, experience a rewarding social life and explore their developing sexuality, they are often without the opportunity to satisfy these desires. Even in late adolescence many teenagers with a physical disability are heavily dependent on parents and other adults for even the most basic of activities of daily living. While a degree of physical dependence may be inevitable, there is no reason why independence of spirit should not be fostered by encouraging teenagers with disabilities to make choices and decisions for themselves. However, problems relating to the way a young person interacts with society are still likely to occur. As Younghusband et al.[34] have pointed out, 'there is a surprising failure to recognize the acute problem of isolation from their peers which confronts many of the more seriously disabled young adults, with the consequence that many experience difficulties in social relationships'.

It is likely that the social problems associated with congenital physical disabilities begin early in a young person's life. For example, Clarke et al.[35] in their work for the Warnock Committee on Special Education found that the social relationships of children with disabilities were frequently impaired. Such children were less likely to communicate with others, more likely to play alone, to engage in passive activities such as listening to, or watching, others, and to have one-way rather than two-way speech patterns. There is also growing evidence that both children and adolescents with physical disabilities are more likely to have difficulties with skilled social behaviour and coping with social situations.[36,37]

The consequences of poor social skills can be substantial and mean, in many cases, that young people with disabilities have difficulties in forming friendships and relationships. For example, 46% of the people with disabilities in Anderson et al.'s study[18] said that they did not have a special friend, yet this was true for only 21% of the able-bodied group. Similarly, of the 76 16 to 27 year olds with either spina bifida or cerebral palsy in Castree and Walker's 1981 study,[13] only 15 had a boy or girl friend. Close friendships, living together and marriage are also less likely for a person with a physical disability.[38,39]

Recreation

Becoming socially isolated from able-bodied society may also become a problem for many teenagers with a disability. Studies by both Dorner,[20,21,40] and Rowe[41] have indicated very high levels of social isolation. For example, in Dorner's 1975 study of 59 13 to 19 year olds with spina bifida, 31 (53%) had had no social or recreational contact with a friend of a similar age for at least a month prior to the interview.[40] An indication of just how restricted a young person's social life can be is provided by Anderson *et al.*[17] Based on the frequency of their social contacts (self- and parental reports), the person's social life was rated as satisfactory, limited, or very restricted. 49% of the able-bodied group were considered to be leading satisfactory social lives, compared to only 21% of those with disabilities. Only 6% of the able-bodied group had limited or very restricted social lives, as against 29% of those with disabilities. These levels of social isolation are borne out in the findings of Thomas *et al.*:[4] young adults with disabilities were almost twice as likely to have indoor hobbies such as watching TV, playing records, etc rather than going out of the home for entertainment and recreation. Levels of recreational activity and the severity of disability were related: the more severe the disability the less likely they were to engage in any recreational activities, particularly activities that took them out of the family home.

Overview

For a young person with a physical disability, the transition to adulthood can be particularly problematic. A range of difficulties are likely to arise: health care, further education, employment, housing, finance, relationships and recreation. There are three main reasons why such problems are likely to occur. First, many teenagers with physical disabilities compete on unequal terms with able-bodied people. They are likely to be less well qualified, less likely to be in work, more likely to find semi-skilled or unskilled jobs, more likely to be poorly paid, and are also more likely to be socially isolated from their able-bodied peers. Second, this group of people are likely to find travel to, and access into, buildings particularly difficult, especially where they have a locomotor problem or use a wheelchair. This means that people with disabilities are more likely to experience difficulties in attending further education courses, finding and maintaining work and enjoying a full social life. Third, the mechanisms by which young people with disabilities move through the health and educational systems become disrupted in the teenage years, yet it is at this time that a continuity of service is paramount if they are to be enabled to enjoy as independent a life as possible.

Having outlined in the previous part the primary needs of young adults with physical disabilities and the difficulties likely to be experienced in meeting these needs, the next part considers the role of the clinician in providing and organizing services to help meet these needs.

The clinician's role

It is clear that young people with physical disabilities have a wide range of needs, many of which are likely to remain unmet. This is for two primary reasons: first, the common practice of treating or dealing with only one aspect of a person's needs; and second, the absence of mechanisms for the coordination of support and care between the three primary services of health, education and social services.

A whole person approach

Many of the needs that young people with disabilities have clearly fall outside the usual remit of the medical clinician. Nevertheless, simply addressing only those issues that are of a medical nature may result in the young person's needs remaining unnoticed by the statutory services. Because of the medical implications of many physical disabilities such as spina bifida and cerebral palsy, for example, the clinician, whether working in a hospital environment or general practice, is in an advantageous position to be able to review the whole range of needs that young people with disabilities are likely to have. By adopting a whole person approach a clinician can ensure that a greater number of needs are likely to be met, with the consequence that people with disabilities are enabled to attain a greater degree of personal autonomy and independence. For the practising clinician, this approach necessitates four key requirements:

- Clinicians need to be able to recognize a wide range of health and non-health needs.
- The ability to meet these needs either by providing a direct service or by referral to other agencies.
- Liaison with other services where medical input might be advantageous in securing those services.
- Regular, periodic checks to ensure that both health and non-health needs are being dealt with.

Providing a service

It would be an inefficient use of resources for a clinician to become actively involved in meeting all of a young person's health and non-health needs. Many of these needs can be adequately addressed by existing services. The problem that continually arises for this client group is finding out about, and accessing, the requisite services. The Royal College of Physicians[42] recommended the creation of regional disability units as a focus of existing services, although these were primarily conceived as medical in nature. In the same year, the Disabled Persons (Services, Consultation and Representation) Act 1986 made it a duty for local education authorities to inform local social services departments when a disabled young person left special education, but the Act stopped short of providing a framework for coordinating the health, social and educational services. The 1986 Act was intended to improve the coordination of resources for people with disabilities, to make further provisions for the assessment of their needs, and establish further consultative processes and representational rights. This Act (amended by the Education Reform Act 1988) requires local education authorities (LEAs) to assess a person's needs where they are the subject of a Statement under the Education Act 1981. It also obliges LEAs to keep under review the dates when disabled children are expected to leave full-time education and to notify social service departments (SSDs) 8 months in advance; within 5 months of receiving notification SSDs are required to carry out an assessment of needs. Where people with a special knowledge of the needs of people with disabilities are being appointed to councils, or similar official bodies, the Act provides for an initial consultation with organizations of disabled people.

Subsequently, Thomas et al.[4] proposed adult disability services whose primary functions included clinical and information services and the coordination of the three major service providers. Despite the absence of a formal method of linking services, it is clear that a clinician has a major role to play in providing services, referral to appropriate agencies, and where necessary, acting as a coordinator of health and non-health services.

In terms of health care, in some areas the handover arrangements from paediatric to adult services have been formalized to some extent through the formation of clinics for young adults with disabilities. Newcastle, for example, has a weekly clinic that acts as a central information, advisory, and coordinating body and has a range of services including those of an orthopaedic surgeon, physiotherapist, occupational therapist and a disability employment advisor (known in the past as the DRO disablement resettlement officer) who provides a specialist information and advisory service.[43] Where such formal arrangements do not exist the clinician has a role to play in the coordination of various health services required by their clients. The type of services likely to be required are detailed in Table 10.11.

For non-health services the clinician can play a key role in informing young people with disabilities of the range of services available to them and providing a means of referral to these services. The types of services likely to be required by this client group and the primary referral agencies are shown in Table 10.12.

Table 10.11 A checklist of health services likely to be required by young adults with physical disabilities

Routine medical assessment
Advice and services for pressure sores, urinary incontinence, bowel management and stoma care
Neurology
Orthopaedics
Ophthalmology
Audiology

Physiotherapy
Mobility specialists
Speech therapy
Occupational therapy

Clinical psychology
Psychiatry

Useful addresses

Family Planning Association
27–35 Mortimer Street
London
W1N 7RJ
Tel: 071 636 7866

SPOD (The Association to Aid the Sexual and Personal Relationships of People with a Disability)
286 Camden Road
London
N7 0BJ
Tel: 071 607 8851

Skill: National Bureau for Students with Disabilities
336 Brixton Road
London
SW9 7AA
Tel: 071 274 0565

The Spastics Society
12 Park Crescent
London
W1N 4EQ
Tel: 071 636 5020   Helpline: 0800 626216

ASBAH (Association for Spina Bifida and Hydrocephalus)
ASBAH House
42 Park Road
Peterborough
PE1 2UQ
Tel: 0733 555988

Remploy Ltd
415 Edgware Road
Cricklewood
London
NW2 6LR
Tel: 081 452 8020

Table 10.12 Primary sources of information and advice for health-related and non-health services

Health education	
Pressure sores/incontinence	clinician
Sex education/contraception/	clinician
Sexual counselling	Family Planning Association
	SPOD (particularly sexual counselling)
Genetic counselling	clinician
	regional genetic centres
	Family Planning Association
	SPOD
Education and training	
Basic and further education	local education authority; Training and Enterprise Councils
Educational psychology	(TEC's)
	specialist careers officers (contact through LEA)
	local colleges of further education (some run 'special needs' courses)
	Skill: The National Bureau for Students with Disabilities
	some of the major charities provide educational courses, including The Spastics Society, ASBAH, etc.
Employment	
Employment training	local colleges of further education
	disability employment advisor (accessed through Jobcentres)
	TEC's
	some major charitable organizations run programmes of employment training
Employment opportunities,	Jobcentres
including sheltered workshops	disability employment advisor (Jobcentre)
and sheltered placements with	some of the major charities provide sheltered employment
commercial organizations	Remploy (sheltered workshops)
	OUTSET (employment for people with disabilities)
Adaptations to the work	Employment service/disability employment advisor
environment	(Jobcentre)
Housing	
Independent/sheltered housing	local authority housing department
	local authority social services department
	local housing associations
	some major charities (e.g. Spastics Society and Cheshire Homes) provide opportunities for independent living as well as sheltered housing
Housing adaptations	local authority social services department
Financial support	
Cash benefits	local DSS (now Benefits Agency)
Housing benefit/council tax benefit	local authority housing department
Advice and help with claiming	local Citizens Advice Bureaux
all types of benefits	local 'money advice' agency
	Disability Alliance
	Disability Rights Handbook (available through Disability Alliance)
Small cash grants	some of the major disability-related charities will provide cash grants towards aids and equipment

Table 10.12 Primary sources of information and advice for health-related and non-health services (cont'd)

Sources of general advice

Most towns have disability advice services (DIALs) that provide advice and help either through a drop-in service or by telephone or post. They are able to provide specialist disability advice (on a voluntary basis) on most subjects – housing, benefits, aids to daily living, transport, holidays, etc.

Citizens Advice Bureaux – particularly benefits and housing

Local authority social work service (through social services departments) – particularly housing, housing adaptations, benefits, and transport.

The Disability Rights Handbook (available from The Disability Alliance) provides detailed information about the benefits available as well as listing a large range of disability-related organizations.

OUTSET
18 Creekside
London
SE8 3DZ
Tel: 081 692 7141

The Disability Alliance
25 Denmark Street
London
WC2H 8NT
Tel: 071 247 8776

References

1 Gloag, D. Unmet need in chronic disability. *Br Med J* 1984; **289**: 211–212.

2 Rowan, P. *What Sort of Life?* Paper for the OECD project. The Handicapped Adolescent. Windsor, Berks: NFER-Nelson, 1980.

3 Hirst, M. Young people with disabilities: what happens after 16? *Child Care Hlth Dev* 1983; **9**: 273–284.

4 Thomas, A.P., Bax, M.C.O., Smyth, D.P.L. The health and social needs of young adults with physical disabilities. Clinics in Developmental Medicine No 106. Oxford: Mackeith Press and Blackwell Scientific Publications, 1989.

5 Thomas, A.P., Ritchie, J., Ward, K. *Meeting the Needs of People with Physical Disabilities: a Review of Social Welfare Centres in Birmingham.* London and Birmingham: Social and Community Planning Research, London, and Community Care Special Action Project, Birmingham, 1990.

6 Finkelstein, V. *Attitudes and Disabled People: Issues for Discussion.* International Exchange of Information in Rehabilitation. Monograph no 5. New York: World Rehabilitation Fund, 1980.

7 Goodall, J. Living options for physically disabled adults: a review. *Disability Handicap Soc* 1988; **3**: 173–193.

8 Davis, K. Notes on the development of the Derbyshire Centre for integrated living. Quoted in Goodall, J. Living options for physically disabled adults: a review. *Disability Handicap Soc* 1988; **3**: 173–193.

9 Department of Health and Social Security. DHSS Minutes of Evidence, 1982. *White Paper: Public Expenditure on the Social Services.* House of Commons Social Services Committee, 31 March 1982.

10 Cooke, K.R., Bradshaw, J., Lawton, D. Take-up of benefits by families with disabled children. *Child Care Hlth Dev* 1983; **9**: 145–156.

11 Greater London Association for the Disabled. *Special School Leavers: the Value of Further Education in their Transition to the Adult World.* London: GLAD.

12 Parker, G.M., Hirst, M. Continuity and change in medical care for young adults with disabilities. *J Roy Coll Physcns Lond* 1987; **21**: 129–133.

13 Castree, B.J., Walker, J.H. The young adult with spina bifida. *Br Med J* 1981; **283**: 1040–1042.

14 Parker, G.M. The case an integrated incontinence service for disabled children. *Comm Med* 1982; **4**: 119–124.

15 Carr, J., Pearson, A., Halliwell, M. The effect of disability on family life. *Z Kinderchir* 1983; **38**, suppl 2: 103–106.

16 Preest, M., Gelbier, S. Dental health and treatment needs of a group of physically handicapped adults. *Comm Hlth* 1977; **9**: 29–34.

17 Cadman, D., Boyle, M., Szatmari, P., Offord, D.R. chronic illness, disability and mental and social well-being: findings of the Ontario Child Health Study. *Pediatrics* 1987; **79**: 805–813.

18 Anderson, E.M., Clarke, L., Spain, B. *Disability in Adolescence.* London: Methuen, 1982.

19 Tew, B.J., Laurence, K.M. Mothers, brothers and sisters of patients with spina bifida. *Dev Med Child Neurol* 1973; **15**, suppl 29: 69–76.

20 Dorner, S. Sexual interest and activity in adolescents with spina bifida. *J Child Psychol Psychiatr* 1977; **18**: 229–237.

21 Dorner, S. Adolescents with spina bifida: how they see their situation. *Arch Dis Child* 1976; **51**: 439–444.

22 Warnock Report. *Special Educational Needs. Report of the Committee of Enquiry into the Education of Handicapped Children and Adults.* Cmnd 7212. London: HMSO, 1978.

23 Inner London Education Authority. Educational opportunities for all? *Report of the Committee Reviewing Provision to Meet Special Educational Needs (Fish Report).* London: ILEA, 1985.

24 Prior, O., Linford, M. *The Young Physically Handicapped in Hounslow: a Study of Adolescents and Young Adults with Severe Locomotor Handicaps.* London: Research and Planning Section, Social Services Department, London Borough of Hounslow.

25 Bookis, J. *Beyond the School Gate: a Study of Disabled Young People aged 13–19*. London: Royal Association for Disability and Rehabilitation, 1983.

26 Stowell, R. *Catching Up? Provision for Students with Special Educational Needs in Further Higher Education*. London: National Bureau for Handicapped Students, 1987.

27 Walker, A. *Unqualified and Unemployed: Handicapped Young People and the Labour Market*. London: National Children's Bureau with Macmillan, 1982.

28 Smith, A.D. Adult spina bifida survey in Scotland: educational attainment and employment. *Z Kinderchir* 1983; **38**: 107–109.

29 Head, P., Griffiths, M. *Report on First Destination of Special School Leavers*. London: Inner London Education Authority, 1983.

30 Hyman, M. *The Extra Costs of Disabled Living*. London: Disablement Income Group, 1977.

31 Baldwin, S. *Disabled Children, Counting the Costs: the Results of a Special Survey in the North and Midlands of Families with a Handicapped Child*. London: Disability Alliance, 1977.

32 Epstein, J. Communicating with the elderly. *J Market Res Soc* 1983; **25**: 239–262.

33 Fox, A.M. Psychological problems of physically handicapped children. *Br J Hosp Med* 1977; 479–490.

34 Younghusband, E., Birchall, D., Davie, R., Kellmer-Pringle, M.L. *Living with Handicap: Report of a Working Party on Children with Special Needs*. London: National Bureau for Co-operation in Child Care and National Children's Bureau, 1970.

35 Clarke, M.M., Riach, J., Cheyne, W.M. *Handicapped Children and Pre-school Education. Report to the Warnock Committee on Special Education*. Strathclyde: University of Strathclyde, 1977.

36 Jowett, S. *Young Disabled People: their Further Education, Training and Employment*. Windsor, Berks: NFER–Nelson, 1982.

37 Thomas, A.P. Social skills and physical handicap. In: Roger, D., Bull, D.E., eds. *Conversation: an Interdisciplinary Perspective*. Clevedon, Avon: Multilingual Matters Ltd.

38 Evans, K., Hickman, V., Carter, C.O. Handicap and social status of adults with spina bifida cystica. *Br J Prev Soc Med* 1974; **28**: 85–92.

39 Laurence, K.M., Beresford, A. Continence, friends, marriage and children in 51 adults with spina bifida. *Dev Med Child Neurol* 1975; **17**, suppl 35: 123–128.

40 Dorner, S. The relationship of physical handicap to stress in families with an adolescent with spina bifida. *Dev Med Child Neurol* 1965; **17**: 765–776.

41 Rowe, B. A study of social adjustment in young adults with cerebral palsy (*BMSc dissertation*). Newcastle: University of Newcastle upon Tyne, 1973.

42 Royal College of Physicians. Physical disability in 1986 and beyond: a report of the Royal College of Physicians. *J Roy Coll Physcns Lond* 1986; **20**: 160–194.

43 Robson, B.J. *Report on the Newcastle Young Adult Clinic for the Disabled*. Newcastle upon Tyne: Orthopaedic Department, Freeman Hospital, 1982.

Chapter 11

Hearing impaired children

11.1 Causes of deafness

Bethan Davies

Types of hearing impairment

1 Conductive

The commonest cause of hearing loss in infants and young children is serous otitis media which typically causes a mild to moderate hearing impairment of conductive nature, often fluctuating in degree and with a tendency to natural resolution (see section 11.2: glue ear).

Other causes of conductive hearing loss are far less common and may not be amenable to surgery. Therefore the management of these conditions may frequently be similar to the management of sensorineural hearing loss. They include:

a Cranio-facial abnormalities affecting the pinna, external auditory canal or middle ear, such as branchial arch disorders including Treacher Collins syndrome or Goldenhar syndrome.[1]
b Cranio-facial abnormalities associated with Eustachian tube dysfunction, including cleft palate,[2] Down syndrome.[3]
c Primary ciliary dyskinesia.
d Congenital ossicular chain defects.
e Traumatic ossicular chain defects.
f A rare form of juvenile otosclerosis.

In some of the above conditions the hearing loss may be mixed (conductive and sensorineural) in nature.

2 Sensorineural

Sensorineural hearing impairment may be due to either cochlear or retrocochlear pathology. Prevalence estimates for sensorineural hearing loss are very varied according to definition of loss and the methodology of the studies. In recent years there has been general agreement that the prevalence is between one and two per thousand live births. However, if those children with moderate hearing losses who need hearing aid provision and other intervention are included, the overall prevalence is more likely to be between two and three per thousand.[4]

Sensorineural loss may be monaural or binaural. Binaural losses may be symmetrical or asymmetrical. The degree of loss may be mild, moderate, severe or profound. The banding currently in use in the UK is as follows:[5]

Audiometric descriptors	Hearing level (dB) or dBHL
Mild loss	20–40
Moderate loss	41–70
Severe loss	71–95
Profound loss	over 95

These measures are calculated on the basis of the average of the pure tone hearing thresholds at 250, 500, 1000, 2000, and 4000 kHz.

The audiometric findings may be of many different shapes:

a Flat.

b Gently sloping with worse hearing at high frequencies.

c Steeply sloping with better (sometimes normal) hearing at low frequencies, and a severe loss at high frequencies.

d An island of hearing at low frequencies only – the so-called left hand corner audiogram.

e Dips of a varying width of frequency band, affecting low, mid, or high frequencies.

f Rarely, no response at maximum output of audiometer (120–130 dBHL).

3   Mixed hearing loss

Mixed conductive and sensorineural loss is very common in children. Most children who have a congenital sensorineural loss suffer from episodes of serous otitis media intermittently and the management of any resulting conductive overlay is of great importance.

Similarly many children with cranio-facial abnormalities also have a mixed hearing loss. In Down syndrome there is a high incidence of conductive loss due to serous otitis media associated with Eustachian tube dysfunction;[3] nor does this have a natural resolution but persists into adult life.[6–8] Improvement after surgical treatment is usually short lived. There is an additional considerable risk of cholesteatoma. Down syndrome children are also at high risk for developing a progressive sensorineural loss as they get older.

In babies and very young children where pure tone audiometry cannot be carried out, it may be difficult when a mixed loss is suspected to measure the level of sensorineural impairment. Removal of the conductive component by surgery, if possible, will usually clarify how much of the loss is sensorineural.

Causes of deafness

Classification can be in a variety of ways:

1   Site of lesion (a) conductive (b) sensorineural.
2   Association with other system defects such as visual, musculoskeletal, neurological.[9]
3   Syndromal or non-syndromal.
4   Genetic or non-genetic.
5   Congenital or acquired.

All such schema have advantages and disadvantages. For the paediatrician the most useful classification is as follows:

1   Genetic (a) syndromal (b) non-syndromal.
2   Non-genetic due to:
  a   prenatal causes
  b   perinatal causes
  c   postnatal causes.

Genetic deafness

Inheritance patterns of congenital deafness may be autosomal dominant, autosomal recessive or X-linked. The autosomal recessive type is very common, the autosomal dominant less so and the X-linked type is relatively rare.[10]

Syndromal deafness, that is where there are stigmata of a recognizable syndrome, is much less common than non-syndromal deafness. A careful search for stigmata, which may be of a minimal nature, is important for the eventual process of genetic counselling. Diagnosis may still be difficult because of the variable penetrance or minimal presentation of some signs within a syndrome. It is important to examine both parents and siblings and, whenever possible, members of the extended family if a syndrome is suspected.

There are many hundreds of recognized syndromes associated with deafness[9] and undoubtedly many as yet unrecognized particularly in children with very severe multiple handicaps in whom it is often difficult to assess hearing. Some of the better known syndromes are:

Waardenburg	Cockayne
Usher	CHARGE
Alport	Refsum
Marshall Stickler	Pierre Robin
Klippel Feil	Osteogenesis imperfecta

Photographs, drawings and clinical data can be obtained from dedicated volumes.[1,9,11]

All dysmorphic or developmentally delayed babies should have their hearing assessed so that any loss can be identified early and appropriate intervention provided. The identification and management of even mild hearing loss in a child with developmental delay or a visual or locomotor defect is important.

The pattern of genetic hearing loss is often although not always similar in siblings. Audiological assessment should be carried out on the siblings of identified hearing-impaired children. Neonatal screening should be offered for new siblings of hearing impaired children and it is necessary to continue to monitor such babies as there may be deterioration from normal or near-normal hearing at birth to a level similar to that of the hearing impaired child over a period of months or years.

Congenital monaural hearing loss, often of a total or subtotal nature, is usually familial and often inherited as a dominant. Binaural deafness may also occur in these families.

It is clear from many studies[10] that non-syndromal deafness of an autosomal recessive nature is the commonest cause of hearing impairment. Such deafness may account for 20% to 40% of cases.[10] It may be that with further genetic research many children who were previously assigned to an unknown aetiology group will be identified as having an autosomal recessive type of deafness.

It is very important in constructing high-risk schedules for neonatal screening of hearing to recognize that many autosomal recessive hearing impaired children will by definition be excluded from such schedules. The necessity for additional screening methods and identification facilities for these children is described elsewhere in this chapter (see Section 11.3).

For professionals involved in the care of families with hearing impaired children it is important to be aware that the birth of a second or subsequent affected child is a time of crisis for the family. In such cases the management of the diagnostic situation is critical and requires the maximum skills of the professionals concerned.

Research on genetic deafness

Carrier detection or prenatal diagnosis has not yet been possible in genetic deafness. However, in recent years, collaboration has developed between clinicians involved in the identification and management of deaf children and scientists involved in gene-mapping. The work has been greatly stimulated by research on syndromes associated with deafness in mice.[12] Gene mapping for deafness in humans is very difficult, especially in the non-syndromal types because of the very large number of gene loci involved. Mapping has already been achieved for Usher type II and Waardenburg type I syndromes.[13,14]

Combined clinics and research projects are now developing and involve audiological physicians, geneticists and microbiologists. Such projects should lead to a rapid expansion of knowledge about genetic deafness and eventually to increased advice being available to hearing impaired families.

Non-genetic deafness

Prenatal causes

RUBELLA

Fifty years ago the association between maternal rubella infection and the subsequent birth of babies with multiple defects was discovered.[15] Thirty years ago, the rubella virus was isolated and antibody detection developed. Following this, immunization became possible and this eventually led to the present measles, mumps, rubella (MMR) vaccination programme. It also made possible the accurate diagnosis of maternal rubella in early pregnancy which gives mothers the opportunity to choose termination when the risks of rubella damage are considered to be high.

There has been a steady downward trend in cases of congenital rubella syndrome over the last 20 years, apart from the epidemic years of 1978–1979, and there has also been a steady fall in the number of terminations for rubella.[16]

The MMR programme appears to be significantly decreasing the risk of exposure of pregnant women to rubella. It is to be expected that there will be a continuing fall, both in the number of terminations and in the number of cases of congenital rubella but continued monitoring of the incidence is necessary.

The risk of multiple defects in the fetus is very much higher if the viraemia occurs in the early weeks of pregnancy. This is demonstrated in data reported in the Public Health Laboratory Service (PHLS) study.[17] This reported on 190 cases of congenital rubella infection. In those cases of infection in the first 19 weeks of pregnancy, 26% were hearing impaired. For those in the first 10 weeks of pregnancy, 90% were affected. The incidence of hearing loss dropped to 50% for infections at 11–12 weeks, and to 33% for infections at 13–16 weeks. Defects following rubella at 17 weeks or later are rare but not unrecorded.

The maternal rubella infection may be of a subclinical nature, although fetal damage may be considerable. Single organ defects, particularly hearing loss alone, tend to occur in the later infections. Often these children are otherwise normal, except for a rubella retinopathy not affecting vision.[18,19] The absence of a rubella retinopathy does not exclude rubella as the cause of deafness.

There is evidence of deterioration of hearing in rubella deafness in many studies.[20,21] The nature of the hearing loss may be from a moderate to a profound level, severe to profound losses being the most common. There is often asymmetry of the hearing loss between the ears.

CYTOMEGALOVIRUS (CMV)

Congenital CMV infection is an important cause of congenital deafness and might account for as many as 12% of cases.[22] The diagnosis of congenital CMV infection is only possible in the *first 3 weeks of life* as, after this period, acquired infection becomes increasingly common and cannot be differentiated from congenital infection. The acquired form is not associated with hearing loss.

Prospective studies have suggested that the probable incidence of deafness is 6% in congenitally infected infants.[23] In a large prospective study in London[24,25] congenital CMV infection was found in 0.3% of live births.

In that study 103 infected babies were identified and followed. Only four of these were symptomatic at birth and all four were eventually shown to have neurological defects and two were hearing impaired.

In the group of 99 asymptomatic babies four had hearing impairment (three bilateral, one unilateral). Two of the children with bilateral loss had cerebral palsy. CMV infection is likely to be the cause of deafness in some of the children previously thought to have deafness of unknown aetiology. It is clear from the data resulting from prospective studies that there is a high incidence of neurological defects, especially cerebral palsy, in children whose deafness is due to CMV infection.

The hearing loss may be of a moderate, severe or profound degree, is usually bilateral and may show unusual audiometric patterns. There is some evidence of deteriorating levels of hearing in some cases and also of late-onset deafness.

Unfortunately this important cause of deafness cannot be identified retrospectively as acquired infection is so common in young children.

OTHER INTRAUTERINE INFECTIONS

Other intrauterine infections resulting in congenital deafness are very rare in the UK. Deafness as a result of syphilis and toxoplasmosis is seen in other countries.

OTOTOXIC DRUGS

Exposure of the fetus to high levels of ototoxic drugs now rarely occurs and is therefore an unlikely cause of congenital deafness. Nevertheless, when the cause of a congenital hearing loss is being investigated, a history should be taken of drugs taken by the mother, especially in the first trimester, with particular reference to ototoxic drugs such as aminoglycosides.

Perinatal causes

The recent rapid advances in neonatal medicine have resulted in an increased survival of very low birthweight babies, especially in large well-equipped units. Many of these babies have suffered a multiplicity of insults in the perinatal period and are at high risk of hearing impairment, as well as other sequelae.

The prevalence of deafness in children who were admitted to special care baby units, has been estimated to be between 0.75% and 9.7%.[4,26] As in all such epidemiological studies it is difficult to compare quoted prevalence rates because of the variations in methodology and the variability of the study populations.

When sensorineural deafness is identified in a high-risk baby it is often very difficult to decide which factors may have been important in causing damage to the auditory system. There is evidence that a preterm baby is more susceptible to the effects of hypoxia than a term baby. In the hearing impaired preterm baby there is frequently a history of birth asphyxia or recurrent apnoeic attacks which have produced hypoxia.

The role of hyperbilirubinaemia in causing sensorineural deafness is uncertain. In the past deafness with cerebral palsy was frequently seen due to rhesus alloimmunization and resulting kernicterus. This condition no longer occurs in the UK. Hyperbilirubinaemia is probably particularly damaging to low birthweight babies, especially those suffering from hypoxia, acidosis and sepsis.[27] Susceptibility to damage from hyperbilirubinaemia increases with decreasing birthweight.

In babies deafened by perinatal insult, the hearing impairment may be moderate to profound and there may be other results of damage, including visual disorders, motor disorders, fits, and severe developmental delay. The assessment of hearing in the preterm infant, especially if multiple problems are present, may be difficult. Maturation of brainstem evoked responses or behavioural responses to sound is sometimes seen, giving a better prognosis for auditory function than originally expected.

Aminoglycosides are frequently used for the treatment of sepsis in neonates and blood concentrations should be carefully monitored. If ototoxic levels are reached it is necessary to monitor the hearing of such babies subsequently although there is little evidence of aminoglycosides causing hearing loss.

Suggested high-risk criteria for neonatal hearing screening are:

1 Family history: parents, siblings or near relatives deaf from infancy.
2 Cranio-facial abnormalities including cleft palate, micrognathia, ear tags, identified syndrome.
3 Prenatal infections especially rubella or CMV.
4 Birthweight below 1500 g or small-for-dates (less than third centile).
5 Hyperbilirubinaemia. Serum level above 200 µmol/l at 34 weeks' gestational age or 250 µmol/l at 36 weeks or 300 µmol/l at 38 weeks.
6 Severe asphyxia: Apgar score of 1–3 at 5 minutes, or clinical indication.

Postnatal causes

Meningitis continues to be an important cause of deafness in children and the loss is often severe to profound. There are variable estimates for the proportion of hearing impaired children who are deafened by meningitis, from 3% to 20%, but many studies quote a level of 6–7%.[28–30] Bacterial meningitis carries a much higher risk for deafness than viral meningitis.[27] Organisms which have been identified as producing meningitic deafness include the pneumococcus *Neisseria meningitidis*, and *Haemophilus influenzae*. The incidence of deafness following meningitis depends on the organism involved; the highest risk is in infections by the pneumococcus, possibly as high as 24%, while the risk with other organisms is probably 7–8%.[31] The degree of deafness is usually bilateral, and severe or profound although occasionally moderate. There is frequently other neurological damage.[32] Temporary vestibular symptoms in the convalescent period are often noted in children deafened by meningitis. *All* children who have sustained a meningitis infection need audiological assessment as soon as they are well.

Measles is now a very rare cause of sensorineural loss in the UK.

Mumps is the commonest cause of sudden onset monaural hearing loss in children. The infection may be of a subclinical nature and the hearing damage is not related to the severity of symptoms. The loss is usually total or sub-total. Bilateral loss from this cause is very rare. Vestibular symptoms may be present in the acute stage.

Other viruses: sudden-onset deafness (binaural or monaural) due to other organisms is rare in children.

Ototoxic drugs: children receiving ototoxic drugs on a long-term basis are usually being treated for severe chronic systemic disease or for a neoplastic disease. Monitoring of the hearing of such children should be carried out so that any resulting deafness can be appropriately managed.

Tumours: children known to have neurofibromatosis need regular hearing screening to identify hearing loss from intracranial tumours. Hearing loss due to other intracranial tumours occurs but is rare in children.

References

1   Gorlin, R.J., Cohen, M.M., Levin, L.S. *Syndromes of the Head and Neck*. Oxford: Oxford University Press, 1990: 641–691.

2   Bluestone, C.D. Prevalence and pathogenesis of ear disease and hearing loss. In: Graham, M.D., ed. *Cleft Palate: Middle Ear Disease and Hearing Loss*. Illinois: C.C. Thomas, 1978.

3   White, B. LeM., Doyle, W.J., Bluestone, C.D. Eustachian tube function in infants and children with Down's syndrome. In: Lim, D.J., Bluestone, C.D., Klein, J.O., Nelson, J.D., eds. *Recent Advances in Otitis Media with Effusion*. Philadelphia: Decker, 1984.

4   Sancho, J., Hughes, E., Davis, A., Haggard, M. Epidemiological basis for screening hearing. In: McCormick, B., ed. *Paediatric Audiology, 0–5 Years*. London: Taylor and Francis, 1988: 1–35.

5   British Society of Audiology. Recommendations for descriptors for pure-tone audiograms. *Br J Audiol* 1988; **22**: 123.

6   Brooks, D.N., Wooley, H., Kanjial, G.C. Hearing loss and middle ear disorders in patients with Down's syndrome. *J Mental Def Res* 1972; **16**: 21.

7   Davies, B. Hearing problems. In: Lane, D., Stratford, B., eds. *Current Approaches to Down's Syndrome*. London: Cassell, 1985.

8   Davies, B. Auditory disorders in Down's syndrome. *Scand Audiol* 1988; Suppl 30: 65–68.

9   Konigsmark, B.W., Gorlin, R.J. *Genetic and Metabolic Deafness*. Philadelphia: Saunders, 1976.

10 Williamson, I., Steel, K. Aetiology of hearing impairment. *Hereditary Deafness Newsletter* no. 5. London: Royal National Institute for the Deaf, 1990: 7–16.

11 Goodman, R.M., Gorlin, R.J. *The Malformed Infant and Child*. Oxford: Oxford University Press, 1983.

12 Steel, K. Human and mouse gene lists. *Hereditary Deafness Newsletter*, no. 1. London: Royal National Institute for the Deaf, 1988: 3–11.

13 Kimberling, W.J., *et al*. Localisation of Usher syndrome type II to chromosome 1q. *Hereditary Deafness Newsletter*, no. 4. London: Royal National Institute for the Deaf, 1990, 35.

14 Steel, K. Editorial note. *Hereditary Deafness Newsletter*, no. 4. London: Royal National Institute for the Deaf, 1990, 2.

15 Gregg, N.M. Congenital cataract following German measles in the mother. *Trans Ophthalmol Soc Austr* 1941; **3**: 35–46.

16 Miller, E. Rubella in the United Kingdom. *Epidemiol Infect* 1991; **107**: 31–42.

17 Miller, E., Waight, P.A., Vurdien, J.E., *et al*. Rubella surveillance to December 1990: a joint report from the Public Health Laboratory Service (PHLS) and National Congenital Rubella Surveillance Programme. *Commun Disease Report* 1981; **1**: R33–36.

18 Roy, F.H., Hiatt, R.L., Korones, S.B., Roane, J. Ocular manifestations of congenital rubella syndrome. *Arch Ophthalmol* 1966; **75**: 601–607.

19 Taylor, I.G. The prevention of sensorineural deafness. *J Laryngol Otol* 1990; **94**: 1327–1343.

20 Sheridan, M.D. Final report of a prospective study of children whose mothers had rubella in early pregnancy. *Br Med J* 1964; **2**: 536–539.

21 Sever, J.L., South, M.A., Shaver, K.A. Delayed manifestations of congenital rubella. *Rev Infect Dis* 1985; **7**, suppl. 1: 5164–5169.

22 Peckham, C.S., Stark, O., Dudgeon, J.A., Martin, J.A.M., Hawkins, G. Congenital cytomegalovirus infection: a cause of sensorineural hearing loss. *Arch Dis Child* 1987; **62**: 1233–1237.

23 Kumar, M.L., Nankervis, G.A., Jacobs, I.B., *et al*. Congenital and postnatally acquired cytomegalovirus infection: long term follow-up. *J Pediatr* 1984; **104**: 674–679.

24 Peckham, C.S., Coleman, J.C., Hurley, R., Chin, K.S., Henderson, K. Cytomegalovirus infection in pregnancy: preliminary finding from a prospective study. *Lancet* 1983; **i**: 1352–1356.

25 Peckham, C.S. Cytomegalovirus in the neonate. *J Antimicrob Chemother* 1989; **23** suppl. E: 17–21.

26 Bergman, I., Hirsch, R.P., Fria, T.J., Shaprio, S.M., Holzman, I., Painter, M.J. Cause of hearing loss in the high-risk premature infant. *J Pediatr* 1985; **106**: 95–101.

27 Newton, V.E. Aetiology of bilateral sensorineural hearing loss in young children. *J Laryngol Otol* 1985, Suppl. no. 10.

28 Das, V.K. Aetiology of bilateral sensorineural deafness in children. *Scand Audiol* 1987; Suppl. 30, 43–52.

29 Flint, E.F. Severe childhood deafness in Glasgow 1965–1979. *J Laryngol Otol* 1983; **97**: 421–425.

30 Taylor, I.G., Hine, W.D., Brasier, V.J., Chiveralls, K., Morris, T. A study of the causes of hearing loss in a population of deaf children with special reference to genetic factors. *J Laryngol Otol* 1975; **89**: 899–914.

31 Gerber, S.E. Review of a high-risk register for congenital or early-onset deafness. *Br J Audiol* 1990; **24**: 347–356.

32 Klein, J.O., Feigin, R.D., McCracken, G.H. Jr. Report of the task force on diagnosis and management of meningitis. *Pediatrics* 1986; **78**; Suppl.

11.2 Glue ear

Anthony Richards

Definition

There has been a very great increase in interest in this condition over the last two decades, as witnessed both by the number of articles appearing in the literature and by the number of surgical procedures carried out to treat it; to the extent that it has been described as a 'modern epidemic'.[1] Yet the disease is certainly not new, and has been recognized for more than 100 years. Some difficulty has been caused by the number of different terms that have been used to describe it. Among the more common current ones are 'otitis media with effusion' and 'sero-mucinous otitis media'. It has been stated that more than 55 terms have been used.[2] A useful definition was given by Paperella: 'an inflammation of the middle ear accompanied by an accumulation of liquid in the middle ear cleft without the signs and symptoms of acute infection.'[3]

Prevalence

Published data on the prevalence of this very common childhood disorder have not been in complete accord; the methods used have varied. A review of 23 studies reported in 24 papers sought to amalgamate these varied findings into a single graph of prevalence against age. The result was a bimodal curve with two peaks at the age of 2 years (approximately 20%) and 5 years (approximately 15%)[4] (Fig. 11.1). It is recognized that the condition is not found in neonates and is relatively uncommon under 6 months of age; there is then an explosive increase in prevalence in babies aged 6 months to one year, followed by a steady increase towards the 2-year peak.[5,6]

Important information on the natural history of the condition has come from longitudinal cohort studies in Denmark.[7–11] Children were tested at intervals of 3 months, and it was found that almost half of the tested ears changed tympanometric type between each visit, lending objective weight to the clinical observation that a great deal of spontaneous recovery, as well as some deterioration, is a feature of this condition. In children below 1 year of age, more deteriorate than improve; from 2 to 5 years of age, the deteriorations roughly equal the improvements, while in the over-5s there were more improvements. This variability and transience make it difficult to represent the

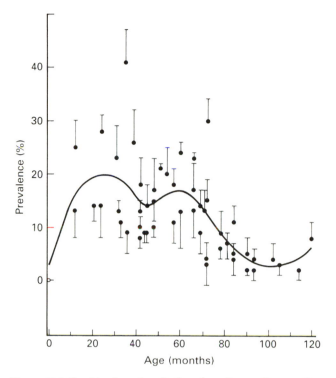

Figure 11.1 Combined results of selected studies on the prevalence of otitis media with effusion with 95% confidence intervals. (Reproduced from G.A. Zielhuis *et al. Clin Otolaryngol* 1990; **15**: 286, by kind permission of the editor.)

course of the typical untreated condition, unless the various patterns are linked to their occurrence rates:

- 15% have a single, or a few short episodes (1–3 months)
- 25% have repeated short episodes
- 15% have a single, or a few longer episodes (3–9 months)
- 15% have repeated, long-lasting episodes
- 10% have extremely prolonged episodes (more than a year)

A Danish study found only 10–20% of children escaped having the condition at least once during their childhood.[12]

The data from studies of epidemiology and natural history will encourage a more conservative approach to treatment. The problem is that confronted with the individual child with glue ear the clinician has no way of knowing the end point – the condition might resolve untreated within a short timespan, or alternatively run a prolonged course over years, and even progress to sequelae.

So far only the otherwise normal child has been considered. There are conditions which predispose to glue ear which, although not common, yield higher prevalence rates of glue ear than those quoted above. Chief among these are Down syndrome,[13] cleft palate (with an incidence of 97%),[14] primary ciliary dyskinesia, and cystic fibrosis.

Pathogenesis

The pathogenesis of glue ear is not well understood. There seems little doubt that Eustachian tube malfunction plays a part in the process. The Eustachian tube has two main functions: to drain the middle ear spaces as part of the mucociliary transport system for this area; and to aerate the middle ear cleft, and keep the pressure there at or close to atmospheric. It is this latter function that seems to be primarily defective in cases of glue ear. In a simple, but well-designed clinical experiment, Sadé demonstrated that if the negative pressure in the middle ear was relieved by myringotomy, the cilia then became capable of draining the mucus into the nasopharynx; defective aeration thus seems to be an important factor. At the same time, there is histological evidence that the mucous membrane of the middle ear is hypertrophic and hypersecreting in children with glue ear, implying that there is oversecretion of mucus as well.[15]

Other aetiological factors have been identified. The incidence of glue ear is increased if the parents smoke, and also if the child attends a day centre. Adenoidal hypertrophy appears to be a factor, although the presence of allergies and genetic predisposition are not.[16]

There appears to be a circular effect operating between the condition of glue ear and that of acute otitis media. There is often a past history of frequent recurrent otitis media in children with glue ear, which suggests that the infections predispose to the formation of the sterile mucus within the middle ear. At the same time, the close correlation between the two is in part because acute otitis is often the *result* of secretory otitis.[17] The constant change from an aerated middle ear cleft to glue ear is thus complemented by a constant change from glue ear to otitis media (Fig. 11.2).

The effects of glue ear

Glue ear typically causes a mild conductive hearing loss, which affects the low frequencies more than the high; this is in contrast with the sensorineural losses, where the high frequencies are most severely affected. The degree of hearing loss associated with glue ear is not consistent. At worst, it rarely exceeds 45 dB

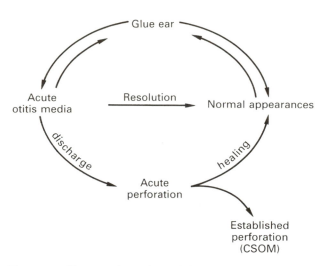

Figure 11.2 The interrelationships of glue ear with acute otitis media and its sequelae.

hearing level; at best, the child may have definite glue ear with hearing which is nearly normal, or possibly varying between this and more marked loss. When the condition is unilateral it is often unsuspected, or revealed only by screening. Its presence will, of course, be less obvious if the child has other congenital problems, global retardation, or sensorineural hearing loss.

Many authors have shown that severe to moderate hearing loss has an important impact on linguistic and intellectual development and on social adjustment; severe or moderate loss in this context implies that the child has an additional congenital or, less commonly, early acquired sensorineural hearing loss. What is less certain is the impact of the milder loss associated with glue ear on these developmental parameters. A review of published literature, which comprises descriptive studies, case control studies, cohort studies and reviews,[18] found that while the older studies had suggested a connection between glue ear and retarded development, the more recent publications found no proven correlation. One problem appears to be that while some children with developmental delay have glue ear, only a small proportion of children with glue ear have developmental problems. In the longer term, it is suggested that any possible slight reduction in development ends when the glue ear disappears and hearing returns to normal.[19]

Of the many difficulties encountered in such studies, the most important are the exclusion of children who have had treatment for long-standing glue ear during the study, and the control of confounding factors that may have a substantial impact on development, especially the social background of the parents, home environment, and exposure to peers at day-care facilities or home. These difficulties, coupled with the relative insensitivity of some of the tests, may imply that the issue of developmental skills and hearing loss is incapable of scientific proof.

Diagnosis

The presence of glue ear should be suspected in otherwise normal children who have recurrent attacks of otitis media or grossly enlarged adenoids causing nasal obstruction; it should be assumed to be present in all cases of cleft palate, and in most cases of Down syndrome, primary ciliary dyskinesia and cystic fibrosis. The commonest presenting symptom is hearing loss. This may be suspected because the parents, relatives or schoolteacher notice either the loss itself, or its secondary effects on behaviour or speech, school or social performance. Alternatively the hearing loss may be found at routine screening in general practitioner or community clinics, or on school entry. In such cases, the parents will either have failed to suspect it, or perhaps will have attributed its secondary effects to inattention, stubbornness, or even low intelligence.

Clinical diagnosis is made more difficult because there is no single diagnostic sign on otoscopy. While the colour of the tympanic membrane may be yellow or bluish, it may be little different from normal. The classically described dullness and loss of light reflex can be misleadingly absent, while the leash of vessels often seen on the malleus handle or periphery of the drum may lead the practitioner to the mistaken diagnosis of acute otitis media, despite the absence of symptoms or other signs of this condition. Retraction of the eardrum is a useful sign, but difficult to elicit. Immobility of the eardrum on pneumatic otoscopy is the single most reliable sign, and can reach detection levels equal to those of tympanometry,[20] but only in the hands of experienced observers equipped with the necessary indirect lighting system.

Increasing use is being made of tympanometry as the gold standard for preoperative diagnosis of glue ear; most community audiology clinics and many GP group practices are able to perform this test, and its use as a screening test has been advocated. The problem is that many more children would fail this screen than the standard audiometric test, leading not only to logistical problems in processing the failures, but also to increased pressure to treat those with glue ear but without significant hearing loss. At a time when criticism has been levelled at over-treatment of the condition, this remains a dilemma.

Treatment of glue ear

Of the treatment options for glue ear, the first is dictated primarily by the known natural history – to watch and wait.[21] Such a policy, at least if conducted over a period of 3 months, would avoid surgery in a substantial proportion of children who would convert naturally from glue ear to normal in such a timespan. For more active medical treatment, the search has centred on antimicrobials, decongestants and antihistamines (often in combination), and steroids. There is insufficient evidence that any of these are effective treatments.[22,23] The same may be said of techniques for auto-inflation of the middle ear by blowing up balloons. The search for an effective medical remedy for this condition continues.

Surgical treatment for glue ear has overtaken adenotonsillectomy as the most commonly performed operation in children. Attention has been drawn to the great variation in rates of surgery between geographically adjacent health districts – differences which cannot be explained on the grounds of prevalence alone, and must reflect professional uncertainty about the indications for surgery, as well as factors of surgical supply, and patient and professional demand.[24] Treatment strategies have included myringotomy, myringotomy plus grommet insertion, adenoidectomy, adenoidectomy in combination with myringotomy or myringotomy with grommet insertion. It has been established that tonsillectomy does not improve the outcome when added to the other treatments.[25] Myringotomy alone produces little or no benefit, while myringotomy and grommet insertion produces an immediate improvement in hearing which is maintained for the 6–12 months that the grommet remains in place, but not beyond this. There seems now to be some evidence that the effusion is resolved for longer when adenoidectomy is added,[26] although the effect on the hearing is insignificant.[27] This is an important distinction on economic grounds, as it is usual in the UK to insert grommets as a day case, whereas at present children for adenoidectomy are usually admitted to hospital for at least one night; this extra cost, and the increased morbidity associated with adenoidectomy, may therefore not be justified unless there is an additional indication, such as post-nasal obstruction, for this procedure.

Ventilation of the middle ear is not without its complications. Tympanosclerosis (calcified thickening of the middle layer of the eardrum) is both more common and more widespread when ventilating tubes have been inserted than when the ear is unoperated and simply subjected to recurrent otitis media. Fortunately, mobile plaques of tympanosclerosis do not adversely affect the hearing, and do not therefore seem to constitute a contraindication to tube insertion. Although the function of grommets is to ventilate, discharge is a recognized sequela of their insertion, especially in long-term aeration such as with the T-tube; a persistent perforation after tube extrusion or removal is also more common with long-term ventilating tubes. The rates of both of these complications vary greatly between reported series.[28]

Treatment policy

A reasonable treatment policy for glue ear would appear to contain the following guidelines:

- To wait for at least 3 months before advising surgery.
- To reserve surgery for bilateral cases unless other factors (poor performance, speech problems) are added.
- In bilateral cases, not to accept the diagnosis alone as an indication for surgery, unless there is also significant (25 dB)[27] hearing loss and associated difficulties.
- To consider grommet insertion as the usual treatment, reserving adenoidectomy for specific indications (nasal obstruction, frequent recurrent otitis).
- To use long-term ventilation (T-tubes) bilaterally in all cases of cleft palate, unilaterally in cases of Down syndrome, and in normal children when grommets have already been inserted twice previously.

References

1   Black, N.A. Surgery for glue ear – a modern epidemic. *Lancet* 1984; **i**: 835–837.

2   Black, N.A. Is glue ear a modern phenomenon? *Clin Otolaryngol* 1984; **9**: 155–163.

3   Paparella, M.M. The character of acute and secretory otitis media. In: Sadé, J., ed. *Acute and Secretory Otitis Media*. Proceedings of the international conference on acute and secretory otitis media, Jerusalem, Israel. Amsterdam: Kugler; 1986.

4   Zielhuis, G.A., Rach, G.H., Van Den Bosch, A., Van Den Broeck, P. The prevalence of otitis media with effusion: a critical review of the literature. *Clin Otolaryngol* 1990; **15**: 283–288.

5   Fiellau-Nikolajsen, M. Tympanometry and secretory otitis media. *Acta Otolaryngol (Stockh)*; Suppl 394, 1983.

6   Haggard, M.P., Hughes, E., eds. Epidemiology of otitis media in children. In: Haggard, M.P., Hughes, E. eds. *Screening Children's Hearing: a Review of the Literature and Implications*. London: HMSO, 1990.

7   Tos, M., Poulsen, G., Hancke, A.B. Screening tympanometry during the first year of life. *Acta Otolaryngol (Stockh)* 1979; **88**: 388–394.

8   Tos, M., Poulsen, G. Tympanometry in 2-year-old children. Seasonal influence of frequency of secretory otitis and tubal function. *J Otorhinolaryngol Rel Specialties* 1979; **41**: 1–10.

9   Tos, M., Holm-Jensen, S., Sorensen, C.H., Mogensen, C. Spontaneous course and frequency of secretory otitis in four-year-old children. *Arch Otolaryngol* 1982; **108**: 4–10.

10   Tos, M. Epidemiology and spontaneous improvement of secretory otitis. *Acta Otorhinolaryngol Belg* 1983; **37**: 31–43.

11   Tos, M. Epidemiology and natural history of secretory otitis. *Am J Otol* 1984; **5**: 459–460.

12   Fiellau-Nikolajsen, M. Danish approach to the treatment of secretory otitis media – frequency and course of the disease. *Ann Otol Rhinol Laryngol* 1990; **99**; Suppl 146: 7–8.

13   Davies, B. Auditory disorders in Down's syndrome. *Scand Audiol* 1988; **30** (suppl): 65–68.

14   Dhillon, R.S. The middle ear in cleft palate children pre- and post-palatal closure. *J Roy Soc Med* 1988; **81**: 710–713.

15   Sadé, J. *Secretory Otitis Media and its Sequelae*. Edinburgh: Churchill Livingstone, 1979: 191.

16   Tos, M., Poulsen, G., Borch, J. Etiological factors in secretory otitis. *Arch Otolaryngol* 1979; **105**: 582–588.

17   Stangerup, S.E., Tos, M. Etiological role of acute suppurative otitis media in chronic secretory otitis. *Am J Otol* 1985; **6**: 126–131.

18   Lous, J. Danish approach to the treatment of secretory otitis media – effect of hearing loss on child development. *Ann Otol Rhinol Laryngol* 1990; **99**, Suppl 166: 14–15.

19   Paradise, J.L. Otitis media during early life. How hazardous to development? A critical review of the evidence. *Pediatrics* 1981; **68**: 869–873.

20   Toner, J.G., Mains, B. Pneumatic otoscopy and tympanometry in the detection of middle ear effusion. *Clin Otolaryngol* 1990; **15**: 121–124.

21   Bluestone, C.D. Management of chronic otitis media with effusion. *Acta Otolaryngol Belg* 1983; **37**: 44–56.

22   Crysdale, W.S. Medical management of serous otitis media. *Otolaryngol Clin N Am* 1984; **17**: 653–657.

23   Cantekin, E.I., Mandel, E.M., Bluestone, C.D., *et al.* Lack of efficacy of a decongestant/antihistamine combination for otitis media with effusion (secretory otitis media). *New Eng J Med* 1983; **308**: 297–301.

24   Black, N. Geographical variations in the use of surgery for glue ear. *J Roy Soc Med* 1985; **78**: 641–648.

25   Maw, A.R., Herod, F. Otoscopic, impedance, and audiometric findings in glue ear treated by adenoidectomy and tonsillectomy. A prospective randomised study. *Lancet* 1986; 1399–1402.

26   Maw, A.R. Factors affecting adenoidectomy for otitis media with effusion (glue ear). *J Roy Soc Med* 1985; **78**: 1014–1018.

27   Black, N. A randomised controlled trial of surgery for glue ear. *Br Med J* 1990; **300**: 1551–1556.

28   Brockbank, M.J., Jonathan, D.A., Grant, H.R., Wright, A. Goode T-tubes: do the benefits of their use outweigh the complications? *Clin Otolaryngol* 1988; **13**: 351–356.

11.3 Screening for hearing impairment

Sarah Sheppard

The need for early detection of hearing loss is now widely accepted.[1-5] In practice it has been difficult to achieve effective screening to lower the age of detection of even severe and profound hearing loss. A study in European Community (EC) countries by Martin *et al.* showed that only 10% of children with hearing losses averaging 50 dB or more were diagnosed by the age of one year.[6] In the USA, Simmons showed the average age of detection of moderate to profound hearing loss to be 2.7 years.[7]

Effective screening tests should have good sensitivity to identify a defined degree of hearing loss and good specificity, that is, to pass correctly unaffected cases. The test technique employed should be of short duration, non-invasive, relatively easy to perform and appropriate to the age of the population to be screened. To achieve effective results screening should be monitored.[8]

Neonatal screening

The earlier screening is carried out, the sooner diagnosis and rehabilitation can occur. Ideally all neonates should be screened but economic and practical constraints currently prevent this. Priority is given to the screening of high-risk groups, most notably preterm babies who have been in special care. This type of targeted screening can be effective in the early detection of approximately half of severe and profound congenital or perinatal hearing losses.[9] Neonatal screening has an additional advantage. Since the majority of births in the UK are in hospital, the babies are accessible for testing without the need to bring them back for screening. Methods of neonatal screening are still being evaluated and it is possible that a combination of techniques may prove to give the optimum results.

The auditory response cradle (ARC)[10] and the crib-o-gram[11] detect a variety of behavioural responses to sound including head turns, changes in respiration rate and startle responses but are not widely used.[12] The ARC has been shown to be less effective with babies in neonatal intensive care units even though a large proportion of those at risk of hearing loss fall within this group.[13] The high intensity stimuli used by both the ARC and the crib-o-gram disturb some babies and result in tests being abandoned. Babies with moderate to severe losses will not necessarily be identified.

Auditory brainstem electric response (ABR) measurements offer a more precise and reliable indicator of hearing sensitivity.[14,15] Electrodes placed on the head detect brainstem responses to sound. The response is a waveform which needs interpretation by a skilled tester. Reliable automatic assessment of the waveform using correlation and amplitude analysis is however now possible.[16,17] Low to moderate sound levels are used which do not disturb the baby. Lack of maturation of the nervous system in babies of less than 37 weeks' gestational age can affect the results.[18]

The measurement of evoked otoacoustic emissions (EOAE) is the most recent technique to be utilized for neonatal screening.[19,20] Stevens has reported an 80% pass rate in a neonatal screening trial suggesting good specificity.[21] A click stimulus is used to evoke an echo or emission from the ear which is recorded as a waveform. The tester must be trained to interpret waveforms with the help of statistical measures to determine the presence or absence of a response. This technique is very sensitive and the response is abolished by mild conductive or cochlear hearing losses. EOAE testing has the advantage of being quicker to perform than ABR measurements. Neither EOAE nor ABR techniques test the entire auditory pathway and thus will not identify central auditory disorders which are thought to be rare. Currently EOAE and ABR measurements are the preferred methods for neonatal screening.

Community screening at 7–9 months

Most babies are not screened for hearing loss neonatally. Other methods must therefore be employed to detect hearing loss in babies who are not considered to be at risk and to detect babies with acquired, progressive or marked conductive hearing losses.[22] For these reasons hearing screening in community clinics by health visitors using the distraction test is still widespread.

When carried out correctly the distraction test has been shown to be effective in detecting hearing loss.[23] If a poor test technique is used, however, few babies will be identified and parents could be given false reassurance about the normality of their baby's hearing. It is therefore vitally important to ensure that health visitors are given adequate training in good test techniques. The introduction of hand-held warblers which produce warble tones at low, middle and high frequency bands at a predetermined screening level helps to standardize the test stimuli.[24] The distraction test has several advantages for hearing screening in that frequency specific sound stimuli are used, the head turn response is behavioural thus testing the whole auditory pathway, and potentially all babies can be tested.

The role of surveillance in early detection of hearing loss

Not all parents notice their baby's hearing loss, but when parental suspicion of a hearing loss is expressed it is generally very reliable.[25,26]

Parental observation has been utilized in the development of the 'Can your baby hear you?' Hints for Parents form by McCormick (Fig. 11.3).[27] Issue of the form by health visitors at their first home visit gives the potential for good population coverage. Guidance is given in a tick sheet format on what type of reaction to sound parents should expect from their baby at various ages up to one year. Unlike single screening tests this inexpensive method utilizes long-term observation and has not generally been found to cause unnecessary parental anxiety. Parental illiteracy or poor motivation can however reduce its effectiveness. The Hints for Parents Form can be used effectively in conjunction with a screening programme to increase parental and professional awareness of hearing impairment.

In West Berkshire, parental observation of babies' responses to sound has been extended using the Hints for parents forms and questionnaires filled out by health visitors to replace screening with the distraction test.[28] In this area neonatal screening is performed on babies at risk of hearing loss and historically the distraction test had not been used effectively. Any parental suspicion or clinician's concern about a child's hearing results in a referral for audiological assessment. An anticipated advantage of this method is that fewer children with mild conductive losses will be referred thus releasing diagnostic services to deal more effectively with more severe cases. The researchers stress, however, that there would be no reduction in cost for this service because health visitors' time would be redirected and training would still be required. Frequency specific hearing loss and moderate hearing losses with abnormal loudness growth or recruitment may not be identified by this surveillance technique until there is a speech or language delay or the child goes to school. The study continues and the effectiveness of this surveillance method has yet to be decided.

Intermediate pre-school screening

Some districts still operate an intermediate screen, usually at the age of 3 years, using behavioural tests of hearing carried out by health visitors. If earlier screening is effective only very few cases of hearing loss except for conductive or acquired hearing losses should be identified. The use of scarce resources to screen all children at this age has to be balanced against the numbers detected. A compromise approach is to test the hearing of children when there is concern about hearing or speech, or language development before referring them for diagnostic testing.[29]

School entry screen

Further screening is carried out almost universally during the first year at school when good coverage should be achieved since all children are required to attend school. Sweep screening using pure tone audiometry is the most commonly used method. This involves testing at a predetermined level, usually 25 dBHL (decibel hearing level), across the speech frequency range of 500 Hz to 4 kHz. As part of an effective screening service sweep screening should not detect severe and profound hearing losses but will, however, identify conductive hearing losses and also mild, high frequency or monaural sensorineural hearing losses. These hearing losses may require intervention and it is therefore valuable to detect them by screening.[30–32]

The possibility of screening for middle ear dysfunction using tympanometry has been considered.[33] This practice could result in unnecessary referrals of children with middle ear dysfunction but with no hearing difficulty and sensorineural losses would remain undetected. Screening of older children is not widely implemented although screening at school leaving age might have public health implications in cases where there is exposure to noise in later life.

Organization of audiological services

Hearing screening programmes are of limited benefit if there are delays in the confirmation of the loss or in the fitting of hearing aids where required. Inefficient referral patterns and poor organization of audiological services can contribute to such delays.

There should be clear guidelines for community health care professionals on how, when and where referrals should be processed. Screening protocols must clearly specify pass/fail criteria and timing of referral and outline a procedure for dealing with cases where the screening test cannot be administered. Service organization and resource allocation should be targeted at identifying and fitting hearing aids to children with severe and profound hearing

Hints for Parents

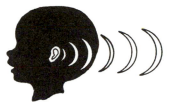

"Can your baby hear you?"

Here is a checklist of some of the general signs you can look for in your baby's first year:-

YES/NO

Shortly after birth
Your baby should be startled by a sudden loud noise such as a hand clap or a door slamming and should blink or open his eyes widely to such sounds.

By 1 Month
Your baby should be beginning to notice sudden prolonged sounds like the noise of a vacuum cleaner and he should pause and listen to them when they begin.

By 4 Months
He should quieten or smile to the sound of your voice even when he cannot see you. He may also turn his head or eyes toward you if you come up from behind and speak to him from the side.

By 7 Months
He should turn immediately to your voice across the room or to very quiet noises made on each side if he is not too occupied with other things.

By 9 Months
He should listen attentively to familiar everyday sounds and search for very quiet sounds made out of sight. He should also show pleasure in babbling loudly and tunefully.

By 12 Months
He should show some response to his own name and to other familiar words. He may also respond when you say 'no' and 'bye bye' even when he cannot see any accompanying gesture.

> Your health visitor will perform a routine hearing screening test on your baby between six and eight months of age. She will be able to help and advise you at any time before or after this test if you are concerned about your baby and his development. If you suspect that your baby is not hearing normally, either because you cannot answer yes to the items above or for some other reason, then seek advice from your health visitor.

©
Produced by Dr. Barry McCormick
Children's Hearing Assessment Centre, General Hospital, Nottingham NG1 6HA
Printed by The Sherwood Press (Nottingham) Limited

Figure 11.3 'Can your baby hear you?' Hints for Parents form. (Reproduced with kind permission from Dr Barry McCormick.)

losses within the first year of life. Referrals of children identified by neonatal or health visitor screening at 7–9 months should be given priority with accelerated access to otological and audiological rehabilitative services where a severe or profound loss is confirmed. At the 7–9 months screen it is common practice for two failures to be required before making a referral to avoid overloading services with children with transient conductive losses. To avoid delay in severe cases, the second test should be carried out no more than 2 weeks after the first test. For cases where there is a history of upper respiratory tract congestion, and there is absence of parental concern the second test can be carried out after 6–8 weeks.

If any parental concern is expressed about the hearing before a screen is carried out, it is advisable to refer immediately. Under certain circumstances older children, for example all children who have had meningitis, require urgent referral for audiological assessment because of the risk of sensorineural hearing loss.[34] Community-based health care professionals play an important role in ensuring that children suspected of having a hearing loss, and those with speech and language delays, are quickly brought to the attention of diagnostic services.

A good quality diagnostic service with a core of trained and experienced paediatric audiological personnel is required for benefit to be gained from screening programmes. Some services operate a middle-tier community clinic to sift out and manage children with mild conductive hearing losses. Such a three-tier system can have the disadvantage of prolonging the route to the diagnostic service and thus introducing delays for the more severe cases. To promote earlier detection of hearing loss and easier access to diagnostic services an open access paediatric audiology service operates in Nottingham.[35,36] Open access enables any professional or parent to refer a child for audiological assessment. The resultant overall increase in referrals to this service has demonstrated a heightened awareness of the need for prompt assessment with a consequent lowering of the age of detection of hearing loss. The referral specificity for this service is high and the respectable false-positive rate for parental referrals is comparable to that of professionals.

Haggard and Pullan[37] have considered the organization, staffing and resource implications of paediatric audiology services in some detail and have proposed a model service structure which incorporates features from the three-tier and open access types of service. The central core of such a service would be the paediatric audiology department (PAD) which would specialize in assessing young children's hearing and those children who are difficult to assess. The PAD would work in conjunction with community clinics but also accept direct referrals for more urgent groups such as neonatal or 7–9 month screen failures. Hearing loss transcends the boundaries of health, education and social services and it is necessary for professionals from these disciplines to work closely together in order to achieve the best service for the child.

Methods of investigation of hearing loss

Investigation of hearing loss should include tests to measure hearing level and indicate whether the hearing loss is conductive, sensorineural or mixed in nature. From birth to 6 months of age it is possible to observe some response to louder sound in the form of startle and stilling responses.[10,38] The auropalpebral reflex (APR) which is a blink in response to intense sound stimuli, can be observed from birth onwards. These responses can given an indication of the presence of some degree of hearing but cannot confirm precise hearing levels.

From a developmental age of 6 months it is possible to obtain frequency specific information about hearing sensitivity using a series of behavioural tests of hearing first described by Ewing and Ewing.[39] The series known as distraction, cooperative and performance tests are suitable for different ages of pre-school children and rely on the child exhibiting a particular behaviour in response to a sound stimulus dependent on the child's developmental age. A reasonably sized room which is fairly quiet and free from visual distractions is needed to carry out behavioural tests of hearing[27] but the tests are not time consuming and do not require expensive equipment. The tests are still widely used but can only be described briefly here. A detailed account of the test technique is given by McCormick.[40]

Distraction test

The distraction test, used from 6 months of age, utilizes the baby's ability to sit unsupported and turn its head to locate quiet sound stimuli presented on a horizontal plane with the child's ear. The baby is seated on the parent's lap with a small table to the front. A tester in front of the child uses small toys to regulate the child's attention to a level between being fully involved in the activity to being free to turn to sound stimuli. This tester watches the child's responses to sound and assesses their reliability.

A second tester is responsible for presenting frequency specific sound stimuli at the appropriate time and in the correct position which is a 45° angle behind the child on a horizontal plane with the child's ear. Low, middle and high frequency sound stimuli across the speech frequency range from 500 Hz up to 4 kHz should be tested independently. To ensure that frequency selective but nevertheless significant hearing losses will not be missed only frequency specific sound stimuli should be used such as warble tones.[27] It is important to note that pure tones are unsuitable for sound field testing because standing waves are created which make accurate measurement of sound levels difficult. The intensity of level of all sound stimuli presented which elicit a reliable response from the baby should be measured using a sound level meter.

Attention must be given to ensuring that there are no olfactory or visual clues given to the baby from the tester at the rear. The position of the parent should be selected so that no shadows are created from behind the parent and baby. It is necessary to look for anticipated or chance head turns of the baby by carrying out no sound trials during which both testers proceed as if a sound were to be presented but do not actually present a sound. The baby should turn its head fully to the sound stimuli to constitute a positive response. A reward in the form of a smile or a tickle of the arm should be given for appropriate responses.

Cooperative test

At a mental age of 18 months, children are normally able to understand simple spoken instructions. In the cooperative test of hearing the child is instructed to give a toy, brick or peg to a choice of at least three recipients which could be 'teddy', 'dolly', 'baby', 'mummy' or 'daddy'. Items with the same number of syllables and with acoustic similarities are recommended. The tester must initially establish that the names of the test items are known to the child and that the child understands the test procedure. This is achieved by the tester demonstrating the task at louder levels and allowing the child to watch them. The tester then returns to a distance of one metre behind the child and out of the child's visual field and gives the instructions in a random order. The level at which two out of three responses are correct should be measured. Incorrect responses can be positively corrected by replacing the brick or peg in the child's hand and repeating the instruction. Correct responses should be praised. Since the stimulus for the cooperative test is a speech signal it is necessary to supplement the test with frequency specific testing. Distraction techniques can be successfully used with this age group but it is often difficult to maintain the child's interest in the sound stimuli. Visual reinforcement audiometry is a useful alternative to distraction testing for this age group.

Visual reinforcement audiometry

The principle of visual reinforcement audiometry (VRA) is to reinforce an observed behavioural response, usually a head turn to frequency specific sounds with a visual reward.[41] VRA can be used with children of a developmental age of 6 months up to 3 years. Research has shown that VRA measurements of children with sensorineural hearing losses relate well to later audiograms.[42] The test arrangement varies in different clinics but commonly two loudspeakers, each with a visual reward, are placed one to each side of the child. Depending on their age, children may be seated on their parent's lap or on a small chair equidistant from both loudspeakers. The test room should be sound treated and have minimal visual interest. There should be a one-way observation window to a second room from where the test is controlled. Two testers usually perform the test with one tester operating the equipment and one tester working in the clinic controlling the child's attention.

Measurements should be made at low, middle and high frequency sound stimuli usually with warble tone stimuli. Initially sound is presented at well above normal hearing thresholds. The visual reinforcer, often an animal with illuminating eyes, is presented simultaneously with the sound stimulus. If necessary the parents' help may be elicited to encourage the child to turn his or her head to the stimuli. Once conditioning is established the level can be reduced to find the quietest level to which the child consistently responds. The visual reward is now presented *after* the child has turned towards the sound and the visual stimulus together with changes in the frequency of the sound stimuli prolongs the child's attention span. Anticipation of either the auditory or visual stimulus by the child is usually eliminated after a period when there is no visual reward.

VRA is a powerful technique for the assessment of hearing sensitivity in young children. The need for calibrated non-portable equipment and a suitable test room usually restricts the use of VRA to diagnostic clinics unlike the more traditional pre-school behavioural hearing tests.

Performance test

The performance test can be used with children of a developmental age of approximately 30 months and above. The children are conditioned to wait until they hear a sound and then carry out an activity such as putting pegs in a board or toy men in a boat. The tester must first demonstrate the task in view of the child with the sound stimuli at a raised level. When the child is conditioned to carry out the task the tester goes out of view of the child. The level of the sound is raised until the child responds consistently and this level is then measured. The sound stimuli must be frequency specific such as warble tones. It is important to vary the length of time between stimulus presentations to ensure that the child is not anticipating the stimulus. True responses should be praised and false responses can be corrected in a positive manner by reversing and repeating the activity for example removing the peg from the board or taking the man out of the boat.

Pure tone audiometry

Having conditioned the child to carry out a performance test, similar conditioning techniques and play activities can be used to obtain a pure tone audiogram.[43] The recommended British Society of Audiology procedure should be employed.[44] Once conditioning is established the stimulus intensity level should be reduced from the suprathreshold level in 10 dBHL steps until there is no response. The stimulus level is then increased in 5 dBHL steps until there is once again a response. This procedure is repeated until the threshold is reached, which is the lowest level, when ascending, at which two out of three responses are obtained. If standard headphones are used the measurement is known as air conduction audiometry because the sound has to be conducted through the whole auditory pathway from the outer ear. Bone conduction measurement refers to thresholds obtained via a bone vibrator placed on the mastoid process.[45] In this case sound is conducted via the bone direct to the inner ear or cochlea thus by-passing the outer and middle ears.

The audiogram is the graphical form of the results of pure tone audiometry. The vertical axis gives the measure of intensity or loudness in decibels for the hearing level (dBHL). The horizontal axis shows the frequency or pitch which is measured in hertz (Hz) (Fig. 11.4). Thresholds are usually measured at 500 Hz, 1 kHz, 2 kHz and 4 kHz bilaterally but other frequencies may also be tested if the child's concentration allows this. Audiograms must be interpreted with care because although headphones allow some separation

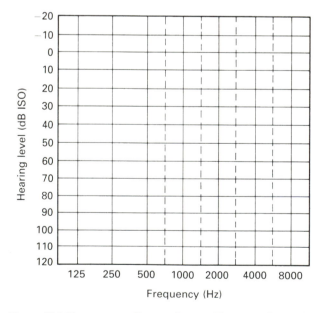

Figure 11.4 Pure tone audiogram format. The vertical axis shows the intensity (loudness) in decibels and the horizontal axis shows frequency (pitch) in hertz.

between the ears, if there is a difference of more than 40 dBHL between the thresholds of each ear, sound will cross over giving rise to a shadow threshold. With bone conduction testing the better ear gives the response regardless of which side the bone conductor is placed on. In order to overcome crossover the technique of masking is used. This procedure introduces a masking noise at specific levels to the non-test ear in a carefully defined way that a true threshold may be obtained.[46] A difference between air and masked bone conduction threshold could indicate the presence of a conductive component to a hearing loss. If masking is not carried out it is not always possible to make accurate interpretations about the presence of a conductive element to a hearing loss.

Speech discrimination tests

Although tests of speech discrimination cannot replace tests which evaluate hearing at specific frequencies, they provide a valuable check on such tests and can be useful in demonstrating a child's hearing sensitivity to parents and teachers. With older children speech discrimination tests designed for use with adults may be used, for example wordlists presented through headphones.[47] For detailed and general information on speech audiometry the reader is referred elsewhere.[48]

Some speech discrimination tests have been designed specifically for children. In these tests age appropriate vocabulary is used often coupled with pictures such as the Reed hearing test[49] which uses monosyllabic words. The Bamford Kowal and Bench BKB sentence tests for children[50] provide a simplified form which relates to pictures of the speech stimuli in the form of sentences.

Picture related tests are generally suitable for children of school age. Speech discrimination tests with toys are more appropriate for pre-school children. The Kendall toy test comprises three lists of 10 items each.[51,52] These items are represented by toys together with another five distractor items to lessen the possibility of chance responses. The child is required to point to the appropriate item when he is instructed to do so. In practice often only one of the three lists is used although the original design of the test was such that each list should be presented at a different listening level.

McCormick has designed a toy discrimination test using seven pairs of items, represented by toys, which have acoustically similar names.[53] Initially the tester must check that the child knows each item by either asking them to say what each item is or by checking with the parent. If a particular toy is not known to the child that toy and its pair can be removed from the test. A minimum of two pairs of items can be used thus making the test versatile and accessible to the very young child. The child is asked to point to the appropriate item when instructed. The level at which the child consistently responds is recorded.

Most speech discrimination tests for young children are carried out using live voice and require the tester to measure levels with a sound level meter. The tester must be careful to keep his voice at the correct level and measure the level correctly. The McCormick toy discrimination test has been automated using microchip technology.[54] The test words are presented with a carrier phrase through a loudspeaker placed in front of the child. The tester controls the test using a key pad which allows for repetitions at the same or louder levels if required. This development has allowed levels to be measured more accurately and frees the tester to concentrate on the child. Results of trials with the automated version of the McCormick toy discrimination test show good correlation with averaged pure tone audiometric thresholds.[55]

Objective measurements of hearing thresholds in children

The hearing impaired child with other problems has been discussed in depth by Mencher.[56] Behavioural tests can often be successfully used by experienced testers with children who are difficult to test, such as those with other disabilities, provided that the test is appropriate to their developmental level. There still remain some children who cannot be tested behaviourally and these children, no matter how young or disabled, should not be denied the opportunity of a hearing assessment. There are also some children with non-organic hearing loss who will not cooperate with behavioural testing. Different methods such as electric response audiometry (ERA) may be required to assess hearing thresholds in these children.

Electric response audiometry

Electric response audiometry (ERA) covers a range of different electrophysiological tests of hearing which are dealt with in depth elsewhere.[57–59] Electrodes placed on the skull are used to record nerve potentials in response to a sound stimulus which is usually a click with centre frequency 2–3 kHz. The responses are very small and computer averaging techniques are required to identify the resultant waveform among other physiological noise. In children ERA measurements are primarily used to determine hearing thresholds, but by analysing the latency and amplitude of the waves it is possible to obtain some indication of the type of hearing loss.

The auditory brainstem response (ABR) has already been discussed in the context of neonatal screening. The ABR is the most suitable of all the auditory evoked potentials for testing young children and infants because the response is resistant to adaptation or habituation effects, is not affected by sleep or sedation

and the technique is non-invasive. Under optimum recording conditions the waveform is stable and can be recorded reliably with stimulus intensities close to zero. The technique does not, however, give ideal low frequency information and may require sedation.

Electrocochleography measures responses derived from the cochlea or auditory nerve. The recording electrode is placed close to or through the tympanic membrane; this procedure requires anaesthesia. This technique is less commonly used with infants and young children than ABR measurements.

The auditory cortical response (ACR) is less reliable in young children owing to a reduction in the amplitude of responses during sleep or sedation. The ACR is more acceptable for children aged 8 years or more where the response stabilizes and becomes easier to identify. The whole auditory pathway must be intact to give normal ACR thresholds. This test is useful when pure tone audiometry does not give reliable thresholds as, for example, in cases of non-organic hearing loss.

Substantial investment in equipment and a test environment with low levels of acoustic noise and electrical inteference are required to carry out ERA measurements. Considerable expertise is necessary to interpret waveform traces accurately. For these reasons ERA testing is normally limited to specialist evoked potential clinics or diagnostic audiology departments but it does, nevertheless, form a valuable and necessary part of a comprehensive audiological service.[60]

Evoked otoacoustic emissions

Emissions or echoes from the ear were first demonstrated by Kemp.[61] Emissions can be evoked by presenting a sound, usually a click, in the ear canal via a small probe fitted with a soft plastic tip which forms a seal in the ear canal. A microphone in the same probe detects the emission in the ear canal. As with the ABR the emission is a very small time-locked response and computer averaging techniques are therefore required to record the response. The waveform recorded is unique to each ear but the pattern of the waveform is linear and highly stable. The presence of an emission is determined by examination of the waveform but should incorporate correlation between replicate traces and some assessment of the signal to noise ratio.[62,63] The presence of an emission is indicative of normal cochlear function but does not give a measurement of hearing thresholds. Most cochlear hearing losses of greater than 20 dBHL or middle ear dysfunction will abolish the emission. Evoked otoacoustic emission measurements are used for neonatal screening and also diagnostically.[64,65] The presence of emissions together with startle responses, auropalpebral reflexes and stapedial reflexes in infants under 6 months of age would suggest near normal hearing sensitivity. The technique is useful for older children where reliable pure tone audiometry is not possible and non-organic hearing loss is suspected because only passive cooperation is required. Evoked emissions testing can help to determine whether a hearing loss is due to cochlear dysfunction or some pathology at a high level of the auditory pathway.[66]

Tests of middle ear function

Given the prevalence of otitis media in children, tests of middle ear function are an important part of a comprehensive audiological assessment. The measurement of acoustic impedance provides a means of investigating the efficiency of the middle ear system in transmitting sound energy entering the ear canal to the cochlea.[67–69] Most impedance meters (also known as admittance meters) employ a probe placed against or just entering the ear canal and forming an airtight seal. The probe comprises a sound transducer which produces a low frequency tone, a microphone to measure sound reflected from the tympanic membrane and a pump to change the pressure in the ear canal. In a healthy middle ear most sound energy is absorbed and transmitted through the system. If there is a difference in pressure between the two sides of the tympanic membrane the mechanism becomes stiff and most of the sound energy is reflected. The process of observing the variation in stiffness or compliance as a function of pressure difference across the tympanic membrane is known as tympanometry. The resulting graph of compliance against pressure is the tympanogram.

Different conditions may cause reduced or high compliance and there is a wide variation in normal values thus making diagnoses difficult. A shallow flat type of curve, however, has considerable diagnostic potential in children since it is usually due to otitis media with effusion. A flat line with a high volume indicates a perforation of the tympanic membrane or the presence of a patent grommet in situ. The volume measured by the probe in these circumstances is the volume of the ear canal and the middle ear cavity.

Acoustic reflex measurements

When a normal ear is stimulated with a fairly intense sound the stapedius muscle in the middle ear contracts thus tensing the ossicles in the middle ear and decreasing the impedance. This is known as the stapedius or acoustic reflex and can be measured on most impedance meters.[69,70] Any disorder of the middle ear results in the suppression of the contraction of the stapedius muscle such that no response can be recorded on the impedance meter. Detectable changes in impedance when an ear is stimulated by a sufficiently loud acoustic signal strongly implies that middle ear function is normal. The presence and threshold of the acoustic

reflex must be interpreted with caution. With profound sensorineural loss the response may be absent even though tympanometry is within normal limits because the stimulus cannot be presented at loud enough levels. In some cases of severe and moderate sensorineural hearing losses the difference between the threshold of hearing and the acoustic reflex threshold, the dynamic range, may be considerably reduced compared with that for normal ears. This phenomenon is known as abnormal loudness growth or recruitment.

Testing for the presence or absence of reflexes is particularly valuable for young infants or children who are difficult to test since only passive cooperation is required. This techique is also helpful is determining whether there is a monaural loss in cases where sound field testing has shown some localization difficulty.

Hearing aids

The early provision of amplification is required to maximize the use of residual hearing. The hearing aid is therefore an important part of a rehabilitation programme aimed at reducing the disability experienced by the hearing impaired child.[71,72] Conventional hearing aids make ambient sound louder across a limited frequency range, and can considerably aid auditory communication, but they do not restore normal hearing. When selecting hearing aids for fitting one should take account of their type and electroacoustic features. These issues can only be discussed briefly here but more comprehensive accounts can be found elsewhere.[73–75]

Types of hearing aid

All hearing aids comprise basically a microphone to detect sound, a variable amplifier, a receiver to convert the amplified signal back into sound and a battery to power the amplifier (Fig. 11.5). The most common type of hearing aid is the postaural or behind the ear aid where all of the components are contained within one case. A plastic hook (elbow) is screwed on to the aid which sits on the ear and connects the aid to the earmould. The microphone is close to the natural position of the ear and, with binaural fitting, localization ability and signal detection in noise are improved.[76,77] Miniature postaural aids which are more suitable for young children are now available. With small babies a more angled ear hook can keep the aid in position. In most cases body-worn aids no longer have significant advantages over the postaural aids in terms of output for profound hearing losses. The receiver is separate from the aid and is connected via a lead. Both of these components are susceptible to damage and the quality of the sound signal is affected by body

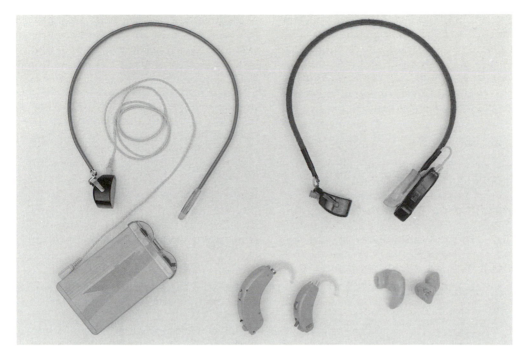

Figure 11.5 Hearing aids. Top left: body-worn conduction aid; top right: postaural bone conduction aid; bottom centre: postaural hearing aids; bottom right: in-the-ear hearing aids.

baffle and the noise of clothes rubbing across the microphone.

In-the-ear aids fit wholly within the concha and ear canal. In-the-ear aids are currently suitable only for people with mild or moderate hearing losses because of their limited amplification. These types of hearing aid are rarely fitted to young children who require new ear moulds at frequent intervals. This usually necessitates sending the whole aid back to the manufacturers for a new case. Postaural, body-worn and in-the-ear aids utilize air conduction of the amplified sound signal. When abnormalities of the pinna or medical conditions of the middle ear prevent the fitting of such aids a bone conduction hearing aid may be required. These aids transmit sound energy to the cochlea by vibration of the skull and can also be used for patients with large conductive losses. They are, however, rather cumbersome because they involve the use of a bone vibrator placed on the mastoid process and held in place by a headband. Hearing aids commonly have some user operated switches including the on/off switch. There may also be internal screwdriver operated switches which are adjusted by the clinician and alter the gain and maximum output of the aid. Many hearing aids have tone controls which allow modifications to be made to the frequency response of the aid. This is the output of the aid at different frequencies for a given input of sound and may be expressed graphically. Some hearing aids have a telecoil (T) setting for use with electromagnetic loop systems or direct input facilities to enable direct coupling of the aid to a radio system.

The output of the hearing aid must lie within the child's dynamic range of hearing. The aid must therefore be sufficiently powerful to amplify sound above the threshold of hearing but the level of amplification must not exceed the child's loudness discomfort level. Many hearing aids have facilities to limit the maximum output by either peak clipping or automatic gain control. Peak clipping involves 'chopping' the peaks off the amplified waveform at varying levels but can introduce marked distortion. Automatic gain control (AGC) operates by compressing the degree of amplification above a certain loudness level. AGC distorts the signal less than peak clipping but the times of activation and cessation of the AGC, known as the attack and release times, must be appropriate so that the early part of a loud sound is not over amplified or that transient sounds do not trigger the AGC unnecessarily.

The earmould

In order to fit a hearing aid an earmould is required to deliver the amplified sound into the ear canal. The earmould anchors postaural aids and the receivers of body-worn aids and forms the case of in-the-ear aids. The earmould must fit well to give a good acoustic seal. Poorly fitting earmoulds give rise to feedback which occurs when amplified sound escapes from the ear canal and is reamplified resulting in a high pitched whistle. The earmould must also be easy to insert and remove, comfortable and cosmetically acceptable. Most earmoulds are made by a two-stage process where an impression of the shape of the ear is made in the clinic and then manufactured into a more permanent earmould. The recommended procedure for impression taking is described by the British Society of Audiology.[78] A variety of materials and styles may be used to make earmoulds depending on the patient's needs, the degree of hearing loss, and the type of hearing aid to be used. Soft materials are often better for young children because they fit better and are more comfortable.[72] Good moulds can be made for babies and young children provided that the impression taker is skilled and experienced. They are discussed further by Nolan.[79] Earmoulds should be replaced as often as necessary, up to every 3–4 weeks for very young children, to ensure a consistently good acoustic seal.

The fitting of hearing aids and the assessment of aided benefit

The fitting of a hearing aid must take into account the information about response levels at specific frequencies obtained during testing which gives the degree and shape of a child's hearing loss. With very young babies below the age of 6 months it may be necessary to rely initially on ABR thresholds for middle and high frequency information supplemented with observation of the child using the aids by parents, teacher and audiologist.[72] Binaural fitting should be routine except where there are contraindications such as a large difference in hearing sensitivity between the ears or where the pinna is absent on one side.[76]

All children fitted with hearing aids should be assessed for aided benefit and reviewed at least yearly. Young children should be reviewed much more frequently in the early stages after fitting to obtain more definitive information about the hearing levels so that appropriate changes in amplification can be made. The electroacoustic features of the aid should be checked against the manufacturers' specifications at the time of fitting and at review appointments. Hearing aid test box equipment can be used to assess the frequency response, maximum output and harmonic distortion of hearing aids. *Real ear insertion gain measurement* is a technique involving the insertion of a thin flexible probe microphone into the ear canal, with or without the hearing aid and earmould in position, to give measurements of the aided and unaided sound field in the ear canal.[80] This can assist in the selection of hearing aids for infants and children who are unable to carry out behavioural tests of hearing, but the child must remain very still. Functional gain, that is how the child responds using behavioural testing with the child wearing the aid, provides vital information about the suitability of aids and their settings.[81]

Aided sound field warble tone measurements provide an excellent measure of functional gain using developmentally appropriate test techniques of distraction, performance testing or visual reinforcement audiometry. Speech tests carried out in noise[82] have also been used to assess aided benefit but require some linguistic ability. The McCormick toy discrimination test can also be used in the automated or live voice format with some children to supplement information from aided warble tone testing and can provide a useful demonstration of the benefit of hearing aids.

When fitting hearing aids, and at subsequent reviews, it is necessary to check for loudness discomfort. If stapedial reflexes are elicited the clinician should be alerted to the presence of abnormal loudness growth and the possibility of loudness discomfort.[81,83] In all cases sound stimuli such as warble tones or narrow band noise should be presented at an intense level to the child wearing the aids. If there is any sign of discomfort such as blinking, flinching or crying it will be necessary to use an aid with output limitation or adjust the level of automatic gain control or peak clipping if the aid already has these facilities.

In addition to the measurements already described, hearing levels should be rechecked in case there has been any change. Tympanometry should be carried out to determine whether there is any conductive component requiring medical treatment. General comments from parents, teachers, or the child regarding the length of time the child wears the aid, responses to sound as well as changes in speech and language development and any signs of intolerance should be noted. Close liaison between audiological, medical and educational personnel and parents is necessary to give optimum support for the hearing impaired child.

Amplification for the educational setting

In classrooms there is often considerable background noise. Sound reflection from hard surfaces such as walls, floors and tables contributes to background noise.[84] By bringing the microphone of an amplification system closer to the speaker speech can be received with less noise contamination. There are various options available for transmitting the signal to the child from a microphone placed close to or worn by the speaker.[75]

Electromagnetic induction involves the use of a wire loop to convert the output from the microphone into an electromagnetic field. A telecoil within the child's hearing aid receives this signal. The hearing aid must have a T or MT setting to receive respectively the signal via the telecoil only or via the telecoil and the hearing aid microphone simultaneously. Owing to variation in the field strength and possible interference, induction loops are not often used in schools now but may be beneficial in theatres and churches or for listening to the television. Infra-red light can be used to transmit the signal from the microphone to the child's receiver. The system is susceptible to strong sunlight and the path between the transmitter and receiver must be free of obstacles.

FM radio transmission is the preferred system for use in schools. The transmitter utilizes a radio frequency carrier wave to bring the signal to the child's receiver. There are two types of radio system; the first being an integral part of a body-worn hearing aid which is often more practical for very young children. With the second type of radio system the receiver is used in conjunction with the child's own hearing aids. A neck loop connection is possible using electromagnetic induction and the telecoil setting of the hearing aid but the output may vary as the child's head moves. A hard wire direct input type of connection provides the most consistent signal. It is, however, important to use leads and connection shoes that are compatible with the child's hearing aids, and to set each individual system to obtain a clear signal.[85] Different transmission frequencies can be used in different classrooms to overcome possible crossover of a signal between two groups. Most systems have a choice of two carrier frequencies which can be used for different purposes, for example, for use in the classroom and in school assembly.

Advances in hearing aid technology

Increasingly sophisticated hearing aids are becoming available. Programmable hearing aids where the electroacoustic features required for an individual patient are stored in the aid are now available.[86] Some programmable aids store more than one programme for different situations such as listening to speech in quiet and noisy locations or listening to music.[87] Implanted bone conduction hearing aids are proving useful for cases of significant conductive loss where there is difficulty in wearing conventional air or bone conduction hearing aids.[88–90]

Research is continuing with signal processing in hearing aids to assist lipreading for profoundly deaf people who only respond to very low frequencies. These aids extract some of the important features of speech and present a simplified signal at frequencies within reach of the patient's residual hearing.[91,92]

Tactile aids also provide an aid to lipreading and give some awareness of environmental sounds for people who derive only minimal benefit from acoustic hearing aids.[93,94] Vibrotactile devices function by producing a vibratory stimulus when a sound is detected via a microphone. These devices are usually single channel, where there is no discrimination between different frequencies of sound, or dual channel where two sites of vibration are activated by two different frequency bands of the auditory signal. Vibrotactile aids provide limited information and an intensive period of training is required, but the instruments are relatively inexpensive and non-invasive. Some users find them very beneficial whereas others do not continue to use them despite intensive rehabilitation.

Cochlear implants

Cochlear implants provide a means of electrical nerve stimulation to produce a sensation of hearing.[95,96,97] Cochlear implants were first carried out in the USA, but considerable advances have subsequently been made in Australia. In the UK, cochlear implants have been used with children who are so deaf that they cannot derive any acoustic benefit from conventional hearing aids.[98] Children below the age of 2 years cannot currently be considered for implantation because of rapid skull growth below this age and the developmental requirements for the child to carry out the tests needed to programme the device. Older children who have been deaf for a long time and congenitally deafened adults appear to derive less benefit from cochlear implants.

Several different types of cochlear implant systems are available. They may be single channel having only one active electrode or multichannel with several electrodes. If the electrodes are inserted inside the cochlea the device is an intracochlear implant, but if the electrodes are placed on the promontory and the cochlea remains intact, the device is extracochlear. Multichannel intracochlear devices have generally been shown to give the most benefit. Intracochlear implants can only be used if the cochlea is patent and CT scans are required as part of the pre-implant assessment to check for ossification as can occur following meningitis. The electrode array is implanted surgically. Externally the patient wears a microphone and a speech processor to process sound so that it can be transmitted to the internal electrode array. Most speech processors are currently about the same size or larger than conventional body-worn hearing aids. The link across the skin from the external to the internal parts of the system may be via a percutaneous plug or an electromagnetic radio link through the intact skin. The latter method is commonly felt to be more suitable for young children. Some speech processors deliver the signal using an analogue system where different frequency bands are delivered to different electrodes. Alternatively the speech processor extracts the important features of speech and some high frequency bands and delivers them to the electrode array in a series of very short fast pulses.

The benefit derived from a cochlear implant is dependent on several factors including the age of the child, the age of onset of the deafness and the duration of the deafness. Young congenitally deaf children have been implanted in the USA, Australia and Europe and although their progress is thought to be more gradual than children with acquired losses the potential for benefit is still considerable.[99,100] The family must be prepared for the lengthy pre-implant assessments, and the time consuming tuning-in or programming of the device coupled with intensive rehabilitation which are vital for successful use of the implant.[101] This is a very exciting and rapidly changing area of development in helping young deaf children.

Acknowledgements

The author would like to thank Dr Barry McCormick for his helpful comments and Mrs Kathryn Beardsley for typing the manuscript.

References

1 Elliott, L.L., Armbrusher, V.B. Some possible effects of the delay of early treatment of deafness. *J Speech Hearing Res* 1967; **10**: 209–224.

2 Gerber, S.E., Mencher, G.T., eds. *Early Diagnosis of Hearing Loss*. New York: Grune and Stratton, 1978.

3 Markides, A. Age at fitting of hearing aids and speech intelligibility. *Br J Audiol* 1986; **20**: 165–167.

4 McCormick, B. Hearing screening for the very young. In: Meadows, R., ed. *Recent Advances in Paediatrics*. London: Churchill Livingstone, 1986: 185–199.

5 Davis, A. A public health perspective on childhood hearing impairment. In: McCormick, B., ed. *Paediatric Audiology 0–5 years*. London: Whurr, 1993: 1–41..

6 Martin, J.A.M., Bentzen, O., Colley, J.R.T., *et al*. Childhood deafness in the European Community. *Scand Audiol* 1981; **10**: 165–174.

7 Simmons, F.B. Identification of hearing loss in infants and young children. *Otolaryngol Clin N Am* 1978; **11**: 19–28.

8 Haggard, M.P. Monitoring the efficiency of hearing screens for the first year of life. *Audiol Pract* 1986; **III/4**: 3–5.

9 Gerber, S.E. Review of a high risk register for congenital or early-onset deafness. *Br J Audiol* 1990; **24**: 347–356.

10 Bennett, M.J. Trials with the auditory response cradle: I neonatal responses to auditory stimuli. *Br J Audiol* 1979; **13**: 125–134.

11 Simmons, F.B., Russ, F.N. Automated newborn hearing screening. The crib-o-gram. *Arch Otolaryngol* 1974; **100**: 1–7.

12 Davis, A.C., Wharrad, H.J., Sancho, J., Marshall, D.H. Early detection of hearing impairment: what role is there for behavioural methods in the neonatal period. *Acta Otolaryngol (Stockh)* 1991; Suppl **482**: 103–109.

13 McCormick, B., Curnock, D.A., Spavins, F. Auditory screening of special care neonates; using the auditory response cradle. *Arch Dis Child* 1984; **59**: 1168–1172.

14 Duara, S., Suter, C.M., Bessard, B.S., Gutberlet, M.D. Neonatal screening with auditory brainstem responses: results of follow-up audiometry and risk factor evaluation. *J Pediatr* 1986; **108**: 276–281.

15 Alberti, P.W., Hyde, M.L., Riko, K., Corbin, H., Abramovich, S. An evaluation of B.E.R.A. for the hearing screening in high risk neonates. *Laryngoscope* 1983; **93**: 1115–1121.

16 Mason, S.M. On-line computer scoring of the auditory brainstem response for estimation of hearing threshold. *Audiology* 1984; **23**: 277–296.

17 Mason, S.M. Automated system for screening hearing using the auditory brainstem response. *Br J Audiol* 1988; **22**: 211–213.

18 Mason, S.M., Barber, C., Davis, A.C., McCormick, B. Evolution and detectability of the neonatal A.B.R: implications for automated screening of hearing. In: Gallai, V., ed. *Maturation of the CNS and Evoked Potentials*. Amsterdam: Elsevier Science Publishers, 1986: 194–203.

19 Stevens, J.C., Webb, H.D., Hutchinson, J., Connell, J., Smith, M.F., Buffin, J.T. Click evoked otoacoustic emissions in neonatal screening. *Ear Hearing* 1990; **11**: 128–133.

20 Bonfils, P., Dumont, A., Marie, P., Francois, M., Narcy, P. Evoked otoacoustic emissions in newborn hearing screening. *Laryngoscope* 1990; **100**: 186–189.

21 Stevens, J.C., Webb, H.D., Smith, M.F., Buffin, J.T., Ruddy, H. A comparison of otoacoustic emissions and brainstem electric response audiometry in the normal newborn and babies admitted to a special care baby unit. *Clin Phys Physiol Measure* 1987; **8**: 95–104.

22 Teele, D.W., Klein, J.O., Rosner, B.A., the Greater Boston Otitis Media Study Group. Otitis media with effusion during the first three years of life and development of speech and language. *Pediatrics* 1984; **74**: 282–287.

23 McCormick, B. Hearing screening by health visitors: a critical appraisal of the distraction test. *Health Visitor* 1983; **56**: 449–451.

24 McCormick, B. Evaluation of a warbler in hearing screening tests. *Health Visitor* 1986; **59**: 143–144.

25 Latham, A.D., Haggard, M.P. A pilot study to detect hearing impairment in the young. *Midwife, Hlth Visitor Commun Nurse* 1980; **16**: 370–374.

26 Hitchings, V., Haggard, M.P. Incorporation of parental suspicions in screening infants hearing. *Br J Audiol* 1983; **17**: 71–75.

27 McCormick, B. *Screening for Hearing Impairment for Very Young Children*. London: Croom Helm, 1988: 27–38, 39–43, 69–79.

28 Scanlon, P.E., Bamford, J.M. Early identification of hearing loss: screening and surveillance methods. *Arch Dis Child* 1990; **65**: 479–485.

29 Hall, D., ed. *Health for All Children: a Programme for Child Health Surveillance*. Oxford: Oxford Medical Publications, 1991.

30 Fisch, L. Development of school screening audiometry. *Br J Audiol* 1981; **15**: 87–95.

31 Martilla, T.I. Results of audiometric screening in Finnish school children. *Int J Paediatr Otorhinolaryngol* 1986; **11**: 39–46.

32 Bess, F.H., Klee, T., Culbertson, J.L. Identification, assessment and management of children with unilateral sensorineural hearing loss. *Ear Hearing* 1986; **7**: 43–51.

33 Brookes, D.N. Impedance in screening. In: Jerger, J., Northern, J., eds. *Clinical Impedance Audiometry*. Massachusetts: American Electromedics Corporation, 1980; 164–182.

34 Dawson, J.A., Wardle, R. Detection and prevalence of hearing loss in a cohort of children following serogroup B, meningococcal infection 1983–1987. *Pub Hlth* 1990; **104**: 99–102.

35 McCormick, B., Wood, S.A., Cope, Y., Spavins, F.M. Analysis of records from an open-access audiology service. *Br J Audiol* 1984; **18**: 127–132.

36 McCormick, B. The development of a model paediatric audiology service. In: *Medicine and Management*. Published proceedings of the fourth Trent Region Seminar, Nuffield Provincial Hospital Trust, 3 Albert Road, London NW1 7SP, 1988: 100–113.

37 Haggard, M.P., Pullan, C.R. Staffing and structure for paediatric services in hospital and community units. *Br J Audiol* 1989; **23**: 99–116.

38 Wharrad, H.J. Neonatal hearing screening tests. In: McCormick B., ed. *Paediatric Audiology 0–5 Years*. London: Taylor and Francis, 1988: 69–79.

39 Ewing, I.R., Ewing, A.W.G. The ascertainment of deafness in infancy and early childhood. *J Laryngol Otol* 1944; **59**: 309–338.

40 McCormick, B., ed. Behavioural hearing tests 6 months to 3.6 years. In: *Paediatric Audiology 0–5 Years*. London: Whurr, 1993: 102–123.

41 Bamford, J., McSporran, E. Visual reinforcement audiometry. In: McCormick, B., ed. *Paediatric Audiology 0–5 Years*. London: Whurr, 1993: 124–154.

42 Talbot, C.B. A longitudinal study comparing responses of hearing impaired infants to pure tones using visual reinforcement and play audiometry. *Ear Hearing* 1987; **8**: 175–179.

43 Wood, S. Pure tone audiometry. In: McCormick, B., ed. *Paediatric Audiology 0–5 Years*. London: Whurr, 1993: 155–186.

44 Recommended procedure for pure tone audiometry using a manually operated instrument. *Br J Audiol* 1981; **15**: 213–216.

45 Recommended procedure for pure tone bone-conduction audiometry without masking using a manually operated instrument. *Br J Audiol* 1985; **19**: 281–282.

46 Recommendations for masking in pure tone threshold audiometry. *Br J Audiol* 1986; **20**: 307–314.

47 Boothroyd, A. Developments in speech audiometry. *Sound* 1968; **2**: 3–10.

48 Martin, M. *Speech Audiometry*. London: Whurr, 1987.

49 Reed, M. *R.N.I.D. Picture Screening Test of Hearing*. Royal National Institute for the Deaf, 105 Gower Street, London, 1969.

50 Bench, J., Kowal, A., Bamford, J. The BKB (Bamford-Kowal-Bench) sentence lists for partially hearing children. *Br J Audiol* 1979; **13**: 108–112.

51 Kendall, D.C. Audiometry for young children. *Teacher of the Deaf* 1953; **306**: 171–177.

52 Kendall, D.C. Audiometry for young children. *Teacher of the Deaf* 1954; **307**: 18–23.

53 McCormick, B. The toy discrimination test: an aid for screening the hearing of children above a mental age of two years. *Pub Hlth* 1977; **91**: 67–73.

54 Ousey, J., Sheppard, S., Twomey, T., Palmer, A.R. The IHR/McCormick automated toy discrimination test – description and initial evaluation. *Br J Audiol* 1989; **23**: 245–251.

55 Palmer, A.R., Sheppard, S., Marshall, D.H. Prediction of hearing thesholds in children using an automated toy discrimination test. *Br J Audiol* 1991; **25**: 351–356.

56 Mencher, G.T., Gerber, S.E., eds. *The Multiply Handicapped Hearing Impaired Child*. London: Grune and Stratton, 1983.

57 Gibson, W.P.R. *Essentials of Clinical Electric Response Audiometry*. London: Churchill Livingstone, 1978.

58 Thornton, A.R.D. Electrophysiological measures of hearing function in hearing disorders. *Br Med Bull* 1987; **43**: 926–939.

59 Mason, S.M. Electric response audiometry. In: McCormick, B., ed. *Paediatric Audiology 0–5 Years*. London: Whurr, 1993: 187–249.

60 Mason, S., McCormick, B., Wood, S. Auditory brainstem response in paediatric audiology. *Arch Dis Child* 1988; **64**: 465–467.

61 Kemp, D.T. Stimulated acoustic emissions from within the human auditory system. *J Acoust Soc Am* 1978; **64**: 1386–1391.

62 Kemp, D.T., Ryan, S., Bray, P. A guide to the effective use of otoacoustic emissions. *Ear Hearing* 1990; **11**: 93–105.

63 Lutman, M.E., Sheppard, S. Quality estimation of click-evoked otoacoustic emissions. *Scand Audiol* 1990; **19**: 3–7.

64 Probst, R., Lonsbury-Martin, B.L., Martin, G.K. A review of otoacoustic em ions. *J Acoust Soc Am* 1991; **89(5)**: 2027–2059.

65 Cope, Y., Lutman, M. Otoacoustic emissions. In: McCormick, B., ed. *Paediatric Audiology 0–5 Years*. London: Whurr, 1993: 250–290.

66 Lutman, M.E., Mason, M., Sheppard, S., Gibbin, K.P. Differential diagnostic potential of otoacoustic emissions. *Audiology* 1989; **28**: 205–210.

67 Jerger, J., Hayes, D. Diagnostic applications of impedance audiometry: middle ear disorder; sensorineural disorder. In: Jerger, J., Northern, J., eds. *Clinical Impedance Audiometry*. Massachusetts: American Electromedics Corporation, 1980: 109–127.

68 Jerger, J., Hayes, D. Clinical use of acoustic impedance testing in audiological diagnosis. In: Beagley, H.A., ed. *Audiology and Audiological Medicine*. Oxford: Oxford University Press, 1981: 707–722.

69 Brooks, D.N. Acoustic measurements of auditory function. In: McCormick, B., ed. *Paediatric Audiology 0–5 Years*. London: Whurr, 1993: 291–311.

70 Djupesland, G. The acoustic reflex. In: Jerger, J., Northern, J., eds. *Clinical Audiometry*. Massachusetts: American Electromedics Corporation, 1980: 65–82.

71 Cunningham, D.R., Ganzel, T.M., Steckol, K.F. Hearing aids for children: a primer for physicans. *J Kentucky Med Assoc* 1986; **84**: 619–623.

72 Wood, S., McCormick, B. Use of hearing aids in infancy. *Arch Dis Child* 1990; **65**: 919–920.

73 Pollack, M. *Amplification for the Hearing Impaired*. Orlando, Florida: Grune and Stratton, 1988.

74 Seewald, R.C., Ross, M. Spiro, M.K. Selecting amplication characteristics for young hearing-impaired children. *Ear Hearing* 1985; **6**: 48–53.

75 Evans, P.I.P. Hearing aid systems. In: McCormick, B., ed. *Paediatric Audiology 0–5 Years*. London: Whurr, 1993: 312–354.

76   Markides, A. *Binaural Hearing Aids*. London: Academic Press, 1977.

77   McKenzie, A.R., Rice, C.G. Binaural hearing aids for high frequency hearing loss. *Br J Audiol* 1990; **24**: 329–334.

78   Recommended procedure for taking an aural impression. *Br J Audiol* 1986; **20**: 315–316.

79   Nolan, M. Earmoulds. In: McCormick, B., ed. *Paediatric Audiology 0–5 Years*. London: Whurr, 1993: 378–401.

80   Dillon, H., Murray, N. Accuracy of twelve methods for estimating the real ear gain of hearing aids. *Ear Hearing* 1987; **8**: 2–11.

81   Green, R. Hearing aid selection and evaluation for preschool children. In: McCormick, B., ed. *Paediatric Audiology 0–5 Years*. London: Whurr, 1993: 355–377.

82   Jerger, S., Jerger, J., Fehah, R. Paediatric hearing aid evaluation: case reports. *Ear Hearing* 1985; **6**: 240–244.

83   Seewald, R.C., Ross, M. Amplification for young hearing impaired children. In: Pollack, M.C., ed. *Amplification for the Hearing Impaired*, 3rd edn. London: Grune and Stratton, 1988: 213–271.

84   Nabelek, A.K. Effects of room acoustics on speech perception through hearing aids by normal hearing and hearing impaired listeners. In: Studebaker, G.A., Hochberg, I., eds. *Acoustic Factors Affecting Hearing Aid Performance*. Baltimore: University Park Press, 1980: 25–46.

85   Wood, S., Cope, Y., McCormick, B. A guide to fitting type 2 radio hearing systems in direct input mode. *J Br Assoc Teachers Deaf* 1990; **14**: 133–141.

86   Staab, W.J. Digital/programmable hearing aids – an eye towards the future. *Br J Audiol* 1990; **24**: 243–256.

87   Ringdahl, A., Erikson-Mangold, M., Israelsson, B., Lindkrist, A., Mangold, S. Clinical trials with a programmable hearing aid set for various listening environments. *Br J Audiol* 1990; **24**: 235–242.

88   Gates, G.A., Hough, J.V., Gatti, W.M., Bradley, W.H. The safety and effectiveness of an implanted electromagnetic hearing device. *Arch Otolaryngol Head Neck Surg* 1989; **115**: 924–930.

89   Roush, J., Rauch, S.D. Clinical application of an implantable bone conduction hearing device. *Laryngoscope* 1990: **100**: 281–285.

90   Bowning, G.G. The British experience of an implantable, subcutaneous bone conduction hearing aid (Xomed Audiant). *J Laryngol Otol* 1990; **104**: 534–538.

91   Rosen, S., Walliker, J.R., Fourcin, A.J., Ball, V. A microprocessor based acoustic hearing aid for the profoundly impaired listener. *J Rehab Res Dev* 1987; **24**: 239–260.

92   Faulkner, A., Rosen, S., Moore, B. Residual frequency, selectivity in the profoundly hearing impaired listener. *Br J Audiol* 1990; **24**: 381–392.

93   Roser, R.J. Tactile aids: development issues and current status. In: Owens, E., Kessler, D.K., eds. *Cochlear Implants in Young Deaf Children*. Boston, Massachusetts: College-Hill Press, 1989: 101–135.

94   Worsfold, S., Day, J. Touching the sound barrier. *Speech Ther Pract* 1991; **6**: 21–22.

95   Cooper, H., ed. *Cochlear Implants: a practical guide*. London: Whurr, 1991.

96   Sheppard, S. Cochlear implants. In: McCormick, B., ed. *Paediatric Audiology 0–5 years*. London: Whurr, 1993: 402–436.

97   Tyler, R.S., ed. *Cochlear Implants: Audiological Foundations*. London: Whurr, 1993.

98   McCormick, B. Paediatric cochlear implants: the Nottingham experience. In: Haggard, M., ed. *Clinical Developments in Cochlear Implants – Current Approaches*. Southampton: Duphar Laboratories Limited, 1990, 75–78.

99   Osberger, M.J., Miyamoto, R.T., Zimmerman-Phillips, S. Independent evaluation of the speech perception abilities of children with the Nucleus 22 channel cochlear implant system. *Ear and Hearing* 1991; **12**: 665–805.

100   Staller, S., Beiter, A.L., Bromacambe, J.A., Mecklenburg, D.J., Arnolt, P. Paediatric performance with the Nucleus 22 channel cochlear implant system. *Am J Otol* 1991; **12**: 126–136.

101   McCormick, B., Archbold, S., Sheppard, S., eds *Cochlear Implants for Young Children*. London: Whurr, 1994.

Chapter 12

Speech and language disorders

Lewis Rosenbloom and Susan Roberts

Language is an acquired skill and the ease with which most children develop linguistic competence by the age of 5 years belies its highly complex and abstract nature.

Language is essentially an interactive system of symbols used for communication purposes. These symbols may be utilized in spoken, written or gestural forms to represent concepts. The interactive nature of language requires a speaker and a listener, or a writer and reader, in order to fulfill the intended communication of concepts or ideas. While the early conceptual use of language is very concrete it assumes more abstraction as linguistic skills develop.

There have been many theories about the manner in which most children acquire language in a rapid and apparently effortless way. The classical explanation was that language acquisition occurred through a process of imitation and reinforcement. Children would copy sounds they heard around them and, after trial and error and reinforcement and reward from adults, would gradually match the normal models of language.

It is clear that imitation cannot be the only explanation, however, since children frequently use many forms of language which they would not hear in adult speech. For example 'mouses' for 'mice', or 'broked' for 'broken'. In the 1960s Chomsky[1] proposed that children are born with an innate capacity for language development. He referred to this as the language acquisition device. This innate structuring device allows the child to recognize grammatical features, for example rules about plurals and verb tenses, or that in the English language the subject always precedes the verb in a sentence. In the previous example the child has recognized the rule that plurals usually have 's' or 'es' at the end, while past tenses usually have 'ed' at the end. After a period of trial and error the child's grammatical forms will match the adult norm.

Although maturation and imitation both contribute towards the acqusition of language, the idea of a language acquisition device goes further towards explaining the rapidity of normal language development.

Components of communication

It is axiomatic that there is much more to communication than talking. Inner languages, symbolic thinking, play and verbal comprehension are fundamental bases for expressive language to develop and be used.

a Inner language

Language is firstly used as a tool for thinking, both in children and in adults. This function is commonly called inner language. The capacity to internalize thought in this way is a crucial cognitive skill which is progressively acquired throughout childhood. For young children it can be illustrated in the way that they play using toys and everyday objects, for example tea sets or dolls, where their imaginative play indicates that they can both understand and use symbols in thought. This can take place without the symbols being translated into words, so that the play sequence can be silent. The observation of symbolic play in childhood forms part of the assessment of linguistic competence.

b Verbal comprehension

The second important aspect of language is the ability to understand the speech of others. This is called verbal comprehension or receptive language.

Verbal comprehension emerges in parallel with inner language. Each reinforces the other. This can be illustrated by a child who is acquiring the symbolic play of putting cups, saucers, forks etc on a table at around the age of 18–24 months. At this stage he should be able to follow a verbal instruction such as 'put the cup on the table'. The more complex and developed a child's play becomes, the more complex verbal instructions he is able to follow.

Inner language and verbal comprehension are more fundamental to cognitive and linguistic competence than is expressive language and normally develop considerably in advance of expressive abilities.

c   Expressive language

Expressive language is a third aspect of language, and is itself composed of several interrelated parts:

    i Semantics
    ii Grammar (syntax)
    iii Phonology (speech sounds)
    iv Pragmatics

Semantics

Semantics is concerned with the meaning of words and is basic to communication. Young children are able to get their message across without the use of correct grammar, although meaningful communication is heavily dependent upon the context in which the exchange takes place, e.g. The child says 'daddy car'. This may reflect one of several situations: daddy's going to work; daddy's arrived home; daddy's washing the car.

It is only with the acquisition of correct grammar that the utterance becomes less reliant on the context or situation.

Up to 2 years of age, 75% of a child's vocabulary is made up of nouns and verbs. These come from common semantic fields, such as food, parts of the body and toys.

Grammar

Grammar consists of two parts: syntax and morphology.

Syntax may be defined as the rules governing the combining of words into sentences and phrases, thus in English the subject always precedes the verb.

Morphology is the term used to define the change within the word itself in order to indicate different grammatical roles, as in plurals and verb tenses – look, looked, looks, looking.

Phonology

Phonology describes the way in which the sound system of language is organized so that contrasts between sounds alter meaning, for example pea/bee. A phonological problem is essentially where there is difficulty in acquiring the rules of the linguistic system, rather than where there is a problem of motor coordination.

Children with language difficulties frequently have phonological problems. By contrast articulation is independent of language and refers to the physical ability to produce sounds. Articulation disabilities are seen for example in children with cerebral palsy and those with cleft palates.

Pragmatics

Pragmatics refers to using language in a social, interactive context. Although the very young child (9–18 months) may only have a limited range of single words, he can use these words for a wide variety of functions – to seek attention, to request objects, to reject, to greet and to name are all examples.

The development of language in childhood

Like other parameters of development the various skills that comprise linguistic competence are progressively acquired from earliest infancy. Smiling and other early social interactions, babbling, understanding tones of voice in play and other situations and progressively the development of the understanding of words and the use of these in speech occur during the first and second years of life. Thereafter increasing sophistication of comprehension and fluency of expression continue to be acquired throughout the remainder of childhood. All of these skills are complemented and fostered when there is concurrent development of physical skills, sensory functioning (especially so far as vision and hearing are concerned) and learning abilities. Problems in any of these areas can produce a knock on effect in all of the others. The obvious link between the normal development of hearing and the acquisition of language skills exemplifies this. Moreover, the child's environment and particularly the opportunities and encouragement given to develop language are all basic to its satisfactory acquisition.

It follows that, whenever communication skills fail to develop satisfactorily, whatever may be the reason for this, children are significantly disadvantaged, not only from the linguistic viewpoint but are also at risk from developing behavioural, social and emotional difficulties.

For these reasons the importance of early screening and the identification of language problems cannot be stressed strongly enough. It has been increasingly recognized over recent years that early intervention is more effective for remediation of language disorders.[2,3] In these circumstances, it is appropriate that screening programmes for communication disorders in childhood require to be developed and applied.

Screening and referral for a speech and language assessment

The successful application of screening to language development is possible only when this is considered within the context of children's development as a whole. While it is easy to measure height and weight, the nature of language precludes such easy measurement. Instead observation of the pre-school child with access to appropriate play materials provides useful information about inner language. Verbal comprehension can be examined by looking at a child's ability to follow verbal instructions, although it is important to avoid the use of gestures, visual cues or too much in the way of situational cues. Expressive language can be looked at in relation to a child's ability to name objects or talk about simple pictures.

The following are broad guidelines for referral to a speech therapy service for more specific assessment of speech and language:

1 A child who has no words at 20–24 months
2 A child who is not speaking in phrases at 28–30 months
3 A child who is unintelligible at 3 years of age or older
4 Parental concern at any stage always needs to be taken into account.

In the UK speech and language therapists provide a service of assessment, diagnosis and treatment for people of all ages suffering from communication problems. The majority of speech and language therapists who work with children are employed within the National Health Service (NHS) but may work in a variety of settings including some locations outside the NHS, such as schools and social service establishments. Most speech therapy services and departments operate an open referral system.

Assessment of speech and language disorders

Assessment is an ongoing and continuous process. The starting point is dependent on what is already known about the child and the presenting problems. The choice of assessment procedures will take into account the child's ability to interact and respond. Formal standardized assessments may be carried out, or more informal observational techniques used; most assessments combine the two.

A speech and language therapist may also record a language sample from the child so that a transcription and analysis can be carried out at a later stage.

Standardized assessments

Many standardized assessments are norm referenced and provide standardized scores which compare an individual child's achievements with those of his peer group within a relevant population. The following are a selection:

1 The Reynell Developmental Language Scales (RDLS) can be used with children aged from 6 months to 6 years.[4] The assessment provides scales for both verbal comprehension and expressive language.
   a Verbal comprehension scale A assesses the child's ability to understand single words by identifying objects or pictures, the ability to relate two objects and to perform increasingly complex activities in response to verbal instructions.
   b Verbal comprehension scale B can be used with both physically handicapped children who have poor motor control, and those children who are shy and withdrawn.
The expressive scale of the RDLS is divided into three sections:
   a Scale 1 assesses early vocal behaviour, use of definite words and word combinations. These can either be accredited from parents' comments or elicited by the assessor.
   b Scale 2 assesses vocabulary through object and picture naming.
   c Scale 3 assesses content and idea through describing pictures.
2 The British Picture Vocabulary Scale (BPVS)[5] assesses the child's receptive vocabulary across the age range from $2\frac{1}{2}$ to 18 years. The child is required to select one drawing from a set of four which best illustrates the meaning of a stimulus word. The final raw score can be converted to a standardized score and a percentile rank.
3 The Pre-School Language Scales[6] are designed to measure receptive and expressive language in children aged 1 to 7 years, this includes items which measure discrimination, grammar, vocabulary, memory, attention span, temporal and spatial relationships. The tasks are developmentally sequenced.
4 The Symbolic Play Test[7] assesses early concept formation and symbolization in children in the age range 1 to 3 years. The child is credited with scores for each response and connection that he or she is able to make when presented with four sets of miniature toys, for example relating a spoon to the cup or saucer.
5 Test for Reception of Grammar (TROG).[8] An individually administered multiple choice test designed to assess understanding of grammatical contrasts in English with an age range 4–13 years. The child is required to select one picture from a set of four

which corresponds to a phrase or sentence spoken by the tester.

6 The Derbyshire Language Scheme.[9] This scheme provides objective measures for evaluating early symbolic abilities, verbal comprehension and expression.

7 The Pragmatics Profile of Early Communication Skills.[10] This profile is used to explore the early communication of children from a pre-linguistic stage of development up to the age of 5 years, in conjunction with parents and carers and in a wide variety of settings.

Informal procedures

Observation techniques need to be used frequently to supplement or confirm the measures derived in the use of standardized assessments. Systematic observation of children's behaviour in both structured and free play situations can provide valuable information and it is also useful to know whether this behaviour can be modified by adult intervention or interaction.

In addition, transcriptions of language samples may be made and analysed for both grammatical and phonological information.

LARSP. The language assessment remediation and screening procedure[11] details the stages of children's syntactic development from 9 months to approximately $4\frac{1}{2}$ years. Following analysis of a language sample an approximate functional age level can be reached. Similarly, phonological development can be assessed from a speech sample following phonetic transcription.

It is also necessary to look at a child's attention capacity, given that many children with speech and language difficulties also have poor attention skills. Levels of functioning attention control can be assessed according to developmental status.[2]

The information gathered from a period of assessment is used to diagnose the nature of an individual child's language problems. These need to be viewed within the context of development as a whole and usually need to be made in conjunction with advice from other professionals.

Disorders of speech and language

Causes

The causative factors of communication difficulties fall into four broad and overlapping areas.

Neurological abnormality

Taking this group at its widest it includes both developmental and acquired neurological disorders. Not infrequently there are associated neurological problems in cerebral palsy, and the neurological basis of the child's speech and language problems is then obvious. When however there are no additional neurological features demonstrable either by examination or investigation, as is so with a majority of children with developmental language disorders, the neurological origin (in its widest sense) has to be assumed. It should be made clear, however, that this neurological basis to developmental language problems does not equate with a label of brain damage. It is more helpful to postulate neurological dysfunction as the cause which may be temporary and recoverable. It is disappointing but not surprising that the increasing availability of sophisticated neurological investigations has not led to a more precise definition of the dysfunction that underlies a variety of developmental disorders of which those affecting speech and language are but one group.

Sensory impairment of hearing and/or vision

These impairments have major effects on language and other aspects of children's development; they are discussed in the relevant chapters in this volume. Intermittent or fluctuating conductive hearing loss may be an important factor in language delay and poor early development.

Emotional disorders

Emotional and behavioural problems are discussed in detail elsewhere in this volume. Delay or difficulty in acquiring language in childhood, when seen in isolation is, for all practical purposes, never caused solely by emotional disturbance in that affected children will always show other behavioural symptoms. This is exemplified in the discussion on elective mutism. The distressing and disturbing effect on children who have language disorders and on their families is also important. It can not only compound the severity of the symptoms but also hinder remedial approaches.

Environmental deprivation

Delay in acquiring a variety of linguistic skills is a concomitant of the other features of environmental deprivation.

Incidence of speech and language disorders

Figures for the incidence of speech and language disorders are scarce and imperfect, coming from a relatively small number of surveys carried out over the past 40 years. These have produced widely varying figures, ranging from less than one in 1000 to more than 20 in 100 children having difficulty with communication at some time in their school life. A useful review of these surveys has been made by Webster and McConnell.[12]

The general picture which emerges suggests that around one child in every 1000 is likely to have severe difficulty in acquiring spoken language; one child in 100 will have difficulties that seriously affect their education and some 10 children in 100 may have difficulties that could interfere with educational progress at some time.

Developmental language delay

This term is often used loosely about any language difficulty. It has a more precise meaning however and should be applied to any child whose overall development is normal but whose language development, which may include both verbal comprehension and expressive language, is progressing at a slower rate. The linguistic stages follow a normal pattern of development. If the level of linguistic functioning is significantly behind developmental norms then some form of therapeutic intervention is likely to be required.

The principal management is to offer specific and structured linguistic programmes of remediation. This may be designed individually for the child, or taken from one of a number of commercially available programmes.

These can be carried out in a variety of ways but it is most important that all those involved with an individual child – parents, carers and teachers – are included. It is important also that there is flexibility in the choice of location for therapy which may be school, nursery, home or playgroup, so that the child is seen in the most appropriate context with the most suitable people. Progress will be dependent not only on what happens during speech therapy sessions, but also on the management of the problem in all other aspects of daily life.

On-going reassessment and review is an important part of the overall management.

If the delayed language development is part of overall or global developmental delay these specific language programmes may be less helpful and a scheme such as Portage might be more useful.[13]

Specific language disorders

The cause of specific language disorders is unknown but as discussed above it is reasonable to assume that their basis lies in a degree of neurological dysfunction or immaturity which may be temporary and recoverable. Children with specific language disorders have normal language learning environments and do not have any of the primary disabilities which may interfere with language development, e.g. hearing loss or learning difficulties. Nevertheless, their language difficulties may be severe enough to persist even given optimum language learning opportunities and strategies.

Although specific language disorder is distinguished from language delay the distinction can often be difficult to make, especially in the early stages, since the first sign of a persistent language disorder is indeed delay in acquiring language.

Presenting problems

Specific language disorders may affect all aspects of language acquisition. Difficulties in expression are most likely to be noticed first, especially in the development of phonology and syntax. There is likely also to be difficulty in acquiring the full range of speech sounds.

The language disordered child's acquisition of grammar commonly shows omission of function words, such as 'a', 'the', problems in acquiring verbs and in using pronouns correctly. Sentences may be telegrammatic and immature. Affected children often make false starts when speaking and have difficulty formulating sentences.

Nevertheless, it has been documented that the difficulties are rarely confined to expressive language.[14] Comprehension difficulties may be masked and attributed instead to poor attention or lack of cooperation. These difficulties may be compounded by associated problems with attention, perception, memory, rhythm, sequencing and motor ability.

Poor auditory memory may lead to processing problems, particularly as children are expected to deal with longer and more abstract messages in the classroom or nursery situation. Recalling words from memory may also be poor so that vocabulary appears limited.

One of the effects of this range of problems is that social skills may be slower to develop in language disordered children due to reduced opportunities for verbal interaction within the peer group. A long-term sequel is that the children may develop inadequate literacy skills in their school careers.[15]

Management

Children with specific language disorders are thought to have difficulties in the language learning process, not only delay but also distortion of their language patterns. They are likely to require intensive and long-term remedial teachers and speech therapists, with individual programmes of work.

Distinguishing language delay and language disorder from the viewpoint of the help required is difficult and it will be argued that the children in these two groups form a continuous spectrum of disability. In practice, the severity of the problems and their failure to resolve with a relatively low level of intervention distinguishes, from a therapeutic viewpoint, the group that requires continuing and intensive help and who without this may well have a poorer prognosis.

Phonological syntactic syndrome[16]

Within the overall umbrella of children with developmental language disorders a number of more specific entities have been described. They are unlikely to be wholly self-contained but are, nevertheless, useful to use from both the diagnostic and intervention viewpoints.

Phonological syntactic syndrome is the most common variety of developmental language disorder. Affected children have difficulty in the acquisition of both phonology and syntax while displaying otherwise normal development and verbal comprehension. There is a wide range of severity, from unintelligibility to relatively minor deviations in the sound system.

Affected children are likely to require regular speech therapy and individual programmes of work designed to help gradual acquisition of the rules of both phonology and grammar. However, children who are functioning at the same age level or who have similar difficulties appear to be helped best in a small group situation.

Semantic pragmatic disorder[16]

The principal difficulty in this type of developmental language problem lies in using language appropriately as a social tool. Difficulties in the semantic field (in understanding meaning) can lead to major comprehension difficulties (in understanding abstract concepts). The difficulties however are more generalized in that affected individuals have problems in comprehending the rules of social behaviour. They not only use their language in a rigid and literal way, while failing to follow the rules of conversation regarding turn taking and changing topic, but also may respond inappropriately to non-verbal cues.

Affected children usually have clear and fluent expressive language hence the synonym for this disorder of 'fluent language disorder'.[17] The relatively good expressive skills are however misleading and may contribute to delayed recognition of the condition.

It is also likely that there is considerable overlap between the condition that psychiatrists now identify as Asperger's syndrome and semantic pragmatic disorder.[18] The differences are likely to be those of emphasis, rather than pathology, with the social functioning difficulties which, in effect, amount to a mild form of autism, being emphasized more when the label of Asperger's syndrome is given.

The management of children with semantic pragmatic disorders is not so well established as it is for those with other specific language problems. Linguistic research into semantics and pragmatics is relatively recent and has not hitherto formed the basis for therapeutic concepts. Experience indicates however that affected children require a specialist teaching approach with much emphasis on social skill training programmes. Nevertheless, the difficulty in learning from social cues and hence in functioning appropriately in society does appear to be long term for more severely affected children.

Autism

The difficulties of using language both as a tool of thought and socially are seen in their most severe degree in children labelled as being autistic. Recent changes in classification have meant that the phrase pervasive developmental disorder is now taken to encompass the whole range of autistic conditions. This is useful in emphasizing how wide the development difficulties are in severely autistic children.

The three main groups of symptoms comprise severe impairment in the development of social relationships, a failure of development of all modalities of communication and a lack of imaginative play.

From a very early age, affected children are isolated with gaze avoidance and an apparent unwillingness or inability to have social contacts with others including their parents. Not only do verbal comprehension and expressive language fail to develop but there is a similar failure of development of symbolic understanding and of gesture when the condition is seen in its most severe form. In parallel to these difficulties is a lack of symbolic and imaginative play with behaviour being compulsive, ritualistic and characterized by obsessions instead.

The majority of autistic children also have severe learning difficulties and are in effect severely mentally handicapped as well as being socially isolated with major linguistic and behavioural difficulties. A minority are not so severely affected however. These children may have isolated skills seen most frequently in a demonstration of perceptual abilities and less often with drawing or musical skills or feats of memory. These isolated abilities may be age appropriate or even more advanced.

This group of autistic children are likely to develop some language which is often clear from an expressive viewpoint but is then used in a superficial and stereotyped way. Their difficulties in social relationships usually remain and could well be considered to be the primary and most major area of dysfunction.

The ultimate ability of autistic children to lead an independent life is determined by their combination of intellectual abilities and potential to mature socially. From the linguistic viewpoint speech and language therapy needs to be offered within a multidisciplinary setting and should be concerned initially with fostering the development of symbolic skills and verbal comprehension.

Learning difficulties

It has been estimated that 55% of all people with a mental handicap will have some associated speech or language difficulty.[19] The range and patterns of linguistic problems are much the same as those seen in children of normal intellectual ability but are often masked and missed because of the associated problems. This is seen for example in two of the most common conditions that are associated with mental handicap, Down syndrome and fragile X syndrome. Many, if not the majority, of individuals with Down syndrome have additional language problems which can make all the difference between their being reasonably competent socially and their being totally dependent. These difficulties include severe phonological syntactic disorders and major comprehension problems that could well be associated with intermittent conductive hearing loss in early childhood. Similarly, boys who have fragile X syndrome not only have a reasonably consistent range of learning and behavioural difficulties but also a range of compounding expressive language problems.

From the diagnostic and therapeutic viewpoints a combination of lack of awareness, interest and resources has led to a frequent failure to recognize and treat the language problems of children with learning difficulties. In theory all children who are recognized as having cognitive problems should have a linguistic assessment and relevant speech and language therapy, usually within a multidisciplinary setting from an early age. In practice this happens infrequently with the inevitable consequence that unrecognized and untreated language problems compound children's learning difficulties. For many this makes the difference between their eventual success or failure in independent functioning as adults.

Elective mutism

Children who appear to choose where and when to speak are seen infrequently and form a particularly taxing diagnostic and therapeutic group. The majority will talk in some specific situations, for example with families at home, but not in other situations, most notably in the infant school. At the more severe end of the spectrum elective or selective mutism can be both prolonged and profound. In such circumstances it is also invariably associated with other evidence of emotional or behavioural disturbance and management needs to be concentrated upon these aspects of functioning.

A proportion of electively mute children appear however to develop this pattern of behaviour secondary to their having inherent language difficulties, usually in the form of an expressive disorder. They then choose not to speak because of shyness, embarrassment or because they know they are likely not to be understood. Linguistic assessment which frequently has to be from secretly recorded tapes should thus always be part of the evaluation of children who refuse to talk and where necessary relevant speech and language therapy programmes should be instituted.

Disorders of fluency

Dysfluency is more commonly referred to as stammering or stuttering.

Many people experience varying degrees of dysfluency at some time during their life, often when tired or under stress. Interruptions to the fluency of speech, ('uhm', 'er') are used to a greater or lesser degree by various people, but are an acceptable part of communication. It is only when the dysfluency disrupts speech to an abnormal degree that it becomes a communication disorder, causing an imbalance in the verbal exchange between speaker and listener.

As children develop their language skills, many will go through a period of dysfluency. This stage usually occurs between the ages of 3–4 years and is referred to as normal non fluency, or *developmental non fluency*. The child tends to repeat whole words e.g. 'can . . . can . . . can I have a drink'. They will not normally be using any associated struggle behaviours.

Although most children will not require any direct form of therapeutic intervention for normal non fluency, an early speech and language assessment is advisable. This would allow for an early differential diagnosis of a more chronic stutter, as recent research recommends.[20] Parents are often very anxious about this problem and should be able to discuss their anxieties with the speech and language therapist.

Over the years there have been countless theories offered as to the cause of dysfluency. It has been viewed at various times as an operant disorder, a disorder of prosody, a cognitive linguistic disorder, a sequencing and timing or temporal programming disorder. Boys are more affected than girls and one current research programme is investigating hormone levels as a causative factor. Dysfluency has been reported in all cultures and across all social groups.

Various estimates have been made as to its incidence. These range from 3.5 per 100[21] to one per 1000.[22] Van Riper[23] surveyed 1000 children from birth to 15 years of age and found that prevalence varied from 0.5% at 3 years of age to a maximum of 1.6% at 8 years of age; by 12 years of age it had stabilized at 1.1%. The great variance between the estimates is probably because of the age differences in the groups studied. If a median point between all the estimates were to be taken, there are likely to be 616 000 people with a disorder of fluency in the UK.

The onset of stammering usually occurs between the ages of 2 and 5 years. The child's speech may be characterized by whole word repetitions, part word repetitions or prolongations of syllables. The child may have associated struggle behaviours. These may result in blocking on the initial sound of a word, or on certain words. Stammerers often have delayed speech and language development and tend to have early difficulties of articulation.[24]

Research indicates that there are different characterizations in the speech of normal non fluent children, compared with those who may go on to develop a stammer. Meyers[25] found that stammerers had more part word repetitions, prolongations and tense pauses, while non stammering children showed more whole word repetitions. A child may be at risk of developing a stammer if any of the following are reported:

1 Any family history of stammering
2 Family pressures
3 High expectations
4 Sibling rivalry
5 Other speech and language problems, e.g. articulatory difficulties.

From the case history taken by the speech and language therapist, a comprehensive profile of the child's personality, background, family status and environment will be compiled. The child's speech will be fully assessed and all stuttering behaviours noted for their frequency and severity.

One current philosophy on the management of dysfluency is to adopt a pragmatic approach, using available and established facts and involving the whole family, not just the child with the presenting problem. Other management approaches advocate more direct methods of modifying the child's stuttering behaviours. This is particularly indicated when the child himself is concerned about the dysfluency and seeking help. There is no single cure for stammering, but the child may be offered the means to understand the problem, and the opportunity to learn techniques to control his speech.

Where direct intervention is recommended, speech and language therapy may be carried out either on an individual basis, or within a group. In addition, many young stammerers have difficulty in asserting themselves and find social interaction problematic. If the dysfluency persists into adolescence, social skills training in addition to speech retraining may be required.

References

1 Chomsky, N. *Language and Mind*. New York: Harcourt Brace Jovanovich, 1968.
2 Cooper, J., Moodley, M., Reynell, J.K. *Helping Language Development*. London: Edward Arnold, 1978.
3 Byers Brown, B. *Speech Therapy Principles and Practice*. Edinburgh: Churchill Livingstone, 1981.
4 Reynell, J.K. *Reynell Developmental Language Scales*. Windsor: NFER, 1977.
5 Dunn, L.M., Dunn, Lesta, M., Whetton, C. *British Picture Vocabulary Scales*. Windsor: NFER, 1982.
6 Zimmerman, I.L., Steiner, V.G. *Pre-school Language Scale*. London: Charles E Merrill Pub. Co., 1979.
7 Lowe, M., Costello, A.J. *Symbolic Play Test*. Windsor: NFER, 1976.
8 Bishop, D. *Test for Reception of Grammar*. Newcastle: Dept of Speech, University of Newcastle, 1983.
9 Knowles, W., Madislover, M. *The Derbyshire Language Scheme*. Ripley, Derbyshire (private publication), 1982.
10 Dewart, H., Summers, S. *The Pragmatics Profile of Early Communication Skills*. Windsor: NFER, 1988.
11 Crystal, D., Fletcher, P., Garman, M. *The Grammatical Analysis of Language Disability: a Procedure for Assessment and Remediation*. London: Edward Arnold, 1976.
12 Webster, A., McConnell, C. *Special Needs in Ordinary Schools: Children with Speech and Language Difficulties*. London: Cassell Educational, 1987.
13 Bluma, S., Shearer, M., Frohman, A., Hilliard, J. *Manual of the Portage Guide to Early Education*. Windsor: NFER, 1976.
14 Bishop, D. Comprehension in developmental language disorders. *Dev Med Child Neurol* 1979; **21**: 225–238.
15 Stackhouse, J. An investigation of reading and spelling performance in speech disordered children. *Br J Disord Commun* 1982; **17**: 53–60.
16 Rapin, I., Allen, D. Developmental language disorders: nosologic considerations. In: Kirk, I., ed. *Neuropsychology of Language, Reading and Spelling*. New York: New York Academic, 1983.
17 Ajuriajuerra, J. de, Jaeggi, A., Guignard, F. *et al*. The development and prognosis of dysphasia in children. In: Morehead, D.M., Morehead, A.E., eds. *Normal and Deficient Child Language*. Baltimore: University Park Press, 1976.
18 Bishop, D., Rosenbloom, L. Childhood language disorders: classification and overview. In: Yule, W., Rutter, M., eds. *Language Development and Disorders*. Oxford and Philadelphia: Mackeith Press, 1987.
19 Enderby, P., Philips, R. Speech and language handicap: towards knowing the size of the problem. *Br J Disord Commun* 1986; **21**: 151–165.
20 Wall, M.J., Myers, P.L. *Clinical Management of Childhood Stuttering*. Baltimore: University Park Press, 1984.
21 Andrews, G., Harris, M. *The Syndrome of Stuttering*. London: Heinemann, 1964.
22 Dalton, P., Hardcastle, J. *Disorders of Fluency*. London: Edward Arnold, 1977.
23 Van Riper, C. *The Nature of Stuttering*, 2nd edn. Hemel Hempstead: Prentice Hall, 1982.
24 Andrews, G., Craig, A., Feyer, A.M. *et al*. Stuttering: a review of research findings and theories. *J Speech Hearing Disord* 1983; **48**: 246–286.
25 Meyers, S. Qualitative and quantative difference of patterns of variability in dysfluencies emitted by preschool stutterers and non stutterers during diadic conversations. *J Fluency Disord* 1986, **11**: 293–305.

Chapter 13

Visual disorders

13.1 Minor visual defects

John Elston

This section covers visual defects of infancy and childhood which are minor in the sense of not interfering with general development or education. They include strabismus, amblyopia, and refractive error. The emphasis is on detection and diagnosis without the use of specialized ophthalmological expertise or equipment.

The development of vision

The visual system at birth is anatomically and functionally immature. The development of high acuity vision and full binocularity begins shortly after birth and continues to the age of about 8 years. This time is known as the sensitive period for the development of visual function.[1] The sensitive period has a sudden onset, probably in the fourth to sixth weeks of life, a period of high susceptibility to disruption in infancy and early childhood and then a slow decline.[2] Interference with normal anatomy, refraction or movements of one eye during this period will result in amblyopia, strabismus and reduced or absent binocularity. Untreated, these defects will be permanent. *Amblyopia* (lazy eye) denotes poor central visual acuity, or fixation not correctable optically. The eye is usually anatomically normal, but amblyopia can be superimposed on for example a developmental anomaly. The pupil reaction, field of vision and colour vision are normal. *Strabismus* (squint) is a misalignment of the visual axes which may be manifest (always present) or latent (revealed only by special tests). If manifest

it is accompanied by degraded or absent binocularity so that the most sensitive test for the presence of strabismus is one that reliably and specifically reveals reduced or absent stereoscopic (three dimensional) vision.[3] Random dot stereograms provide this information and, if positive, indicate the presence of full sensory binocularity (sensory fusion). Motor fusion is indicated by the ability to maintain full stereopsis in the face of prismatic deviation of the visual axes by up to 40 prism dioptres base out (temporal) and 10 dioptres base in (nasal).

The neurological substrate of binocularity is the primary visual cortex, where 85% of cells are binocularly driven. There is experimental and clinical evidence indicating that during the sensitive period the two eyes are in competition with one another.[4] Any factor, for example a ptosis, that interferes with the afferent visual system of one eye results in a progressive reduction in its input to the binocular cells in the visual cortex, which become responsive only to the normal eye. There are also histological changes in the lateral geniculate body (part of the afferent visual system) where the number of cells driven by the deprived eye falls.

The possibility of limited recovery of neuronal structure and visual function if the disruption is not too severe or for too long emphasizes the importance of the early diagnosis of strabismus and amblyopia. Patching of the normal eye to promote visual development in the amblyopic eye is most effective early in the sensitive period and is the necessary preliminary to surgical re-alignment of the visual axes if a strabismus is present.

Examination of the infant's visual system

Healthy neonates may have either straight eyes or, in up to 60%, a divergent strabismus, which may be intermittent. Over the first 4–6 months of life, the prevalence of divergence lessens and deviations become smaller.[5] A large persistent divergent strabismus suggests an underlying central nervous system disorder. Convergent strabismus is not seen in normal neonates but may develop between 2 and 4 months of age. This is the age at which normal alignment of the eyes and stereoscopic vision begin to develop and the fundamental defect may be a failure of maturation of binocular cells in the visual cortex. Convergent strabismus is always abnormal and, since it may be intermittent at onset, repeated examinations may be necessary to confirm its presence.

Examination of an infant's visual system is important to exclude the surgically treatable causes of severe visual handicap, particularly congenital cataracts and congenital glaucoma. It is possible to establish the anatomical normality of the eyelids and external eye, including the clarity of the cornea using a pen torch. In *congenital glaucoma* the cornea is hazy or opaque and enlarged. Photophobia and tearing are prominent.

The most common cause of a persistently watery eye in infancy is an imperforate nasolacrimal duct. It may be accompanied by mucous discharge. There is no interference with the development of vision and, in 90% of cases, the problem resolves spontaneously in the first year of life. Massage of the sac may help to speed the process and antibiotics drops should only be used if infection supervenes.

Congenital cataracts may be seen as a white spot in the pupil. If not, they can be visualized by the light reflected from the retina. The observer looks along the ophthalmoscope beam which is aimed at the pupil at arm's length with all the dials turned to zero. A visually significant cataract will show as a black shadow against the red reflex and can be seen before the development of nystagmus, or the behavioural characteristics of poor visual function. This test is therefore an important part of the examination of every neonate. The earlier the cataracts are treated, the better the visual outcome; most early treated children will develop better than 6/18 vision.[6] Because of the profound amblyopia that accompanies unilateral congenital cataract, surgery is not usually recommended.[6]

Visual function is difficult to assess clinically in infants. However, mothers who complain that their infant either squints or cannot see properly, are very rarely wrong. The majority of minor visual defects, as defined at the start of this chapter, will be noticed by the child's parents.

Maternal concern about poor eye contact can be investigated by holding the baby with the head supported, and face to the examiner's face. The examiner then spins, for example in a swivel chair, on his own axis through 90°. The acceleration will drive the infant's eyes in the opposite direction (vestibulo-ocular reflex) and if vision is normal the infant will refixate with a fast eye movement onto the examiner's face. If vision is poor the eye movements will tend to be much more random. The infant should also fixate steadily on a bright light source.

There is evidence that infants prefer to fixate on a card or screen filled with a grating of regularly spaced bars, in preference to a blank of the same luminosity.[7] The width and contrast of the grating bars against the background can be varied and an attempt made thereby to measure the visual function objectively (grating acuity). The monocular grating acuity can be assessed in the clinic with cards (for example Teller grating acuity cards) or using computer generated displays. Photorefraction is another method that may enable the identification of *hypermetropia* (long sightedness) and *myopia* (short sightedness) in preverbal children.[8] Those at risk of developing amblyopia and strabismus may thereby be identified.

Infantile esotropia is a large angle convergent strabismus usually, or at least initially, without amblyopia. The cause is not known; although convergent strabismus occurs commonly in conditions such as hydrocephalus and in very low birthweight infants with periventricular haemorrhage, infantile esotropes typically are developmentally and neurologically normal. Refractive error is not usually an aetiological factor. The treatment is surgical after alternate eye patching to protect against amblyopia, and theoretically the best results in terms of the development of binocularity will be achieved if the visual axes are re-aligned by the age of 18 months to 2 years. High grades of binocularity are never achieved in infantile esotropes. Some children may develop some stereopsis, accompanied by a small convergent strabismus (micro-esotropia) which will ensure stability of the visual axes.

Infantile convergent strabismus may also be the result of a unilateral or asymmetric developmental abnormality of the afferent visual pathway, such as congenital cataract or optic nerve hypoplasia. Acquired pathology including, importantly, retinoblastoma may present as unilateral strabismus. A fundus examination through a fully dilated pupil is therefore mandatory in all cases.

Delayed visual maturation (DVM) is a relatively common failure of normal visual development characterized by anatomical normality of the eyes, including the retinae and optical nerves, but poor visual function in infancy. The parents notice poor eye contact and a lack of visual interest. The child is otherwise neurologically and developmentally normal; electrophysiological examination is mandatory – an electroretinogram (ERG) to exclude a retinal dystrophy or dysplasia, and a cortical visual evoked potential (VEP) to establish the normality of the visual pathways. In DVM the VEP may be normal or have a somewhat reduced amplitude.[9] Isolated DVM has an excellent prognosis and affected infants have normal vision by the age of 4 to 6 months. DVM may also occur in association with structural, ocular or neurological abnormalities involving the visual system.

Spontaneous nystagmus developing in infancy or early childhood even if intermittent is always abnormal. The development of normal stable ocular fixation is critically dependent on a normal afferent visual system, and nystagmus may be the presenting sign of a visual defect due for example to bilateral congenital cataracts or retinal dystrophy. In children with cone dystrophy the nystagmus will be accompanied by photophobia and tearing.

Idiopathic congenital nystagmus is not present at birth, but develops in the first few months of life. The movements are conjugate (i.e. the same in both eyes) usually pendular and horizontal; they increase on full lateral gaze when a jerk component becomes obvious, and often decrease in an eccentric gaze position (the null zone) and for near fixation. The neurological substrate is not understood. The amplitude of the nystagmus often reduces in late childhood and visual function is usually reasonably good, especially for near vision (for example 6/18 and N6).[10]

Ocular and oculocutaneous albinism are always accompanied by nystagmus and strabismus. The diagnosis, especially in ocular albinism which is inherited by X-linked transmission, may be difficult and require slit lamp examination. *Nystagmus with a vertical or torsional element* (a twisting of the eye around its anteroposterior axis) may be the presenting sign of serious neurological disorders such as chiasmal glioma and craniopharyngioma, in which see-saw nystagmus is seen. All cases of nystagmus should therefore be referred for specialist assessment.

Congenital Horner syndrome (a 1–2 mm ptosis with relative pupillary constriction) is associated with failure of development of iris pigmentation, most noticeable in dark-eyed children. An *acquired Horner syndrome* may indicate serious underlying pathology such as neuroblastoma. A more severe *congenital* ptosis or one that is acquired during the sensitive period will, by occluding the pupil, cause amblyopia and subsequent strabismus (usually convergent). The ptosis may be due to mechanical factors, for example capillary haemangioma (which will resolve spontaneously), or be dystrophic, when it may be accompanied by superior rectus underaction. Treatment consists of patching for the amblyopia and subsequently, in some cases, surgery for the strabismus and the ptosis. Serious neurological disease, for example third nerve palsy or myasthenia gravis, may also present with ptosis in childhood.

Examination of children of 2 years and older

With increasing age, more objective and reliable methods of vision testing are applicable. Letter matching tests such as the Sheridan-Gardner can be used successfully in most 3–4 year olds. However, a child with an amblyopic eye may be able to read single letters down to 6/6 size, but only 6/24–6/18 when rows of letters are presented.[11] Where possible, testing should therefore be carried out with Snellen acuity charts where rows of letters or symbols, e.g. Landolt c rings, are used or, for the younger child, the Sonksen-Silver test.

The gross appearance of ocular alignment is an unreliable guide to the presence or absence of manifest strabismus, since orbital, facial and ocular factors may mimic or mask a squint. An example is hypertelorism in which the eyes and orbits are widely separated thus simulating a divergent strabismus. A symmetrical corneal light reflection excludes a large manifest strabismus, but this test cannot reliably detect small deviations. Testing the vision in each eye separately using either letter charts, matching techniques or contrast sensitivity is important to exclude amblyopia, but equal vision does not exclude strabismus.

Random dot stereo tests, for example the Lang Test,[12] are applicable after the age of 3 years and are being developed for younger children. At all ages the cover test is the most practical diagnostic arbiter for the presence or absence of strabismus. In experienced hands, that is those of an orthoptist or ophthalmologist, it is very accurate. The child is asked to fixate a target at distance (6 m) or near (33 cm); the eye that appears to be viewing the target is covered and any movement of the apparently non-viewing eye to take up fixation is noted. As the child gets older it becomes easier to carry out the tests. An appropriate accommodative target (that is small letters, animals etc., not a light) must be used for near vision testing. Alternative cover testing is used to demonstrate a latent deviation (phoria).

Accommodation develops over the first few months of life and becomes an important factor in the aetiology of strabismus. Accommodative convergence is the amount of binocular convergence of the visual axes necessary for viewing a near object. Its normal development may be disturbed and excessive convergence may be elicited by appropriate accommodation, leading to a convergent strabismus on near fixation.

The near convergence may be due to or associated with hypermetropia in which case the full spectacle correction (measured after cycloplegic refraction) may control the strabismus by reducing the accommodation necessary for near vision. This is termed a fully accommodative convergent squint.

Refraction is also important in the convergent strabismus that develops in childhood for both near and distance fixation (concomitant convergent squint). Unlike a fully accommodative esotropia, amblyopia is common in such cases. The poor vision is associated with a refractive error, usually unequal hypermetropia with astigmatism in the amblyopic eye. Genetic factors governing the development of hypermetropia, anisometropia and astigmatism are important in these cases and a family history of strabismus or amblyopia should prompt careful examination.[13] An accommodative element to the convergence is often present, i.e. the strabismus is greater for near than distance fixation (partly accommodative convergent squint). Treatment involves spectacle correction and occlusion therapy: the older the child and the poorer the vision when the defect is detected the more patching is required. Surgical re-alignment of the visual axes is delayed until the maximum visual acuity has been achieved, but in older children binocularity may not develop. Divergent strabismus in childhood is much less common than convergent. It also differs in being less often associated with amblyopia, more common in girls than boys and characteristically intermittent. Binocular functions therefore tend to be reasonably well developed. A further unexplained characteristic which may be useful diagnostically is the tendency for the child with a divergent strabismus to shut one eye in bright sunlight. Some exo-deviations improve spontaneously with age, and orthoptic exercises may be helpful: surgery is less often required than in eso-deviations.

A subgroup of children have a relatively small degree of anisometropia (1 or 2 dioptres) or unilateral or unequal astigmatism and become amblyopic with reduced binocular functions but no obvious manifest strabismus (a microconvergence may be present). This group notoriously slip through the screening net and often do not present until their vision is screened at the age of 5 years. The parents do not notice any abnormality and the children may have passed vision tests with both eyes if single letters were used, e.g. the Sheridan Gardner test, due to the crowding phenomenon (see above). Tests of stereoscopic vision however will be negative in this group and will detect these children. By the time of presentation, spectacle correction and patching treatment of the amblyopia does not usually produce much visual improvement and may precipitate an obvious manifest strabismus.

Myopia may start to develop in 3–4-year-old children especially if there is a family history. Myopia in infants and younger children is often associated with ocular, especially retinal pathology. In 3–4 year olds, the parents notice the child peering closely at, for example, television or narrowing (squinting) the eyes. Because near vision is good even if the myopia is asymmetric, amblyopia is uncommon. Divergent strabismus for distance fixation may be seen. The full myopic correction should be prescribed otherwise accommodative convergence will not develop normally. Early onset myopia often progresses in childhood but it must be emphasized to parents that it is a variant of normality and not a disease.

The majority of children with defective *colour vision* are boys with congenital red/green colour 'blindness' (deuteranomaly) who have difficulty distinguishing between red and green. This is a static condition of no educational significance, although it does impose some career limitations. An acquired defect of colour vision is rare and invariably accompanied by visual failure or other symptoms. It may be seen, for example, in retinal dystrophies or anterior visual pathway pathology.

Colour vision testing is included in many vision screening programmes; the most commonly used test (Ishihara colour plates) can only give reliable results over the age of 7 or 8 years. There is no justification for repeated testing.[14]

If the visual axes are aligned in certain positions of gaze but not in others, then *incomitant strabismus* is present. It is usually due to developmental abnormalities of the ocular motor system, either central or peripheral and in an otherwise normal child may present with an abnormal head posture (AHP). The child uses a head turn (ocular torticollis) if horizontal eye movement is defective or a head tilt if cyclo-vertical eye movement is abnormal, to maintain binocularity. Very rarely an AHP may be due to a homonymous hemianopia (the head is turned to bring the intact hemifield field into the primary position), an inability to generate horizontal eye movements (ocular motor apraxia), or more commonly due to sternomastoid torticollis or structural abnormalities of the cervical spine. Acquired ocular motor palsies (for example sixth nerve palsy) may also be responsible.

The most common developmental abnormality causing ocular torticollis is Duane syndrome in which the normal nerve supply from the sixth cranial nerve to the lateral rectus muscle on one side (usually the left) does not develop, and the lateral rectus is innervated from the third nerve (oculo-motor nerve). The result is a failure of abduction, with retraction of the globe (due to co-contraction of the lateral rectus and medial rectus) on adduction. Rarely the condition is familial; it may also be bilateral. Associated abnormalities include sensorineural deafness, the Klippel-Feil anomaly (short neck and low posterior hair line) and the first arch (Goldenhar) syndrome. Amblyopia may develop but only rarely is surgery required.[15]

In Brown syndrome the anterior portion of the superior oblique tendon is congenitally short and will not allow the eye to elevate in adduction. The child therefore turns the head away from the affected side. Frequently the condition improves spontaneously, but surgery may be required.[16] Moebius syndrome is due to agenesis of the VIth and VIIth cranial nerve nuclei bilaterally presenting with facial weakness, a bilateral horizontal gaze palsy and often partial atrophy of the tongue. Vertical eye movements are normal but the child has to turn the head to achieve lateral gaze.[17]

Congenital underaction of the superior oblique muscle, probably due to an incomplete congenital fourth nerve palsy, presents with a turn and tilt of the head to the opposite side. Tilting the head to the affected side causes the eye to elevate excessively, producing an obvious vertical strabismus (positive Bielschowsky head tilt test). If the ocular torticollis is marked, surgical weakening of the ipsilateral inferior oblique is required.

Isolated ocular motor palsies in childhood are uncommon but can present with an abnormal head posture, shutting of one eye, the observation of abnormal eye or eyelid movements or pupillary dilatation. In general, development of a IIIrd, IVth or VIth nerve palsy indicates a serious underlying problem and requires full neurological examination and investigation. The differential diagnosis includes myasthenia gravis which can present in infancy and childhood with ophthalmoplegia and ptosis. Orbital disease should also be considered; metastatic neuroblastoma can present with proptosis and mechanical restriction of eye movements.

References

1 Hubel, D.N., Wiesel, T.N. The period of susceptibility to the physiological effects of unilateral eye closure in kittens. *J Physiol* 1970; **206**: 419–436.
2 Von Noorden, G.K. Factors involved in the production of amblyopia. *Br J Ophthalmol* 1974; **58**: 158–164.
3 Fox, F., Albin, R.N., Shea, S.L., Dumais, S.T. Stereopsis in human infants. *Science* 1980; **207**: 323–324.
4 Kratz, K.E., Speer, P.D. Effects of visual deprivation
and alterations in binocular competition on responses of striate cortex neurons in the cat. *J Comp Neurol* 1976; **170**: 141–152.
5 Nixon, R.B., Helverston, E.M., Miller, K., Archer, S.M., Ellis, F.D. Incidence of strabismus in neonates. *Am J Ophthalmol* 1985; **100**: 798–801.
6 Hing, S., Speedwell, L., Taylor, D. Lens surgery in infancy and childhood. *Br J Ophthalmol* 1990; **74**: 73–77.
7 Teller, D.Y., MacDonald, M.A., Preston, K. Assessment of visual acuity in infants and young children: the acuity card procedure. *Dev Med Child Neurol* 1986; **28**: 779–798.
8 Atkinson, J., Braddick, O.J., Dunton, K., Watson, P.G. Refractive screening of 6–9 month olds using photorefraction. *Br J Ophthalmol* 1984; **68**: 105–12.
9 Fielder, A.R., Russell-Eggitt, I.M., Dodd, K.L., Millar, D. Delayed visual maturation. *Trans Ophthalmol Soc UK* 1985; **104**: 653–661.
10 Dell-Osso, L.F., Schmidt, D., Daroff, R. Latent, manifest latent and congenital nystagmus. *Arch Ophthalmol* 1979; **97**: 1877–1885.
11 Youngson, R.M. Anomaly in visual acuity testing in children. *Br J Ophthalmol* 1979; **59**: 168–170.
12 Lang, J. A new stereotest for strabismus. *J Paediatr Ophthalmol* 1983; **20**: 72–74.
13 Graham, P.A. The epidemiology of strabismus. *Br J Ophthalmol* 1974; **58**: 224–231.
14 Stewart-Brown, S.L., Haslum, M. Screening of vision in school: could we do better by doing less? *Br Med J* 1988; **297**: 1111–1113.
15 Kirkham, T.H. Duane's syndrome and familial perceptive deafness. *Br J Ophthalmol* 1970; **53**: 335–339.
16 Brown, H.W. True and simulated super oblique tendon sheath syndrome. *Documenta Ophthalmol* 1973; **34**: 123–136.
17 Henderson, J.L. The congenital facial diplegia syndrome: clinical features, pathology and aetiology. *Brain* 1939; **62**: 381–403.

13.2 Severe visual impairment

Patricia Sonksen and Mary Kingsley

To be born with severely defective vision is a developmental emergency; sometimes it is also a visual emergency. The latter is the first priority of management because physiological and morphological development of the visual nervous system is greatest and most rapid during the first 6 months after birth and is dependent upon the quality of visual input. Only a few of the severe visual disorders which affect western societies are amenable to treatment – cataract, glaucoma, high refractive error, retinoblastoma and some grades of retinopathy of prematurity. Prompt diagnosis and instigation of surgical, medical and optical treatment offer these babies the best chance to attain

their limited visual potential. Urgent referral to an ophthalmologist is recommended whenever severe visual impairment (SVI) is suspected.

Early consideration of the visual diagnosis in a wider paediatric perspective is important for several medical, developmental and counselling reasons. In western societies aetiology is genetically determined in 50–60% of cases[1] and between 50–75% have additional disabilities or associated diseases.[2] Early identification of inherited conditions such as the recessively transmitted congenital retinal dystrophies permits timely genetic counselling. Subgroups with distinct visual, developmental and medical prognoses can now be identified using electrophysiological techniques complemented by careful paediatric and developmental assessment for additional disabilities and associated medical disorders.[3,4] These and similar advances are gradually providing a firmer base for counselling parents about these aspects.[5] Higher resolution cytogenetics and the advent of gene probes make precise diagnosis and prenatal screening available for an increasing number of visual disorders, e.g. Norrie's disease;[6] definition of an interstitial deletion of the short arm of chromosome 11 is of assistance in planning follow up for Wilms' tumour[7] in cases of aniridia.

Experienced developmental assessment and counselling provides an opportunity to prevent or minimize many of the potentially disastrous effects of SVI on early development.[8] Some, such as failure of the infant to develop awareness and interest in his environment and family, tend to be resistant to intervention at a later date; recognition of additional impairments of learning, hearing and neuromotor control permits a comprehensive evaluation of the constraints they collectively impose on development and this facilitates the planning of developmental intervention strategies, medical treatement and therapy.[9,10] Referral to a developmental, community or general paediatrician with experience of severe visual disorder is recommended as soon as SVI is diagnosed or suspected.

Prevalence, causation and detection

The prevalence of SVI is approximately one per 1000 children. Accurate epidemiological data are not available because the criteria for classifying children of different ages as SVI have not been agreed and data on the visual status of the multiply disabled and the mentally handicapped sections of the population are fragmentary. Some studies provide useful information.[11–13] Evidence suggests that the prevalence of SVI among children who have experienced prenatal, perinatal and postnatal cerebral insults and those with syndrome complexes involving the nervous system is much higher; Warburg's study[14] suggests that approximately 7% of children attending institutions and schools for the severely learning disabled are SVI. Ideally children in these categories should all have the benefit of a specialized visual assessment. Currently resources for this are not widely available in the UK. Genetic diseases of the eye such as some forms of cataract, retinal dystrophy and albinism together with intrauterine infections are the most common prenatal causes of SVI. Complications of prematurity, neonatal asphyxia and severe infections dominate the perinatal list of causes while trauma, tumour and infection head the postnatal one.

Criteria for defining severe visual impairment where the child is able to cooperate with tests of visual acuity are relatively straightforward: the category includes any child with corrected binocular acuity of 6/18 or worse as these children will all have special educational needs. Children with acuity better than this, who have restricted fields and/or oculomotor dyspraxia, may effectively be severely visually impaired and therefore also have special educational needs. The Department of Health's new BD8 form (BD8, 1990) and revised procedures for certification of blind and partially sighted people take breadth of field as well as acuity into account.[15]

Defining criteria for severe visual impairment in babies and pre-school children is much more difficult because all aspects of visual function including acuity are still continuing to develop. Moreover, the visual problems need to be set in a framework of evolution, integration, functional growth and specialization of the whole central nervous system rather than upon a mature non-pliant system. Thus the degree of disability resulting from a particular level of visual impairment is itself not static; it changes as development proceeds, and is influenced in many babies by other additional clinical problems. Objective measures such as grating acuity using a preferential looking technique are not practical in many SVI and multiply disabled infants. Measures derived from one technique are not strictly comparable with others and certainly do not reflect the perspective and complexity of the situation outlined above. Rather than attempting to define a series of objective criteria to span the early years, it would perhaps be more sensible to base registration upon a comprehensive ophthalmological and developmental paediatric opinion reviewed at regular intervals until the age of 7 years; a single category – severely visually impaired – rather than partially sighted and blind, would suffice. At present registration of adults, children and babies is done by an ophthalmologist. The advantages of registration to a family are that they become eligible for the attendance allowance and access to educational and social support services is facilitated.

Eyes and visual behaviour should be carefully examined at birth, at the 6-week medical check and immediately if any concern is voiced by parents or primary care professionals. The examination includes an enquiry into occurrence of SVI in family members and the presence of factors during the antenatal, perinatal and neonatal periods which predispose to SVI, such as intrauterine infection, prematurity, smallness for dates, birth asphyxia and serious or complex medical events.

Signs which alert the clinician to the possibility of SVI include abnormal appearance or asymmetry of the globes, nystagmus, roving eye movements, persistent squint in any position of gaze (particularly divergent), interference with the red reflex and less than age appropriate visual behaviours.

Elicitation of selected visual behaviours from a developmental sequence is the most accessible method for hospital or community paediatricians and general practitioners to examine an infant's vision. Like other physical signs the early visual behaviours should be elicited using a standard technique and interpreted according to strict criteria. Each therefore requires a precise statement of:

1 The visual attribute measured, e.g. spatial resolution (acuity), fixation of single small round objects (SROs), tracking behaviour, convergence skills, fields.
2 Physical properties of the test material.
3 Technique used to elicit the behaviour.
4 Quantative and qualitative response criteria.
5 Guidelines for interpretation which include developmental status as well as chronological age.

Many statements surrounding old and current developmental tests of vision are poorly thought through. Tests using small sweets are a good example.[16] The attribute is defined vaguely as 'vision for sweets' or with false precision as 'acuity'. In sighted babies macula vision is used to fixate a sweet (direct pupil to target gaze). Spatial resolution of two points as such is not required but is embodied in the definition of acuity. The importance of shape is not emphasized or explained; sweets should be round otherwise the longer dimension impinges on the retina and becomes the effective size of stimulus. Similarly, the importance of using a baize cloth to suppress auditory stimuli from the surface on which the sweet lies, and advice on the position of the tester in relation to the child are not explained. Instructions frequently suggest 'scattering hundreds and thousands', although this introduces several errors; moving objects stimulate strips rather than points of the retina and scattered sweets tend to coalesce into groups and thus effect a larger target. The most commonly given pass/fail criteria are 'pokes at' or 'picks up' sweet; both skills embody aspects of motor and cognitive development in addition to vision and serve to take the attention of the tester from the child's eyes to his hands. The purely visual components of the behaviour should be observed first and then other features such as index finger approach and mode of pick-up provide valuable additional information about general development. The chronological age at which a normal baby exhibits the visual behaviour is usually given without any qualitative guidelines or advice to consider it in the context of the child's level of general development; the latter can help distinguish between SVI and global retardation.

Good test descriptions should specify with explanation, as follows:

- Test title: foveal function, fixation of SROs.
- Material: 1 mm sweet – hundreds and thousands.
- Technique: sit facing the child at a table. Choose a sweet which contrasts strongly with the baize cloth.

Encourage interest in the sweet and once engaged move hand smoothly across the table surface releasing the sweet imperceptibly en passant. Observe child's eyes throughout.

- Response criteria: brisk fixation of sweet from full sitting distance.
- Age criteria: developmental age of more than 9 months.
- Interpretative guidelines: any quality of gaze, other than the brisk fixation described above is always suspicious of SVI, e.g. visual awareness with or without fixation after searching or peering. Lack of visual engagement of the sweet in a baby with a developmental age of under 9 months does not necessarily imply visual impairment. It is important to remember children who are visually aware of a 1 mm sweet from table top distance may still have distant acuities worse than 2/60.

Once SVI is suspected, specialized investigations assist the clinician in making a precise visual diagnosis, for instance preferential looking techniques (Acuity Card Tests),[17,18] photorefraction,[19] flash and patterned visual evoked potentials.

In older children SVI presents under a variety of guises. These are often complaint by the child of difficulty in seeing the blackboard, double vision, or headaches. Parents or teachers may have noticed a squint, headturn, peering, proneness to minor accidents or deterioration in school work or behaviour. Such symptoms should always receive serious consideration and prompt examination of the eyes, nervous system and blood pressure.

From the age of $2\frac{1}{2}$ years children achieve the developmental skill to match optotypes (black on white representations of letters, geometric shapes or objects used in acuity tests) and cope with a linear display. The developmental content of tests varies so age-related compliance data are required for each test. An optotype test should only be incorporated into visual surveillance at an age when 90% can cooperate, otherwise too high a proportion of children will fail for developmental rather than visual reasons. However, the value of a measure of acuity is sufficiently great for clinicians to attempt optotype tests in children of $2\frac{1}{2}$ years and over who present with visual symptomatology. Tests for children under 7 years should incorporate a matching facility, control crowding, adhere to Snellen specification of optotypes and contain displays for 3 m and 6 m test distances. Suitable ones are the Sonksen-Silver Acuity System (S-SAS),[20] the Cambridge Crowding Cards (CCC),[21] the Egan-Calver Chart (E-CC)[22] and the LH test.[23] The S-SAS uses a flip-over booklet system to present one line of optotypes at a time; compliance data and age-related standards for acuity are available for the S-SAS.[24] The S-SAS, the CCC and the LH tests include displays for testing at both 3 m and 6 m. Symbols in the LH test are geometric shapes. The S-SAS and the LH test include a test of near vision. The CCC effects crowding by surrounding each test letter with four others rather than linearly. The E-CC can only be used at 6 metres and requires an illuminated display box.

The Sheridan-Gardner seven letter chart[25] is widely used in the UK. Unfortunately, although letters are to Snellen specification, crowding is not controlled; spacing between letters varies and is too wide thus introducing considerable errors. Many tests available use pictograms instead of letters;[26,27] the symbols often deviate considerably from Snellen specifications in overall and integral dimensions and crowding is poorly controlled. This introduces further errors to the measure. Pictograms are graphically more complex than the seven capital letters researched by Dr Mary Sheridan[28] and thus more difficult to match; the level of symbolic understanding and vocabulary required to name them is higher than generally realized. Children with SVI have particular difficulty in understanding symbolic representations in miniature and picture form so pictogram tests are not suitable for them.

Single optotype (SO) tests introduce even greater optometric errors than charts with poorly controlled crowding. The SO acuity is often one or two sizes better than a linear finding. Personal experience suggests that in children with SVI the discrepancy may be even greater. The SO measure may grossly underestimate difficulty with reading and diagram work and even place a child in an incorrect educational category; it may also lead to failure to recognize the true nature of secondary behaviour and learning difficulties. Every effort should be made to obtain a measure of linear acuity in children suspected of having a visual disorder; in this context the S-SAS has advantage because it contains linear displays of size 60 m, 36 m and 24 m. Only when a child cannot see the linear size 60 m display at 1 metre should an SO measure be substituted. In such instances the patient's problem is more realistically represented if acuity is recorded as: Linear < 1/60; SO 3/36.

In visually disordered children, the linear acuity recorded is often the size of display for which some, rather than all, the optotypes are seen; true acuity is the smallest size of display seen in its entirety. Although this practice is emotionally comforting for professional, older patient and parent, it ill serves a young child with respect to the educational provision he requires. Another common practice which has a similar disadvantage is zealous encouragement to 'look harder' and to 'have a go' which in the context of a limited choice (of six or seven optotypes) can boost the acuity measure by a couple of lines. More often than not inattention or lack of cooperation reflects difficulty in seeing. Instead of prolonged encouragement a return to a larger display or stepping a metre closer will quickly clarify whether the reason is behavioural or visual. Common sense dictates that acuity in the visually impaired should, as it does in the more fully sighted, reflect what can be seen 'at a glance', that is what is clearly or easily seen, because this is the level required to function successfully.

In surveillance work a measure of distant acuity takes priority over near because only 0.5% of individuals with normal distant acuity have errors of near acuity.[29] In children with SVI it is essential to obtain both measures for optimal prescription of spectacles, optical aids and educational materials. A near test display conforming to the Snellen Standard should be used and the acuity recorded at a test distance of at least 30 cm not only because this is the standard test distance but also the optimal one for perusing text. The S-SAS and LH test both have suitable near displays for young children. The arguments pertaining to pictograms, single optotypes, widely spaced displays and to part and over zealous measures are equally relevant. The use of near and distant linear measures in the context of making recommendations for classroom reading material is discussed further.

Impact on development
The global phase: 1–4 months

SVI curtails development by its effect upon parents as well as baby. Shock and sadness reduce the ability of the former to promote development.[8,30] The depth of these emotions is particularly great when the impairment is visual and is compounded by the complexity of coping with all the paediatric issues discussed at the beginning of the chapter. Response to social overtures is altered; passive expression and failure to look into parents' eyes are easily misinterpreted as lack of interest. Saddened, parents withdraw and unwittingly deny desperately needed experience to a blind neonate. Vision presents the world in a lively and fascinating perspective so that interest, drive, and awareness of physical and communicative potential blossom. These attributes are in jeopardy in SVI; they are the driving force of future development; experience suggests that the early months are critical for their emergence.

Emotional support for parents together with developmental counselling is therefore a priority of service provision. The doctor responsible for the initial paediatric and developmental assessment and counselling, or the ophthalmologist can ensure that support is ongoing by requesting the advisory or peripatetic teacher of the visually impaired from the local education authority (LEA) to visit the family. Most advisory or peripatetic teachers wish to be involved from the earliest opportunity. A specialist health visitor from the Wolfson Centre of the Institute of Child Health attends the ophthalmology clinic at the Hospitals for Sick Children, London. She provides parents with support and early developmental guidance and she contacts the appropriate advisory teacher, community paediatrician and local health visitor. This scheme could prove a useful model for services delivered regionally.

The integrative phase: 4–14 months

Vision provides perspective and meaning to inputs from the other special senses. It thus promotes localization skills (hearing and touch) and the emergence of the postural and saving mechanisms necessary for mobility; similarly it promotes the development of concepts which underlie communicative skills, comprehension of language, spatial relationships, cause and effect and smoothly coordinated movement (manipulation and locomotion).[9,31] Delay in any one aspect will compound developmental delay of other areas. Babies with SVI are at risk of entering the second year ill-equipped in comparison to their sighted peers, since the latter understand how they and the world around them work, and are ready to develop basic skills and understanding towards mastering their environment and creativity within it.

Assessment of babies with SVI with a view to developmental intervention requires insight into constraints imposed by poor vision and other disabilities, familiarity with special methods of assessment and knowledge of the responses of SVI babies. This approach has been pioneered in the UK in a research and service clinic known as the Developmental Vision Clinic at the Wolfson Centre, London.

The Reynell-Zinkin scales of (mental) development for young visually impaired children[32] can be used to explore levels of understanding in five areas: social adaptation; sensorimotor understanding; language (comprehension and expression); and exploration of the environment. Methods for the assessment of hearing and language behaviours and of fine and gross motor function need adaptation.[9,33] Skills not usually included in test batteries for sighted children but of particular value to visually impaired children, such as tactile discrimination and scanning strategies, also require assessment and intervention.[9]

The pattern of constraints and levels of function found in each child with SVI are different so intervention needs to be designed individually. Blind babies, like their sighted peers, develop and learn through everyday family events and interactions. At the Wolfson Centre the team consider the current level and possible progress of each developmental field within the constraints imposed by the visual impairment. The goals are simply explained to parents and practical ideas are generated which optimally use alternative input channels plus any residual vision to help the baby achieve the next stage.[9] For example, a totally blind baby of 10 months does not turn towards, nor reach out for, a favourite rattle but stills and then smiles when he hears it, and grasps and shakes it

when the assessor touches his hand with it. The baby hears the rattle and understands that the noise is made by shaking it. He has not realized that he can reach for the source of the sounds or where the sounds are located in relation to himself. Explanation of his difficulties and advice to guide his hand to the sound-making source, rather than moving the source into his hand, will facilitate these aspects of learning. Neurological examination is normal but propping and saving responses in sitting may be absent with the baby sitting with a rounded back apparently hugging himself. The baby has not realized that the floor is all around him and provides a surface which he can use for stabilization. Once the reason for the delayed motor development is understood parents can be given ideas for play activities which teach the baby the concept underlying these responses.

Guidance literature for parents and professionals caring for SVI babies and young children is available.[34-38]

Functional assessment of vision

The functional assessment of vision has two objectives:

1 To provide the basis for a programme to promote visual development.
2 To formulate guidelines which ensure that maximal use of residual vision is made in all learning situations.

1 Promotion of visual development

During the first 6 months of life, control of the neuro-motor mechanisms involved in fixation, following, tracking and convergence, and the development of peripheral and foveal acuity, and of binocularity reach good functional levels in sighted babies. Evidence suggests that this period is the biological and probably critical one for neuronal networks and coding templates subserving these processes to be laid down.[39] Impoverished visual images constrain all these developments through many interwoven mechanisms. As a result vision may remain suboptimal throughout the period and possibly never fully reach its limited potential in infants with SVI.

Recently, a developmentally based programme for visual development (PVD) has been designed and evaluated at the Wolfson Centre on 58 babies in their first year of life.[40,41] The evaluation showed that the PVD was extremely effective in promoting all the aspects of visual development mentioned above.

Assessment for a PVD

First, a lure is identified for which the baby shows visual awareness. If there is no awareness of a $2\frac{1}{2}$ inch

(6 cm) red spinning ball then a 5 inch (12 cm) coloured ball or one with reflecting surfaces and a glowing light source ('oogly' on a pen torch) are tried in turn, the last in a darkened room if necessary. The level of neuro-motor competence (fixation, following, tracking and convergence) and the sphere of visual attention for this lure are noted at different distances and speeds.

The PVD is developed from the findings. The visual properties of appropriate targets are enhanced as necessary; looking is encouraged by reinforcing visual experience through touch and sound, and the concepts and motor skills inherent in visual behaviours are actively taught. Details of the programme are published as an appendix to the scientific paper reporting the evaluation study and in the Developmental Guide.[35,41] Like the programme for general aspects of development and the use of residual vision the PVD is demonstrated to parents and uses materials and intervention strategies which have natural appeal to babies and parents and can be incorporated into daily routines and interactions.

Several points of clinical import emerged from the evaluation study. Babies with a combination of learning, physical disabilities or hearing impairments were able to benefit visually from a PVD, as did many babies with minimal or no apparent vision when first seen. The prospect for visual progress was generally good for babies with treated cataracts, cortical visual impairments, malformations of the globe (unless very gross), lesions of the optic nerve and dysplastic or dystrophic disorders of the retina with the exception of Norrie's disease and Leber's amaurosis. The PVD favourably influenced visual progress when introduced at any time during the first year. The advantage of earlier introduction is that vision of higher quality is made available sooner to all aspects of general development and learning, and fosters development of the visual nervous system during the period of its greatest pliancy. Several schemes to improve visual efficiency in nursery and school age children are available.[42-44]

2 Use of residual vision

Vision is the major input modality for so many aspects of development that maximal use of residual vision is a priority of any programme to promote general development.

Assessment and programme development for use of residual vision

The assessor sets out to demonstrate how well a child can see what is needed to achieve each priority of current development.[40] The quality of vision in different fields and at different distances is also studied. Test materials of standard size, shape, colour and luminance are used initially at standard test distance, e.g.

smartie, a $2\frac{1}{2}$ inch (6 cm) red ball on a string. The physical properties listed above of the visual lures are enhanced and the distance adjusted stepwise until visual awareness is noted at a distance which is suitable to train the developmental skill concerned.

The findings are then developed into guidelines for use of residual vision[9,35,40] and as such become an important component of each aspect of the developmental programme. For example, if a baby is unable to see a $2\frac{1}{2}$ inch (6 cm) red ball spinning 10–12 inches (25–30 cm) from its eyes but is visually aware of a 5 inch (12 cm) bright yellow and red ball at this distance, guidance for sound localization would prescribe the latter visual characteristics for rattles. Had the baby been able to see the 5 inch ball only in the temporal field of the left eye, guidance would prescribe a 5 inch rattle to enhance training of sound localization to the left and guiding the baby's hand to the sound source to the right. In the context of saving reactions in sitting, the baby's vision for large coloured sheets at a distance of 15–18 inches (38–46 cm) (sitting height) would have been assessed. Had the baby shown visual awareness of red and yellow but none for beige or brown, the colour of floor coverings at home would be discussed and a brightly coloured playmat advised.

Good visual acuity is required to discriminate the fine details for identification of real objects and pictures;[45] the relative effect of an uncorrected refractive error upon the clarity of a picture of an orange and upon a much smaller Snellen optotype, is shown in Figure 13.1. The orange is much larger than the letter, but the contrast between component parts and the background is much less than the 90% contrast of black and white optotypes.

Toddlers and pre-school children learn from everyday items and realistic coloured pictures. Once able to express through word or gesture what they see, it becomes both possible and important to assess qualitative

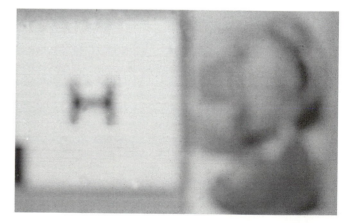

Figure 13.1 The relative effect of an uncorrected refractive error upon the clarity of a picture of an orange and upon a much smaller Snellen optotype.

and quantitative aspects of vision for these materials. Sets of pictures, the Sonksen Picture Guide to Visual Function (SPGVF), and of objects have been developed for this purpose.[40,45] Assessment aims to establish three levels of vision.

Level 1   reflects capacity to resolve fine detail and defines the maximum distance at which a child can learn from materials of visual complexity similar to that of the test items.
Level 2   reflects capacity to resolve gross visual characteristics and defines the maximum distance at which a child can recognize familiar objects and pictures of visual complexity similar to the test items.
Level 3   reflects capacity to resolve presence, but insufficient to recognize even familiar items, and defines the maximum distance of visual awareness for items with gross visual characteristics similar to those of the test item.

Method of assessment: the breadth of a child's vocabulary should be established; the actual test items should *never* be used for this purpose as the opportunity to distinguish between level 2 and level 1 vision will be lost. Only gross visual clues such as colour, size and shape are needed to recognize items at greater distance once they have been viewed close to. The test object/picture is presented at 3 metres, then at 2 m, 1 m, 0.5 m and <0.5 m until correctly identified. Objects not identified after peering may be explored tactilely as this demonstrates the characteristics of items that the child is unable to resolve visually at any distance. The identification distance defines Level 1.

Some of a child's own belongings (or the now familiar test items) are then presented, in a similar way, to define level 2.

One of the child's own belongings should then be used to define level 3; care should be taken to mask placement of the item.

The levels provide a basis for prescription of practical guidelines for teachers and parents to use in the classroom and home environment.[40,45] In some children it will be necessary to evaluate field as well as distance parameters in order to define optimal guidelines. After observing the assessment many parents comment that it has helped them to understand their child's vision.

The relationship between acuity for Snellen optotypes and the pictures from the SPGVF was investigated in children with induced refractive errors,[45] the pictures fell into three grades of visual complexity. Subsequently, the relationship has been further studied in a series of children with SVI and other disabilities. Pictures were presented from each grade of visual complexity at a distance of 3 metres. Provisional analysis suggests that the severity (mild, moderate or severe) of visual impairment can be gauged from test findings.

Children unable to see Grade I pictures at 3 metres are likely to have a severe visual impairment.

Children unable to see Grade II, but able to see Grade I pictures at 3 metres are likely to have a moderate visual impairment.

Children unable to see Grade III, but able to see Grade II pictures at 3 metres are likely to have a mild visual impairment.

Children able to see Grade III pictures at 3 metres are unlikely to have a significant impairment of visual acuity.

The Grade III pictures have recently been evaluated as a screening test, the Sonksen Picture Test (SPT) to identify children of 21 months and over with minor errors of visual acuity.[46] The test was within the communicative capability of 98% of 837 children aged 21–60 months. It was five times quicker to administer to children over $3\frac{1}{2}$ years of age, than the Sheridan Gardiner (SG) 7 letter test. The findings, tabulated below, in a 4-year-old illustrate the importance of using a linear display of optotypes, spaced according to the Snellen Standard, and the potential of the SPT method.

Infant school children need to see clearly what they are writing in order to monitor their work. The contrast of pencil against school exercise book paper is much less than that of optotype tests. A near acuity measure may be misleadingly good and it is helpful to observe a child's ability to see handwritten material of different contrasts and sizes in order to make practical recommendations for classroom work.

A child's vision for communication aid displays, for picture books, bliss boards, computer programmes and concept keyboards, is often overestimated. Vision for these materials also requires assessment using the principles described.

The functional assessment of vision is time consuming and both experience and ingenuity are required in

Test distance	Sonksen-Silver Acuity System (S-SAS)	Sheridan Gardiner (SG)	Single optotype (SO)	Sonksen Picture Test (SPT) Grade III	Sonksen Picture Test (SPT) Grade II
6 metres	6/12	6/9	6/6	–	–
3 metres	3/6		3/3	unable to see 3 of 6	able to see all 6

its execution and in design of the practical prescriptions based upon it.

Low-vision aids

Low-vision aids (LVAs) are traditionally prescribed for visual difficulties expressed by the patient; the population served is therefore adults and older children who have lost vision. The most frequent reason for seeking a low-vision aid consultation is difficulty with reading in the context of work or leisure.[47,48] Young children cannot express their needs and may not even appreciate a difficulty which is congenital. They learn from real life situations and play with materials with quite different visual properties to print.

Although Barraga suggested in the sixties[49] that optical aids as a method of training vision in children could usefully be researched, and Silver in the late seventies[50] suggested that their earlier introduction to younger children might serve as a familiarization exercise for their later use with reading, there have been no systematic studies to evaluate the use of optical aids in augmenting the learning experiences of pre-school children. With the latter in mind a research service low-vision aid clinic was set up in 1985 at the Wolfson Centre for children between the ages of 18 months and 7 years.[51] In order to evaluate optometric factors in the context of developmental and visual status and the visual attributes of the learning environment, a developmental paediatrician and ophthalmic optician saw children together during the 3 years of the research. This practice proved so valuable that it is now continued in the service clinic.[52] A variety of near and distance optical magnifiers and closed circuit television systems (CCTVs) were investigated each with a range of pre-school learning materials and learning situations. Many young patients were able to use a variety of LVAs with benefit during their pre-school years.[51] The developmental and visual criteria for doing so are summarized below.

Near stand magnifiers such as the lobster pot are mechanically and conceptually the simplest and were successfully introduced at a younger age than monocular or binocular telescopes. Developmental levels in language, performance and attention control of sighted 2 to 3 year olds were sufficient for success with a lobster pot, but those of a 3 to 4 year old were required for the distance aids. Children needed sufficient vision to see a 1.5 cm sweet or resolve a size 12 m Snellen distance letter at 10 cm to benefit from the lobster pot and to see a three quarter of an inch stationary Stycar ball or resolve a size 60 m Snellen distance letter at 2 metres to benefit from the monocular and binocular telescopes. A degree of synergism between visual and developmental levels operated so that children with poorer vision needed to be slightly more mature developmentally

to succeed. In many cases use of the aid during a 6-week trial period at home was associated with an improvement in unaided visual acuity and appeared to have promoted further visual development in addition to providing wider visual horizons for development.

Experience of younger patients with CCTVs is still relatively limited, but the enthusiasm and quick mastery of the mechanical aspects by 3, 4 and 5 year olds augurs well for their use with this age group. The higher magnification capacity of CCTVs in comparison to simple optical magnifiers could further enhance the opportunities of very young children with SVI to learn from nursery age material and possibly also from tasks like bead threading and tracing, although the latter still needs further research.

Service provision

The model of assessment and developmental support described above is currently only provided in full by the Wolfson Centre where it was developed and where it is still being further researched. Other large centres offering specialized developmental and social support for families of young children are Moorfields Eye Hospital, the Donald Winnicott Centre, London and the Alder Hey Hospital in Liverpool. Regional or subregional rather than district services are realistic in the context of the incidence of congenital SVI and the level of experience required and they can provide the eye team with developmental support and the developmental team with ophthalmological support. The exact composition of the vision team in addition to the paediatrician, should probably vary in accordance with existing expertise and interest. Input from the disciplines of psychology, health visiting, therapy, optometry, teaching and social work are all pertinent.

Children with a dual-sensory impairment

A child with a dual-sensory impairment has multisensory deprivation and should not be considered as a deaf child who cannot see or a blind child who is unable to hear. Learning ability, communication skills and perceptions of the world are degraded and distorted. The impairment of vision and hearing may both be congenital and occur in the CHARGE association (coloboma, congenital *heart* disease, chonal *atre*sia, *r*etarded growth and development, *g*enital hypoplasia and *e*ar abnormalities and/or deafness) or as a result of intrauterine infection. Visual impairment may precede the onset of hearing loss, e.g. Norrie's disease; conversely, congenital hearing impairment may be followed by visual deterioration, e.g. Usher syndrome. In some neurometabolic disorders or following severe anoxic episodes, both are acquired.

The developmental and educational implications for children with a dual-sensory impairment are enormous; it is essential for the development of early learning and social skills to make maximal use of residual vision and hearing.[53] McInnes and Treffry[54] also stress that these children need to be taught to use and integrate their degraded sensations meaningfully. Without such help many continue to function at a level far below their inherent ability.

Assessment is a highly skilled process requiring great experience. Families with deaf-blind children should be referred to specialist centres as soon as possible. Such help is available through Sense, the National Deaf-Blind and Rubella Association. Facilities are available for assessment at their centres and are complemented by domiciliary visits by a qualified teacher of the deaf-blind. The Wolfson Centre can provide assessment of additional disabilities and medical problems.

Education needs careful and specialized supervision from educational and medical professionals. Specialist deaf-blind education will remain necessary for those unable to gain sufficient information through residual vision and augmented hearing. A deaf-blind child who learns to use his residual vision sufficiently well to establish lip-reading or to see manual signs may best be educated through deaf methods, whereas one with sufficient hearing to learn speech may benefit most from education using methods for the visually impaired.

Independence and employment prospects are particularly limited for this group and placements for life often need to be arranged for young adults. Sense, the Royal National Institute for the Deaf (RNID) or the Abbots Leigh Centre offer this service.

The education services

Advisory teacher

These teachers have an additional professional qualification in the education of the visually impaired. Courses are now available at universities and institutes of education in Birmingham, Cambridge, Edinburgh, London, Manchester and Swansea. Advisory teachers visit schools and homes to offer advice to parents and professionals, e.g. nursery teachers and health visitors. They advise on resources which are available locally and discuss the educational implications of a child's visual disability. Their responsibility also embraces SVI in special schools both within and without the home local education authority (LEA). An important aspect of their work is to develop a network of links with other professionals to promote continuity and consistency of care and advice.

Peripatetic teacher

Some, but not all, peripatetic teachers have the additional professional qualification mentioned above. Peripatetic teachers are particularly concerned in teaching specific skills, such as braille. For this purpose they may visit a child's school daily.

Support teacher

These teachers do not usually have the additional qualification. They spend a high proportion of each day with one child. This support may be in class, for example sitting next to the child dictating work from the blackboard or out of class by enlarging or adapting teaching materials.

Non-teaching aides or welfare assistants

Aides or assistants work under the direction of the class teacher and usually help with tasks of a more practical nature, e.g. setting up equipment, focusing on LVA and daily living skills.

The statement of special educational needs

Severe visual impairment is associated with many long-term special educational needs. For this reason a child with SVI should have the protection of a statement of educational needs as defined by the 1981 Education Act which entitles them to receive the resources, both human and material, which they require.

The statementing process

The statement is prepared by the LEA following a multidisciplinary assessment which includes the opinions of the parents. The head teacher will have consulted the specialist teacher of the visually impaired before constructing his or her report. In practice, the advisory teacher usually submits a separate report. Parents are asked if they would like the opinions of any other professionals who have been involved with their child to be obtained, e.g. hospital ophthalmologists, or developmental paediatricians.

This advice is considered by a placements panel consisting of the advisor for special education, the principal educational psychologist, the assistant education officer with responsibility for special needs, and the statementing officer. The panel specifies the provision required by the child and recommends suitable school placement. This draft statement is then sent to the parents. As with all statements of special educational needs parents can disagree with the proposed provision and the draft statement may be revised in consultation with them. Parents who remain dissatisfied after the statement has been signed can appeal to the LEA. Local Tribunals are the final arbiters.

Factors to be considered

Parents make a vital contribution to the preparation of the statement. Gaining parental confidence in school placement is essential for its success and consideration of their opinions is a very important part of the decision making process.

Advisory teachers arrange for parents to visit schools making the necessary introductions to staff. They often accompany parents and child on the visit and are thus available to discuss resources available in the context of a particular child. Parents are thus helped to come to a realistic decision.

The distance of a school from a child's home needs to be considered. The debilitating effect of long journeys may outweigh the benefit for very young children and those who are sickly. The layout of school buildings is also important. Dark stone staircases and long distances between split site school buildings can increase the anxiety level for a partially sighted child.

Personality is important. A child who is shy, retiring or introverted may find the bustle of a mainstream school more stressful than the family-like atmosphere in a special school. In contrast, extrovert children are more likely to find mainstream school invigorating and stimulating. Some SVI children worry more than their sighted peers about the minor social disasters which happen to all children. Learning ability is another consideration. Children with general or specific learning disability often thrive best in a smaller group with a higher teacher–pupil ratio, whereas children with above average ability may find the experience of a large group stimulating.

The enthusiasm with which the headteacher and staff receive the challenge of a handicapped child in a mainstream school makes a vital contribution to the success of the placement. This aspect should be taken into account by the placement panel. The availability of advisory and specialist teaching time is crucial, particularly when skills such as keyboarding, or mobility need to be taught. Specialist equipment, its provision and management in the classroom, are additional factors to consider.[55]

Children with similar acuities often function very differently in the same school setting; impairment of other visual attributes (such as colour and control of eye movements), personality and learning ability exert a cumulative influence which needs to be taken into account.

Educational options

Education is a preparation for life within the community; for any child with special needs it is a matter of compromise.

Special schools

Special schools for children with visual impairment give parents and children a choice of educational placement. In recent years most of the schools for partially sighted children have closed and the choice is becoming more restricted. Currently Exhall Grange School in Coventry caters for the more academically able partially sighted child and has residential facilities. Joseph Clarke School in Waltham Forest has day facilities only and takes children within its catchment area. With the trend towards integration some of the specialist schools for the blind are on the point of closure. Currently, alternative placements are being debated and the outcome of integration needs to be properly evaluated. Studies are few[56,57] and as yet no controlled longitudinal ones have been published.

Many schools for children with SVI offer particular areas of specialist help, e.g. The Royal National Institute for the Blind (RNIB) New College Worcester is a secondary school for academically able pupils. The Sunshine House Nursery Schools at Northwood, East Grinstead and Southport cater for children between 3 and 8 years of age who have additional handicaps. The Royal School for the Blind at Wavertree in Liverpool, Rushton Hall School, Northants and Condover Hall in Shropshire provide for children with additional handicaps. The Pathways Unit at Condover has facilities for children with a dual sensory impairment. For children in integrated settings short courses at special schools and RNIB centres could provide a valuable resource not available at present. A list of specialist schools catering for children without other serious disabilities can be obtained from the RNIB. Many have facilities for residential or day placement.

Material resources

Alteration or adaptation of the working environment, the input modality and the method of output used by a child to express himself all require material resources.[58] The provision of window blinds may help a child with cone dysfunction syndrome; a desk lamp may provide a child who has retinitis pigmentosa with the additional lighting necessary for specific tasks. A sloping desk top may improve illumination and the posture of children who read or write with their nose almost on the page.

Written material can be presented in a variety of forms depending on the child's needs, e.g. braille, cassette tape, talking book or compact disc (CD). Kurzweill, Delta and Optacon machines all have optical character recognition; the Kurzweill has voice output, the Delta a refreshable braille output, and the Optacon a tactile output using sighted letter shapes. Some partially sighted children can use large print, others, especially those with restricted fields (tunnel vision), will not find large print beneficial. Reading speed is invariably slower than normal with these methods. The use of braille and print are not necessarily exclusive; some children use braille to read large quantities of text and access references by print methods.

Pictorial material is increasingly used in school because pictures stimulate, motivate and reward children; partially sighted children may prefer a written description to a confusing indistinct picture.

Low vision aids are another way of improving input for older partially sighted school children. These are obtained through a regional LVA clinic in close liaison with the advisory teacher. Motivation is an important factor determining success and it is sensible to use material the child longs to read, such as the football results. CCTVs enable text or pictures to be enlarged onto a television monitor. Some of these reverse the image so that black text appears as white on a black background making it easier to see. Ease of use and facilitation of specific tasks are important considerations for the prescribing team.

Handwriting, typescript, braille and speech are the four basic methods used for expression. A child's own handwriting can be made easier for him to read if he is allowed to use a black felt pen or 2B pencil on good white matt paper. Typescript produced by a portable lap-top computer, or a printer receiving input from a word processor, are alternatives. Braille'n'print and Emprint machines produce a print output from a braille input. Braille output can be produced as hard copy braille or as soft refreshable braille. The former is produced by Perkins and Mountbatten braillers. In a refreshable braille system plastic pins rise through a platen in response to an electrical impulse; the pins form the shape of braille letters. Once read the pins can be withdrawn and new text presented. Versabraille and Delta machines use this system. Speech output can be recorded onto cassette tape or dictated to an amanuensis who then writes or types the content.

A child's self-esteem and self-worth are of paramount importance. A child who finds aids and equipment an unbearable embarrassment should be encouraged to understand their potential rather than be forced to use them. Once motivated confidence will follow.

Young people with special educational needs are eligible for full-time education until the age of 19 years. The RNIB student support service offers advice and limited financial help to those over 16 years in training placements. Some further education colleges specialize in visually impaired students.

Employment prospects for visually impaired people are changing. As automation advances, opportunities in repetitive jobs are decreasing, e.g. packaging, but openings in clerical, administrative and computer fields are increasing with advances in information technology.

Useful addresses

Royal National Institute for the Blind
224 Great Portland Street
London W1N 6AA

Royal National Institute for the Deaf
105 Gower Street
London WC1

Sense
National Association for the Deaf, Blind and Rubella Handicapped
311 Grays Inn Road
London WC1

Abbots Leigh Centre
2 The Gables
Street Road
Glastonbury
Somerset BA6 9EG

The Wolfson Centre
Mecklenburgh Square
London WC1N 2AP

References

1 Robinson, G.C., Watt, J.A., Scott, E. A study of congenital blindness in British Columbia: methodology and medical findings. *Can Med Assoc J* 1968; **99**: 831–836.

2 Robinson, G.C. Epidemiological studies of congenital and acquired blindness in blind children born in British Columbia 1944–1973. *Proceedings of First Multidisciplinary Conference on Blind Children*, Vancouver, Canada, 1974; 1–21.

3 Black, M.M., Sonksen, P.M. The congenital retinal dystrophies: a study of early cognitive and visual development. *Arch Dis Child* 1992; **67.3**: 262–265.

4 Lambert, S.R., Kriss, A., Taylor, D., Coffey, R., Pembury, M. Follow-up and diagnostic reappraisal of 75 patients with Leber's congenital amaurosis. *Am J Ophthalmol* 1989; **107**: 624–631.

5 Goodyear, H.M., Sonksen, P.M., McConachie, H. Norrie's disease: a prospective study of development. *Arch Dis Child* 1989; **64**: 1587–1592.

6 De la Chapelle, A., Sankila, E.M., Lindlof, M., Aula, P., Norio, R. Norrie's disease caused by a gene deletion allowing carrier detection and pre-natal diagnosis. *Clin Genet* 1985; **28**: 317–320.

7 Riccardi, V.M., Sujansky, E., Smith, A.C., Franke, U. Chromosomal imbalance in aniridia: Wilms' tumour association, 11p interstitial deletion. *Pediatrics* 1978; **61**: 604.

8 Sonksen, P.M. A developmental approach to sensory disabilities in early childhood. *Internat Rehab Med* 1985; **7**: 27–32.

9 Sonksen, P.M., Levitt, S.L., Kitzinger, M. Identification of constraints acting on motor development in young visually disabled children and principles of remediation. *Child Care Hlth Dev* 1984; **10**: 273–286.

10 Sonksen, P.M. Vision and early development. In: Wybar, K., Taylor, D., eds. *Paediatric Ophthalmology: Current Aspects*. Ch 8, 85–95. New York: Marcel Dekker, 1983.

11 Williamson, W.D., Desmond, M.M., Andrew, L.P., Hicks, R.N. Visually impaired infants in the 1980's: a survey of aetiologic factors and additional handicapping conditions in a school population. *Clin Paediatr* 1987; **26**: 241–244.

12 Bryars, J.H., Archer, D.B. Aetiological survey of visually handicapped children in Northern Ireland. *Trans Ophthalmol Soc, UK* 1977; **97**: 26–30.

13 Schappert-Kimmijser, J., Hansen, E., Haustrate-Gosset, M.F. *et al.* Causes of severe visual impairment in children and their prevention. *Doc Ophthalmol* 1975; **39**: 213–241.

14 Warburg, M. Blindness among 7700 mentally retarded children in Denmark. In: Smith, V., Keen, J. eds. *Visual Handicap in Children*. Clinics in Developmental Medicine, no 73. London: Spastics International Medical Publication, 1979.

15 Certification of blind and partially sighted people: revised form BD8 and procedures. HN (90)5, HN(FP)(90)1, LASSL(90)1: Dept of Health, Health Publications Unit, Lancashire.

16 Bellman, M., Cash, J. *The Schedule of Growing Skills in Practice*. Windsor: NFER-Nelson, 1987.

17 Teller, D.Y., McDonald, M., Preston, K., Sebris, S.L., Dobson, V. Assessment of visual acuity in infants and children. *Dev Med Child Neurol* 1986; **28**: 779–787.

18 Keeler Acuity Cards. Keeler Ltd., Windsor, Berkshire.

19 Atkinson, J., Braddick, O.J., Durden, K., Watkinson, P.G., Atkinson, S. Screening for refractive errors in 6–9 month old infants by photorefraction. *Br J Ophthalmol* 1984; **68**: 105–112.

20 Sonksen-Silver Acuity System and Manual. Windsor, Berkshire: Keeler Ltd, 1988.

21 Cambridge Crowding Cards. London: Clement Clarke International Ltd.

22 Egan-Calver Chart. Windsor, Berkshire: Keeler Ltd.

23 Hyvarinen, L., Nasanen, R., Laurinen, P. New visual acuity test for pre-school children. *Acta Ophthalmol* 1980; **58**: 507–511.

24 Salt, A.T., Sonksen, P.M., Wade, A., Jayatunga, R. The maturation of linear acuity and compliance with the Sonksen-Silver Acuity System. Submitted to *Dev Med Child Neurol*, March 1994.

25 Sheridan-Gardiner 7 Letter Test. Windsor, Berkshire: Keeler Ltd.

26 BUST Test. Stockholm, Sweden: Elisyn.

27 Kay-Picture Test. Windsor, Berkshire: Keeler Ltd.

28 Sheridan, M.D. *Manual for the STYCAR Vision Tests*. Windsor, Berkshire: NFER, 1976.

29 Peckham, C.S. Vision in childhood. *Br Med Bull* 1986; **42**: 150–154.

30 Sonksen, P.M. Constraints upon parenting: experience of a paediatrician. *Child Care Hlth Dev* 1989; **15**: 29–36.

31 Fraiberg, S. *Insights from the Blind*. London: Souvenir Press, 1977.

32 Reynell, J., Zinkin, P. Reynell-Zinkin development scales for visually handicapped children. *Manual Part I, Mental Development*. Windsor, Berkshire: NFER, 1979.

33 Sonksen, P.M. A developmental reappraisal of clinical tests of hearing for normal and handicapped children. Part III: the handicapped child. *Maternal Child Hlth* 1984; **10**: 170–174.

34 Scott, E.P., Jan, J.E., Freeman, R.D. *Can't your Child See?* Baltimore, London and Tokyo: University Park Press, 1977.

35 Sonksen, P.M., Stiff, B. *Show Me What my Friends Can See*. A developmental guide for parents of babies with severely impaired sight and their professional advisers. London: The Wolfson Centre, 1991.

36 Reid, C.A. *One Step at a Time*. London: RNIB, 1989.

37 Series of five leaflets. Talk to me I and II, heart to heart, move with me, learning to play. Blind Children's Center, Los Angeles, California.

38 Hyvarinen, L. *Vision in Children*. Meaford, Ontario, Canada: Oliver Graphics, 1988.

39 Atkinson, J. Human visual development over the first 6 months of life: a review and hypothesis. *Hum Neurobiol* 1984; **3**: 61–74.

40 Sonksen, P.M. The assessment of 'vision for development' in severely visually handicapped babies. *Acta Ophthalmol* 1983; Suppl **157**: 82–91.

41 Sonksen, P.M., Petrie, A., Drew, K.J. Promotion of visual development in severely visually impaired babies: evaluation of a developmentally based programme. *Dev Med Child Neurol* 1991; **33**: 320–335.

42 Hull, W., McCarthy, D. Supplementary program for pre-school visually handicapped children. *Educ Vis Handicapped* 1973; **5**: 97–104.

43 Chapman, E.K. *Look and Think: a Handbook for Teachers*. Visual perception training for visually impaired children (5–11 years). London: RNIB, 1989.

44 Barraga, N. *Program to Develop Efficiency in Visual Functioning*. Louisville, Kentucky: American Printing House for the Blind, 1980.

45 Sonksen, P.M., Macrae, A.J. Vision for coloured pictures at different acuities: the Sonksen picture guide to visual function. *Dev Med Child Neurol* 1987; **29**: 337–347.

46 Hodes, D.P., Sonksen, P.M., McKee, M. Evaluation of the Sonksen picture test for detection of minor visual errors in preschool children. *Dev Med Child Neurol* 1994; **36**: 16–25.

47 Silver, J.H. Low vision aids in childhood. In: Wybar, K., Taylor, D., eds. *Paediatric Ophthalmology, Current Aspects*. New York: Marcel Dekker, 1983.

48 Faye, E.E. Identifying the low vision patient. In: *Clinical Low Vision*, 2nd edn. Boston: Little, Brown, 1984.

49 Barraga, N.C. *Increased Visual Behaviour in Low Vision Children*. Research Series 13. New York: American Foundation for the Blind, 1977.

50 Silver, J.H. The visually handicapped child; techniques for prescribing and assisting. *Ophthal Optic* 1979; **24**: 897–900.

51 Ritchie, J.P., Sonksen, P.M., Gould, E. Low vision aids for preschool children. *Dev Med Child Neurol* 1989; **31**: 509–519.

52 Gould, E., Sonksen, P.M. A low-vision aid clinic for pre-school children. *Br J Vis Impairment* 1991; **9**: 1–3.

53 Freeman, P. *The Deaf/Blind Baby. A Programme of Care.* London: William Heinemann Medical Books, 1985.

54 McInnes, J., Treffry, J.A. *Deaf-blind Infants and Children: a Developmental Guide*. Milton Keynes: Open University Press, 1982.

55 Chapman, E.K., Stone, J.M. *The Visually Handicapped Child in Your Classroom*. London: Cassell, 1988.

56 Jamieson, M., Partlett, M., Pocklington, K. *Towards Integration: a Study of Partially Sighted Children in Ordinary Schools*. Windsor, Berkshire: NFER-Nelson, 1977.

57 Stockley, J. *Vision in the Classroom*. London: RNIB, 1987.

58 Jan, J.E., Freeman, R.D., Scott, E.P. *Visual Impairment in Children and Adolescents*. New York: Grune and Stratton, 1977.

Chapter 14

Learning disorders

14.1 Developmental delay and learning disorders

Ian McKinlay

What is normal?

The population mean predicts the number of deviant individuals, whether the characteristic under study is blood pressure, obesity, sodium or alcohol consumption[1] and this applies to learning and development. The normal range can change as the population acts to promote its health and well-being. There has been a substantial upward change in the normal range of British children's height in the 20th century, though disadvantaged children still lag by one standard deviation.

In 1870 it was normal for British children to be unable to read. Then universal education became available and the considerable majority of children now read fluently by the age of 9 years. There has been a general improvement in the normal range of cognitive attainments with better health, nutrition, schooling and introduction of social programmes. An illustration of this process is the difference between the prevalence of epilepsy in special schools for children with moderate learning difficulties in northern Sweden (18%)[2] and Manchester (5.5%).[3] In the Manchester special schools at least one-third of the clinical workload for the school doctor relates to child protection. More Manchester children are in special schools because of social disadvantage than in Sweden where biological disorders account for a much higher proportion of a smaller total.

Who knows what is normal?

There are developmental achievements which all parents anticipate, for instance smiling, walking or talking. When children attain these it brings pleasure to their families, especially if this occurs quickly. However, knowing what is normal may be a problem for parents and professionals.

As family size becomes smaller there is less opportunity to observe the development of young children. With greater mobility and less stability of families there is likely to be reduced contact and support from grandparents and other close relatives.

Cross-sectional developmental surveillance programmes tend to encourage a checklist approach among professionals. If it is known that *average* children, that is more than half, smile by 6 weeks, sit by 8 months, walk by 13 months and begin to talk by 18 months, it is difficult to know when development becomes abnormal. It is more helpful to know about normal ranges.

Familial effects

Families have their own rates of normal development. Whereas most children crawl then go on to walk between 10 and 18.5 months,[4] about 10% of normal children do not crawl but move around by shuffling on their bottoms, creeping on their bellies or rolling over. They begin to walk between 13 and 27 months. A few get up and walk without having moved around before. They often do this before their first birthday but normally before 15 months. These familial variants of normal development are associated with lower muscle tone but are of no long-term pathological significance. Some bottom shufflers become professional athletes. Failure to obtain a full family history for a child with apparent developmental delay may generate undue worry and subject children to unnecessary tests.

Cultural effects

Early motor development is affected by culture but the effects are small. Parents need to go to some trouble to prevent their children from becoming mobile at a normal age. Wrapping them in swaddling bands or winter coats and laying them in mangers, cots, pushchairs or papooses in the early months of life does have measurable effects on early motor development.[5] However, the effects are small and not of lasting consequence[6,7] provided that the children are fed adequately, kept in good health and do not have sensory defects, especially of vision. Locomotor development is largely an expression of inbuilt mechanisms rather than learned behaviour.

Likewise early babble emerges at a normal time in children who receive little stimulation, even in children with severe sensorineural hearing loss. It is in progression to organized language that inbuilt potential is affected by sensory input and nurture.

Ethnic effects

Some ethnic differences influence normal development of which the best known is the more rapid early locomotor attainments of black-African children.[8,9] Differences in later development such as in academic and sporting achievements are likely to reflect an interaction between constitutional influences and learning opportunities.

Sex effects

Girls have a small advantage in early development.[10–12] In addition boys are more susceptible to insults before, during and after birth leading to developmental delay and neurological disability. Some lesions are sex-linked recessive disorders and others are environmental. In consequence there are about 50% more boys than girls with severe mental retardation or cerebral palsy.

There are also more boys than girls with developmental delay and learning difficulties. Expectation may lead to greater concern being expressed about a boy with problems than a girl. Also boys tend to show more conspicuous behavioural reactions to frustration than girls and so come to attention. Boys are four times more likely than girls to be referred to specialist services because of learning or behaviour problems. They are more than twice as likely to be referred for the same degree of difficulty.[11,13]

Care effects

It is common for doctors to be asked whether a child's developmental progress is being impaired avoidably by lack of care. Usually there are other grounds for concern about care as well as the child's development. The child may have been left unattended, illnesses may have been neglected, physical abuse may have occurred or the parent(s) may be known to abuse drugs or alcohol. Hygiene may be unsatisfactory and clothing may be inappropriate. The home may not be heated adequately. Furnishing such as bedding and floor coverings may be lacking. Safety hazards may cause concern.

The long-term consequences of early under stimulation[14,15] may be of less significance than was thought a generation ago. Probably continuing physical and emotional care is of more importance and can compensate for deprivation.[16] In a special school for children with moderate learning difficulties in Salford in 1988, of 124 pupils, 15 were or had been on the child protection register (compared with 2.14 per 1000 in the authority), 21 had mothers receiving current psychiatric treatment, 19 had suffered parental bereavement, 12 had mothers who acknowledged a long-standing lack of attachment and four had mothers with major chronic illness such as renal dialysis, cardiac disease and paraplegia.

Judgement about the quality of care is a matter for social services and the courts. In preparing medical advice it is wise for doctors to confer with the family health visitor who knows about the child's development and conditions in the home over a period of time.

The child's growth is an important factor. Decelerations in growth rate and thinness for height and head circumference are consistent with insufficient food intake provided there is no evidence of serious chronic illness such as renal failure, cyanotic congenital heart disease or malabsorption. Some children of mothers who abused alcohol or drugs in pregnancy are short with small heads, irritability and slow development, including motor difficulties.

Behaviour is another factor. A child who is lethargic or apathetic is more worrying than a child who is active. The possibility of a biological disorder causing mental retardation or a specific learning difficulty must be considered.[17–19] Children who have not received consistent discipline and care are often unruly. It can be difficult to distinguish between a child with constitutional hyperactivity and one who is receiving inadequate care, such as from a depressed mother. However, the former show more continuously deviant behaviour whereas the latter are more dependent on circumstances. Advice from a child psychiatrist and a clinical psychologist is appropriate if there is any doubt.

The family history is relevant, particularly insofar as there may have been abuse or neglect of older children. Examination for past or present signs of physical abuse is appropriate as many neglected children have also been assaulted.

A medical opinion on the cause of developmental delay contributes to the multidisciplinary process of child protection, particularly in the context of the Children Act 1989. Even if a child has a constitutional disorder of development it may be decided that care is unsatisfactory also. It is important to know about such a condition in planning future services. There are times when it is difficult to distinguish between effects of poverty and limited parental cognitive ability and those of neglect. The child's needs are paramount but support for the family should normally be offered and the response to that monitored before considering alternative care. Nonetheless some children make remarkable progress after being taken into care. We have been too cautious about this issue in the past to the detriment of many children.

Specific developmental delay or disorder

Most children develop consistently. Social responsiveness, mobility and language may all develop early, in an average way, or all may be slow. Developmental rate may accelerate or decelerate in later months or years. However it is interesting how often children fulfil early predictions. For instance language development by the age of 3 years has good predictive value for later educational attainment.[20] However, some children show specific developmental delay in social behaviour, vision, hearing, mobility or language. This may lead to a mistaken attribution of global developmental delay, especially if more than one component is affected. It is common, for instance, for children with specific language problems to have fine motor difficulties also.

Suspicion of developmental delay

It may be clear at birth that a child has a disorder, such as Down syndrome, which is very likely to lead to developmental delay. Some newborn infants have illnesses, for instance symptomatic asphyxia, seizures, periventricular leukomalacia, meningitis, which put them at high risk of developmental delay. Usually

such children will be followed up by a paediatrician so that help can be offered if difficulties emerge.

Such surveillance can be traumatic for parents. They are aware of the perinatal concerns and are anxious about the outcome. At a time when it is not possible to give clear answers, doctors may be pressed to speculate on this. It is appropriate to share knowledge of diagnoses with parents when there can be reasonable certainty. Such counselling should be given in an unhurried way by an experienced, sympathetic doctor to both parents together with the child present.[21] If both are not available, the parent who attends should be able to bring another adult relative or friend. An adult interpreter may be needed. The parents may be pleased to have a social worker, therapist or a nurse present so that the consultation can be discussed at home later and the next appointment can be prepared for. The consultation should include discussion of a plan to help the child and parents, including contact with other agencies.

More commonly, the identification of developmental delay emerges as the result of increasing suspicion on the part of parents and/or professionals. Parents are the main authorities on their children's progress. They are usually right to be concerned and professionals have been guilty of inappropriate reassurance at times. However, it can be that the child is developing normally but in a different way from siblings. When parents have not formed a close attachment to a child they may be critical, even hostile, when the child is normal. Both problems need to be addressed.

Professionals can become concerned about children whose parents have not expressed suspicion of a problem. It may be that the child's progress is typical for that family whose history is not fully known by the professional. Alternatively the parents may be so preoccupied by other problems or so inexperienced in child-rearing that it has not occurred to them that the child is not doing well. There may be such an emotional investment in the child's normality that the parents deny the significance of their observations. For instance the extended family may have been critical of the pregnancy or the child may be the first to a couple who have abandoned other partners or who have experienced prolonged infertility or loss.

Doubtful development

To describe a child as showing developmental delay initiates a process with substantial consequences. It is a cue for health professionals to investigate the possible medical causes and genetic implications. Remediable disorders such as sensory impairments, poor health, metabolic defects or seizure activity may be explored. If a diagnosis is made this is helpful. If the degree of developmental delay leads to attribution of mental retardation, or the quality of disordered posture, movement and tone allow the description of cerebral palsy, this may lead to provision of supportive services and benefits.

If, however, tests draw a blank and the deficit is not such that a precise classification can be given, the position is a difficult one for families. Their concern has been aroused but not explained. The child and family may not qualify for help.

It may be suggested (understandably but incorrectly in particular cases) that lack of care has been a factor and child protection services have become involved provoking resentment on the family's part. Especially when the concern was first raised by professionals, the identification of developmental delay may have been counterproductive unless counselling is given for the parents. It is not only major disabilities which provoke grief reactions.

Developmental surveillance

It is of benefit to children and families that remediable sensory defects are identified as soon as possible so that parents may be taught skills to optimize their children's progress and aids can be provided. In order to make best use of limited resources, more evaluation of the benefits of early intervention programmes such as the Portage schemes is needed. There is some evidence for benefit from *head-start* programmes for children from disadvantaged backgrounds and for children with developmental disorders.[22] Nonetheless there are doubts as to whether surveillance programmes lead to sufficient benefit for the right children to justify continuation of the programmes in their present form.

This has implications for policy (who should carry out surveillance?), for in-service training (what should be taught and by whom?) and for audit (sensitivity/specificity/cost-benefit).

In Britain attempts are being made to combine child health services and to rationalize child health surveillance.[23] General practitioners (GPs) who are interested in developmental work may either review their child patients opportunistically or in regular clinics. There are many advantages in this. GPs have greater knowledge of families. The small number of children involved (about 100 pre-school) make it easier to sustain enthusiasm. As GPs tend to stay in post for long periods there is continuity for stable populations. Medical problems such as infections detected during surveillance can be treated immediately thus combining preventive with therapeutic work. Involvement in surveillance gives opportunities to maximize immunization and vice versa. There are benefits from being able to see children when they are well.

Doctors in community child health services also offer developmental screening services. These are best suited to deprived areas where the population is highly mobile, registration with general practitioners is incomplete and consultation rates with all health services are low. Close liaison with general practice should be encouraged. Health visitors, orthoptists and audiometricians work closely with both services.

Practical implications of the evolving system need to be considered. A general practitioner will be responsible for a newborn child with Down syndrome once in a professional career. A child with severe mental retardation will be born once in 10 years and a new child with cerebral palsy, severe sensorineural hearing loss or severe visual impairment will arise every 20 years. Appropriateness of referral of a child to a speech therapist will be considered twice a year and to the education authority for assessment of special educational needs once every year or two.

To maintain clinical skills in assessment of children with possible developmental delay, collaboration between primary care staff and community paediatric services are needed. This happens already in many districts. There needs to be an understanding of how orthoptic and audiometric services run, how to obtain therapy advice and social work support, how to alert the education authority and to provide parents with information about self-help organizations.

Child development centres

Most districts have an outpatient multidisciplinary assessment, diagnostic and rehabilitation clinic called a child development centre (CDC). It may be hospital or community based. The facility may not be for developmental work exclusively, it is sometimes associated with an educational or even a care facility. These centres were set up as the result of pressure from parents and voluntary organizations to create a more coordinated secondary care service for children suspected of developmental delay or neurodevelopmental disability. Where such centres involve consultants in developmental paediatrics, or other senior doctors from the community service, there is an opportunity to organize efficient policies. Referral practices can be agreed and audited. More needs to be learned about such services which are quite diverse and not universally available. Some CDCs only offer services for pre-school children, but others advise school children also, backing up the primary care school services.

Alerting the education authority

The ways in which education services become aware of developmental or sensory problems in children requires consideration when surveillance has been the responsibility of GPs. Especially in large towns or cities, each school will have pupils registered with many GPs. The school health service is likely to remain a responsibility of the community child health doctors except for private schools. Information could be passed on through parent-held records or computerized records, such as the pre-school module and the school health module. The school is able to obtain advice through a school nurse or doctor with such information available to them. There is work to be done in coordinating the system.

When it is appreciated that a child under 5 but over 2 years of age may have special educational needs the health services are obliged to inform the local education authority. It would seem to work best if GPs agree to do this through the community child health service.

Learning difficulties

Many children in whom learning difficulties emerge in school have been identified as having developmental problems. For instance it is characteristic of children with developmental spoken language delay or articulation problems to have literacy difficulties. Children who are clumsy at school entry tend to remain clumsy relative to their peers and often show difficulties with maths as they grow older. Both may be associated with visual and spatial perception disorders.[13]

Some children seem to overcome early delay and do well at school (late developers). Others who have normal early development turn out to have learning difficulties, especially if other family members have struggled with literacy, there are few books in the house, frequent changes of address or poor school attendance.

Dyslexia

Learning difficulty for written language is often referred to as dyslexia.[24] Some professionals include difficulties with handwriting (dysgraphia) within that term. Distinctions have been drawn between backward readers who are of lower general cognitive ability and children with a specific literacy difficulty but at least average general ability.[25] The term *dyslexic* has been reserved by some authors for a subgroup of children, mostly boys, with literacy difficulties in association with problems of orientation, sequencing and motor organization.[26] However, evidence that such distinctions are of practical importance for teaching are controversial.[27–29] It has been suggested that dyslexia is a middle class term used by parents who are intolerant of their children's learning difficulties. However, specific literacy difficulties are more common in children from less affluent backgrounds.[26] Articulate parents are more likely to demand extra help for their children.

In some inner city primary schools one-third of 7 year olds have barely made a start at reading and writing and one third of 11 year old secondary school entrants have a reading ability below that of an average 9 year old. Parents of children of good general ability may seek the help of doctors in disputes with education authorities about remedial provision. While it is appropriate for the doctor to give medical advice to the education authority's assessment process, such as checking for sensory defects and associated motor learning difficulties,[30] it is unwise to become engaged in a dispute with educationalists and their specialist advisers.

Undoubtedly children respond to understanding, support and a curriculum which is appropriate to their needs and teachers benefit from expert teaching advice as to how to provide for pupils with problems, but evidence for the long-term effectiveness of remedial teaching is lacking.[28,31,32] If the child or family is experiencing distress over the learning problem, this deserves to be treated in the same way as any other disability, with involvement of psychological services where appropriate.

Dysgraphia

Interest in the mechanical skills of handwriting as opposed to the content of written material has fluctuated over the 550 year history of European public education.[33] For centuries it was possible for teachers to make a living as a handwriting specialist and children spent hours every week practising writing. This must have been boring and, for most children, unnecessary. However there are children for whom writing does not come easily and who do not pick it up by copying.[34–36] They need specific help.[13,37,38] From a teacher's perspective children are most conspicuous through their behaviour and their written work. In a time when the emphasis is on content (appropriately for most children) there is a risk that those who find graphomotor skills difficult to learn will be underestimated or left behind.

For many children, particularly those with comprehensible spelling ability, there are advantages in considering the use of a word processor with a spellcheck, especially for writing important documents such as assessed school work, job applications and even examination papers (by agreement with examining boards and with the support of the school). However, for this to be a success, the child and parents have to be motivated, a teacher has to be available, the school needs to be willing to cooperate and resources are required for suitable equipment. Thought needs to be given to the equipment chosen. Schools are developing use of word processors, which is of general benefit to children as well as those with problems, but this equipment is not portable. Access to equipment at home will be helpful but the cost may be beyond the means of some families.

Dyscalculia

Difficulties with maths have attracted less attention than literacy problems yet they are quite common and of practical importance in everyday life. Calculators and cash registers have made life easier in many ways but it is an advantage to be able to check results by rough estimates if gross errors are not to occur. In adults, specific dyscalculia has been known to occur after strokes but in children it is exceptional to be able to find specific lesions and not justified to look for them.[39] Ability in maths underlies physics, music and technical drawing so choice of career needs to take this into account.

Children who find mental arithmetic difficult to conceptualize may benefit from extended use of concrete equipment as used in infant classes. However, this can make a child conspicuous, leading to embarrassment, and skilled educational advice may be required.

Motor learning difficulties

Central motor deficits have been identified in children for many years and described in a variety of ways. Dupre referred to *debilité motrice* in 1907 but the term became too diffuse to be useful.[40] Authors such as Orton[41] described the children in terms of *minimal brain damage*, acknowledging the constitutional nature of the disability. However, the term has a pejorative flavour and damage is not usually demonstrable or worth seeking, though medical conditions such as hydrocephalus, congenital hypothyroidism, intrauterine growth retardation or posttraumatic state can cause motor difficulties. The alternative term of *minimal cerebral dysfunction*[42] has an honest intention but has not been a success – the difficulties are often more than minimal and cerebral dysfunction is hardly a popular term. *Clumsy* also has a pejorative quality, being used to describe gaucheness and carelessness as much as immature motor ability. *Developmental dyspraxia and agnosic ataxia*[43] is a fair neurological designation for some of these children but is rather technical. However the self-help organization for families of children with motor learning difficulties has opted to call itself The Dyspraxia Trust so the term is likely to become more widely used even though not all children with motor problems would be described as dyspraxic by clinicians.

Most of all, children with motor learning difficulties need to be accepted as they are and ways must be found for them to experience success and relaxation in contrast to their many frustrations in everyday

life. Practice will only be beneficial if the child is ready to benefit from that. Often the child with difficulties will lack confidence and will accept inability to perform having failed at the first attempts; and will not make further attempts even though developmental progress has brought achievement within reach. The successes of therapists are often at that stage by remotivating the child to try with a short course of pragmatic treatment.[23,37] There is no evidence for benefit from remedial therapy techniques such as sensory integrative therapy[44] which enjoys a vogue among many occupational therapists. For children with speech dyspraxia a short course of intensive therapy can be very beneficial when the child is mature enough to cooperate (usually 7–9 years old). Involvement in group activities, such as summer clubs or youth clubs, can prove successful and enjoyable but requires a high ratio of adults to children as many children with motor problems are lacking in social skills or confidence.

The psychological characteristics of children with motor difficulties are as important as their physical characteristics. Shaffer and colleagues[12] showed that the existence of motor difficulties and anxiety had high predictive value for the need for psychiatric help for anxiety, depression or withdrawal in adolescence. However, motor difficulties alone (or anxiety alone) were usually overcome.

The condition known as Asperger's syndrome[45,46] is infrequent, occurring in about 1:2000 children, and is still not sufficiently well known. These children have average intelligence, marked motor difficulties, pedantic, sometimes inappropriate, monotonous speech, autistic features such as obsessional interests, mannerisms and an inability to understand social relationships, no sense of humour, a literal conception of language ('Give me your hand' might provoke a tantrum), poor understanding of maths and social isolation. Psychiatric help in diagnosis and treatment should be considered.

Conclusion

As the major nutritional and infectious illnesses have been controlled, developmental problems have assumed greater importance and cause more distress to families and children. Their ascertainment and management require clinical skill, organizational ability and a willingness to work with other agencies. Increased alertness to child protection issues has placed new responsibilities on professionals to distinguish between constitutional and environmental causes. There is no greater challenge for cooperation between all aspects of child health services than to create a sensitive, efficient and effective service for children whose development causes concern.

References

1 Rose, G., Day, S. The population mean predicts the number of deviant individuals. *Br Med J* 1990; **301:** 1031–1034.

2 Blomquist, H.K. *Mental Retardation in Children. An Epidemiological and Ethological Study of Mentally Retarded Children Born 1959–1970 in a Northern Swedish County.* University of Umeå, Sweden: Umeå University Medical Dissertations, New Series 76, 1982.

3 McKinlay, I.A., Bradley, G., Hindle, A., Ehrhardt, P. Motor co-ordination of children with mild mental handicap. *Upsala J Med Sci* 1987; **44** (Suppl): 129–135.

4 Robson, P. Shuffling, hitching, scooting or sliding: some observations in 30 otherwise normal children. *Dev Med Child Neurol* 1970; **12:** 608–617.

5 Hayashi, K. The influence of clothes and bedclothes on infants' gross motor development. *Dev Med Child Neurol* 1992; **34:** 557–558.

6 Kagan, J., Klein, R.E. Cross-cultural perspectives in early development. In: Leiderman, H., Tulkin, S., eds. *Cultural and Social Influences in Infancy and Early Childhood.* Stanford: Stanford University Press, 1975.

7 Touwen, B.C.L. The neurological development of the infant. In: Davis, J.A., Dobbing, J., eds. *Scientific Foundations of Paediatrics,* London: William Heinemann, 1981: 830–842.

8 Super, C.M. Environmental effects on motor development: the case of African precocity. *Dev Med Child Neurol* 1976; **18:** 561–567.

9 Capute, A.J. Normal gross development: the influence of race, sex and socio-economic status. *Dev Med Child Neurol* 1985; **27:** 635–643.

10 Eme, R.F. Sex differences in childhood psychopathology: a review. *Psychol Rev* 1979; **86:** 574–595.

11 Drillien, C., Drummond, M., eds. Frequency and distribution of neurodevelopmental disability. In: *Development Screening and the Child with Special Needs.* London: Spastics International Medical Publications, 1983: 55–89.

12 Shaffer, D., Schonfield, I., O'Conner, P.A. *et al.* Neurological soft signs: their relationship to psychiatric disorder and intelligence in childhood and adolescence. *Arch General Psychiatr* 1985; **42:** 342–351.

13 McKinlay, I.A., Gordon, N.S., eds. Motor learning difficulties: 'clumsy children'. In: *Neurologically Handicapped Children: Treatment and Management.* Oxford: Blackwell Scientific Publications, 1986: 183–203.

14 Bowlby, J. *Maternal Care and Mental Health.* World Health Organization Monograph Series, 179. Geneva: World Health Organization, 1952.

15 Rutter, M. The long term effects of early experience. *Dev Med Child Neurol* 1952; **22:** 800–816.

16 Kolvin, J., Miller, F.J.W., Scott, D.McI., Gatzanis, S.R.M., Fleeting, M. *Continuities of Deprivation?* Aldershot: Avebury, 1990.

17 Hagberg, B., Hagberg, G., Lewerth, A., Lindberg, U. Mild mental retardation in Swedish school children. II etiological and pathogenetic aspects. *Acta Paediatr Scand* 1981; **70:** 445–452.

18 Costeff, H., Cohen, B.E., Weller, L.E. Biological factors in mild mental retardation. *Dev Med Child Neurol* 1983; **25:** 580–587.

19 Hagerman, R.J., Silverman, A.C. *Fragile X Syndrome: Diagnosis, Treatment and Research.* Baltimore: Johns Hopkins Press, 1991.

20 Fundudis, T., Kolvin, I., Garside, R.F. *Speech Retarded and Deaf Children: their Psychological Development.* London: Academic Press, 1979.

21 Cunningham, C.C., Morgan, P.A., McGucken, R.B. Is dissatisfaction with disclosure inevitable? *Dev Med Child Neurol* 1984; **26:** 33–39.

22 McKinlay, I. Child development and learning disorders. *Current Opinion Neurol Neurosurg* 1988; **1:** 1027–1036.

23 Hall, D.M.B. *Health for all Children.* 2nd edn. Oxford: Oxford University Press, 1992.

24 Farnham-Diggory, S. *Learning Disabilities.* London: Fontana, 1978.

25 Rutter, M., Graham, P., Yule, W. *A Neuropsychiatric Study in Childhood.* Little Club Clinics in Developmental Medicine, 35/36. London: William Heinemann, 1970.

26 Miles, T.R., Haslum, M.N. Dyslexia: anomaly or normal variation? In: *Clumsy Children, Child Health and Education Study. Third Report to the Department of Health and Social Security on the 10 year Follow-up,* Paper 6. London: HMSO, 1985.

27 Hulme, C. *Reading Retardation and Multisensory Teaching.* London: Routledge and Kegan Paul, 1981.

28 Leatherbarrow, A. Remedial teaching for literacy. In: Gordon, N.S., McKinlay, I.A., eds. *Neurologically Handicapped Children: Treatment and Management.* Oxford: Blackwell Scientific Publications, 1986: 235–254.

29 Bradley, L. Reading, spelling and writing problems: research on backward readers. In: Gordon, N.S., McKinlay, I.A., eds. *Helping Clumsy Children* revised edn. Edinburgh: Churchill Livingstone, 1989: 135–154.

30 Gordon, N.S., McKinlay, I.A., Rosenbloom, L. Medical contributions to the management of dyslexia. *Arch Dis Child* 1984; **59:** 588–590.

31 Yule, W. Issues and problems in remedial education. *Dev Med Child Neurol* 1976; **18:** 674–682.

32 Hewison, J. The current status of remedial intervention for children with reading problems. *Dev Med Child Neurol* 1982; **24:** 183–186.

33 Jarman, C. *The Development of Handwriting Skills.* Oxford: Blackwell Scientific Publications, 1979.

34 O'Hare, A.E., Brown, J.K. Childhood dysgraphia. Part 1: An illustrated clinical classification. *Child: Care, Hlth Dev* 1989a; **15:** 79–104.

35 O'Hare, A.E., Brown, J.K. Childhood dysgraphia. Part 2: a study of hand function. *Child: Care, Hlth Dev* 1989b; **15:** 151–166.

36 Alston, J., Taylor, J. *Handwriting: Theory, Research and Practice.* London: Croom Helm, 1987.

37 McKinlay, I.A. Children with motor learning difficulties: not so much a syndrome, more a way of life. *Physiotherapy;* 1987. **73:** 635–638.

38 Alston, J., Taylor, J. *The Handwriting File.* 2nd edn. Wisbech: Learning Development Aids, 1988.

39 O'Hare, A.E., Brown, J.K., Aitken, K. Dyscalculia in children. *Dev Med Child Neurol* 1991; **33:** 356–361.

40 McKinlay, I.A. Clumsy children *Update* 1987; **35:** 243–249.

41 Orton, S.T. *Reading, Writing and Speech Problems in Children*. New York: Norton, 1937.

42 Bax, M.C.O., MacKeith, R. *Minimal Cerebral Dysfunction*. Little Club Clinics in Developmental Medicine. London: William Heinemann, 1963, no 10.

43 Gubbay, S.S., Ellis, E., Court, S.D.M. Clumsy children: a study of developmental apraxia and agnosia. *Brain* 1962; **85:** 603–612.

44 Ayres, A.J. The development of perceptual motor abilities: a theoretical basis for treatment of dysfunction. *Am J Occup Ther* 1963; **18:** 221–225.

45 Bishop, D.V.M. Autism, Asperger's syndrome and semantic-pragmatic disorders: where are the boundaries? *Br J Disord Commun* 1989; **24:** 107–121.

46 Wolff, S. Asperger's syndrome. *Arch Dis Child* 1991; **66:** 737–741.

14.2   Psychological tests

Jane Lethem

Introduction

Psychological tests are tools for quantifying or categorizing certain attributes of the individual who is to be tested.[1] The aim of psychometric testing of a child is to yield information that is as accurate and objective as possible, which can contribute to an assessment of the child's functioning. Use of such instruments can assist in answering questions like, 'Is my son slow at learning or just lazy?'; 'Is this little girl globally delayed, or delayed only in language development?'; 'Do most children of this age have as many problems remembering what they are told as this one does?'; 'How much improvement has there been in this young patient's ability to cope with a painful medical treatment?'. These questions and others like them are complex. Testing alone cannot provide the answers but forms part of a clinical process which may also include interviewing the child, parents, other family members, teacher or carers, and carrying out observations of the child in a number of possible settings such as the home, nursery, or hospital.

Production, updating and marketing of psychological tests of all kinds is a growth area.[2,3] This chapter emphasizes tests that are of use in answering the kinds of clinical questions that will be familiar to professionals working in the area of community child health.

Characteristics of psychological tests

The medium of the test

The medium of the test may be a task or set of tasks given to the child by the psychologist, a checklist completed by the psychologist while observing the child, a structured interview of the child or parent(s) by the psychologist, a questionnaire for a parent or teacher to answer about the child or a self-report questionnaire to be filled in by the child. Some scales combine several media such as tasks plus psychologist's observations.

Illuminating comparisons

A test can only provide useful information if it enables a comparison to be made of the child's performance on the test either with other children of the same age, or with the child's own performance on a different occasion. Tests may be norm-referenced or criterion-referenced.[4] Most psychological tests require that deductions be made about an abstract quality such as intelligence or personality, on the basis of responses to questions or concrete tasks. The results of norm-referenced tests are scaled in such a way that the child's score may be represented in relation to the statistical range of scores expected for children of the same age.[5] Scaled results may be expressed in a number of ways, such as quotients as in intelligence quotient or IQ, and centiles or age equivalents as with mental age, reading age. In contrast, criterion-referenced tests relate the child's performance to specific behavioural goals without reference to the performances of other children. Examples of this are feeding self with a spoon, or performing long division.

Standardization

For any given psychological test, materials and procedures need to be as similar as possible each time the test is given. Testers are usually provided with a standard set of equipment and/or record sheets for noting the child's responses, together with detailed instructions for administering, scoring and interpreting the results obtained. Usually specialized training is required and testers should demonstrate competence in giving the test in the appropriate standardized manner before using it clinically.

Sample population

The development of a scale involves standardized administration of the new test to a large and representative sample of children. The resulting scores will tend to follow a normal distribution.[6] The mean of the distribution is calculated by dividing the sum of all the scores by the number of scores. The term standard deviation refers to a measurement of the extent to which scores vary from the mean. An individual's scores on two tests which have different means or standard deviations may be compared by calculating how many standard deviations the individual's scores are away from the mean, known as standard scores.

The British Ability Scale sample[7] totalling 3435 children between 2 and 17 years of age, grouped in six age bands, and drawn from 11 regions in Britain, corresponded closely to the British population as a whole in terms of gender, occupation of parents and urban or rural place of residence. Data from the sample were used to generate tables of norms with which the scores of individual children could subsequently be compared.

Validity and reliability

If their results are to be meaningful, psychological tests need a high degree of validity and reliability.[6] A test is valid if it measures what it purports to measure, that is if its results correlate highly with some other current criterion of the attribute it was designed to measure or with the occurrence of a future event, such as high correlation between intelligence test scores and future examination performance. A reliable test shows consistency of results when given by different testers, or on different occasions. The standard error of measurement describes an estimate of reliability. The term generalizability[1] refers to the extent to which comparable results may be obtained by the same test under different conditions.

Selection of tests

In each case, a test should be chosen with a particular hypothesis about the child in mind, such as that lack of cooperation with adults results from an inability to understand instructions and requests or that poor performance in school is due to a specific learning difficulty. However, given the enormous number of scales on the market, a psychologist's training, views about theories of development and access to test equipment, are also likely to play a part in determining the selection of tests for a particular assessment. A small sample of scales is highlighted below.

Cognitive assessment

The majority of standardized psychological tests are concerned with aspects of cognitive functioning. Results can contribute to the understanding of a child's developmental status, pattern of abilities or problems, or overall intellectual level. Depending upon the reason for the assessment, interpreting the results may enable the psychologist to give an opinion about the probability of the child being gifted, showing a global or a specific learning disability or having brain damage.[8] Advice may follow concerning educational needs, vocational aptitude or the likely benefits of therapeutic intervention.

Tests of early development

Scales for the under fives such as the Bayley Scales of Infant Development,[9] the Griffiths Scale,[10] the Merrill Palmer Scale[11] usually combine items which test motor, social, communicative, and non-verbal cognitive abilities. Some scales such as the McCarthy Scales of Children's Abilities,[12] for $3\frac{1}{2}$ to $8\frac{1}{2}$ year olds and the British Ability Scales,[7] for $2\frac{1}{2}$ year olds to 17 plus year olds have an age range which begins at the pre-school level.

Tests for school age children

The Wechsler Intelligence Scale for Children – Third UK Edition (WISC-III UK)[13] consists of subtests of verbal ability and non verbal ability. Results are processed into verbal IQ, performance IQ and full scale IQ. Scaled subtest scores yield a profile of the child's abilities on a range of verbal and non-verbal tasks. The British Ability Scales (BAS)[7] are grouped by cognitive processes: speed, reasoning, spatial imagery, perceptual matching, short-term memory and retrieval and application of knowledge. Each process is represented by one or more test presented to the child through either visual or verbal stimuli, to which the child's response will be in either a motor or verbal modality. The result of each test can be transformed into a centile score. Provided that a selection of tests appropriate to the age of the child has been administered, general IQ, visual IQ and verbal IQ can be calculated.

Some children have disabilities which make it difficult or impossible to make certain kinds of responses. The psychologist must take such limitations into account when choosing tests to administer. The Peabody Picture Vocabulary Test[14] yields an IQ which correlates well with other tests of intelligence and requires the child simply to be able to point to one of four pictures on a page, or to vocalize one of four numbers in response to verbal instructions by the tester. During administration of the Leiter International Performance Scale Battery for Children[15] neither the tester nor the child is required to use language. It is a non-verbal performance scale yielding IQ and mental age. Raven's Coloured Progressive Matrices[16] is a non-verbal measure of general ability which requires the child to point in response to a visual stimulus.

Tests of educational attainments

The Schonell Word Reading Test and Schonell Spelling Test[17] yield a reading age and spelling age respectively. Measurements of both reading ability and comprehension of written passages can be obtained by employing the Neale Analysis of Reading Ability Revised British Edition.[18] The WISC-III UK and BAS include tests of mathematical ability. The Graded Arithmetic-Mathematics Test[19] comprises two forms, for use with primary and secondary school age groups respectively.

Neuropsychology

Results of the WISC-III UK and BAS can provide clues to a child's neuropsychological status. For example poor performance on tests which depend upon memory or a discrepancy between WISC-III UK verbal IQ and performance IQ larger than 15 points[8] may suggest brain damage. As there may be other explanations for such scores on intelligence tests, further investigation should be carried out. The Luria-Nebraska Neuropsychological Battery: Children's Revision[20] identifies brain damage and enables the psychologist to describe cognitive deficits in detail.

Measuring emotions and behaviour

Questionnaires and structured interviews make use of the knowledge that a child's parents, teacher or psychologist have acquired through observation. Richman and Graham[21] developed a screening questionnaire for pre-school children which highlights behavioural and emotional difficulties such as tempers, fears, soiling, worries and mood. The Vineland Adaptive Behaviour Scales[22,23] assess communication, daily living skills, socialization, motor skills and maladaptive behaviour. They are helpful in assessing the independence of children and adolescents with learning disability. The Observational Scale of Behavioural Distress[24,25] is an example of an instrument for use in a specific situation. It is used to assess and to monitor changes in the distress shown by children during medical treatment. It can provide an objective measure of changes in distress following an intervention designed to help the child to cope with painful or invasive medical procedures.

Interpretation

The test in context

The psychologist who is using a test as part of an assessment needs other information which may be of relevance to the hypothesis to be tested as well as knowledge of the immediate context of the administration of the test. Information should be sought from the parent(s) and referrer about the child's developmental and medical history, family background, their opinions about the child's strengths and their current concerns. Whenever possible, the child's views should also be elicited. Parental permission is sought to contact the child's school or nursery in order to learn about the child from the perspective of a teacher, nursery nurse or other carer.

The purpose of testing should be explained to the parent(s) and whenever possible to the child, in an age appropriate way. While testing is taking place, the psychologist should make a note of the child's emotional state, social skills, attention, concentration and cooperation. Any interruptions or other deviations from standardized procedure should also be recorded.

Limitations of testing

A child's performance on a test may be influenced by factors other than ability to respond. These include the child's physical well-being, attention, concentration and cooperation. The interaction with the tester is important and is likely to be influenced by the child's previous experience of adults. Anxiety and fear of failure may interfere with a child's performance.

Language, ethnicity and culture are important factors to take into account. It is often difficult to decide whether to use a test when the child's first language is not English or when the child's ethnic and cultural background differs from that of the population of the standardization sample and from that of the psychologist. It may be argued in such cases that testing should not be carried out. However that may result in the child receiving only a subjective assessment and being deprived of the opportunity to demonstrate abilities. Two case examples illustrate the dilemma facing the psychologist.

A 6-year-old girl of Asian descent whose parents speak English as their second language was referred in relation to severe communication problems and unusual behaviour. Although her parents and teachers suspected that her non-verbal abilities were considerably greater than her verbal abilities, there was little concrete evidence. However, as part of a thorough assessment, the Leiter Scale was administered and her results indicated that her non-verbal abilities were close to age appropriate.

A 4-year-old boy with cerebral palsy, of a family of African origin who speak English as a second language, was seen for an opinion about his level of intellectual functioning, adjustment to his disability and prognosis. In the context of a detailed assessment, the Peabody Picture Vocabulary Test was used because the child was capable of the pointing response required. His scores suggested a below average performance for his age. However, his parents explained that several of the items depicted were unfamiliar to him and that some of the words used would not usually be spoken at home.

Had a psychological test not been employed in the first example, the girl's non-verbal potential might have been underestimated. In the second case, results were inconclusive as there were a number of possible explanations for a lowered score. In cases like these, when a psychologist does decide to test, it is vital to report the limits of the test for the particular child and possible alternative explanations for the child having made errors.

Drawing conclusions

It is sometimes said that intelligence tests only measure the ability to do intelligence tests. Test scores are meaningless, for clinical purposes, until their implications are explained. The task of test interpretation includes deciding whether its administration was standardized or whether particular characteristics of the child or the situation might have influenced the scores in an unusual way. Data from the test should be related to the expected performance of children of the age of the child tested and to data about the child from other sources. An opinion should be reached concerning the original hypothesis and appropriate recommendations made.

Sharing conclusions with child, parent(s) and referrer

The child, parents and referrer each require feedback of a slightly different kind. Children are often relieved to have a simple explanation that gives them some insight into past difficulties plus an outline of the sort of help from which they might benefit. Parents are likely to have many questions, about the meaning of the assessment and implications for the immediate and longer term future. They need time to express these. After discussing the interpreted results with parents it is usually helpful to summarize them on paper, in the form of a letter or report. A copy of the report should be sent to the referrer. The psychologist should exercise caution in including test scores in reports as children may be labelled inappropriately if such scores are quoted out of context.

Summary

Psychometry can play an important part in assessing or monitoring a child provided that interpreted results are integrated with other forms of information about the child, including developmental and medical history, family background and observations by parents, teachers or other carers as well as by the psychologist. Norm-referenced psychological tests provide a method for the standardized collection of raw data which can be transformed into a form which enables a comparison to be made between the child tested and other children of the same age. Test results have the attraction of appearing objective; however they can only be meaningful if issues of the reliability and validity of a test, together with its suitability for the individual child, have been taken into account.

References

1 Cronbach, L.J. *Essentials of Psychological Testing*, 3rd edn. New York: Harper and Row, 1970.
2 NFER-Nelson. *Catalogue for Occupational Therapists, Community Medical Teams, Psychologists, Social Workers, Health Visitors, Speech and Language Therapists, Care Managers, Researchers, Trainers and Doctors*. Windsor, Berks: NFER-Nelson, 1992.
3 The Psychological Corporation. *Psychological Assessment Catalogue*. Sidcup, Kent: Harcourt Brace Janovich, 1991/92.
4 Popham, W.J., Husek, T.R. Implications of criterion-referenced measurements. *J Educ Measurement* 1969; **6:** 1–9.
5 Anastasi, A. *Psychological Testing, 5th edn*. New York: Macmillan, 1982.
6 Maxwell, A.E. *Analysing Qualitative Data*. London: Methuen, 1961.
7 Elliot, C.D. *British Ability Scales: Technical Handbook*. Windsor, Berks: NFER-Nelson, 1983.
8 Kaufman, A.S. *Intelligence Testing with the WISC-R*. New York, Toronto: John Wiley and Sons, 1979.
9 Bayley, N. *Bayley Scales of Infant Development*. New York: The Psychological Corporation, 1969.
10 Griffiths, R. *The Abilities of Babies*. London: University of London Press, 1954.
11 Stutsman, R. *Guide for Administering the Merrill-Palmer Scale of Mental Tests*. New York: Harcourt, Brace and World, 1948.
12 McCarthy, D.A. *Manual of the McCarthy Scales of Children's Abilities*. New York: Psychological Corporation, 1972.
13 Weschler, D. *Weschler Intelligence Scale for Children Third UK Edition (WISC-III UK)*. London: The Psychological Corporation, 1992.
14 Dunn, L.M. *Peabody Picture Vocabulary Test*. Minnesota: American Guidance Service Inc, 1965.
15 Leiter, R. *Leiter International Performance Scale Battery for Children*. Chicago: Stoetling Co, 1979.
16 Raven, J.C. *Raven's Progressive Matrices and Vocabulary Scales*. Oxford: Oxford Psychological Press, 1991.
17 Schonell, F.J. *Reading and Spelling Tests: Handbook of Instructions*. Edinburgh: Oliver and Boyd Ltd, 1950.
18 Neale, M.D. *Neale Analysis of Reading Ability Revised British Edition*. British adaptation and standardization by Una Christophers and Chris Whetton. Windsor, Berks: NFER-Nelson, 1989.
19 Vernon, P.E., Miller, K.M. *Graded Arithmetic-Mathematics Test, Metric edition: Manual of Instructions*. London: Hodder and Stoughton, 1976.

20 Golden, C., Hammeke, T., Purisch, A. *Luria-Nebraska Neuropsychological Battery: Children's Revision*. Windsor, Berks: NFER-Nelson, 1990.

21 Richman, N., Graham, P. A behavioural screening questionnaire for use with 3 year old children. *Assoc Child Psychol Psychiatr* 1971; **12:** 5–33.

22 Doll, E.A. *The Measurement of Social Competence. A Manual for the Vineland Social Maturity Scale*. Minneapolis: Educational Publishing, 1953.

23 Sparrow, S., Balla, D., Cicchetti, D. *Vineland Adaptive Behaviour Scales*, American Guidance Service. Windsor, Berks: NFER-Nelson, 1986.

24 Jay, S.M., Elliot, C.H. Behavioural observation scale for measuring children's distress: the effects of increasing methodological rigor. *J Consult Clin Psychol* 1984; **52:** 1106–1107.

25 Sylva, K. Behaviour measurement review: No. 3: observational measures for assessing distress during medical treatment. *Assoc Child Psychol Psychiatr: newsletter* 1992; **14:** 24–27.

Chapter 15

Orthopaedic problems

David Hunt

Introduction

The whole range of orthopaedic problems are encountered in paediatric practice in the community. Sorting out those problems which are significant from those which will resolve can be difficult and confusing. Reassuring anxious parents requires confidence in the natural outcome of each condition.

The aim of this chapter is to indicate the common, significant conditions: to show how the diagnosis and the natural outcome can be assessed by a few simple rules. The list is not comprehensive, but is based on those conditions which constitute the commonest reasons for referral to a paediatric orthopaedic clinic.

Congenital dislocation of the hip

Until Ortolani described a test for the diagnosis of the congenitally dislocated hip (CDH) in the newborn infant in 1937,[1] it was generally believed that this condition could not be diagnosed until the child started walking. When Ortolani's test was shown to be effective, particularly when modified by Barlow[2] who also added his own test, the possibility of screening all newborn children for dislocation of the hip became a reality.

Screening programmes were then introduced and are now standard practice in developed countries. Many different professionals are involved: paediatricians, midwives, health visitors, clinical medical officers, community physicians, general practitioners, and orthopaedic surgeons.

Neonatal screening programmes have established the incidence of hip instability. This can vary according to the experience and expertise of the examiner, but some degree of instability can be detected in 9 per 1000 live births among Caucasians.[3,4]

At least 80% of congenitally dislocatable hips stabilize spontaneously. Of these, 50% do so in the first few days of life.[5] The true incidence of congenital dislocation of the hip is then 1.6 per thousand births. Clinical examination and ultrasound have reduced this incidence by half, but not eliminated it. It remains to be shown whether or not a comprehensive screening programme combining both these techniques will lower the incidence of late diagnosis further.

The incidence of missed diagnosis varies from 0.07 to 0.17 per 1000 live births.[3,4] In other words, one in 100 dislocated hips will be missed by a screening programme. Nevertheless, if the diagnosis is made up to one year old, 90% of infants can be treated by simple conservative means, and will have normal hips. Even up to 18 months, conservative treatment will succeed in more than 50%.[6]

The structure of a neonatal screening programme is largely determined by locally available resources. The principles have been the subject of much debate,[7] but in setting up or reviewing such a programme, there are fundamental principles which should be followed.

Consistency

It is the responsibility of each health authority to define local policy. Professional training or speciality are not so important. Junior members of staff have to be trained, and they change frequently so that while they can screen, responsibility for the programme cannot be delegated to them. A designated officer must be responsible for the implementation of the programme in each district and should be a permanent member of staff.

Uniformity

Every infant must be screened at the same ages. It is now recommended that this should be done within 24 hours of birth, and again before leaving the maternity unit. With early discharge, the second examination is more difficult. The baby is next examined at 6 weeks, between 6 and 9 months, and finally between 18 and 24 months.

Other aetiological factors

Where there is suspicion of an abnormal hip, extra care must be given and investigation considered, even if the hips are normal on examination. Predisposing factors include it being more likely with a first born baby, a breech presentation, caesarian section, the female gender and a strong family history. The presence of other deformities such as plagiocephaly, infantile scoliosis or talipes equinovarus should also raise suspicions.

Technique of examination

Ortolani described an examination of both hips simultaneously. Barlow's modification was to apply a posterior force through the hips examining each individually while using the other hand to hold the opposite femur, and thus the pelvis, steady. It is essential in any screening programme that all examiners should test the hips in exactly the same way. A suggested technique is as follows:

The child is laid supine on a firm surface. With the legs together, the hips and knees are flexed fully (Fig. 15.1). It is important to hold the tibia in the web between the index finger and thumb, with the thumb on the femur and middle finger on the greater trochanter. Pressure is applied into the examining couch. In the mind's eye, one can imagine that this maneouvre tends to push a loose hip posteriorly out of the socket. This is after all how hips dislocate. It may be possible to feel the hips slide up over the posterior lip, and out

of the acetabulum. This is the first part of Barlow's modification of Ortolani's test.

Both hips are then abducted, still with the middle finger on the greater trochanter (Fig. 15.2). This finger lifts the trochanter forward as the hip is abducted. If the hip is dislocated, the first thing that will be noted is limitation of abduction on the affected side. If the hip is irreducible, this is all that will be observed, and so is a vital sign; it is an indication for further investigation and particularly significant at the 6-week check when it is easier to observe than at birth.

It is now important to repeat the examination, one hip at a time. Barlow's test is reapplied by flexing the hips and knees, and applying a posterior force through both hips to see if either hip may be felt to move up over the posterior rim of the acetabulum and so dislocate. Holding one hip like this to stabilize the pelvis, the other hip is examined by abducting and lifting the trochanter forward as before (Fig. 15.3). If a hip is reducible, it will now relocate with a deep clunk. This is distinct from the ligamentous click, which

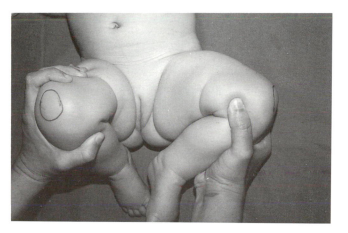

Figure 15.2 Examination of hips in newborn child. Both hips abducted. This is Ortolani's test.

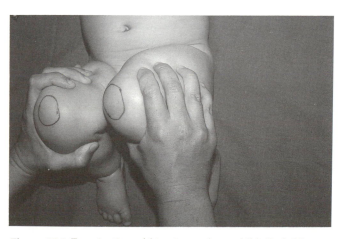

Figure 15.1 Examination of hips in newborn child. Both hips are flexed. This is Barlow's test.

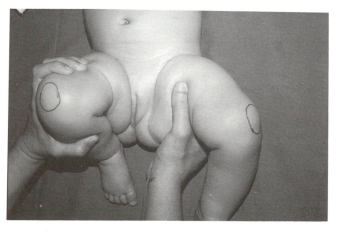

Figure 15.3 Examination of hips in newborn child. One hip is examined at one time.

will be found frequently, but is not necessarily significant. The clunk on relocation is Ortolani's test. Finally, in full abduction, the leg is released; the head of the femur, held between finger and thumb, is rocked backwards and forwards. Occasionally, a hip which may have been considered normal up to this point can be rolled in and out of the acetabulum posteriorly by this manoeuvre. This is the final part of Barlow's test. The same is now done to the other hip. Other signs, particularly asymmetry of skin creases, are unreliable in the newborn, and only become significant when the child is walking. These tests apply to newborn children only and are useless after the age of three months.

Ultrasound examination

The failure of screening programmes to eliminate late diagnosis of congenital dislocation of the hip has sustained research into alternative diagnostic techniques. Ultrasound technology has advanced to provide high resolution images of the developing femoral head and acetabulum, so that all degrees of instability and dysplasia can be imaged (Fig. 15.4a,b). It is now possible to classify the newborn hip into four grades on the ultrasound appearance, from normal (grade I) through grades of dysplasia and subluxation (grades II–III) to frank dislocation (grade IV).[8]

Ultrasound is now an alternative method of screening for congenital dislocation.[9] It is possible to detect the dysplastic hip which is likely to progress to dislocation in spite of being clinically normal. Similarly, a hip which is dislocatable clinically may be shown on ultrasound to be the type which will stabilize spontaneously, and does not need treatment. However, as yet, the addition of ultrasound to the armoury of screening techniques for congenital dislocation has not succeeded in fully eliminating the late diagnosed or *missed* CDH.

Follow up and treatment

When any abnormality is detected in a newborn hip, immediate referral to an orthopaedic surgeon with an interest in paediatrics is recommended. Treatment may be started sometime in the first month, usually at 2 weeks old. At least 50% of hips will stabilize in the first few weeks, so many will be treated unnecessarily if treatment is started early. Treatment involves splintage of the hips in reduction (Fig. 15.5). Any form of splintage carries an incidence of damaging the growing hip, which may be as high as 10%.[10] Thus unnecessary splintage should be avoided.

The treatment of congenital dislocation causes much confusion. The treatment method is determined by the age at diagnosis, and the efficacy of the technique used. It is not always straightforward, even when the diagnosis is made early. Methods are summarized in the flow chart in Figure 15.6.

(a)

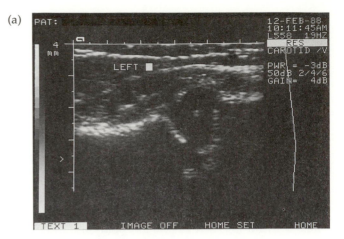

(b)

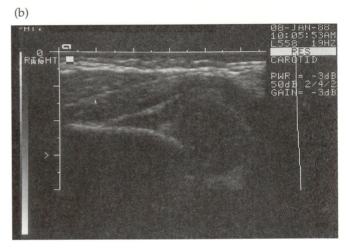

Figure 15.4 (a) Ultrasound of a normal hip. The femoral head is seen clearly as a dark shadow with a central white spot. It makes a deep indentation in the dense white line which is the bony pelvis. (b) Ultrasound of a dislocated hip. The femoral head does not make a significant indentation in the bone, i.e. it does not lie in the socket.

Between the age of 6 months and 1 year the risk of avascular necrosis of the femoral head from over-zealous attempts to reduce and hold the dislocated hip is at its highest. This must be carefully explained to the parents, and all treatment abandoned until one year of age if avascular necrosis occurs. The chances of achieving a reduced hip by traction alone are as good at 1 year as at 6 months. The risks of operative reduction before 1 year old are high.

Late presentation

In spite of screening and ultrasound examination, cases of congenital dislocation are still missed. Any child who walks with an asymmetrical, waddling gait when starting to walk must be suspected of having a dislocated hip. Examination shows shortening of the affected leg with external rotation, asymmetry of skin creases and limitation of abduction (Fig. 15.7a,b).

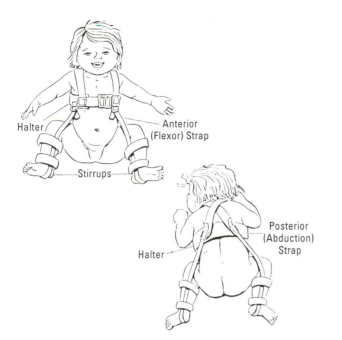

Figure 15.5 Diagram of a Pavlik harness, a commonly used technique for splinting dislocatable hips.

Surgical treatment

For the established dislocation, at or beyond 1 year old, treatment is by an initial period of traction followed by either a trial of splintage in a plaster cast, or an open reduction. Gallows traction is commonly used, the hips being abducted over 3 weeks (Fig. 15.8). Tight adductor muscles may need to be released during this period. At the end of this time an X-ray is taken, and the hip examined under anaesthesia. If it is widely dislocated, an open reduction will be performed. If it is apparently located, a trial of reduction is carried out by placing the hips in a plaster hip spica and maintaining that for 6 weeks (Fig. 15.9).

The temptation to manipulate a dislocated hip back in must be resisted. It is certain to result in permanent damage, even if it were to succeed in relocation of the hip.

After 6 weeks in plaster, or earlier if the hip is not fully reduced, an arthrogram is performed under anaesthetic. This will clearly define the containment of the femoral head in the acetabulum (Fig. 15.10). If there is significant soft tissue obstruction, open reduction is performed. The capsule of the hip is opened, the soft tissue obstruction excised, and the femoral head

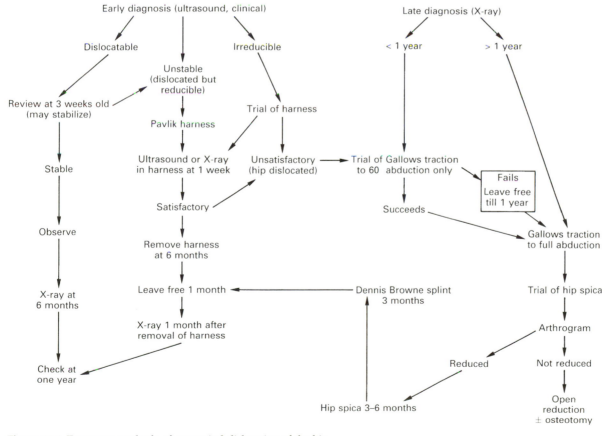

Figure 15.6 Treatment methods of congenital dislocation of the hip.

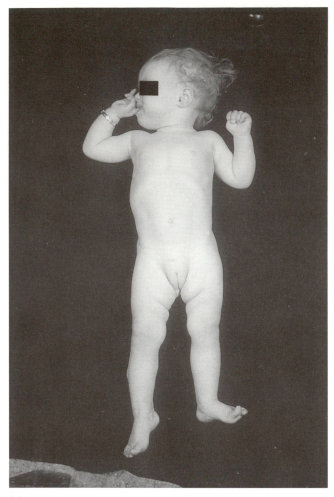

(a)

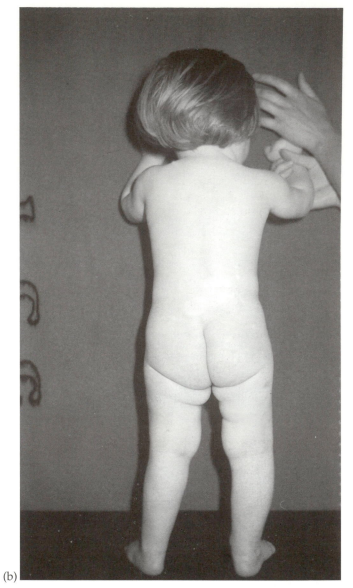

(b)

Figure 15.7 (a,b) Late presentation of congenital dislocation of the hips showing asymmetry of the legs and skin creases. The left hip is dislocated.

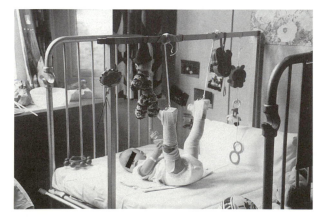

Figure 15.8 Gallows traction.

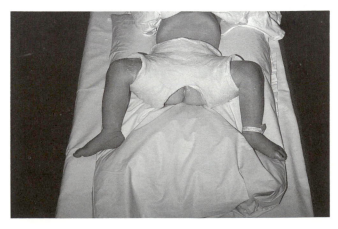

Figure 15.9 Plaster of Paris hip spica.

relocated. It is certain to be unstable, as the acetabulum has not developed sufficiently to contain the head. The Salter innominate osteotomy can be carried out at the same procedure (Fig. 15.11). By making a transverse cut across the ilium, the acetabulum can be turned downwards and forwards over the femoral head, preventing it dislocating upwards and backwards.[11] Postoperatively the hip is held in a plaster splint for 6 weeks, when the hip is examined again under anaesthetic. If it feels unstable, it is then necessary to perform an upper femoral osteotomy to re-align the femur at the hip. The hip is then held for a further 6 weeks in a plaster, followed by a further 3 months in a suitable abduction splint, such as a Dennis Browne (Fig. 15.12).

The clicking hip

The significance of the ligamentous click which can be detected in up to 20% of newborn hips has not been fully established.[12] These are otherwise normal hips clinically, with a full range of movement and no dislocation, or subluxation. In the past these hips have been followed up and X-rayed at 6 months or 1 year. It is in this group that ultrasound examination is likely to prove of most value, eliminating the need to follow

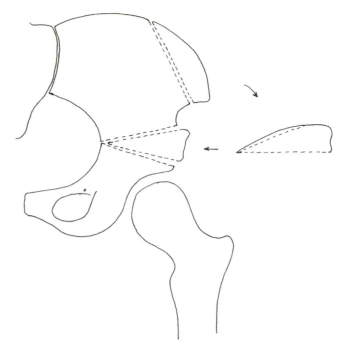

Figure 15.11 Salter innominate osteotomy. This operation constructs an acetabulum which will cover over the femoral head preventing it slipping out of the back or the top.

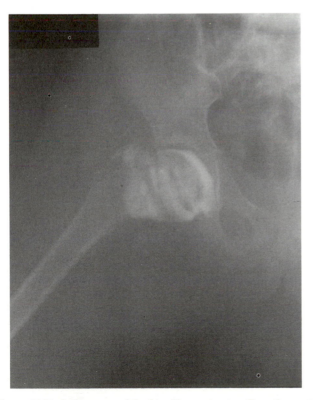

Figure 15.10 Arthrogram of the hip. The contrast outlines the cartilaginous femoral head indicating containment of the head in the acetabulum.

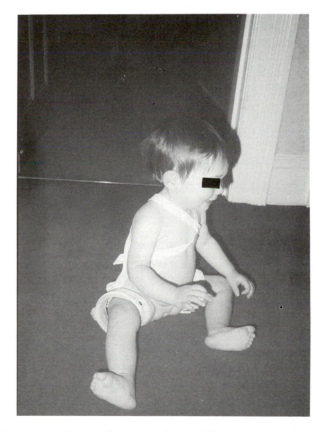

Figure 15.12 Dennis Browne splint holding the legs widely abducted.

up many of these hips and identifying those which are at risk of progressing to full dislocation.

Results of treatment

When the diagnosis is made early, conservative treatment with simple splintage will result in normal hips in over 90%.[6] Of these, 10% will not be treated successfully, and may need open reduction later. When the diagnosis is made at 1 year, 80% will have a satisfactory outcome treated by conservative means. However, 20% will require an open reduction. Over the age of 18 months, the figures are reversed, less than 20% achieving satisfactory hips by conservative means. Above the age of 3 years, the wisdom of treating at all must be questioned.

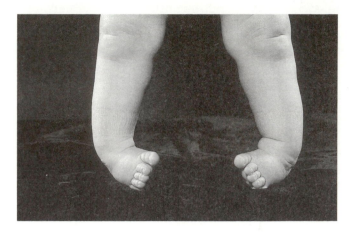

Figure 15.13 Typical appearance of talipes equinovarus.

Club foot: talipes equinovarus

This is the most common congenital foot deformity, and is the deformity known as *club foot*. It occurs 2.29 times per 1000 births.[13] It is slightly more common in boys. It is due to a number of causes, such as heredity,[14] intrauterine moulding, or a neuromuscular disorder.[15]

The deformity is a consequence of soft tissue contracture and bony abnormality. This produces the typical small foot, held in equinus or plantar flexion with the heel rotated inwards and the forefoot also twisted medially (Fig. 15.13).

Classification of the deformity at birth and relating this to prognosis is difficult. All degrees of deformity are seen, from the mild, correctable positional talipes, to the severe, fixed deformity suggesting neuromuscular abnormality. With treatment, sometimes quite mild deformities, although correctable, keep recurring, whereas some severe deformities can correct surprisingly well quite quickly. However, available classifications are based on the degree of correction possible at birth.[16] This is summarized in Table 15.1.

Treatment

Correction of the deformity should be started as soon as possible after birth. There is a lot of benefit to be obtained from early conservative treatment. Stretch-

ing and strapping, or serial plaster casts are equally commonly used and are equally effective (Fig. 15.14). It is simply dependent on the local policy, but either method must be started early. Strapping must be changed every 48 hours. Plasters need to be changed once a week. There is no evidence that early surgical correction improves the results of treatment.

Conservative treatment needs to be continued for between 3 and 6 months. If the foot corrects, treatment is either discontinued or a splint is provided for the child to wear at night for 2 or 3 years (Fig. 15.15). This usually takes the form either of night splints or bootees, connected by a bar (the Dennis Browne splint) and is all that is required for the mild grade I club foot.

Surgical treatment

There are many differing views on the timing and technique of surgical treatment. For the intermediate group or grade II, the deformity is a result of tendon, ligament and capsular contracture. The main deforming force is due to tethers in the posterior and lateral part of the foot, i.e. in the heel. Release of these tethers by a simple posterior release at about 6 months of age is effective, and can dispense with the need for the more extensive surgery that group III requires. For

Table 15.1 Classification of talipes equinovarus.

Grade I Mild or positional talipes	Grade II Moderate talipes	Grade III Severe talipes
Correctable	Partially correctable	Uncorrectable
No contracture	Soft tissue contracture	Soft tissue contracture and bony abnormality
No fixed plantar-flexion	Plantar flexed <20°	Plantar flexed >20°
No fixed inversion	Inverted <20°	Inverted >20°

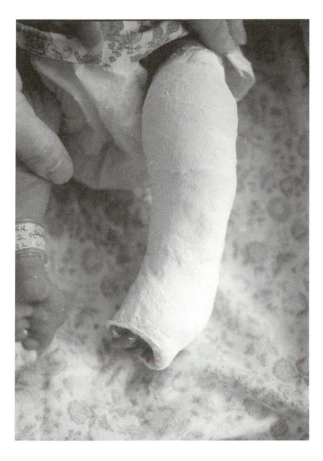

Figure 15.14 Plaster cast for talipes.

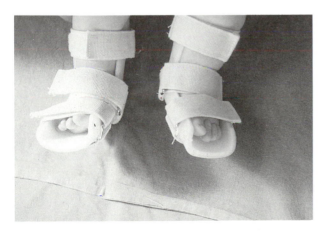

Figure 15.15 Night splints.

the severe grade III club foot the standard method is, at the age of approximately 9 months, when the structures are larger and the wounds more likely to heal, a full release of the tight structures both posteriorly and medially. This includes:

Lengthening of the Achilles tendon
Lengthening of flexor hallucis longus

Release of posterior capsule
Release of talo-navicular joint
Release of tibialis posterior

Postoperatively, the foot is again held corrected in plaster for 3 months, followed by splints at night.

Outcome and later surgical treatment

With this regimen, 90% will achieve excellent results. Approximately 15% of cases treated surgically will relapse at about 18 months. Often this is mild and does not require treatment. If the main problem proves to be forefoot adduction, treatment should be resisted, as this tends to improve with maturity and is not a problem in the adult. If further intervention is however required, conservative treatment has no place and further surgical correction in the form of repeat soft tissue release, tendon transfer such as a lateral transfer of tibialis anterior to give active eversion or, much later, bony procedures to improve the shape of the foot may rarely be indicated.

Minor deformities of the lower limb

Approximately 20% of children referred to an orthopaedic clinic come because of minor deformity of the lower limb. Conditions such as in-toeing, bow legs and knock knees (genu valgum) are the most commonly seen. They cause a lot of anxiety in both patients and doctors because, although we believe they usually get better naturally, how do we reassure the parents? There is then a need to know what the diagnosis is, and how to make it. What is the incidence, what percentage get better without treatment and finally, what are the indications for treatment, if any?

Angular deformities

Diagnosis of angular deformities such as bow legs (genu varum) or knock knees (genu valgum) is relatively easy to make. Bow legs are defined as a deformity of the legs in which standing with the feet together, the knees are wide apart and cannot be brought together. Knock knees are the opposite deformity such that when standing the knees are together and the feet are wide apart. Angular deformities do tend to correct spontaneously (providing underlying rickets is excluded as the cause) but not necessarily completely. Genu valgum is occasionally treated surgically as is genu varum. The cut off point is an angle of 30° between the line of the femur and the line of the tibia. If the angle is more than 30° when standing the deformity will tend to worsen rather than correct.

Rotational deformities

Rotational deformities are less easy to diagnose and require specific methods of examination to do so. They can give rise to bow legs or knock knees as secondary deformities. An understanding of normal parameters is important when considering rotational deformities.

Under 3 years, the normal child has no rotatory deformity. When standing, feet point straight forward or are slightly externally rotated. There is mild genu valgum and the feet are slightly flat. Physiological flat feet are the norm.[17] The hips in extension have 60° of internal and 60° of external rotation. The normal adult tibia is twisted laterally at approximately 20°.[18] There is a tendency for skeletal posture to improve up to age 8 years after which there is secondary compensatory deformity up to the age of maturity.

There are basically four common combinations of femur, tibia and foot rotational deformities (primary deformity) and these are given in Table 15.2, but there is little evidence regarding the aetiology of these groups. There is a racial or inherited contribution, and in part the findings are also a consequence of fetal moulding. Any of the individual deformities can occur in isolation in which case they will be very mild.

The clinical presentation of the child is typical (Figs 15.16–15.19) but it is not possible to make the diagnosis of a primary rotational deformity on appearance alone. Simple specific tests for the primary deformity need to be undertaken.

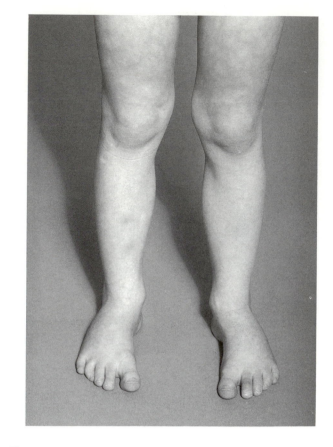

Figure 15.16 Rotational deformities group 1: femoral retroversion, internal tibial torsion and metatarsus adductus.

Anteversion of the femoral neck

The angle subtended by the femoral neck and the femoral shaft is normally 20° to the coronal plane (Fig. 15.20). This is normal anteversion. In persistent fetal anteversion the neck is twisted forward more than normal. The foot lies internally rotated. There is excessive internal rotation and reduced external rotation. This is the commonest cause of in-toeing.

Retroversion of the femoral neck

Retroverted hips lie in external rotation, and internal rotation is limited. If the normal arc is 50° internal and external rotation, retroverted hips will have less than 50° internal rotation but more than 50° external. This deformity is uncommon, affecting less than 1% of children.

Table 15.2 Patterns of lower limb deformity

Rotational or primary deformity	Clinical appearance

1 Retroversion of the femoral neck
    Medial tibial torsion
    Metatarsus adductus
	Normal legs
	Neutral or in-toeing

2 Retroversion of the femoral neck
    Lateral tibial torsion (normal)
    Flat feet
	Normal legs
	Out-toeing

3 Anteversion of the femoral neck
    Medial tibial torsion
    Metatarsus adductus
	Knock knees
	In-toeing

4 Anteversion of the femoral neck
    Lateral tibial torsion (normal)
    Flat feet
	Knock knees
	Neutral feet

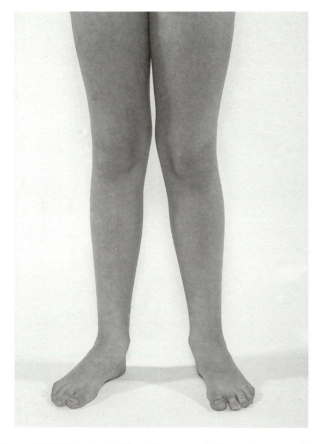

Figure 15.17 Rotational deformities group 2: femoral retroversion, lateral tibial torsion and flat feet.

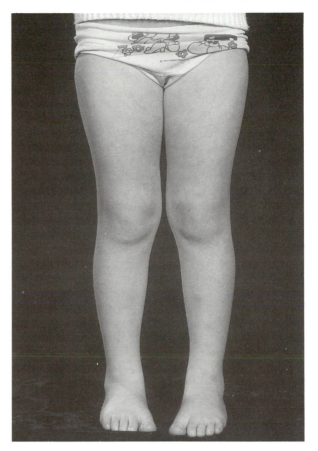

Figure 15.18 Rotational deformities group 3: femoral anteversion, internal tibial torsion and metatarsus adductus.

Tibial torsion

Medial or internal tibial torsion means the tibia is laterally rotated less than the normal 20°. To test this, the child sits on the side of the couch with the knees bent. Then looking straight down the tibia it can be seen whether the foot turns out 20° (normal), more than 20° (external tibial torsion), straight ahead, or even inwards (internal tibial torsion) (Fig. 15.21).

Metatarsus adductus

When the hindfoot is normal and there is no talipes equinovarus or calcaneovalgus, approximately 5% of children will have turned-in or adducted forefeet.[19] This is metatarsus adductus and is commonly seen with rotational lower limb deformities (see Fig. 15.16). It is essential to differentiate this from other foot deformities and this is easily done by looking at the hind foot. The heel is in the normal position, all the deformity is distal to the mid-tarsal joint. If it is passively correctable, which it is in 95% of cases, it will correct spontaneously without treatment. For the few that cannot be corrected, serial plasters or occasionally release of the abductor hallucis is required.

Treatment

Treatment for rotational deformities can be clearly stated. Apart from serial plasters for metatarsus adductus, there is no evidence that conservative treatment makes any difference to the outcome and may even be harmful. If a deformity is severe enough, surgical correction by osteotomy of the affected bone is the only method of treatment. Needless to say, the deformity must be very severe before such treatment is justified.

Scoliosis

Scoliosis is tilting or curving of the spine in the lateral plane. The normal spine is straight in the lateral plane but curved in the anteroposterior plane. This is the normal thoracic kyphosis and cervical and lumbar lordosis.

There are a number of causes of scoliosis. Differentiating the significant curves from the insignificant is essential, as this indicates the prognosis and the need for treatment.

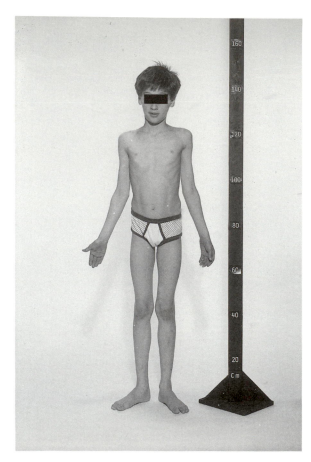

Figure 15.19 Rotational deformities group 4: femoral anteversion, lateral tibial torsion and flat feet.

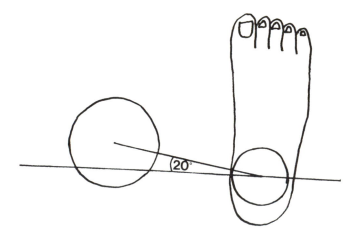

Figure 15.20 Femoral anteversion. The circle on the left is the femoral head. The circle on the right is the femoral shaft. The line between the two is the femoral neck. It is lying 20° forward of the coronal plane.

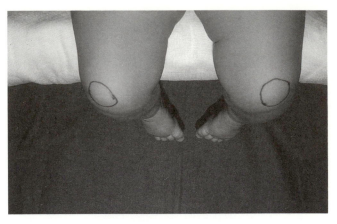

Figure 15.21 Assessment of tibial torsion. This child has internal tibial torsion. The feet turn in.

Classification

A practical, working classification of the important types of scoliosis is as follows:

1 Postural
2 Structural
    a) congenital
    b) paralytic
    c) idiopathic.

Postural scoliosis

Clearly it is possible for the normal spine to produce a scoliosis simply by bending to one side. However, in some children, a curve is seen for which there is no obvious cause. It may be habit. Postural curves disappear on sitting or lying down, and there is no rotation of the spine associated with the curve. Occasionally, postural curves are secondary to another condition, such as shortening of one leg causing the pelvis to tilt, or generalized hypotonia as seen in some children with developmental delay. For this reason the child must be fully examined and kept under observation, with posture training, until the curve has disappeared and primary causes have been eliminated.

Structural scoliosis

All forms of scoliosis other than postural can be classified as structural. This means the scoliosis cannot be eradicated by altering posture. It is a fixed deformity. The curve does not disappear on lying down or sitting, and there is rotation of the spine in addition to the curve. This means there is a rib hump with asymmetry of the thoracic cage.

a CONGENITAL

True congenital scoliosis is always associated with vertebral abnormalities. The incidence of vertebral abnormalities is approximately 0.5 per thousand births. Not all congenital vertebral anomalies are accompanied by a scoliosis just as they are not all accompanied by neurological abnormalities.

Congenital abnormalities of the spine can be simply classified:[20]

1 Failure of formation e.g. hemivertebra.
2 Failure of segmentation e.g. vertebral fusions.
3 Mixed.

CLINICAL FEATURES   The problem with congenital spinal anomalies is that in the very young infant, no curve is present and so the diagnosis is not made. Often the spinal anomaly is seen on an incidental X-ray, but this is usually when the child is older. It may not be visible on X-ray in the newborn.

A spinal anomaly must always be considered in a child with an unusual foot anomaly such as a cavus foot or clawing of the toes, suggesting a mild neurological defect.

MANAGEMENT AND PROGNOSIS   Congenital scoliosis associated with multiple anomalies tends to progress steadily, but sometimes rapidly, with development of neurological signs, particularly at the time of the growth spurt. It is now recommended that these curves are treated surgically at a young age – about 5 or 6 years – in order to prevent neurological complications and cardiopulmonary problems, which are often associated with these severe deformities.

b PARALYTIC SCOLIOSIS

Any severe neurological or neuromuscular disorder, such as cerebral palsy, poliomyelitis, muscular dystrophy or myelomeningocele, may be associated with scoliosis. It is a direct consequence of abnormal muscle innervation and consequent muscle imbalance. The curves associated with poliomyelitis or myelomeningocele may be very severe, especially if the lesion is high in the spine and the curve starts at an early age. Scoliosis is present in 15% of children with cerebral palsy, but it is rarely severe, the asymmetric spastic quadriplegics being worst affected. However, surgical treatment is rarely required.

c IDIOPATHIC SCOLIOSIS

This is the largest group of scoliosis. It is probably present in 1:200 children.[21] Three types are recognized according to the age of onset:

Infantile: 0–3 years
Juvenile: 4–9 years
Adolescent: 10 years–end of growth.

The cause of these curves is unknown, but there is an increased family incidence.

Infantile scoliosis

This type of curve is normally noticed at some time during the first year of life. It is more commonly a left-sided curve (convexity is to the left) and is more common in boys. It is associated with plagiocephaly and sometimes torticollis. Ninety per cent of these curves resolve without treatment.[22] The remaining 10% progress.

Juvenile and adolescent scoliosis

In general terms, these curves can be considered together. They are both more common in girls and a right-sided thoracic curve is the commonest pattern. The curve can be lumbar or thoraco-lumbar, in which case the cosmetic deformity is much less severe.

The thoracic curve is easily noticed because of the prominence of the shoulder on the same side as the curve and of the hip on the opposite side. These curves are likely to progress. Untreated, 25% will develop respiratory problems.[23] Progression is related to the age of onset. The earlier it presents, the more likely it is to progress and require treatment (Fig. 15.22).

Screening for scoliosis

Screening to detect adolescent idiopathic scoliosis has been tried extensively, particularly in the USA. The use of a simple, forward-bending test, observing the child from behind, demonstrates the rib hump caused by rotation of the rib cage. This can be calibrated by using a scoliometer which indicates the size of the rib hump and correlates with the extent of the curve. Curves are measured and monitored by measurement of the Cobb angle from the anteroposterior X-ray (Fig. 15.23). However, screening has now been discontinued, as it has resulted in a false-positive detection rate almost ten times the natural incidence. This has produced excessive anxiety among children and parents. Appropriate education and general awareness of the condition is at present all that is required.

Treatment of scoliosis

The principles of treatment are conservative or surgical. Conservative treatment in the form of bracing is appropriate for controlling an early idiopathic curve. Modern bracing techniques have made available lightweight, polythene or thermoplastic braces which are more acceptable to patients (Fig. 15.24).

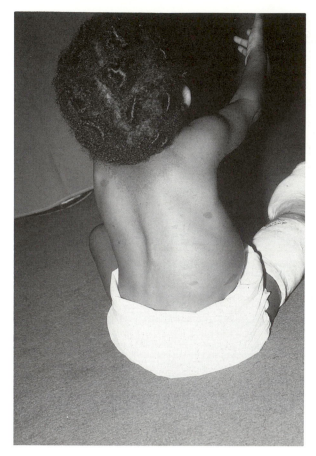

Figure 15.22 The appearance of a thoracic scoliosis in an infant. In this case associated with neurofibromatosis.

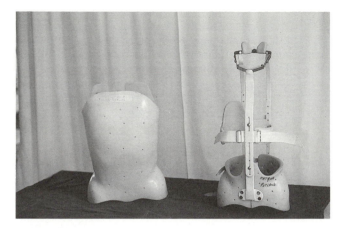

Figure 15.24 The Boston brace for control of scoliosis on the left, compared with the older style brace on the right.

Similarly, advances in internal fixation devices have improved the correction possible and the stability of surgical treatment by spinal fusion (Fig. 15.25).

The limping child

The child that limps causes great anxiety in the parents, and diagnostic confusion for the doctor, and often the cause is not obvious. Limp may be caused by a problem in the foot, lower leg, knee, thigh, hip or the spine, or even centrally. Thus, a logical diagnostic process must be followed, taking the history and examining each part individually.

The causes of limp are listed as follows:

Congenital dislocation of the hip
Irritable hip syndrome
Inflammatory arthritis
   septic
   rheumatoid
Perthe's, Severs, and Osgood-Schlatter's diseases
Osteochondritis dissecans and chondromalacia of the patella
Slipped upper femoral epiphysis
Foreign body e.g. glass in the foot
Fractures, dislocations and ligament injuries
Leg length discrepancy
Neurogenic
   spinal cord anomalies
   cerebral palsy
   neuromuscular disease
   focal brain lesion
Psychological

It is not possible to give a full description of each of these causes here but the list illustrates the diagnostic difficulty with the limping child. Congenital dislocation of the hip has been fully considered in this chapter. That it is included as a cause of limp only

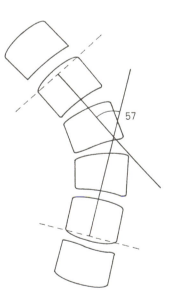

Figure 15.23 The Cobb angle. The angle between a perpendicular dropped from the vertebral plates of the vertebrae which show the greatest deviation on either side of the apex of the curve on an anteroposterior X-ray.

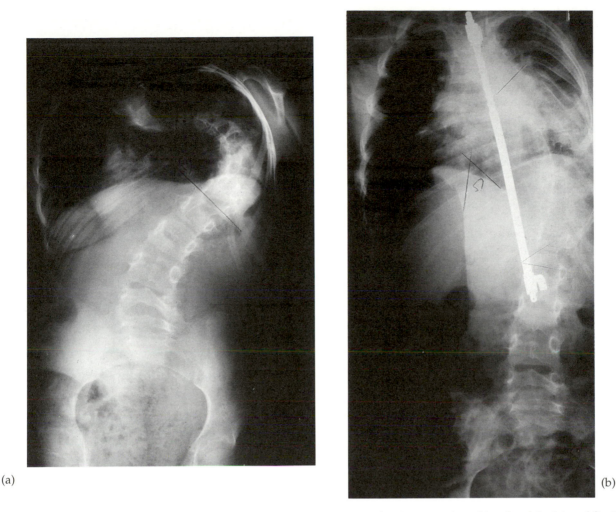

(a)

(b)

Figure 15.25 (a) Preoperative X-ray of severe scoliosis. (b) Postoperative X-ray showing correction achieved and the internal fixation device.

underlines the fact that it still presents late, and the typical Trendelenberg or waddling gait when the child first walks may be the first sign. Inflammatory arthritis, both acute or chronic, infective or juvenile chronic arthritis are conditions which may present with deceptively mild physical signs, and are diagnoses to be considered but not described further here.

Irritable hip syndrome

This is the clinical term used to describe transient synovitis of the hip. It is a common condition, and thought to be related to a viral upper respiratory tract infection, though no specific viral antibodies have as yet been identified[24] and there is a history of viral infection in less than 50%. There is no relationship with Perthe's disease. All movements of the hip are restricted and painful, with inability to weight-bear, and therefore a limp. The X-ray is typically normal,

but ultrasound scanning of the hip commonly shows an effusion which is too small to show on X-ray.[25] The sedimentation rate and C-reactive protein may be temporarily elevated. The condition settles with bed rest and skin traction, usually within a few days. The limp may persist for some weeks, but if the clinical examination, sedimentation rate and check X-ray are normal, strong reassurance is all that is required.

Perthe's disease

This condition, which is not common but well-recognized, causes confusion in diagnosis and management. It occurs between 1 in 5000 and 1 in 9000 children, varying according to social status. It is more common in deprived children and is four times as common in boys as in girls. It usually presents between the ages of 4 and 9 years. It presents as a painful limp with restricted hip movement, particularly loss of abduction in flexion. Pathologically, there is ischaemic necrosis of part of the growing capital epiphysis of the femur, followed later by revascularization and resumption of growth.

Perthe's disease is diagnosed radiologically. The X-ray appearances are typical, but a great range of severity of the changes affecting the femoral head are observed (Fig 15.26). The degree of change and the age of onset correlate with the prognosis, and the treatment can thus be determined at the outset.[26] However, in practice, the application of a complete classification to this relatively uncommon condition is very difficult. Furthermore, Perthe's disease has to be viewed in perspective. Not only is it uncommon, but the number of patients requiring active treatment is very much the minority. Most patients recover completely with rest during the episodes of irritability. It is then possible to simplify the criteria for treatment into two groups.

The first group is the younger child (under 6 years) with minimal involvement (less than half the head involved on X-ray). In this group, the radiological diagnosis is an incidental finding, and the prognosis is excellent without treatment of any form. At the other end of the spectrum is the second group. This is the older child of 6 years or more with involvement of more than half the head. This child requires treatment. This classification may be regarded as an oversimplification, but in practice it has been shown to be effective. Of course, two other subgroups must be recognized: first, the young child with total involvement of the head. Here, the age is the relevant factor, and the prognosis is good without treatment. Second, there is the older child with partial involvement. This is the problem group, such a hip needs careful assessment and probable treatment.

The overriding principle of treatment for Perthe's disease is to contain the head of the femur in the acetabulum, until the head has revascularized. Under normal weight-bearing conditions, the femoral head is only partially contained. By abducting and internally rotating the hip, the head is fully and concentrically contained, and so as it reforms with revascularization, it will mould to the shape of the cup, regaining its normal shape.

This may be achieved by a non-weight-bearing approach with bed rest, splintage in abduction or by operation in the form of femoral osteotomy (Fig. 15.27) as is usually practised in the UK. Though at first surgical re-alignment seems more drastic, it provides the most effective means of containment, and avoids the need for prolonged bed rest or splintage, and the results are simply better.

Limp associated with trauma

Minor trauma or repetitive injury is a common cause of a limp. The history of injury is usually obvious. It is self-limiting and rarely presents to doctors. The conditions included in this category range from simple pulled muscles or sprained ankles, to traction apophysitis, stress fractures and slipped epiphyses or fractures and dislocations.

Slipped upper femoral epiphysis

This common condition requires special consideration because it is so often misdiagnosed. It is the commonest cause of limp in early adolescence. Although considered a traumatic condition, very often there is no history of trauma. Typically, the overweight, hypogonadal boy in whom it is most commonly, but not always, found, complains of intermittent episodes of pain in the affected hip or, classically, in the knee. This condition, above all, bears out the dictum that no knee examination is complete until the hip has been examined. With repeated, minor trauma, the proximal epiphysis of the femur slips off the back of the femoral shaft. Clinical examination may not reveal

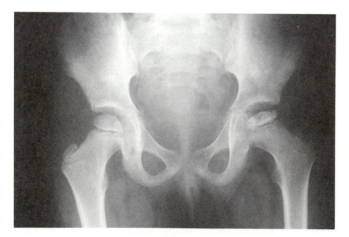

Figure 15.26 Perthe's disease. Collapse of the femoral head.

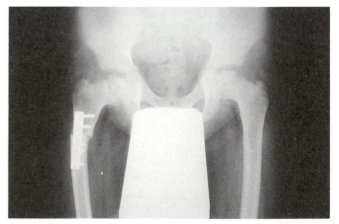

Figure 15.27 Perthe's disease. Containment of the head by femoral osteotomy.

clear physical signs, but there is always increased external rotation of the affected hip compared to the normal one, and this may be painful. This condition is also missed on X-ray when the slip is minimal. Even the smallest difference between the position of the proximal femoral epiphysis on both sides is indicative of a slipped epiphysis (Fig. 15.28).

Treatment is complex and a subject of intense surgical debate. It is aimed at prevention of further slip by placing pins up the femoral neck, and into the head of the femur when the slip is minimal (Fig. 15.29) and realignment of the head on the shaft of the femur, either by an osteotomy of the neck of the femur[27] or below the level of the greater trochanter[28], when the slip is more than 50%.

Foreign bodies

The child who stands on a needle which breaks may have little in the way of physical signs apart from a limp. An X-ray is always required and the finding of a piece of needle in a foot can cause surprise to a parent and doctor.

Leg length discrepancy

The short leg gait due to difference in leg lengths is typical and obvious. There is the dipping on the shorter side without the waddling associated with paralysis of the hip, or dislocation.

There are numerous causes of limb length irregularity, ranging from congenital absence or shortening of bone, soft tissue abnormalities such as arteriovenous malformations, inherited disorders of bone, trauma or infection causing growth arrest, and neurological abnormalities such as cerebral palsy or poliomyelitis.

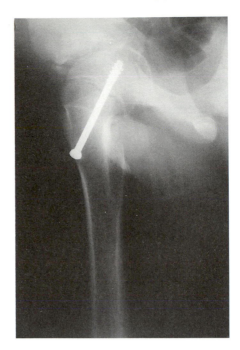

Figure 15.29 Pinning of the femoral head.

Technical advances in surgery have made equalization of leg lengths safer and more satisfactory. In general terms, the options are either to shorten the long limb by growth arrest or by excision of part of a long bone, or to lengthen the short limb using an external fixation device, which allows gradual stretching of callus as it forms across an osteotomy.

Neurogenic causes of limp

Neuromuscular imbalance between the two sides of the body, whatever the cause, will produce a limp. Therefore, full neurological examination is part of the assessment of the limping child. Limping associated with a tight Achilles tendon and an equinus foot may be the first presentation of a spastic hemiplegia associated with cerebral palsy, or be secondary to weakness due to a focal motor lesion in the brain.

Psychological

Habitual limp following an episode of limping due, for example, to an irritable hip is so common as to be considered normal. It is a mild way of seeking attention and with reassurance it soon resolves. However, abnormal gait associated with hysterical symptoms does occur, and causes diagnostic difficulty and anxiety, which may compound the problem. The question is always how far to go with investigations, such as spinal X-ray examinations, CT scans, even myelograms. The importance of a full physical and neurological examination cannot be over-stressed.

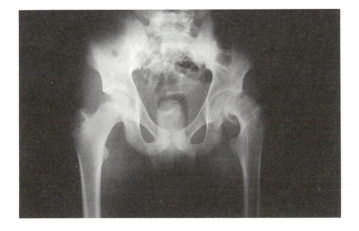

Figure 15.28 Slipped upper femoral epiphysis affecting both sides but more obvious on the left.

Sport and children

Injuries

How important are sports injuries to children when the average child spends less than one hour per week doing sports and the overall incidence of injury sustained doing sport is no different than injury in the playground? The answer is that it is an important topic because a number of risk factors can be identified and, if observed, a lot of suffering and disability associated with sport can be prevented.

Sports related injuries in children and adolescents can be tabulated under certain identifiable risk factors with the associated injury (Table 15.3). These are self-explanatory and most are related to overuse. Too much activity in tired children increases the risk of accidental injury. A full description of each condition is not possible here and standard works of orthopaedics or sports injury medicine are recommended. Two conditions are common but not widely known. Shin splints are well known among athletes. There is pain on the medial side of the lower tibia due to increased pressure in the posterior or deep muscle compartment of the lower leg. Compartment syndrome affects the anterior compartment lateral to the tibia and gives rise to cramp felt in this area after activity. Both conditions are treated by fasciotomy which is simply incising the investing fascia of the affected compartment to relieve the pressure. However, some general points can be made which are largely common sense. It is predictable that intensive training in children or adolescents will damage growing tissues. It is sadly often forgotten that the damage done may be permanent. The importance of rest cannot be overstated. Young people do not need to get fit as do adults; they can reach peak performance with surprisingly little training. It is not only unkind but unwise for the overweight, flat-footed child to go running, for example, when the same child would get better exercise and more satisfaction from swimming.

Drugs

The use of drugs in sport is not confined to adults and great harm can be done if the skeletally immature take drugs. The effect of anabolic steroids can be premature closure of the epiphyses.[29] However, there is no good evidence that anabolic steroids actually improve performance. The only demonstrable effect is weight gain which may be of short-term benefit in some sports. Amphetamines do enhance aggression which in itself may increase the risk of injury. Vitamin supplements have no effect on sporting performance.

Trauma

Birth injuries

The child is still subject to injury during birth, in spite of modern maternity care. Fractures, dislocations or displacement of the epiphysis all present straightforward orthopaedic problems as long as the possibility of serious injury is recognized, and the diagnosis made.

That there are still a significant number of birth injuries to the brachial plexus each year in the UK is perhaps even more alarming. This devastating injury, leaving the child with a paralysed arm, has received little attention because it is widely believed that the prognosis is good, and the functional recovery is excellent with conservative treatment in the form of physiotherapy.

Table 15.3 Sports injuries in children

Risk factors	Possible injury/outcome
1 Training and overuse	Stress fractures
	Shin splints
	Compartment syndromes
2 Muscle/bone imbalance	Osgood-Schlatter's disease
	Chondromalacia patellae
3 General physique	Slipped epiphysis
e.g. Flat feet	Ligament injuries
obesity	e.g. plantar fasciitis
4 Footwear	Tendonitis
5 Playing surfaces	Fractures
6 Other diseases	Acute exacerbation
e.g. Diabetes	
asthma	
7 Growth	Osteochondritis dissecans
	Slipped epiphysis
	Osteoarthritis

However, at least one-third of these children have a very significant disability, particularly of the shoulder. Recently, encouraging results have been achieved by surgical exploration, excision and grafting of the damaged plexus, but this must be done early, between 3 and 6 months of age.[30]

Child abuse

Orthopaedic surgeons are often asked if a particular fracture could be a result of child abuse. Taken in isolation it is not possible to be definitive. However, there are indicators, from the fractures alone, which can be helpful in establishing the diagnosis. For example, in any child under 1 year old, one in 10 fractures is non-accidentally induced.[31] An epiphyseal injury under 1 year, not occurring at birth, is always non-accidental.[32] Multiple fractures, in different stages of healing, particularly when epiphyseal injuries are found, are virtually diagnostic of physical child abuse when bone dysplasias such as osteogenesis imperfecta can be excluded (Fig. 15.30).[33]

References

1 Ortolani, M. Un segno polonoto e sua importanza per la diagnosi precoce di prelussazione congenita dell 'anca. *Paediatria* 1937; **45**: 129.

2 Barlow, T.G. Congenital dislocation of the hip in the newborn. Early diagnosis and treatment of congenital dislocation of the hip in the newborn. *Proc Roy Soc Med* 1966; **59**: 1103.

3 Fredensborg, N. The results of early treatment of typical congenital dislocation of the hip in Malmo. *J Bone Joint Surg* 1976; **58B**: 272.

4 Artz, T.P., Levine, D.B., Lim, W.N., Salvati, E.A., Wilson, P.D. Neonatal diagnosis, treatment and related factors of congenital dislocation of the hip. *Clin Orthopaed Rel Res* 1975; **110**: 112.

5 Rosen, von S. Diagnosis and treatment of congenital dislocation of the hip in the newborn. *J Bone Joint Surg* 1962; **44B**: 284.

6 Wilkinson, J., Carter, C. Congenital dislocation of the hip: the results of conservative treatment. *J Bone Joint Surg* 1960; **42B**: 669.

7 Department of Health and Social Security. *Screening for the Detection of Congenital Dislocation of the Hip*. London: HMSO, 1986.

8 Graf, R., Schulen, P. Sonographie in der Orthopadie. In: Braun, Gunter-Schwerk, eds. *Ultradiagnostik* 4, Ecomed

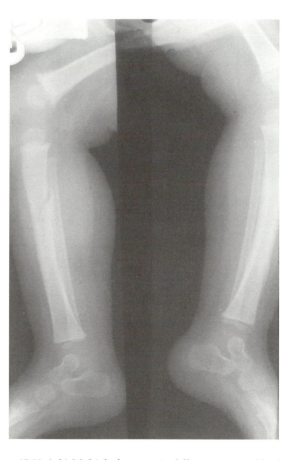
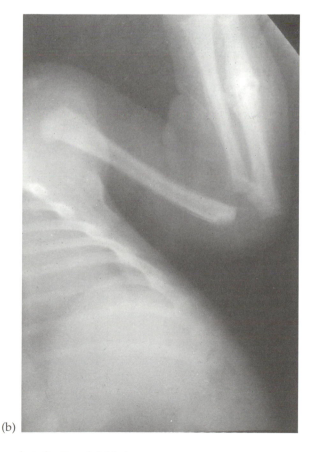

(a)　(b)

Figure 15.30 (a,b) Multiple fractures in different stages of healing, strongly indicative of child abuse.

Verlag, 1986, 7.

9   Clark, N.P., Theodore, Harke, H., et al. Real time ultrasound in the diagnosis of congenital dislocation and dysplasia of the hip. *J Bone Joint Surg* 1985; **67B**: 406–421.

10 Kalamachi, A., MacFarlane, R. III. The Pavlik harness: results in patients over three months of age. *J Paediatr Orthopaed* 1982; **2**: 3.

11 Salter, R.B. Innominate osteotomy in the treatment of congenital dislocation and subluxation of the hip. *J Bone Joint Surg* 1961; **43B**: 518.

12 Allan, D.B., Gray, R.H., Scott, T.D., Tonkin, M., Hughes, J.R., Evans, G.A. The relationship of ligamentous clicks arising from the newborn hip and congenital dislocation. *J Bone Joint Surg* 1985; **67B**: 491.

13 Congenital Malformations Surveillance. Atlanta: US Department HEW Public Health Service, 1977.

14 Wynne Davies, R. *Heritable Disorders in Orthopaedic Practice*. Oxford: Blackwell Scientific Publications, 1973.

15 Turco, V.J. *Clubfoot*. Edinburgh: Churchill Livingstone, 1981.

16 Harrold, A.J., Walker, C.J. Treatment and prognosis in congenital club foot. *J Bone Joint Surg* 1983; **65B**: 8.

17 Morley, A.J.M. Knock knee in children. *Br Med J* 1957; **2**: 976.

18 Staheli, L.T., Engel, G.M. Tibial torsion: a method of assessment and a survey of normal children. *Clin Orthopaed Rel Res* 1972; **86**: 183.

19 Rushforth, G.F. The natural history of the hooked fore foot. *J Bone Joint Surg* 1978; **60B**: 530–532.

20 MacEwen, G.D. Congenital scoliosis with a unilateral bar. *J Bone Joint Surg* 1967; **49A**: 1–1014.

21 Wynne Davies, R. Familial idiopathic scoliosis. *J Bone Joint Surg* 1968; **50B**: 24.

22 Lloyd-Roberts, G.C., Pilcher, M.F. Structural idiopathic scoliosis in infancy: a study of the natural history in 100 patients. *J Bone Joint Surg* 1965; **47B**: 520.

23 James, J.I.P *Scoliosis*. Edinburgh: Churchill Livingstone, 1967.

24 Blockey, N.J., Porter, B.B. Transient synovitis of the hip: a viralogical investigation. *Br Med J* 1968; **4**: 557.

25 Bickerstaff, D.R., Neal, L.M., Booth, A.J., Brennan, P.O., Bell, M.J. Ultrasound examination of the irritable hip. *J Bone Joint Surg* 1990; **72B**: 549–553.

26 Catterall, A. The natural history of Perthe's disease. *J Bone Joint Surg* 1971; **53B**: 37.

27 Dunn, D.M., Angel, J.C. Replacement of the femoral head by open operation in severe adolescent slipping of the upper femoral epiphysis. *J Bone Joint Surg* 1978; **60B**: 394–403.

28 Southwick, V.O. Osteotomy through the lesser trochanter for slipped capital femoral epiphysis. *J Bone Joint Surg* 1977; **49A**: 807–835.

29 Busch, M.T., De Haven, K.E., Pannis, A.S. Two to ten-year results of lateral retinacular release for patellofemoral pain. Presented at American Academy of Orthopaedic Surgeons 56th Annual meeting, Las Vegas, Nevada 1989.

30 Hunt, D.M. Surgical management of brachial plexus birth injuries. *Dev Med Child Neurol* 1988; **30**: 821–828.

31 Worlock, P.H., Stower, M.J., Barbor, P. Fracture patterns in child abuse. *J Bone Joint Surg* 1987; **69B**: 154.

32 Sharrard, W.J.W. *Paediatric Orthopaedics and Fractures* vol 2, 2nd edn. Oxford: Blackwell Scientific Publications, 1979.

33 Kleinmann, P.K. ed. *Diagnostic Imaging of Child Abuse*. Baltimore: Williams and Wilkins, 1987.

Chapter 16

Physical illnesses

16.1 Blood disorders

Nellie Adjaye

1 Haemoglobinopathies: thalassaemia and sickling disorders

The major haemoglobinopathies that occur in the UK have high incidence in the ethnic minority groups who total approximately 3.5 million persons. These include mixed races, many Jews, Italians and Turkish Cypriots.[1] (The ethnic minority groups are described elsewhere in this book.) Sickling disorders affect mainly the peoples of African extraction; the Afro-Caribbean population in the UK is estimated to have a carrier rate of the sickle gene of 8–25%. Other groups who carry the sickle genes have originated from the Middle East (Arabia and Iran), the mediterranean basin (Turkey, Greece, and Italy) and the Indian sub-continent (Fig. 16.1).

Thalassaemias are found mainly in the peoples of mediterranean or Asian descent. In this population between 3 and 17% of the population may carry the gene for one of these conditions. β-thalassaemia gene is widespread in the world (Fig. 16.2) and where there is an overlap of these two genes, it is not unusual to find sickle-thalassaemic syndromes in ethnic minority groups who originate from these areas.

Other abnormal haemoglobinopathies that may be found in the ethnic minority groups in the UK are HbC, HbD, HbE and thalassaemia traits. Table 16.1 illustrates the frequency of haemoglobinopathy traits detectable by routine haemoglobinopathy screening in ethnic minorities in the UK compared with the indigenous British population. Figure 16.3 shows areas of the world where Hb C D E originate.

In both sickle cell and thalassaemic conditions, the inheritance follows the simple mendelian laws, and the risk of producing an affected child is one in four for a couple who are heterozygotes. It is estimated that about 100 infants are born annually in the UK with sickle cell disease (SCD), i.e. HbSS, SB°, SB+ and SC−, but the birth rate of infants with thalassaemia major is falling through screening, counselling and prenatal diagnosis. Estimates put the annual figure at less than 30 per year.[2]

In *thalassaemia major*, there is inherited quantitative defect in the synthesis of the β globin chain. The homozygous infant usually presents between the ages of 6 and 12 months with pallor, listlessness, anaemia (haemoglobin in the region of 5–6 g/dl (0.8–0.9 mmol/l)), abdominal distension due to hepato-splenomegaly, or failure to thrive. Diagnosis is confirmed by blood film which shows numerous target cells and on electrophoresis there is a high concentration of fetal haemoglobin (HbF), almost complete absence of HbA, and a normal or slightly raised HbA_2. Treatment is best undertaken by specialist centres or in close collaboration with them. It consists of a regular monthly blood transfusion regimen with infusions of the chelating agent desferrioxamine to reduce the iron overload that otherwise causes endocrine disturbances such as growth retardation, failure of puberty and diabetes. Provided the

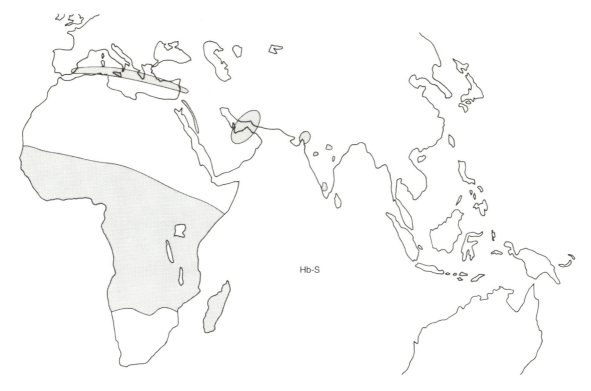

Figure 16.1 The areas of the world where haemoglobin-S occurs commonly: migration and the slave trade have carried the gene to the Americas, northern Europe including Britain, Australia and elsewhere. (From Flemming (Ed.) *Sickle Cell Disease: A Handbook for the General Clinician*. Edinburgh: Churchill Livingstone, 1982; by kind permission of the publishers.)

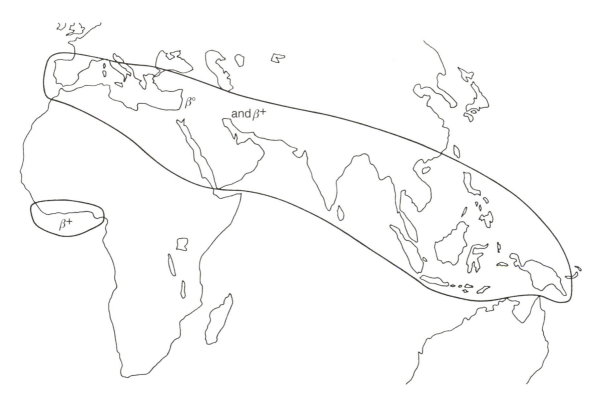

Figure 16.2 The areas of the world where the β-thalassaemias occur commonly. (From Flemming (Ed.) *Sickle Cell Disease: A Handbook for the General Clinician*. Edinburgh: Churchill Livingstone, 1982; by kind permission of the publishers.)

Table 16.1 Frequency of haemoglobinopathy traits detectable by routine haemoglobinopathy screening in ethnic minorities in the UK

	Per cent of population carrying:									
	Thalassaemia traits			Abnormal haemoglobins					Total	
Population	β	α	Homozygous α^+	HbE	HbS	HbC	HbD	All	Pathological
Mediterranean									
Cypriots	16	1	2	0	1	0	0	20	18
Others	1–10	0–1	?2	0	+	0	0	1–14	1–12
South Asians									
Sindi	10	0	6	?	?	0	+	16	10
Gujarati	6	0	6	+	+	0	+	12	>6
Other Indians	3	0	6	+	+	0	+	9	3
Pakistani	5–6	0	6	0	?	0	+	12.5	6.5
East Asians									
(e.g. Hong Kong)	3	3	?	+	0	0	0	6	6
West Indians	1–2	0	?5	0	6–12	1–3	+	>16	>11
Africans	1–2	0	?5	0	12–20	0–15	0	>25	>20
'Native' British	0.1–0.2	+	0	0	0	0	+	0.1–0.2	0.1–0.2

Reproduced by kind permission of the authors and publishers: *Ethnic Factors in Health and Disease*, edited by Cruickshank & Beevers, 1989.

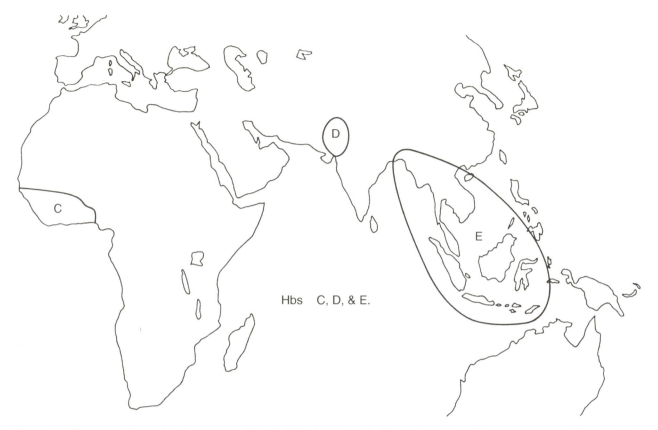

Figure 16.3 The areas of the world where haemoglobin-C, D-Punjab (also called D-Los Angeles) and E occur commonly. (From Flemming (Ed.) *Sickle Cell Disease: A Handbook for the General Clinician*. Edinburgh: Churchill Livingstone, 1982; by kind permission of the publishers.)

haemoglobin is not allowed to fall below 11 g/dl (1.7 mmol/l), regular transfusion preserves good health. The iron chelating agent is administered by subcutaneous infusion by a small syringe-driver during an 8–12 hour period overnight at least five nights per week. The recommended management of thalassaemia has been summarized by a World Health Organization group.[3] Without treatment by regular blood transfusion, early death from chronic anaemia and heart failure ensues. The prognosis is improved with early treatment of regular blood transfusion and chelating agents as patients reach the reproductive age group, without the severe complications of endocrinopathy from haemosiderosis.

Sickle cell disease (SCD) (the homozygous SS, heterozygous SC, S Bthal) rarely presents before the age of 3 or 4 months because the high fetal haemoglobin interferes with the sickling phenomenon. Thereafter the classical vaso-occlusive crises and infective complications occur increasingly. However, the condition is highly unpredictable. The natural history varies with the ethnic origin of the group at risk, the environment, the level of awareness of the disease and its hazards. Ethnic minorities of African descent seem to carry the more severe form of the disease while the

peoples originating from the Middle East tend to have a milder form. The natural history of the disease in the UK has not been fully studied, because of the lack of regional *or* national integrated approaches to the haemoglobin disorders. However, the recent recognition of the Brent Sickle Cell Centre in the Central Middlesex Hospital, London, as a regional haemoglobinopathy centre for the North West Thames Region affords an opportunity for such a study, by a longitudinal follow up of children diagnosed with SCD in the neonatal period.

Sickle cell disease, with at least 4000 cases, is one of the most common inherited diseases in Britain. In some urban areas, it accounts for up to 40% of all haematological hospital admissions.[4] Although painful vaso-occlusive episodes (crises) is the most common cause of acute admissions in the school child, morbidity and mortality from acute splenic sequestration or fulminant pneumococcal infections occur more frequently in children under 5 years. Murtaza *et al.* in their follow up of 171 children in South London encountered six episodes of acute splenic sequestration and five episodes of pneumococcal meningitis.[5] Asplastic crisis is another specific serious complication of SCD; it usually occurs in later childhood. This sudden cessation of intense erythropoietic activity with a progressive drop in haemoglobin level is usually attributed to the human parvovirus.[6]

Community care

Evidence is accruing that the general prognosis of sickle cell disease can be improved if families and doctors are aware of the diagnosis in early life. This permits proper immunization, regular monitoring in sickle cell clinics, education of the family and of the doctor, and earlier diagnosis and therapy of complications. Parental education to test for pallor and splenomegaly significantly reduces the mortality from acute splenic sequestration.[7,8] The longitudinal study from the Children's Hospital in Oakland also indicates that newborn screening when coupled with extensive follow up and education will significantly decrease patient mortality.[9] In the UK, the comprehensive care of children and their families with these major haemoglobinopathies has been haphazard. It requires the concerted efforts of the statutory agencies of health, social services and education, working in collaboration with the voluntary sector or charities. Community education, initially to improve awareness of the condition, researching into the needs of the families affected by SCD and thalassaemia, and provision of supportive care at home are some of the activities undertaken by the charities to complement the overall care of the children with SCD or thalassaemia. An example is the Sickle Cell Society's report *Sickle Cell Disease: The Need for Improved Services*[10] which made 24 recommendations for better services for people affected by SCD; this formed the basis of the Runnymede Survey in 1984.[11] The Runnymede Trust investigated the provision of screening and counselling services for SCD in 101 health authorities in England. The report highlighted the need for neonatal screening and better counselling services for SCD within the National Health Service. Since then, sickle cell and thalassaemia centres are now gradually being established within the NHS. A list of currently available centres is produced as Appendix 16.1. The role of a sickle cell and thalassaemia centre, such as that in Brent, is to give specialist counselling to parents of affected children as well as individual patients at all levels – pre-pregnancy, post-pregnancy, care of the affected child, and so on. The centre also runs courses for would-be counsellors in the health professions. Close collaboration with the local haematologists and paediatricians, as well as charities and statutory agencies, ensures that the essential follow up of newly diagnosed patients is effected. A suggested model of this approach of care of the haemoglobinopathies in Brent appears in Figure 16.4 as a way forward to achieving satisfactory care of children with chronic haemoglobinopathies in the community while collating information on the epidemiology of the diseases. Details of the Brent Sickle Cell Centre activities have been reviewed elsewhere.[12] The community care of thalassaemia has followed a similar history to that of SCD. In the past, genetic counselling of the couple has followed the birth of a thalassaemic child – after the event. The UK Thalassaemia Society has encouraged the development of screening and education on counselling for the condition at all levels. However, because of the different religious beliefs of the different ethnic groups affected by thalassaemia in the UK, the success in reducing births of thalassaemia has been variable.[13]

Glucose-6-phosphate dehydrogenase (G-6-PD) deficiency

G-6-PD deficiency is the most common of the enzyme deficiences of the erythrocytes resulting in abnormal energy metabolism within the red blood cells, and giving rise to haemolysis. The disorder is caused by an X-linked trait, with the gene located on the long arm of the X chromosome. There are two types of G-6-PD: types A and B. Type A is confined to the black population; affected individuals may have 10–15% of the normal enzyme activity. The enzyme deficiency in the black population is nearly always associated with a variant of the A enzyme (A minus). This variant is unstable and is more rapidly degraded as the red blood cell ages. Thus a haemolytic reaction in a black patient is usually self-limiting since a young cell population with newly synthesized A-minus enzyme appears in the peripheral blood.[14] Type B G-6-PD, the normal enzyme, is found in all populations. The non-black variety of G-6-PD deficiency is widespread in the mediterranean, Middle Eastern and oriental populations. Affected males have very low or absent activity in their red blood cells. Several variants of G-6-PD have been isolated, but they are not always associated with enzyme deficiency. Clinical features of G-6-PD deficiency are drug-induced haemolytic anaemias usually caused by sulphonamides and antimalarials such as primaquine and chloroquine, chronic haemolytic anaemias in certain families and neonatal jaundice, particularly in the oriental and mediterranean populations. In the Netherlands, it is frequently the sole cause of neonatal jaundice in non-Caucasian neonates requiring exchange transfusion for hyperbilirubinaemia.[15] G-6-PD deficiency should be considered in neonatal jaundice in babies of the appropriate racial background as should drug-induced haemolytic anaemias. General counselling on avoidance of the offending drugs, preferably giving the parents a list of such drugs to carry and show to a pharmacist, whenever they have to purchase drugs, has proved helpful.

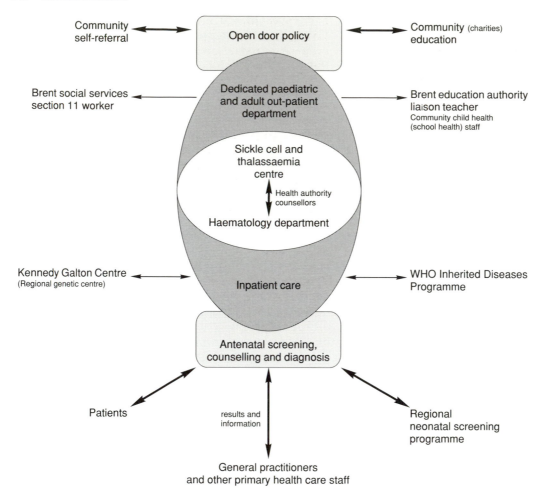

Figure 16.4 Comprehensive care for the haemoglobinopathies: the Brent approach. (Courtesy of Dr S.C. Davies, Consultant Haematologist, Central Middlesex Hospital.)

Iron deficiency anaemia

Iron deficiency anaemia in children has been recognized for many years in the UK.[16] It is more prevalent in the underprivileged and in ethnic minorities. In the 1960s, Davis et al.[17] found that the mean corpuscular haemoglobin concentration levels in Afro-Caribbean children were significantly lower than in matched white children of the same age groups from 5 months to 23 months. The prevalence of iron deficiency anaemia in the two groups were 54% and 22% respectively. De Lobo found that 24% of 3 year olds born to mothers of Asian origin in Luton had haemoglobin concentration of 10g/dl (1.55 mmol/l) or less.[18] Thus the incidence of iron deficiency in the toddler population depends on the population studied. In more recent times, several papers have reported relatively high frequency of dietary iron deficiency particularly among children of Pakistani muslims,[19,20] and Bangladeshi children in London.[21] Inadequate dietary content of foods containing iron, and the early use of fresh cow's milk are some of the causes. Chronic iron deficiency anaemia is an important medical problem in children. There is some evidence that it is a contributory factor to delayed language and cognitive development.[22] Attention deficit disorder and impaired school performance and clumsiness have also been attributed to iron deficiency anaemia.[23] Aukett and his team in a well-planned, double-blind, randomized intervention study of 97 toddlers with anaemia showed a direct relation between iron deficiency, physical growth and delayed psychomotor development[24] and called for early identification and treatment of the condition within the community. Since then, the debate has centred around the feasibility of screening for iron deficiency at the primary care level as part of routine surveillance.[25] It is interesting to note that the recent publication of a programme for child health surveillance in the UK,[26] while accepting that screening for iron deficiency was possible and desirable, did not firmly recommend routine screening, but suggested further research into its acceptability to parents. James *et al.* have shown that routine screening for iron deficiency anaemia is possible within general practice in an inner city with high social deprivation and a high ethnic minority population.[27] When testing for iron deficiency in the 1–4 year age group, they found a high prevalence of anaemia in black children (25%) compared with white children (8%). They now offer routine screening at 14 months to all children in their practice with appropriate health education on diet and intervention as necessary. The procedure seems very well accepted by parents, and thus the authors recommend that screening for iron deficiency be part of routine child health surveillance.

Outpatient care of leukaemia and other cancers

Acute lymphocytic leukaemia and malignant solid tumours in childhood are still a major cause of morbidity and mortality in children in the age range 1–14 years, ranking third after accidents and congenital malformations.[28] Although there has been marked improvement in the prognosis of children with cancer over the last 30 years, in particular over the last decade,[29] it is still the cause of death in some 400 children per year in the UK.[30] The increased survival rate has been attributed to the development of better accurate diagnosis and effective multi-agent chemotherapy, centralization of care, and treatment by multidisciplinary teams.[29]

As more children survive previously fatal cancers and leukaemia, so the need for the multidisciplinary hospital teams involved with the treatment of the children to develop effective communication with primary health care teams has become urgent. The role of the hospital team and the primary health care team in the management of childhood malignancy was questioned in the early 1980s in an anonymous paper from a general practitioner.[31] Since then some centres of excellence have conducted research into the wider aspects of the treatment and care of children with malignancies in the community, paying particular attention to the management of the one third or so cases who will need terminal care. The Paediatric Oncology Team at the Bristol Royal Hospital for Sick Children have developed an information pack covering important aspects of paediatric oncology for general practitioners. The contents of this pack which include the appropriate treatment protocol, their side effects and management of infections, pain and emesis have improved communications between the oncology unit and general practitioners.[32] General practitioners find it helpful and patients can be treated at home with all the *supportive care* available. Such support to families of children with malignancy should be carefully coordinated at all levels so that the wide-ranging medical

and psychological needs of the patient can be met. The hospital team should help the family find what support networks are available and establish links where appropriate. Social workers, health visitors and the community child health service are in the best position to do this. Recent research funded by the Cancer Research Campaign has highlighted the problems faced by family and school following a child's return to school after treatment for malignancy.[33] Resource material titled *Welcome Back* has been prepared for teachers in response to teachers' requests to help children with reintegration into schools.

The development of a symptom care team within the Department of Haematology and Oncology at the Hospital for Sick Children, Great Ormond Street, London in 1986 is another good example of outreach care provision from a specialist centre to the community. The team consists of a paediatrician with experience of paediatric oncology working with two nursing sisters. Based in the hospital, it extends into the community and provides supportive care at primary care level and all stages of the illness from diagnosis, during treatment, relapse, and the terminal stage. They also provide bereavement counselling when needed. This team has shown that *outpatient* care can be provided on a 24-hour basis while keeping the child at home. This enhances the family's confidence and ability to look after their child successfully even in the terminal stage.[34]

Haemophilia

Haemophilia A (factor VIII deficiency) and haemophilia B, (factor IX deficiency) are bleeding disorders that are inherited as X-linked recessive traits. Thus both affect males exclusively and females are carriers. Clinically, the two conditions are indistinguishable, but can be differentiated by factor VIII and factor IX activity assays. There are about 4000 cases in the UK. The diagnosis can be suspected at birth in male babies who develop unusually large cephalhematoma or bleed for long periods after circumcision. The infant with haemophilia generally has few problems during the first year of life though excessive bruising may be noted when the child begins to walk. Acute haemarthroses secondary to trauma or spontaneous bleeding into muscle mass begin to occur from about the second year of life, then continue on an episodic basis throughout life. Diagnosis is confirmed by factor VIII or factor IX assay.

Community care

Treatment of haemophilia is by replacement therapy with factor VIII or IX during acute bleeding episodes into joints or muscles. In recent years, because of the risk of transmission of viral hepatitis and HIV in cryoprecipitates, centres treating haemophiliacs now use the heat-treated lyophilized factor VIII and IX concentrates. An added advantage of this product is the ease of storage reconstitution and administration. Since the early 1970s, the concept of home care for haemophiliacs has steadily gained popularity with patients and health workers alike. This has been encouraged by the Haemophilia Society. This charity has spearheaded the development of haemophiliac centres throughout the National Health Service. To date, there are about one hundred such treatment centres in the UK. Like the Sickle Cell Society, they complement the NHS resources. Each centre has a director who may be the local haematologist or who liaises closely with a regional centre of excellence. The local treatment centre often has a team including a social worker and a psychologist for support to the patient and the family. Where possible, close liaison with the charity ensures that educational material is made available to the NHS, including the primary health care team – the general practitioner and school health service. It is the aim of the haemophiliac centres that each patient will receive an annual comprehensive multidisciplinary assessment or review. Such a review consists of paediatric haematological and rheumatological assessment of the large joints, review of psychological support needed by the family, the community support, genetic counselling, family planning for the teenagers and so on. Prenatal diagnosis coupled with expert counselling is now routinely offered to female carriers of the haemophiliac gene.

Appendix 16.1

Major Sickle Cell and thalassaemia centres in the UK

London Borough of Brent
Brent Sickle & Thalassaemia Centre
Central Middlesex Hospital
Acton Lane
London NW10 7NS
Tel: 0181 965 5733 Ext. 2685

London Borough of Hackney
St. Leonards Hospital
Nuttal Street
London N1 5LZ
Tel: 0171 601 7762

London Borough of Haringey
The George Martin Sickle & Thalassaemia Centre
St. Ann's Hospital
St. Ann's Road
London N15 3TH
Tel: 0181 442 6230
      0181 442 6575

London Borough of Islington
Sickle Cell Centre
Royal Northern Hospital
Holloway Road
London N7 6LD
Tel: 0171 272 7777 Ext. 351

London Borough of Newham
Plaistow Hospital
Samson Street, Plaistow
London E13 9EH

London Borough of Southwark
The Lenny Henry Sickle Cell Centre
Haematology O/P Department
Kings College, Denmark Hill
London SE5 9RS
Tel: 0171 737 4000

Birmingham
Sickle Cell & Thalassaemia Centre
Ladywood Health Centre
395 Ladywood Middle Way
Ladywood
Birmingham B1 2TP
Tel: 0121 454 4262

Cardiff
Sickle & Thalassaemia Centre
Butetown Health Centre
Loudoun Square
Cardiff CF1 5UZ
Tel: 01222 488026/471055

Liverpool
Sickle Cell Centre
Abercromby Health Centre
Grove Street
Liverpool L7 7HG
Tel: 0151 708 9370

Manchester
Sickle Cell & Thalassaemia Centre
Moss Side Health Centre
Monton Street
Manchester M14 4PG
Tel: 0161 226 8972 Ext. 213

Nottingham
Sickle Cell & Thalassaemia Centre
Victoria Health Centre
Glass House Street
Nottingham NG1 3LW
Tel: 01159 480500 Fax: 01159 413371

Southampton
Haemoglobinopathy Counsellor
Southampton Central Clinic
East Park Terrace
Southampton SO0 4NN
Tel: 01703 634321 Ext. 289

References

1 Estimating the size of the ethnic minority populations in the 1980's. *Population Trends 44*. London: HMSO, 1986.

2 Royal College of Physicians of London. *Prenatal Diagnosis and Genetic Screening: Community and Service Implications*. London: RCP, Chapter 4: Ethnic minorities.

3 A short guide to the management of thalassaemia. In: Sirchia, G., Zanella, G., eds. *Thalassaemia Today: the Mediterranean Experience*. Milan: Centro Transfusionale, Ospedale Maggiore Policlinico di Milano, 1987: 635–670.

4 Brozović, M., Anionwu, E. Sickle cell disease in Britain. *J Clin Pathol* 1984; **37**: 1321–1326.

5 Murtaza, L.N., Stroud, C.E., Davies, L.R., Cooper, D.J. Admissions to hospital of children with sickle cell anaemia: a study in South London. *Br Med J* 1981; **282**: 1040–1050.

6 Serjeant, G.R., Topley, J.M., Mason, K., *et al*. Outbreak of aplastic crises in sickle cell anaemia associated with parvovirus-like agent. *Lancet* 1981; ii: 595–597.

7 Emond, A.M., Collis, R., Darvill, D., *et al*. Acute splenic sequestration in homozygous sickle cell disease: natural history and management. *J Pediatr* 1985; **107**: 201–206.

8 Grover, R., Shahidi, S., Fisher, B., Goldberg, D., Wethers, D. Current sickle-cell screening program for newborns in New York City, 1979–1980. *Am J Pediatr Hematol* 1983; **73**: 249–252.

9 Vichinsky, E., Hurst, D., Earles, A., Kleman, K., Lubin, B. Newborn screening for sickle cell disease: effect on mortality. *Pediatrics* 1988; **81**: 749–755.

10 Sickle Cell Society. *Sickle Cell Disease: the Need for Improved Services*, 2nd edn. London: Sickle Cell Society, 1983.

11 Prasher, U., Anionwu, E., Brozović, M. *Sickle Cell Anaemia: Who Cares?* London: Runnymede Trust, 1985.

12 Anionwu, E.N. Running a sickle cell centre: community counselling. In: Cruickshank, J.K., Beevers, D.G., eds. *Ethnic Factors in Health and Disease*. Chapter 14. Oxford: Butterworth-Heinemann.

13 Modell, B., Petrou, M. Thalassaemia screening: ethics and practice. In: Cruickshank, J.K., Beevers, D.G., eds. *Ethnic Factors in Health and Disease*. Chapter 13. Oxford: Butterworth-Heinemann.

14 Weatherall, D., Hatton, C.S.R. Congenital haemolytic anaemias. *Med Int* 1987; **2**: 1712–1713.

15 Wolf, B.H.M., Schultgens, R.B.H., Nagelkerke, N.J.D., Weening, R.S. Glucose-6-phosphate dehydrogenase deficiency in ethnic minorities in the Netherlands. *Trop Geogr Med* 1988; **40**: 322–330.

16 MacKay, H.M.M. Anaemia in infancy: its prevalence and prevention. *Arch Dis Child* 1928; **3**: 117–144.

17 Davis, I.R., Marden, R.H., Sarkany, I. Iron deficiency anaemia in European and West Indian infants in London. *Br Med J* 1960; **2**: 1426–1428.

18 de Lobo, E.H. *Children of Immigrants to Britain: Their Health and Social Problems*. London: Hodder and Stoughton, 1978.

19 Ehrhardt, P. Iron deficiency in young Bradford children from different ethnic groups. *Br Med J* 1986; **292:** 90–93.

20 Goel, K.M., Logan, R.W., House, F., *et al*. The prevalence of haemoglobinopathies, nutritional iron and folate deficiencies in native and immigrant children in Glasgow. *Health Bull Edinb* 1978; **36**: 176–183.

21 Harris, R.J., Armstrong, D., Ali, R., Laynes, A. Nutritional survey of Bangladeshi children aged under 5 years in the London Borough of Tower Hamlets. *Arch Dis Child* 1983; **58**: 428–432.

22 Walter, T., Kovalskys, J., Stekel, A. Effect of mild iron deficiency on infant mental developmental scores. *J Pediatr* 1983; **102**: 519–522.

23 Pollitt, E., Soemantri, A.G., Yunis, F., Scrimshaw, N.S. Cognitive effects of iron deficiency anaemia. *Lancet* 1985; **i**: (8421) 158.

24 Aukett, M.A., Parks, Y.A., Scott, P.H., Wharton, B.A. Treatment with iron increases weight gain and psychomotor development. *Arch Dis Child* 1986; **61**: 849–858.

25 Editorial. Iron deficiency: time for a community campaign? *Lancet* 1987; **i**: 141–142.

26 Hall, D.M.B., ed. *Health for All Children: a Programme for Child Health Surveillance*. Oxford: Oxford University Press, 1989: 34–36.

27 James, J., Evans, J., Male, P., Pallister, C., Hendrikz, J.K., Oakhill, A. Iron deficiency in inner city pre-school children: development of a general practice screening programme. *J Roy Coll Gen Practit* 1988; **38**: 250–252.

28 Office of Population Censuses and Surveys. *OPCS Monitor: Deaths by Cause, 1985*. DH2 86/2. London: HMSO, 1986.

29 Birch, J.M., Marsden, H.B., Morris Jones, P.H., Pearson, D., Blair, V. Improvements in survival in childhood cancer: results of a population based survey over 30 years. *Br Med J* 1988; **296**: 1372–1376.

30 Office of Population Censuses and Surveys. *Mortality and Statistics in Childhood: Review of Registrar General on Deaths in England and Wales, 1985*. London: HMSO, 1987.

31 Anonymous. City practice revealed: malignant disease and the child, the family and the GP. *Update* 1981; 1st December: 1667–1669.

32 James, J.A., Harris, D.J., Mott, M.G., Oakhill, A. Paediatric oncology information pack for general practitioners. *Br Med J* 1988; **296**: 97–98.

33 Larcombe, I.J., Walker, J., Charlton, A., Meller, S., Morris Jones, P., Mott, M.G. Impact of childhood cancer on return to normal schooling. *Br Med J* 1990; **301**: (6744) 169–71.

34 Goldman, A., Beardsmore, S., Hunt, J. Palliative care for children with cancer: home, hospital or hospice? *Arch Dis Child* 1990; **65**: 641–643.

16.2 Childhood diabetes

Daniela Lessing and David Harvey

Introduction

True estimates of the prevalence of childhood diabetes are not available because of inadequate data. The prevalence from studies of cohorts[1] and from general practice[2] suggest that between 1 and 2 per 1000 children under 16 develop diabetes. Some studies have shown an increasing incidence,[3] however a comparison of the age-specific prevalence of juvenile-onset diabetes between the 1946 and 1958 British cohort birth studies suggested that the overall prevalence had not increased, but that the disease was occurring at an earlier age.[4] A national survey of childhood-onset diabetes was carried out in the British Isles in 1988 and the results showed an incidence of 13.5/100 000/year in children under 15 years of age; a total of 1600 children was identified.[5] This incidence falls midway between the highest and the lowest reported by international studies; there is a 16-fold difference between Finland (28.6) and Japan (1.7); it is higher than the incidence of 7.7/100 000/year ascertained in 1973–74 from the British Diabetic Association Register. In the 1973–74 data, 19% of all new cases were under 5 years of age; whereas, in the recent survey, 26% of new cases were under 5 years.[5]

Aetiology

Environmental factors contribute 60–90% and genetic factors 5–40% of the risk.[6] The seasonal variation in the incidence of diabetes, with peaks at 5 years and 11 years of age point to infections having a role in precipitating diabetes. Viruses which have been implicated include cytomegalovirus[7] and reovirus.[8] The role of diet remains, at the moment, controversial. Family studies have shown that diabetes in children is associated with particular antigens of the human leucocyte A system (HLA). The HLA region is found on chromosome 6, suggesting that a disorder of immune regulation is closely associated with the diabetogenic process. Ninety-five per cent of white people with insulin-dependent diabetes have HLA-DR3 or DR4, whereas these are found in 50% of the general population. The initial trigger for the immune-mediated destruction of islet beta cells is unknown but during the process a variety of islet-cell antibodies appear and are found in 18–20% of new diabetics before insulin treatment. Histological studies show that the islets become infiltrated with lymphocytes and polymorphs but, at the same time, there may be an element of regeneration.

Management of diagnosis

Diabetic symptoms need to be recognized promptly by the primary care team or parents, so that immediate referral can be made. Ketoacidosis at presentation is now unusual, except in the very young child, so admission to hospital is often not necessary, but if needed should be brief. Initial insulin treatment can be given either by a continuous insulin infusion at the rate of 0.1 unit/kg/hour or by twice-daily injections using a combination of long-acting and short-acting insulins. The initial dose is based on 0.5 unit/kg/day; two-thirds of this is given in the morning. It has been reported that more aggressive treatment may produce a higher remission rate,[9] and work is in progress on the use of cyclosporin, which is capable of modifying the immune system in children.[10]

The aim of admission is to give the child and family intensive involvement and education in all the practical aspects of diabetes care and it is essential that ward, clinic and community based staff adopt a unified approach to teaching methods. The dietitian introduces the family to the principles of measured carbohydrates and the importance of good nutrition and with the parents and child will draw up an appropriate plan of meals. A member of the community team supervises the transition from hospital to home and school, and provides the parents with some of the commercially available booklets,[11] a diary, and a contact number. Hypoglycaemia is discussed before the child goes home, but it is not now the policy to provoke an attack in hospital.

In the first days following diagnosis, the family are often very upset. There is a need for plenty of time for discussion, simple explanation, support and questions.

Role of the community team

Discharge from hospital is a time of great anxiety for most families and early visiting by a member of the community team may help the transition from hospital to home by offering practical and emotional support. The family have many adjustments to make in learning to live with a child with diabetes and must strike the right balance between living as normal a life as possible and the restrictions imposed by the condition.[12] A well-functioning family improves a child's well-being by providing emotional support, advice, and practical help;[13] conversely family problems can have deleterious effects on metabolic control.[14,15] There is no standard approach to the care of the child with diabetes; in common with other chronic diseases, care is life long, with the patient and family responsible for day-to-day control. Education forms a vital part of the programme and is a continuous learning process. The ultimate outcome must be a balance between the current decrease in quality of life by the measures needed to obtain good blood glucose levels and the risk of severe impairment of quality of life that may occur through blindness, leg amputation, and other complications.[16]

The organization of services for children with diabetes in the UK has recently been studied.[17] The majority of paediatricians (293, 81%) work in districts where there is at least one diabetes nurse specialist, liaison nurse or specialist health visitor. Several districts now have home care teams who offer a flexible service designed to meet the needs of each child and his family.[18] It is important, however, to realize that an authoritarian approach should be avoided and that, for a variety of reasons, perfect control may not be achieved.[19] The community teams must form a partnership with the family and together must act in the child's best interest. They provide clinical supervision of day-to-day problems through telephone advice or domiciliary visiting and are responsible for education and support. It has been reported that parents who have access to specialist nurses have greater needs and concerns and this may be the result of the nurses' role in helping families achieve good metabolic control and the consequence of greater parental awareness and increased vigilance.[20]

Management of established diabetes

Insulin

The majority of children in our care receive a combination of short-acting and medium-acting insulin given twice a day before breakfast and the evening meal. The dose varies between 0.7–1 unit per kilogram per day with two-thirds of this being given in the morning. The medium-acting insulin usually forms two-thirds of the total dose. Twice-daily insulin allows more flexible adjustment and late complications may be reduced,[21] but data are limited. Adolescents have greater insulin requirements due to increased growth hormone secretion and may need up to 1.5 units per kilogram per day.

Human insulin was first produced commercially in the early 1980s by recombinant DNA technology or enzymatic conversion of porcine insulin; it is now used routinely. In October 1989, the Committee on Safety of Medicines announced that, with the British Diabetic Association, it would be urgently investigating reports of sudden death and loss of the usual warning symptoms of hypoglycaemia. There is no convincing evidence implicating human insulin as the cause of these problems and it should continue to remain the standard treatment for diabetes in childhood.[22,23]

Other more intensive regimens can be used for insulin delivery, particularly in teenagers. The introduction of insulin pens has been the most recent development for use with multiple daily injections. These pen-like devices contain prefilled disposable cartridges of short-acting insulin and disposable needles. They remove the need for drawing up insulin and therefore increase accuracy. Many adolescents accept multiple daily injections[24] and the greater freedom they offer them in daily life. Some centres are actively promoting the use of the pen-based regimens among older children and adolescents. Short duration insulin is given before main meals with about 30% of daily requirements given as medium-acting or long-acting insulin before bed. Improved control may occur, but in some children the flexibility of this method leads to dietary non-compliance.[25]

Continuous subcutaneous insulin infusion has been used successfully in adults, but has limited use in children. Insulin is delivered through an infusion catheter and a subcutaneous needle, usually placed under the abdominal skin, throughout the day including during moderate exercise. It must, however, be removed when the child has vigorous exercise, for example during football and swimming. The pump is attached either to a belt or a shoulder holster and delivers a constant basal rate of insulin with a bolus 15–20 minutes before meals.

Monitoring control at home

The purpose of monitoring is to assess daily diabetic control of the child and as a result to change treatment, if necessary. The cornerstone of control is the documentation of results in a diary. At every home and clinic visit the results must be reviewed and the findings discussed in an uncritical and unhurried manner. Parents are allowed to express their concerns about monitoring and the programme is altered to meet the family's needs.

The ability to measure blood glucose at home has many advantages for the family in the management of their child. Testing can be done at different times of the day to show the peaks and troughs of blood glucose and, with the help of telephone links or the visiting community team, stabilization can be achieved. Parents are encouraged to use the results to make their own adjustments to the dose of insulin. The number of blood glucose estimations expected from the family vary from clinic to clinic and also on the compliance of the parent and child, but a minimum of one reading every other day at different times (before and mid-way between main meals and before bed) gives a seven-point profile once a fortnight. Many parents find blood glucose testing extremely valuable, especially when on holiday or during an intercurrent illness accompanied by vomiting, or if the child has signs of hypoglycaemia. They can act immediately and appropriately on the results. Many finger pricking devices are on the market, and individual preference dictates the choice. Blood glucose meters are not essential but families who do regular blood glucose testing find them useful, as it removes the uncertainty when reading strips.

Blood glycosylated haemoglobin (HbA$_1$) measurement (normal range up to 8%) remains the gold standard of diabetic control and needs to be assessed every 3 months. It is a measure of glycaemia over a period of time, so high results indicate poor control. It is our experience that increasing age and duration of diabetes is associated with higher HbA$_1$ values, and therefore greater attention should be focused on these children.

Urine testing is non-invasive and indirectly estimates blood glucose values. Interpretation of results is not accurate as a negative test does not mean that the blood glucose level is normal at the time of testing and a positive result is dependent on a child's renal threshold. Since the average renal threshold is about 10 mmol/l, negative urine tests are necessary for good control. The presence of ketones and high urinary concentrations of glucose can be used as a sign to the parents that extra insulin or urgent medical advice is required.

Diet

One of the objectives in the care of children with diabetes is to ensure that a healthy and appropriate diet for the needs of a growing child is supplied at home. In some families complete alteration of diet is required while in others only minor changes are necessary. The emphasis should be on healthy eating for the whole family and everyone at home needs to be encouraged to eat the same food. Different problems occur at varying ages, for example, the faddiness of the toddler and the school child surrounded by sweet-eating friends. The British Diabetic Association have recently published dietary recommendations.[26]

The function of a diet in diabetes is to reduce hyperglycaemia and hypoglycaemia and to minimize obesity and long-term diabetic complications. In general, children with diabetes have the same nutritional requirements as other children, but energy requirements vary widely, so the energy content of the diet needs to be based on how much the child usually eats and must be regularly reviewed. The traditional diabetic diet consists of meals and snacks taken regularly throughout the day, thereby avoiding swings in blood glucose levels. The distribution of food is based on a carbohydrate exchange system and typically consists of three main meals and three snacks per day. On average, 25% of the total daily carbohydrate is given at each main meal and 5–10% for each snack. In school-aged children, fats should provide 30% and carbohydrates around 50% of the energy requirements. A high-fibre diet is encouraged with adjustments for changes in physical growth and food preferences which occur frequently in the adolescent period. Young adults should follow the recommendations for alcohol consumption given for the non-diabetic population. They should be advised of the risks of hypoglycaemia, particularly occurring some hours after intake, as well as reduced awareness of the symptoms. Specialized diabetic foods are not generally recommended. Booklets are available on the carbohydrate content of the various foods, and include *Countdown* prepared by the British Diabetic Association.

Education in the home

Continuing education of the child and family is an important part of care. Improved metabolic control is not always achieved but there may be other potential benefits. These include increased self-confidence leading to a greater awareness and earlier recognition of problems, such as hypoglycaemia and ketoacidosis, improved technical skills and as a consequence of these factors fewer hospital admissions. Motivation of the families must be maintained and this is often achieved by the community team discussing recent and innovative advances in diabetes care. There are many programmes used in diabetes education which may be carried out either in group settings or individually.[27,28] The age at which a child is able to give his own injections is very variable, and must be judged on an individual basis; in our experience, it can be as young as 5 years.

Schooling

Management and control of diabetes in a child is required throughout the day; since much time is spent in school, it is important to ensure that teachers are given adequate information and knowledge about diabetes. Problems arising in school, such as hypoglycaemia and emotional difficulties, may adversely affect a child's academic performance. In one survey, it was found that 75% of teachers had inadequate understanding of diabetes and little knowledge of the recognition and treatment of emergency diabetic problems, and aspects of diet.[29] Where community teams exist it should be the policy to visit the school of a newly diagnosed child to prepare the teachers, and to contact the school nurse and doctor. A simple explanation of diabetes is given including the recognition of hypoglycaemia and its causation, for example during exercise, its effects on the child's academic performance and its prevention and treatment. The older child should always carry glucose tablets with him, but for a younger child supplies must be left in strategic places, so they are easily available to staff. Dietary explanations need to be given to the school catering staff to ensure that no special tray is prepared and that yogurts or fruit are substituted for sweet puddings. Some parents feel happier if they are given the weekly school menu and mark in what the child can have. Follow-up visits by the community team should be yearly, when the child changes schools, or if problems arise.

Difficulties encountered in diabetes

Most children develop hypoglycaemic symptoms if their blood glucose falls below 2 mmol/l. Hypoglycaemia can occur during the remission phase, the so called 'honeymoon period' when the child retains the ability to produce endogenous insulin. The symptoms are variable and include irritability, sweating, feeling faint, headache, stomach ache, blurred vision or hunger. The child may look pale and sweaty and his behaviour may be erratic. Some children have obvious symptoms, while in others, progression to coma or convulsions is rapid. Treatment consists of raising the blood glucose by oral means such as dextrosol tablets or by glucose gel absorbed through the buccal mucosa. If the child is unable to ingest sugar, intramuscular glucagon (0.5 mg for children under 6 years, 1 mg for older children) must be given. Nocturnal hypoglycaemia causes major parental concern and late evening blood tests may be necessary. Anticipation of the causes of hypoglycaemia can reduce the attacks.

Fasting hyperglycaemia can occur in otherwise well controlled children and is due to a waning of the medium duration insulin and nocturnal surges of growth hormone. This is known as the 'dawn phenomenon' and can be reduced by giving the medium-acting insulin at bedtime instead of before the evening meal.

Brittle diabetes is occasionally a major problem[30] and can be due to intercurrent illness, disturbed family dynamics or failure of diabetic management.

Complications

These are generally not apparent in the paediatric age group, but the aims of control are to minimize retinopathy, neuropathy and nephropathy. Some clinics have computer-based patient record systems that ensure regular procedures. These include annual eye examination with dilatation after 10 years, annual blood pressure, urinalysis for infection and protein, skin state, liver size, and assessment for flexion deformity of the finger joints.[25] A combined clinic with both the paediatrician and the adult diabetologist helps with the transfer of children to the adult services at a time convenient to the patient.

The British Diabetic Association (BDA)

Parents should be encouraged to join the association located at 10 Queen Anne Street, London W1M 0BD. They produce a monthly magazine, *Balance*, and various information books and packs including a school pack. BDA holidays are organized for various age groups throughout the country as well as weekends for families.

The future

Work is in progress to replace insulin injections and research has swung between the artificial pancreas, insulin infusion pumps, islet transplantation, pancreas transplantation, immunomodulation, pen injectors and glucose sensors. Great advances have been made, but pen injectors have made the greatest impact on the majority of insulin-treated patients. Research is continuing to find more convenient ways of giving insulin, including new types of insulin, different insulin regimens and longer acting insulin with less variable absorption.[31]

References

1 Stewart-Brown, S., Haskim, M., Butler, N.R. Evidence for increasing prevalence of diabetes mellitus in childhood. *Br Med J* 1983; **286**: 1855–1857.

2 Williams, D.R.R. Hospital admissions of diabetic patients. Information from hospital activity analysis. *Diabetic Med* 1985; **2**: 27–32.

3 Burden, A.C., Hearnshaw, J.R., Swift, P.G.F. Childhood diabetes: an increasing incidence. *Diabetic Med* 1989; **6**: 1–3.

4 Kurtz, Z., Peckham, C., Ades, A. Changing prevalence of juvenile onset diabetes mellitus. *Lancet* 1988; **ii**: 88–90.

5 Metcalfe, M.A., Baum, J.D. Incidence of insulin-dependent diabetes in children under 15 years in the British Isles during 1988. *Br Med J* 1991; **302**: 443–447.

6 Diabetes Epidemiology Research International. Preventing insulin-dependent diabetes mellitus: the environmental challenge. *Br Med J* 1987; **295**: 342–345.

7 Pak, C.Y., Eun, H.M., McArthur, R.G., Yoon, J.W. Association of cytomegalovirus infection with autoimmune type 1 diabetes. *Lancet* 1988; **ii**: 1–4.

8 Cambell, I.L., Harrison, L.C., Ashcroft, R.G., Jack, I. Reovirus infection enhances expression of class 1 MCH proteins on human pancreatic beta and rat insulinoma (RIN-m5F) cells. *Diabetes* 1988; **37**: 362–365.

9 Ludvigsson, J., Heding, L.G., Larsson, Y., Leander, E. C-peptide in juvenile diabetics beyond the postinitial remission period. *Acta Paediatr Scand* 1977; **66**: 177–184.

10 Bougeneres, P.F., Carel, J.C., Castano, L., *et al.* Factors associated with early remission of type 1 diabetes in children treated with cyclosporin. *N Engl J Med* 1988; **318**: 663–670.

11 Kinmonth A-L., Greene, S., Todd, L., *et al. An Introduction to Diabetes.* Slough: Ames Division, Miles Laboratories, 1982.

12 Thomas, D. Living with a diabetic child. In: Baum, J.D., Kinmonth A-L., eds. *Care of the Child with Diabetes.* Edinburgh: Churchill Livingstone, 1985: 3–11.

13 Newbrough, J.R., Simpkins, C.G., Maurer, H. A family development approach to studying factors in the management and control of childhood diabetes. *Diabetes Care* 1985; **8**: 83–92.

14 Waller, D.A., Chipman, J.J., Hardy, B.W. Measuring diabetes-specific family support and its relation to metabolic control: a preliminary report. *J Am Acad Child Adolesc Psychiatr* 1986; **25**: 415–418.

15 Marteau, T.M., Bloch, S., Baum, J.D. Family life and diabetic control. *J Child Psychol Psychiatr* 1987; **28**: 823–833.

16 Home, P. Towards the ultimate outcome. *Diabetic Med* 1989; **6**: 11.

17 British Paediatric Association. *Report of a BPA Working Party.* London: BPA, 1989.

18 Mair, E.J. Paediatric home care: a flexible approach to the family centred care of children with diabetes mellitus. *Practical Diabetes* 1989; **4**: 173–176.

19 Andel, M., Tattersall, R. Authoritarianism in diabetology. *Diabetic Med* 1989; **6**: 471.

20 Moyer, A. Caring for a child with diabetes: the effect of specialist nurse care on parents' needs and concerns. *Advanced Nursing* 1989; **14**: 536–545.

21 McNally, P.G., Burden, A.C., Hearnshaw, J.R. What causes diabetic renal failure [letter]. *Lancet* 1988; **i**: 501–502.

22 Pickup, J.C. Human insulin. *Br Med J* 1989; **299**: 991–993.

23 Gale, E.A.M. Hypoglycaemia and human insulin. *Lancet* 1989; **ii**: 1264–1266.

24 Jefferson, I.G., Marteau, T.M., Smith, M.A., Baum, J.D. A multiple injection regime using an insulin pen with prefilled cartridged soluble human insulin in adolescents with diabetes. *Diabetic Med* 1985; **2**: 493–497.

25 Johnston, D.I. Management of diabetes mellitus. *Arch Dis Child* 1989; **64**: 622–628.

26 Kinmonth, A-L., Magrath, G., Reckless, J.P.D. Dietary recommendations for children and adolescents with diabetes. *Diabetic Med* 1989; **6**: 537–547.

27 Baksi, A.K., Hide, D., Giles, G., eds. *Diabetes Education.* Chichester: John Wiley & Sons, 1984.

28 Court, S., McCowen, C., Hackett, A.F., Parkin, J.M. Experience with running a programme of education for diabetic children and their parents. *Diabetic Med* 1989; **6**: 366–368.

29 Bradbury, A.J., Smith, C.S. An assessment of the diabetic knowledge of school teachers. *Arch Dis Child* 1983; **58**: 692–696.

30 Tattersall, R. Brittle diabetes. *Br Med J* 1985; **291**: 555–557.

31 Home, P. Replacing insulin injections. *Diabetic Med* 1989; **6**: 289–290.

16.3 Asthma and allergic disorders

Brent Taylor

Asthma is the most common chronic disorder of childhood and causes much disability and occasional deaths. Conditions like eczema and hay fever cause much discomfort and occasional handicap. Food allergies remain contentious; a variety of symptoms and conditions are blamed on dietary and other environmental 'allergies'.

Asthma

Asthma, a condition characterized by hyperreactive airways and frequently associated with atopic reactivity, is very common and appears to be an increasing problem. There are, however, many gaps in our understanding of the condition. There is no agreed diagnosis, the aetiology remains largely unknown, the pathogenesis is poorly understood, the natural history is unclear and management is controversial.

Asthma, bronchial hyperreactivity and atopy

Over 90% of children attending asthma clinics can be shown to have hyperreactive airways, either on exercise testing or by the inhalation of controlled amounts of bronchoconstricting agents such as histamine or acetyl choline. Compared with normals, most children with asthma demonstrate a fall in respiratory function within a minute or two of provocation, a fall which lasts between 20 and 60 minutes unless reversed by a bronchodilator drug. Not all individuals with hyperreactive airways have asthma. The phenomenon can be demonstrated in relatives of asthma suffers and in others.[1]

Most children with asthma, up to 90% of those attending asthma clinics, also demonstrate skin prick test reactivity to aero-allergens, (particularly the house dust mite, grass pollens and cat fur in the UK). There is often no relationship between skin test sensitivities and asthmatic symptoms on exposure to the allergens. Such skin test reactivity (atopy) occurs in a high proportion of the population, with reactivity increasing with age. Some 30% of normal British school children have been shown to react to one or more allergens[2] and over 50% of an American population aged between 20 and 30 years have been shown to react, with subsequent decline of reactivity into the eighth decade.[3] College students, medical students in particular, have a high rate of atopy.[4]

Not all asthmatic children have atopy or bronchial hyperreactivity or both. Some have one or the other, but most have both. Some, especially younger asthmatics, have neither. The pathophysiological basis of atopy and bronchial hyperreactivity is poorly understood. Neural and humoral mechanisms are involved. There is an inherited tendency, apparently independent for both. Teleologically these phenomena may provide resistance to parasites and, in the case of bronchial hyperreactivity, tuberculosis.

Epidemiology

The prevalence of asthma is unclear with reported rates in childhood varying from 0.1% to 21% in different populations. This variation probably reflects differing diagnostic criteria between studies and different countries. In general, point prevalence and cumulative prevalence rates have been lower in developing than in developed countries suggesting some environmental causal or triggering factors associated with western lifestyles.

There is quite good evidence, if not conclusive, that both the prevalence and overall severity of asthma is increasing. Certainly the number of children admitted to hospital has increased dramatically over the last 20 years in the UK and in New Zealand. Alternative explanations for this might reflect changes in the organization of medical care or in the behaviour of families with the illness. Anderson,[5,6] assessing all age groups, has demonstrated an increase in the rate of asthma admissions (of at least equivalent severity) between 1970 and 1985 in a London region. Burr and coworkers[7] demonstrated an increased reporting of asthma and wheeze together with an increased prevalence of exercise-induced bronchospasm in Welsh school children using identical methodology in 1973 and 1988.

Asthma is more common in childhood than in adult life, with boys being twice as liable as girls. The sex ratio equalizes in the late teenage years and may reverse with older females being more likely to have the condition. These facts suggest that many children, especially boys, are likely to grow out of the disorder. However, there are no adequate longitudinal studies on representative populations to provide a clear picture of the natural history. One study in Melbourne, Australia, following up children identified as asthmatic at the age of 7 years together with a control population,[8] demonstrated considerable variability in outcome according to the initial severity of asthma. Overall, at the age of 21 years,[9] some 70% of boys and 50% of girls who had mild or moderate asthma at the age of 7 were symptom free, compared with only about 30% of boys and 20% of girls with severe asthma at 7 years of age.

The spectrum of asthma

The severity of asthmatic attacks varies from very occasional mild wheeze often accompanying respiratory virus infection, through increasingly severe, and frequent episodes (still triggered in many cases by respiratory viral infections especially in younger children), to a group of children with frequent asthma either moderate continuous, severe but intermittent, or severe chronic asthma. The latter group constitute about 5–10% of children between 5 and 10 years of age. Children with asthma at the severe end of the spectrum may show growth retardation or chest deformity or both, and are likely to lead restricted lives.

Wheezy bronchitis and asthma

Occasional episodes of wheezing accompanying respiratory viral illnesses may be labelled *wheezy bronchitis*. There is no intrinsic objection to the use of this label as many such infants or young children have no further episodes. However it is usually helpful, certainly from an epidemiological point of view, to diagnose asthma from the third such attack. Wheezing is very prevalent with up to 40% of infants having at least one episode.[10] The original Melbourne study[8] demonstrated close similarities between children labelled wheezy bronchitis and those labelled asthma at the age of 7 years. However, for younger children under the age of 2 years, episodes of wheezing in most cases are not a bad prognostic feature. Few go on to have further wheeze or to develop asthma. Recent prospective studies[11] suggest there may be at least two groups of wheezy children: one with associated atopy and ongoing asthma; and another not developing atopy and with no wheeze after the early toddler stage. Reported 'wheezing' and reported 'asthma' do not appear to be the same condition in most epidemiological studies.

Asthma and the environment

Asthma is unique among respiratory illnesses, particularly in childhood, in having no clear relationship to socioeconomic deprivation. This may reflect preferences in diagnostic labelling with asthma being acceptable to socially advantaged families. However almost all population studies have shown reported 'asthma' to be equally prevalent across social class and related markers of social disadvantage, whereas reported 'wheezing' shows a strong correlation with disadvantage. Parental, especially maternal, smoking is a major contributor to wheeze and bronchitis but not, apparently, to asthma.

The factors causing the (probable) increased rate of asthma in industrialized countries over recent years remain unclear. Many asthmatic children, as well as adults, may develop symptoms when exposed to air pollution or particular environments, but this may be a non-specific reaction.

The primary prevention of asthma

There is little that can be done with present understanding to prevent the development of asthma. The inheritance pattern of asthma is unclear. There are no definite genetic markers. Only about 50% of diagnosed asthmatic children have a family history of eczema, asthma or hay fever. Asthma is more likely if one or both parents have severe asthma. The relationship between asthma in the child and a family history of hay fever and eczema is less consistent.[12]

Breast feeding does not prevent asthma. There is a statistical association between breast feeding and a reduced likelihood of other wheezing disorders in early life, but this reflects the accompanying social disadvantage of non-breast-fed children, especially maternal smoking, rather than any specific protective effect from breast milk.

The role of allergy in the initiation of the asthmatic process is poorly defined. Avoiding pets, even in families predisposed to asthma, eczema and hay fever, does not appear to reduce the likelihood of chil-dren developing asthma in the first 8 years.[12] The role of heavy exposure to house-dust mite and related allergens is controversial. Mould spores have been incriminated as a factor in the increased likelihood of asthma with damp housing,[13] but there is no agreement on this.[14]

Immunization against the viruses causing respiratory illness in early life remains only a preventive possibility.

Clinical presentation

The characteristic symptoms of asthma are: *cough*, *wheeze* and *breathlessness*. The triggers to an attack may be a respiratory viral infection, rarely exposure to an allergen. In most cases no identifiable factor can be found. Episodes can last minutes or days, occasionally longer. Remission of symptoms can occur spontaneously or in association with drug therapy.

Severe episodes may be associated with cyanosis, severe breathlessness and pulsus paradoxus. Individuals with chronic severe asthma may wheeze most of the time with exacerbations. Individuals with asthma at the less severe end of the spectrum may be symptomless between attacks or may manifest evidence of bronchial hyperreactivity: shortness of breath; cough; or wheezing on exercise, emotional upset or laughing on going into a cold wind or with other changes of temperature. As with laboratory-induced bronchospasm, this manifestation of increased bronchial lability passes off usually within minutes.

There may be nocturnal symptoms, particularly cough. Some children, particularly between the ages of 2 and 5 years have asthma presenting with the predominant symptom of *nocturnal cough*. The child wakes sometimes once sometimes more frequently usually between the hours of 11 p.m. and 5 a.m., and such episodes may progress to wheezing and severe breathlessness. Sometimes the child does not wake but the family do.

A diagnostic trial of anti-asthma therapy can be helpful. Responsible improvement in respiratory function following bronchodilator therapy is highly suggestive for the diagnosis of asthma.

Social effects

Children with asthma, particularly severe asthma, may lead socially blighted lives with frequent absences from school, problems with games and other activities, cossetting by the family and inability to enjoy holidays or other absences from the family.

The aim of modern asthma treatment is to enable the sufferer to lead a normal life. Advances in treatment allow this in the vast majority of cases.

Management

A Drugs

1 ACUTE ASTHMA

Acute wheezing and breathlessness caused by asthma can usually be relieved by bronchodilator therapy. The proper mode of administration is critical to ensure that an effective dose of bronchodilator to relieve symptoms is delivered to the airways. Few children under the age of 7 years can manage the required respiratory gymnastics to use reliably a standard *metered dose aerosol* (MDA). Various forms of *spacer* are available. These include various plastic extensions to the metered dose aerosol, use of a plastic coffee cup as a mask with a hole punched in the bottom to take the MDA and large independent plastic devices with one-way valves, e.g. the Nebuhaler, which enable metered dose aerosol therapy to be used by children as young as 2 years.

Inhaled bronchodilator can also be delivered in various *powdered formulations*. Devices requiring minimal inspiratory effort are the most effective, such as the Bricanyl Turbohaler. Solutions of bronchodilator through a *nebulizer* provide optimal bronchodilatation. However the machines are expensive and inconvenient. Spacer devices are satisfactory in most instances.

Oral bronchodilators can provide useful therapy and as background therapy may enhance the efficacy of inhaled bronchodilators. Salbutamol and terbutaline syrups are widely available and may provide longer duration of bronchodilatation if not to the same peak of relief as can be obtained with inhaled therapy.[15]

Oral theophylline has a long and somewhat disputed history as therapy for asthma. The ability to monitor blood levels optimizes efficacy and provides a check on compliance with therapy. However some 10% of children are unable to tolerate even low doses of theophylline with gastrointestinal or psychological side effects and there has been recent concern about the effects of these medications on children's ability to concentrate, with implications for learning.

Anticholinergics have been used as bronchodilators. Although they may have a part to play in the management of very young children with wheezing they have not proved widely popular in the paediatric age range.

Summary of bronchodilator therapy for acute asthma

Age 7 years or more: try metered dose aerosol – check adequacy of inhalation technique. Change to spacer if inadequate.
Age 5–7 years: try powder inhalation, e.g. Turbohaler.
Age 2–5 years: try spacer, e.g. Nebuhaler.
Age 0–2 years: nebulizer if very bothered, oral sympathomimetic otherwise.

Nebulized bronchodilator may be required for very severe symptoms at any age. *Oral steroids* e.g. prednisolone 0.5–2.0 mg/kg 6 hourly for two to 10 doses controls symptoms within 6–12 hours in most episodes of severe asthma and may reduce the need for frequent bronchodilator therapy during an acute attack. Admission to hospital, particularly for oxygen therapy or fluid management may occasionally be required. There is evidence that 'enriched' community care of asthma, especially by interested general practitioners can reduce the need for emergency admission to hospital. Some hospitals offer an open-door policy for certain children with asthma. The indications for and benefit from such a policy have not been clearly identified.

2 CHRONIC ASTHMA

Secondary prevention (stopping established asthma from being symptomatic, i.e. becoming a disability) is possible with either inhaled steroids, e.g. beclomethasone dipropionate, or disodium cromoglycate. The latter drug, administered by an inhalation device, the Spinhaler or by an MDA, is helpful in some cases of moderate asthma in childhood but needs frequent inhalations – three to six per day for best effect. Many children and families find this frequency difficult. *Inhaled steroids* provide reliable relief in most children with moderate to severe asthma with a twice a day regimen, one to four puffs each dose. Both disodium cromoglycate and inhaled steroids seem remarkably safe with over 20 years' experience. There have been reports of adverse effects from inhaled steroids on the hypothalamo-pituitary-adrenal axis. However there appear to be no long-term effects on growth, certainly no more than can result from severe uncontrolled asthma. No specific changes have been identified with long-term use of topical steroid therapy although the possible growth effects, and other potential side effects, remain a long-term concern. Pharyngeal thrush is an occasional finding, but rather less frequently than in adults. It has been suggested that there may be long-term benefits associated with the use of inhaled preventative therapy with reduced inflammation leading to a reduction in adult chronic respiratory illnesses.[16] Consensus statements on the management of asthma in childhood now support the earlier introduction of inhaled steroids.[17]

B Other management

1 ALLERGY/ENVIRONMENTAL MANIPULATION

Much effort is put into anti-house dust mite measures. Families are recommended to render bedrooms in particular dust free by frequent vacuuming or removal of carpets and dust collecting curtains. Mattresses are enclosed in plastic wrappings. Feather pillows and dusty blankets are banned. The benefits of these procedures have not been confirmed in any properly conducted control trial. Studies have demonstrated no consistent change in respiratory function, asthmatic symptoms or drug usage with anti-house dust measures.

Neither does removing pets reliably benefit asthma. Subjects with seasonal symptoms related to various pollens or other spores are sometimes recommended to relocate to different parts of the country or world. There are no consistently predictable benefits from such a dislocation. Generally speaking there is a poor correlation between allergen exposure including pollens and the symptoms of asthma.

2 PHYSICAL

Physical fitness is recommended for individuals with asthma. There is some evidence that general fitness training reduces bronchial hyperreactivity but the results are unpredictable in individuals and there have been no properly controlled studies. It may be that only individuals with less severe asthma can complete an exercise programme, more severely affected individuals being unable to do so. Physiotherapy – postural drainage and various breathing exercises – have been recommended for asthma. Again, there are no controlled trials demonstrating benefit.

3 PSYCHOLOGICAL

Many families and children with asthma have psychological problems, especially dependency. This is understandable as asthma is an unpredictable condition which can be life-threatening. However there is no evidence of a predisposing psychological type for asthma and psychological problems in families with asthmatic children are similar to those where children have other chronic, severe problems such as cancer or renal failure. Such families may benefit from support irrespective of the condition.

Hypnosis can be useful therapy. Family therapy has been shown to benefit asthma in children with severe symptoms.[18] In general, however, apart from general support and education about the condition, there is no consistent place for psychological treatment in most cases of asthma.

C   Management in the community

1   GENERAL PRACTICE

Most asthma requiring medical attention can be managed by the primary health care team. Many general practitioners are establishing asthma clinics, sometimes with specialist nurses to advise on drug administration, to record respiratory function and generally oversee the adequacy of control. Many health centres have a

nebulizer and some general practitioners carry a portable nebulizer for home visits. Possible indication for referral to a hospital paediatrician for a second opinion or on-going help with management include severe asthma poorly controlled, sudden severe attacks, persistent symptoms, continuing parental or doctor concern. Admission to hospital may be required for very severe attacks.

2   SCHOOL

The role of the school health service is to ensure that children with chronic disorders like asthma attend school regularly and are enabled to lead a full life. School teachers are sometimes wary about accepting their responsibilities to act *in loco parentis* (usually delegated from the head teacher) in relation to apparently unpredictable and occasionally life-threatening conditions like asthma. Few teachers have had training in conditions like asthma, even though in the average class of 30 children there are likely to be two or three children with the condition few teachers have much understanding of factors which might trigger an exacerbation or understanding of the common drugs used to treat the condition.[19] As well as supporting general training for teachers, the school health service has a responsibility to ensure that the individual school child's needs are being met. This includes ensuring that individual teachers are not unnecessarily restricting asthmatic children's activities, that children (certainly from the age of 7 or 8 years) have their drug therapies with them for self-administration when required, particularly before activities likely to induce bronchospasm, and that there are no other unnecessary restrictions. This may involve the school nurse or doctor liaising with the family and perhaps a home visit, as well as with other involved doctors or health workers.

3   OTHER

Community child health staff and the general practitioner may find it helpful to discuss individual children's health needs with other child care groups, e.g. nurseries or youth clubs. This can often be undertaken by health visitors or other community nurses dealing with children.

Eczema (atopic dermatitis)

This common skin disorder of unknown aetiology is often associated with asthma and other atopy-associated conditions. Rashes are common in early life. Atopic eczema can be confused with other rashes, particularly seborrhoeic dermatitis or asteatotic eczema. It is possible to distinguish these conditions.[20] The diagnosis of eczema requires that a rash of characteristic appearance and symptoms persists for at least 3 months. The lack of understanding regarding aetiology means that management is symptomatic.

Natural history

There is good evidence that the prevalence of atopic eczema has increased considerably since the second world war.[21] The mechanisms are obscure but may reflect environmental contaminants entering the food chain. Eczema is most common in early life. Fortunately 90% of children with infantile eczema grow out of the disorder by the age of 10 years.[22] There is some evidence that more severe eczema is likely to be associated with conditions like asthma although there is not universal agreement on this point.[11] Eczema tends to run in families but the inheritance pattern is not clear.

Clinical presentation

Eczema commonly presents with the itch-scratch-itch cycle. This is associated with redness, and subsequent damage from the scratching including scaling, thickening and lichenification. In infancy the face and trunk are most commonly affected. Unlike seborrhoeic dermatitis, atopic eczema does not usually involve the flexures in the nappy area. In older children, when the condition persists, limb flexures, particularly the elbows and knees and the ankle area, are the most commonly affected sites. Secondary bacterial infection with weeping and cracks in the thickened dermis is not uncommon.

Social effects. The scratching and itching tends to be bothersome at night with effects on the child's and family's daytime performance through loss of sleep. Some children with severe eczema are treated as infectious or otherwise unacceptable by playmates, or their care givers. There may be associated asthma and allergic rhinitis.

Management

1 Emollients

These are the mainstay of eczema treatment. Emulsifying ointment is cheap and effective. It should be applied as often as necessary to keep the skin moist. A tablespoonful of ointment held under the hot tap while the bath is running results in an emulsion which leaves a greasy ring around the bath and the child. There are occasionally problems resulting from the deteriorating effect emulsifying ointment has on elastic, e.g. in underwear.

There are numerous alternative preparations, many very expensive, for general emollient use or as bath oils. In general, for eczema treatment, ointments are preferred to creams which can have a drying effect.

The lanolin or other components in creams can be irritating in their own right.

2 Anti-itch

Oral antipruritics, e.g. antihistamines such as chlorpheniramine maleate (Piriton) or trimeprazine tartrate (Vallergan) can be effective especially with their associated sedative action to reduce itching at night. Non-irritating clothing, most often recommended as cotton garments, can help, as can the avoidance of irritating soap powders.

3 Anti-infective

Obviously infected eczema, with cracking and weeping, benefits considerably from a 7–10 day course of oral antibiotics, usually selected as having an anti-staphylococcal action. Erythromycin or flucloxacillin are suitable in an appropriate dose for the child's size. Topical antibiotics are not recommended.

4 Anti-inflammation

Topical steroids are widely prescribed. The more potent varieties can cause permanent thinning of the skin, which is undesirable for what is usually a self-limiting condition. Most children requiring topical steroids can be controlled with hydrocortisone 1% ointment applied sparingly as necessary and preferably not on the face.

5 Other management

Many recommend a trial of dietary manipulation, particularly excluding eggs and milk. There is little objective evidence of benefit from controlled trials to justify this approach. There is no convincing evidence that breast feeding prevents eczema. Indeed some studies have shown more eczema in breast-fed babies.

Management in the community

Most cases of eczema requiring medical attention are managed by general practitioners. Indication for referral to a specialist includes unusually severe eczema or when the condition is not responding to orthodox management. The community child health service has a limited role to advise and support parents in the care of their child's eczema.

Hay fever/allergic rhinitis

This inflammatory condition of the upper airways may be perennial, or may be seasonal (hay fever) associated with high pollen or spore levels. Perennial rhinitis can often be shown to result from sensitivity to the house dust mite or other likely allergens. However, in some cases, no allergic factors can be demonstrated.

Natural history

Hay fever and allergic rhinitis, like eczema, appear to be increasing. Some infants have symptoms – blocked nose and sneezing – blamed on allergic rhinitis, but the condition, in general, develops during late childhood, early adolescence or early adult life and is often burnt out by middle age. Strachan[23] has produced evidence that reduced family size and increasing domestic hygiene play a part in the increased prevalence of the condition.

Clinical presentation

Sneezing, blocked nose, red itching conjunctivae and occasionally throat irritation are the dominant symptoms. Symptoms can be quite disabling and, because of the seasonal association around educational examination times, can have a marked influence on children's lives.

There is generally a close association between symptoms of hay fever and the appropriate pollen or mould spore count. High pollen counts are likely to produce symptoms in hay fever sufferers. However there is some variability in an individual's response at different times during one season and between seasons. Occasionally seasonal allergic rhinitis and hay fever can be associated with an exacerbation of wheezing and asthma but this is unusual.

Management

1   Antihistamines

Modern long-acting antihistamines, e.g. terfenadine, which appear to have reduced sedative action, are preferred by many sufferers of hay fever and allergic rhinitis when they feel they need such treatment.

2   Topical inflammatory agents

Intranasal disodium cromoglycate is sometimes helpful but the most effective relief can be obtained from intranasal topical steroids such as beclomethasone dipropionate. This is available either in a metered dose aerosol formulation, as a spray or as drops. As with other intranasal medications drops are best administered by someone else with the subject hanging down forwards to enable the liquid to run down from the top of the nasal space to ensure maximum mucosal coverage. Only very occasionally are oral steroids required. Some recommend oral steroids for children sitting important examinations but such therapy should only be considered for cases who are severely disabled.

3   Hyposensitization

This involves repeated injections of increasing amounts of the incriminated allergen in the hope of producing blocking antibodies or some other influence on the immune system. This can be effective, but is not widely available in the UK at present because of the risks. There have been a number of reported deaths from the treatment, which can now only be undertaken in a centre with comprehensive resuscitation equipment and where the individual being treated can wait for at least half an hour after receiving a dose.

Food intolerance

Intolerance to food includes allergic reactions, presumed allergic reactions and other responses to dietary constituents including the bowel damage associated with coeliac disease.

1   Anaphylaxis

A few individuals demonstrate a shock response to certain specific foods. Strict avoidance, probably on a lifetime basis, is required.

2   Definite allergic reactions

Certain individuals may manifest immediate reactions (5–30 minutes), intermediate reactions (3–18 hours) or delayed reactions (1–7 days) to certain specific foods. Egg, fish and nuts can cause immediate reactions including anaphylaxis, urticarial skin rashes, angio-oedema. Various foods including cow's milk can cause intermediate reactions, e.g. vomiting or diarrhoea. Lactose intolerance, or toxin or infectious food poisoning need to be excluded. Delayed reactions to foods are difficult to confirm.

In general, in vitro tests are unreliable. History is usually sufficient for the diagnosis of immediate reactions. Great care in a supervised environment is required for challenge tests for less life-threatening suspected food allergies or intolerance. Challenge tests, preferably placebo-controlled, are required for accurate diagnosis.

3   Possible allergic reactions

A variety of conditions, including migraine and hyperactive behaviour, can in a proportion of cases be triggered by certain foods. The mechanism of action is unclear and although avoidance of identified causes can help individuals, the majority of sufferers from the condition are not benefited by exclusion diets.

There is evidence that soya milk is more allergenic than cow's milk. Preservatives and additives are widely blamed for a variety of conditions. There is little or no objective evidence of direct harm from these substances. Often there are difficulties within the family where minor or even more serious disorders are blamed on an external cause like foods. In many chronic diseases there is a strong placebo effect from any new treatment particularly if applied with enthusiasm in circumstances where the parents believe it will help.

Various unorthodox allergy procedures are available.[24] Even conventional allergy tests are not particularly useful from a clinical perspective.[25] Management of children and families where food intolerance is suspected but cannot be confirmed can be very difficult. Specialist referral, which may include psychological and psychiatric involvement, may be necessary.

References

1 König, P., Godfrey, S. Prevalence of exercise-induced bronchial lability in families of children with asthma. *Arch Dis Child* 1973; **48**: 513–518.

2 Godfrey, R.C., Griffiths, M. The prevalence of immediate skin tests to *Dermatophagoides pteronyssinus* and grass pollen in school children. *Clin Allerg* 1976; **6**: 79–82.

3 Barbee, R.A., Lebowitz, M.D., Thompson, H.C., Burrows, B. Immediate skin test reactivity in a general population sample. *Ann Intern Med* 1976; **84**: 129–133.

4 Taylor, B., Broom, B. Atopy in medical students. *Ann Allerg* 1981; **47**: 197–199.

5 Anderson, H.R. Increase in hospital admissions for childhood asthma: trends in referral, severity and re-admissions from 1970 to 1985 in a health region of the United Kingdom. *Thorax* 1989; **44**: 614–619.

6 Anderson, H.R. Is the prevalence of asthma changing? *Arch Dis Child* 1989; **64**: 172–175.

7 Burr, M.L., Butland, B.K., King, S., Vaughan-Williams, E. Changes in asthma prevalence: two surveys 15 years apart. *Arch Dis Child* 1989; **64**: 1452–1456.

8 Williams, H., McNichol, K.N. Prevalence, natural history, and relationship of wheezy bronchitis and asthma in children: an epidemiological study. *Br Med J* 1969; **4**: 321–325.

9 Martin, A.J., McLennon, L.A., Landau, L.I., Phelan, P.D.F. The natural history of childhood asthma to adult life. *Br Med J* 1980; **2**: 1397–1400.

10 Fergusson, D.M., Horwood, L.J., Shannon, F.T., Taylor, B. Breast feeding, gastrointestinal and lower respiratory illness in the first two years. *Aust Paediatr J* 1981; **176**: 191–195.

11 Sporik, R., Holgate, S.T., Cogswell, J.T. Natural history of asthma in childhood: a birth cohort study. *Arch Dis Child* 1991; **66**: 1050–1053.

12 Horwood, L.J., Fergusson, D.M., Shannon, F.T. Social and familial factors in the development of early childhood asthma. *Pediatrics* 1985; **75**: 859–868.

13 Burr, M.L., Mullins, J., Merrett, T.G., Stott, N.C.H. Asthma and indoor mould exposure. *Thorax* 1985; **40**: 688.

14 Strachan, D. Damp housing and ill health. *Br Med J* 1989; **299**: 325.

15 Grimwood, K., Johnson-Barrett, J.J., Taylor, B. Salbutamol: tablets, inhalation powder or nebulizer? *Br Med J* 1981; **282**: 105–106.

16 Barnes, P.J. A new approach to the treatment of asthma. *N Engl J Med* 1989; **321**: 1517–1527.

17 Asthma: a follow-up statement from an international paediatric consensus group. *Arch Dis Child* 1992; **67**: 240–248.

18 Lask, B., Matthew, D. Childhood asthma: a controlled trial of family psychotherapy. *Arch Dis Child* 1979; **54**: 116–120.

19 Bevis, M., Taylor, B. What do school teachers know about asthma? *Arch Dis Child* 1990; **65**: 622–625.

20 Yates, V.M., Kerr, R.E.I., Mackie, R.M. Early diagnosis of infantile seborrhoeic dermatitis and atopic eczema: clinical features. *Br J Dermatol* 1983; **108**: 634–638.

21 Taylor, B., Wadsworth, J., Wadsworth, M., Peckham, C. Changes in the reported prevalence of childhood eczema since the 1939–45 war. *Lancet* 1984; **ii**: 1255–1257.

22 Vickers, C.F.H. The natural history of atopic eczema. *Acta Dermatovener (Supplement)* 1980; **92**: 113–115.

23 Strachan, D. Hayfever, hygiene and family size. *Br Med J* 1989; **299**: 1259–1260.

24 David, T.J. Unorthodox allergy procedures. *Arch Dis Child* 1987; **62**: 1060–1062.

25 David, T.J. Conventional allergy tests. *Arch Dis Child* 1991; **66**: 281–282.

16.4 Cystic fibrosis

John Dodge

Incidence

Approximately 250–300 babies with cystic fibrosis (CF) are born to British parents every year, and nearly 6000 patients with CF were known to the UK Cystic Fibrosis Survey in 1993.[1] This makes it the most common serious genetic disease of children among those of European descent and, because the treatment of CF is so complex and expensive, it makes demands on health service resources which are far greater than its frequency would suggest. The life expectancy of affected individuals has been greatly extended by treatment, and the task of paediatricians is to deliver young adults into the care of physicians in the best shape possible. Because the number of infants born with CF exceeds the number of adults dying with it by 100 or more each year, the total number of affected individuals will continue to rise, even if there are no further developments in treatment, and the relative numbers of child and adult patients should be roughly in balance before the next century is far advanced.

Genetics

Inheritance of CF is autosomal recessive, and carriers are about 1 in 25 of the healthy population. Like some other common genetically-determined disorders, such as thalassaemia, the clinical severity of the condition varies between patients, and these variations relate to differences in the precise mutation at the gene locus. The affected gene is carried on the long arm of chromosome 7. The most common mutation, which, when homozygous, produces a severe form of CF, is deletion of three bases at position number 508 which code for a single phenylalanine molecule. The mutation is described as $\Delta F508$ and it is present in about 70% of carriers of CF. It is therefore present in homozygous form in about half of all patients, the remainder either carrying one $\Delta F508$ and another mutation, or two other mutations. This heterogeneity means that so far no single genetic test can identify all carriers; as we still do not know the exact function of the corresponding protein, which has been designated cystic fibrosis transmembrane regulator (CFTR), we cannot detect carriers by identifying a functional abnormality. Sequencing of the gene and its related protein was reported in 1989[2,3] and with the rapid pace of research in molecular biology it may be that a simple and generally applicable test for carrier detection will become available over the next few years. Such a test, offered to couples in the whole population before or soon after conception and linked with a programme for prenatal diagnosis and, if requested, termination of affected pregnancies, could substantially reduce the future incidence and prevalence of the disease. Until now, carrier detection has been limited to families who already have an affected child.

Neonatal screening

It is possible to detect CF in up to three-quarters of affected newborns by measuring the level of trypsinogen in dried blood spots similar to those obtained for detection of phenylketonuria or hypothyroidism. Although CF is accompanied in most cases by pancreatic insufficiency, residual pancreatic function is generally present at birth. The earliest pathological changes in the pancreas include small duct obstruction, which, together with cell damage, leads to trypsinogen reabsorption and increase in the serum concentration to above normal levels. The technique used is either a radioimmunoassay (immunoreactive trypsin (IRT)) or an enzyme-linked assay (ELISA), and the units of measurement vary according to the particular commercial kit and local methods employed.

Some health authorities screen neonates by using one or other of these tests. Although most affected babies will be detected, neonatal screening is not completely sensitive and some will be missed. This means that clinicians in those districts must still remember CF as a possible cause of symptoms in young children, and cannot assume that it would have been automatically picked up by the newborn Guthrie programme. Also, a significant proportion of normal infants have a transient rise in serum trypsinogen levels in the first week of life, and therefore give false-positive results. A normal result on a repeat blood test will eliminate most of these from further investigation, and CF is not diagnosed in any screened babies until they have had two elevated trypsinogen levels and a positive sweat test. Health visitors or general practitioners need to be particularly careful not to arouse undue anxiety in the parent when asking for a repeat blood test, because the majority of those babies with an initial suspicious result will prove *not* to have cystic fibrosis.

The benefits of early detection of CF have not yet been generally accepted as proven, at least in terms of subsequent morbidity and survival. However, many babies detected by screening already have symptoms such as loose stools, slow weight gain or cough, which have not necessarily been recognized as abnormal either by the parents or their medical advisers but which indicate malabsorption or early bronchial obstruction and possible infection. In the absence of neonatal screening, diagnosis is frequently delayed and may not be made until permanent lung damage has occurred. Parents of such children are understandably angry and resentful towards the medical profession in general and their own doctors in particular. Conversely, detection of the disease in its early stages, perhaps before any symptoms have developed, is perceived as offering the child the best chance of avoiding or postponing serious complications.

Clinical features

Most of the symptoms and signs of CF can be explained on the basis of abnormal exocrine secretions in various organs. In the small intestine, neonatal obstruction may result from inspissated meconium

(meconium ileus) and similar retained masses in the ileum and proximal colon may cause pain and obstructive symptoms in older children and adults. Retained bronchial secretions are responsible for progressive obstructive lung disease complicated by infection leading eventually to widespread bronchiectasis, pulmonary fibrosis and respiratory failure. Obstruction to small pancreatic ducts and retention of proteolytic and other enzymes leads to destruction of the exocrine pancreas and in some cases the pancreatic islets also become involved with consequent diabetes mellitus. A consistent abnormality in sweat glands is defective chloride permeability in the ducts leading to excessive sodium chloride loss in the sweat. The precise relationship between the regulation of sweat chloride channels in epithelial cells and the CFTR gene product is not entirely clear, nor has any treatment aimed at curing or controlling the fundamental intracellular problems yet been developed.

The clinical picture in individual patients will be determined by the severity of the lung disease, malabsorption and malnutrition on the one hand and the success or failure of treatment and preventive measures on the other. Some children may be indistinguishable from their healthy friends, while others may be puny, wasted respiratory invalids. Happily, increasing numbers of patients are able to enjoy reasonably good health throughout childhood and to take part in the full range of school activities. The underlying disease has not changed and this improvement is the result of aggressive treatment, most effectively delivered by an expert team.

Management

Although it is generally accepted that the wide range of skills and experience required for the optimum care of children with cystic fibrosis, along with the authoritative advice which their parents require, can only be offered by large specialist centres, much of the day-to-day care can be given at local or community level. The most important therapists are the parents, who need to learn techniques of physiotherapy, the importance of regular surveillance, the need to treat infection early and to recognize minor degrees of clinical deterioration. The specialist clinic should decide overall management policy. The early intensive counselling of parents is best carried out by someone with a major involvement in CF care, who will best be able to handle the unexpected questions and discuss prognosis and new developments in treatment from the strong ground of personal experience. Parents of newly diagnosed children need the security of an accessible clinic where everything possible can be done for their child. They also need detailed genetic counselling; with the advent of carrier detection and prenatal diagnosis, this

is now becoming a task for geneticists rather than CF specialists.

In some regions, paediatricians from the CF centre hold joint clinics in peripheral hospitals with local consultants; others prefer to see the child at the regional or specialist centre, the frequency depending upon the severity of the illness. Between visits to the centre the child may or may not be seen by another paediatrician at his local hospital. If care is shared between hospitals there is obvious need for direct and prompt communication between the professionals involved.

Many general practitioners with CF children on their lists do not wish to become involved in their treatment beyond prescribing antibiotics as advised by the hospital and in urban areas with easy access to the hospital the family doctor is often bypassed. The increasing tendency to keep patients out of hospital as much as possible means that primary care and community staff are likely to have a larger role in the future, but local demographic and other factors will determine the particular patterns of care.

Nutrition and digestion

Most patients need to take pancreatin with their meals, and modern formulations are reasonably effective. However, every meal and snack must be accompanied by capsules which may number ten or more. It is important that teachers and others supervising school meals are aware that the child is not taking a drug but a necessary aid to digestion.

Frequent or persistent abdominal pain (meconium ileus equivalent or distal intestinal obstruction syndrome) is usually an indication that the dose of pancreatin should be increased. It is important to distinguish it from acute appendicitis and thus avoid an unnecessary operation and a possible harmful anaesthetic. If *any* unusual and possibly serious symptom develops, every effort should be made to refer the child to his regional specialist clinic.

If normal growth is to proceed in the presence of unavoidable calorie losses in the stools and increased demands for coping with infection, nutritional requirements must be increased to 120% or more of the recommended daily allowance for age and sex. This can be very difficult to achieve and some children take special high calorie supplements. There is a close relationship between the nutritional state and the patient's well-being and survival, and apparently drastic measures are sometimes used to maintain or restore weight gain. Impressive results have been achieved by supplementary nasogastric or gastrostomy feeding, given overnight. Community services may be asked to supply the necessary equipment, including infusion pumps.

Physiotherapy and exercise

Regular physiotherapy is a cornerstone of treatment. Its object is to help the child cough up retained secretions, and it is normally carried out two or three times a day or even more frequently during exacerbations of infection. Older children can learn techniques of forced expiration and postural drainage but if treatment is to be carried out during school hours they need a private place and sometimes the help of the school nurse. Participation in games and physical exercise should be strongly encouraged and it is important to avoid overprotection. However, encouragement must be tempered with common sense and an appreciation that the child's performance may be limited by fatigue or breathlessness.

Respiratory infection

Although physiotherapy is started from the time of diagnosis, and prophylactic antibiotics may be used in the early years of life, sooner or later most patients develop chronic bronchial infection. Initially this is likely to be with *Staphylococcus aureus* or *Haemophilus influenzae*, but eventually most patients become colonized with *Pseudomonas aeruginosa*. However, chronic infection is compatible with many years of good health. A recently recognized pathogen which may colonize older patients is *Pseudomonas cepacia*. It was initially believed to have sinister significance, but subsequent experience has shown that it is not always associated with an accelerated decline in respiratory function or worsening prognosis. Antibiotics should be used early and in generous dosage during upper and lower respiratory infections. Exacerbations of pseudomonas infection require intravenous antibiotics, and some centres believe that regular 10–14 day courses of such antibiotics should be given to colonized patients whether or not they have an increase in cough and sputum. In the past these courses of treatment have required admission to hospital but parents can be taught to give the antibiotics through implantable intravenous lines, thus allowing the child to stay at home or attend school. The indwelling catheters may be of the Broviac or Hickman type, with an exposed port to which a syringe or infusion set can be attached, or a fully covered implantable port (e.g. Portacath) which is subcutaneous and entered with a needle.

Younger children often show signs such as wheezing and pulmonary hyperinflation indistinguishable from bronchial asthma, and may require home nebulizers for delivery of bronchodilator drugs. Intervals between pulmonary exacerbations can be extended by the use of nebulized antibiotics such as gentamicin, ceftazidime, carbenicillin and colistin. Provision of nebulizers, infusion pumps and related equipment may be through the hospital or community services.

Smoking is discouraged as strongly as possible. This ban also extends to passive smoking and the parents must be told unequivocally that the child should be kept out of smoke-filled rooms.

Cystic fibrosis is not a contraindication to standard immunizations: on the contrary, it is particularly important to immunize these children against pertussis and measles. So far, no successful immunization against *Pseudomonas aeruginosa* has been developed.

School activities

Children with CF should join in all school activities so far as is possible, and teachers and other children must know that the condition is not infectious even when a child has a severe cough. A CF teenager in good health could go on overseas trips without the family but would probably require a medical certificate for customs to allow import of regular medication. Summer camps for groups of children with CF have great value for developing independence, but carry a definite risk of cross-infection with different strains of *Pseudomonas aeruginosa* or *Pseudomonas cepacia*. However, this risk is present to a greater extent in hospital wards which treat CF patients and is usually small. On balance, the advantages of such holidays probably outweigh the potential risks, but patients with *Ps. cepacia* should not be allowed to attend.

Psychological problems

Adolescents with CF often become depressed. Males in particular often worry about small stature and delayed puberty. The discovery that nearly all infected males are infertile, as a result of blockage of the vas deferens, is a source of much distress and it needs to be clearly pointed out that infertility does not mean impotence. The realization that life is likely to be curtailed by CF may be followed by a fatalistic approach to treatment and a refusal to carry out physiotherapy or take medication. Typically, CF children and adolescents are very conformist but occasionally they act out their feelings of anger and resentment. In girls there is sometimes a strong wish to become pregnant before their health deteriorates. Not uncommonly the stresses of coping with CF are sufficient to disrupt the parents' marriage, and this adds further to the burden carried by affected children.

Social support

The social worker and the specialist CF nurse have an important role in helping parents of the newly diagnosed child to come to terms with the implications of the diagnosis. Families in difficult economic circumstances can be helped to obtain special benefits. The criteria for attendance allowances are not usually met in childhood although this rule seems to vary in different parts of the UK.

Local branches of the Cystic Fibrosis Trust* offer advice and support for families, while the central office sends out regular newsletters and publishes a useful range of information booklets. Older patients may join their own organization, the Association of Cystic Fibrosis Adults (ACFA)† which is affiliated to an international organization of the same name. Both these patient associations also publish newsletters and hold regular meetings.

New directions in treatment

There is an active heart–lung transplant programme in the UK and early results of this procedure have been very encouraging. In numerous instances the CF patient has been the recipient of heart and lungs as a single unit and become a donor of a healthy heart to a third party.

Experience of transplants in children is fairly limited but some spectacular successes have been achieved. Nevertheless, this will be predominantly a technique applicable to adults, because children can generally be maintained in reasonable condition by conventional treatment, because supply of donor lungs for children is severely limited, and because the survival rate of transplanted hearts and lungs after a few years is not yet known.

Terminal care

In spite of rapidly increasing medical knowledge and imaginative developments in treatment, some CF patients still die in childhood. Whenever possible the children should be allowed to die in the familiar and comforting surroundings of their own home.

General practitioners and community nurses have professional experience and often personal knowledge of the family, which gives them a central role in the management of terminal illness and the aftercare of the family. After an interval of 6–8 weeks parents may appreciate the opportunity to review their child's life and illness with one of the senior CF doctors. This allows them to ask questions about aspects of care which may have been bothering them, and to obtain reassurance that they were in no way to blame for their child's death. Those who have come through bereavement of a child and regained a positive approach to life can be of enormous help to other young parents.

References

1 Dodge, J.A., Morison, S., Lewis, P.A. *et al*. Cystic fibrosis in the United Kingdom, 1968–1988: incidence, population and survival. *Paediat Perinat Epidemiol* 1993; **7**: 157–166.
2 Rommens, J.M., Ianuzzi, M.C., Kerem, B.-S., *et al*. Identification of the cystic fibrosis gene: chromosome walking and jumping. *Science* 1989; **245**: 1059–1065.
3 Riordan, J.R., Rommens, J.M., Kerem, B.-S., *et al*. Identification of the cystic fibrosis gene: cloning and characterization of complementary DNA. *Science* 1989; **245**: 1066–1073.

Further reading

1 Goodchild, M.C., Dodge, J.A. *Cystic Fibrosis: Manual of Diagnosis and Management*, 2nd edn. London: Baillière Tindall, 1989.
2 The Cystic Fibrosis Research Trust publishes a wide range of booklets for parents, teachers and other interested persons. Topics include immunization, social work support, school, nutrition, physiotherapy, genetics, attendance allowances, bereavement, and a guide to government and voluntary help.

16.5 HIV infection

Jacqueline Mok

Introduction

Infection with the human immunodeficiency virus (HIV) is now known to be a leading cause of immune deficiency in infants and children. The virus is transmitted during sexual intercourse, parenterally through blood and blood products, and by vertical transmission from an infected mother to her child. The majority

*The Cystic Fibrosis Trust, Alexandra House, 5 Blyth Road, Bromley, Kent, BR1 3RS.
†The Association of Cystic Fibrosis Adults (ACFA) c/o Cystic Research Trust, above address.

of infants and children with HIV infection have been born to infected mothers, and with control of blood-borne spread, transmission from mother to child will be the predominant route of infection. Current estimates are that the acquired immunodeficiency syndrome (AIDS) in children accounts for about 2% of the total AIDS cases but, with the increase in numbers of infected women, there will be a concomitant increase in children with HIV infection.

The child at risk

A child may be suspected to be at risk of HIV infection for the following reasons:

1 Mother with a known or suspected risk activity: injecting drug use; sexual promiscuity; sexual partner of HIV-infected man; past history of blood transfusions before routine screening of donors.
2 Past history of blood tranfusions prior to routine screening, or treatment with blood products.
3 Sexual abuse by an HIV-infected person.
4 History of promiscuity or drug use in older children.

Often, social workers refer children who are considered to be at risk of HIV infection, usually in the context of placement in care or for adoption. Community paediatricians who are medical advisers to adoption panels will have to decide whether further action is required. The issue of testing for HIV infection is discussed later, but the parents should always be counselled before blood is drawn, as well as after the result is known, on the implications of the results both for the child and for the family.

Diagnosis of HIV infection

The cornerstone of diagnosis of HIV infection in children rests on the suspicion of infection based on the clinical presentation or epidemiological risk, and confirmed by laboratory testing. The standard laboratory criterion for diagnosing HIV infection in adults is serological testing for the presence of HIV-specific IgG antibodies. Passive transfer of maternal antibodies, which can persist for up to 18 months,[1,2] means that antibody testing alone is an unreliable method of diagnosis. Also, negative results can be found despite other evidence of HIV infection, in the early stages of infection prior to an antibody response; where the child is hypogammaglobulinaemic;[3] and with disease progression when loss of antibody may be associated with antigenaemia.[4,5] While the detection of the HIV core antigen may be an indicator of advanced disease, some infected children remain free of antigen.

Techniques which attempt to quantify the infant's response to infection include antibody production in vitro by peripheral blood lymphocytes,[6] the detection of IgM or IgG subclass antibodies,[7,8] and sequential comparisons of HIV protein bands in maternal and infant sera by Western blotting.[9] Virus culture, often considered the gold standard for confirming the diagnosis, is available in only a few centres and may lack sensitivity. The polymerase chain reaction (PCR), a gene amplification technique, has not been properly evaluated; PCR-positive antibody-negative children, and vice versa, have been reported.[10-12] None of the laboratory tests have stood the test of time, and it is important that laboratory results are correlated with eventual clinical outcome. The European Study[2] has also found that hypergammaglobulinaemia was the most sensitive and specific early marker for HIV infection. Guidelines for the diagnosis of HIV infection in children under 13 years of age are shown in Table 16.2.

Clinical spectrum of HIV infection

The initial definition of AIDS in children required documentation of a previous opportunistic infection or associated malignancy, with exclusion of second-

---

Table 16.2 Definition of HIV infection in children under 13 years

1   Children under 18 months at risk of perinatal infection must have *one* of the following:

   a   HIV cultured from peripheral blood lymphocytes or other tissue
   b   Clinical signs and symptoms meeting the Centers for Disease Control (CDC) criteria for AIDS
   c   Positive HIV antibody test *and* evidence of cellular and humoral immune deficiency *and* symptoms (class P-2)

2   Children who have been infected by other means, or older children at risk of vertical infection, must have one of the following:

   a   Positive HIV culture
   b   Repeatedly positive HIV antibody test
   c   Symptoms meeting CDC criteria for AIDS

Modified from[13]

ary causes of immune deficiency. This restrictive definition only identified about 25% of infected children, at the extreme end of the disease spectrum. Prospective studies of children born to HIV-infected mothers have revealed a bimodal distribution of disease presentation, with a severe rapidly progressive infantile form and a more slowly progressive form which is compatible with survival into adolescence. With longer survival, a wider clinical spectrum is apparent, where HIV is seen to affect every organ. The classification of HIV infection in children is shown in Table 16.3.

Most children present with clinical disease at a median age of 8 months, with only 21% presenting after the age of 2 years. The survival of children varies with the disease pattern, the best outcome being seen with lymphoid interstitial pneumonitis with a median survival of 72 months following diagnosis, while children with *Pneumocystis carinii* pneumonia rarely survive beyond 1 month from diagnosis.[14] It follows, therefore, that paediatricians in the community will see children with disease patterns which are compatible with longer survival, such as lymphoid interstitial pneumonitis, static encephalopathy or recurrent bacterial infections. With early therapeutic intervention, it is conceivable that even children with severe disease will be surviving to school age.

Care of the infected child

At present, treatment is supportive and aimed at the symptoms of HIV disease. Until more is known about the natural history of HIV infection in children, many families live with a disease which has an uncertain future, knowing that the outcome is usually fatal. Support for the child and family must therefore be of a consistent nature, bridging the gap between hospital and community services. Services are best coordinated by a paediatrician, and core members of the multidisciplinary team should include nurses, counsellors, and staff from the social work and education departments. Where necessary, the advice and help of dietitians, physiotherapists, occupational therapists, speech therapists, and psychologists should be sought.

Co-trimoxazole (Septrin) prophylaxis

Guidelines have been published[15] for the use of prophylaxis against *Pneumocystis carinii* pneumonia (PCP) for children infected with HIV. Although PCP can occur at any age, mortality is at its highest in those less than 6 months old. At least half the children who developed PCP were not recognized to be infected with HIV before the diagnosis of PCP, although some had had earlier HIV associated symptoms. Ideally, prophylaxis should be administered only to those children with proven HIV infection, although in practical terms this is difficult because the youngest patients are those who are least easy to diagnose to be HIV infected due to the presence of maternal antibody. No data have emerged to define the predictors of PCP among HIV infected children, but correlates of PCP include age under 1 year, reduction in CD4 lymphocyte numbers, and HIV-related symptoms. Recent studies of lymphocyte subsets among healthy infants and young children have demonstrated that these counts are much higher, compared to healthy adults. Current guidelines for PCP prophylaxis in paediatric HIV infection relate to the

Table 16.3 Classification system for HIV infection in children

---

P-0 Indeterminate infection. Children under 18 months old who have maternal antibody and no other tests performed.

P-1 Asymptomatic infection
    A   normal immune function
    B   abnormal immune function
    C   immune function not tested

P-2 Symptomatic infection
    A   non-specific findings, e.g. lymphadenopathy, hepatosplenomegaly, failure to thrive, diarrhoea
    B   progressive neurological disease, e.g. loss or plateau of developmental milestones, impaired brain growth, progressive symmetrical motor deficits
    C   lymphoid interstitial pneumonitis – persistence of abnormal chest X-ray for at least 2 months despite appropriate antimicrobial therapy; this may require histological confirmation
    D   secondary infectious diseases – includes children with those opportunistic infections listed in the CDC surveillance definition for AIDS, those with unexplained recurrent serious bacterial infections (two or more within a 2-year period), and other infectious diseases such as oral candidiasis persisting for more than 2 months, two or more episodes of herpes dermatitis within a year, or multidermatomal or disseminated herpes zoster infection
    E   secondary cancers
    F   other diseases possibly due to HIV infection such as hepatitis, cardiopathy, nephropathy, haematological disorders and dermatological diseases.

age appropriate CD4 count. Many paediatricians, however, commence Septrin prophylaxis in any child who has evidence of HIV infection, irrespective of CD4 count, and this is particularly appropriate for children under 18 months of age. Some paediatricians feel it is safer to recommend that all babies of indeterminate status are started on PCP prophylaxis until infection status is proven to be negative.

Recurrent infections

Children with HIV infection have defects in their humoral as well as cellular immune systems. Humoral defects manifest as recurrent bacterial infections, which can be treated with broad-spectrum antibiotics or regular infusions of gammaglobulin.[16,17] Defective immune responses mean that trivial childhood illnesses such as measles and chicken pox could have devastating results. Close monitoring of such infectious diseases in the classroom requires tactful working relationships between the parents, medical and teaching staff. It is important to protect confidentiality while ensuring the safety of the immune-compromised child.

Nutrition

Failure to thrive is usually the combination of poor appetite, recurrent infections and a direct effect of HIV on the gut. Added to these, parents from deprived areas are usually unable to afford foods with high nutritional values. The child's weight should be monitored on a regular basis, and dietetic advice sought at the first sign of poor weight gain. Some children need parenteral nutrition and the home care team may be able to teach parents how to manage indwelling catheters and the administration of intravenous solutions at home. The home care team should always be on the alert for misuse of needles and syringes in households where drug use is prominent.

Encephalopathy

Involvement of the central nervous system can manifest as loss or plateau of developmental milestones, progressive motor difficulties, impaired brain growth or rarely, with seizures.[18,19] Although earlier retrospective studies[19,20] reported the prevalence of HIV encephalopathy to range from 50 to 90%, analysis of cohorts of children followed prospectively suggests a lower incidence of 20%.[21] However, children in prospective studies were under the age of 2 years, and it is possible that they will show evidence of neurological involvement later. The true extent of central nervous system involvement is, as yet, unknown.

Regular reassessment will reveal delay or regression in milestones. Secondary microcephaly will be obvious with sequential measurements of the head circumference, and poor brain growth can be confirmed by imaging techniques. The child suffers both physical and mental handicaps, and is likely to require referral to the physiotherapist, speech therapist and occupational therapist. The paediatrician must liaise with education and social work staff as the child will have special educational needs.

Lymphoid interstitial pneumonitis

This is slowly progressive, and the child presents insidiously with cough and breathlessness. Symptoms and radiological findings persist despite adequate therapy with antimicrobials. With progressive lung involvement, hypoxaemia is present which may require supplemental oxygen therapy. Parents can be taught the management of oxygen therapy in the home, and some children may only require oxygen intermittently. Severe limitation of respiratory function may result in special educational help being sought for the child, ranging from a modified school programme to the provision of a teacher in the home.

Immunization

The immune dysfunction associated with HIV infection has led to caution among paediatricians when considering immunization procedures for infected children. Vaccine efficacy is reduced compared to that seen in immune-competent individuals. Also, vaccination itself could accelerate progression of the disease by antigenic stimulation. Live attenuated vaccine viruses could replicate excessively in immune-deficient individuals and result in disseminated disease. There is also a danger that excretion of oral polio vaccine virus will be prolonged, and cause vaccine-related paralysis in other immune-compromised persons in the household.

However, review of patient records revealed that some children had received immunization with live vaccines, including oral polio, measles, mumps and rubella vaccines, after the onset of HIV-related symptoms. Although the follow up of the children was limited, there were no reports of serious adverse events such as paralytic poliomyelitis, atypical measles, or aseptic meningitis in the month following vaccination.[21] Review of surveillance records for adverse vaccine reactions also confirmed these findings; no report of a vaccine-associated illness occurred in a child with HIV-related disease.

Moreover, it can be argued that there is good reason to offer immunization as soon as is practicable, before the onset of immune deficiency.

The serological response to most inactivated and live vaccines is reduced in HIV-infected persons and is related to the degree of immune suppression present. Therefore, paediatricians looking after HIV-infected children should monitor the response to immunization. With deterioration in immune function, consideration should be given to the use of hyper-immune globulin following exposure to chicken pox or measles, despite a history of immunization.

In the UK, the Joint Committee on Vaccination and Immunization has recommended that HIV-positive individuals, with or without symptoms, should receive the following as appropriate:[22]

Inactivated vaccines: diphtheria, tetanus, pertussis, polio, Hib (*Haemophilus influenzae* type b), typhoid, cholera, hepatitis B.

Live vaccines: measles, mumps, rubella, polio.

Because live polio virus may be excreted for prolonged periods in HIV-infected patients, with the risk of infecting other family members who may be immune deficient, the clinician may choose to use inactivated polio vaccine. For practical purposes, it is unlikely that the child at risk of HIV infection will be symptomatic when presented for immunization and the normal programme should be offered. There is no case for testing the child's HIV status, or withholding immunization, on the grounds that the child might be HIV positive. In Edinburgh, where children of HIV-infected mothers have been given live polio vaccine, no adverse reaction has been noted in either the child or mother.[23] The parents, who may be immune deficient, should be warned of the risk of prolonged faecal excretion of polio vaccine virus, and of the need for handwashing after changing the nappy of the infant given live polio vaccine. Uninfected siblings of known HIV-infected children should be immunized routinely, unless the infected child was severely immune deficient when again use of inactivated polio vaccine (IPV) should be considered. As HIV-infected parents become severely immune compromised, their children should be offered IPV. This will necessitate close liaison between the physicians looking after the parents and children.

There have been reports of local reactions and dissemination of BCG vaccine in HIV-infected patients. Where the risk of tuberculosis is small, BCG should not be given to HIV-positive children. In many developing countries, the risk of contracting tuberculosis with its complications outweighs the risk of dissemination of BCG vaccine. Studies of tuberculosis among adults in the USA and some parts of Africa suggest an increased incidence of overt disease in HIV-infected individuals. The severity of tuberculosis can also be increased in HIV-infected children. The World Health Organization has therefore recommended that BCG vaccination should be offered, regardless of the HIV status.[24]

Implications for the family

Approximately 80% of HIV-infected children come from families where one or both parents are also infected. The diagnosis of AIDS in a young child usually implies that the mother is herself infected. The majority of the mothers in Edinburgh have been infected during needle-sharing drug use, or were sexual partners of HIV-positive drug users.

Paediatricians working with HIV-infected children must be prepared to address issues beyond the medical management of the disease in the child, for the families usually come from areas of severe deprivation. HIV infection is one more problem the family has to cope with, along with homelessness or suboptimal housing, imprisonment, unemployment, the effects of drug use, or problems faced by refugee families.

HIV disease in the parents

There are few chronic conditions of childhood where there is concomitant illness in the child and parents. HIV infection occurs in young parents who may be ill, dying or dead from AIDS and therefore unable to care for the child. Often, drug use has alienated other family members so that support from the family is non-existent. In addition, the stigma and fear provoked by HIV and AIDS may mean that the parents opt not to disclose the diagnosis to close family members, thus limiting potential sources of emotional and practical assistance. The paediatrician will have to be aware of the resource needs of the family, and be able to identify agencies which might be able to offer practical as well as emotional help.

Where the parents have difficulties in transporting the child to hospital, members of volunteer groups sympathetic to the needs of HIV-affected families have fulfilled the role of driver or babysitter. Parent-support or self-help groups are usually poorly attended because of the stigma of HIV and the fear of breach of confidentiality.

Other siblings in the family

There may be more than one child infected with HIV. At present, no clear pattern of vertical transmission can be predicted for HIV-infected women, nor is much known about maternal factors which might contribute to this risk. The latest analysis on risk factors from the European Study suggests that the sicker woman is more likely to pose a greater risk to her child.[2]

When more than one child is infected, this leads to increased stresses within the family. The pattern of disease does not always run true in any family, with children from the same family suffering more than one disease manifestation and with varying outcomes. Often the uninfected siblings have to bear the family secret, or the hysterical reactions from family members, friends and others in the community. The uninfected children will have to cope with the loss of siblings and parents due to HIV disease. In Edinburgh, the social work department is already identifying families to work with the family affected by HIV and to provide respite care for children during times of parental illness. This flexible care system prepares children for the eventual loss of parents.[25]

Drug use in the parents

Some local authorities automatically put the children of drug-using parents on the child protection register. As a result, many mothers who use illegal drugs do not approach social workers for help. With the spread of HIV infection among drug users, it is crucial that services reach as many users as possible. While there is a statutory duty to investigate any child believed to be at risk, drug use in itself should never be the sole reason for taking a child into care in the absence of other anxieties.

It can be more difficult for parents who use drugs to discontinue their habit than users without children. Few residential rehabilitation facilities enable the mother to detoxify while retaining direct responsibility for her children. Some drug users find it difficult to look after their children while undergoing intensive therapy. In these circumstances, alternative care arrangements for the children have to be sought, either with family members or foster parents.

Placement in foster care

In Edinburgh, before the emergence of the HIV problem, the Lothian Region Social Work Department already had a clear policy of family placement as the optimum care for most children, especially those under 12 years. This resulted in foster families who had been trained and supported in the care of children and families with a wide range of emotional or physical problems. With the arrival of HIV infection in the city, this commitment to children with special needs was extended.[25]

Social work staff will have anxieties about personal and family safety which can be alleviated by training sessions where information on HIV and its recognized modes of transmission should be discussed. Medical advisers to adoption panels may be asked to fulfil this training role. Due to the difficulties in interpreting an HIV antibody test result in young children, the routine testing for HIV antibody is not recommended for the placement of children in foster care.

Experience in Edinburgh has shown that with thorough preparation, families can be recruited who are prepared to care for children who have been considered at risk of HIV infection. The children are not routinely tested for the presence of HIV infection, although it may sometimes be necessary to check whether the child is a risk for hepatitis B infection. Many local authorities offer immunization against hepatitis B to foster families who care for these children.

As part of preparation, foster parents should have an opportunity to discuss in greater detail specific issues about HIV infection in children. Although the outlook is uncertain, the need for regular medical follow up should be stressed, as well as the possibility of a compromised immune system so that trivial infections may need prompt medical attention. Attention to good hygiene practices such as hand washing and covering open wounds with waterproof dressings must be emphasized. Most families welcome leaflets which provide simple explanations and reassurances. Mutual support among the foster families has been invaluable, both to share experiences in caring for the children as well as to protect themselves against the insensitivities of others.

Adoption

Regulations for adoption agencies outline the need for comprehensive medical reports on the child and each birth parent. Details should include the history of genetically transmitted disease in the family as well as the presence of significant illness in either the mother or father. A report with the medical background of the child and family must be available to prospective adoptive parents.

All prospective adopters will need to understand the limitations of HIV antibody testing in infants. However, the natural mother should be asked about activities which might place her at risk of HIV infection – needle-sharing drug use, sexual intercourse with an HIV-infected man, or a history of sexual promiscuity. If risk activities are identified, the woman should be counselled about the possibilities of HIV infection, and testing offered. A physician knowledgeable in the interpretation of the test result should be asked to advise on the usefulness of the result.

Where the woman refuses to be tested, the adoption agency should proceed to place the baby for adoption, and the adoptive parents be informed about the child's background. Testing of the child could be performed at the request of the adoptive parents, after the adoption order is granted. Where prospective adoptive parents seek absolute guarantees about freedom from HIV infection, their suitability as parents must be questioned.

HIV in schools

The infected child

The issue of school attendance by children with HIV infection has created hysteria in many communities. It must be emphasized that such children have the same needs and rights as other children. This includes the protection of confidentiality and privacy of the family while acting in the best interest to protect the child's well-being. Decisions regarding school attendance rest on the risk to the health of the HIV-infected child, and on the risk posed to other children by the infected child. Thus the health care team is involved in the decision-making process regarding the best educational placement. This could be in a mainstream school with or without some modification to the school programme or in a special school. Among the issues to be considered are the health of the child, socialization skills such as the ability to control body secretions and biting behaviour, and the presence of oozing skin lesions or transmissible diseases such as tuberculosis.

Who needs to know

Guidelines from the Departments of Education of Scotland, England and Wales state that there is no need for staff of educational establishments to know the HIV status of any child at school.[26] No case of HIV infection has been documented to have been transmitted in the school or day-care setting. There is also a danger that a false sense of security could arise from knowing about one particular child, with no attention paid to general infection control policies for all children.

In principle, there is no necessity for the identity of an HIV-infected child to be disclosed, but this policy must go hand in hand with policies for good hygiene practices in all schools. Guidelines must be available to enable staff to deal with spillages of blood and other body fluids, to dispose of infected material and to disinfect soiled surfaces. Where educational staff feel supported in the management of all issues surrounding HIV-infected children in schools, there is usually a positive attitude towards these children.

As with all children with special educational needs, it is sometimes essential to disclose the diagnosis to the teachers.

The child may be severely immune depressed, and the parents need to be warned about infectious diseases such as measles or chicken pox. Teachers may be the first to pick up signs of learning difficulties which may be related to encephalopathy. The difficulties usually lie not with informing the teacher, but which teacher to inform. Some head teachers feel they should hold that information, which may never be passed on to the relevant class teacher, while others feel the need to inform all staff in the school including the janitor. The parents should always be part of the decision about who should receive information on their child's HIV status. They should be persuaded that it is in the child's interest that the teaching staff be aware of the diagnosis; but their wishes and rights should be respected should they decide not to disclose the information.

HIV education in schools

HIV infection is still a relatively new disease. The absence of a specific cure engenders fear and panic in the minds of most people. Also, at present, the disease is seen to affect groups which are socially disenfranchised, such as homosexuals and intravenous drug users. There is therefore a need to raise awareness and develop basic knowledge about the disease, especially among youngsters at school, in an attempt to dispel myths and anxieties which exist. By disseminating the correct information, it is hoped that individual behaviour and lifestyle can be modified and the spread of HIV infection limited.

For the above reasons, education on HIV and AIDS must never be taken out of the context of health education, sex education, or the social education curriculum. Even primary school children can be taught about HIV in the context of hygiene and healthy lifestyles. Coordinated and realistic strategies can only be achieved by close cooperation between health, education and social services.

The future

With steps taken to screen donors of blood and the use of heat-treated blood products, cases of children with transfusion-acquired HIV infection should diminish. The prevention of most cases of AIDS in children will depend on decreasing the numbers of births to HIV-infected women. Unfortunately, self-identification of risk activities, and voluntary testing often fail to detect infected women. Also, the potential spread of HIV to sexually active or intravenous drug using adolescents merits grave concern.

The education of children and adolescents about the avoidance of risk behaviours is an activity which should be awarded top priority by paediatricians who work in schools.

At present, several studies are in progress to examine the risk of vertical transmission of HIV, to elucidate the natural history and clinical spectrum of infected children, as well as to identify factors in the mother or child which might affect the outcome. It is hoped that with better understanding of the disease, along with more effective therapy for infected children, the care of these children will be improved. All paediatricians must develop at least a basic understanding of this new and important disease of childhood.

References

1 Mok, J.Y.Q., Hague, R.A., Yap, P.L., *et al.* Vertical transmission of HIV: a prospective study. *Arch Dis Child* 1989; **64**: 1140–1145.
2 The European Collaborative Study. Children born to women with HIV-1 infection: natural history and risk of transmission. *Lancet* 1991; **i**: 253–260.
3 Pyun, K.H., Ochs, H.D., Wedgwood, R.J., Marshall, G.S., Barbour, S.D., Plotkin, S.A Seronegativity and paediatric AIDS. *Lancet* 1987; **i**: 1152–1153.
4 Borkowsky, W., Krasinski, K., Paul, D., *et al.* Human immunodeficiency virus type 1 antigenemia in children. *J Pediatr* 1989; **114**: 940–945.
5 Epstein, L.G., Boucher, C.A.B., Morrison, S.H., *et al.* Persistent human immunodeficiency virus type 1 antigenemia in children correlates with diseases progression. *Pediatrics* 1988; **82**: 919–924.
6 Amadori, A., DeRossi, A., Giaquinto, C., Faulkner-Valle, G., Zachello, F., Chieco-Bianchi, L. In vitro production of HIV-specific antibody in children at risk of AIDS. *Lancet* 1988; **i**: 852–854.
7 Pyun, K.H., Ochs, H.D., Dufford, M.T.W., Wedgwood, R.J. Perinatal infection with human immunodeficiency virus: specific antibody responses by the neonate. *New Engl J Med* 1987; **317**: 611–614.
8 Slade, H.B., Pica, R.V., Pahwa, S.G. Detection of HIV-specific antibodies in infancy by isoelectric focusing and affinity immunoblotting. *J Infect Dis* 1989; **160**: 126–130.
9 Johnson, J.P., Nair, P., Alexander, S. Early diagnosis of HIV infection in the neonate (letter). *New Engl J Med* 1987; **316**: 273–274.
10 DeRossi, A., Amadori, A., Chieco-Bianchi, L., *et al.* Polymerase chain reaction and in-vitro antibody production for early diagnosis of paediatric HIV infection. *Lancet* 1988; **ii**: 278.
11 Laure, F., Rouzioux, C., Veber, F., *et al.* Detection of HIV-1 DNA in infants and children by means of the polymerase chain reaction. *Lancet* 1988; **ii**: 538–541.
12 Rogers, M.F., Ou, C.Y., Rayfield, M., *et al.* Use of the polymerase chain reaction for early detection of the proviral sequences of human immunodeficiency virus in infants born to seropositive mothers. *New Engl J Med* 1989; **320**: 1649–1654.
13 Classification system for human immunodeficiency virus (HIV) infection in children under 13 years of age. *Morbidity and Mortality Weekly Report* (Centers for Disease Control) 1987; **36/15**: 225–236.
14 Scott, G.B., Hutto, C., Makuch, R.W., *et al.* Survival in children with perinatally acquired human immunodeficiency virus type 1 infection. *New Engl J Med* 1989; **321**: 1791–1796.
15 Centres for Disease Control. Guidelines for prophylaxis against *Pneumocystis carinii* pneumonia for children infected with HIV. *Morbidity and Mortality Weekly Report* 1991; **40**: 1–13.
16 Hague, R.A., Yap, P.L., Mok, J.Y.Q., *et al.* Intravenous immunoglobulin in HIV infection: evidence for the efficacy of treatment. *Arch Dis Child* 1989; **64**: 1146–1150.
17 The National Institute of Child Health and Human Development Intravenous Immunoglobulin Study Group. *New Engl J Med* 1991; **325**: 73–80.
18 Belman, A.L., Diamond, G., Dickson, D., *et al.* Pediatric acquired immunodeficiency syndrome: neurologic syndromes. *Am J Dis Child* 1988; **142**: 29–35.
19 Mintz, M., Epstein, L.G., Koenigsberger, M.R. Neurological manifestations of acquired immunodeficiency syndrome in children. *Int Pediatr* 1989; **4**: 161–171.
20 Epstein, L.G., Sharer, L.R., Goudsmit, J. Neurological and neuropathological features of HIV infection in children. *Ann Neurol* 1988; **23(suppl)**: 19–23.
21 The European Collaborative Study. Neurologic signs in young children with human immunodeficiency virus infection. *Pediatr Infect Dis J* 1990; **9**: 402–406.
22 Department of Health, Welsh Office, Scottish Home and Health Department. *Immunisation Against Infectious Diseases*. London: HMSO, 1992.
23 Mok, J.Y.Q., Hague, R.A., Taylor, R.F., *et al.* The management of children born to human immunodeficiency virus seropositive women. *J Infect* 1988; **18**: 119–124.
24 Tarantola, D., Mann, J.M. *Acquired Immunodeficiency Syndrome and Expanded Programmes on Immunization: Special Programme on AIDS*. Geneva: World Health Organization, 1987.
25 Mok, J., O'Hara, G. Placement of children from HIV-affected families: the Edinburgh experience. *Pediatr AIDS HIV infect – fetus to adolescent* 1990; **1**: 20–22.
26 Department of Education and Science and Welsh Office. *Children at School and Problems Related to AIDS*. London: HMSO, 1986.

16.6 Skin diseases

Helen Goodyear and John Harper

This section is a pot-pourri of common skin disorders that may be encountered by doctors and other health workers in community practice.

Some dermatological terms in this text are defined as follows:

Macule: a circumscribed flat area of discolouration.
Papule: a small raised area. A maculo-papular rash is thus both raised and discoloured.
Nodule: a palpable mass larger then 1 cm in diameter.

Plaque: a large well-demarcated raised irregular area of affected skin.

Vesicle: a small blister (less than 0.5 cm in diameter).

Congenital skin lesions

Salmon patch (stork bite)

This is the most common vascular lesion of infancy and appears as a flat pink lesion on the nape of the neck, the upper eyelids or the glabella. Most of these gradually fade and disappear in childhood, although those on the back of the neck may persist.

Strawberry naevus (capillary haemangioma) (Fig. 16.5)

This is a common abnormality which arises from immature angioblastic tissue and develops as a protruberant nodule during the first few weeks of life. It slowly increases in size, reaching a maximum in the first year, and then tends to remain static for a 6–12-month period before spontaneous involution. Multiple lesions are sometimes seen.

Management is usually conservative with the reassuring knowledge that over 90% of these lesions resolve by the age of 7 years. Indications for active treatment are those lesions which, by virtue of their size and site, compromise vital structures, such as the airway or the eyes. In this situation the treatment of choice would be either a slowly reducing course of oral prednisolone (2 mg/kg body weight/day initially) or intralesional steroids.

Larger haemangiomas may be complicated by traumatic bleeding although it is uncommon for significant blood loss to occur. Local pressure is usually sufficient to stop the bleeding. Ulceration sometimes occurs especially in the anogenital area or on the ears, nose or lips. Treatment includes potassium permanganate soaks and oral antibiotics if there is a suggestion of secondary infection. A rare complication of one or more large haemangiomas is thrombocytopenia due to platelet trapping (Kasabach-Merritt syndrome).

Port wine stain (naevus flammeus)

This is present at birth as a large, irregular, deep red or purple flat area of skin, which is often unilateral and on the face. It represents a vascular malformation involving mature capillaries. This birthmark persists; there is no tendency to fade or spread. As the child grows older and becomes more self-conscious, camouflage make-up is useful. Recently, the use of a tunable pulsed dye laser for the treatment of port wine stains has shown excellent results. Rare associations include meningeal involvement (Sturge-Weber syndrome) and gross hypertrophy of a limb (Klippel-Trenaunay-Weber syndrome).

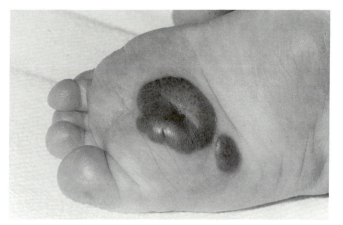

Figure 16.5 Strawberry naevus.

Pigmented naevi

These naevi may be evident at birth, but most appear during childhood and adolescence. In childhood they are usually flat or only slightly elevated. Histologically they show junctional activity, but malignancy is extremely rare, and with maturation the majority become intradermal and are benign. In contrast, a giant pigmented naevus (an extensive pigmented hairy lesion usually of the bathing trunk area) does have a significant recognized predisposition to malignant melanoma. Treatment for these lesions is dermabrasion which involves planing down of the skin by a high-speed wire brush or diamond fraise. The earlier dermabrasion is performed the better; good cosmetic results can be obtained in the first few weeks of life.

Café-au-lait patches are hyperpigmented oval macules which are found in 10–20% of normal individuals. The presence of six or more lesions greater than 1.5 cm in diameter is suggestive of neurofibromatosis. Café-au-lait patches are also seen in McCune-Albright syndrome and tuberous sclerosis.

Mongolian spots are bluish-black macules, due to melanocytes located deep in the dermis, often seen in the lumbrosacral area and buttocks. They are seen in black babies of African or Asian descent and can be mistaken for bruising leading to an unjust suspicion of non-accidental injury. They fade gradually as the child grows older.

Depigmented lesions

Multiple oval hypopigmented ash leaf macules are present at birth or in early infancy in tuberous sclerosis. They are best diagnosed with the aid of a Wood's lamp.

Incontinentia pigmenti achromians of Ito (hypomelanosis of Ito) is characterized by depigmented areas with a whorled appearance. These white streaks are usually present at birth, vary in extent and may be unilateral or bilateral.

There is a marked dilution of pigmentation of the skin, hair and eyes in all variants of *oculocutaneous albinism*.

Piebaldism (white spotting) presents with a white forelock of hair and patches of skin without pigment at birth which remain unchanged throughout life. This is not to be confused with vitiligo in which irregular ivory-white depigmented patches, often symmetrical, develop and may slowly extend before the lesions become static.

Voigt's or Futcher's lines are sharply demarcated bilateral lines of pigmentation corresponding to a dermatome, usually found on the upper arms. The presence of these lines is proportional to the degree of pigmentation of an individual.

Other common causes of patchy hypomelanosis are: post-inflammatory lesions, pityriasis alba (a mild type of eczema predominantly on the face and upper trunk), and pityriasis versicolor which is due to a yeast-like organism. The patchy hypopigmentation of pityriasis versicolor is more noticeable after suntanning.

Transient rashes of the newborn

Milia (milk spots)

These are tiny white or yellow papules, particularly prominent on the face and occasionally on the upper trunk and limbs. They are due to blockage of the sebaceous glands by keratin and sebaceous material. Milia can be very conspicuous in the first few days of life but tend to disappear spontaneously by 3–4 weeks, although they may persist into the second or third month.

Miliaria

Miliaria are caused by blockage of sweat ducts and are precipitated by the tendency to overheat babies. *Miliaria crystallina* are tiny clear vesicles, without erythema, occurring on the head, neck and trunk of the newborn. *Miliaria rubra* (prickly heat) are tiny papulovesicles surrounded by erythema occurring particularly in flexural areas, such as the neck, groins and axillae, following excessive sweating. The lesions clear in a cool environment. Both forms of miliaria may become secondarily infected with *Staphylococcus aureus*.

Erythema toxicum neonatorum

This presents in the first week of life as a generalized blotchy macular erythema with tiny yellow or white papules which sometimes progress to pustules. It is present for one to two days and then clears spontaneously. Histopathology reveals an accumulation of eosinophils.

Cutis marmarata

This is a reticulate bluish mottling of the skin on the trunk and extremities, seen as a physiological response to the cold. It is usually of no pathological significance and tends to disappear gradually, although in a few it may persist into childhood.

Nappy rash

Nappy rash is usually due to the occlusive contact of urine and faeces with the skin and may be seen at any time until the child is continent. It is usually bound by the margins of the nappy with sparing of the inguinal folds. Simple measures are usually effective: to leave the nappy off when possible; frequent nappy changes; avoidance of plastic pants; and the use of a protective cream such as zinc and castor oil or metanium (titanium in a silicone base) after each nappy change. Secondary infection by *Candida* is common and causes the skin to be bright red and scaly, with surrounding discrete satellite lesions and involvement of the skin folds. Treatment comprises an anti-candidal/hydrocortisone application – for example nystatin and hydrocortisone (Nystaform HC) or miconazole and hydrocortisone (Daktacort). An attempt should also be made to clear the gut reservoir with the use of oral nystatin (Nystan) suspension or miconazole (Daktarin) gel.

Differential diagnosis of nappy area eruptions include infantile seborrhoeic eczema, atopic eczema, scabies, acrodermatitis enteropathica or acquired zinc deficiency, Wiskott-Aldrich syndrome, Letterer-Siwe disease, psoriasis and Kawasaki's disease.

Infantile seborrhoeic eczema

This is an acute, self-limiting, erythematous scaly eruption of unknown cause affecting infants under the age of 3 months. It starts as thick yellow scales on the scalp (cradle-cap) and may spread behind the ears, and to the folds of the neck, the axillae and the nappy area. The rash may be extensive in an otherwise healthy child. Often no treatment is required apart from reassurance and a bland emollient such as aqueous cream. For the more severely affected it may be necessary to use 1% hydrocortisone alone or in combination with miconazole (Daktacort) or clotrimazole (Canesten-HC). The thick scaling of cradle-cap can be removed using coconut or soya oil massaged into the scalp before washing with a mild baby shampoo.

Although infantile seborrhoeic eczema has been regarded as a disease distinct from atopic eczema, there is undoubtedly an overlap between these two conditions.

Atopic eczema

Atopic eczema in the UK affects around 10% of children under the age of 5 years. The onset is usually between 3 and 18 months. About 70% have a positive family history of atopy (eczema, asthma, hay fever). There is a general tendency towards spontaneous improvement throughout childhood and over 90% will clear by the age of 15 years. The predominant symptom is itching which often makes the child fretful. The disease typically waxes and wanes and an acute exacerbation is frequently related to skin infection. Clinical features vary from an acute weeping erythematous papulovesicular eruption to a chronic dry scaly thickened skin. Atopic eczema often starts on the face and can affect any area with a predilection for the flexures, especially the antecubital and popliteal fossae (Fig. 16.6). Although skin prick tests for specific allergens are often positive, they provide little guide to clinical management as multiple factors are usually involved.

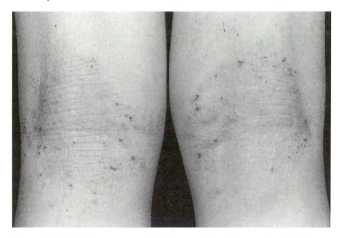

Figure 16.6 Atopic eczema affecting popliteal fossae: typical site.

Treatment

1 *Emollients*: a bath oil (such as Oilatum, Balneum or Alpha Keri) with once or twice daily baths as necessary; a soap substitute (such as aqueous cream); and a moisturizer applied frequently to all areas of the body.

2 *Topical steroids*: application of a mild potency topical steroid (such as 1% hydrocortisone) is usually sufficient, although occasionally a moderately potent topical steroid may be necessary.

3 *Antibiotics*: an acute exacerbation of eczema is often associated with secondary bacterial infection (usually *Staphylococcus aureus* or beta-haemolytic streptococcus or both) and broad spectrum antibiotics (flucloxacillin and penicillin V, or erythromycin) are needed. Skin swabs for bacterial culture and sensitivities should be taken prior to therapy as resistant strains of staphylococci on the skin surface are common in this group of children.

4 *Antihistamines*: an antihistamine elixir, such as trimeprazine (Vallergan) or promethazine (Phenergan), is helpful at night.

5 *Diet*: routine exclusion diets are usually unhelpful. They should be reserved for the very young with severe eczema who have not responded to conventional therapy and for those who have a clear history of specific food intolerance. The diets employed tend to avoid dairy products and use a cow's milk substitute based on soya protein (such as Formula S and Wysoy), casein hydrolysate (such as Nutramigen and Pregestimil) or whey protein (such as Pepti-Junior). They should be supervised by a dietitian to ensure the child is not at risk of nutritional deficiency.

6 *General measures*: the most important part of management is supportive care emphasizing the good prognosis. Excessive heat should be avoided and the child should be dressed in cool, loose cotton clothing. Other factors which are known to aggravate eczema include synthetic fabrics, clothes washed in biological detergents, irritant foods (for example, citrus fruits or tomatoes) causing perioral eczema, cigarette smoke, dander from pets and the house dust mite.

7 It is important that the school leaver with atopic eczema is given career guidance to avoid contact with chemical irritants which would aggravate and possibly potentiate the eczema, as for example in hairdressing, catering, nursing and engineering.

Infections

Viral infections

Many systemic viral infections cause a rash, including measles, rubella, chicken pox, and enteroviruses. It is important to distinguish exanthem due to viruses from those due to bacteria and *Mycoplasma pneumoniae*. *Exanthem subitum* (roseola infantum) is characterized by fever for 3–5 days and discrete rose-pink maculopapules on the neck and trunk spreading to the arms, face and legs. It typically affects children under 3 years. Human herpes virus type 6 has been reported as the causal agent of exanthem subitum. *Erythema infectiosum* (fifth disease), due to human parvovirus causes an erythematous rash which often begins on the face giving the so-called slapped cheek appearance. The rash on the trunk and extremities has central fading giving a reticulate appearance.

Warts

Warts are very common in school children and are caused by the human papilloma virus (HPV). There are a number of strains of HPV giving rise to different clinical types of wart – the common type, plantar, plane, filiform and genital warts. Most warts disappear spontaneously, although this can take from a few weeks to a number of years. Children who are immunosuppressed and those with atopic eczema are especially susceptible to warts and mollusca contagiosa.

Treatment

1 Common warts: the daily application of a keratolytic wart paint such as 16.7% salicylic acid with 16.7% lactic acid (Salactol) or 10% glutaraldehyde (Glutarol). It is important to rub the surface of the wart with a manicure emery board or pumice stone until the wart becomes flat prior to application of a drop of wart paint to the centre of the wart. This may take up to 12 weeks, or in some cases even longer. Cryotherapy using liquid nitrogen is used to treat persistent warts.

2 Plantar warts (verrucae): similar to the treatment of common warts (as above) using wart paints and regular paring. For more extensive plantar warts (mosaic warts), formalin soaks (4% formaldehyde in normal saline) are useful. Cryotherapy may be used to treat plantar warts but repeated treatment is often required and it can cause severe pain for a few days afterwards.

3 Genital warts: in young children, genital and perianal warts are usually acquired non-sexually. However, the possibility of sexual abuse should always be considered. They respond to treatment with podophyllin (15%, 20% or 25% in benzoin compound tincture) applied once weekly, under medical supervision, for up to 6 weeks. Cryotherapy is also an effective treatment for these warts. Large persistent perianal warts, particularly if they involve the anal canal, usually require surgical removal under a general anaesthetic.

Mollusca contagiosa (water warts) (Fig. 16.7)

These are smooth translucent papules with a characteristic central punctum, caused by a pox virus. They are common in children, tend to occur in crops and seed by autoinoculation with lesions typically occurring on adjacent skin surfaces. As a large proportion of them resolve spontaneously, over a period of a few weeks to several months, no treatment is required initially, especially in young children. Cryotherapy with liquid nitrogen is an effective form of treatment.

Herpes simplex infection

There are two types of herpes simplex virus (HSV). The majority of infections in children are due to HSV type 1. Genital disease and perinatally acquired infection are often caused by HSV type 2. Primary herpes simplex infection usually develops before the age of 5 years. It is often mild and goes unnoticed. Recurrent herpes is usually seen in older children and may affect

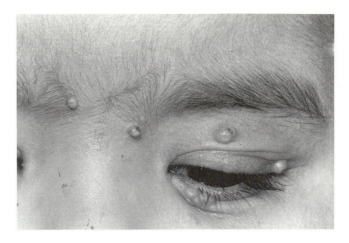

Figure 16.7 Mollusca contagiosa.

any site, most commonly the skin and mucous membranes around the mouth. Gingivostomatitis tends to present as a sore mouth with pyrexia, decreased appetite and drinking. The number of lesions is extremely variable. Primary gingivostomatitis is a self-limiting disease and treatment with analgesics and fluids is usually sufficient. Occasionally, in severe cases, intravenous fluids may be required. Acyclovir (suspension or tablets) may shorten the course of the illness but only if given soon after the appearance of lesions. Herpetic whitlow is an infection of the skin of the nail fold, usually as a result of finger sucking. Herpetic eye infection may occur at any age. Vesicles are seen on the eyelids and occasionally dendritic ulceration of the cornea may occur. Neonatal herpes simplex is acquired from the mother's genital tract during delivery and may cause a severe generalized infection with high mortality. Genital herpes is usually sexually transmitted, but in young children with either oral or finger infection the virus may be transmitted by touch. Children with atopic eczema may develop a severe widespread infection with HSV known as eczema herpeticum. This should be treated with intravenous acyclovir in the same dose as for an immunocompromised child (500 mg/m^2 8-hourly).

Herpes zoster (shingles)

This painful blistering rash, caused by the varicella virus, is typically unilateral and limited to the area of a dermatome. Following chicken pox infection, the virus remains dormant in the dorsal root ganglion until reactivated when it causes an attack of herpes zoster. There may be a prodromal period of pain 24–48 hours before the appearance of vesicles. Lesions usually heal within 10–21 days and post-herpetic neuralgia is rarely seen in children. Treatment is usually symptomatic with rest and analgesia.

Hand, foot and mouth disease

This infection affects young children and is caused by a coxsackie virus, most commonly A16. It tends to occur in minor epidemics and produce tiny vesicles on the buccal mucosa, palms and soles. Lesions fade after 2–3 days and resolution of the illness occurs within 7 days. Infants may have a more extensive exanthem with lesions on the buttocks.

Impetigo

This is a contagious superficial skin infection with a yellow exudate that dries and forms a honey-coloured crust. It may present as fragile blisters, particularly in neonates and infants. The condition is caused by *Staphylococcus aureus*, beta haemolytic streptococcus or a mixed infection. Impetigo may occur as a secondary infection of a pre-existing skin condition such as atopic eczema or an infestation such as scabies or head lice.

Treatment

1   *Soaks*, either normal saline or potassium permanganate, to remove the crust, two or three times daily.

2   *Topical antibiotics* such as chlortetracycline (Aureomycin), fusidic acid (Fucidin) or mupiricin (Bactoban) are useful for the treatment of early minor infections, applied three or four times daily.

3   *Systemic antibiotics*: most cases of impetigo require a course of oral antibiotics, such as flucloxacillin, penicillin V or erythromycin. This is especially important for the treatment of streptococcal infections to prevent the serious complication of glomerulonephritis.

4   *Hygiene*: the child should have a separate towel and should be kept away from school until the lesions have healed.

5   In patients with recurrent staphylococcal infections, a search should be made for nasal carriers. Nasal swabs should be taken not only from the patient, but also from the whole family and close friends. Treatment with a nasal cream containing chlorhexidene and neomycin (Naseptin) or mupirocin (Bactroban Nasal) is important to eradicate the focus of infection.

Staphylococcal scalded skin syndrome is a rare serious complication which occurs as certain phage types of staphylococci produce an exotoxin, causing widespread toxic epidermal necrolysis. The focus of infection is usually the upper respiratory tract, otitis externa or conjunctivitis and it develops within a few hours to a few days. It is important to recognize this potentially life-threatening condition because it responds well to intravenous anti-staphylococcal antibiotics.

Superficial fungal infections (ringworm infection)

Infection of the scalp (tinea capitis) is seen as one or more patches of hair loss with broken hairs of different lengths (Fig. 16.8). Some species (in particular *Microsporum*) fluoresce green under Wood's (long-wave ultraviolet light) lamp. Treatment is with griseofulvin (10 mg/kg/day) for 4–6 weeks. Infection of the trunk (tinea corporis) characteristically appears as annular lesions with central clearing and an itchy, palpable, erythematous edge. It is usually caught from pets. Tinea pedis (athlete's foot) usually presents as macerated painful skin between the fourth and fifth toes and may spread as an acute vesiculopustular eruption, to the sole and dorsum of the foot. Samples of skin scrapings or plucked hairs should be sent to the laboratory for culture. Localized infections can be treated with topical therapy alone using imidazole agents (for example clotrimazole (Canesten), miconazole (Daktarin)), whereas more extensive involvement requires the addition of griseofulvin.

Infestations

Scabies

This is a highly contagious disorder caused by the mite, *Sarcoptes scabiei*. The infection is transmitted by close physical contact, although the incubation period can be as long as 2 months. The typical eruption consists of intensely pruritic papules, vesicles and burrows. The distribution tends to favour the finger webs, wrists and genitalia. In infants, lesions are commonly found on the palms and soles and around the axillae (Fig. 16.9).

Treatment

1   All members of the household and close contacts should be treated at the same time, whether they are apparently infected or not.

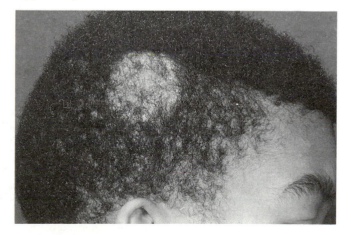

Figure 16.8 Tinea capitis.

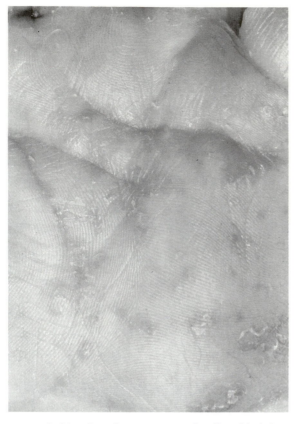

Figure 16.9 Scabies: the palms are commonly affected in infancy.

2   Gamma benzene hexachloride (Quellada) or mono-sulfiram lotion applied to the whole body from the chin downwards, including the fingers and toes, the soles of the feet and the genitalia by the following protocol: first day bath and apply lotion; and after 24 hours repeat the application without a bath; third day bath and wash all bed linen, underwear and night-clothes that have been used.

3   After treatment, itching may take several weeks to settle; for this use calamine lotion. Occasionally nodular lesions persist after successful therapy.

Lice (pediculosis capitis)

Head lice are common in school children. The nit is a head-louse egg which is firmly attached to scalp hair; nits are readily recognizable as small white adherent grain-like particles. Transmission is by direct head contact. Head lice cause severe scalp irritation and secondary bacterial infection. Treatment is with malathion (Prioderm, Derbac) or cabaryl (Carylderm, Derbac) to be applied to the entire scalp and left on for 12 hours. The hair should then be washed and the dead nits removed with a fine-tooth metal comb.

Other common skin disorders

Psoriasis

This is a chronic, relapsing, inflammatory skin disorder, characterized by plaques covered with silvery scales. It is primarily a disease of young adults but can develop for the first time at any age. A common presentation is as guttate psoriasis: a shower of small, discrete, red, scaly lesions, predominantly on the trunk, often seen following a streptococcal sore throat. This requires appropriate treatment with penicillin or erythromycin.

Treatment of chronic plaque psoriasis should be kept to a minimum with the application of 2% sulphur and salicylic acid ointment or coal tar and salicylic acid ointment. For more difficult and extensive psoriasis, dithranol is the treatment of choice. A course of ultraviolet light therapy is often helpful. Topical steroids should not be used in the treatment of stable plaque psoriasis, except in special circumstances.

Pityriasis rosea

This disorder is characterized by the appearance of a single lesion called the herald patch, followed 1–7 days later by an eruption of numerous smaller discrete lesions on the trunk, upper arms and thighs. Typically the distribution is along the lines of the ribs, giving a christmas tree appearance. It is thought to be due to an infectious agent, although this has not yet been proven. The rash clears spontaneously in 6–8 weeks and no treatment is usually required beyond reassurance.

Granuloma annulare

These lesions consist of asymptomatic skin-coloured ring-shaped papules typically on the dorsal aspect of the hands and feet. The cause is unknown. Multiple lesions are considered to be associated with diabetes mellitus, although this is not well established. Resolution may be slow, taking years rather than months.

Alopecia areata

These are areas of well-circumscribed hair loss on the scalp which have characteristic exclamation mark hairs. The cause is unknown, although there is an increased incidence of vitiligo and other autoimmune diseases in affected individuals and their families. It should be distinguished from habitual hair-pulling (trichotillomania) and ringworm of the scalp. There is no specific treatment for this condition. Alopecia areata is usually self-limiting. Occasionally the whole scalp is bald with loss of eyebrows and eyelashes (alopecia totalis) and rarely there is complete loss of all body hair (alopecia universalis).

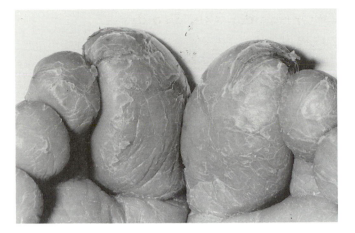

Figure 16.10 Juvenile plantar dermatosis.

Acne

This is principally a problem of adolescence, although acneiform lesions can be seen in neonates or infants. Treatment is directed at removing the keratin plugs using a chemical peeling agent, such as benzoyl peroxide, available as a gel, cream or lotion in 2.4%, 5% and 10% concentrations. This is applied once daily after washing, preferably at night. For moderate or severe acne, long-term low-dose antibiotic therapy is required, usually with minocyclin, oxytetracycline or erythromycin.

Juvenile plantar dermatosis (Fig. 16.10)

This is a very common disorder of school children, related to the wearing of occlusive synthetic shoes or trainers. It is usually localized to the feet which have a glazed appearance and are dry, slightly scaly, or often with painful fissures. There is a high incidence of atopy in these children or their relatives. Sweating and friction are thought to be important factors. Treatment includes emollients and advice on footwear. Topical steroids are unhelpful; useful advice includes wearing two pairs of thin cotton socks to reduce fric-

tion and the liberal application of dusting powder (talc) to keep the feet dry.

Skin care

Dry skin

This responds well to treatment with emollients; a bath oil, soap substitute and moisturizer applied as needed to areas of dry skin.

Sunbathing

Sunbathing (erythema, heat, pain and swelling) and skin damage can be avoided by covering up and applying an ultraviolet-A and ultraviolet-B (UVA/UVB) sunscreen with a high sun protection factor. Chronic UVB and to a lesser extent UVA exposure can lead to the development of skin cancers later in life.

Black skin

Post-inflammatory hypopigmentation is more noticeable with dark skin. Erythema is less obvious which may alter the appearance of some inflammatory rashes.

Bath water additives

The use of bubble bath, scented soaps and detergents to clean the bath can lead to an irritant reaction of the skin and aggravation of pre-existing skin conditions. They may also cause vulvovaginitis in girls.

Bibliography

Harper, J.I. *Handbook of Paediatric Dermatology*, 2nd edn. London: Butterworths, 1990.
Rook, A., Wilkinson, D.S., Ebling, F.J.G., Champion, R.H., Burton, J.L., eds. *Textbook of Dermatology*, 5th edn. Oxford: Blackwell Scientific, 1992.

Chapter 17

Behavioural problems and psychiatric disorders

M. Elena Garralda

Introduction

Transient periods of behavioural and emotional change are common in children: they can be regarded as part of the growing-up process. For a considerable minority of children however they are marked enough to constitute a problem, and if sufficiently severe and handicapping they constitute psychiatric disorders, causing distress and disruption and deserving assessment.

Young children often react to stress by changes in recently acquired biological habits – sleep, feeding, continence – or by an increase in oppositional attitudes characteristic of the toddler stage. Both intrinsic factors in the child, for instance health and developmental progress, and in the family, including the parents' psychiatric adjustment, influence these reactions. Rarely, children present with mental disorders characterized by profound changes affecting several areas of personality development as in infantile autism.

Other symptoms acquire increased relevance in older children. Particularly of concern because of their severe implications are those involving suicide acts or which are part of psychotic states. They characteristically become manifest in adolescence.

Sleep disorders

A regular and social pattern of prolonged uninterrupted night sleep is one of the first developmental tasks for the infant. Settling, or the progressive physiological and psychological maturation that results in the establishment of a pattern of wakefulness during the day and sleep at night from midnight till early morning is already present in most infants by 3–6 months of age and by about 8 months most are likely to have an uninterrupted period of sleep throughout the night. Before 6 months of age, whether the infant is breast or bottle fed may contribute to settling since breast-fed

babies tend to sleep through the night at a later age than bottle fed babies. Large night-time feeds can create or compound problems by leading to wet nappies, discomfort and wakings. Similarly cow's milk intolerance is associated with persistent tendency to wake in some infants.[1] Settling is helped by parents using a standard pre-sleep routine, but sleep is easily disrupted by the internal and environmental stresses that are part of growing up and sleep disturbances are common in childhood. Their main features change at different ages and range from mild responses to inevitable stress to severe disturbance which alters markedly the child and family life.

In infants under one year, night waking is one of the most common problems reported by parents about their offspring. About 20% of 1–2 year olds wake most or every night according to their parents and the poor sleeping pattern tends to be persistent through the early years. In one survey 41% of children waking at night repeatedly at 8 months of age still had a problem at 3 years. Probably many more infants wake during the night but this goes unrecognized.[2–4]

Problems in getting off to sleep and to a lesser extent sleeping with parents are common, associated problems and severe sleeping problems (that is waking at least five nights a week, and waking three or more times a night for more than 20 minutes or going to the parents' room) occur in 6–10% of 1–2 year olds.

Most problems in infants are isolated and circumscribed but in older pre-school children there is a link with behavioural problems and about a third of sleep problems are likely to occur in the context of generalized behavioural difficulties, with poor concentration, being difficult to manage and frequent temper tantrums.[3]

Developmental considerations

It has been pointed out that in the second year of life falling asleep entails loosing the child's ties to the very people and outside world which have only recently become increasingly appreciated and valued as part of the process of attachment and social development. Toddlers are deeply attached to their mothers, but when the mother is out of sight they cannot maintain a sufficiently stable internal image of her so that they cannot reassure themselves of her continued existence. As a result, they are reluctant to go to sleep or procrastinate at bedtime. Or they use transitional objects to which they get attached and which partially substitute symbolically the image of the mother as a way of managing the separation anxiety of going to sleep in a separate bedroom from the parents. During the second half of the second year, separation anxiety decreases as object permanence becomes more established and verbal skills develop and the sleep process becomes more smooth.[5]

Toddlers are also in the phase of development when they are establishing autonomy and control over their parents and when specific show of aggression against them is most marked. The psychoanalytic exploration of the nightmares of toddlers is said frequently to reveal anxiety over losses of control and aggressive feelings. The physical presence of the parents, their calm and affection, may reassure the child that aggressive wishes have not magically harmed them.

Older children find it difficult sometimes to fall asleep for fear that they might die and never awake, following explanations by adults that dying is like sleeping forever. This can be a special worry to children admitted to hospitals for operations.

Aetiological factors

Sleep changes in young children are frequently related to over-stimulation or frightening experiences that have occurred during the day. Injuries, operations or prolonged separations can be particularly stressing and this may become expressed in dreams of being chased or attacked by animals, monsters or witches.

The causes of persistent sleep problems in children are many and varied, from states of internal discomfort such as those due to illness, for example eczema, severe asthma or obstructive sleep apnoea, to inherent peculiarities and temperamental styles (adverse perinatal events, easily irritated babies, children who are less malleable, rhythmic and consistent in their behaviour than other children).

Environmental factors become increasingly important in the older children. Parental confidence and competence in parenting are important and sleep problems in 1–2 year olds are more common in only children – though this might only be the case for low socioeconomic families – in first and second borns, or if there is a history of a sibling with a sleeping problem. As with other behavioural problems, the parents' ability to provide a generally emotionally secure, stable, warm and responsive approach devoid

of strain and the absence of family and marital psychopathology are also important. Maternal depression is linked to sleep problems in the child and their persistence.

Cultural factors have a role to play. In some societies, children are not expected to go to bed by themselves nor to sleep alone, but an over-busy and over-scheduled western lifestyle may foster sleep problems by creating false parental expectations and anxieties about children's sleep.

Treatment

Transient sleep problems can be successfully managed by many parents without assistance or with routine health visiting advice. In infants, the problem can often be remedied by parents seeing to it that the bodily needs of the child are met in a gratifying and relatively consistent manner, and by an empathic appreciation of the parent's anxieties and stresses, often by friends or relatives. Moving the child from the parents' bedroom or avoiding over-stimulation at bedtime can be helpful. Leaving the toddler's bedroom door partially open at night is often reassuring.

For more severe difficulties, a number of measures have been tried all with varying degrees of success. Medication (trimeprazine tartrate, 30–60 mg at night) for 1–2 year olds can result in parents reporting improvements with children waking less often or for shorter periods, but generally it has few long-term beneficial effects.[2] It is best used for limited periods in order to decrease maternal distress and increase confidence and to allow more efficient methods to become instituted.

The use of behavioural techniques can be effective and is becoming increasingly popular.[6,7] The basic features of the treatment consist of:

- Extinction: gradually reducing the amount of attention given on waking by the parents.
- Reinforcement: using star charts as praise for desired behaviour such as staying in bed.
- Shaping: gradually making bedtime earlier.
- Cueing: establishing a bedtime routine.

Therapy is contingent upon parents being willing and having the necessary motivation to embark on a suitable programme. In some surveys only about half of those offered the treatment are able to carry it through, but of these children three-quarters improve significantly. Even if the children do not improve, parents often find the support provided by therapists useful.

Nightmares and night terrors

Nightmares occur universally throughout childhood. They consist of a dream which arouses sufficient anxiety and fear to awaken the child at least partially. They are frequent in the pre-school child and decrease in number after the age of 6 years, but they can occur in children of all ages. As with other sleep disorders of childhood, they are more common when the child has been over-excited during the day, when under stress or after frightening experiences. In a minority of children they are part of a more generalized behaviour disorder. The cognitive ability to distinguish dreams from reality matures at about 7 years of age and alongside this the difficulty of falling asleep because of fear or nightmares subsides.

Nightmares can be differentiated from night terrors, characterized by intense anxiety and piercing screams, because of the psychophysiological concomitants. In nightmares there is little autonomic disturbance. They occur during REM sleep, there is richness in dreams, awareness on waking up, and only partial retrograde amnesia for the episode. In contrast, in night terrors there is marked autonomic disturbance, unawareness by the child of his surroundings, and total retrograde amnesia. Night terrors are not accompanied by dreams, they occur in a psychological void, and EEGs show arousal from the slow wave phase four of sleep.[5] Occasionally complex partial seizures may be mistaken for bizarre types of dreaming, sleep walking or night terrors.[8]

The treatment of choice is avoiding over-stimulation, reassuring the child by giving him extra attention at night at times of stress, and seeking a psychiatric opinion if the sleep problem is part of a behaviour disorder. Drug therapy, for example diazepam as an hypnotic in doses of 1–5 mg for night terrors (diazepam suppresses stage four sleep which is involved in terrors) is seldom indicated. When sleep walking is part of the sleep disorder, sensible protective measures to ensure the child's safety need to be considered and implemented by the parents.

It has been suggested that parents should resist awakening the child *during* night terrors or sleep walking as this may increase the child's disturbance. Regular night terrors can be broken by waking the child before each episode is due and keeping him awake for a few minutes.[9]

Temper tantrums

Temper tantrums – outbursts of bad temper, irritation, anger or petulance – are a common unsophisticated way of expressing marked displeasure. They are characteristic of early childhood and peak during the second year of life as the child learns to exercise autonomy and control over others. Gradually they become substituted by sulking, whining or brooding and eventually by more mature ways as verbal skills and understanding of situations increase. It has been estimated that about 10% of 5 year olds have tantrums

at least once a week, boys more than girls. A further 10% have tantrums less than once a week and 18% less than once a month.[10,11]

Outbursts do not usually last longer than five minutes and extremes, as when children throw themselves to the floor or have breathholding attacks, are rare. In the pre-school child over half the outbursts arise from some conflict with parental authority, for example over issues of toilet training in the toddler, and later over refusal to put toys away or clashes over clothing. Disagreements with playmates increasingly become the precipitant for outbursts as a child grows older. In some cases, however, temper tantrums can be an expression of anxiety and insecurity. They are more frequent when children are physically unwell, hungry or tired, at the end of the morning or afternoon.

The methods of control vary with age, with decreasing use of physical force, coaxing, diversion of attention and ignoring, and more scolding, threatening and isolation. On the whole, more bribery, spanking, threatening and isolation are used for boys and more ignoring for girls. Tempers are more common when there is family psychosocial disadvantage (including low social class, absence of father figure, three or more other children in the household, residence in a poor urban area).

A number of children with temper tantrums are psychologically vulnerable from infancy. They display more crying, feeding or sleeping problems than other babies. In these children the tantrums are commonly part of behavioural and developmental problems such as feeding and sleeping difficulties and incontinence. They can also be linked to speech disorders, when an inability to communicate might lead to frustration and tantrums.

Association with general behavioural problems

Tempers are relatively common among children with clinically relevant and general behavioural problems: in an epidemiological study,[12] about 19% of disturbed 3 and 8 year olds but only 5% of non-disturbed children had the symptom. Disturbance in this context meant that a child had a disorder which caused significant social or psychological disability to himself or to others. The most common clinical picture in the younger children was of a child who was active, attention-seeking, disobedient and difficult to manage. It must be noted that temper tantrums were not one of the most common symptoms in these children and that they were not associated with persistence of the behavioural problem.

In older children, tantrums can be seen in association with antisocial symptoms such as destroying belongings, frequently fighting, taking things that belong to others, disobedience, telling lies and bullying and irritability. They can also be at times, however, an expression of anxiety and distress.

Treatment

The treatment of temper tantrums is dependent on the associated clinical picture. When they are part of a more widespread behavioural disturbance, attention needs to be given to the understanding of the associated features, temperament and development in the child, family and social issues, and to the relative part played by each of those, so that the intervention can be targeted most profitably. In severe problems, referral to child psychiatric clinics will be indicated.

In some cases it is possible to identify a main underlying cause amenable to intervention. Tantrums might primarily be:

1 An expression of frustration over communication difficulties in a child with speech delay. It will be helpful to try to improve the efficiency of the child's communications.
2 The result of difficulties in parent–child communication or of maternal depression, with poor responsiveness by mothers to the child's needs, and escalation of the child's demands for attention into tantrums. Treatment should address mother–child communication and the mother's mental state.
3 In anxious, dependent children, a reflection of difficulty in coping with situations demanding increased independence, for example, using his own bedroom at night or starting school. Anxiety management and assertiveness training may be the preferred treatment option.
4 An expression of deep insecurities in the child, perhaps due to deprivation and early stressful experiences. Consideration should be given to referral for psychotherapy.

Whatever the underlying causes and primary interventions, direct intervention for the tantrums themselves is likely to be needed at some point in treatment. Behavioural techniques are generally useful.[13] The general principle is that the child's natural tendency to express displeasure in this way should be curtailed and that the ability of tantrums to achieve his aims (for example increased attention from others, getting his own way) should be reduced, while the child should be helped to find alternative ways in which to exercise his autonomy. A variety of techniques may be used, from restraining the child to the use of time out. A young child may be restrained by being held until the tantrum subsides. This is best done by holding the child from behind as it has the overall effect of reducing eye-contact, achieving a certain distance, and halting the overall escalation of mutual anger and destruction.

Time out means ensuring that the child has as little social reinforcement and social contact as possible. It does not necessarily mean exclusion from the room though this is often needed. The child should know exactly what the parent's expectations are and a clear command should be followed by a time-out threat and its implementation. The procedure should be used consistently, for a length of about five minutes and be progressively faded out.

It is important to link the here-and-now procedures with longer-term ones including the withdrawal of privileges and the reinforcement of good behaviour. The use of a star chart is helpful for the latter. Stars are given for tantrum-free days or for tantrum reduction. They are a graphic way of sharing pleasure in the child's achievement and drawing attention to it. Treats may be gained for several tantrum-free days. The child is generally rewarded for learning to control his anger and frustration and for using alternative and more appropriate ways. In older children, counselling the child to use simple self-control manoeuvres (such as counting up to ten before responding to frustration), to remove himself from the fraught situation, or to gain relief from strain by physical activity are also useful.

Feeding and eating disorders including anorexia nervosa

If the development of a social sleep pattern is an early important task for the infant, feeding is of course basic for survival and an activity which if disturbed may give rise to particular stress in parents and strain in the mother–child relationship.

The newborn baby comes into the world with a considerable skill at finding and sucking from the nipple or the bottle: if his face close to the mouth is stroked he will turn towards the stimulus with open mouth and this rooting reflex is following by a placing reflex. He fastens onto the stimulus and begins to suck. Sucking responses adapt very quickly to differences in the way the milk is provided, whether breast or bottle, whether the baby is fed on demand or not.[14]

The child may take up to 12 feeds a day during the first fortnight. Over the next few weeks he settles to a regular routine of 4-hourly feeds, and eventually moves on to three meals a day. By 3–4 months, if solid food is placed on the back of his tongue, he can successfully pass it backwards and swallow it.

Feeding problems in young children

More anxiety is expressed over the infant's feeding problems by mothers, in routine contact with health visitors, than any other topic. The percentage of mothers reporting feeding problems retrospectively for the child in infancy is 13%. There is an association with sleeping problems, and 39% of children with feeding difficulties also had sleeping difficulties as babies.[4]

The frequency of feeding problems in pre-school children varies in different surveys and this is probably due to sampling and methodological differences. Golding[4] in a British national survey of 5 year olds found that 36% of children were reported as having eating or appetite problems, usually faddiness or not eating enough, though the problems were severe in only 1%. Overeating was also uncommon and present in 1%. In a longitudinal study of London children aged 3–8 years, there was poor appetite in 19% of 3 year olds and 13% of 8 year olds, with similar rates for faddiness, though there was a tendency for faddiness to peak at 4 years and subsequently to decline.[12]

There are continuities in these problems throughout childhood and babies with eating problems are twice as likely as other babies to have feeding difficulties at 5 years of age. The magnitude of this association is however less than for sleeping problems. The continuities are stronger with older children and of 3 year olds with feeding difficulties about two-thirds will continue to have difficulty one year later. Feeding problems are often an isolated problem but they are also found in association with other behavioural symptoms.

Aetiological factors

Individual differences are relevant. Babies differ from the start in terms of regularity of bodily function but also in feeding and sleeping. Variations between babies in sucking – more or less vigorously or placidly – are marked from birth.[14]

Feeding difficulties in infants are linked to both biological and environmental factors. There is an association with low birthweight in infants but not in older children. As for the influence of early experiences in mother–child contact, these probably have only a short-lived effect on feeding. The nature of the continuing mother–child relationship has long been regarded as crucial, but it is often difficult to know to what extent any difficulties in this area are primary or secondary to the strain caused to mothers by a poorly eating baby or child.

There are family associations. For example, children with feeding difficulties tend to come from families with fewer children in the household, either being an only child or having one other sib. This in turn is linked to younger maternal age and is probably related to experience and confidence in parenting. Feeding problems in infants have been found not to be related to social class, maternal smoking, parental situations or type of neighbourhood.[4]

In a number of children, feeding disorders are an expression of childhood behavioural disturbance. They may then be linked to developmental problems in the child, mainly speech delay, and to family factors. This will not uncommonly include maternal depression, a strained parental marital relationship, negative parental attitudes towards the child, and external stress (such as severe financial problems, or housing stress with poor physical environment).[12]

Psychological aspects of non-organic failure to thrive

Non-organic failure to thrive (also see Section 9.5) is often associated with feeding problems, but in contrast with the frequency of the latter it is a rare problem. About 1–5% of paediatric admissions are for failure to thrive, and less than one-quarter of those brought to hospital for investigations have an important organic disease. In over a half, the problem is regarded as non-organic in origin.[15] In older children, failure to thrive is often associated with behavioural and developmental problems.

Aetiological factors

As regards temperamental features, children with non-organic failure to thrive fall into two broad groups: those who are irritable and non-cuddly babies and those who, often at a slightly older age, seem apathetic, withdrawn and apprehensive and lack vocalization.[15]

The assumption that non-organic growth retardation stems primarily from inadequate caretaking and uninvolved mothers has been criticized as an oversimplification. Much about the mother's attitude is probably related to temperamental difficulties in the child. Mothers with demanding, growth-retarded babies are observed to be often tense and anxious, handling them aggressively, whereas slow apathetic infants tend to be ignored. The concept of a maternal deprivation syndrome or psychosocial dwarfism is highly problematic. In a number of cases the problem can be better understood as difficulties in the mother–child relationship derived from a temperamental mismatch and developmental delays in the child.

However in some instances environmental neglect and gross family and social dysfunction including marital friction, poor housing, overcrowding and poverty, can be identified as having a primary influence. In these children other features of the emotionally rejected, socially deprived toddler, such as indiscriminate friendliness, might be apparent. Crucially, there are links between non-organic failure to thrive and physical abuse, and there is a substantial risk for continued growth retardation.

Treatment

Whether due to temperamental or environmental problems, inadequacy of nutrition and feeding difficulties are central to the development of the disorder, and in treatment primary importance should be given to the child's nutritional intake and growth. It is important to consider also the parent–child interaction, the quality of general care provided and, as for feeding disorders generally, emphasis should be put on reducing the strain and stress focused on feeding.

Anorexia nervosa

The International Classification of Diseases, 9th edition (ICD-9)[16] defines anorexia nervosa as a disorder in which the main features are persistent active refusal to eat and marked loss of weight. The level of activity and alertness are characteristically high in relation to the degree of emaciation. Typically the disorder begins in teenage girls but it may sometimes begin before puberty and rarely it occurs in males. In some general population surveys the accumulated frequency up to 15 years of age is 0.8%, with a peak age of onset at 14 years.[17]

Amenorrhoea is usual and there may be a variety of other physiological changes including slow pulse and respiration, low body temperature and dependent oedema. Unusual eating habits and attitudes towards food are typical and sometimes starvation and self-induced vomiting or laxative use follows or alternates with periods of overeating. There are often associated psychiatric symptoms, notably depression.

It is important to state that the cardinal feature of anorexia nervosa is not lack of appetite but rather an implacably disturbed attitude towards weight, shape and fatness, so-called weight phobia, fear of fatness and relentless pursuit of thinness with weight loss of at least 25% of body weight.[18,19]

The patients are often described as well-behaved, compliant and good before the onset of the illness. They may express the wish never to grow up. They are hard working and perfectionist, but sensitive and unsure of themselves. A number have been premorbidly obese. Obvious precipitating events occur in perhaps over half the cases. They include being teased for size or shape, puberty, separation from family or loss of family member, parental conflicts, entering a new school and sexual conflicts.

Starvation, and bulimia and vomiting, can combine to produce profound metabolic and endocrine disturbances due to changes in hypothalamic function and peripheral hormone metabolism. The consensus of opinion is that such changes are reversible with weight gain.

Aetiological theories

In common with many other psychiatric disorders, anorexia nervosa is an illness of unknown aetiology and many theories have been put forward to explain its development:

- Socio-cultural: several studies have shown a high proportion of schoolgirls to be weight-conscious and embarking on some form of dieting. The socio-cultural emphasis on slimness may play an aetiological role since the incidence of anorexia is higher among cultural groups where this is prevalent, for example in ballet schools and private schools.
- Psychodynamic: the condition represents a struggle for control, for a sense of identity, competence and effectiveness.
- Developmental psychobiological: it represents a psychobiological regression to childhood in face of mounting conflict during the adolescent phase of development.
- The family pathology theory: family characteristics of enmeshment, over-protectiveness, rigidity and lack of conflict resolution are predisposing factors. The anorexia has an important function in maintaining the family homeostasis.
- Hypothalamic dysfunction: the basic dysfunction is a morbid fear of fatness and hypothalamic dysfunction.

Treatment

Compliance is often a problem in treatment. If the anorexia is mild, outpatient intervention can be tried with the establishment of weight goals. Family therapy is indicated in prepubertal or young anorectics and can result in marked improvements in the parents' confidence and control and a decrease in the child's anxiety. In older adolescents individual counselling is more effective.

If the problem is severe, inpatient admission is required, with close nursing supervision over food intake, the setting of target weights and the use of behavioural reinforcing techniques to encourage weight gain. Psychotherapy and family therapy are helpful in correcting underlying conflicts and ensuring a permanent resolution. Antidepressants are sometimes indicated in the presence of severe depressive symptoms.

Treatment usually has good short-term effects. After 4 years follow up, half the patients can be expected to have recovered fully and another quarter to have improved. A quarter have persisting severe problems with weight and menstruation. The mortality is now described as below 5%: predictors of death are the patient's lowest reported weight and repeated hospital admissions, but half of those who die kill themselves through overdoses.[20] There is uncertainty as to whether anorexia nervosa has a better outcome in younger prepubertal children.

Encopresis and enuresis

Encopresis

Encopresis is a disorder in which the main manifestation is the persistent voluntary or involuntary passage of formed motions of normal or near-normal consistency into places not intended for that purpose in the individual's own socio-cultural setting. Sometimes the child has failed to gain bowel control and sometimes the encopresis occurs after a period of continence.

The condition is not usually diagnosed under the age of 4 years. Although there are cultural variations, in British samples more than half the toddlers of 18–24 months of age have achieved bowel continence and almost all children aged $2\frac{1}{2}$ years are continent by day and night. Among 5-year olds, 96% are said by their mothers never to soil or make a mess in their pants, 3% say that this happens occasionally and in only 1% does it occur at least once a week.[21] Boys are twice as likely to have this history as girls.

Encopresis has traditionally been divided into three groups:

1 Continuous: these children have never achieved continence and have not learnt to control their bowels. Some children will suffer from mental retardation or neurological disorders such as cerebral palsy or spina bifida which impair the capacity to learn bowel control; or they may come from socially disadvantaged families with parents who are limited in personality and intellect.
2 Discontinuous: these children can control the process of defecation, have had periods of continence; but stressful events may precipitate the soiling.
3 Retentive: associated with constipation and overflow, excessively fluid faeces and faecal impaction.[22]

In practice, the above categories rarely present as separate entities with characteristic associated clinical, aetiological or prognostic factors.

Aetiological factors

The problems noted above under the three traditional subgroups may all be represented singly or in combination. Constipation, anal fissure leading to painful defecation and retention and spina bifida play a part in some children. Hirschsprung's disease is a rarely associated condition.

Psychological problems with (1) major battles over control at the time of toilet training with later negative interactions focused on soiling; (2) major life events disrupting the normal progress of acquiring bowel control; (3) fears of the toilet; and (4) discouragement and shame by the child over incontinence, can all play a part in the genesis or continuation of the problem. In some children the soiling is part of a general developmental delay or of disorganized personal style with overactivity, distractibility and impulsivity. In others no clear aetiological factors are convincingly present.

Some children present with isolated encopresis and yet in others it is part of a severe psychiatric disorder with behavioural and emotional symptoms and associated family psycho-social disadvantage. Clinically, careful history taking, both medical and psychiatric, is necessary to decide on these alternatives.

Assessment and treatment

The possibility of contributing organic factors should always be considered. A careful physical investigation combined with a detailed history of toilet use, frequency and precipitants for episodes of soiling as well as of parents' reactions to the symptom are mandatory. When there is constipation, the first line of treatment is to clear the blockage of feces in the bowel. Then the child is put on a regular bowel-training programme using senna laxatives usually with a stool softener such as lactulose. Suppositories may be used to aid defecation and consideration should be given to the content of fibre in the diet.

A simple behavioural programme to assist with toilet training can include regular sitting on the toilet, for example three times a day after meals, combined with regular checking of the cleanliness to promote awareness in the child, and the use of star charts for successful defecation in the toilet. A special treat can be exchanged for stars. When there is associated child and family pathology, other child psychiatric techniques such as psychotherapy or family work are indicated.

An outpatient treatment programme employing the above strategies is helpful for many children and can result in improvements not only in soiling but also in the associated behavioural problems which in many cases are secondary to shame and family discord resulting from the symptom. In some difficult and stubborn cases however the resources of a day hospital or inpatient psychiatric unit are required.

Enuresis

Enuresis is defined as involuntary urinary incontinence in the absence of any organic abnormality after the age at which bladder control is ordinarily attained (usually by 4 years of age). It has several forms: nocturnal and diurnal, primary (never having achieved continence) and secondary (after a period of continence). In British surveys it has been found that 5% of 7 year olds, 2% of 10 year olds and 0.8 of 14 year olds are incontinent at least once a week. It is thus more common than encopresis but, as in soiling, it is more frequent in boys than in girls.[23,24]

Aetiological factors

Enuresis can be due to a number of factors and a single cause is seldom identified for an individual child. In some cases no obvious cause can be found. The aetiological factors to be considered are in the following areas:

- Genito-urinary tract disorders: infections, particularly in girls with diurnal incontinence, and diminished functional capacity of the bladder.
- Neurological disorders: in spina bifida, epilepsy, diabetes.
- Stressful life events occurring at the time of toilet training or just afterwards (3–4 years of age): family break-up, prolonged mother/child separations, admissions to hospital, accidents and surgery, moving home, birth of a sibling.
- Social disadvantage: poverty, overcrowding, parental criminality, low social class.
- Mental retardation, with general immaturity.
- Current psychosocial stresses.
- Coercive toilet training.
- A family history of enuresis.

Enuretic children are more likely than other children to suffer psychiatric disorders but the prevalence is not high, particularly if the enuresis is primary. Children who develop secondary enuresis sometimes become incontinent again after a stressful event, having previously been nervy children. The low self-esteem and confidence of some enuretic children is often confined to the embarrassment of the symptom and the result rather than the cause of the incontinence.

Assessment and treatment

When physical causes are involved, medical and or surgical treatment of the underlying problem is necessary. Diurnal enuresis in girls can be associated with urinary tract infections requiring investigation and treatment. However, the most common types of enuresis are developmental or associated with stress and psychological symptoms.

Relatively few children with bedwetting receive treatment and many families probably accept bedwetting as part of growing up and wait for natural resolution. A number of common sense measures such as night lifting and fluid restriction before bed are adopted by many parents. There is little evidence for their efficacy in clinical psychiatric samples but they may be more effective for less complex cases.

Drug treatments (imipramine, DDAVP or desamino-D-arginine vasopressin) can be effective: however, they only suppress and do not cure the symptom and are best used for short periods when continence is particularly important: for example, for going away on a camp holiday. Amphetamines and anticholinergic drugs do not have beneficial effects. When imipramine is used, at adequate doses of 1–2.5 mg/kg, the effect is usually noted within one week of starting treatment with few side effects. However, tolerance may develop 2–6 weeks after treatment is commenced.

A simple behavioural treatment of star charts with stars gained for dry nights is a good way of commencing long-term treatment. If this is not successful, the bell-and-pad technique is the most effective way of achieving continence. The device consists usually of an auditory signal linked to electrodes in the form of perforated metal or foil sheets upon which the child sleeps. The sheets are separated by an ordinary cotton sheet: when the child passes urine, contact is made between the two electrodes, this sets the auditory signal into motion and wakes up the child. It is unclear why this technique works; cure varies between 50% and 100% and is usually reached during the second month of treatment. A major problem however is the high number of parents who discontinue the treatment prematurely. This is due to technical faults, failure of the child to wake up, false alarms and disturbance to other family members. A good deal of support from clinics is required to anticipate these problems and intervene so as to avoid discouragement and discontinuation of treatment.

Recognition of autism and other psychotic disorders

Infantile autism and psychotic states such as schizophrenia are the more profound and severe psychiatric disorders of childhood. They affect personality functioning in an all-encompassing and bizarre way. They are both rare and although having a number of features in common they differ substantially.

Infantile autism

Infantile autism is a rare condition. It affects two to four children in every 10 000 and as with many other developmental problems is more common in boys than in girls. Earlier reports of increased rates in middle-class and professional families have not been confirmed in recent epidemiological surveys.

Although the syndrome is present from birth it only becomes manifest as the child develops the skills that are primarily affected to a sufficient extent for deficits to be apparent. This is usually the case by 30 months of age, but onset of the condition can be seen in later childhood.

The main features include severe problems in the understanding of spoken language.[25] Speech is delayed and if it develops, which it never does in a considerable percentage of children, it is characterized by echolalia, the reversal of pronouns, immature grammatical structure and inability to use abstract terms. Non-verbal speech, the use of gesture and inner speech, as manifested by the active pretend games of the pre-school child and by imaginative play, are also affected. In the more able children speech is stereotyped, it lacks inflection and repetitive questions are often asked.

There is in autism a particularly profound failure in the development of social relationships. This is most marked before the age of 5 years, with impairments in the development of eye-to-eye gaze, social attachments and cooperative play. There is a general lack of reciprocity and empathy. Children may fail to go to their parents for comfort although they can enjoy physical contact and games. They appear to treat people as objects, handling and examining the face or hair of their parents. Intense attachments can be formed to bizarre objects. Many of these features, for example gaze avoidance, become less marked as children become older.

Stereotyped, rigid, non-functional, non-social play behaviour and routines are common. In later childhood there may be preoccupations with bus routes or numbers. There is often insistence on sameness or resistance to changes in the environment. Obsessive–compulsive rituals can develop in some children. Stereotyped mannerisms, for example flicking fingers in front of the face repeatedly or flapping of hands, are seen particularly in the less intelligent children. Associated behavioural problems, with tantrums, hyperactivity, sleeping and feeding difficulties are common and may be the presenting feature in the less severely affected children.

Cognitive development is often affected and three-quarters of children show some degree of intellectual impairment. They have special deficits in verbal IQ scores, and in measures of sequencing, abstraction and coding.

Aetiological factors

The earlier descriptions emphasized anomalies in the parents' affective contact and parent–child relationships. It has however become apparent that the latter cannot explain the basic features. Autism is now seen as the result of brain dysfunction and genetic influences. It can occur in association with a variety of disorders affecting the brain: tuberous sclerosis; congenital rubella; infantile spasms; encephalitis; to quote but a few. There is a tendency to develop epileptic fits in adolescence. Other non-specific biological and structural brain anomalies have also been noted.[26]

There is established evidence that genetic factors play a part, with increased rates for autism in families of affected children, and, in twins, a clearly higher monozygotic than dizygotic concordance for both autistic and other cognitive deficits. More recently, high rates of social gaucheness as well as a tendency to be intellectual have been noted in the parents of autistic children; they may be a marker for one of the genetic determinants of autism.

Recognition of autism

The syndrome at its most typical is easy to recognize. However, atypical forms appear to be particularly frequent and there are a number of features which commonly lead to diagnostic uncertainty:

- In severely handicapped children, it can be difficult to know to what extent the social and communication anomalies represent a specific deficit over and above existing generalized developmental delays.
- In intelligent children, the deficits may be mild and not immediately apparent when first meeting the child. Some of these children, for example those with Asperger's syndrome, may have apparently normal speech development but dysfunctional non-verbal or visual-spatial skills, or they may present with antisocial and sometimes grossly callous aggressive behaviour; careful assessment is sometimes needed to identify the underlying empathic and communication deficits.
- Many parents give a history of normal early development with sudden change in behaviour after some psychological or physical stress. There is then a picture reminiscent of disintegrative psychosis, Heller's syndrome or of speech regression with or without a cluster of epileptic seizures in the Landau-Kleffner syndrome. It is difficult to know whether this is due to a lack of awareness of early anomalies by parents, whether the condition is indeed stress triggered, or whether this is simply a reflection of the fact that developmental regression and unevenness across the developmental domain appear to be particularly associated with autism.[27]
- Some children fail to display social avoidance. They take affection and cuddles, although usually quite passively. It may take some time before the lack of empathic relating is manifested to the observer.

Outcome

Autism is a persisting disorder: about two-thirds of children become severely handicapped adults in mental institutions and only about 10% are working and self-supporting, with intellectual level and speech competence being the best prognostic indicators.

Although there is no cure, behavioural and drug treatments can lead to symptomatic improvements and reduce associated troublesome behaviours. Placement in a school with appropriate expertise in dealing with autistic children is highly desirable.

Psychotic states of childhood

Schizophrenia and manic-depressive illness are very rare before adolescence. Occasionally, prepubertal children without any or with only mild pre-morbid anomalies in personality development manifest a major behavioural change – with delusional beliefs and perceptual symptoms such as hallucinations, disorganized/incoherent/laconic speech, odd and inappropriate affective states, bizarre behaviour, changes in level of activity with either hypoactivity or hyperactivity – generally compatible with a schizophrenic diagnosis.

The condition is difficult to diagnose before 7 years of age because a certain level of cognitive development is necessary for children to communicate verbally such symptoms as hallucinations. The nature of delusional beliefs changes with age: the younger the child, the less structured they are. For example, children under 10 years tend to express abnormal ideas about identity changes through identification with inanimate objects or animals, or have irrational fears of the cosmic content or transitory paranoid delusions. In prepubertal and pubertal children, delusions become progressively more persistent and complex with paranoid and hyperchondriacal ideas, and later with religious and depressive themes. By adolescence these are mostly paranoid or persecutory in content.[28] Non-psychotic symptoms also can be present. Irritability, obsessions, school refusal, aches and pains and problems in relationships can be very disturbing.

The differential diagnosis between psychotic and other severely disturbed (but not psychotic) adolescents may be difficult in inarticulate youngsters who have erratic, impulsive behaviour and odd and unusual ideas, or in severe histrionically elaborated conduct or emotional disorders. In these cases careful observation may be needed to establish the loss of contact with reality and profound breakdown in personality functioning which are characteristic of psychotic states.

It can also be difficult to differentiate between types of psychotic states in adolescence since mixed schizophrenic and manic depressive, or non-elaborated clinical pictures, appear to be more common in this age group. Prolonged observation and follow up may be needed to allow a definite diagnosis to be made. Acute organic psychoses, phenomenologically very similar to the functional psychoses, are seen after ingestion of drugs, such as amphetamines, or in the course of acute toxic delirious states as part of severe systemic physical illness. There is often associated clouding of consciousness and subsequent total recovery. Careful enquiry and screening about drug intake or physical illness is important in all psychotic states.

Aetiological factors

The aetiological factors which contribute to the development of psychotic states in adults (for example genetic influences) are also relevant for the psychotic states of children and adolescents. But there are indications that biological predisposing and precipitating factors such as early neurodevelopmental deficits (clumsiness, learning difficulties, abnormal personality developments), viral infections or other brain changes such as brain tumours may be more common in schizophrenic conditions starting in childhood or adolescence.

Treatment

When a child or adolescent presents with psychotic symptomatology, admission to a psychiatric unit is highly desirable for careful observation and sometimes for the child's safety. However, with appropriate home support, outpatient or day-patient monitoring can also be appropriate. Treatment usually involves the use of antipsychotic medication (phenothiazines, butirofenones, lithium carbonate), and parental and educational support. About one-fifth of youngsters can be expected to recover, half to improve but with the possibility of further relapses and the rest remain ill. Good premorbid personality and higher intelligence as well as post-pubertal onset all carry a better prognosis.

Psychological disorders in the family

It has long been recognized that children of parents with psychiatric problems have themselves an increased risk of psychiatric disorders. In surveys of parents ill enough to require psychiatric assessment, one-third of the children are found to have persistent psychological symptoms with a further third showing transient difficulties.[29]

For some rare conditions such as schizophrenia the link has genetic components, but even then only a small percentage of children of schizophrenic parents will suffer the condition. Parental psychiatric disturbance more commonly acts as an environmental influence and this is particularly so when it affects the parents' ability to provide a secure, consistent, loving environment, devoid of major strains in the relationships between family members and adequate care and discipline. More than in psychotic conditions such as schizophrenia and manic-depressive illness, this is affected by parental histories of personality disorders and depressive illness.[29]

Personality disorders

Personality disorders indicate persistent patterns of maladaptive behaviour generally recognizable by the time of adolescence or earlier and continuing throughout most of adult life. They involve suffering by the patient, or others have to suffer and there is an adverse effect upon the individual or on society. Problems in inter-personal relationships, within the family, at work, or in a wider social context, are commonly a feature, and there are often associated depressive episodes.[16] These can be compounded by alcohol or other substance abuse and the development of dependency states.

Child abuse is a problem which has been found to be related to personality problems in parents.[30] In a survey, as many as one-third of abusing fathers and 13% of mothers had aggressive psychopathy and convictions for violent crimes were also frequent. Marital violence has been reported in about one-third of families.

There are indications that adverse earlier experiences in the parents – for example illegitimacy, separation and abandonment, exposure to aggression – contribute. Abusing mothers tend to show high levels of self-criticism, hostility and guilty feelings on questionnaire enquiries. Guilt, excessive identification with the child, displacement of aggression from self or others onto the child and paranoid feelings, or feeling got at by the child, probably play a part in many aggressive acts. Drug intake and alcohol further impair self-control and lead to violence.

Formal psychiatric disturbance is usually not involved in abuse but it is a factor in fatal cases.[31] Schizophrenia is diagnosed in one-fifth of mothers sent to prison for killing children, and this is an underestimate because some mothers commit suicide after killing the child. Psychotic mothers are often well adjusted personally and socially prior to the onset of the illness or between episodes. They can respond to psychiatric treatment, whereas mothers with severely affected personality disorders are usually difficult to help through psychiatric intervention.

Maternal depression

Depression is a ubiquitous psychiatric disorder. It is common; up to 40% of young mothers in difficult social circumstances are depressed. It often has an effect on the children. Although the puerperium is a time when depressive feelings are common, depression is also common at times other than childbirth.

Many recently delivered women experience transient episodes of tearfulness and mild depression 4–5 days after the birth of the child and the incidence of depression is believed to be raised during the first few months after childbirth.[32] The condition usually remits within a few months and this process can be facilitated by supportive measures, for example reduction of isolation, identification of sources of stress and correction of these. Maternal depression can be indicated by a mother who consults repeatedly on behalf of her healthy baby. In these instances, paediatric–psychiatric liaison is particularly appropriate to ameliorate the mother's symptoms and attend to the needs of the child. In severe cases, marked improvements can be obtained with antidepressants.

Puerperal psychoses and severe psychiatric conditions starting in the puerperium are rare. They may take the form of an affective disorder, either manic or depressive, or of a schizophrenic illness or they may be mixed, so-called schizo-affective. The treatment involves the use of medication, either neuroleptics or antidepressants, but many severely depressed women eventually require ECT. Ideally, mothers should be admitted to specialized mother-and-baby units where particular nursing skills are available and attempts can be made to preserve mothering capabilities or to foster the development of the mother–child bond. Special attention needs to be given to mothers who express infanticidal impulses or when they are in acutely disorganized states.

Depressed mothers' styles of interaction with their children are altered by their condition.[33] They are less expansive than other mothers in their communications with their babies and more critical. The babies are less alert and engaged with their mothers. Infants of postnatally depressed mothers perform less well than other infants on measures of cognitive, social and behavioural development.[34]

Insecure attachments are observed in toddlers of depressed mothers, particularly with the more negative maternal interactions. Pre-school children of depressed mothers have an increased risk of intellectual deficits, especially if there is associated marital conflict and also psychiatric problems in the fathers. The children have more accidents and contacts with medical services. In school children, maternal depression is linked to depression in the child, but also to conduct disorders and hyperactivity and to learning difficulties in the children. There are indications that when pre-school children of depressed mothers develop psychological problems, disturbance in the child becomes a problem in its own right in that it tends to persist even after the mother's mental state improves. It is possible that interactions with depressed mothers in children who themselves are temperamentally vulnerable may, because of increased maternal criticism, lead to more negative self-concept in the children. This may be a mechanism contributing to the development of psychiatric disturbance in children of depressed mothers.

Suicide

Suicide is an act of deliberate self-harm resulting in death. It is very rare in childhood and only exceptionally reported in under 12 year olds. The rates increase gradually with age to about 30 cases per million per year in 15–19 year olds. In the USA it is considered to be the third most common cause of death in 15–24 year old white young men. It is more common in male than in female adolescents.

Completed suicide

The methods used in completed suicide are often violent and involve hanging, shooting, suffocation, car fumes, or jumping from high places. In the histories of youngsters with completed suicide it is common to find a prior mixture of both depressive and conduct symptoms. The suicidal act tends to be precipitated by an immediate emotional crisis involving a family dispute or a disappointing or humiliating experience, for example a particularly bad school report. Many of these children are of high intelligence although not particularly good achievers. It is not uncommon for adolescents to have had a history of suicidal ideas, threats and attempts, although it is important to note that, overall, suicidal thoughts and even threats rarely result in suicide. It has been noted that antisocial behaviours and an inhibited personality, or youngsters who are very quiet, lack friends, do not talk openly about their problems, who are lonely and extremely sensitive, feature specially frequently among youngsters who commit suicide. In psychiatric adolescent inpatients with histories of attempted suicide who later commit suicide, 'fears of losing one's mind' as well as feelings of hopelessness have been noted at the index admission to hospital. An evaluation of disturbed adolescents' ability to communicate openly, truthfulness and clarity of thinking seems relevant when assessing the probability of future suicidal actions.[35]

A factor that deserves attention in relation to suicide in childhood is the effects of imitation. Suicide rates have been found to increase after newspaper reports, and the more famous the person the greater the increase in rates appears to be.[35]

Attempted suicide

Attempted suicide, or act of self-injury with a suicidal intention but a non-fatal outcome, is considerably more common. It is estimated that for every suicide there are at least 100 adolescents, more commonly girls, attempting suicide.

The majority of cases are due to drug overdoses, for example analgesics or psychotropic medication. They range from the medically trivial to those requiring intensive care treatment. They are often precipitated by disputes over discipline, by arguments with friends or family members and preceded by threats.

Attempted suicide is a behaviour rarely seen before adolescence and developmental considerations are pertinent. Adolescents question and criticize established views and parental authority and they go through a considerable inner emotional turmoil while their own sense of identity is consolidated. Experimenting with potentially dangerous behaviours such as the use of drugs is in a number of cases part of the process. Feelings of depression and of self-deprecation are also common and one in twelve 14-year-olds in general population surveys admits to occasional suicidal ideas. This inner turmoil often goes unrecognized by adults and an emotional gulf as well as altercations can develop between parents and children. Close, intimate friendships with peers are common but breakdown in these can be a further source of pain and alienation. Within this context, attempted suicide may be regarded as a dysfunctional way of expressing despair, loneliness, alienation and experimentation with danger.[36]

About half the youngsters who take overdoses are found to suffer psychiatric disorders with symptoms of depression: this is usually acute and reactive to stresses or difficulties, but in some cases it is part of chronic psychiatric disturbance and disturbed behaviour.[37] It may be part of a pattern of drug and alcohol abuse. Chronic physical health problems contribute in a number of children. Children who have attempted suicide are more likely than other children to make further suicidal attempts.

Aetiological factors

A number of family and social features usually in various combinations are associated with attempted suicide in adolescence. These include:

1 Parental psychiatric problems with depression and personality difficulty: not uncommonly this is linked to a family atmosphere of discord and tension and there may be a family history of suicidal attempts.
2 Marital strain.
3 Inconsistent parental discipline.
4 Poor family communication of feelings and information.
5 Social isolation of the child. For a minority of children, there is a history of physical or possibly sexual abuse.

Assessment and treatment

It is important that an assessment of every child and family is made as soon as possible, when the child is medically fit and prior to discharge, by someone capable of assessing the risk of recurrence or the need for intervention. An evaluation by a psychiatrist is desirable although not always necessary. Both children and parents should be interviewed. The following information is relevant:[38]

- Details of the attempt: number and type of tablets taken, how acquired, where taken, likelihood of being found, notes left.
- Precipitating circumstances, suicidal intention.
- Any emotional and behavioural changes in the months prior to the overdose, any changes and stresses in the child's life.
- Child's mental state, with special emphasis on depressive symptomatology.
- Quality of family relationships and of the social network of the child; previous involvement with helping agencies (e.g. social services, general practitioner).
- How the attempt has changed the circumstances which precipitated it.

Special concern about future attempts is needed when the attempt has been serious, the child is depressed, the precipitating circumstances are unresolved or the social support for the child is poor. In a minority, obvious psychiatric disorder will call for inpatient psychiatric treatment. When there is a serious breakdown in the family circumstances, social services involvement and admission into care may be necessary. In a few cases, observation on the paediatric ward will be required to clarify the clinical and social picture.

For the majority of cases, return home following a psychiatric assessment and crisis intervention is indicated. Psychiatric follow up and the use of family therapy techniques or individual counselling for the child will be needed where there are continuing difficulties.

References

1 Horne, J. Sleep and its disorders in children. *J Child Psychol Psychiatr* 1992; **33**: 473–487.
2 Richman, N. Prevalence and treatment of sleep problems in young children. In: Stevenson, J.E., ed. *Recent Research in Developmental Psychopathology*, Oxford: Pergamon Press, 1985.
3 Zuckerman, B., Stevenson, J., Bailey, V. Sleep problems in early childhood: continuities, predictive factors, and behavioural correlates. *Pediatrics* 1987; **80**: 664–671.
4 Golding, J. Feeding and sleeping problems. In: Butler, N.R., Golding, J., eds. *From Birth to Five: a Study of the Health and Behaviour of British Five Year Olds*. Oxford: Pergamon Press, 1986.
5 Luria Ablon, S., Mack, J.E. Sleep disorders. In: Noshpitz, J.B., ed. *Basic Handbook of Child Psychiatry: volume 2, Disturbances in Development*. New York: Basic Books, 1979.
6 Richman, N., Douglas, J., Hunt, H., Lansdown, R.,

Levere, R. Behavioural methods in the treatment of sleep disorders: a pilot study. *J Child Psychol Psychiatr* 1985; **26**: 581–590.
7 Seymour, F.W., Brock, P., During, M., Poole, G. Reducing sleep disruptions in young children: evaluation of therapist-guided and written information approaches: a brief report. *J Child Psychol Psychiatr* 1989; **30**: 913–918.
8 Stores, G. Confusions concerning sleep disorders and the epilepsies in children and adolescents. *Br J Psychiatr* 1991; **158**: 1–7.
9 Stores, G. Sleep disorders in children. *Br Med J* 1990; **301**: 351–352.
10 Goodenough, F.L. *Anger in Young Children*. Minneapolis: University of Minnesota Press, 1931.
11 Golding, J., Rush, D. Temper tantrums and other behaviour problems. In: Butler, N.R., Golding, J., eds. *From Birth to Five*. Oxford: Pergamon Press, 1986.
12 Richman, N., Stevenson, J., Graham, P.J. *Pre-School to School: a Behavioural Study*. London: Academic Press, 1982.
13 Hill, P. Behaviour modification with children. *Br J Hosp Med* 1982; **27**: 51–60.
14 Dunn, J. Feeding and sleeping. In: Rutter, M., ed. *Developmental Psychiatry*. London: Heinemann Medical, 1980.
15 Skuse, D.H. Non-organic failure to thrive: a reappraisal. *Arch Dis Child* 1985; **60**: 173–178.
16 World Health Organization (WHO). *Mental Disorders: Glossary and Guide to the Classification in Accordance with the 9th Revision of the International Classification of Diseases*. Geneva: WHO, 1978.
17 Rastam, M., Gillberg, C., Garton, M. Anorexia nervosa in a Swedish urban region: a population-based study. *Br J Psychiatr* 1989; **155**: 642–646.
18 Crisp, A.H. Anorexia nervosa. In: Silverstone, T., Barraclough, B., eds. *Contemporary Psychiatry. Selected Reviews from the British Journal of Hospital Medicine*. Ashford: Headley, 1975.
19 Hsu, L.K.G. *The Development of the Concept of Anorexia Nervosa*. London: Smith, Kline & French Laboratories, 1980.
20 Patton, G. The course of anorexia nervosa. *Br Med J* 1989; **299**: 139–140.
21 Golding, J., Tissier, G. Soiling and wetting. In: Butler, N.R., Golding, J., eds. *From Birth to Five*. Oxford: Pergamon Press, 1986.
22 Anthony, E.J. An experimental approach to the psychopathology of childhood: encopresis. *Br J Med Psychol* 1957; **30**: 146–175.
23 Kolvin, I., MacKeith, R.C., Meadow, J.R., eds. *Bladder Control and Enuresis*. London: Heinemann Medical for Spastics International, 1973.
24 Shaffer, D. Enuresis. In: Rutter, M., Hersov, L., eds. *Child and Adolescent Psychiatry*, 2nd edn. Oxford: Blackwell Scientific, 1985.
25 Rutter, M. Infantile autism and other pervasive developmental disorders. In: Rutter, M., Hersov, L., eds. *Child and Adolescent Psychiatry*, 2nd edn. Oxford: Blackwell Scientific, 1985.
26 Garralda, M.E. Autism, language disorders and psychosis in children. *Curr Opinion Psychiatr* 1989; **2**: 472–475.

27 Burack, J.A., Volkmar, F.R. Development of low- and high-functioning autistic children. *J Child Psychol Psychiatr* 1992; **33**: 605–616.

28 Garralda, M.E., Ainsworth, P. Psychoses in adolescence. In: Coleman, J.C., ed. *Working with Troubled Adolescents*. London: Academic Press, 1987.

29 Rutter, M., Quinton, D. Parental psychiatric disorder: effects on children. *Psychol Med* 1984; **14**: 853–880.

30 Smith, S.M. *The Battered Child Syndrome*. London: Butterworths, 1975.

31 d'Orban, P.T. Women who kill their children. *Br J Psychiatr* 1979; **134**: 560–571.

32 Kumar, R. Reproduction and psychiatric disorders in women. In: Lader, M.H., ed. *Handbook of Psychiatry, 2: Mental Disorders and Somatic Illness*. Cambridge: Cambridge University Press, 1983.

33 Puckering, C. Maternal depression. *J Child Psychol Psychiatr* 1989; **30**: 807–817.

34 Murray, L. The impact of postnatal depression on infant development. *J Child Psychol Psychiatr* 1992; **33**: 543–561.

35 Pfeffer, C.R. Suicide: In: Hsu, L.K.G., Hersen, M., eds. *Recent Developments in Adolescent Psychiatry*. New York: John Wiley, 1989.

36 Rutter, M., Graham, P., Chadwick, O., Yule, W. Adolescent turmoil: fact or fiction. *J Child Psychol Psychiatr* 1976; **17**: 35–56.

37 Taylor, E., Stansfield, S.A. Children who poison themselves. I. A clinical comparison with psychiatric controls. *Br J Psychiatr* 1984; **145**: 127–135.

38 Hawton, K., Catalan, J. Psychiatric management of attempted suicide patients. *Br J Hosp Med* 1981; **25**: 365–372.

Chapter 18

Death at home

18.1 Care of the dying child

Danai Papadatou and Costas Papadatos

Introduction

Until the beginning of this century, home was the traditional site for the care of the sick and the dying. However, with the progress of cure-oriented medicine and a sophisticated technology-based system, dying and death began to occur more and more in a hospital setting. This led to major problems, since hospital personnel were not adequately educated and prepared to assume the responsibility for meeting the needs of an increasing number of dying patients. In recent years, a movement in death and dying developed, and the concept of hospice care for the terminally ill received considerable attention.[1] Cicely Saunders, a nurse, social worker and physician, was the first to recognize the inadequacy of the care that the general hospital offered to the dying and developed, in England, the first hospice programme – St Christopher Hospice – which served as a model for many similar programmes that were later established in the USA and around the world.[2]

The concept of a hospice does not refer to a facility or institution, but rather to a philosophy. It is an approach focused on comfort care when cure is no longer a reasonable expectation, and addresses the psychological, social and spiritual needs of the dying individual, of the family and of the care givers involved in patient care. The ultimate goal of the hospice approach is to maximize the quality of life, by affirming life, so that individuals who are dying may live as fully and comfortably as possible. The hospice approach extends even after the patient's death and provides support to the family during the period of bereavement.[3,4]

The majority of hospice care programmes serve an adult population, but there is a growing trend to develop similar programmes for dying children. Most of these programmes, however, focus on institutionalized care[5–7] rather than home care. In 1976, Ida Martinson was the first to examine the feasibility and desirability of a home care alternative to hospitalization for children dying of cancer.[8]

Within this alternative the parents were the primary providers of the child's care. They were assisted by community nurses who offered guidance, supervision and support, while the child's physician served as a consultant to the family and to the nurse. Findings of her study suggest that a programme of home care is a viable and feasible alternative to traditional hospitalization. Families, one month and one year later, reported feeling satisfied with the overall experience.[8] Similar results are supported by other studies which stress that the rewards of the home care experience are significant for the dying child who feels more secure and loved in his or her natural environment, for the parents who derive satisfaction from being the primary care givers and from fulfilling their child's wish to remain at home, and for the siblings who are involved in the whole experience of care.[9–12] Adjustment following the death of the child has been observed to be more effective for families whose child died at home than for families whose child died in the hospital.[12,13] In addition, financial benefits are significant, since home care has repeatedly been found to be less expensive than a similar level of care provided in the hospital.[11,14]

Participation in a paediatric home care programme

Every home care programme needs to be carefully designed in order to meet the particular needs of families with terminally ill children in the community.[15-17] Frequently, a home care coordinator (usually an experienced paediatric nurse) acts as a liaison between the hospital staff, the family and the available community resources and services. The hospice team adopts an interdisciplinary approach for the management of the dying child and the care of the family as a whole. Depending on the programme, the team may include nurses (community or hospital-based), general practitioner, paediatrician, pharmacist, social worker, family therapist or psychologist, physiotherapist and volunteers who are trained to deal with the complex issues of separation preceding death and grief during the period of bereavement.

As an alternative to hospitalization, home care may not be desirable or appropriate for every family. Hutter and his colleagues[18] stress that, when a child is dying, the decision to provide care at home or in the hospital needs to be individualized with full participation of both the family and the child. Families must first recognize that no treatment can control or cure the disease and accept that death is imminent. Major factors affecting their decision for home care are: the child's wish to be at home; the parents' desire to care for the child at home; the willingness and ability of family members to care for and meet the needs of the sick child; and the availability of adequate resources to support the family. These include the presence of a supportive extended family and the availability of a team of professional care givers who provide assistance and consultation on a 24-hour, 7-days-a-week basis. Rehospitalization should always remain as an option and be possible at any time. Moreover, the eventual occurrence of death within the hospital setting should not be interpreted by the family members or the home care team as a failure. Recently, a group of experts and members of the International Work Group on Death, Dying and Bereavement have identified a set of assumptions which serve as guidelines, across cultures, in the care of children with terminal illness and their families, regardless of whether dying occurs in hospital or at home.[19]

Palliative care

The three essential components of palliative care are: physical comfort and symptom control; support for the dying child; and support for the family members. The effectiveness of palliative care depends on the knowledge and team work spirit assumed by professionals of various disciplines.

Physical comfort and symptom control

The period surrounding the child's terminal care and death is a very stressful time for family members. Not only do they have to deal with their own intense emotions, but they have also to assume full responsibility for their child's terminal care. Parents are anxious about the dying process, the physical changes and medical complications which may arise. Members of the hospice team need to address these issues and teach parents certain specific skills, such as how to ensure the child's physical comfort (e.g. mouth washing, bathing, skin care, providing liquids etc), when to administer analgesic drugs, or how to apply certain techniques and procedures (e.g. oxygen administration, tracheopharyngeal suction, intravenous feeding etc). Procedures requiring specialized skills (e.g. urinary catheterization) are managed by team members who are also responsible for providing equipment and the medical supplies necessary for the child's comfort and the enhancement of the quality of his or her life.

In terms of the hospice concept, the pain experienced by a dying child may be either physical, psychological, social or spiritual or any combination of all four.[20] Consequently, pain management involves intervention on several levels and aims to keep the child pain-free, comfortable and fully alert until the moment of death. Team members need to possess extensive education in pain control, so as to avoid underprescribing or overprescribing medication, and use effective communication skills and psychological techniques which help children cope with pain, anxiety and distress.[21-23]

According to reports of parents whose family participated in a home care programme, the two most salient variables determining the degree of their satisfaction were the ability to control effectively the child's pain and the access to prompt professional services when requested.[11,24]

Support for the dying child

In addition to the physical comfort of the child, attention must be directed to his or her psychological well-being. This requires a deep knowledge of the child's emotional needs and recognition of his or her understanding of impending death. All dying children need to be recognized as alive, involved in living experiences, and as being close to death. Acknowledging both aspects is crucial in providing effective support during the terminal phase. Dying is a period of emotional fluctuation for the child who is pulled in opposite directions.[25] Even though these may seem contradictory they are, nevertheless, part of the same process.

All terminally ill children know to a greater or lesser degree that they are dying but fluctuate between awareness and denial. Denial differs from avoidance of discussions of death-related topics and from pre-tending that everything will get better; a child may use the latter in an effort to protect loved ones who have difficulty accepting his or her awareness of dying. Children, like adults, may not possess a knowledge of death, since no human has such knowledge, but they have emotions, beliefs, and needs in relation to dying and death which are usually expressed on a symbolic level.[26–31] Being consciously or intuitively aware that they are dying does not imply that they always come to peaceful terms with this reality. Some children may experience anger, a sense of injustice, or anxiety that is usually related to the process of separation from their loved ones, rather than with death itself. When these feelings are openly or symbolically addressed and worked through, children may feel freer to live more meaningfully their remaining life. Their will to live may coexist with their awareness of dying.

Children also experience a conflict between a need to maintain a sense of belonging among their loved ones, and a need to withdraw emotionally as death approaches. Dying does not remove their desire to have a special and unique place within the family environment. Sometimes older children or adolescents strive to maintain their belonging by accomplishing something for which they will be remembered. However, at the same time, dying children tend to withdraw, in an attempt to decrease the emotional energy required in dealing with too many painful separations. Not unlike adults, children also experience a grieving process. Adolescents, in particular, grieve not only over the life they have lived, but also over the life they have *not* lived;[25] their developmental process of identity formation and projection of self into the future is invested with dreams, expectations and goals.

Interestingly enough, children's withdrawal does not lead to total detachment from others. They often form a symbiotic relationship with a person (usually a parent) who is able and willing to accompany them. This relationship provides them with the illusion that they will carry the loved one along to death and beyond, and provides them with a sense of security and self-worth.[32,33]

Professional intervention should facilitate the expression of fears, concerns and conflicts that children are often unable to verbalize. A trained carer can use art, creative play, story telling, guided imagery or relaxation techniques to tap into the dying child's inner world, reduce stress and anxiety, help the patient gain a better control over the dying conditions, and give a personal meaning to his or her experiences.[30,31] The child's participation in such creative and symbolic activities often generates a healing process and releases much of the inner pain which otherwise remains unexpressed. In addition, the professional may serve as an interpreter of symbolic language, so that family members respond to the child's needs and communicate more honestly and effectively with him or her. Clinical experience suggests that careful listening to the child's non-verbal and symbolic communication may allow a better understanding of when and how he or she chooses or wishes to die.

Support for the family members

In order to provide psychological care to the family, hospice care providers need to understand the complex, multidimensional process which is experienced in response to the awareness of the child's impending death.[34–37] This grieving process is usually referred to in the literature as *anticipatory grief*. However, some experts argue that such a term is a misnomer, since family members do not only grieve over a major loss they expect to occur in their lives. According to Rando[37] they grieve over *past losses* (e.g. a mother may grieve over the lively, healthy and dynamic child she has lost due to a terminal illness and over the dreams she had for him or her), *present losses* (e.g. a child may grieve over the altered relationship with his or her dying sibling who is now very sick, sleeps most of the time and does not want him or her around) and *future losses* (e.g. a father may grieve over losing his child, and over the losses that may happen in the family prior to the death or after). The nature of these losses and the meaning attributed to them by family members, the dying child, or even care givers themselves, affect the way each experiences grief.

With death approaching, family members not only grieve for the forthcoming loss of their child, but also for themselves, and for their family as a unit which will never be the same again. Grieving over these losses evokes feelings of depression and disorganization which are necessary and adaptive. The breaking down of old patterns of behaviour allows family members to develop new patterns.[38] Experiencing a grieving process for an impending death generates intense anxiety, feelings of anger, hostility and guilt. Anxiety stems from a sense of helplessness and insecurity caused by the unknown and the uncertain demands of the terminal illness, while anger and hostility are experienced as a response to the threat of being deprived of their child. Anger may be directed at others significant in the child's care, God, or even at the dying child for abandoning the family. As a result, it is not uncommon for family members to feel worthless and guilty. Their guilt is intensified by the occurrence of ambivalent feelings, such as: wanting the child to live despite the pain and anguish, and wanting the child to die; wanting to care for him or her, and wanting to run away. Thus, they are pulled in opposing directions: a move towards the dying child, attending to his or her needs, and a move away from him or her. The challenge for each family member is to find a balance between these conflicting pulls. When this is achieved, a process of *decathexis* develops – a relaxation or withdrawal of emotional energy focused on the child. Decathexis is not from the dying child, but from the *image* of the child as someone who will be present in the future; decathexis is from the hopes, dreams and expectations held for him or her. Contrary to popular misconception, this detachment does not prevent family members from supporting the child and being involved in meaningful interactions.[37,38]

Professional intervention should address and facilitate the expression of these natural emotions and thoughts, and support behaviours such as discussing the death of their child, making funeral preparations or thinking what the future will be like without their child, etc which are all integral to the grief experience when death is imminent. However, a caution should be drawn to the detrimental effect of too much or too little grief.

It has been found that too much grief, experienced for a long period, compromises the parents' ability to care and interact with their dying child who is left feeling abandoned and emotionally isolated. On the other hand, too little or absence of grief when death is imminent results in intense reactions at the moment of death, and predisposes family members to poor bereavement outcomes. Research findings[39] suggest that there is an optimum amount of so-called anticipatory grief that is therapeutic and associated with fewer atypical grief responses following the death of a child; however, further research is needed to determine more precisely the amount which has greater therapeutic value.

Intervention during the terminal phase should be family-oriented, since this period is both extremely difficult and significant for all individuals involved in the child's care. When adopting a family network model, people who have a major relationship to the nuclear family at the time of initial crisis (relatives, friends, priest, teacher, etc) are invited by the family and the health care professionals to assume a supportive role.[18,40] This support network is usually established shortly after the diagnosis of a chronic and life-threatening disease and provides assistance throughout the course of the child's illness, during the terminal phase, and the bereavement period.[18]

Bereavement follow up

Home care does not end when the child dies. The team provides the family with bereavement counselling for a few months following the death. However, since the period of bereavement is long-lasting, families who have difficulties in adjusting to the loss may be encouraged to seek additional support from existing agencies and bereavement associations in the community.

When the child dies, family members are faced with a double loss: not only are they confronted with the loss of their child, but also with the loss of their family unit as they have always known it. Despite the fact the same child has died, each family member is actually mourning a different loss. Each parent and sibling grieves over the loss of a unique relationship he or she held with that particular child. This explains why family members have difficulty grieving at the same time, in the same way, for the same things.[41] In fact, grief is an individual journey and, although family members are encouraged to share their grief, they also need to give each other space, and be able to respect their personal differences in handling emotions. There is not a single correct way to grieve. Recent findings suggest that family members respond to the feeling of emptiness caused by their child's death after a chronic illness with basically three different patterns of grieving:[42]

1 *Getting over it* – by accepting death and giving some kind of explanation and meaning to it.
2 *Feeling the emptiness* – by keeping busy or involved in various projects, activities and interests.
3 *Keeping the connection* – by maintaining a sense of empty space, integrating it in everyday life and cherishing recollections of the child.

These patterns – none of which is superior to the other – have been found to persist as long as 7 to 9 years after death. This suggests that bereavement over the loss of a child is a long-term process and emphasizes the need to reconsider theories which suggest that grief is resolved within 2 years.

The death of a child has diverse effects on family members and their relationships. Communication problems may arise as roles are redistributed within the family unit, priorities are re-ordered, and family relationships are changed. Recognizing these changes and integrating them into a new reality constitutes a challenge for every bereaved family.

Parental bereavement

It is suggested that parental bereavement appears to be more traumatic, complicated, intense and long-lasting, when compared to other bereavements. Rando provides new insights in understanding the uniqueness of parental bereavement, which fails to be adequately explained by available models and conceptualizations held for grief and mourning.[41] This uniqueness is due to the closeness and intensity of the relationship that exists between a parent and child. The child's death affects the parents' innermost selves. A part of them dies too. Feelings, hopes, dreams and expectations projected by parents onto this particular child (who symbolized different things for each of them) die too. As a result, parental identity is affected and intense guilt is experienced.

Guilt feelings are caused by a set of ideal standards and unrealistic expectations parents hold for themselves, such as to be all loving, all giving, totally selfless, protective and supportive at all times to their child. Recalling times they did not meet these irrational standards and when they experienced ambivalent feelings toward their child generate a sense of having failed in their parental role, which in turn affects their self-image. These feelings are intensified by additional guilt for having survived their own child and for not being able to prevent his or her suffering and death. These reactions are absolutely normal and need to be confronted and examined within the reality of the situation. If, however, negative evaluations last for a long period of time, parents resort to self-punishing or non-adaptive behaviours which require professional intervention. Major complications in adjustment may also occur if parents overprotect their surviving children from fear of losing them too, or if they try too quickly to replace the child who died by giving birth to a new one, or by expecting that one of their surviving children will assume the role, characteristics and identity of the child who died. It is widely supported that such replacements may be harmful and hinder adjustment.[43,44]

Surviving sibling's bereavement

Special consideration should be addressed to surviving children who are confronted not only with the loss of their sibling, but with the loss of their parents' attention, care and support. For bereaved parents the surviving children may serve as reminders of the one who died. Sometimes surviving siblings are resented for being alive, or for being less than perfect when compared to the deceased child, or for having adjusted too quickly to the loss. It is only with time that parents find the energy to relate to and reinvest their love into their other children.

The responses of surviving children to their sibling's death are profound and long lasting. Seven to 9 years after the death they continue to display a range of behaviours which are attributed to the loss. These, basically, include a tendency to withdraw socially and experience feelings of loneliness and sorrow. Nevertheless, they are reported to have gained maturity as a result of their loss.[45] Findings suggest[46] that the two major variables affecting their responses to bereavement are: the emotional closeness they shared with their ill sibling (the greater the degree of closeness, the more behaviour problems surviving children experienced after the death); and the cohesiveness of the family environment (the greater the degree of cohesiveness, the fewer behaviour problems were reported). Of particular importance also is the message they received from their parents about their

worth and place in the family unit, and occasionally from their dying sibling.

Bereavement counselling should be extended to other family members. Grandparents are frequently ignored. Nevertheless they suffer deeply for the loss of their grandchild, as well as for the pain experienced by their own bereaved children.

Health care professionals trained in bereavement counselling and family therapy may facilitate communication among family members.[47,48] Interventions are basically aimed at encouraging them to express and accept their personal, subjective, and unique way of grieving; to develop an altered sense of self and find a new balance within the family unit; to give meaning to their experience; and invest energy and love into new relationships. Professionals may mobilize the family network to provide constant care and support during a normal, long-lasting journey. According to parents' reports, 7 to 9 years after their child's death, the most prevalent factor contributing to their survival is 'close family ties'.[49]

Caring for the care provider

Professionals are also vulnerable to suffering from an accumulation of grief. As stated by one, 'Death is like a Sun: It may bring light to deeper levels of awareness and enhance the purpose of our life, but it may hurt the eyes and blind the soul when we are exposed to it for too long.'[33]

If the resulting stress that care providers experience remains unrecognized and no attempt is made to decrease it, they are most likely to develop symptoms leading to 'burnout'. By acknowledging their feelings and grief reactions, care givers may develop effective ways for dealing with stress, thereby preventing their feelings from interfering with their ability to provide care.[33,50] Professionals need the time, space and support to grieve over the loss of a particular child with whom they had been intimately involved. The existence of a staff support network is extremely significant and an integral part of the hospice concept. Death education and planned support meetings give care providers the opportunity to air their feelings, work through their grief, and find creative ways to care for themselves.

It has been frequently argued that an attitude of detached concern allows professionals to protect themselves from burning out, while providing care for their patients. This, however, becomes particularly difficult when the professional is involved in the care of a particular child for long periods of time and is deeply affected by his or her death. The concept of *mature concern*[32] may better describe the challenge for any care provider: to be able to identify with the pain of the other, but not with the other; to participate in the family's journey, and be affected by it, yet recognize that he or she cannot experience the family's journey, life and death as if they were his or her own; and to be willing to be personally challenged and grow as a human being.

References

1 Campbell, L. History of the hospice movement. *Cancer Nursing* 1986; **9**: 333–338.

2 Saunders, C. A therapeutic community: St. Christopher's Hospice. In: Schoenberg, B., Carr, A.C., Peretz, D., Kutscher, A.H., eds. *Psychosocial Aspects of Terminal Care*. New York: Columbia University Press, 1972.

3 International Work Group on Death, Dying and Bereavement. Assumptions and principles underlying standards for terminal care. *Am J Nursing* 1979; **79**: 296–297.

4 Saunders, C., Summers, D.H., Teller, N., eds. *Hospice: The Living Idea*. London: Edward Arnold, 1981.

5 Wheeler, P.R., Lange, N.F., Bertolone, S.J. Improving care for hospitalized terminally ill children: A practical model. In: Corr, C.A., Corr, D.M., eds. *Hospice Approaches to Pediatric Care*. New York: Springer Publishing Company, 1985, 43–60.

6 Dominica, F. Helen House: A hospice for children. *Mat Child Hlth* 1982; **7**: 355–359.

7 Siegel, R., Rudd, S.H., Cleveland, C., Powers, L.K., Harmon, R.J. A hospice approach to neonatal care. In: Corr, C.A., Corr, D.M., eds. *Hospice Approaches to Pediatric Care*. New York: Springer Publishing Company, 1985, 127–152.

8 Martinson, I.M., Moldow, D.G., Armstrong, G.D., Henry, W.F., Nesbit, M.E., Kersey, J.H. Home care for children dying of cancer. *Res Nursing Hlth* 1986; **9**: 11–16.

9 Martin, B.B. Home care for terminally ill children and their families. In: Corr, C.A., Corr, D.M., eds. *Hospice Approaches to Pediatric Care*. New York: Springer Publishing Company, 1985, 63–86.

10 Lauer, M.E., Mulhern, R.K., Bohn, J.B., Camitta, B.M. Children's perception of their sibling's death at home or in the hospital: the precursors of differential adjustment. *Cancer Nursing* 1985; **8**, 21–27.

11 Duffy, C.M., Pollock, R., Levy, M., *et al.* Home-based palliative care for children: the benefits of an established program. *J Palliative Care* 1990; **6**: 8–14.

12 Lauer, M.E., Mulhern, R.K., Wallskog, J.M., Camitta, B.M. A comparison study of parental adaptation following a child's death at home or in the hospital. *Pediatrics* 1983; **71**: 107–112.

13 Mulhern, R.K., Lauer, M.E., Hoffmann, R.G. Death of a child at home or in the hospital: subsequent psychological adjustment of the family. *Pediatrics* 1983; **71**: 743–747.

14 Moldow, D.G., Armstrong, G.D., Henry, W.F., Martinson, I.M. The cost of home care for dying children. *Med Care* 1982; **20**: 1154–1169.

15 Wilson, D.C. Developing a hospice program for children. In: Corr, C.A., Corr, D.M., eds. *Hospice Approaches to Pediatric Care*. New York: Springer Publishing Company, 1985, 5–29.

16 Martinson, I.M., Martin, B., Lauer, M., Birenbaum, L.K., Eng, B. *Children's Hospice/Home Care: an Implementation Manual for Nurses*. Washington: Children's Hospice International, 1991.

17 Martin, B.B., ed. *Pediatric Hospice Care: What Helps?* Los Angeles: Children's Hospital of Los Angeles, 1989.

18 Hutter, J.J., Farrell, F.Z., Meltzer, P.S. Care of the child dying from cancer: home vs hospital. In: Papadatou, D., Papadatos, C., eds. *Children and Death*. Washington: Hemisphere Publishing Corporation, 1991, 197–208.

19 International Work Group on Death, Dying and Bereavement. Position statement: palliative care for children. *Death Studies* 1993; **17**: 277–280.

20 Woodson, R. Hospital care in terminal illness. In: Garfield, G.A., ed. *Stress and Survival*. St. Louis: The C.V. Mosby Company, 1979.

21 Lipman, A.G. Drug therapy in cancer pain. *Cancer Nursing* 1980; February: 39–46.

22 Eland, J.M., Anderson, J.E. The experience of pain in children. In: Jacox, A.K., ed. *Pain: A Source Book for Nurses and Other Health Professionals*. Boston: Little, Brown and Company, 1977, 453–473.

23 Swafford, L.I., Allen, D. Pain relief in the pediatric patient. *Med Clin North Am* 1968; **52**: 131–136.

24 Martinson, I.M., Geis, D., Anglim, M.A., Peterson, E., Nesbit, M., Kersey, J. Home care for the child. *Am J Nursing* 1977; **77**: 1815–1817.

25 Papadatou, D. Caring for dying adolescents. In: Pritchard, A.P., ed. *Proceedings of the Fifth International Conference on Cancer Nursing*, London 1988. London: Macmillan Press, 1989, 34–37.

26 Bluebond-Langner, M. *The Private Worlds of Dying Children*. New Jersey: Princeton University Press, 1978.

27 Kübler-Ross, E. The dying child. In: Papadatou, D., Papadatos, C., eds. *Children and Death*. Washington: Hemisphere Publishing Corporation, 1991, 147–160.

28 Raimbault, G. *L'Enfant et la Mort*. Toulouse: Editions Privat, 1983.

29 Furth, G. *The Secret World of Drawings: Healing Through Art*. Boston: Sego Press, 1988.

30 Baker, S.R. Utilizing art and imagery in death and dying counseling. In: Papadatou, D., Papadatos, C., eds., *Children and Death*. Washington: Hemisphere Publishing Corporation, 1991, 161–175.

31 Papadatou, D. The dying adolescent. *Acta Oncol* 1988; **27**: 837–839.

32 De M'Uzan, M. Le travail du trépas. In: *De l'Art A La Mort*. Paris: Editions Gallimard, 1977, 182–202.

33 Papadatou, D. Working with dying children: a professional's personal journey. In: Papadatou, D. Papadatos, C., eds. *Children and Death*. Washington: Hemisphere Publishing Corporation, 1991: 285–292.

34 Friedman, S.B., Chodoff, P., Mason, J., Hamburg, D.S. Behavioral observations on parents anticipating the death of a child. *Pediatrics* 1963; **32**, 610–625.

35 Futterman, E.H., Hoffman, I. Sabshin, M. Parental anticipatory mourning. In: Schoenberg, B., Carr, A.C., Peretz, D., Kutscher, A.H., eds. *Psychosocial Aspects of Terminal Care*. New York: Columbia University Press, 1972, 243–272.

36 Fulton, R. Gottesman, D.J. Anticipatory grief: a psychosocial concept reconsidered. *Br J Psychiatr* 1980; **137**: 45–54.

37 Rando, T.A., ed. A comprehensive analysis of anticipatory grief: perspectives, processes, promises and problems. In: *Loss and Anticipatory Grief*. Massachusetts: D.C. Health and Company/Lexington, 1986, 3–37.

38 Rando, T.A. ed. Understanding and facilitating anticipatory grief in the loved ones of the dying. In: *Loss and Anticipatory Grief*. Massachusetts: D.C. Health and Company/Lexington, 1986, 97–130.

39 Rando, T.A. An investigation of grief and adaptation in parents whose children have died from cancer. *J Pediatr Psychol* 1983; **8**: 3–20.

40 Speck, R., Attneave, C. *Family Networks*. New York: Vintage Books, 1973.

41 Rando, T.A. Parental adjustment to the loss of a child. In: Papadatou, D., Papadatos, C., eds., *Children and Death*. Washington: Hemisphere Publishing Corporation, 1991, 233–253.

42 McClowry, S.G., Davies, E.B., May, K.A., Kulenkamp, E.J., Martinson, I.M. The empty space phenomenon: the process of grief in the bereaved family. *Death Studies* 1987; **11**: 361–374.

43 Cain, A.C., Cain, B.S. On replacing a child. *J Am Acad Child Psychiatr* 1964; **3**: 443–456.

44 Pine, V.R., Brauer, C. Parental grief: a synthesis of theory, research and intervention. In: Rando, T.A., ed. *Parental Loss of a Child*. Champaign, Ill: Research Press, 1986, 59–96.

45 Martinson, I.M., Davies, E.B., McClowry, S.G. The long-term effect of sibling death on self-concept. *J Pediatr Nursing* 1987; **2**: 227–235.

46 Davies, E.B. The family environment in bereaved families and its relationship to surviving sibling behavior. *Child Hlth Care* 1980; **17**: 22–32.

47 Grebstein, L.C. Family therapy after a child's death. In: Rando, T.A., ed. *Parental Loss of a Child*. Champaign, Ill: Research Press, 1986, 429–449.

48 Davies, B., Spinetta, J. Martinson, I.M., McClowry, S., Kulenkamp, E. Manifestations of levels of functioning in grieving families. *J Fam Issues* 1986; **7**: 297–313.

49 Martinson, I.M. Grief is an individual journey: follow-up of families post death of a child with cancer. In: Papadatou, D., Papadatos, C., eds. *Children and Death*. Washington: Hemisphere Publishing Corporation, 1991, 255–265.

50 Vachon, M.L.S., Pakes, E. Staff stress in the care of the critically ill and dying child. In: Wass, H., Corr, C.A., eds. *Childhood and Death*. Washington: Hemisphere Publishing Corporation, 1984, 151–182.

18.2 Sudden infant death syndrome

Pamela Davies

Introduction

Sudden, unexpected and *unexplained* deaths of infants now form the most substantial part of post-neonatal mortality in many industrialized countries. They have been recognized in the medical literature for well over a century, but have reached prominence with the prevention or successful treatment of previously lethal illnesses. Only in the last decade or so have general practitioners and community and hospital paediatricians become more aware of the profound impact of these deaths on individual families. The great majority occur at home, unseen and unheard, making them a particular cause for community concern. They are often referred to as cot deaths, a description originally intended to include those sudden unexpected deaths for which a cause might be found at necropsy. The term *sudden infant death syndrome* (SIDS) was defined at an international conference in 1969 as 'the sudden death of any infant or young child, which is unexpected by history, and in which a thorough post mortem examination fails to demonstrate an adequate cause for death'.[1] A US working party has lately expanded this to include an examination of the death scene, and a review of the case history, while limiting the deaths to the first year of life. It is a difficult subject to write about succinctly as it is not a single entity, and its ramifications encompass almost all aspects of paediatrics.

Incidence

Sudden infant death syndrome as defined above is a diagnosis of exclusion. The numbers so classified will be dependent on the thoroughness of the post-mortem examination, on pathologists' understanding of what constitutes an adequate cause of death, and on whether or not a comprehensive enquiry into family circumstances is made at the time of death. Unfortunately, uniformity in these matters between regions and countries cannot be taken for granted. However SIDS was accepted as a registrable 'cause' of death in England and Wales in 1970; and was included in the International Classification of Diseases in 1979. An official rate for England and Wales can be compiled from figures provided in good faith by the Office of Population Censuses and Surveys. It had hovered close to 2 per 1000 live births until 1988, since when it has apparently more than halved. Rather similar figures have been reported from Northern Ireland and Scotland, and from areas of Australia, Canada and the USA. Lower rates might be expected in countries with much lower overall infant mortality rates than the UK. This is borne out by a post-perinatal SIDS rate of 0.94/1000 for four large urban areas of Sweden during the years 1984–86,[2] and a post-neonatal rate of 0.3/1000 for Hong Kong for 1986–89.[3] The latter's astonishingly low figure contrasts starkly with that given for the southern island of New Zealand, 6.3/1000 between 1979 and 1984.[4] Ethnic differences in rate inside a single country have also been reported. Lower post-neonatal rates of sudden infant death were found in England and Wales between 1982 and 1985 in infants of mothers born in Asia and Africa when compared with those for infants of mothers born in the UK or Irish Republic. These figures were standardized for maternal age, parity and social class.[5] Blacks in the USA have a rate twice that of whites.[6]

Epidemiology

If there are difficulties in ascertaining true SIDS rates, so-called proven epidemiological associations must also be regarded warily for a condition that has so many facets. What seems undisputed is that disproportionately few of the deaths occur in the neonatal period, and very few after about 8 months of age. Most occur between 2 and 6 months with a peak around 3 months. A similar age pattern, at much lower rates, is seen only for the injury and accident category of infant deaths. When all registered SIDS deaths are considered with all other infant deaths from known causes, there are few distinguishing features. Thus they occur relatively more commonly in infants born to young, unsupported mothers who have received antenatal care late or not at all, to mothers who smoke, and to those with husbands in social classes IV and V. The deaths are relatively more common in infants of low birthweight (whether due to preterm birth or intrauterine growth retardation), among multiple births, among artificially fed babies, and among those who are seen irregularly or not at all at child health clinics. Second or subsequent births in a family are more frequently involved than the first. Although some of the infants have died before immunization schedules were due to start, when a comparison has been made with age-matched controls, SIDS infants are less likely to have begun or completed their schedules. It must always be emphasized that many of the categories mentioned above are minority ones, and deaths occur in infants of normal birthweight, born to non-smoking, breast-feeding women of social class I

and II families who have had early and regular antenatal care, and who attend regularly with their infants at child health clinics. Two-thirds of the deaths occur in the winter months, October to March; and two-thirds are discovered between 0400 and 1200 hours. The male:female ratio is 1.4:1.[6,7]

Clinical features

This may seem an anachronistic heading as by definition the deaths are traditionally thought of as sudden and unexpected. But it is worth emphasizing that signs of illness, often minor, are frequently present in young infants. A prospective Cambridge study of 298 infants less than 6 months old seen at home revealed, after direct questioning, that 81% of mothers reported such signs within the last 24 hours.[8] The largest study in which the history of SIDS infants has been compared with that of controls was organized by the US National Institute of Child Health and Human Development; 757 SIDS infants and two sets of living controls, each with an equivalent number, one matched for age, the other for age, birthweight and race (black or non-black) but neither for season, were included. Diarrhoea and vomiting, and a 'listless or droopy' appearance were highly significantly more likely in the SIDS victims in the 2 weeks before their death (including the last 24 hours), though numbers involved were small. Colds and coughs were not more common.[9] A smaller but prospective 2-year case-controlled study based on a geographically defined area (four health districts in Avon and North Somerset) reported 95 sudden infant deaths (seven of them explained at post-mortem examination, the remainder classified as SIDS). They were compared with 190 living controls matched for age, time of year and area. Major signs* of illness occurred in 21% of the index cases in the 24 hours before death compared with 9% of controls. Minor signs† were significantly more common 2 weeks (39% versus 23%), one week (33% versus 16%) and 24 hours (23% versus 5%) before death among the 95 index infants compared with the 190 controls. Three times as many index cases were seen by their family practitioners in the week before the death (18% versus 6%).[10]

The mode of death

The nature of the deaths means that the exact sequence of events has rarely been recorded; and it is unlikely to be the same in all cases. Biochemical evidence of terminal hypoxia is suggested by raised lactic acid and

---

* Difficulty in breathing, wheezing, repeated coughing, drowsiness, missing more than one feed, vomiting more than half a feed, pyrexia, diarrhoea and irritability.
† Snuffles, occasional cough, off feeds but taking most of them, grizzly.

hypoxanthine levels in vitreous humour[11,12] and by raised brain lactate levels with low pH[13] in a proportion of cases. And although a sudden lethal cardiac arrhythmia has to remain a possibility in those not apparently terminally hypoxic, respiratory failure has certainly claimed more attention. However, deaths associated with profound hypoglycaemia or fits due to other central nervous system causes could also be associated with terminal hypoxia.

A previous episode of apnoea – the cessation of respiratory air flow – is reported by fewer than 10% of parents of SIDS infants. Apnoea may be central (breathing movements cease), obstructive, usually upper airway obstruction (ineffective breathing movements continue) or mixed. Those investigating *observed* episodes point out that they occur in the same age range as SIDS, and share some other associations. They are more likely to be seen between 0800 and 2000 hours.[2] The provoking causes are various, mainly involving the cardiorespiratory and central nervous systems, though occasionally none can be found.[14] It is natural to infer that had they occurred when the infant was *unobserved*, and appropriate prompt resuscitation unavailable, death might have followed in some cases. But recent evidence suggests that apnoea is not the immediately initiating event, but rather terminal; and that prolonged severe hypoxaemia – possibly caused by upper or lower airway obstruction, intrapulmonary shunting or both – and leading to bradycardia comes first.[15] The patency of the upper airway is ensured by the normal tone of various muscles. Thach has described a number of ways in which sudden airway obstruction can occur but which would be undetected at necropsy.[16] The intrathoracic petechial and blotchy haemorrhages seen on thymic, pleural and pericardial surfaces at post-mortem examination in a majority, though not in all, SIDS infants have been interpreted by him as evidence of increased negative intrathoracic pressure associated with upper airway obstruction.

Possible factors contributing to sudden infant death

Physiological vulnerability

In 1971 Froggatt and colleagues, investigating the epidemiology of sudden unexpected infant deaths in Northern Ireland, came to the conclusion that they were most likely explained by some critical combination of intrinsic and extrinsic factors proving lethal at a period of increased physiological vulnerability.[17] This hypothesis has not really been supplanted in the intervening 20 years. However, it would obviously be inapplicable to those infants (the exact proportion is uncertain and may vary in different parts of the country) who die at their parents' hands by smothering; the

evidence is often difficult or impossible to detect at post-mortem examination, but comes to light later.[18] The hypothesis too perhaps does not explain the paucity of unexplained deaths in the first 4 weeks of life, for the period of increased physiological vulnerability must surely start with the abrupt change from dependent to independent existence consequent on birth. But sleep states, metabolic rate, temperature regulation and cardiorespiratory control are certainly continuing to mature towards the adult pattern in an integrated way between 2 and 6 months.[19] Some intrinsic factors might be linked with the less favourable intrauterine environment suggested by some of the epidemiological associations. Central nervous system myelination for example has been shown to be just significantly delayed in SIDS infants compared with other carefully selected infant deaths matched for post-conceptional age.[20] Matthews has reviewed the likely role of the autonomic nervous system in SIDS;[21] and others have recorded that the higher heart rates and reduced heart rate variation found in infants subsequently dying suddenly without apparent cause compared with those in living controls, suggest alterations in autonomic control of the heart.[22] Some of the possibly relevant extrinsic factors are considered below.

Perception of symptoms

An adequate cause for death may be found at post-mortem examination in a proportion of infants who die suddenly and apparently unexpectedly. Serious bacterial or viral infection, unsuspected congenital abnormality or metabolic disease are among illnesses accounting for most of these. They were found in 19% of 134 such deaths between 1 week and 2 years of age in the DHSS Multicentre Study conducted between 1976 and 1979 in eight urban areas;[23] and in 7% of 95 in the Avon Study.[10] The frequency of signs of illness in early infancy has already been referred to. Mothers' appreciation of these, and their consequent actions have also been studied.[24–27] Whereas most parents seem competent in perceiving when a child is unwell,[24,26,27] a proportion apparently fail to recognize the importance of some signs or act inappropriately as also do some general practitioners (these proportions were 24% and 64% respectively in the Multicentre study[23]) and they may also fail to use available medical services.[28] Spencer has discussed how far this latter failure can be laid entirely at the feet of parents and concludes, from a personal survey and a review of the literature, that while factors inherent in the parents and their environment are partly responsible there are undoubted barriers erected by the primary health care services which are too difficult for many parents to surmount.[25] Field trials of a scoring system for symptoms and signs that can be used by mothers in the home, and by health professionals, suggest that its use would be mutually helpful in the assessment of the severity of illness.[29-32]

Sleeping position and clothing (see also infection)

Surveys which have compared the normal sleeping position in deaths registered as SIDS and in living controls have suggested the prone position is a risk factor.[10,33,34] Infants settled to sleep thus will not be able to roll over on to the side or back in the first months; a New Zealand survey showed that, for the majority, the waking position was still prone at 4 months of age. Infants settled for sleep on their sides on the other hand may roll over on to their backs during sleep.[35] Guntheroth states that a quarter of the dead babies are found face down with their airway against bedding, so that suffocation has to be a possibility.[6] It has also been suggested that heat loss is less effective in the prone position as more of the body's surface area is in contact with underbedding.[4] It has been shown that many mothers in the UK over-clothe and overwrap their offspring at night, sometimes to a marked degree.[36,37] Mothers in social classes IV and V tended to do this most commonly, particularly if they thought the infant was unwell; they also kept the room temperature higher. The Avon study too showed that overheating and the prone sleeping position were independently associated with an increased risk of sudden unexpected infant death.[38] These practices may stress the infant's temperature regulating ability and alter the subtle balance of other factors such as metabolic rate and cardiorespiratory control mechanisms. Beal and Porter have hypothesized that winter death rates from SIDS could be substantially reduced if infants under 6 months of age were tied into swaddling and slept supine as in Asia and Czechoslovakia where SIDS is uncommon; and if older infants who might resent such restriction had their cots made up so that their feet touched the lower end, making it less easy for them to burrow under blankets and reduce heat loss.[39]

Infection

The winter clustering of sudden infant deaths is the same as for first year deaths from proven respiratory infection.[40] While viruses from upper respiratory tract and gut were isolated more frequently from babies with sudden deaths than from controls in the Avon study, the difference was not significant, and the range of infecting organisms was similar. However, a combination of viral infection and wrapping in excess of 10 togs (a tog is a unit of thermal resistance) greatly increased the risk of death compared with wrapping of less than 6 togs.[41] Major signs (see section on clinical features above) were significantly more common among those unexpected deaths in whom non-polio

viruses were isolated than in those who were virus negative.[10]

Evidence of infection in the upper and lower respiratory tract is frequently found at post-mortem examination in deaths registered as SIDS, though by definition it is insufficient to account for them. Watkins and colleagues investigated patterns of respiratory illness in the first year of life. They found episodes of lower respiratory illness (defined as those with adventitial sounds present at one or more consultations) were particularly frequent in children of manual workers, yet this could not be explained by factors such as over-crowding, parental smoking habits and respiratory symptoms, or predominance of artificial feeding. They felt there was a need to consider nutrition and immunity more than environmental pollutants in future aetiological surveys.[42] Asian children in the UK are less likely to die from respiratory infection than other UK infants, and less likely to die sudden, unexpected and unexplained deaths.[5] Watkins and colleagues felt the relative freedom from respiratory illness in the first 3 months of life and its seasonal incidence made an infective rather than an allergic aetiology more likely. The possibility of an acute pulmonary anaphylaxis, first postulated by Coombs as a cause of sudden infant death, is again under investigation with the more sophisticated diagnostic tools now available,[43] and may explain a small proportion of cases. While Coombs considered cow's milk to be the likely allergen, viral antigens are also a possibility. The US study suggested gastrointestinal symptoms were more common in index cases than controls.[9] Evidence of some metabolic upset which might accompany gut infections was present in a small proportion of the DHSS survey infants.[23] The infant variety of botulism has been suspected as a cause of sudden infant deaths in the USA[44] and in some parts of Europe,[45] but has not been confirmed elsewhere.[46]

Metabolic disease

The extent to which undiagnosed inborn errors of metabolism might cause sudden unexpected death has come under scrutiny.[47] Certain disorders of fatty acid oxidation, notably medium-chain acyl-CoA dehydrogenase deficiency, have been incriminated by some[48] but not others.[49,50] So too has type 1 glycogen storage disease.[51] Profound hypoglycaemia would probably cause death. In this context it should be noted that in the Multicentre study 32% of infants dying at home had received their last feed 10 hours or more before death.[23]

Nurture

Despite acknowledged difficulties regarding uniformity of agreement on SIDS figures, it does appear there may be real ethnic differences in susceptibility.

While this could be due to differences in immunity were infection to be an important factor, the possible importance of subtle differences in nurture, including closeness of surveillance, is suggested. The very low rate among Hong Kong infants, if genuine, is the most striking.[3] It seems likely that babies there are rarely, if ever, left alone. The Multicentre study reported that 12% and 24% of infants dying at home had last been seen alive 10 hours or 8 hours or more respectively before the death was discovered.[23] Other such aspects of infant care are in need of careful prospective study.

The post-mortem examination

As the deaths have not occurred under medical care, they are by law reported to the coroner (procurator fiscal in Scotland). His officer, often a uniformed policeman, may visit the home, inspect the infant's bedding and question the parents about the circumstances of the death. No systematic details of such items as normal sleeping position, position when found, position of the cot in the room, temperature and ventilation of the room, or time and nature of last feed are routinely recorded. These details might be of relevance to the post-mortem examination which is conducted by a pathologist chosen and paid by the coroner. This may be an individual whose main interest is forensic, aiming only to exclude an unnatural form of death, rather than one knowledgeable about the developmental pathology of infancy and keen to exclude as far as possible its common and more esoteric disorders. Watson investigated 98 deaths registered as SIDS in Inner North London and West London during 1982 and 1983. She found that no histological examination of tissues had been made in 14%. Viral or bacterial cultures were made in under half of the cases, and the same applied to investigations for chromosomal, toxicological and radiological abnormalities.[52] Low standards of post-mortem examination are disheartening and must surely cast doubt on the validity of collected statistics. Wigglesworth and colleagues have drawn up a basic minimum of investigation of apparent SIDS cases, to be expanded as time and facilities permit or as specific research is being undertaken.[53] In contrast to most perinatal and neonatal deaths, sudden infant deaths occurring at home have only rarely been the subject of detailed enquiry by those involved in the family's care, once the pathologist's examination is complete. It is hoped that, in future, this may become routine; hitherto unsuspected clues about the deaths may be revealed, or the primary health care team could be alerted to the special needs of the family.[54]

Impact of SIDS on families

This has been poignantly described by affected parents.[7,55] It seems unlikely that time could ever obliterate completely the shocking memory of the moment of discovery of the death of an apparently thriving and cherished infant – a discovery often made by one or other parent who occasionally may be the only adult in the house at the time. Sometimes the infant may be just alive, and resuscitation is attempted. The intensity of the emotions experienced may well be greater than that following infant death occurring during hospitalization for illness, especially if a supportive staff there have been able to prepare parents and answer all their questions. The nature of SIDS entails the involvement of the coroner and the home visit of his officer; the non-contributory nature of the post-mortem examination, and possible publicity surrounding the occasional inquest make it small wonder that this 'distressing aftermath of official enquiry' is accompanied by such feelings of 'bewilderment, recrimination and frustration' as Jepson aptly puts it.[56] Guilt too, often irrational, is felt especially by mothers and may cause tension between spouses and members of the wider family. Paediatricians also have to be aware of the impact of the deaths on surviving siblings. The permanence of death is appreciated only by older children, but the tragedy will affect children of all ages in some way, as will their parents' ensuing grief and often depression.

The role of voluntary organizations

Bereaved parents in many parts of the world have formed themselves into voluntary organizations, and through these have been largely responsible for creating the (artificial) entity of SIDS, and for bringing the subject to the attention of governments and of doctors. The latter in turn have gradually come to realize the size of the problem, and the intensity of the shock, bewilderment, grief, anger and guilt engendered by the deaths; to acknowledge that health professionals have a vital role to play in helping affected families back to near normality and to support them before and after the birth of subsequent siblings. The longest established of these organizations* in Great Britain is the Foundation for the Study of Infant Deaths, started in 1971. Its three aims – to provide support for bereaved parents, to act as a centre of information, and to fund research into sudden infant death – have been largely followed by other groups set up later. The charities have provided the bulk of the money and impetus for research into the subject and have been a

---

* The Foundation for the Study of Infant Deaths, 35 Belgrave Square, London SW1X 8QB; The Scottish Cot Death Trust, Royal Hospital for Sick Children, Yorkhill, Glasgow G3 8SJ; and Irish Sudden Infant Death Association, 13 Christchurch Place, Dublin 8.

source of comfort for many families. They have organized a network of bereaved parents in many areas of the country who have come to terms with their own grief and who are able to befriend and support the newly bereaved.

As a result of her many years work with the Foundation and with health professionals, Limerick has summarized the management of sudden infant death which can be adapted to health care and legal systems in various countries. Her recommendations include 'speedy notification of the death to the family's normal health care advisers, and guidelines for immediate management by hospital accident and emergency staff. Parents need written information and the opportunity to talk with someone compassionate and informed about sudden infant deaths. Suggestions for doctors and nurses stress the importance of immediate support, early explanation of the post-mortem report, and continued befriending by other suitable parents. Later counselling should be offered to discuss the care of future children and re-build parent confidence.'[57]

Education about sudden infant death has been necessary not only for community and hospital paediatricians, obstetricians, general practitioners, health visitors, midwives, and the staff of accident and emergency departments, but also for coroners, coroner's officers, ambulance crews, the police, ministers of religion and funeral directors – in short all those coming into immediate contact with the families. The widely circulated Department of Health leaflet *Reducing the Risk of Cot Death* is for all in contact with, or caring for babies.[58] Such education has to be a continuing process because of rapid staff turnover in some categories. As the deaths receive more and more publicity and the organizations endeavour to protect parents from the more sensational claims about causation, they gain more respect from health professionals by acknowledging that some infants dying suddenly and unexpectedly do so at their parents' (usually the mother's) hands, and perhaps in the future may consider ways in which such deaths might be reduced. Child abuse has all too many aspects, and in another context it has been said there are forces in society denying it as a possibility and preventing exploration of the issue.[59] It would be sad if the organizations concerned with sudden infant death were ever to be seen in this light.

Recurrence risks

The low frequency of recurrence of SIDS within families, and a similar rate for monozygous and dizygous twins do not suggest genetically determined disorders commonly cause sudden unexpected deaths.[6] A small proportion of families do have a significantly increased risk. Thus Beal and Blundell studying 187 SIDS infants in South Australia found this to be true

of 8% of the total.[60] Roberts and colleagues identified 160 families through a sibling who had been abused before the age of 1 year. Infant deaths from all causes in the 332 other children from these families were three times those expected when correction was made for legitimacy, social class, maternal age and parity distribution. Deaths registered as SIDS too were about four times those expected.[61] Emery has investigated families with a previous death registered as SIDS, and in whom a further one or more siblings died suddenly and unexpectedly. Two main groups seemed to emerge. One consisted of infants in whom a variety of conditions were found at post-mortem investigation, most familial, suggesting the original death may well have been inadequately investigated and wrongly designated as SIDS. The other group consisted of deaths in which there was either proven evidence or strong suspicion of filicide.[18]

Prevention

A wider community approach

Infant mortality rates are generally agreed to be an important indicator of the well-being of a nation. The UK's position in the world rankings has not been an enviable one for many years. While perinatal and neonatal rates have shown a continuing significant fall in the last two decades, the same is not true of those first year deaths occurring after the first week or month of life. With so many of the latter occurring apparently suddenly and unexpectedly in the home, the onus for improvement must fall heavily on those concerned with community care.

This onus is particularly great in deprived inner city areas and, with the experience of one such area in mind, Polnay has argued cogently for the integration of hospital and community-based services for children into a combined district paediatric service; one which has the added benefit of preventing the isolation felt by many working in the community services.[62] But the child health clinic is surely the linchpin of paediatric services, whether in an urban or rural area. However, as we have seen, deaths registered as SIDS occur relatively more commonly in those who have been brought to their clinic irregularly or not at all. This usually means that mothers do not see the clinics as attractive, welcoming or conveniently sited places, and may find the staff censorious and unduly critical. Jenkins has emphasized the need for flexibility of approach and for consistency of advice offered by those working in child health clinics. The meeting of social needs, and the provision of health education within the clinic complex for a variety of groups are also stressed.[63] Perhaps the whole ethos is best summed up by Spencer: 'lasting improvements in child health demand the strengthening of primary care by both parents and services based on an effective, mutually respecting partnership of parents and professionals. Awareness and respect for parental skills would be a step in the right direction.'[25] One hopes that the greater involvement of primary care teams in the provision of child health services previously delivered from community clinics will promote these improvements.

Sleeping position and bedding

Evidence reviewed here, and more widely elsewhere with regard to the apparent recent fall in incidence[64] suggests that unless there is a very clear-cut medical indication (such as the Pierre Robin syndrome), small babies should be settled for sleep on their back (preferably, or sides) rather than prone. Care should be taken to see that they are not overwrapped, particularly when unwell. Coverings with a high tog value such as duvets should be avoided.

Risk scoring system

Carpenter and colleagues have developed, and used for intervention over many years, a risk scoring system for the identification of infants at high risk of dying suddenly and unexpectedly. Total scores have been calculated at birth and at 1 month of age from a number of differently weighted variables. Infants with scores above 800 are at very much greater risk of dying than those with scores below 400. Family doctors and health visitors have been alerted to high-risk families, and health visitor intervention has included an increased number of home visits and naked weighing of the infant there five times in the first 6 months of life. It is claimed that mortality in the high risk group has been reduced by more than 50%.[65] The sensitivity and specificity are insufficiently high, and critics have argued that application of the Sheffield scoring system to other populations has not always given similar results.[66] Only a very large randomized controlled trial with careful control of the nature of the health visitor input and rigorous standardization of postmortem findings could decide whether this form of intervention is of value.

Smoking

Parental smoking is an acknowledged risk factor for infant death. Measurement of nicotine and its major metabolite cotinine in pericardial fluid at autopsy in 24 sudden infant deaths, both SIDS and non-SIDS, showed environmental exposure to tobacco in over two thirds.[67] Parents all too rarely get the constructive and practical help needed to overcome their addiction.

Apnoea monitors

Increasing awareness of SIDS and ill-informed publicity about apnoea monitors, whether respiratory, cardiorespiratory or transcutaneous, create difficulties for parents and health professionals alike. Yet there is no scientifically validated evidence to show that their use does, or does not, prevent SIDS. Again a randomized controlled trial involving many thousands of infants would be needed to prove efficacy or otherwise, and is unlikely to be mounted in the UK. The monitors at present in widest use in the home here are respiratory monitors, detecting central apnoea only. Elsewhere cardiorespiratory monitors have been used to signal the bradycardia that may accompany obstructive apnoea while ineffective breathing movements continue. None of the respiratory monitors currently available is entirely satisfactory. The same is true of cardiorespiratory monitors. Little is known about harmful aspects of home monitoring, for adequately conducted surveys are few. Their results suggest some stress is always apparent, and further studies are needed.

Some infants who have had life-threatening apnoeic episodes may need some form of monitoring if the nature of the provoking event can be accurately identified. As already stated, the evidence that apnoea is the final pathway to death in a proportion, even a majority of sudden unexplained deaths is tentative only; and the obstructive (upper airway) variety rather than central apnoea has more proponents. Parents who have had a sudden unexpected infant death are often acutely anxious when subsequent siblings are born. Comprehensive support over the ensuing months is important for those families, and at present this often seems to include a monitoring device of as yet unproven benefit and for which there may be little rationale. If such alarms are used it should be under close professional supervision with technical backup, and accompanied by instruction in infant resuscitation technique.

Perhaps in view of reported ethnic differences in SIDS, more notice should be taken of the fact that small infants in some cultures never sleep alone in the first months of life.[68]

Conclusions

Sudden, unexpected infant deaths which are unexplained and therefore registered as SIDS are not a single entity. As the majority occur at home they must particularly concern doctors working in the community. While more searching investigations at postmortem examination, sometimes involving specialist laboratories, may uncover illnesses at present undiagnosed, there is also need for a searching but sensitively conducted enquiry at the scene of death, and as soon as possible after it, into the infant's immediate environment. Later, when pathological investigations are completed, there should be a thorough review of all information relevant to the previous history and death of the infant, and to the wider family circumstances. When this is done it is likely that far fewer of the deaths will be unexplained.

The intensity of the emotions engendered by the deaths, and the families' need for immediate and continuing support and explanation should be appreciated. The problem of post-neonatal mortality in general rests mainly with the primary health care services. The more flexible these can be in allowing and encouraging ready access for parents of young children at all times, and the more ready they are to foster good and skilful professional relationships with them, the more successful will they be in reducing the present unnecessary toll of deaths.

References

1 Beckwith, J.B. In: Bergman, A.B., Beckwith, J.B., Ray, C.G., eds. *Sudden Infant Death Syndrome*. Seattle: University of Washington Press, 1970, 18.

2 Wennergren, G., Milerad, J., Lagercrantz, H., *et al*. The epidemiology of sudden infant death syndrome and attacks of lifelessness in Sweden. *Acta Paediatr Scand* 1987; **76**: 898–906.

3 Lee, N.N.Y., Chan, Y.F., Davies, D.P., Lau, E., Yip, D.C.P. Sudden infant death syndrome in Hong Kong: confirmation of low incidence. *Br Med J* 1989; **298**: 721.

4 Nelson, E.A.S., Taylor, B.J., Weatherall, I.L. Sleeping position and infant bedding may predispose to hyperthermia and the sudden infant death syndrome. *Lancet* 1989; **i**: 199–201.

5 Balarajan, R., Raleigh, V.S., Botting, B. Sudden infant death syndrome and postneonatal mortality in immigrants in England and Wales. *Br Med J* 1989; **298**: 716–720.

6 Guntheroth, W.G. *Crib Death: the Sudden Infant Death Syndrome*. 2nd edn. Mount Kisco, NY: Futura Publishing Company, 1989.

7 Golding, J., Limerick, S., Macfarlane, A. *Sudden Infant Death: Patterns, Puzzles and Problems*. Somerset: Open Books Publishing, 1985.

8 Thornton, A.J., Morley, C.J., Hewson, P.H., Cole, T.J., Fowler, M.A., Tunnacliffe, J.M. Symptoms in 298 infants under 6 months old seen at home. *Arch Dis Child* 1990; **65**: 280–285.

9 Hoffman, H.F., Damus, K., Hillman, L., Krongrad, E. Risk factors for SIDS: results of the National Institute of Child Health and Human Development SIDS Cooperative Epidemiological Study. *Ann NY Acad Sci* 1988; **533**: 13–30.

10 Gilbert, R.E., Fleming, P.J., Azaz, Y., Rudd, P.T. Signs of illness preceding sudden unexpected death in infants. *Br Med J* 1990; **300**: 1237–1239.

11 Sturner, W.Q., Sullivan, A. Suzuki, K. Lactic acid concentrations in vitreous humor: their use in asphyxial deaths in children. *J Forensic Sci* 1983; **28**: 222–230.

12 Rögnum, T.O., Saugstad, O.D., Øyasaeter, S. Olaisen, B. Elevated levels of hypoxanthine in vitreous humor indicate prolonged cerebral hypoxia in victims of sudden infant death syndrome. *Pediatrics* 1988; **82**: 615–618.

13 Buttterworth, J., Tennant, M.C. Postmortem human brain pH and lactate in sudden infant death syndrome. *J Neurochem* 1989; **53**: 1494–1499.

14 Simpson, H., MacFadyen, U. Near-miss of sudden infant death syndrome: a clinical approach. In: Meadow, R., ed. *Recent Advances in Paediatrics*, 1986; **8**: 201–216.

15 Poets, C.F., Southall, D.P. Recent developments in research into sudden infant death. *Thorax* 1994; **49**: 196–197.

16 Thach, B.T. The potential role of airway obstruction in sudden infant death syndrome. In: Culbertson, J.L., Krous, H.F., Bendell, R.D., eds. *Sudden Infant Death Syndrome: Medical Aspects and Psychological Management*. London: Edward Arnold, 1988, 62–93.

17 Froggatt, P., Lynas, M.A., MacKenzie, G. Epidemiology of sudden and unexpected death in infants ('cot death') in Northern Ireland. *Br J Prev Soc Med* 1971; **25**: 119–134.

18 Emery, J.L. Infanticide, filicide, and cot death. *Arch Dis Child* 1985; **60**: 505–507.

19 Johnson, P. Airway reflexes and the control of breathing in postnatal life. *Ann NY Acad Sci* 1988; **533**: 262–275.

20 Kinney, H.C., Brody, B.A., Finkelstein, D.M., Vawter, G.F., Mandell, F., Gilles, F.H. Delayed central nervous system myelination in the sudden infant death syndrome. *J Neuropathol Exp Neurol* 1991; **50**: 29–48.

21 Matthews, T.G. The autonomic nervous system: the role in sudden infant death syndrome. *Arch Dis Child* 1992; **67**: 654–656.

22 Schechtman, V.L., Raetz, S.L., Harper, R.K., *et al*. Dynamic analysis of cardiac R–R intervals in normal infants and in infants who subsequently succumbed to the sudden infant death syndrome. *Pediatr Res* 1992; **31**: 606–612.

23 Knowelden, J., Keeling, J., Nicholl, J.P. *Post Neonatal Mortality: a Multicentre Study undertaken by the Medical Care Research Unit, University of Sheffield*. London: HMSO, 1985, 1–52.

24 Pattison, C.J., Drinkwater, C.K., Downham, M.A.P.S. Mothers' appreciation of their children's symptoms. *J R Coll Gen Practit* 1982; **32**: 149–162.

25 Spencer, N.J. Parents' recognition of the ill child. In: Macfarlane, J.A., ed. *Progress in Child Health, volume I*. Edinburgh: Churchill Livingstone, 1984, 100–112.

26 Campion, P.D., Gabriel, J. Illness behaviour in mothers with young children. *Soc Sci Med* 1985; **20**: 325–330.

27 Cunningham-Burley, S., Irvine, S. 'And have you done anything so far?' An examination of lay treatment of children's symptoms. *Br Med J* 1987; **295**: 700–702.

28 McWeeny, P.M., Emery, J.L. Unexpected postneonatal deaths (cot deaths) due to recognizable disease. *Arch Dis Child* 1975; **50**: 191–196.

29 Morley, C.J., Thornton, A.J., Cole, T.J., Hewson, P.H., Fowler, M.A. Baby Check: a scoring system to grade the severity of acute systemic illness in babies under 6 months old. *Arch Dis Child* 1991; **66**: 100–105.

30 Thornton, A.J., Morley, C.J., Green, S.J., Cole, T.J.,

Walker, K.A., Bonnett, J.M. Field trials of the Baby Check Score Card: mothers scoring their babies at home. *Arch Dis Child* 1991; **66**: 106–110.

31 Morley, C.J., Thornton, A.J., Green, S.J., Cole, T.J. Field trials of the Baby Check Score Card in general practice. *Arch Dis Child* 1991; **66**: 111–114.

32 Thornton, A.J., Morley, C.J., Cole, T.J., Green, S.J., Walker, K.A., Rennie, J.M. Field trials of the Baby Check Score Card in hospital. *Arch Dis Child* 1991; **66**: 115–120.

33 Beal, S. Sleeping position and SIDS (letter). *Lancet* 1988; **i**: 512.

34 Dwyer, T., Ponsonby, A-L.P., Newman, N., Gibbons, L.E. Prospective cohort study of prone sleeping position and sudden infant death syndrome. *Lancet* 1991; **337**: 1224–1247.

35 Hassall, I.B., Vandenberg, M. Infant sleeping position: a New Zealand survey. *N Z Med J* 1985; **98**: 97–99.

36 Bacon, C.J. The thermal environment of sleeping babies and possible dangers of overheating. In: David, T.J., ed. *Recent Advances in Paediatrics*. Edinburgh: Churchill Livingstone, 1990, 123–136.

37 Bacon, C.J., Bell, S.A., Clulow, E.E., Beattie, A.B. How mothers keep their babies warm. *Arch Dis Child* 1991; **66**: 627–632.

38 Fleming, P.J., Gilbert, R., Azaz, Y., Berry, P.J., Rudd, P.T., Stewart, A. Interaction between bedding and sleeping position in the sudden infant death syndrome: a population based case-control study. *Br Med J* 1990; **301**: 85–89.

39 Beal, S., Porter, C. Sudden infant death syndrome related to climate. *Acta Paediatr Scand* 1991; **80**: 278–287.

40 Limerick, S. Sudden death in infancy (cot death). Hugh Greenwood Lecture, University of Exeter, 1987.

41 Gilbert, R., Rudd, P., Berry, P.J., *et al*. Combined effect of infection and heavy wrapping on the risk of sudden unexpected infant death. *Arch Dis Child* 1992; **67**: 171–177.

42 Watkins, C.J., Sittampalam, Y., Morrell, D.C., Leeder, S.R., Tritton, E. Patterns of respiratory illness in the first year of life. *Br Med J* 1986; **293**: 794–796.

43 Coombs, R.R.A., Holgate, S.T. Allergy and cot death: with special focus on allergic sensitivity to cows' milk and anaphylaxis. *Clin Exp Allergy* 1990; **20**: 359–366.

44 Arnon, S.S., Midura, T.F., Damus, K., Wood, R.M., Chin, J. Intestinal infection and toxin production by *Clostridium botulinum* as one cause of sudden infant death syndrome. *Lancet* 1987; **i**: 1273–1277.

45 Sonnabend, O.A.R., Sonnabend, W.F.F., Krech, U., Molz, G., Sigrist, T. Continuous microbiological and pathological study of 70 sudden and unexpected infant deaths: toxigenic intestinal *Clostridium botulinum* infection in 9 cases of sudden infant death syndrome. *Lancet* 1985; **i**: 237–241.

46 Byard, R.W., Moore, L., Bourne, A.J., Lawrence, A.J., Goldwater, P.N. *Clostridium botulinum* and sudden infant death syndrome: a 10 year prospective study. *J Paediatr Child Hlth* 1992; **28**: 156–157.

47 Emery, J.L., Howat, A.J., Variend, S., Vawter, G.F. Investigation of inborn errors of metabolism in unexpected infant deaths. *Lancet* 1988; **i**: 29–31.

48 Howat, A.J., Bennett, M.J., Variend, S., Shaw, L., Engel, P.C. Defects of metabolism of fatty acids in the sudden infant death syndrome. *Br Med J* 1985; **290**: 1771–1773.

49 Miller, M.E., Brooks, J.G., Forbes, N., Insel, R. Frequency of medium-chain acyl-CoA dehydrogenase deficiency G-985 mutation in sudden infant death syndrome. *Pediatr Res* 1992; **31**: 305–307.

50 Holton, J.B., Allen, J.T., Green, C.A., Partington, S., Gilbert, R.E., Berry, P.J. Inherited metabolic diseases in the sudden infant death syndrome. *Arch Dis Child* 1991; **66**: 1315–1317.

51 Burchell, A., Bell, J.E., Busuttil, A., Hume, R. Hepatic microsomal glucose-6-phosphatase system and sudden infant death syndrome. *Lancet* 1989; **ii**: 291–294.

52 Watson, E. Changes in verdict of sudden infant death [letter]. *Lancet* 1985; **i**: 631.

53 Wigglesworth, J.S., Keeling, J.W., Rushton, D.I., Berry, P.J. Pathological investigations in cases of sudden infant death. *J Clin Pathol* 1987; **40**: 1481–1483.

54 Taylor, E.M., Emery, J.L. Trends in unexpected infant deaths in Sheffield. *Lancet* 1988; **ii**: 1121–1123.

55 Luben, J. *Cot Deaths: Coping with Sudden Infant Death Syndrome*. London: Bedford Square Press, 1989.

56 Jepson, M.E. *Community Child Health*. London: Hodder and Stoughton, 1983, 60.

57 Limerick, S. Family and health-professional interactions. *Ann NY Acad Sci* 1988; **533**: 145–154.

58 Department of Health. *Reducing the Risk of Cot Death*. London: HMSO, 1992. (Leaflet BTS 1/E).

59 Fulginiti, V.A., Krugman, R.D. Cleveland, England: child abuse in the public eye. *Am J Dis Child* 1989; **143**: 651–652.

60 Beal, S.M., Blundell, H.K. Recurrence incidence of sudden infant death syndrome. *Arch Dis Child* 1988; **63**: 924–930.

61 Roberts, J., Lynch, M.A., Golding, J. Postneonatal mortality in children from abusing families. *Br Med J* 1980; **281**: 102–104.

62 Polnay, L. The community paediatric team: an approach to child health services in a deprived inner city area. In: Macfarlane, J.A., ed. *Progress in Child Health, Vol 1*. Edinburgh: Churchill Livingstone, 1984, 187–198.

63 Jenkins, S. The functions of child health clinics. In: Macfarlane, J.A., ed. *Progress in Child Health, Vol 1*. Edinburgh: Churchill Livingstone, 1984, 199–212.

64 Guntheroth, W.G., Spiers, P.S. Sleeping prone and the risk of sudden infant death syndrome. *JAMA* 1992; **267**: 2359–2362.

65 Carpenter, R.G., Gardner, A., Harris, J., *et al*. Prevention of unexpected death: a review of risk-related intervention in six centres. *Ann NY Aca Sci* 1988; **533**: 96–105.

66 Madeley, R.J., Hull, D., Elwood, J.M. Evaluation of the Nottingham Birth Scoring System. *Ann NY Acad Sci* 1988; **533**: 106–118.

67 Milerad, J., Rajs, J., Gidlund, E. Nicotine and cotinine levels in pericardial fluid in victims of SIDS. *Acta Paediatr* 1994; **83**: 59–62.

68 Davies, D.P., Gantley, M. Ethnicity and the aetiology of sudden infant death syndrome. *Arch Dis Child* 1994; **70**: 349–353.

Chapter 19

Community child health in developing countries

Michael Chan

Introduction

Three-quarters of the world's five billion people live in developing countries. Each year the world's population increases by more than 80 million, 40 million die and more than 122 million are born. Over half the births, 73 million, take place in Asia, 20 million are born in Africa and 12 million in Latin America. Only 15 million births take place in the industrialized world.

Children form a substantial proportion, between 35 and 50%, of the population in most developing countries. Together with their mothers they are in the majority but the health care system is not geared primarily to their needs. The mother and child constitute a biological and social dyad; therefore it would be inappropriate to discuss child health problems without mentioning the mother, particularly in developing countries where the infant's survival depends to a large extent on mother's care.

Most people in developing countries live in rural villages without the benefits of clean piped water, sanitation and electricity. Children are therefore expected to assist their parents in collecting fuel and fetching water for domestic use. Rural communities suffer other disadvantages such as poor roads and transport, and inadequate access to health facilities and schools. The combination of these adverse factors with diminishing agricultural yields has prompted rural people to migrate to the cities, a growing phenomenon called the *urban drift*. When they arrive in the city, these migrants usually find themselves worse off because they are forced to live in peri-urban slums. The plight of children in these insanitary slums is grim. They are exposed to communicable diseases that are rife because of the appalling overcrowding and the septic environment. Facilities for health care and education are even scarcer in the slums than in rural areas of developing countries. Poverty forces parents to send their children to work in factories where their labour is exploited and their health put at high risk. There are about 140 million children working, from weaving carpets to humping bricks, in the developing world. Some 30 million children are forced to live on the streets of Latin America, Asia and Africa. This is the depressing reality in most of the developing countries of the tropics.

Health indicators in tropical developing countries are very poor when compared with those of industrialized countries, in spite of the decline of mortality in recent decades. Child death rates in Africa, for example, have dropped by 40% since 1950 when one child in every three died before reaching 5 years of age and many others were crippled for life from a variety of causes. In 1990, high infant mortality rates above 100 per 1000 live births were found in 33 countries all in sub-Saharan Africa and Asia, while the lowest rates of 5 to 17 per 1000 included only nine countries outside Europe and North America. Infectious diseases including malaria contribute substantially to infant mortality in the tropics with measles accounting for one million deaths and neonatal tetanus, pertussis and polio another million deaths in 1990. It has been estimated that diarrhoeal diseases are responsible for as many deaths in pre-school children as acute respiratory infections, i.e. about four million every year. Infants of low birthweight are at higher risk of disease and death than normal babies; and 90% of the world's low birthweight babies are born in developing countries. The major causes of infant mortality in developing countries are similar to those which prevailed in industrialized countries at the beginning of this century. This similarity suggests that socioeconomic factors rather than climate are significant contributors to infant mortality in the tropics. Higher death rates are recorded in rural than urban communities reflecting the lower socioeconomic status of agricultural workers.

A strong association between declines in infant mortality rates and improvements in basic sanitation and health services has been shown in some developing countries such as Brazil.[1] Surveys revealed this reduction in infant mortality was achieved despite any measurable improvement in the socioeconomic conditions or nutritional status of children in cities, e.g. São Paulo. Specific technologies widely recommended by the World Health Organization (WHO) and United Nations International Children's Emergency Fund (UNICEF) in the 1980s have had a significant impact on reducing infant mortality rates in developing countries. According to UNICEF, an estimated three million children in 1991 have been saved through national immunization programmes, oral rehydration therapy, and health education campaigns including breast feeding and growth monitoring, in the absence of social or economic change. As a result of these interventions, infant mortality rates are no longer an indicator of change in social development.

The Convention on the Rights of the Child, after a decade of detailed negotiations, was brought for adoption to the General Assembly of the United Nations at the end of 1989. This Convention aims to set universal standards for the defence of children against neglect, exploitation and abuse. It, therefore, should be of great importance for the well-being of children in the developing world. The provisions of the Convention apply to three main areas of children's rights: survival, development, and protection; but it also covers economic, sexual and other forms of child exploitation, and requires that appropriate measures be taken to protect children from the use and sale of drugs. The Convention recognizes the right of access to health care services, and to an adequate standard of living, including food, clean water, and a place to live. Many of the Convention's provisions are designed to provide protection for children in a wide range of circumstances. Some deal with mentally or physically disabled children, others with refugees or parentless children, or with children who are separated from their parents. More than 100 countries ratified the Convention by September 1990 at the World Summit for Children. The Convention includes follow-up measures designed to encourage compliance with its provisions by governments, private organizations and individuals. A Committee on the Rights of the Child has been established with ten experts serving in their personal capacities, and countries which ratify the Convention will report to the Committee on steps they have taken to comply with its provisions. It is expected that the Convention will provide a universally valid basis for advocacy on behalf of children everywhere.

Lack of resources for health

The experience of countries such as China, Costa Rica and Cuba, among others in the developing world, show that it is possible significantly to improve child survival with limited financial resources, if there is strong political will to implement effective policies in health and education, particularly of women. These have included primary health care interventions, community participation and development programmes. However, these measures have had limited impact on neonatal and perinatal mortality which account for about half the infant mortality of the developing world.

Notwithstanding the observations made about China, Costa Rica and Cuba, there has been a genuine lack of resources in the 1980s when global economic difficulties affected Africa most severely. Average incomes have fallen by 10 to 25% throughout most of Africa and much of Latin America. In 1986, Africa's earning from exports fell by US$19 billion. Debt repayments and falling commodity prices are the two main causes of economic decline in much of the developing world. Debts owed to industrialized countries totalled more than US$1000 billion. In 1988, debt and interest payments made by developing countries were US$178 billion or three times as much as all the aid received. On average, debt repayments claim almost 25% of the developing world's export revenues. Most debtor nations have been forced to adopt economic adjustment policies in an attempt to stave off balance-of-payments crises while meeting debt obligations, maintaining essential imports, and struggling to return to economic growth. Adjustment policies have taken the form of a dampening of demand, a devaluation of the currency, a withdrawal of subsidies on fuel and staple foods, and deep cuts in government spending. More than 70 developing nations are now adjusting their economies by such methods. Africa, afflicted by wars, drought and recession has been hardest hit. Military spending by developing nations amounted to US$145 billion in 1988, but there are signs that this expenditure is falling in China, India and Pakistan for the first time in 50 years. Total military expenditure in both industrialized and developing countries exceeds the combined annual incomes of the poorest half of humanity. The developing world spends about 30% more on the military than on health and education combined. Current annual expenditure on training a soldier amounts to $20 000 while only $350 is spent on educating a child.

Government expenditure on health in the 1980s fell in most countries of sub-Saharan Africa, in more than half the countries of Latin America and the Caribbean, and in one third of the nations of Asia. UNICEF reported that in the 37 poorest nations of the world, per capita expenditure on health fell by 25% and on education by 50% in the past decade. Over the last 5 years hundreds of health clinics have been closed down, and many that remained open are understaffed and lack essential supplies. For example, in the first part of 1989 the health services of Ecuador, Panama, Paraguay and Peru were unable even to buy vaccines.

Deterioration of child health

Infant mortality has risen in parts of Latin America and sub-Saharan Africa and the incidence of low birthweight has increased in some Latin American countries. These indicators reflect the deterioration of nutrition and health suffered by women and children in the 1980s. The impact of AIDS, particularly in Africa, cannot be overemphasized. An estimated 6–11% (3.1–5.5 million) of children will be orphaned in Central and East Africa during the 1990s as their parents die of AIDS. Pregnant women in Zaire and Uganda have a high incidence of HIV infection. Of more than a thousand women attending antenatal clinics in Kampala, Uganda, 13.4% were HIV-positive in 1986, but the proportion had risen to 24% by 1988. In the Rakai province of Uganda one in seven children has lost its mother.

Health care services for children

Common causes of ill health in children of developing countries, such as diarrhoea and acute respiratory infections, usually require hospital admission if early treatment is not available in the home or community. The absence or neglect of health care in the community has led to crowding of hospitals with very ill children who are not given optimum treatment because of the heavy call on inadequate resources of medical staff and drugs. Complications and death from these preventable diseases are frequent. Shortage of doctors nationally and their concentration in cities of developing countries where medical care is provided on payment makes hospital care an inefficient and expensive basis of health services for children. Current economic problems have brought further deterioration of hospital services. Therefore a hospital-based service is not a viable basis for the health care of children in developing countries, although the hospital is an essential component of a health service.

Primary health care

The health care needs of people in developing countries was the focus of the Alma Ata meeting in 1978.[2] Primary health care was the means by which health for all was to be achieved by the year 2000. The Alma Ata Declaration stated without ambiguity that primary health care 'involves, in addition to the health sector, all related sectors and aspects of national and community development – in particular, agriculture, animal husbandry, food, industry, education, housing, public works, communications – and demands the coordinated efforts of all those sectors.' Collaboration between the health service and other development sectors was seen as a vital basis for successful primary health care.

The essential components of primary health care outlined in the Alma Ata Declaration are:

1 Education of the people about prevailing health problems and methods of preventing and controlling them.
2 Promotion of food supply and proper nutrition.
3 Adequate supply of safe water and basic sanitation.
4 Maternal and child health care and family planning.
5 Immunization against major infectious diseases.
6 Prevention and control of locally endemic diseases.
7 Appropriate treatment of common diseases and injuries.
8 Provision of essential drugs.

However, this has not been achieved in many developing countries where the expectation for improvement in health has been exclusively placed on limited primary care. Funding of primary health care has come from financial cuts made at district level. Therefore, the implementation of the Alma Ata recommendations in most developing countries has been to the detriment of district health services and without reference to intersectoral development in the community. The consequence of this narrow approach to health care has been heavy reliance on simple technologies such as oral rehydration therapy and immunization without strengthening of the health service infrastructure. These interventions have been promoted with funding from foreign and international agencies that provide training and supplies for a maximum of 5 years after which the national budget is usually unable to maintain the service. Another disadvantage of this approach has been the lack of collaboration of these programmes and their non-integration into the national primary health care system. Short-term gains in improved child survival have occurred but continuing health care of children has been compromised.

The national financing of primary health care was addressed by a meeting of African health ministers in 1987 in Bamako, Mali. At this meeting UNICEF outlined a proposal for an imaginative solution to the problems of providing essential drugs and basic mother and child (MCH) facilities in sub-Saharan Africa: this proposal has become known as the Bamako Initiative. In essence, the Bamako Initiative suggested that essential drugs should be sold to patients at prices above cost price. The income generated thereby would be used to establish a revolving fund for drugs and to provide income for the local community to maintain and develop primary health care facilities. So far the implementation of this method of financing in some countries indicates that the poorest families in need of health care have been reluctant to attend health centres. Also the income generated is insufficient to buy drugs, most of which are manufactured outside Africa.

Integrated mother and child services

As the health of the young child is intimately bound up with that of the mother, a child health service in developing countries should cover a range of related activities, from family planning and antenatal care to the supervision of health of school children and adolescents. The reasons for this priority to be given to mothers and children were described by Cecily Williams in 1964.[3] They include: integrated comprehensive services optimize the interdependence of mother and child, and provide continuity of care; prevention and intervention during pregnancy, infancy, and childhood reduce morbidity and mortality; preventive services decrease childhood disability and the resulting social burden; the needs of women and children are often not understood because they are the least powerful members of society; providing women with the choice of child-spacing results in better health of mother and infant; and, new knowledge indicates that problems in childhood result in poor health in adulthood. In 1992, the government of India declared that mother and child health (MCH) would be its only health service priority for the next 5 years. Implementation of this policy will be based on the WHO's recommendations for the Safe Motherhood and Child Survival programmes.

In many developing countries MCH services are usually geared to young children under 5 years of age because they are at highest risk of disease and death. A comprehensive service should include treatment and prevention of disease, and the promotion of health. These must be incorporated in training, teaching, and research concerned with practical, fact-finding evaluation and improvement of services. There is a danger of dividing services for mothers from those that are primarily aimed at children and making accessibility difficult for women and their children. The Integrated Child Development Service (ICDS) in India is a good example of an integrated service for mothers and children which is built on existing infrastructure. It operates from a community centre and services are delivered by *anganwadi* (courtyard) health workers. The ICDS has been successful in reducing infant and child mortality, and in urban slums and rural areas malnutrition has been halved. The success of this programme has been attributed to the following factors:

1 Integration of nutrition, health and educational services.
2 Inclusion of services to mothers and pregnant women.
3 Supply of nutritional supplements for consumption in the centre for children (up to 6 years of age), and for pregnant and lactating women.
4 Delivery of services by female workers trained for the job and receiving in-service training.
5 Monitoring, evaluation, continued education and supervision by the academic community.

The programme is reviewed annually and improved by solving problems of service delivery and coverage. For example, the reasons for some children remaining unimmunized and malnourished include recurrent diarrhoea, parental suspicion of the services and inadequate supplies of food, and these are receiving attention. The ICDS programme demonstrates the importance of continuity of services and intersectoral cooperation for a successful health service for children in developing countries. It began in 1975 and is expected to be available to all mothers and children in India by the end of the 1990s.

Community health workers

The key to a successful MCH service for rural people or to dwellers of crowded slums is the health centre. This centre should be located for easy access to the community and serve a defined area for home visiting by health centre staff. It may have some beds for inpatient care and for childbirth. Community cooperation is essential for home visits to achieve the aim of identifying all mothers and children at high risk in the village or slum. Therefore health workers must collaborate with various community organizations. This would be made easier if health workers chosen by the community were trained and appointed to serve at the local health centre. Training of these community health workers (CHWs) is usually for short periods of 3 months and they are more economical to produce than nurses or midwives. They are a useful cadre of health service personnel to provide a grassroots service.

Community health workers provide essential basic health services at the village level. They operate from home, a health post or from a dispensary. Each community health worker would be responsible for about 100 to 200 families depending on terrain, population density and number of workers available. The CHW provides a limited curative service and also promotes health through a range of activities from advocating simple preventive measures to fostering wider community development of direct relevance to health, such as literacy, housing and water supply. In the Indian subcontinent, CHWs, usually women, are trained to provide advice on contraception and on feeding and weaning babies, to register births and deaths, to distribute oral rehydration solution for children, and iron and folic acid tablets to pregnant women, to treat minor ailments and to refer seriously ill and malnourished children to the primary health centre.

In 1987, a WHO study group[4] was convened because the community health workers programme in many countries was in crisis. Inadequate planning and strategy implementation, lack of specific and regular budget, and recruitment problems were some of the reasons for failure. The recommendations that emerged from the study included the following principles, chief of which was a commitment to provide and maintain support for the CHW programme. Other recommendations covered details of the CHWs' duties within the district health system; strengthening of the district health system; using different types of workers in the CHW programme to respond to particular local needs and resources; remuneration of CHWs; joint selection of CHWs by the community and health officers; training programmes for CHWs in line with national primary health care strategies based on community needs and conditions; monitoring, supervision and support of CHWs; and a career scheme for CHWs. The involvement of non-governmental organizations to support and develop innovative strategies to help government community health workers' programmes was also recommended.

Community health workers cannot function without the support of a network of health posts or subcentres, primary health centres, and district level facilities with their staff. This link for continuity, referral and supervision is necessary if hospitals are not to be inundated with children suffering from conditions that are preventable and better treated at the health centre. An example of a community health service is shown in Figure 19.1. A health post serves 1000 to 2000 people, and five health posts should have one subcentre. A primary health centre (PHC) serves a population of 80 000 to 100 000. In each district of 1.5 million, eight to fifteen health centres are serviced by one district hospital. This is the goal in many countries but coverage is still limited. At the health post or village level in India, there are one or two CHWs as well as a traditional birth attendant (TBA). The TBA is usually given 6 weeks part-time training in hygiene, simple midwifery care, and aseptic care of the neonate's umbilical cord. The subcentre has a staff of two: a male and a female health worker who are responsible for registration of births and deaths, the treatment and control of malaria, tuberculosis and leprosy, family planning including the insertion of intrauterine devices and motivating women for sterilization, immunization of women and children, and the treatment of common illnesses. A supervisor of health workers and CHWs is based either at one in four subcentres or at a PHC. Two doctors are based at the PHC to provide consultation and treatment of outpatients, visit subcentres 2 days a week to conduct clinics, care for up to six

inpatients at the PHC, and provide supervision of health personnel. Other staff at the PHC are the pharmacist, laboratory technician, records clerk, driver, and cleaners. Another tier between the PHC and the district hospital exists in India; it is the upgraded PHC with ten beds, an operating theatre, two staff nurses and two specialists (an obstetrician and a paediatrician). The district hospital with 50–100 beds is the base for specialists, medical officers, and public health doctors.

Prevention of mental handicap and developmental disabilities

There are no accurate statistics of children with disabilities and handicapping disorders in developing countries because these problems are given low priority. It is estimated that there are some 400 million persons with handicap in the world; four out of five live in developing countries and one-third are children under 15 years. The impression gained from visiting hospitals in the tropics is that of children whose disabilities have developed from a lack of appropriate care, and children with severe disabilities who are long-stay patients. There is usually an absence of parental involvement in management, dependence on appliances from developed countries, and a shortage of therapists. However, there are signs that the needs of disabled children have begun to attract the attention of concerned nationals, and groups catering for the blind, deaf and physically and mentally handicapped now exist in most cities in Asia, Africa and Latin America. These groups are linking with appropriate agencies, such as the International League of Societies for Persons with Mental Handicap, that aim to provide help to the disabled, their families and specialists, to assist them to lead as close to normal lives as possible.

Mental handicap is the most frequent disability and affects about 100 million. Surveys in India have shown that the frequency of severely mentally retarded persons is about 13 per 1000, four times more than the prevalence rate in developed countries. There is also a growing awareness that prevention and treatment at its earliest stages of development are preferable alternatives to the provision of long-term care and rehabilitation. Major causes of mental handicap in developing countries include infections, nutritional deficiencies, genetic disorders, perinatal problems, and head injuries. Infections of the central nervous system that afflict children and present as meningitis or encephalitis are detailed in Table 19.1. Of these, measles and tuberculosis are preventable by routine vaccination, and malaria by vector control, chemoprophylaxis, and anti-mosquito measures such as bed nets. Vaccines are also available for protection against *Haemophilus influenzae*, and *Neisseria meningitidis*.

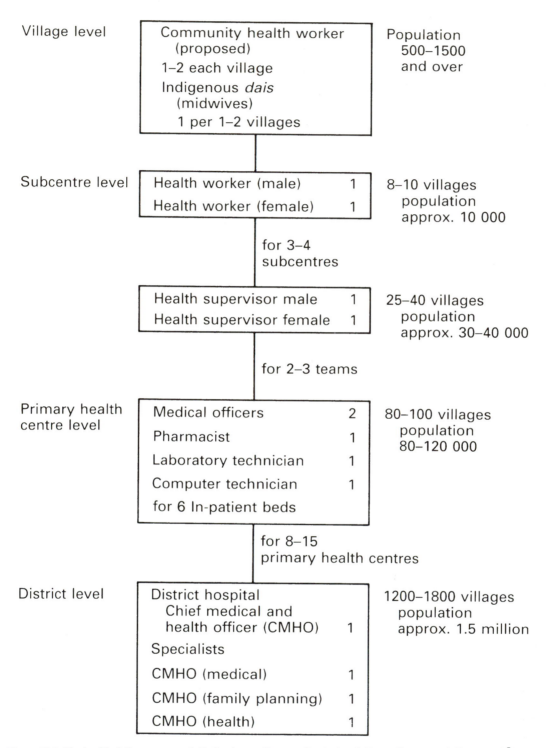

Figure 19.1 The health delivery system in India: from village to district level. (From Sharma and Chaturvedt[5] by kind permission of the authors and publishers.)

Table 19.1 Infectious agents for meningitis and encephalitis

Meningitis	Encephalitis
Escherichia coli	Measles virus
Proteus spp.	Arboviruses
Klebsiella spp.	Eastern equine encephalitis virus
Group B streptococcus	Western equine encephalitis virus
Haemophilus influenzae type b	Venezuelan equine encephalitis virus
Neisseria meningitidis groups A, B, C	Japanese B encephalitis virus
Streptococcus pneumoniae	St Louis encephalitis virus
Tuberculosis	Malaria

From: Chan[6] by kind permission of the author and publisher.

Diarrhoea with severe dehydration or hypernatraemia from incorrect reconstitution of rehydration fluids may also cause brain damage. Nutritional deficiency of iodine found in some highland areas of Asia, Africa and South America contributes to mental handicap during early childhood. Down syndrome is as common in the tropics as it is in temperate lands. Communities where large families are the norm and contraception is not practised will see more affected children, particularly of multiparous older mothers. Consanguinity is high in parts of the Middle East, North Africa and the Indian subcontinent with partnership between first cousins, or between uncles and nieces occurring in half of all marriages. Congenital microcephaly and hydrocephalus have been reported to be frequent with consanguinity although published evidence is largely anecdotal. Perinatal problems contributing to mental handicap range from intrauterine infections with toxoplasma and rubella to birth asphyxia and trauma, and low birthweight. In parts of the world (SE Asia, West Africa, in particular) where the sex-linked red cell disorder of glucose-6-phosphate dehydrogenase (G-6-PD) deficiency is common, kernicterus from severe haemolytic jaundice is another important cause of cerebral palsy and mental retardation. A service to provide care to women during pregnancy, labour and delivery, and to newborn infants will lead to prevention of perinatal brain injury. Head injuries may arise from road traffic accidents, and falls from trees, while brain damage can occur from drowning and poisoning from chemicals (kerosene and insecticides), drugs (iron), and unripe fruit such as ackee in the West Indies (hypoglycaemia). Dangerous customs such as the administration of cow's urine mixture, a potent hypoglycaemic agent, to West African children with convulsions add to the many causes of mental handicap in developing countries. Prevention of brain damage from these causes can be achieved by public education, a reliable health care service with trained personnel, and public health measures.

The Commonwealth Association for Mental Handicap and Developmental Disabilities made recommendations at its meeting in 1985 for the prevention of mental handicap in developing countries. They included iodization of salt for regions with congenital goitre, avoidance of pregnancies in older women, active immunization of pregnant women against tetanus, training programmes for birth attendants, use of the cervicograph (partogram) as a simple graphic method of recording labour, resuscitation of the newborn, long-term follow up of low birthweight infants, prevention and early treatment of infections in children, avoidance of the use of eye cosmetics containing lead, the creation of genetic counselling units, and further studies to determine the prevalence and aetiology of mental handicap with a view to promoting practical programmes of prevention. The meeting in 1986 added more recommendations such as the prevention of kernicterus in the neonate, and emphasized health education and training of professional carers.

Physical handicap affecting the limbs is more common in developing than in industrialized countries because of the prevalence of poliomyelitis, accidents involving motor vehicles, heavy loads, burns and scalds, falls from trees, and war. Despite efforts to improve routine immunization coverage, poliomyelitis exists in many developing countries. In India about 350 000 children annually are victims of poliomyelitis, with paralysis of one or both lower limbs. Deformities are correctable by physiotherapy or surgery followed by orthopaedic calipers and shoes. However, they are best prevented by vaccination. Education of parents and children about preventing accidents in the home and avoiding road or industrial injury have to be implemented to reduce the burden of physical handicap.

Visual handicap, with varying degrees of disability including blindness, afflicts about one million children in the tropics, principally because of malnutrition. Vitamin A deficiency is common in Asia in spite of abundant supplies of vitamin A-rich fruit and vegetables. Food taboos due to ignorance of nutrition are a major cause of blindness in 200 000 Indian children every year; a disability that is eminently preventable at no extra cost to the health system or the family. Many more children have ocular signs of keratomalacia which are reversible with vitamin A treatment. Deficiency of vitamin A is also a significant factor in the deaths of Asian and African children with measles who succumb to overwhelming bacterial infection such as pneumonia. Trachoma causes blindness in some six million people, mainly adults in developing countries. Children, particularly neonates, are at risk of ophthalmia from *Neisseria gonorrhoeae* and *Chlamydia trachomatis* (a different subtype from that which causes trachoma). If untreated, neonatal ophthalmia may cause permanent visual handicap. Tetracycline eye ointment is effective treatment for most causes of neonatal ophthalmia, while silver nitrate eye drops instilled at birth are effective for *Neisseria gonorrhoeae* only. *Toxocara canis* infection also contributes to visual impairment and blindness.

Deafness is the hidden handicap whose existence and incidence are often unrecognized. It is estimated that five million in the world are so profoundly deaf that speech will not develop without special education. A further 200 million or more are partially deaf. Two-thirds of people with hearing disabilities live in the developing world. Prevention of profound deafness must be a part of national and international health planning. This can be achieved through obstetric and neonatal care, immunization against measles, rubella and meningitis, and prevention and prompt treatment of enteric disease. The early and effective treatment of middle ear infection is a priority for prevention of deafness in children.

Information about the prevention of blindness, deafness, mental and physical handicap disseminated widely throughout the community by health workers at all levels of the primary health care system is the most important method of reducing the burden of these problems. For children who have disabilities and handicap, a multidisciplinary support team must be trained to help parents and families to encourage them to lead as normal a life as possible. Strengthening of the infrastructure for integrated primary and district level health care must remain a priority for governments of developing countries.

References

1 Monteiro, C.A., Benicio, M.H.D'A. Determinants of infant mortality trends in developing countries – some evidence from São Paulo city. *Trans Roy Soc Trop Med Hyg* 1989; **83**: 5–9.
2 Alma-Ata Declaration 1978. *Primary Health Care.* Geneva: World Health Organization, 1978.
3 Williams, C.D. Maternal and child health services in developing countries. *Lancet* 1964; **i**: 345.
4 World Health Organization. Community health workers – strengthening community health workers for health for all. *Weekly Epidemiol Rec* 1988; **35**: 265–268.
5 Sharma, R., Chaturvedt, S.K. In: Hetsel, B.S., ed. *Basic Health Care in Developing Countries.* Oxford: Oxford University Press, 1978: 97.
6 Chan, M.C.K. Severe childhood infection. In: Hosking, G., Murphy, G., eds. *Prevention of Mental Handicap: a World View.* London: Royal Society of Medicine Service, 1987, 79.

Chapter 20

Professionals in the community

20.1 Introduction

Many different professionals operating from a wide variety of sites may be involved in the care and development of children. This may result in working in relative isolation. Yet traditionally, the various disciplines have recognized the need to work closely together in order to achieve the best results for children. This need is reinforced by the Children Act 1989 which stresses the importance of inter-agency cooperation in the planning and delivery of services to children and their families.

Since close communication may be difficult, it is important to strengthen good working relationships by other routes. An understanding of the background and training of the different professionals is useful to this end, facilitating optimal multidisciplinary care which in turn benefits the child.

The following sections discuss many of the skills and training of the professionals who contribute to the well-being of children.

20.2 Child health doctors

Leon Polnay

For the first 60 years of the child health services, the child health clinics and school health services were staffed almost exclusively by clinical medical officers and senior clinical medical officers. These were career grade posts which were responsible to community physicians, originally to the medical officer of health, and for which there was no recognized training grade. The last 20 years has seen an increasing pace of change: child health doctors have changed from being a third force aligned to community medicine to become a part of paediatrics; the service is now largely led by consultant paediatricians in community child health; training posts from senior house officer (SHO) to senior registrar have been established; and family doctors are taking a major role in child health surveillance. The grades of clinical medical officer and senior clinical medical officer may soon begin to change to staff grade or

associate specialist and thus align with the grading of posts with similar responsibility in other parts of the health service.

The work fits into three tiers of activity. Tier one is at the primary care level and encompasses the child health surveillance programme which is directed at all children. This is the essential foundation of the service. The medical input is from family doctors and clinical medical officers, but also involves more senior doctors and those in training grades. The senior doctors are involved in liaison, training, policy and audit of child health surveillance. The number of family doctors carrying out pre-school child health surveillance has rapidly expanded since the new general practitioner (GP) contract in 1990. Community nurses, health visitors and school nurses provide the largest part of the tier one service. Tier two level deals with the secondary management of problems identified by child health surveillance programmes. Activity is in pre-school referral clinics, school clinics, day nurseries, special schools and special education assessments. Tier two clinics need not be limited to advice on development, behaviour, child care and children with special needs but may also include the investigation and treatment of any paediatric problem in a community setting. Examples would include failure to thrive, asthma, enuresis and middle ear disease. This work is carried out by consultants, senior clinical medical officers, experienced clinical medical officers, registrars and senior registrars. Tier three is the management of children with severe and complex problems (medical and psychosocial) with a large multidisciplinary element. Examples would be work in a child development centre or the investigation of child sexual abuse. This work is, in general, carried out by consultants, senior clinical medical officers and doctors receiving higher clinical training. In addition, tier three includes management and policy making, information systems and training. Skills in epidemiology and public health issues as they relate to children often fall within the tier three activity.

Community paediatricians work on a geographical basis with a team being responsible for a particular community. Many of the teams are consultant led and the number of such teams is expanding. The teams consist of senior and junior doctors with the former carrying the tier two and tier three responsibility. Very important is the team's local knowledge of the population and the close working relationships that develop with local family doctors, community nurses, schools and social services. This local interdisciplinary organization is the key to an effective community service. It is not rapidly established, but facilitates understanding of the breadth of a family's life experience, to provide a genuinely integrated service and to give a long-term perspective on children's development. The relationship between health, education and social services in a community is a delicate and fragile ecosystem in which the balance, communication and understanding among its component parts is essential.

Training programmes for doctors in community child health have only been established in the last 10–15 years. They are still in a phase of development. Prior to this, doctors gained their skills by experience, and by attendance on the occasional course. There was no structure for training, though there was one for career progress. This disassociation had an adverse effect on the respect and status of the service and the quality and sophistication of the work.

Doctors working at tier one to tier two levels require a 3-year general professional training. For full-time doctors and ideally for general practitioners, this should include SHO posts giving experience of hospital paediatrics, community paediatrics and of paediatrics in general practice. A suitable postgraduate qualification for these doctors is the DCH examination. Training programmes must include not only paediatrics, but also an appreciation of the roles of other professionals who work with children in the community. This is essential if they are to work effectively with other disciplines.

For doctors working at tier two to three levels, the desired qualification is the MRCP examination. The core paediatric knowledge required is the same for all doctors practising paediatrics whether in hospital or in the community. Some doctors share a hospital and community component to their jobs. For all, the vision of a combined child health service requires that training programmes should not suffer from narrow compartmentalization. A common training at SHO and registrar level is needed that gives all trainees experience in both hospital and community. The MRCP examination should be passed before the end of this period. At senior registrar level, a modular system is valuable, with a team responsibility involving all general aspects of community paediatrics (clinical, management, work within tiers one and two) and modules in tier three specialities such as the child development centre and paediatric neurology, child psychiatry and child protection. Social paediatrics and educational medicine are important subjects that are central to the day-to-day work of the community paediatrician. Several MSc courses in community paediatrics are now available to provide academic training, a bridge for some from hospital to community and for others an enlargement of postgraduate educational experience.

Continuing medical education and peer group review are important for all groups of doctors. The individual nature of the work in schools and clinics means that it is easy to become isolated in clinical practice compared to the work of the hospital. Continuing education in the form of clinical meetings, team meetings, journal clubs and individual liaison is therefore most important.

In summary, the community paediatrician is a doctor well trained in paediatrics, locally based in a community, integrated into its service networks, with a broad clinical remit from tier one to tier three and also a responsibility to take an overview of the health of all children.

20.3 Health visitors

Margaret Ayton

Health visiting has a different focus from other community health care disciplines since health visitors work with the apparently well population to promote good health and prevent ill health. This approach has been fundamental to practice since the public health origins of health visitors in the last century.[1] The emphasis on maternal and child health created at this time was reinforced by legislation contained within the National Health Service Act 1946, and by demands from practitioners for a greater role in child health surveillance following the findings of child death inquiries as well as demands from practitioners to have their practice legitimized.[2] The current NHS legislation introduced in the National Health Service and Community Care Act demands a service which meets the identified needs of the population; it has allowed health visitors to reconsider their public health origin and to work specifically with individuals and groups within the community with recognized specific health needs.

These developments have influenced the education and training of health visitors. Today's practitioner is a registered general nurse who has completed a further year at an institute of higher education. The curriculum, based on a philosophy of promoting health, explores concepts such as health assessment, primary prevention, public health, human development and most importantly health promotion. Tannahill[3] provides a model for health promotion with three overlapping spheres of health education, screening and health protection. These frequently provide the focus for the training course content. The disciplines of social and developmental psychology, sociology and epidemiology are used to clarify some of the complexities involved within these concepts. The curriculum also provides the opportunity to develop the practical skills necessary for effective health promotion. These include health counselling, facilitating group work, networking and community outreach work.

However, health visiting has been criticized for its rather nebulous nature of practice and lack of clearly defined boundaries. In an attempt to overcome this the following principles were developed by a group of educationalists, managers and practitioners:[4]

- The search for health needs.
- The stimulation of the awareness of health needs.
- The influence of policies affecting health.
- The facilitation of health-enhancing activities.

Integrated with the described concept of health promotion these principles provide the framework for health visiting practice, and promote work with a range of client groups in different settings. These settings include work in the client's home with groups within the wider community and in clinic settings within the primary health care services. Regardless of the setting it is essential that health visitors work in partnership with clients. Although some practitioners appear reluctant to adopt this approach, the success of parent-held records clearly demonstrates the benefits of working in this way.[5]

Until recently the contextual setting of health visiting was determined by client groups. Traditionally this involved working with families with young children. Although the child still provides the focus for practice, the importance of women's health to the family has received much more attention and health visitors play an important role in contributing to women's psychological health in particular. The early identification of postnatal depression is an example of this.[6] The work of the child development programme demonstrates the importance of the support provided by health visitors in developing parenting skills.[1] Health visitors provide support to women at particularly vulnerable times by offering antenatal and postnatal support groups.

In the past, the health visitor's role with children has focused on child health surveillance programmes. Although surveillance is frequently broadly defined, Hall[7] suggests that health promotion is a more appropriate description of the service needed by this client group. The promotion of breast feeding, the prevention of childhood accidents and the undertaking of developmental screening programmes at the recommended ages are examples.[7] However, with the changing emphasis in health visiting practice, and the introduction of GP contracts, the health visitor's role in developmental screening is also changing. Where practice nurses are suitably trained they may participate in screening, allowing health visitors to spend greater time working with more vulnerable clients or developing new strategies in health promotion.

An important emphasis of work has been child protection and the recommendations of some of the child death inquiries have suggested greater health visitor involvement.[8] Although there is obviously a need for the protection of vulnerable children and for the requirements of the Children Act 1989 to be met, health visitors are facing conflict within this area of practice. In particular they question whether they are carrying out preventive work or merely propping up social services. There is a risk that child protection work may take up so much time that little time is spent with equally vulnerable groups such as elderly people. However, it is a requirement that commissioning authorities recognize the need to purchase advice on child protection from provider units[9] and in this way health visiting retains a role within this important area.

Until recently little attention was given to health promotion in men; however it is now acknowledged that men have specific health needs and frequently have difficulty in accessing preventive health care. The setting up of well-men clinics, including screening for testicular cancer, is an important development in health visiting practice.[10]

It is these more innovative approaches to practice, coinciding with the demands of the National Health Service and Community Care Act 1990, which has led to a changing emphasis in health visitor practice. Many health visitors have extended the principle of searching for health needs into health profiling. This involves practitioners in collecting objective and subjective data to identify and rank the health needs of a specific population. In this way clearly defined practice objectives are established. Where this approach has been adopted health visitors have been able to demonstrate practice outcomes and evaluate health visiting intervention.[11] The process has also identified the need for a much greater emphasis on public health within health visiting; the incidence of coronary heart disease, accident rates and people who are HIV positive highlights the need for effective health promotion strategies within the public health arena.

These problems demonstrate the need for health visitors to work closely with other health care professionals and voluntary and statutory organizations. Collaborative work to improve the health status of homeless families provided a good example.[12] To achieve effective outcomes in health promotion in public health, intersectoral work is essential and highlights the important role health visitors play in referral and liaison with other agencies and workers. Collaboration among the disciplines within community nursing is particularly important.

The evidence suggests that the health visitor's role in the community varies between both provider units and practitioners and is continually developing to meet new health needs. Where practitioners have adopted health profiling as a framework for practice it provides the opportunity to develop a service which is proactive and responsive to the health needs of the population; it also allows practitioners to manage the changes required in practice in a positive way giving greater client satisfaction. In order to achieve this, health visitors must be encouraged and facilitated by their managers to adopt innovative approaches to

practice rather than be constrained by the demands of outdated traditions.

The demand for a cost effective service with demonstrable practice outcomes is a further major change influencing the health visitor's role within the community. Health visitors must provide a service which commissioning authorities wish to purchase, but this may be restricted to traditional roles if the purchasers and their advisers have only a limited understanding of the contribution that health visitors make to client care. The publication of the recent government white paper, *Health of the Nation*,[13] may help to influence these demands but it is also important that health visitors play a role in demonstrating the contribution they can make in identifying health needs and ensuring these are included with business contracts and specifications.

Although the many changes currently facing practitioners make it particularly difficult to give a comprehensive account of the role of health visitors in the community their expertise in identifying and developing strategies in health promotion remains constant. It is merely the target groups which change. The evaluation of practice should ensure that appropriate groups and individuals are identified and that effective health visiting intervention provides a high level of client satisfaction.

References

1 Barker, W. *Early Child Development Project*. Bristol: University of Bristol, 1984.
2 Robinson, J. *An Evaluation of Health Visiting*. London: Council for the Education and Training of Health Visitors (CETHV), 1982.
3 Tannahill, A. What is health promotion? *Hlth Educ J* 1985; **44**: 167–168.
4 Council for the Education and Training of Health Visitors (CETHV). *An Investigation into the Principles of Health Visiting*. London: CETHV, 1977.
5 Jackson, C. Power to the parent. *Health Visitor* 1991; **64**: 340–341.
6 Taylor, E. Postnatal depression: what can a health visitor do? *J Advanced Nursing* 1989; **14**: 866–877.
7 Hall, D. *Health for All Children*, 2nd edn. Oxford: Oxford University Press, 1991.
8 London Borough of Brent. *A Child in Trust*. Middlesex: London Borough of Brent, 1985.
9 Department of Health. *Working Together: a Guide to Arrangements for Inter-agency Cooperation for the Protection of Children from Abuse*. London: HMSO, 1991.
10 Brown, I., Lunt, F. Evaluating a 'well-men clinic'. *Health Visitor* 1992; **65**: 12–14.
11 Health Visitor Development Group. *Oxfordshire's Strategy for Health Visiting*. Oxford: Oxfordshire District Health Authority, 1988.
12 Health Visitors Association, General Medical Services Committee. *Homeless Families and their Health*. London: HMSO, 1988.
13 Department of Health. *The Health of the Nation*. London: HMSO, 1992.

20.4 School health nurses

Pippa Bagnall

School nurses are registered general nurses, many of whom will have undertaken the certificate in school nursing. Some school nurses may have completed further training in subjects such as health education, counselling, children with special needs and child protection.

Most school nurses are based in a child health clinic or health centre. However, some may have a permanent base at a special school or within a secondary school. The workload varies widely across the country and this is an area which must be reviewed in order to ensure all children have access to and benefit from the school nursing service.

School nurses are employed by the health authority as part of the community nursing team. Due to current changes in the management structure within community nursing services there may not be a clear line of management between the field workers and senior managers. However, there should be a senior nurse with expertise in school nursing to coordinate and develop this service. School nurses work as part of a team in a close liaison with health visitors, community medical officers, teachers, education social workers and social workers. Unfortunately, communication is not always as it should be and this can provide a stumbling block to meeting children's health needs.

The role of the school nurse has developed rapidly over the last decade and a similar growth is likely to occur during the next few years. The school nurse is emerging as a member of the primary health care team whose ultimate goal is the promotion of children's health by identifying and meeting their health needs. She is a vital link between the child, the home and the school.

Identification of needs

There are three ways in which a school nurse identifies and meets children's needs.

1   Assessment

On school entry, the school nurse collects together all the information available on each child. In health authorities where school entry medicals are selective, the school nurse and school doctor assess the needs of each child and decide which children will have a medical examination. If there is no record of a child's previous health care a medical examination should be compulsory.

Once a child has been assessed by the school health team a plan of care is made and this should be evaluated at appropriate intervals. Ideally, children are interviewed by the school nurse or school doctor at least every 3 years and more frequently when there is any cause for concern.

2   Screening

School nurses carry out screening procedures according to local health authority policy. Instead of a mechanical task orientated approach school nurses adopt a more flexible attitude in order to be more available to those who really need the care. Routine screening includes vision and hearing testing and growth measurements.

3   Health promotion

The education and community nursing services have undergone enormous changes and the role of the school nurse as health promoter has been recognized and firmly established. School nurses should ensure children have access to information on all aspects of health, 'answering their questions fully and providing advice and counselling in confidence where appropriate.'[1]

Opportunities arise informally and formally. An example of an informal occasion is the health interview between child, parent and school nurse. This gives the opportunity for discussion on subjects such as diet, teeth, personal hygiene, sleep and exercise. More formal health education takes place in the classroom. Health education is now continuous throughout the school curriculum and there are subjects which can be covered by a school nurse in cooperation with the class teacher. Some school nurses' health education programmes have been formally included in the school curriculum after careful discussion and planning between the school nurse, the teachers and governors. The importance of promoting children's health must not be underestimated.

In identifying and meeting children's health needs there are two areas which require more school nursing time then ever before. The school nurse has a prominent part to play in the care of children with special educational needs and those who have suffered from any form of abuse.

Children with special educational needs

Since the 1981 Education Act more children with moderate and severe special needs are being educated alongside their peers in ordinary schools. The extended role of the school nurse ensures that these children are supported. In addition, the school nurse is involved in identifying and sometimes providing the care. 'School nurses should prepare all concerned for their admission to school, provide reports for the Statement of Special Educational Needs and act as a resource for and support to the child, the family and the school staff.'[2]

Victims of actual or suspected child abuse

School nurses aim to be available and readily accessible to children so they can discuss anything causing them concern, confidentiality being assured except in a few circumstances. On some of these occasions

children will admit to suffering from some form of abuse. It is then necessary for the school nurse to explain to the child the need to seek further help and investigation and to follow the formal procedures for pursuing a case of suspected child abuse.

Additionally, school nurses have an important role to play in supporting and monitoring these children at regular intervals, but they will also communicate with other professionals either informally or at a case conference.

Recent developments in community care mean that the service provided by school nurses will play an increasingly important part in the prevention of illness and the promotion of health.

References

1   Health Visitors Association. *Meeting School Children's Health Needs: The School Nurse's Role*. London, 1988, 15.
2   Health Visitors Association. *Meeting School Children's Health Needs: The School Nurse's Role*. London, 1988, 17.

20.5 Community nurses

Mark Whiting

There has been a striking proliferation of paediatric community nursing services in recent years. A major source of impetus for this development has been the changing face of health care provision in the UK and, in particular, the increasing emphasis upon the community as providing a major focus for care. The fundamental explanation for the surge in paediatric community nursing provision, however, has been the increasing recognition that the complex health-related needs of children demand the expertise of appropriately trained and experienced nursing staff regardless of the setting in which care is to be provided.

The notion that the community should play such a central role in the care of the sick child is not, however, a new one. Our present district nursing (DN) and health visiting (HV) services (whose respective roots lay in the squalor and social deprivation of the mid-19th century industrial towns of Liverpool and Manchester) have, in the past, contributed significantly to improvements in sanitation, health and mortality rates among the child population. Historically, it must be acknowledged that the work of DNs and HVs has contributed significantly to the care of the sick child in the community. Over the years, the role of these professionals in the care of sick children has become somewhat limited. The work of the DN is now concentrated largely in the care of the adult, increasingly

elderly, population.[1] Although the work of HVs is predominantly concerned with young children and their families,[2] health education and health surveillance, rather than specific, practical nursing care activities, form the basis for current health visiting practice.

A formal paediatric community nursing scheme was first introduced in the UK in 1949, in Rotherham. This was soon followed by developments, in 1954, in Birmingham and Paddington in London. At this time, much of the paediatric community nurses' work involved the care of children with acute infectious diseases, predominantly of the respiratory and gastro-intestinal systems. The care of such children demanded close cooperation between the hospital and community-based medical teams; the nursing staff provided a vital link in the integration of services.

In 1969, in order to facilitate the development of a children's day surgery unit, a team of paediatric community nurses was introduced in Southampton. In the same year, a community nursing team was linked to the outpatient department of the Royal Hospital for Sick Children, in Edinburgh. These developments provide further illustration of the key role that such schemes have played historically in the integration of hospital and community-based services at a local level.

It is somewhat surprising, therefore, to note that despite the strongest of recommendations from the

Platt[3] and Court[4] Committees, paediatric community nursing developed at a painfully slow pace and, by 1980, only a handful of district health authorities boasted such services. However, during the 1980s and early 1990s, there has been a tremendous proliferation.[5] The Department of Health has warmly welcomed this progress.[6] A further significant development in the recent past has been the growth in the numbers of paediatric clinical nurse specialists. Many of these nurses work as outreach nurses based at regional referral centres, providing both clinical expertise for other professionals and practical care to children with specific medical problems. The combined effect of these two areas of development has been to allow for the balance of care to begin to shift away from hospital and towards the community.

The impact that this has had upon the lives of many children has been dramatic, and has contributed significantly to reducing the lengths of hospital stay for children suffering from many medical conditions and with a wide range of health care needs.

A number of specific groups of children have provided a focus for care by paediatric community nurses. It is useful to discuss each group in turn.

1 Children with acute medical problems

The availability in the community of nurses with expertise and knowledge of the traditional hospital-based management of children with acute medical problems, such as gastroenteritis, urinary or respiratory tract infections, has allowed many such children to be discharged from hospital at an early stage in their recovery and, in some instances, has provided an alternative to admission for children whose illness was mild. The provision of such an alternative has demanded the development of imaginative admission policies, with nursing staff being able to draw upon the expertise of both hospital- and community-based medical staff to enable parents to be supported in the care of their child at home.

2 Children with chronic medical problems

Paediatric community nurses are increasingly called upon to play a key role in the care of children suffering from a wide range of chronic medical problems. Specific local initiatives have been launched in the care of children suffering from asthma, cystic fibrosis, diabetes mellitus, cancer and leukaemia, and eczema. The intervention of the paediatric community nurse in the management of such problems may facilitate early discharge from hospital and reduce the likelihood of recurrent admission. The key role, with this group, is as a support agent, providing a vital link between the long-term management regimens advocated by hospital-based paediatricians and those agencies which provide support for the families of such children in the community. The paediatric community nurse is also able to provide hands-on nursing care and to play a major part in the process of teaching children and their families about the impact of chronic disease upon the family unit. Such teaching is vital if families are to comply with often very complicated regimens of care, and if sick children are to attain their maximal potential within the limitations imposed by chronic disease.

3 Care of the child undergoing planned surgery

The introduction of structured preoperative preparation programmes and the facilitation of early post-surgical discharge has been possible in a number of areas of the UK in which paediatric community nursing teams have been introduced. Day surgical provision is an area that is likely to benefit significantly from the ready availability of an experienced paediatric nurse in the community. The closeness of relationship between the nurses themselves and the in-hospital team allows for the establishment of comprehensive packages of perioperative care which are likely to prove very reassuring for both the parents and the children themselves. Ready communication between the paediatric community nurses and members of the primary health care team, including the general practitioner, health visitor and school nurse, is vital.

4 Care of the child requiring emergency surgery

Follow-up care in the community for children who have required emergency surgery has been a particularly valuable innovation in many areas. Such a facility has been provided for children who have undergone a wide variety of emergency surgical and orthopaedic interventions, including appendicectomy, and stabilization of lower limb fractures. The availability of early discharge for such children has contributed to both a reduction in the length of postoperative stay and a minimization of the disruption caused to family life by the unexpected hospitalization that emergency surgery often requires.

5 The child with disabilities

The roles of paediatric community nurses in the care of the child with disabilities are many and varied. Intervention may be required on many fronts but, almost without exception, the role of the nurse is that of enabler and facilitator. The parents of children with disabilities very rapidly acquire the mantle of the expert in the care of their child. Although many health care professionals may, from time to time, make a contribution to meeting the complex needs of such children, the identification of a key health worker is vital. The paediatric community nurse is often uniquely placed to be such a person.

As can be seen above, the caseloads of paediatric community nurses are extremely diverse. An analysis of the nature of the care provided by these nurses[5] has indicated that its content is equally diverse. In supporting such an array of activity, the development of paediatric clinical nurse specialists has proved of immense value. The increasing availability of such specialists has facilitated the development of a complex network of community nursing expertise for children whose care needs are often being managed, in part at least, at regional or supra-regional referral centres.

In many areas of the UK, the paediatric community nurse is a relative newcomer. Furthermore, it must be acknowledged that many districts do not yet employ such nurses. Despite this, the innovative nature of much of their work would indicate that the potential for service development is immense. It would appear reasonable to assume, therefore, that the demand for paediatric community nursing teams is likely to increase significantly over the next decade as pressure on inpatient accommodation becomes ever greater, as medical science provides ever wider care options and as family-centred home care becomes the accepted norm for the sick child.

References

1 Office of Population Censuses and Surveys. *Nurses Working in the Community*. Dunnell, K., Dobbs, J. eds. London: HMSO, 1982.
2 Clark, J. *What do Health Visitors Do? A Review of the Research 1960–1980*. London: Royal College of Nursing, 1981.
3 Ministry of Health. *The Welfare of Children in Hospital: Report of the Committee*. Chairman: Sir H. Platt. London: HMSO, 1959.
4 Department of Health and Social Security. *Fit for the Future. Report of the Committee on Child Health Services*. Chairman: S.D.M. Court. London: HMSO, 1976.
5 Whiting, M. *Community Paediatric Nursing in England in 1988*. Unpublished MSc Thesis, University of London, 1988.
6 Department of Health. *Welfare of Children and Young People in Hospital*. London: HMSO, 1991.

20.6 Social workers

Sue Brock

Other sections in this book describe the role of some of the specialist social workers, including those working for voluntary organizations. This section deals with general aspects of social workers' training and role with children.

A professional social worker is recognized by the training body CCETSW (Central Council for Education and Training in Social Work). The professional qualifications of some social workers are earlier than the foundation of CCETSW (1971), and may be, for instance, a Home Office Certificate in Child Care, or a membership of the Institute of Almoners. More recent qualifications include CSS (Certificate in Social Service) and CQSW (Certificate of Qualification in Social Work). These are basic qualifications to which people may subsequently add training modules, such as Approved Social Worker, an additional qualification in mental health.

The new professional qualification is the Diploma in Social Work. There has been for some time a Masters Degree in Social Work. This involves a three year course, as does the professional training of social workers in some continental countries. In England, at present, most social workers have a two year training course for their basic qualification. Many go on to add to this in a modular fashion. Modules may include those on management; child protection; treatment of mentally disordered offenders; research methods; philosophical issues in social work; care of the dying person and their family; groupwork, etc. At the moment, a training in the specialization of practice teaching is being introduced. This training may lead to an MA. A professional training and qualification in social work is one of the prerequisites of many schools of psychotherapy.

Paediatric social work used to be a well-known and understood specialization of those working with children and their families. The training equipped workers with a thorough understanding of the impact of illness and handicap on the child and the family. Paediatric social workers worked as members of a multidisciplinary paediatric team. Then came generic training, which equipped people for working across a wider range of social work, as recommended in the Seebohm Report (1970). Recently social work, including hospital-based work, has become increasingly based in a social services department of the local authority. The work has become more task-focused. The assimilation of the paediatric social worker with the hospital-based social worker and now care manager has not been easy. At the same time as these developments in social services departments, there has been an upsurge of voluntary developments where client-centred work is the focus – a different part of the continuum of work with people, being less task-focused and more geared to working at the individual pace of the client. The history of the voluntary worker goes well back into the past; statutory work is a more recent development.

Perhaps paediatric social work can now best be seen in oncology units, where some Malcolm Sargent social workers are based, straddling the divide between social services and voluntary organizations. The Malcolm Sargent social workers, within a hospital team specializing in malignant conditions, work very much with the children and their families, and with the GP and community-based nurses. They all ensure that much long-term treatment and terminal care can be carried on at home. This idea can also be seen in the development of hospital-at-home teams.

General social workers, as their title indicates, are those whose work is not specialized into the fields of child abuse, family work, or voluntary social workers. This leaves few who work with children and families except, perhaps, the intake workers of the social work department of a hospital or the short-term assessment workers of social services departments of local authorities. These social workers are the contact point with the department, and refer families to other colleagues after assessment. Perhaps assessment is the main skill of a general social worker, and no more so than in a Child Development Centre where children with multiple difficulties are assessed by a multidisciplinary team of professionals, and coordinated treatment plans are made and reviewed. The term Assessment Centre is applied within social services departments, where care plans for a child in care are made through a system of multidisciplinary recommendations to case conferences and reviews. The multidisciplinary approach which thrives in paediatric departments of hospitals is developing in social services departments, especially and significantly in community mental handicap teams, and in the education field, especially since the Disabled Persons Act of 1986. Young people are discussed and statemented after the age of 14 years, if they have needs requiring special services and adaptations, or if disability occurs before the age of 19 years, or eight months before leaving full-time education, whichever is the earlier.

Working together is the trend for the future – between the NHS and social services departments, between education, medicine and social services, and between colleges and social services departments in the training of social workers.

Group work provides a very useful way of enabling people to work through difficulties. Young people in particular may find it less threatening than one-to-one individual work.

Many social workers are trained as group workers. They become highly skilled and use this method to help young people. Much of the work in family centres and project centres is done in groups.

In 1982, the Criminal Justice Act made it mandatory for local authorities to provide intermediate treatment centres as an alternative to custody. Since 1986, these have become project centres and recently worked cooperatively with the juvenile justice team to enable young persons to continue to live within their communities, and to live cooperatively. The trend is toward inter-agency resource centres. From 1992 many project centres are being closed because of the cost of funding them and because of the development of juvenile justice teams. In many areas, staff no longer have the opportunity to offer a group experience for the older age range.

It has been said that delinquency, like adolescence, is something you grow out of. The effects of abuse, however, need to be addressed as soon as possible. Indeed, abuse may be prevented in many instances, if the indicators have been recognized early and urgently addressed. Many children and young people attending family centres and project centres have been victims of abuse and are in danger of family breakdown. It helps if the child's needs can be met in the community.

Family centres cater for parents, and children under 5 years; project centres are for those aged 7–17 years. Both offer a range of facilities – group work, holiday groups, parents' groups, educational programmes, interpersonal skills development programmes, recreational opportunities, and a rich source of opportunities for play. Referrals are made by the local authority and may also come by self-referral.

Facilities for children aged 5–7 years are extremely variable according to the policies and resources of the local authority. This matter has been addressed in the Children Act 1989. Often the needs of this age group are met by voluntary organizations and volunteers.

Acknowledgements

Brian Pereira, Staff Development Consultant, Berkshire Social Services; Margaret Anne Howard, formerly of Social Services Inspectorate; Ray Johns, Director, The Castle Priory (Spastics Society); Geraldine Deith, Training Tutor, Lord Mayor Treloar College, Alton; Mikki Coleman, Tutor, Bracknell College, Woodley Hill House, Reading, Berkshire. (Correct at time of writing.)

20.7 Educational social workers

Bryan Wadland

Education social workers (ESW), or education welfare officers (EWO) as they used to be known, are employed by local education authorities (LEA) and their training is the same as that of any social worker – the certificate of qualification in social work (CQSW) which became the Diploma in Social Work in 1994. In some LEAs, the education social work service includes social workers employed in child and family guidance centres where, as members of a multidisciplinary team, they use systemic or psychoanalytic approaches. In other authorities, social workers based in clinics are from social services. Not all ESWs are qualified in social work, as they come from varied backgrounds, but those in child and family guidance centres are. Education social work teams are led by a team leader who provides professional guidance and supervision. Team ESWs are usually responsible for one or more schools depending on size and geography. The ESW has a high level of contact with the schools, their pupils and teachers, so is well placed to deal with most referrals.

Normally referrals are made to education social work teams by the headteacher of a nursery or primary school, or year head of a secondary school. The ESW needs to be in the school regularly, perhaps weekly, and to have regular times with the pastoral staff to review properly cases referred or in progress. The ESW needs a fixed place in the school to see parents and pupils where both know they can make contact with the social worker. The aim of all education social work is to enable children and young people to get the maximum benefit from their educational provision and to function comfortably in school.

Clearly regular attendance and the ability to participate fully in school activities and relationships is essential. The causes of poor or non-attendance are not simple, but a useful classification is:[1]

Medical: health needs
Psychological: problems range from extreme phobia to nervousness
Institutional: here the cause is from within school (curriculum, school structure or fellow pupils)
Cultural: pupils are kept away from school for family needs
Generic: a combination of several causes.

In considering referrals made by schools the widest perspective is necessary to understand the problem. Mortimore and Blackstone noted the association between poor school attendance and certain family factors.[2] Furthermore they found 'pupils with poor attendance records are likely to suffer as a result of having less direct instruction'. Close working with parents and the pastoral staff of the school is vital for progress to be made. Precision in referral, in continuing liaison and feed back is important. ESWs work closely with educational psychologists, child guidance professionals and the whole range of education-based support services. The contribution made by education social work is one way of overcoming the effects of disadvantage and deprivation, thus giving a greater equality of opportunity. Education is about horizons, and education social work is much about enhancing opportunity. The school community is about both learning and care and as such the community must be aware of its more vulnerable members who need extra help.

Education social work has a distinctive and independent role in relation to school, the LEA, parents and pupils. Its task is to analyse a situation, seek the causes and decide how it can be dealt with. Changes may be needed through work with the family, the pupil, the school or by involving other agencies. While respecting confidentiality, ESWs will help school staff to understand family backgrounds. An illustration of the independent role is where the pupils, parents and school may each have differing and conflicting views when a pupil is excluded from school. The governors and LEA will also have their views. An ESW can have an independent opinion, seek the best way forward for the pupil and at the same time the parents can be helped to express their feelings and views, even if they are inarticulate or have language difficulties. Such independence should be expected by the LEA.

Schools are well placed to be aware of pupil needs and the means by which these can be met. These needs may not obviously be to do with learning (although many learning problems are emotional in origin), but meeting needs is an integral part of the concept of a complete and broad education. Children and young people who have been abused need protection and may express this within the security of a school setting. They are likely to remain in that school setting and need the continuing pastoral support of the school where they felt confident enough to seek help in the first place.

Children with evolving behaviour problems will be evident and the school can do much to influence their development. The ESW's role is an essential support to the school with such children. Many pupils value the opportunity to talk with an experienced and sympathetic adult as a counsellor outsided the home.[3] Support by ESWs is vital for children with special educational needs in mainstream or special schools, boarding schools or special units.

Health factors are important in school children, particularly for those with special needs and those where health is affected by disadvantaged circumstances and conditions, especially in the inner city areas. Close links are therefore necessary with health professionals to enable such children to maximize their educational opportunities. The Children Act 1989 brings new liaison and cooperative working requirements for LEAs, health and social services over a wide range of services. For the ESW, the Act, implemented in 1991, brings the responsibility of education supervision orders made in a family proceedings court on nonattending children. ESWs also exercise, on behalf of LEAs, the regulatory and protective functions for children and young people in employment and entertainment. The positive role in this is that work experience may complement curriculum needs for many pupils.

Thus the ESW represents the independent social work component in the education system relating with school, education, support services, pupil, parent, community and outside agencies.

The thrust of the work is to ensure and promote opportunity which would otherwise be denied, and enable pupils to achieve through education (schools and support services) the ability and confidence to function successfully as stable and fulfilled adults. The process is a dynamic and cooperative exercise with parent, pupil and school.

References

1 Reid, K. *Truancy and School Absenteeism*. London: Hodder & Stoughton, 1985, 48–50.
2 Mortimore, P., Blackstone, T. *Disadvantage and Education*. London: Heinemann Educational Books, 1982, 83, 85.
3 Davis, L. *Caring for Secondary School Pupils*. London: Heinemann Educational Books, 1985.

20.8 Probation officers

Lennox Thomas

The title of probation officer replaced that of police court missionary in the second half of the 19th century. At a time of many social reforms, the police court missionaries campaigned for reform of the criminal justice system and were, in the main, natural heirs of Elizabeth Fry and John Howard. Probation work was then, as it is now, centred around magistrate courts. The Victorian workers rescued young artisans and petty thieves from a life of crime. Their work became statutory with the passing of the Probation of Offenders Act 1907. This act introduced the Probation Order, a contract requiring the offender to make him or herself available to the officer for a specified time. The act also introduced probation officers to the juvenile courts. An early account of the work of probation officers can be found in Holmes.[1]

Probation officers along with others continued to have an influence on government policies as a result of their direct work with children and their families. They were involved with the mass movement of children evacuated in the Second World War. From this experience, they came to learn of the extent of social deprivation and the condition of children. Probation officers made a contribution to the drafting of the 1944 Education Act and later the Curtis Committee which presided on the health and welfare of children

at risk of harm and abuse. The role of the probation officer expanded in the post-war period to have direct influence on the lives of children and indirectly through supervising their parents. Since the Children and Young Persons Act 1969, probation officers have reduced the role they play in direct work with children who appear before the courts. Their previous work with 9 year olds and older has been passed to the local authorities. It is more likely that probation officers work with children from the age of 13, and in the metropolitan areas from the age of 15 years.

Civil work

Probation officers, under the title of welfare officers when reporting to magistrates domestic courts, or divorce courts have the duty to inform the court of the effect of parental separation and divorce on children.

The officer has a therapeutic role to play as well as helping parents to agree on the provisions made for their children. Civil work is the term given to cases which come from courts in non-criminal proceedings. The courts have the power to request reports in these cases under the Guardianship of Minors Act 1971, the

Domestic Proceedings and Magistrates' Court Act 1978, and the Children Act 1975. In the adoption of children, probation officers and social workers, as members of guardian ad litem panels, established by local authorities, can act as guardian ad litem with the duty of safeguarding the interest of children.[2]

Children are supervised by probation officers as a result of orders made in matrimonial proceedings at the magistrate's court, the divorce court, and in guardianship and wardship proceedings. The probation officer has responsibility for promoting and overseeing the health and welfare of these children. Probation officers have powers through the court to make referrals to paediatricians over health or developmental concerns. The Children Act 1989, introduced in October 1991, has brought about comprehensive changes in the way that children are dealt with by the various statutory agencies. The Act does not only seek to simplify existing complex legislation but also to introduce new principles. For example, the child's welfare must be the paramount consideration and courts shall not make an order unless they consider that doing so would be better for the child than making no order at all. This is based on the principle of parental responsibility, that parents have a duty to look after their children. Civil work has become increasingly specialized in the probation service and separated out from the criminal work with offenders which forms the major part of the service's work. Since the Home Office's 1984 statement of national objectives and priorities for the probation service, civil work has been seen as having a slightly reduced level of future resources.

Work with offenders

While civil work and direct therapeutic intervention in the lives of children forms a small but important part of the probation officer's task, more day-to-day contact is made with children on probation or other statutory orders through supervision of their parents or carers. The probation service sees itself as an agency concerned with the protection of children not only through the influence on their parents, but by working together with other professionals with child health and child protection functions. The professional network exists for probation officers and others to share their concerns over aspects of their work with clients as well as to help provide additional services for clients. Many people who come to the attention of the courts and the probation service experience some form of social deprivation, homelessness or long-term unemployment. Others might be in the grip of an addictive or habit forming behaviour or experiencing psychiatric or psychological problems. There are many complex and varied reasons why people appear before the criminal

courts. The search for the causes of persistent delinquent behaviour has puzzled both practitioners and academics for many years. In general, law breaking has been viewed in many ways as part of a developmental phase from adolescence to adulthood, as a social norm in response to peers, as social and psychopathology, and as a response to poverty among others. Methods of engaging in work with the supervision of offenders have changed according to the ways in which the current causes of delinquency have been explained. The probation order is a fixed period within which the offender by contract at court seeks to refrain from lawbreaking and be of good behaviour, to be industrious or find employment and to keep appointments given by the probation officer in the office or at the offender's home. Apart from the legal responsibilities and duties the officer performs in relation to the client, he or she undertakes to advise, assist and befriend and offender.

Traditional psychodynamic methods of work with offenders and their families provided useful skills for working with and understanding defensive structures and the functioning of the ego. This method also provided a professional bedrock of understanding the forces of unconscious motives and importantly which aspects of this could be legitimately engaged within a social casework relationship. This method coupled with developmental theories was extended into working with offenders and their families. Other contributions to the understanding and treatment of clients have been structural and systemic family therapy, client advocacy, and offending behaviour models. Clients attend group or individual sessions and are sometimes seen in family groups or with partners. There has been a greater emphasis in recent years on concentrating on the offending behaviour patterns of clients. While this has always been given emphasis, the route towards change had been through the client gaining insight into his or her problems. Change in client behaviour to non-offending alternatives is now not seen as necessarily requiring insight, but education of the choices.

The forces for change in the probation service have led to a move away from its early roots in social work towards fulfilling its role as an arm of the criminal justice system. Along with these changes the probation service, like other public service agencies, has had to consider the issues of race and gender for practice. The social forces of racism and sexism affect the work of the probation service in as much as probation officers are raised in society. It is a difficult task for individuals to disentangle themselves from negative social values which might affect their work. When negative stereotypes affect individual clients and play some part in shaping their lives it is important that the professional does not help to perpetuate this.[3–5] The probation officers have a powerful role and they are learning to acknowledge and use this in the service of clients particularly the young who themselves have little power.

References

1 Holmes, T. *The London Police Courts*. London: Thomas Nelson & Sons, 1900.
2 Weston, W.R. *Jarvis's Probation Officers' Manual*. London: Butterworths, 1987.
3 Thomas, L.K. Racism and psychotherapy. In: Kareem, J., Littlewood, R., eds. *Working with Racism in the Consulting Room – an Analytical View in Intercultural Therapy: Themes, Interpretations and Practice*. London: Blackwell Scientific Publications, 1992.
4 Thomas, L.K. Race training: politics, prejudice and practice. In: *Right or Privilege*. Study Paper 10 of Post-qualifying Training with Special Reference to Child Care. London: Central Council for Education and Training in Social Work, 1991.
5 Thomas, L.K. *Race and Culture: Some Psychoanalytic Insights*. London: Tavistock Clinic Gazette, 1987.

20.9 Residential care staff

Sue Brock

Approximately 40% of staff working with children as care staff were in 1990 unqualified. General assumptions about the role include: 'Anyone can do it', and 'It's just common sense'. It is true that care workers need an abundance of common sense, but not everyone can be, or would want to be, a care worker. They are a large body of people who are currently unrepresented by a training body or union. Their work is extremely varied, and ranges from the very domestic, to the responsibilities of key worker to children in their care. They may be employed by voluntary or by statutory organizations, and they may work in residential or day-care settings. For most, there is little supervision of their work: for some, there will be in-house or group supervision.

Care staff are those people who have a day-to-day interest and role in caring for children. Some used to be called houseparents, which gives some indication of the nature of their work. It is a job where initiative and perseverance are required. The work is usually undertaken in shifts, with the care worker acting as a member of a team. Care workers often do night shifts, and may be required to do domestic duties, such as laundry work or cooking. Care workers often act as key workers and link workers for the children in their care, acting as advocates for the children, and reference points for the children's contacts, for example with families, dentists, or schools.

Care workers also include those unqualified staff working within family centres, or with the home care service run by the local authority. They may be in paid employment with voluntary organizations, such as the Spastics Society, National Childrens Homes, Family Service Unit, or Barnardo's, or for I CAN which runs schools for children with special educational needs. They work voluntarily, for organizations such as Home Start, where the volunteer works with new or unsupported parents who have very young children and are experiencing the frustration and difficulties often involved. Here the difference between care worker and volunteer becomes blurred.

Although unqualified in the professional sense, care workers may have attended in-house training courses, or courses run by the Spastics Society at Castle Priory for care staff working with children with special needs. They may have attended a group to study the Open University pack *Caring for Children and Young People*. They may be active members of Mencap or the Samaritans which helps them to keep in touch with developments in child care.

There have been many changes in the recruitment and training of care staff in recent years. Many trained staff working with children have the Certificate of Residential Care of Children and Young People. Senior staff working in residential and day-care settings may have a Certificate in Social Service (CSS) or Certificate in Qualification in Social Work (CQSW). Many have qualifications in management. The rate of change is increasing. The White Paper, now the Community Care Act 1990, *Caring for People, Community Care in the Next Decade and Beyond*, promoted domiciliary, day and respite care to enable people to live in the community. Since 1991 there has also been an innovation in social care training – the National Vocational Qualification (NVQ). This national qualification will value people's ability to do the job, and show competence in prescribed areas. There will be particular emphasis on equal opportunities and anti-discriminatory practices and an employment-based assessment. The qualification will be closely related to jobs and employers in social care, and will facilitate the flexible transfer of staff. A system such as this is already in operation in many European countries.

The NVQ competences for social work practice are due to be completed in 1995. This will strengthen the strands of training in social work – the NVQ, Dip.

Social work and post-qualifying courses. In addition, for those with a lot of relevant experience and training these are schemes for assessment of prior learning and credit accumulation and transfer.

In addition to the NVQ, the new Diploma in Social Work, and the growth of modular training at all levels, is also quality assurance, described in the White Paper, to develop and maintain high standards of practice. Many care workers keep in touch with developments through TV programmes and video training packs, through in-house training, and journals.

The NHS Community Care Act has been implemented. Among its many objectives is that no child should grow up in a mental handicap hospital. The new role of care manager has developed with budgeting responsibilities. In the future the care worker will no longer be untrained and unrepresented, but identified, empowered, and recognized. Further trends lie in more shared care within the community. Concurrent with the changes in existing services, new initiatives are developing, some of them national and some regional, such as the Post Adoption Centre and Parent Link, a support network with a central office, and the development of services for abused people such as Child Line – a phone-in service staffed by highly trained and specialist professional people.

20.10 Family aides (community support workers)

Sue Brock

'As a family aide I feel as if I'm going up a descending escalator and never reaching the top.' This quotation says a lot about the role of the family aide. The job attracts people with considerable experience of life, an abundance of energy, a high degree of common sense and competence, an enthusiastic interest in people, an optimistic outlook, a sense of humour and of the ridiculous, an ability to assess realistically the possibilities for change, and a determination to help the clients achieve this by frequent very small steps.

Family aides work within the local authority social services department. They work alongside the social worker (now often known as a care manager) designated to the client's family, and are supervised by a senior person in a managerial position.

A family aide may be known as a community support worker, or by a similar title, varying from area to area. Broadly, the job is to give assistance, guidance, and practical help to clients to look after themselves and their families. They visit selected clients regularly, and report back to the social worker handling the case. The aides help in financial planning, in home-making, and child care. They enable families to meet otherwise conflicting demands, such as hospital visits, staying at home with a new or sick child, taking different children to various schools or playgroups, attending interviews, and shopping.

The family aide gets to know the family well. In time, the aide is likely to know the relatives and contacts, and may be in touch with different generations of the family spread over her divisional area. An aide is, therefore, a source of useful information and help.

As with other jobs, the actual need to be met may not be apparent at the outset, and the presenting problem and referral may be only a starting point, or tip of the iceberg. The family aide 'gets right in under the grit and grime', and likes to be involved from the begin-ning in order to work in prevention of problems rather than be used as a last resort. Along with all staff in the caring services, their job is changing.

A family aide's work ranges over a wide area: helping families where there is a sick or disabled child or children, where there has been a death in the family, doing a school run as part of a more complex package of help for the family, helping with budgeting and living with the consequences of debt, scrubbing the floor or doing the ironing, always modelling the way to do the task and helping the client to develop their own skills. In many families, the clients learn to do the home-making, and like to get it done before the family aide arrives, so that they get the pleasure of recognition of their efforts, and can spend the time on what they know they really want and need, that is to be listened to and to have time to talk. Many of the tasks of the family aide are aimed at helping people to look after themselves, to get a better self-image, and to be able to offer a better home for their children.

A family aide may well be involved in working with others in families where there is suspected or proven child abuse. The family aide will let the family know that she or he has no authority and cannot remove children from the home, but that the relationship with them is not confidential, and that everything is reported. Family aides may work with others when a parent has supervised access to a child, and may take a child to a neutral place to see the parents; they may work with parents from whom a child has been removed, to enable them to change, with a view to having their child returned.

Family aides may meet one another to arrange a regular outing for their clients, such as a coffee morning, during which the mothers can meet one another, have their hair done, talk about such matters as clothes, children, families, and make-up; they obtain mutual support and a change of scene. This provides an opportunity for the children to play with others and the staff to see their clients socializing outside their own homes.

Communication with other professionals is a vital part of the work, and there is a strong link here with health workers, such as health visitors, hospital social workers, and the staff to see their clients mixing socially outside their own homes.

Communication with other professionals is a vital part of the work, and there is a strong link here with

health workers, such as health visitors, hospital social workers, and doctors.

Acknowledgements

With special thanks to Cath Tilley whose quotes I used. Yvonne Smith for the speedy response to my query with information; and to many family aides on whose inspiration I have drawn.

20.11 Physiotherapists

Diana Kverndal

The Chartered Society of Physiotherapy is the sole recognized examining and professional body for physiotherapists in the UK. The minimum requirement for entry to physiotherapy training is five 'O' Levels and two 'A' Levels. Courses are a minimum length of 3 years, including 1000 clinical hours and are run by schools of physiotherapy in the National Health Service (NHS) although many are now degree or diploma courses attached to universities or polytechnics, with close clinical links with local health districts.

After 2 years of general clinical practice, the physiotherapist may then choose to follow a speciality such as paediatrics, gaining the necessary experience and knowledge with the help and supervision of senior paediatric physiotherapists. A paediatric clinical interest group arranges post registration courses, study days and newsletters for its members. The majority of senior paediatric physiotherapists will have also completed an 8-week post registration course, studying the Bobath approach to paediatric physiotherapy for children with neurological problems. Many therapists are also showing an interest in visiting Hungary to study the Peto approach to treatment for children with handicaps.

Paediatric therapists are usually employed by the NHS and based in hospitals, child development centres or special schools, depending on each local health authority, although some are employed by voluntary or charity agencies such as The Spastics Society or Bobath Centre. As it is now generally agreed that paediatric physiotherapy should involve as much care in the community as possible, the physiotherapist will aim to visit and treat children in their homes, at their schools, childminders and nurseries, regardless of their base.

Paediatric physiotherapists in the community are involved in the care of children from birth to 18 years, with physical and mental handicaps of varying degrees and a variety of chronic illnesses. This

includes such conditions as cerebral palsy, spina bifida, Down syndrome, poliomyelitis, global developmental delay, muscular dystrophy, Erb's palsy, cystic fibrosis, and juvenile chronic arthritis.

The role of the paediatric physiotherapist is to teach the child and family by means of a variety of physical methods, ways of overcoming or minimizing handicaps or illnesses, stimulating gross motor development thereby encouraging global development to reach maximum potential. This may involve for example, teaching home chest physiotherapy, fitting and use of calipers or splints; teaching the family and carers ways of handling, positioning, carrying and playing with the child that best stimulates development; preventing development of abnormal postures, contractures and patterns of movement. The paediatric physiotherapist needs to have a detailed knowledge of normal and abnormal development, pathology, and available treatments and management of the above conditions as well as of the many acute illnesses encountered in the hospital, special care baby units and clinics. The physiotherapist often becomes closely involved with a child and the family, becoming an important support for them. This role needs to be fulfilled within the framework of the many other professionals involved.

Generally, children must be referred to the physiotherapist by a doctor, although this need not necessarily be a consultant; referral is usually accepted from the whole range of doctors in the community and hospital services. Early referral is essential for a number of reasons. Extensive myelination is still occurring in the first years of life when it is easier to intervene to help develop correct movement patterns before incorrect ones are learnt and established. Parents spend a large amount of time with a young baby and find it easier to control a baby's positions and movement than those of an active toddler. Having a physical and positive task to do for their child often helps parents begin to accept their child's illness or handicap, thereby facilitating development of a good parent–child relationship. The experienced paediatric physiotherapist can also contribute to diagnosis, or indeed to the reassurance of normality when a problem is only suspected or very mild. Teamwork and trust are essential in management.

After referral, a full clinical assessment is made and copies of findings are sent to the health professionals involved. This provides a baseline for later assessments of the child's gross motor progress. Regular reports are made over the years. Videos are a useful way of recording the child's abilities and can also function as teaching aids for both parents and other members of staff.

Treatment will vary for each child and family on account of both the illness or handicap, and also the individual circumstances and outlook on life held by the family. A weekly physiotherapy session is usually less appropriate for a child with special needs than aiming to teach parents and carers the necessary daily physiotherapy management. This must be done without putting an impossible added burden onto the family, and by fitting it as far as possible into their everyday lives and routines. When treatment sessions take place at the child's home, school or nursery the family is saved the difficulties of travel with their child, and it is also easier for the physiotherapist to give appropriate advice and suggestions. The parents are less likely to dismiss them as impractical when they are actually seen carried out in their own home or surroundings.

20.12 Occupational therapists

Inga Warren

Occupational therapy uses purposeful activity to develop the skills which are necessary for independence at school, work and play. Techniques are found to overcome or manage disabilities and to help the child and family successfully adapt to their physical, social and cultural environments.

The paediatric occupational therapist combines neurophysiological, sensory, cognitive, psychodynamic, behavioural and technical approaches. Children with physical disabilities, psychological disorders, developmental problems or specific learning difficulties may benefit from occupational therapy. A referral to an occupational therapist is appropriate for children with sensorimotor problems which prevent them from performing motor skills as well as their peers, for children who have difficulty caring for themselves, or with learning, work or play tasks, moving their limbs for functional use, or who have impaired cognitive behavioural skills. Poor handwriting, feeding difficulties, inability to master dressing and undressing, immature play skills, poor attention or limited parent–infant interaction are a few examples of problems that can be treated.

Intervention is planned after a wide range of skills have been assessed using standardized tests, observation and information given by the child, parents or other carers. So far as possible assessment and treatment are located where most suitable for the child. This may be the home, nursery or school. There are many advantages to seeing the child in familiar home surroundings: the child may feel more secure, the home environment can be assessed and use made of existing resources there. The occupational therapist works directly with the child and also indirectly by advising, directing and encouraging parents and teachers. In practice interventions involving both child and family are most likely to be successful. The occupational therapist may be requested by the local education authority to assess a child and make recommendations as part of the formal statementing procedure of a child with special educational needs.

Treatment activities are aimed at stimulating the child to explore and initiate appropriate activity independently. Emphasis is placed on the child gaining self-confidence through achievement, and activities may be modified to ensure that they are rewarding. Similar principles apply to working with parents and other carers and it is important to recognize they will find it easier to support activities which are consistent with their own values and standards. Helpful daily routines and habits are important for organizing occupational behaviour.

Guidance with regard to activities of daily living (ADL) such as feeding, dressing, writing and toileting helps to promote independence. Functional improvement is facilitated by use of specialized equipment or adapted techniques. Occupational therapists also undertake assessment of need for a wide range of equipment and adaptations designed to help children to live at home with their families, be integrated into local schools and the community, and enhance performance in any setting. Such adaptations range from feeding and writing aids to wheelchairs and architectural alterations. Much equipment is available commercially but individual pieces may need to be designed. Orthoses such as hand splints may be provided to maintain or improve function or safety.

Treatment will vary a great deal from child to child. Some children may have problems in only one performance area but many have difficulties in several areas which overlap and interact, creating complex problems. A 7 year old with poor coordination and attendant emotional and behavioural problems may benefit from outpatient psychomotor therapy, a home programme of pencil control exercises, and be taught to use a keyboard. A severely multiply handicapped child may need a specialized wheelchair, adapted toilet and bath seats, alterations to the home, and splints which prevent deformity. In addition parents may be advised about play and helped to achieve specific goals such as head control or independent feeding; similar help may be offered at the child's school. A 1 year old with delayed development may be seen regularly at home where play and learning techniques can be demonstrated to the parents, who then work to incorporate the ideas into daily life. A 4 year old with a hemiplegia can be shown optimum techniques for dressing, positions to encourage normal and discourage abnormal movement and play which promotes perceptual skills. The child's nursery school teachers will need similar advice.

Occupational therapists complete a 3- or 4-year diploma or degree programme. The syllabus includes biological, sociological, psychological and medical studies, occupational therapy theory and clinical training placements. Occupational therapists are trained for work in physical or psychological medicine, in hospitals or in the community and develop specialized skills, such as in paediatrics, through supervised work experience and postgraduate courses and degrees. Most paediatric occupational therapists providing community services are employed by health authorities and work with district child development teams. They are often based in child development centres or special schools. In some areas occupational therapists attached to child and family psychiatric services also provide community-based programmes. Social services also employ occupational therapists (but these are often not paediatric specialists) who provide equipment and adaptations for management of a disabled child at home. Local arrangements vary greatly and referral may be to the local paediatric department or child development centre, or to social services. Occupational therapists are also employed by agencies providing specialist regional or national services such as the Spastics Society, Bobath Centre, ACE, Wolfson Centre and the Disabled Living Foundation.

Collaboration with other professionals working with children, many of whom will have overlapping roles, is essential. Occupational therapy is a broad based discipline and readily lends itself to working with the transdisciplinary models so much a part of community paediatrics. Family members are part of the team too and have a unique opportunity actively to influence their child's emerging occupational skills. It is through such skills that human beings adapt to their environment.

Further reading

Dunn, W. (ed). *Pediatric Occupational Therapy: Facilitating Effective Service Provision*. Thorofare, NJ: Slack, 1991.

20.13 Speech and language therapists

Jean Cooper Robinson

Communication skills permeate the nature of man. They comprise all processes associated with the comprehension and production of oral, written and nonverbal language. Their universal application belies their incredible complexity often only recognized when the process breaks down. A multitude of problems can impair the ability to communicate and disorders are not respectful of age or sex. The young are particularly susceptible.

Inability to communicate has attracted attention since earliest times and possibly the oldest reference is in a papyrus of the middle Egyptian dynasty approximately 2000 BC. However, it was not until the 19th century that the first real advances were made in the study and treatment of human communication disorders and not until early in this century did a related profession take shape, when communication became more important and the telephone and gramophone were in wide use. Interest in communication disorders began to flow from several disciplines, particularly psychology and education, and, partly because of the effects of war, various branches of medicine. Later other disciplines joined in contributing to the mainstream of speech and language pathology. This upsurge of interest was apparent internationally, although to some extent the profession has developed with different biases from one country to another.

The strength of the profession is its multiple roots, but this has contributed to its major dilemma –

terminology. For example, what is meant by the terms communication, language and speech? What is understood by the terms disorder, defect and disability? What does therapy denote? These linguistic or terminological questions have been the basis of much discussion nationally and internationally, as has also been the name of the profession and what its practitioners should be called. In the USA the terms speech clinician and speech pathologist are widely used; in Europe, logopedist and phoniatrist and in the UK speech and language therapist. There are limitations to each of these titles and the issues involve identity, academic orientation and financial rewards. Undoubtedly the discussion will continue for some time to come. But what is more important is to understand the nature of the work of the professional concerned with habilitation and rehabilitation of the communicatively disordered.

For the purposes of this article the term *speech and language therapist* will be used for the professional practitioner and *speech and language pathology* as the core subject of the discipline.

Speech and language therapists are specialists in human communication disorders, involved in their prevention, assessment, intervention, scientific study and research. They observe the code of ethics of their national professional body and/or as prescribed by their national/state government. Their remit also extends beyond the direct care of the communicatively disordered person. For example:

1 Teaching other professionals and non-professionals (including the general public) about the nature of communication disorders and the facilities for helping them.
2 Teaching students of the profession to gain clinical experience and expertise.
3 Informing their governments or other policy making bodies about the needs of the communicatively disabled.
4 Assisting voluntary organizations whose work relates to the communicatively disordered.
5 Improving the provision of services for the communicatively disordered.

The work is based in hospitals, community clinics, schools, homes and private offices and involves a consultative not a prescriptive relationship, with almost all health, education and welfare professions.

An integral part of speech and language therapy is an understanding of the behavioural aspects of human communication. It also requires an awareness of the role and findings of other clinical disciplines and so speech and language therapy is an applied interdisciplinary behavioural science.

There are many models of professional training. In the UK and other English speaking countries speech and language therapy education provides a generic qualification and the professional body, e.g. The College of Speech and Language Therapists (CSLT) in the UK and the American Speech-Language & Hearing Association (ASHA) in the USA, assumes responsibility for certification of clinical competence.

The CSLT has drawn up guidelines for the courses at universities, polytechnics and other higher educational institutions. These guidelines establish course requirements but allow for variety and flexibility to meet the changing needs of the profession. There is variable emphasis on biological, physical, behavioural and linguistic contributions. However in order for graduates to gain official recognition by the CSLT for certification to practise, all courses include teaching in anatomy, physiology, phonetics, linguistics, psychology, audiology, child development, neurology and related medical subjects, speech pathology, therapeutics and a substantial amount of clinical practice.

Advanced specialist and postgraduate courses, also opportunities to study for the M Phil and PhD awards, have been developed as part of a continuing education programme.

The current rapid development of technology and greater emphasis on multidisciplinary team work is having and will continue to have a profound effect on the study and practice of the profession.

In the lifespan of clinical professions maturity is when the clinical outcome becomes predictable, and patients have access to high quality, effective services. It is when the profession respects both its own expertise and the roles and responsibilities of other professions, and cooperates on standards of inter-professional service delivery. In many countries the profession is now reaching maturity. To ensure long-term viability, its members must continue to contribute new as well as use existing knowledge. It is essential that the profession continues to recruit and retain high quality personnel who have academic backgrounds compatible with the needs of the profession and those it serves.

20.14 Orthoptists

Diana Thornhill

Orthoptics (from the Greek *orthos* = straight, *optikos* = sight) is concerned with squint (see Appendix 20.1) and disorders of binocular vision, eye movements and visual acuity – their prevention, diagnosis and treatment. It has expanded to include glaucoma and visual field testing, also biometry and fundus photography, and will extend further with changes in training.

The orthoptist's training

Training is now a 3-year degree course at Liverpool and Glasgow universities, attached to the faculties of medicine and combined with clinical study at certified hospital centres.

The orthoptist's work

The orthoptist works in liaison with consultant ophthalmologists and ophthalmic teams in hospitals and in the community.

Patients of all ages are seen, but children form about 60% of the workload.

1 In hospitals and paediatric units

In routine eye clinics, orthoptists undertake the diagnosis and treatment of amblyopia (see Appendix 20.1) and squint in otherwise healthy children, hold visual screening sessions, and see patients referred from other clinics. Occasionally, the orthoptic findings are the first presenting sign of a systemic disease or neurological problem.

Orthoptists also take part in the management of amblyopia and motility disorders in premature babies and children with developmental abnormalities, cerebral palsy, hydrocephalus, Down syndrome, and congenital cataract, in order to achieve the best possible vision and straight eyes.

2 In the community

Visual screening

Pre-school programmes are designed for the earliest reliable detection of subnormal vision or squint. Prevention or early detection of amblyopia is vital because treatment is more effective and easier to carry out before school age; early treatment of squint

is preferable so that, where possible, a child has straight eyes before starting school.

Routine screening sessions are held in health clinics, family doctor practices and schools; screening at second tier level is undertaken when health visitors, school nurses, family doctors or parents are anxious about a particular child's eyes. Ideally all children under school age should be screened by orthoptists. In some areas orthoptists operate mobile screening services, using fully-equipped vans which are large enough for vision-testing to be carried out inside. Any children with visual defects are referred on to an ophthalmologist.

Handicapped children

Orthoptic investigation is essential in the multidisciplinary assessment of mentally and physically handicapped children, of whom about 35% have visual problems. The orthoptist can supervise the children's use of spectacles, advise on occlusion (see Appendix 20.1), give exercises in some cases, and discuss squint surgery with the ophthalmologist and the parents where appropriate.

Treatment and follow-up involve liaison and mutual support between the orthoptist, other therapists, the child and family.

Follow up

The orthoptist checks that those referred for treatment are receiving it and are keeping their appointments.

Diagnosis

Investigation of a squint, eye muscle problem or amblyopia involves:

1 General examination of the eyes by the ophthalmologist.
2 Ordering of glasses if needed.
3 Testing of visual acuity of each eye by the orthoptist using methods suited to the child's age and ability. Qualitative tests can be recorded for babies.
4 The orthoptist also tests for the presence and type of squint, measures the deviation, examines the ocular movements and evaluates binocular vision and stereopsis, selecting appropriate tests for each child.
5 Visual field testing may be included.

From these findings plus the ocular history a diagnosis can be made and the prognosis and management discussed with the ophthalmologist and parent.

Treatment

The aims of treatment are:

1 To obtain and preserve normal vision in each eye.
2 To restore comfortable binocular single vision (see Appendix 20.1) and stereopsis.
3 To restore normal appearance of the eyes.

A good prognosis depends on early diagnosis and treatment – no child is too young.

Amblyopia is treated by occlusion which can be total, by covering the better eye with an adhesive patch to enforce use of the amblyopic eye; or partial, using translucent film or graded filters on one lens. Drugs are also used as drops to blur the sight of the better eye temporarily.

The orthoptist can advise on the type of occlusion, monitor progress and work by close cooperation with the child and family to gain all possible improvement in vision.

Squint can be managed after treatment for amblyopia by surgery to re-align the visual axes, in order to restore binocular vision, or for cosmetic purposes. Orthoptic exercises before and after surgery can improve binocular function. Drugs (in the form of drops) and prisms are useful temporary adjuncts to treatment.

Non-surgical treatment is also used. A small number of squints, in which the eyes become straight with glasses worn to correct hypermetropia (long sight), can be controlled by exercises. Close-work problems due to inability to converge the eyes comfortably are treated with exercises. Children with symptoms caused by intermittent squints may be given exercises and temporary prisms, but may also need surgery.

Specific reading difficulty

Children having an educational psychologist's or remedial teacher's diagnosis of specific reading difficulty (dyslexia) may be referred via the ophthalmologist or family doctor to the orthoptist. The purpose of referral is to look for visual or movement defects and investigate binocular vision, convergence and the reference eye (the eye which is dominant in the central field while the two eyes are functioning together).

Children may be helped to overcome the problem by treatment for convergence weakness or by occlusion of one eye to encourage establishment of a preferred reference eye.

The success of orthoptic diagnosis and treatment in children depends entirely on their early referral, so that re-education of visual functions can be provided from the earliest opportunity to achieve equal vision in the two eyes, binocular single vision and an acceptable cosmetic appearance.

Recognition of the orthoptist's role and cooperation from medical colleagues in the multidisciplinary team are very important.

Appendix 20.1

Glossary

Amblyopia is defective visual acuity which persists after correction of the refractive error and the removal of any pathological obstacle to vision.
Binocular single vision is the ability to use both eyes simultaneously so that each eye contributes to a common single perception.
Occlusion is the embarrassment of the vision of an eye in order to prevent or reduce visual stimulation.
Squint is a condition in which one or other visual axis is not directed towards the fixation point.

20.15 Play specialists

Pamela Barnes

Our knowledge about the unfortunate effects which children may experience as a result of illness has increased considerably. This has enabled those working in hospital and community services to look at the ways in which to address this problem, and achieve a more integrated approach.

A real step forward in the overall care of children is an increased awareness of the importance of play in the development of children. Play is a way 'in which a child may develop a capacity to deal with the stresses and strains of life.'[1] Play is not just a way of passing time, it is a valuable provision for therapeutic reasons, and has a vital function in health care. Play has therapeutic and diagnostic qualities which are particularly important for those children who are admitted to hospitals, or attending outpatient and accident and emergency departments.

Alongside the importance of play programmes within the hospital has been the growth of the way in which play can be used, positively, within the community services. 'The success and quality of play indulged in by children, however, is dependent on the presence of the aware adult.'[2] This has led health services to employ a designated member of staff – a play specialist (PS) – to engage children in appropriate play activities when attending health service facilities.

In hospitals

The role of the PS has been developing and evolving over the last 25 years. Medical and nursing staff have now recognized the essential role of play in the treatment of sick children and not only promote the presence of parents in hospitals but also the provision of play under the guidance of professional PSs. Through the use of appropriate materials, activities and toys related to age and ability, the PS enables children to regain their self-confidence. The therapeutic qualities of paint, dough, water and sand, assist children to cope with the anxiety and stress of illness and the management of feelings.

In hospitals, which have formal routines, and are often intimidating for parents under considerable stress, the PS can take a key role in improving communication between the parents and professionals. The PSs should use their skills to encourage parents to join in play with their child, creating a more relaxed and informal atmosphere on the ward.

The role of the PS cannot be over-emphasized. It is a highly demanding role requiring considerable skills and expertise, making play available to a wide range of children and ensuring continuity of care. The PS must provide a service to other professionals in an informal way, by preparing children through play for operations and aiding recovery. For instance, a child recovering from cardiac surgery can be encouraged to take part in water play and blowing bubbles, so helping with breathing exercises and mobility.

The PS can give valuable contributions at case conferences, not only by providing up-to-date developmental play assessments but also acting as a source of information regarding the child's interaction with peers, patterns of appropriate or inappropriate behaviour, and general state of health. The PS is in a key position to observe family interaction and communication.

An area of expertise that is offered by PSs is their knowledge of normal development, thus allowing identification of a child's difficulties which may differ from the actual reason for admission, for example vision problems detected in play but not related to the acute illness.

The diagnostic value of play is considered to be highly informative. 'The study of spontaneous play can provide a rich source of information about the nature of the child's competence.'[3]

Play is a key issue in the study of child development, and the failure of sequential stages of abilities, both physical and cognitive, can signal emotional and developmental problems ahead. Children admitted to hospital with failure to thrive can be more fully assessed with observations made by the PS in the play setting, allowing for a more detailed picture of the child.

In outpatient departments

The outpatient department is often the child's first contact with the hospital. Here the PS helps to create a more positive experience for the child and family through a suitable environment and appropriate play. The play specialist can initiate ideas, help parents with suitable play materials for their children, and be a point of contact for the chronically ill child and family.

When the consultant decides to admit a child to hospital, the PS can offer help to parents and child with preparation for admission. Specialist children's clinics will benefit from appropriate play activities provided by the PS, for example a diabetic clinic where suitable games are provided in an educational attempt to improve an understanding of dietary needs by the child and the family (Fig. 20.1).

Child assessment units

In a child assessment unit, play and the role of the play specialist can be seen as part of the services provided, giving support in all areas of assessment and treatment. As health services for children move away from hospital towards outpatient and day facilities, the need to use play effectively and efficiently will become even more apparent, if we are to provide an integrated service.

Outreach work – hospital/community

A development in some hospitals has been to use their play schemes to evaluate the problems of children and their families suffering the consequences that can be exacerbated by inner city life, such as stress from marital breakdown, violence within the family, and teenage pregnancy. Children may be seen in structured play programmes either as inpatients or as outpatients with their families. The mode of a child's play can indicate sibling rivalry, aggression, and even

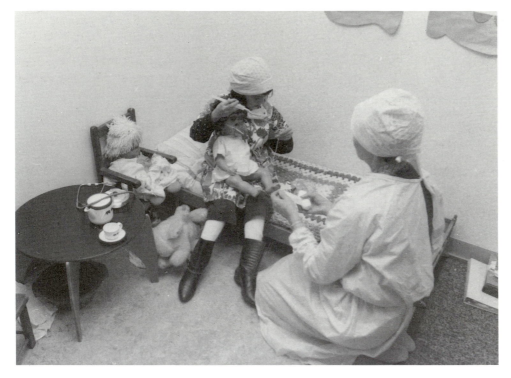

Figure 20.1 Role play for needle phobia in an outpatient clinic.

abuse by an adult. Thus a play scheme and a trained PS can be valuable to the paediatric team.

Arising from the information gathered is a heightened awareness that some children can be involved in inappropriate play. This can be highlighted by the play specialist, and together a psychologist and PS might deal with these problems through joint play sessions. Working with the psychologist in play therapy is a new venture extending the existing role of the play specialist, but does require further training.

Member of the paediatric team

It is essential for the PS to develop a role as a member of the multidisciplinary team. The value of play and the understanding of the ways in which children use play require a high level of knowledge and training for those involved in caring for children. Play allows for the understanding of the normal social, emotional, intellectual and physical development through sequential stages. Play helps children with an understanding of their identity, culture and environment, allowing children a way in which they can communicate and express themselves. The trained PS can assist the paediatric team in identifying these needs of children and through play programmes help in meeting some of these needs. An example was James, who needed to wear spectacles, but would not comply. Through appropriate play ses-

sions of making spectacles for dolls, other children and adults, James was eventually able to come to terms with wearing spectacles himself. An activity like this takes time, sensitivity, and knowledge of working with children.

Training for play specialists

The need for training PSs was identified as early as 1973. Four colleges set up courses for hospital play specialists but it was not until 1985, encouraged by the Department of Health and Social Security and the British Paediatric Association, that the National Association of Hospital Play Staff founded the Hospital Play Staff Educational Trust and the Hospital Play Staff Examination Board. This was planned to ensure a national standard of training for play specialists. The Board designed courses for persons experienced in caring for children to develop their skills in the field of therapeutic and diagnostic play. The units of study on these courses validated by the Board included:

1 Developmental patterns and play of children from birth to adolescence.
2 Play provision for children in hospital including the effects of hospitalization and illness on children and their families.
3 Working alongside others with an understanding of community services, both statutory and voluntary.

4 Organizational, management communication and teaching skills.

At the same time, the Board set down the criteria for approval of courses leading to the award of the Board's certificate. Only students who have followed a course approved under Board regulations and have successfully completed Board assessment are entitled to hold a certificate issued by the Board. The Board is now looking at ways in which to extend the training for hospital PSs into higher level qualifications. New methods of training could enable this to happen through a modular system.

Future

The emphasis for the future is on continued and improved support for parents and children both in hospital and the community, calling for a far-sighted multidisciplinary approach. The play specialist's knowledge of play and development could assist in achieving a more integrated service. Education of parents as to the significance of play in early development of children needs promoting. Parents need to have a greater understanding of the importance of play so that they may encourage their children in achieving full individual potentials.

In the community, a PS should be able to support the community paediatric team and help to prevent admission to hospital, support a child on return home, or prepare a child for treatment or admission to hospital, through play.

With the emphasis on quality assurance in the new approach to health services a good play service should be able to demonstrate its cost effectiveness. Although the emotional well-being of a child cannot be costed, it can be demonstrated that a play service can speed recovery and reduce length of stay for children in hospital.

This can only be achieved by the recognition of the role of PSs backed up by appropriate training and qualifications.[4] Everyone must strive to improve the care of children[5] including the provision of play with the employment of trained professional play specialists.

References

1 UK National Committee (Harvey, S., Chairman). *Play in Hospital*. London: Organisation Mondiale de l'Education Préscolaire (OMEP), 1966.
2 Tizard, B., Harvey, D. *Biology of Play*. London: William Heinemann, 1977.
3 Garvey, C. *Play: the Developing Child*. London: Fontana, 1977.
4 Hogg, C., Rodin, J. *Quality Management for Children: Play in Hospital*. London: Play in Hospital Liaison Committee, Serve the Children, 1990.
5 Department of Health. *Welfare of Children and Young People in Hospital*. London: HMSO, 1991.

Further reading

Barnes, P.A. *Let's Play in Outpatients*. Leaflet No. 3. London: National Association of Hospital Play Staff.
Barnes, P.A. *Hospitals where Healing is Child's Play*. Manchester: South Manchester Health Authority, 1987.
Einon, D. *Creative Play*. Harmondsworth: Penguin, 1985.
Harvey, S. The value of play therapy in hospital. *Pediatrician* 1990; **9**: 191–197.
Hospital Play Staff Examination Board. *Regulations for Courses*. London: Thomas Coram Foundation, 1990.
Jolly, J. *The Other Side of Paediatrics*. London: Macmillan, 1981.
Millar, S. *The Psychology of Play*. Harmondsworth: Pelican, 1968.
Rodin, J. *Will This Hurt?* London: Royal College of Nursing, 1983.

20.16 Music therapists

Alison Levinge

The ability to appreciate and respond to music is an inborn quality which seems to remain despite handicap, illness, or injury. The understanding and acknowledgement of this ability has led to the development of the creative use of music in a clinical setting, and to its recognition as a therapeutic medium. Music therapy is now established as a profession, and recognized in many countries throughout the world. In the UK, music therapists work with:

- learning disabilities
- the mentally ill
- the physically handicapped
- the visually impaired
- the deaf and hearing impaired
- the socially and emotionally deprived
- children of all ages with special needs
- the elderly

- HIV patients
- prisoners

Referral: appropriate uses

Having formal musical training or ability is *not* a requirement for referral. It is rather that, as a universal language, music can be used as an effective therapeutic medium for those children presenting with difficulties in one of the three following areas.

1 Physical difficulties

For the child with physical difficulties, music may be used in order to:

a define movement sequences.
b coordinate muscle pattern.
c provide an enjoyable medium, in which spontaneous movements can be encouraged.
d lead to the experience of holding and doing; cause and effect.

2 Language and communication problems

Music can encourage the development of pre-language skills in the important areas of:

a listening
b turn-taking
c imitation
d pitch discrimination
e shaping auditory sequencing
f rhythmic awareness.

Deafness

Music therapy can help those children diagnosed as deaf or suffering from hearing impairment. Music therapists working in this area have demonstrated that music can help to stimulate responses and encourage children to make sounds.

Autism

The autistic child may seem locked in his or her own world and have specific difficulties in communication, particularly in the areas of language and both visual and physical contact. Music therapy can allow the autistic child to become aware of his or her surroundings, and may facilitate the transition from a world of isolation to a world of meaning.

3 Emotional difficulties

For those children with disturbed and difficult behaviour, making relationships can be confusing and painful. The musical relationship, however, may hold and contain difficult feelings and can match and support the child by providing a non-threatening medium. The child can then begin to explore what it means to be with an other in a more positive way.

Method of referral

Referrals can be made directly to a music therapist, or through agencies such as school, GP, health visitor, etc. The child may then be seen in a school or an establishment such as a child development centre.

Assessment

In an assessment, emphasis is placed upon practical music making. The child is presented with a variety of instruments, usually percussion, and encouraged to explore, play and express him- or herself in sound. The therapist accompanies and supports the child's play, which may also include vocalization, thus allowing a musical picture to build up. For the purpose of the assessment, the child's play is heard in terms of those elements within music identified as: rhythm, pitch, timbre, dynamic, duration. Through the expression of the child's unique musical personality, the music therapist comes to understand his or her difficulties and needs, and appropriate recommendations for treatment can be made.

Treatment

The creative use of music in the clinical setting provides the framework within which therapeutic goals may be pursued. Treatment is based upon shared music making, and the therapist seeks to establish a connection with the child through the musical medium.

The relationship between the child and music therapist begins to develop, with the therapist using a variety of musical responses, which may incorporate elements of the child's play. The therapist uses his or her own music to define, shape and structure, to provide meaning, and to help the child to feel secure enough to explore his or her own difficulties. The therapist's music will also reflect the character and quality of both the musical and non-musical events which develop within the session.

The importance of sound to the infant's development is well recognized, and it is possible to see parallels between the elements of music and some aspects of the early mother–infant interactions. The essential nature of music is interactive, and can therefore enable the therapist to recreate early experiences of relating.

Training

To become a qualified music therapist in the UK it is necessary to complete one of the training courses which have been recognized by the Department of Education and Science. Each course requires a high level of musicianship, and students are normally accepted only if they have a musical ability which is of degree or diploma standard.

Further information regarding music therapy can be obtained from the British Society of Music Therapy, Tel: 0181 368 8879.

20.17 Audiological scientists

Sarah Sheppard

Audiology, the study of hearing and balance disorders, is a rapidly developing field. In the UK the graduate professional scientist in audiology is the audiological scientist. This term was coined by an ACSHIP subcommittee report in 1975.[1] The audiological scientist works as a member of a team which includes medical, scientific, technical and educational personnel. Most audiological scientists are graduates in science and all have studied audiology to the MSc level. During their first year in service audiological scientists complete a further programme of training and assessment known as the certificate of audiological competence.

Most audiological scientists work within hospital audiology departments or community audiological services. Audiological scientists may be involved in providing a service for all ages or specialize in one area, for example, diagnostic neuro-otological assessments, aural rehabilitation, or paediatric audiology. The main responsibilities of audiological scientists include the following:

- A commitment to deliver a clinical audiological service.
- Ensuring that reliable and valid techniques are used and that the results of these are correctly interpreted.
- The development and evaluation of new test techniques.
- Management of the scientific aspects of the service including monitoring and evaluating the standard of the clinical service.
- Responsibility for a wide range of sophisticated test equipment.

- Training of staff.
- Service orientated research.

Audiological scientists are also essential members of the multidisciplinary cochlear implant teams, both in assessing the audiological suitability of prospective candidates for implantation and also in ensuring that these devices are properly set up, evaluated and maintained after fitting.

Audiological scientists who specialize in paediatric audiology are concerned with the audiological assessment and management of children including the very young and those with multiple disabilities. They select and fit hearing aids for children who require them and provide on-going audiological and hearing aid reviews to monitor the hearing status and ascertain any changes in amplification required. Many hearing impaired children use special systems such as frequency modulation (FM) radio aids to help them in the educational setting and the audiological scientist can give expert advice on the fitting and use of such aids. They may also participate in the establishment and monitoring of screening programmes and referral patterns. This work may include specific staff training and a wider role in the dissemination of information about early detection of hearing loss and its management.

Reference

1 ACSHIP DHSS Advisory Committee on Services for Hearing-impaired People. *The Role of the Graduate Scientist in Audiology*. London: HMSO, 1975.

20.18 Specialist teachers

Molly Moodley

Specialist teachers are teachers first and then specialists. Except in a few areas of special education, these teachers serve their apprenticeship in mainstream schools.

They come to special education via many routes. Some make this choice for personal reasons. They either know of, or have intimate experience of, someone with special needs. This motivates them to teach a particular group of children. Others meet children with special educational needs in the hurly-burly of mainstream schools and develop an interest. These children cause their teachers concern and can be the source of irritation and frustration. They are viewed as clumsy, slow, naughty, disruptive, antisocial and poorly motivated. Teachers, while enjoying a challenge, prefer their pupils to be uncomplicated, easy to teach and receptive to learning. The imparting of knowledge to pupils with normal learning curves is their main task. To the specialist teacher this hints at boredom and they look to special education to make teaching more meaningful.

Others choose to work in this area from the knowledge of educational and psychological theories of learning. They too find children with special educational needs challenging and seek job satisfaction in this field. Many of these children are the subjects of the statementing procedure under the Education Act 1981.

Specialist teachers are to be found in the most extraordinary settings. They work in organizations and institutions that at first appear unlikely places for the education of children. Such teachers are found in health authority and social services provisions.

A teacher is sometimes a member of the child development team of a district health authority. The teacher's contribution to the team is in the area of play, and speech and language development. This information forms an invaluable part of the diagnosis and treatment of the child and the family.

The teacher working in a hospital school or tuition unit has an important role in giving sick children a normal experience in an alien and frightening environment. Teachers are not trained to deal with the sick and dying; but the hospital teacher develops a sensitivity in dealing with children's questions and fears on these issues. These teachers are much valued by parents, nurses and the medical staff for the normality they create and the lessening of anxiety which hastens recovery.

As in hospital settings, in special schools for children with medical problems teachers must acquire relevant medical knowledge. They become aware of medical procedures and the effects of medication on children's personality, attitudes and learning behaviour. These observations are critical in the medical management of these children.

In psychiatric settings, the treatment of the young includes education. By providing a secure environment and a framework for learning, the teacher allows the child space to explore fears, doubts, aggression and other emotions in safety. The teacher must develop skills in dealing with childhood psychiatric disorders. As the non-medical member of the team, the teacher is dependent on her colleagues to diagnose and prescribe a course of treatment. However, it is the teacher who has day-to-day contact and responsibility for the child. The success of an intervention programme is often dependent on her to ensure it is carried out, and that sensitive, informed observations are recorded and shared.

Specialist teachers are also drawn from the fields of art, music and drama. They use their subjects to work with a variety of children with special educational needs. They aim to give them the pleasure of expressing themselves through these subjects or use them as therapy.

Recently there has been greater awareness of child sexual abuse. It is often the class teacher, through observation of children at work and play, who alerts other professionals skilled in working with these children. A teacher attached to an assessment or therapeutic team may have particular skills to enable a child to communicate painful, traumatic experiences. This may be achieved through structured play, drawing, writing and talking, all within a safe learning environment.

The majority of specialist teachers are found in a variety of special schools. In some of these schools there are children and youngsters with profound and multiple handicaps. The emphasis of the teaching is on motivation, communication, self-help and independence skills. All this is done in a caring environment. Where there are children with physical disabilities there is the same emphasis on teaching and they are encouraged to take part in the mainstream curriculum.

Teachers for children with sensory impairment receive specialist training. They become skilled in the technological requirements of their craft and help the hearing-impaired and visually-handicapped children to lead successful lives.

There are some teachers who work with children who fail to acquire language and literacy skills. They have devised programmes collaboratively with colleagues to help these children.

Working with parents is intrinsic to the job of the specialist teacher. Without parental cooperation and investment, programmes to manage children's behaviour and learning would fail. These teachers have developed ingenious ways of involving reluctant parents in true partnerships. In the area of under-five education a valuable link is the home-school liaison teacher. She supports parents in dealing with their feelings and makes them aware of available provisions to help their child.

The skills that specialist teachers have include those to be found in the best of our teachers. The best teachers inspire children to learn. Over and above this inspirational quality the specialist teacher needs knowledge, sensitivity, patience, dedication and resilience.

The most successful teachers are those who remain clearly teachers and do not confuse their roles with those of doctors, therapists or social workers.

The specialist teacher aims above all to help children in his or her charge to make sense of the world, to manage their emotions and behaviour in socially acceptable ways; to reach their potential as human beings; to have autonomy and a sense of purpose; to find pleasure in literature, art, music, science etc, and to be motivated to continue learning.

20.19 Clinical psychologists

Richard Lansdown

In the 1940s clinical psychology was an infant profession, its role limited to the production of test results and its autonomy curtailed by its location within psychiatry. The 1960s and 1970s saw a shift: an interest in behaviour therapy led to a much broader approach which came to encompass family therapy, group work and more general consultation. Inevitably, this phase had characteristics of the rebellious adolescent and the break from psychiatry was at times painful. Now most health districts have independently organized psychology departments and early adulthood has been attained.

Training follows a straightforward path. A good degree in psychology is a prerequisite and it is now expected that this will be followed by at least 2 years' work in a health-related field, possibly on an assistant psychologist grade. This allows would-be psychologists not only to have early hands-on experience, but acts also as a crude sift giving trainees an opportunity to make up their mind about whether to proceed in clinical psychology.

Postgraduate training consists of a 3-year course in a university or in-service setting leading to a doctor's or master's degree or to a diploma awarded by the British Psychological Society. There is emphasis on practical work in varying fields and placements are obligatory in adult mental health and child services. Other placements can include neurology, the elderly or community work. There is great pressure on training courses with between 20 and 40 applicants for every place. At present about 80% of candidates are women.

A good idea of psychologists' present perception of roles comes from the language they use. 'Patient' has been frequently replaced by 'client', the underlying notion being that the people one helps are essentially equal. The focus on handicap and psychopathology that was once so prevalent has given way to a realization that there is nothing necessarily abnormal in certain responses to environmental stresses. A recent proposal[1] to rename the profession 'Healthcare Psychology' bears this view out. This trend towards normalization is consistent with the focus of a first degree in psychology, only a small segment of which deals with the abnormal.

Although a small number of psychologists work in social services departments and as community psychologists, the vast majority are employed within the Health Service. About 300 of the 1700 qualified clinical psychologists working in the UK offer child work, and specialist services are provided in about 85% of health districts. In some districts this service is, however, no more than very limited.[2]

Clinical psychologists working with children do so in a number of settings which include hospitals, children's homes, nurseries, drop-in clinics and general practice health centres. Referrals include common disorders such as bed wetting and sleep problems, emotional and behavioural problems and developmental disorders. A significant number of children will be seen because of psychological problems arising from physical disabilities which can include depression in chronically sick children (and their parents), a refusal to cooperate with treatment and learning difficulties of iatrogenic origin.[3,4]

Children are seen individually or in groups, with and without their parents. While a small proportion of psychologists have a psychoanalytic orientation most use broadly behavioural techniques. When working with families, a theory which sees each family member as part of an overall system is probably the most commonly adopted approach. Much of the help offered goes not directly to children and their families but to others looking after them, for example via consultation on wards or in nurseries.

A small proportion of time is spent in formal testing; clinical psychologists are generally more willing than their colleagues in education to use developmental or intelligence tests, but these are invariably only part of a more global assessment.

The Portage schemes for developmentally delayed children are an example of the use of criterion referenced (as opposed to norm referenced) tests and of the indirect way in which much psychological work is done. A check list of attainments is completed by mothers who are helped to play with their children in a way designed to promote a specific piece of behaviour. Parents are visited at home by a variety of people who work under the supervision of a professional, usually a psychologist.

A similar working-via-parents model can be seen in sleep clinics which are now held in a number of areas. Here psychologists will discuss sleep problems, one of the most common difficulties presented by pre-school children, and will work with parents to reach a behavioural approach which will allow a resolution to the problem satisfactory to both parents and children.

Drop-in services have also been found to be popular with some parents. There is a minimum of paper work and formality involved, thus a service is offered to some parents who are wary of going on record or who are intimidated by hospitals and doctors' surgeries.

There is a good deal of support for the effectiveness of psychological intervention with children. Two recent meta-analyses[5,6] conclude that those who have received intervention fare better than those who are not treated or are treated by other means.

So far the picture has been given of psychologists working single handed. While much community work does follow this pattern it is by no means exclusive. Child development teams are an example of how a psychologist can join a multidisciplinary setting; the attachment of a psychologist to a general practice is another. In the latter it is rare to have anyone specializing only in child work.

The picture is not, however, totally rosy for there is a chronic manpower shortage. Overall some 15% of posts established for child work are unfilled and about 20% of newly qualified postgraduates elect not to join the Health Service. There are plans to increase the numbers of places on training courses but this is only part of the story. Nevertheless, clinical psychology is an exciting profession, it has made enormous strides over the past 20 years and there is every sign that, staffing permitting, it will continue to grow conceptually and effectively.

References

1 Management Advisory Service to the NHS. *Review of Clinical Psychology Services* Cheltenham: 1989.
2 British Psychological Society Special Interest Group (Children and Young People). *Preliminary Report Concerning Child Clinical Psychology Services in Great Britain*, 1989, (unpublished).
3 Lansdown, R. *More than Sympathy*. London: Tavistock Publications, 1980.
4 Garrison, W.T., McQuiston, S. *Chronic Illness During Childhood and Adolescence*. London: Sage Publications, 1989.
5 Casey, R.J., Russo, D.C. The outcome of psychotherapy with children. *Psychol Bull* 1985; **98**: 388–400.
6 Weisz, J.R., Weisz, B., Alicke, M.D., Klotz, M.L. Effectiveness of psychotherapy with children and adolescents: a meta-analysis for clinicians. *J Consulting Clin Psychol* 1987; **55**: 542–549.

20.20 Educational psychologists

Patrick Fletcher

Educational psychologists are usually employed by a local education authority (LEA), as part of a team led by a principal educational psychologist. Typically, the psychologist would have a geographical patch and offer a service to children in schools and of pre-school age within that patch. The work involves psychological consultations, assessments of individual children, and advice to teachers and parents on how to help children with learning and behaviour problems.

There is an increasing emphasis on providing support and advice to teachers and other professionals to help improve their skills. This can be done through consultation where the psychologist and teachers work together in a problem-solving way. The concern may be about an individual child, a difficult class of children or an aspect of the school organization. An example of the latter would be a psychologist working with the school to develop a whole school policy on behaviour. They also provide in-service training for teachers and other professionals.

Educational psychologists mainly spend their time in schools as this is the source of most of their work. Often they will visit their schools on a regular pre-arranged basis.

Training

Before undertaking specialist training an aspiring educational psychologist obtains a degree in psychology followed by a minimum of 2 years' teaching experience. A typical training course would cover a wide range of psychological theories and research and their application in practice. Training is geared towards enabling psychologists to work effectively with individual children, groups of children, families, teachers and schools as organizations. Examples of skills that have to be developed are those of interviewing, consultancy and applied problem solving.

Work with children with special educational needs

Most of the work a psychologist does at an individual level in schools involves children with special educational needs. There is an emphasis on early intervention, that is, tackling learning difficulties before they become too entrenched. Strategies worked out by the child's teachers and the psychologist, often involving the parents, will be reviewed over time. If the child fails to make progress and serious learning difficulties remain, the school having used all additional resources available to it and adopted a variety of strategies (after completing the School-based stages of assessment 1–3), an assessment under the 1993 Education Act would normally be carried out.[1]

Educational psychologists and the 1981 Education Act

In many LEAs the psychologist is asked to advise on whether or not a child should be subject to a statutory multidisciplinary assessment under the Act. If a statutory assessment goes ahead, an educational psychologist will carry out an assessment and provide advice as a statutory part of the process. They may also be involved in the planning to implement the recommendations made in the statement of educational needs especially if the child is being maintained in an ordinary school. The psychologist would also have an important part to play in the annual review of such children.

Psychological assessment

Often this will involve observation of the child in the classroom looking at how the child copes with school work and how he or she relates to the teacher and peers. Observation of children at play would be crucial for very young children attending a nursery. Relevant aspects of the child's communicative skills with others would be important as well as the quality of their play.

If assessing a child with a disability the psychologist may complete a developmental checklist (such as the PIP developmental charts) with those adults who know the child best.[2]

Where it seems helpful and appropriate, standardized tests of ability may be used to obtain a profile of children's abilities, for example, The British Ability Scales.[3] Tests specifically designed for use with children with a particular disability are also available, for example the Snijders-Oomen Non-verbal Intelligence Scale for Young Children,[4] which is constructed for use with deaf children.

For children with significant learning difficulties documentation of the pattern of the child's development through the comparison of the slowly developing areas with more rapidly developing areas provides crucial information. A child with severe learning difficulties is likely to show delayed development in all areas whereas an autistic child may show an uneven pattern of development.

The aim of the assessment is to obtain as accurate a description as possible of the child's strengths and weaknesses. Through the psychologist's knowledge of the learning processes involved the child's strengths or abilities can be used constructively to promote future learning. Areas where the child needs specific help can be identified. Under Section 167 of the 1993 Education Act an accurate assessment of the child's educational needs is necessary to ensure that the appropriate provision is made by the LEA to meet the child's needs.

Parents

Educational psychologists strive to work in partnership with parents, sharing information and endeavouring to be as frank as possible. Often they have the difficult task of counselling parents to help them come to terms with the consequences of their child's learning difficulties. Psychologists may be involved in Portage schemes[5] where they help parents of young children with serious learning difficulties to develop learning programmes for use at home.

Contact with other professionals

In many areas community child health doctors and psychologists meet regularly to discuss special needs provision and to plan for specific children. There is also frequent contact between psychologists and other health authority personnel such as speech therapists treating young children with significant language difficulties or occupational therapists treating children with perceptual difficulties which affect their learning.

References

1 Education Act 1993: Draft Code of Practice on the Identification and Assessment of Special Educational Needs, DFE.
2 Jeffree, D.M., McConkey, R. *P.I.P. Developmental Charts*. Hester Adrian Research Centre, University of Manchester: Hodder and Stoughton Educational, 1976.
3 Elliott, C.D. *British Ability Scales: Handbook and Technical Manual*. Windsor: NFER-Nelson, 1983.
4 Snijders, J.Th., Snijders-Oomen, N. *Snijders-Oomen Non-Verbal Intelligence Scale for Young Children*. Groningen: H.D. Tjeenk Willink, 1976.
5 Cameron, R.J. *Working Together: Portage in the UK*. Windsor: NFER-Nelson, 1982.

20.21 Child psychotherapists

Judith Elkan and Mirjana Renton

Child psychotherapy is a method of treating problems in children, adolescents and families based on psychoanalytical principles and techniques. Psychoanalytical therapy aims to help the child to understand conscious and unconscious conflicts, anxieties and inhibitions which are unreachable by ordinary logic and advice.

Child psychotherapy is a distinct profession. Training requires a minimum of 4 years, following an honours degree in psychology or its equivalent, and experience of work with children and families. The professional body to which child psychotherapists belong is the Association of Child Psychotherapists.

The work of the child psychotherapist

Child psychotherapists work with child psychiatrists, psychologists, social workers and other professions in multidisciplinary teams within child guidance clinics, hospital departments of child psychiatry, schools for emotionally and behaviourally disturbed children, GP clinics, mother and baby clinics, walk-in clinics for adolescents, and in private practice.

There are three basic areas of work:

Therapy

The specific contribution of child psychotherapy is to focus at depth on understanding the child's disturbed emotional experiences in relation to himself, his family and his surroundings. By helping children to understand the anxieties and conflicts underlying their troubles psychotherapy can prevent the worsening of difficulties and promote a process of recovery and healthy development.

Consultation

Children with problems create difficulties both in their families and among other professionals caring for them: the child psychotherapist's work extends to consultation with professionals, and institutions that deal with babies, children and adolescents under stress.

Teaching

Child psychotherapists also engage in teaching professionals in allied disciplines about child development, with emphasis on the interrelationship of emotional, intellectual and social factors.

Referral

Problems may arise as a result of inadequacies of care, stress, the child's temperament or a combination of these. Experiences such as prolonged separation, illness, death, neglect or abuse of any kind, and traumas due to accidents or disasters can inflict overwhelming emotional pain which may severely disrupt the child's development and functioning. Psychotherapeutic intervention may be essential to help children make sense of these distressing experiences. While some children will manifest overt disturbance, others will appear to be functioning almost 'too well': the latter are a cause for special concern, for they may conceal emotional scars which can have seriously disabling effects later in life.

What problems to refer

Disturbances in children express themselves in a wide variety of symptoms. These range from disturbance in eating and sleeping, problems of wetting and soiling, psychosomatic complaints, speech and learning difficulties, inhibitions, anxieties and phobias, violence, delinquency and ill-controlled behaviour to depression, self-injury and psychotic disorders.

When to refer

Some emotional problems in infancy and childhood are transitory and part of normal development, but when problems persist and are severe it is appropriate to make a referral. Early intervention can prevent problems from becoming more severe.

Who refers

Referrals usually come from doctors, nurses, health visitors, physiotherapists, speech therapists, social workers, educational psychologists, teachers and others of the helping professions. Parents and adolescents can also initiate referral.

What happens on referral

Assessment and diagnosis precede recommendations for treatment. The patient and his family are usually seen by one or more members of the clinic team. Following discussion by the team, recommendations are made either for psychotherapy or some alternative course. The frequency of psychotherapy is usually once a week, (but may be up to five times a week), and therapy can last from one to several years.

Individual psychotherapy for the child, and therapy for parents or family may be needed, but cannot always be carried out because of unstable circumstances or lack of cooperation from the family. In these situations consultation is offered to the referrer and may lead to recommendations for special schooling, placement in care, remedial teaching or support and advice on management for those who continue to care for or have charge of the child.

What happens in therapy

The setting

The therapist works in a consulting room which is plainly and simply furnished. It is arranged to ensure that the patient (child or adolescent) can express himself in safety. Each patient is provided with a box of toys for his exclusive use, available during his session time. The toys are small and are selected for their expressive potential; they comprise a small-sized doll family, sets of little animals, cars, bricks, fences, small containers, balls, plasticine, string, scissors and drawing material. At the outset the therapist explains to the patient that he will be seen regularly, that the session is 50 minutes long and that there will be planned holiday breaks.

This simple, regular and constant setting provides safe boundaries within which the patient can gradually communicate his difficulties and allow feelings about loving, hating, fear, rage, aggression, rivalry, stupidity, goodness, badness, excitement, depression, grief and hope to surface. Children show astonishing capacity to dramatize through play the complexities of relationships in their inner and outer worlds.

Method of work

The therapist does not offer suggestions or take initiatives; the patient is left free to express himself as he wishes at his own pace. The therapist watches and listens, comments and interprets to the patient about the meaning of his particular activities.

The process of understanding the underlying forces determining the patient's life requires the therapist to attend closely to the child's communications, verbal and non-verbal, and to be a recipient of all kinds of powerful feelings, positive and negative, which gradually emerge during the therapy and are often directed at the therapist. By thinking about and finding patterns in the patient's behaviour and showing connections between his inner and outer reality, the therapist helps the patient to understand and accept his conflictual and unwanted feelings and integrate them. This enables the patient to make fuller and more constructive use of his capacities.

This process may best be exemplified through an extract from a first session with a 9-year-old boy who had learning difficulties, was truanting and beginning to steal. In this session he drew a boat at sea with the shore and lighthouse in the background. He said the boat was a drifter and in danger of going on the rocks and breaking up, but the lighthouse might help the boat reach safety. The therapist spoke about the boy's hopes and fears; she said the picture showed something about his problems – how he felt himself, like the boat, to be drifting into trouble, but was hoping that someone, perhaps the therapist, would be like the lighthouse and guide him onto a safer course. The therapist also pointed out the conflict between the side of himself which chose to drift into trouble, and another side which could see the danger but was unable to deal with it on his own, and hence was searching for help.

The images of the boat/boy drifting revealed some recognition of the risk at hand, but not the nature and power of the forces which pulled him off course. The danger is that, without therapy to help him understand the underlying reasons, these forces could continue to operate destructively throughout his life.

The process of therapy is lengthy and requires the cooperation of parents. But parents also need help in understanding the child and their relationship to him, and therapeutic support offered to them contributes to the process of recovery.

Further reading

Daws, D., Boston, M. eds. *The Child Psychotherapist and Problems of Young People*. London: Wildwood House, 1977.

Szur, R., Miller, S., eds. *Extending Horizons: Psychoanalytic Psychotherapy with Children, Adolescents and Families*. London: Karnac Books, 1977.

20.22 Dietitians

Carol Atkins

The dietitian working in community paediatrics is an important member of the community child health service whose aim is to promote normal growth and development in all children. The dietitian's role is varied and constantly expanding to incorporate new areas of education and preventive treatment. The work involves the provision of dietary advice from infancy to adolescence for children with normal nutritional requirements and those with special dietary needs.

The training is comprehensive and thus suited to the dietitian's many professional roles. It includes such disciplines as biochemistry, medical and social sciences, nutrition and psychology. Dietetics is now an all graduate profession and dietitians qualify either after a 4 year BSc degree course in nutrition or a 3 year BSc degree in a scientific subject (often nutrition); the latter being followed by a Diploma in Dietetics to complete qualification for status as a State Registered Dietitian. During training a dietitian is seconded to a hospital dietetic department for 7 months to receive practical training and to develop skills in the application of nutritional knowledge to patients of all age groups and different medical conditions. After qualification the majority of dietitians take up a hospital dietetic post to gain further experience in a wide range of conditions before specializing in one particular area, which may be paediatrics. The British Dietetic Association runs training courses for dietitians who work with children. The 'Introduction to Paediatric Dietetics' is a 5-day intensive residential course which covers infant nutrition, enteral feeding, gastroenterology, food intolerance, vitamin and mineral supplementation, cystic fibrosis, lipid disorders and diabetes. There is an examination at the end of the course, and a 4000 word case study is also assessed. The advanced course is a 6-day course – usually held at the Institute of Child Health, London – which includes inborn errors of metabolism, renal disease, liver disease and preterm infants.

The majority of paediatric dietitians are hospital based but dietitians based in health centres in the community or attached to general practices may also spend a large proportion of their time working with children.

The role of the dietitian

Dietary assessment

Common referrals to a community based dietitian are children with poor growth rates, anaemia or feeding difficulties. The dietitian assists the paediatrician by taking a dietary history to determine the child's average daily nutritional intake, thus identifying if the problem is one of inadequate nutrition or possibly malabsorption. The dietitian is practised at obtaining the details of feeding regimens, frequency and duration of feeds and types of food preferred; all necessary information on which to base dietary advice. Standard measurements of the child such as height, weight, anthropometric measurements and plotting of percentile charts are done as required, enabling the dietitian to calculate the normal nutritional requirements of the child.

Provision of special diets

Some patients require specific dietary treatment and referrals should include a brief medical history and diagnosis where appropriate. The dietitian provides the appropriate dietary advice and the practical details of how to achieve the dietary modifications. Standard diet sheets have only a limited place in dietetics today as the dietitian uses skill and expertise to devise a diet specific to the individual's needs. The child's individual nutritional requirements are influenced by the type of diet indicated, social status of the family, the money available for food, and dietary habits – all these factors must be taken into consideration in order to provide a diet that is both appropriate to the child's condition and acceptable to the child and family. To achieve dietary compliance the advice must be practical and the family can be helped by the provision of special recipes, details of suitable manufactured foods such as milk-free foods and available proprietary dietary products, lists of shops where certain items can be purchased, contact with specialist organizations such as the British Diabetic Association, liaison with social services, schools and nurseries particularly regarding provision of suitable dietary meals and liaison with other health professionals.

Following initial consultation with the dietitian the child is offered follow-up appointments either at home or in a hospital clinic to assess the effect of the diet, to reduce problems encountered and to modify the dietary treatment in line with changing nutritional requirements. A dietitian is involved with the treatment of a wide range of conditions such as allergies, cystic fibrosis, weight reduction and inborn errors of metabolism, e.g. phenylketonuria. A very important role of the dietitian is providing support and encouragement to the child and family to maintain the required dietary control.

Follow up of hospital patients

A community-based dietitian is often involved with children on special diets who have been discharged from hospital. This necessitates close liaison with the hospital dietitian and then dietary follow up of the child at home with suitable modification to the diet to take account of the child's improving appetite, changing social life and nutritional requirements. Children discharged on parenteral or nasogastric feeding regimens, or newly diagnosed diabetics for example, would normally be under the care of the dietitian in the community.

Education

Health education about nutrition is particularly important in paediatrics as the children of today form the adult population of tomorrow. Dietary practices learnt in childhood are taken into adulthood and onto the next generation. The role of the dietitian is to provide practical advice which will promote optimal growth and development in children, and encourage healthy eating habits that can be easily incorporated into family life.

Education is offered through visual displays, videos, leaflets, or in discussion groups with mothers, teachers, children and other health professionals. Liaison with other health professionals is particularly important when drafting nutritional guidelines and food policies for all members of the community child health service to use.

The current high profile in the press given to nutritional regimens provides the opportunity both to educate and clarify good dietary practice. The dietitian should be seen as an important member of the community child health service without whom the proper nutritional care of many patients would be impossible.

20.23 Dientists

James Hogan

In Geoffrey Slack's collection of drawings by children on *My Visit to the Dentist*, the dentist is represented as a sleek, leering man in a white coat with predatory hands, against a background usually interpreted by psychoanalysts to be symbolic of pain, blood and electronic assault. This manifest dislike of dentists shocked students and teachers of dentistry at the London Hospital in the late 1960s. Although it was attributed by some to the theory of the 'oral sadistic phase' in child development, when 'the first teeth are coming through, thus providing the baby with weapons to express its aggression',[1] dentists recognized that here was the truth about their profession they had always feared. Certainly, dental training, and most dentists, in recent decades have tried hard to reverse the Big Bad Wolf image. This has been helped by the increase in female dentists (now over 20%), and in the commercial development of more refined and patient-friendly dental equipment and surgery design.

In little over 150 years, dentists have advanced from an unregulated band of itinerant tooth-pullers, working largely as less-than-respectable artisans in the marketplace or in backstreet 'tooth-booths', to the status of an established, respected, and influential scientific profession.[2] In a Gallup survey in 1989 of professionals in the USA, dentists came out top in the professional popularity stakes, easily beating doctors and bankers. This even surprised dentists.

Since ancient times, there have always been some practitioners providing high-quality dental services, and dentistry has an impressive scientific history in Europe from Hippocrates, through Fauchard and

Hunter in the 18th century, to the present. Nevertheless it cannot be denied that until the 20th century the impact has been solely on an elite minority of the population.

The emergence of dentistry as an effective and responsible profession is not unrelated to the government realization that an alarming amount of the invalidism among troops in the Boer War (1899–1901) was due to widespread dental disease. A subsequent national enquiry revealed very high levels of dental disease among school children in the UK. The Interdepartmental Committee on Physical Deterioration recommended the creation of a school medical service, and particularly drew attention to the need to inspect eyes, ears and teeth. In 1918, the School Dental Service was established and in 1920 the practice of dentistry was regulated by a professional register.

In the 19th century the majority of dentists were tradesmen who combined dental work with selling patent medicines, wig-making, barbering, and minor surgery. Many developed considerable skills in restoring damaged dentitions. However, the emphasis was on mechanical craft, rather than health care.

In 1910, the British surgeon William Hunter, eager to turn dentistry into a scientific-based discipline, denounced the widespread practice of 'concealing gross untreated problems of oral sepsis under a facade of dental reconstruction'. His theory of focal infection maintained that gross decay and rotting gums produced foci, which were thought to be involved in a wide range of disorders, including arthritis.

Registered dentists were strongly influenced by this theory and a mass extraction boom occurred in dentistry between the Wars. It was not until the 1940s that the focal infection theory was finally discredited using the scientific methods Hunter himself advocated. But there is no doubt that it contributed, overall, to bringing dentistry into the scientific and professional mainstream of medicine.

About 20 000 dentists now work in the UK. There are 22 dental schools offering training which includes a thorough grounding in basic and applied medical sciences during a 5-year course.[3] The newly qualified dentist is now competent to perform most of the treatments patients are likely to need. Increasingly, vocational training in particular specialities is undertaken along the dentist's career pathway.

Over 86% of dentists work in the general dental service (GDS) spending about one-tenth of their time on private treatment.[4] Dentists who undertake only private work are still rare although there is a growing movement towards independent practice by dentists working in a deregulated variant of the GDS. Only 6% of the remaining dentists are employed in the hospital service. The community dental service (CDS) employs 7% of dentists. There is reorientation of roles within the CDS and the GDS.

Usually, however, the GDS treats families while the CDS is concerned with epidemiology, dental health promotion and the treatment of special needs groups. The hospital dental service takes referrals from doctors and dentists. However, collaboration between the three sectors has developed dramatically over the past decade and it is not uncommon for dentists to work in two or even three sectors. The development makes it easier to coordinate the care of children, particularly those with special needs. When the dentist in the hospital emergency service is also the community dentist who visits the local school, and is able to talk directly to the family dentist, the full circle of dental contacts is complete. The contracts of service recently introduced for the GDS and CDS encourage both sectors to become complementary services. Already, in many health districts, community and hospital services work together exchanging skills and facilities.

There are other employment options for dentists – in the armed forces, in university teaching, in research, and increasingly in industrial dentistry (running a practice within a large company). Nevertheless, dentistry is going through a critical manpower review. The changing patterns of distribution of dental disease in advanced industrial countries is altering manpower needs.[5] Fewer dentists will probably be required, but more dental auxiliaries. The team approach, with specialist dentists as leaders, is professionally and economically preferable. Full integration of dental teams into primary health care systems in the 21st century is undoubtedly desirable, and probably inevitable.

To date in the UK only the recruitment of dental students has been reduced. However, the inquiry by the Nuffield Foundation into dental auxiliaries reported in 1993 and recommended a radical redefinition of dental manpower and its composition.

Since then, the Mouatt Report (1994) on the future of dental training introduced recommendations that are likely to alter the interface between primary and secondary dental care, substantially increasing the proportion of specialist treatments and training provided in the community.

References

1 Pond, D.A. The tooth and the psyche. *Br Dent J* 1968; **125**: 457–460.

2 Davis, P. *The Social Context of Dentistry*. London: Croom Helm, 1980.

3 *Careers in Dentistry*. London: General Dental Concil, 1989.

4 Medical and dental staffing prospects in the NHS in England and Wales. *Health Trends* 1991; **23**: 4.

5 Sheiham, A. Future patterns of dental care – manpower implications for industrial countries. *Br Dent J* 1989; **166**: 240–243.

20.24 Dental hygienists and dental therapists

Judith Peers

There are two types of operating dental auxiliaries in the UK – dental hygienists and dental therapists – both have important roles in the prevention of dental disease and dental health.

Dental hygienists and therapists, like dentists, are regulated by the General Dental Council (GDC).

Dental hygienists are trained to carry out dental work of the following kinds: to scale, clean and polish teeth, to administer local infiltration analgesia (under direct supervision of a registered dentist), to apply preventive materials such as fluorides and fissure sealants; to motivate and educate patients to maintain their oral health; and to carry out domiciliary visits.

Dental therapists are trained to carry out the above and, in addition, extractions of deciduous (milk) teeth, undertaking simple fillings in both permanent and deciduous dentition and administering local infiltration analgesia for these procedures.[1,2]

The course of instruction for student hygienists and therapists should extend up to 12 months for hygienists and 2 years for dental therapists. Subjects included on both courses must relate to basic clinical sciences, operative and preventive dentistry and dental health prevention. Students have the opportunity of treating and caring for children, adults and special needs groups. They are also given the chance to observe all aspects of a wide variety of working conditions for example in general hospitals and community dental clinics. In addition to this training the student therapist course includes closer links with dental undergraduates in specialized areas such as community dentistry, paedodontics, child psychology and child health. At the end of their training the students must pass a qualifying examination (examination for the certificate of proficiency in dental hygiene or certificate of proficiency as a dental therapist) before they are allowed to enrol with the GCD.[3]

Hygienists are currently trained in either dental schools or the armed services. The training facilities for therapists are somewhat limited in comparison after the closure of the one school for dental therapists in New Cross London in 1983; students are now being trained in smaller numbers at the Royal London Hospital Therapist school. After completing their 2-year training and examination they leave the school duly qualified as dental hygienist and therapist.

Hygienists may be employed in the armed services, or in the community and hospital dental services, but most work in the general dental services. Dental hygienists carrying out dental work in any situation are required to work under the direction of a registered dentist who has examined the patient and prescribed treatment. Therapists are restricted to salaried employment in the hospital and community dental services. They are under the direction of a dentist who gives the therapist a written prescription.[4,5]

Role in the community

Hygienists are employed in the general dental service, so it is the dental therapist who is recognized as the main operating dental auxiliary in the community dental service. Nevertheless apart from the therapists' broader paediatric training, there is some overlap between the two professionals in the community.

The hygienist or therapist aims to improve and maintain oral health and prevent or reduce the incidence of dental disease (tooth decay and gum disease). This can be carried out through primary or secondary prevention.

The operative skills of both professions are still used in community dental clinics for pre-school and school-aged children, but the role of the community dental service is changing. The role of both professionals is moving towards the prevention approach and health promotion.

Work for children with special needs is important, especially the physically and mentally handicapped for whom dental treatment might be hazardous or difficult. Preventive measures are often needed such as the use of systemic or topical fluorides to reduce tooth decay. Fissure sealants are used as another method of reducing stagnation areas by applying resins to the tooth surfaces which are likely to develop tooth decay. Both these methods of treatment are painless and relatively simple to apply. Maintaining good oral hygiene can prove difficult with these children who often do not have the dexterity or the ability to brush adequately. Toothbrush adaptors can be made to improve grip and parents shown how to assist the child with toothbrushing. This involves the demonstration of correct positioning and handling of the brush.

School daily toothbrushing programmes set up for the children, supervised by the school nurses, welfare staff or teachers are very useful. Dental health education sessions for the children's parents, carers, teachers, welfare staff and school nurses can also contribute to the dental health of these children.

Most of this work takes place at the schools and centres for special needs children. The children are therefore among familiar surroundings with an atmosphere that is non-threatening. A hygiene room, medical room or even a classroom can provide the simple facilities that are required to set up portable dental equipment, such as mechanical handpieces for prophylaxis, oral irrigators, dental instruments, materials and toothbrushes.

A good rapport is important before any attempt is made to treat children, especially those who are anxious. Sometimes simply stroking the filaments of the toothbrush on their skin or merely handling the brush can be their initial start to dental treatment, until the child gains more confidence, after which other forms of treatment can be carried out.

It is important for the hygienist or therapist to report back to the prescribing dental officers to keep them informed of progress and to discuss any complications or queries regarding changes in treatment.

Coordinating and implementing dental health programmes within the community is another role of hygienists and therapists. Programmes can be found in day nurseries, mother and toddler groups, family centres, and mainstream and special schools. Depending on the age range, the form of dental health education delivered will vary although the ultimate goal is to modify behaviour through education. For example, a puppet show with a dental health message or role play using dentists' and nurses' uniforms can prepare pre-school children for dental inspections.

Project work with school children and teaching staff on diet-related subjects can include modifying school tuck shops, collecting food packages for ingredient checking, and calculating the sugar content of certain foods. This often fits in very well with other health-related topics in the national curriculum. Also oral hygiene instruction using disclosing agents to show the presence of plaque on the dentition with classes of children can relate well to science-related subjects.

All these activities can take a visual form which can be home produced and include audio-visual aids, such as videos, posters, diagrams models and activity sheets. These require regular modification and re-evaluation to ensure that they convey an up-to-date message which is easily understood by the children.

Sensitivity towards aspects of social, cultural, racial and religious differences within a group of children is very important. Therefore, hygienists and therapists must have a knowledge of religious practices, ethnic backgrounds and beliefs in the community where they work.

Hygienists and therapists are often involved in community-based programmes such as implementing and maintaining fluoride schemes set up in nurseries, special schools and health centres. The teaching staff and school nurses can distribute daily fluoride tablets to children who are at particular risk of tooth decay. Keeping health visitors informed of current advice ensures a mother with a new child can be confident of receiving correct information on dental health from the start. A dental representative, such as a hygienist or therapist, would be an important member of working parties to drawing up policies on food and health issues such as school meals. The importance of sugar reduction could be stressed when menu planning with the working party. These activities give the hygienists and therapists the opportunity to work with other paediatric professions.

References

1 General Dental Council. *Dental Auxiliaries Regulations* (reg 25 and 26). London: GDC, 1986.
2 General Dental Council. *Dental Auxiliaries (Amendment) Regulations*. London: GDC, 1991.
3 General Dental Council. *Recommendations Concerning Courses of Instruction for Dental Hygienists and Dental Therapists*. London: GDC, 1989.
4 Woolgrave, J., Boyle, J. Operating dental auxiliaries in the UK: a review. *Commun Dent Hlth* 1984; **1**: 93–99.
5 British Association for the Study of Community Dentistry. *The Future Role of the Dental Auxiliary Personnel in the UK*. London: BASCD, 1983.

20.25 Orthotists

Chris Drake

The orthotist is a qualified professional who has expertise in the application of orthopaedic appliances and apparatus (orthoses). Their role is to assess, design, make, fit and supply an effective, practical device (orthosis) acceptable to the patient and fulfilling therapeutic criteria of the clinical team involved in treatment. The integration of the orthotist into the clinical team is of vital importance if orthoses are to be used effectively.

With some diseases and conditions, such as poliomyelitis, spina bifida, cerebral palsy and muscular dystrophy, the application of an orthosis plays a major part in controlling deformities and maintaining limb function. An ankle foot orthosis (AFO) can be used to prevent excessive plantar flexion in a child with hemiplegic cerebral palsy, who toe-walks. The use of a spinal orthosis will help to prevent scoliosis in muscular dystrophy. The level to which orthoses are used depends upon the severity of the condition for which the child needs specific treatment; it ranges from a simple foot orthosis preventing eversion of the longitudinal arch, to a full walking orthosis extending from axilla to feet.

Each child is assessed by the clinical team, which usually includes an orthopaedic surgeon, a paediatrician, therapist and orthotist with parents present. Assessment is vitally important, and difficult for the orthotist to carry out in isolation. Involvement of as many members of the clinical team as possible is preferable, allowing for full discussion and interchange of ideas. The design, choice of materials, fabrication and supply are for the orthotist to carry out, but they can refer back to the clinical team at any time.

To achieve this, the orthotist needs to have knowledge of pathology, anatomy, physiology, biomechanics, engineering and material science and understanding of other treatment regimens. It is essential to be able to communicate with the child and also with the parents or carers, who may feel that the need for their child to have an orthosis highlights that their child has a physical problem or is handicapped. Children usually take the application of an orthosis in their stride and it is the parents who need psychological guidance in adapting to the orthosis. The ultimate success or failure of an orthosis is often dependent upon the initial approach at assessment.

Most orthotic design work is based on an external mechanical approach using Newton's third law of motion: *to every action there is an equal and opposite reaction*. This basic biomechanical function is present, in one form or another, in almost every orthosis manufactured. Orthoses are aimed to control, correct or enhance limb function, whether based on an exterior metal framework construction or an all-contact orthosis, where thermoplastics are used. Many factors are taken into account when designing an orthosis – choice of materials, amount of force used to control or correct the limb, weight, appearance and practicality. The overriding factor to consider is the final comfort and function of the orthosis and other points may have to be sacrificed to achieve a satisfactory end result.

An orthosis fitted and supplied correctly becomes an extension of the therapist's programme when the child is in school and daily life. It complements the orthopaedic surgeon in maintaining limb function and

movement preoperatively and enhances his work postoperatively. An orthosis may also be useful when surgical intervention is contraindicated or unnecessary. Used at the right time a good orthosis may prevent the onset of many disabling deformities and the need for surgery in the future, whereas a badly designed and ill fitting orthosis may cause severe distress and complications to both child and parents. Once an orthosis has been supplied, the orthotist in conjunction with the clinical team must constantly reassess its effectiveness, adjust it to accommodate changes in the child's growth and development, ensure it is in good serviceable order and monitor duration and correctness of use. Failure to maintain follow up may lead to failure of treatment.

Orthotic training in England comprises a 4-year sandwich course, leading to the award of a Business and Education Council (BTech) Higher National Diploma and the subsequent award of a Diploma in Orthotics by the Orthotic and Prosthetic Training Education Council (OPTEC), after which the orthotist is allowed to practise. In Scotland, Strathclyde University offers degree-level training and this is now the case in England at Salford University. In both circumstances theoretical and practical training is given in medical sciences, biomechanics, gait analysis and rehabilitation to allow understanding of other professional fields, training in fabrication, application, design, psychology and allied engineering sciences, enabling the student to put theory into practice. At various stages throughout training, the student has the opportunity for valuable practical experience in patient contact in order to understand the practical problems involved with the supply of orthoses. After graduation, the orthotist makes the decision to practise within either the National Health Service (NHS) or the private sector. The majority of orthotists in the UK are employed by private companies who have contracts for the supply of orthoses to the NHS.

Unfortunately no specific paediatric postgraduate training is available in England, and specialization develops from the orthotist having a flair and the interest to learn more, although there are a number of short courses available at various centres, mainly the Centre for Prosthetics and Orthotics, Strathclyde University in Scotland.

Orthotists employing their skills effectively can play a major part in treatment and rehabilitation by assisting and improving limb function, independence and mobility, but it is vital they communicate well with child and parents and fully integrate themselves with the whole clinical team if the objectives set are to be achieved.

Chapter 21

The parent

Berry Mayall

Introduction

Other chapters in this book deal with interventions by health staff in the lives of children and their parents. These interventions aim at curing children, preventing ill health and promoting good health. In most encounters between children and health staff, a parent is present.

This chapter considers parents' perspectives on child health services. Its justification lies in the fact that, since virtually all child health care, say 99%, is carried out by parents, their views on how health services provide the final 1% are very important.

This chapter draws on many sources of data, including my own two studies which focused on parental and health staff perspectives on child health care and the services.

I start with the well-known proposition that the medical service, like education and welfare services, constitutes a form of social power.[1-3] Medical discourse establishes certain standards of health status, certain health behaviours and lifestyles, and urges people both to accept these intellectually, and to act within that acceptance. This immediately raises the issue of people's levels of responsibility for their health and for their health behaviour. There may be latent or overt disagreement between paid health workers and the unpaid health workers – citizens, including parents. But social approbation will rest with the paid workers' ideology of good health care and, therefore, of responsible behaviour.

In the case of child health, mothers are asked to carry that responsibility. There is powerful pressure on them to conform with medical models. For, whilst the charge of neglecting your own health may be serious, the charge of neglecting your child's health is clearly damning. In addition, the mother has already gone through pregnancy and childbirth, where the medicalization of care has been accomplished,[4] so we might expect her to be thoroughly conditioned to accept what doctors and nurses propose. However, it can be argued that it is precisely because responsibility for the child's health and welfare is ascribed to the mother, together with the powerful emotional bond that ties mothers into fighting for their children's welfare, that gives mothers uniquely strong reasons for relying on their own ideas about how to achieve good child health. Thus, child health care presents an interesting case of the more general, but often muted, argument that goes on about health care behaviour between health staff and citizens.

In proposing what constitutes good child health and how to achieve it, paediatric health staff are concerned not only with technical matters; inevitably also they enter complex moral arenas: these concern goals and methods of child-rearing, the social context of child-rearing, definitions of responsible parenthood, what weight to ascribe to material and behavioural factors as affecting good health. Here the aim is to outline some issues in these areas, in order to provide a basis for consideration of parental perspectives on health services for their children, and of implications for health staff and services.

Children, mothers and fathers

Integral to people's perspectives on child health care are their models, or social constructions, of children and of parents – mothers and fathers. Thus the sort of health care people perceive children as needing derives from their ideas about what sort of people they think children are, what they want their children to be both now and when they grow up, and from their ideas about how children become healthy and maintain their health. People's models of good parenting derive partly from conceptions of what children need, but also from other common assumptions, rooted in tradition and social conventions, about characteristics of a good parent.

Models of childhood

Parental and professional talk about children suggests two basic models of childhood: the child as person and the child as project.[5–7] Mothers perceive children as people having their own characters, wishes and rights. They are seen as active participants in learning and indeed as initiators in learning speech, physical skills and social behaviours. Children learn through the ordinary give-and-take of life with their parents, other adults, and children; they are social beings, who enjoy and have the right to take their place in social relationships in the family, with the wider family and with their peers. From birth, children express wishes and wants, and later on they articulate views on how their lives should be lived; mothers tend to think children's views and wishes should be listened to, responded to and taken into account. Parents are concerned for the happiness of their children both now and in the longer term.[7,8] Mothers set great store by establishing their children's normality and they do this through comparison with other children, through talk with other mothers, and through contact with health staff.[9]

By contrast, health staff are encouraged, by the remit of their job description, and through their training and its accompanying textbooks, to conceptualize the child in another way, essentially as a project. They have borrowed from psychology the notion of the child as pre-social, and of childhood as presenting a socialization task to adults. Learning takes place through stimulation and interaction, initiated and encouraged by the mother. Children must be moulded to fit into the social and moral world around them.[10] Further, childhood is a series of developmental stages, each presenting inherent, latent or overt problems: the normal problems of the normal child.[11]

This contrast is given schematically here as a framework for thinking about understanding between parents and health staff. Whilst each side may recognize the other's perspectives, they approach negotiations with each other with different emphases as regards parental life with children, as well as from different social contexts. Health staff (like other welfare staff) may propose parental life with children largely as child-rearing tasks, carried out under their benevolent guidance. Health staff consider their work includes educating mothers about how best to develop and socialize their children. They aim, through regular surveillance, to prevent, detect and manage child problems; enlisting appropriate maternal behaviour is seen as important in prevention and management. Mothers, operating on a different model of childhood, will not see it as appropriate to define living with their children mainly as a socialization task,

though they do recognize and accept that task. They do not think that health staff knowledge is necessarily superior to their own; yet they do find health staff knowledge useful and take it into account along with other people's knowledge. They prefer to use curative and preventive services when they see a need; yet they also know about and accept the health and welfare surveillance remit of health staff.

As regards children's part in health care, we may note here that possibly both staff and parents underplay children's contribution during tri-partite meetings. It has been observed that, during consultations, children are often spoken about, rather than communicated with;[12] and that children find it difficult to take an active part in discussion in the rather daunting social and psychological climate of the clinical setting.[13] However, our studies suggest that mothers perceive children as young as 2 years old are interested in self-care.

Models of motherhood and fatherhood

Health, welfare and education staff often refer to 'parents',[14–16] rather than distinguishing between parents according to gender. This practice obscures the clear, gendered division of labour and responsibility traditional and current in UK society.

In social policies, in the media, in the behaviour of paid health, education and welfare staff and in the delivery of services, we see the assumption that mothers do, will and should take ultimate responsibility for their children's health and welfare and also shoulder the day-to-day responsibility and labour of child care work and decision making. This includes making and maintaining contacts with health, education and welfare services. We have very clear inflexible sets of assumptions about mothers and motherhood. For instance, our social policies and practices that affect mothers' and fathers' behaviour (employment, parental leave, day-care and after-school care for children) assume a traditional division of labour and responsibility.[17] Mothers who live away from their children meet incomprehension and outrage, which may be contrasted with the common acceptance that many fathers do. It is normal, statistically and morally, for single-parent households to be headed by mothers.[18] Mothers are expected to shoulder the extra care a disabled child requires, and to give up employment to do so.[19]

By comparison, we do not have a ready definition of a good father.[20,21] For most fathers, and most mothers, accepted definitions of fatherhood stop at providing financial support for the family and supporting the mother's child care work. Though there has been a lot of rhetoric about the new father, all the evidence suggests he is largely a mirage:[22,23] most fathers are not increasing their share of the labour and responsibility of child care.

The education, welfare and health services may use the term 'parents', but they address themselves to mothers. It is mothers who are expected to negotiate with agencies about children; to become involved in managing and running services and to work unpaid to sustain poorly funded services, such as playgroups, and schools.[24,25] Social workers work with mothers, both in their ascribed roles as emotional centre and manager of the household, and as the parent held responsible for child welfare.[26,27] Doctors and health visitors conceptualize parenting as mothering and services are designed and offered with mothers, not fathers, in mind.[28,29] Staff feel uneasy in the presence of fathers; they cannot call on socially legitimated assumptions about fathers as child carers.[21] The health services, it seems, have not adopted policies aimed at helping fathers who do participate in child care or at promoting father-participation. For instance, antenatal literature and classes marginalize the father's role in child care.[30,31]

The socioeconomic context of mothering

As regards factors affecting the quality of maternal child care, it is important for health staff to consider the social and economic contexts within which mothers do the caring and weigh these against behavioural explanations for quality of child care.

The designation of women as responsible for children within a condition of dependency on the father or the state,[32] constructs them both within households and in the wider society as a social and political minority, subject to disadvantage and discrimination. It is integral to the common unwillingness to recognize this power structure, that social policies and practices have long centred on maternal behaviour rather than material disadvantage as the principal explanatory factor in child health and the principal focus for intervention.

Both in the past[33,34] and today, policies and practices in the health and welfare services show this focus clearly. Financial support for households with dependent children has always been grudging. Organizational links between the medical and nursing services, and housing, social security, employment and social services are poor. Whilst the medical profession pays lip service to poverty, poor housing and social decay as factors in poor child health,[14] neither the profession nor the service addresses these issues adequately. Some doctors specifically define social issues as outside their remit.[8] The history of health visiting shows an early concern for public health issues,[35,36] but its main thrust in recent years has been on individualistic health education, emotional support, and child surveillance.

Yet there is massive evidence, not only of links between material deprivation and ill health, but of how these linkages are forged. The evidence is overwhelming that those in the lowest social classes have much poorer chances of good health than other people, and this is true throughout adulthood. Child ill health throws long shadows forward.[37–39] In the last 10 years the divide between the reasonably well-off and the poorest in our society has widened and the health chances of the poor have become worse.[40,41] There is a mounting literature on how material deprivation inhibits mothers from good child care.[8,42–45] As study after study has documented, good child health care cannot be achieved without the money to resource the essentials: good food and clothing; warm, safe spacious housing in which to run, explore and play; enough care givers to ensure their safety, provide physical care for them, and to interact with them.

Poverty drives women to compromise, and to rank one health choice over others. For instance mothers tell of not taking the toddler to the clinic in cold weather because their younger baby is ill. A family living in damp housing with only one heater sleeps together to keep warm, though they know the risks of cross-infection.[8,44]

Children's health may suffer when their principal care giver – the mother – is not in charge of family resource decisions and allocations. For instance, a mother who wanted safer heating appliances was told by the father that, since child safety depended on maternal supervision, paraffin heaters would suffice. Socially accepted power relations within families may lead to poor health care for children, and their mothers. Thus mothers report feeding themselves and their children on cheap food and giving the better food to the father.[46] It is striking that mothers with past experience in two-parent households, but now managing alone, report satisfaction at their newly gained power to spend wisely, for household health and welfare.[42]

Material deprivation casts its shadows over children's health beyond the home; from the fact that poor people live in low-quality housing and neighbourhoods, near dangerous roads, in areas with poor services, such as playgrounds, pre-school services and schools. The fact that child pedestrian deaths from traffic accidents are seven times higher in class V than in class I is a grim and not coincidental statistic. Both the physical conditions in the neighbourhood of poor children's homes, and the inability of poor parents to provide a high enough level of protection to their children, are implicated.[38]

I have suggested that the designation of poor maternal behaviour as a principal explanation for poor child health is consistent with the social and political positioning of mothers as dependants. An important feature of this denigration of mothers is the routine devaluing of mothers' knowledge by health and welfare and education staff.[4,47,48] The social legitimation for the intervention of health, welfare and education staff into parental child-rearing provides a further incentive for staff to propose their own knowledge as superior. Data show that neither high social class nor ethnic majority status fully protect mothers from denigration, although the character of criticism varies according to how staff define mothers' social and ethnic group.[8]

The assumption by health staff that mothers lack good health care knowledge and do not behave responsibly as regards their children's health care[49] is part of a much wider and long-established myth among health staff that people in general are irresponsible and that it is part of the function of health staff to teach them higher standards of morality. A report of the Royal College of General Practitioners (RCGP) notes in chapter 4 that the promotion of health 'entails helping people to learn and to accept responsibility for their own well-being', and goes on: 'many people still believe that responsibility for their health can be left to professionals.'[50] The point is echoed in chapter 6 of another RCGP paper on child health services.[14] A recent report (from a high-level working group) on child health surveillance has minutely referenced statements throughout (330 for 100 pages of text), except as regards parental attitudes, where the authors assert, without supporting evidence: 'Changes in attitude and behaviour are more likely to be achieved by parents [sic] who have been helped to accept responsibility for their own and their children's health.'[51]

Child health services for mothers, fathers and children: a summary

The foregoing sections suggest a number of general points which relate to the provision of child health services suitable for parents and their children.

A comprehensive integrated service

First we may note a topic which will not be examined here. A number of recent reports have considered the child health services as a whole, in the wake of governmental proposals and legislation.[16,49,51–53] These studies, like others over the years, take up the perennial demand by parents for accessible, integrated and coherent services – a demand which has still not been met.

Thus, mothers in every study on the subject indicate that they need a comprehensive and integrated service, which would provide good liaison between types of health staff, and which would present common policies and practices. Integration and liaison are key words as regards linkages between health services and other services and systems that impinge on the health of children and their parents: housing; social services; social security; employment; education; and pre-school and after-school systems. Parents need easy

access on a 24-hour basis to services for children: convenient physical access (local services, ramps, parking for cars and pushchairs and prams); and a welcoming, pleasant atmosphere.

I go on here to note four interlinked areas, where health staff may respond to provide appropriate services. My final section expands these themes.

Resources

I have noted the connections between adequate material resources and good child health care. From the parental point of view, due recognition of these linkages should be part of the service provided by health staff.

Partnership

The character of staff–parent relationships critically affects the quality of child health care. Parents, mostly mothers, do almost all the health care of children, but the small extra amount – the advice, diagnosis, treatment given by health staff – is important and can be crucial. Furthermore, in most cases, health staff have to enlist the labour of mothers in order to achieve the desired outcome for child health.

Gender issues

An essential prerequisite of attempts towards partnership on the part of health staff must be recognition of both the common interests and problems of mothers, and the importance of interacting with mothers as individuals rather than as members of class or ethnic groups. Mothers have some common interests, as a class of people assigned the major responsibility for child care within a condition of economic and social dependency and suspected of being irresponsible and insufficiently knowledgeable. However, their social class and ethnic group will be mediating factors in their negotiations with health staff. We know relatively little about what fathers want from services. But we do know that some feel marginalized; they are not viewed as responsible for the child, as having knowledge, as being an appropriate discussant on child-care matters. At a more general level, fathers find that child health services are a world of women – staffed by women, provided with women in mind, and used by women.

Children's perspectives

I have suggested some differences between parents and health staff as regards models of childhood, motherhood and fatherhood. In addition, these models may not fit with children's own perception of their role in health care and in meetings with health staff. Perhaps both parents and health staff pay insufficient attention to children's perspectives on their participation in meetings with health staff.

The child health service response

Resources

Health staff – especially those in community health services – may play an important part in giving active recognition to the influences of social, economic and political factors on the maintenance and restoration of good health. This they can do: in face-to-face meetings with parents and children; in their relationships with other local services; and as occupational groups with civic responsibilities.

Health staff should make it part of their work to listen to parental accounts of how child-care work is contextualized and structured by socioeconomic factors. Only in this way, can there be shared understanding on which to base advice. In addition, health staff should do their part to help individual people improve their resources for child care. Whilst doctors may find it easier to designate these two tasks as appropriate for health visitors or social workers, these tasks should be a constituent, central part of their own work for child health.

It is also desirable that health staff, both management and field staff, continue the establishment and maintenance within districts of adequate coordination, within the health service and with other services. Here, the establishment of community paediatric services and the devolvement to neighbourhood health services should make such linkages easier to forge and strengthen. For users of services, clusters of services grouped together (housing, social services, health) present a more usable package than services scattered across an area.

As influential occupational groups, health staff can contribute to pressure on governments to improve the socioeconomic conditions in which parents rear children. They have work to do through their policy and practice documents, issued by professional bodies and working parties. Such documents generally do allude to such factors as housing, unemployment and poverty, but are weaker on pressing for change. Indeed, in continuing to work within an individualistic, behaviour change paradigm, occupational groups reinforce the traditional view that health status and health care are only weakly related to social conditions. A sterling model here was the Black Report, with its emphasis on the necessity for socioeconomic reform;[38] in particular the emphasis on improving services and on raising standards of living for families with children. A further role for health staff is to argue through their professional organizations and unions, locally, regionally and nationally, for social reform. Finally, health staff organizations could press for a health impact statement in policy proposals across a wide spectrum of areas: transport, housing, education, health, employment, social security. The goals may be Utopian; the work towards them is useful and positive.

Partnership

In a range of services – health, education, welfare, housing – the concept of partnership between providers and users has been developed, over the last few years, in order to secure cost effective and socially-appropriate services. Yet, in these services, there is a huge imbalance in the power and status of the providers, compared to the users, and especially compared to mothers, who do much of the negotiating. It is debatable whether true partnership is attainable, where the power resides so heavily with one side. However, a range of strategies by health staff may lead to constructive relationships.

Treating people as experts is the first essential. This may not come easily to health staff, but it should be at its easiest when they deal with mothers. Probably, of all social groups, they are the most aware of, and most knowledgeable about, health issues, and the keenest to promote good health.

As I have suggested earlier, mothers come to health staff with their own models of childhood and parenthood and with their own knowledge of child care. So they seek a service which respects their perspectives and their knowledge. Providing such a service is not merely a matter of social convention or politeness, but it is an essential basis for a successful health service. Since most health service interactions with people are about helping people make a decision, it is essential that the health staff establish the person's diagnosis and views on treatment as a basis for adding in the health staff contribution: information and advice.[54]

Providing adequate information to people is an important constituent of partnership. It is also a means of achieving accountability to the public. The evidence suggests that what mothers mainly seek from health staff is information. Mothers welcome hearing the biomedical side, the technical points, and the views, formal and less formal, of health staff. Furthermore, mothers, whatever their class or ethnicity, include books, magazines and leaflets in their sources of information.[8] Health services could harness these points more than they do. Much more written information could be provided, on both preventive and curative services; for instance, detailed accounts of the aims and methods of immunization and developmental assessments; leaflets on particular conditions, especially chronic ones; fact sheets on local health services.

The function of health staff as information purveyors leads us on to health education within the context of partnership. If the provision of a health service can be conceptualized as a means of controlling the behaviour of the population, health education is the more overt side to this enterprise and may meet resistance. Health visitors have, by tradition, seen themselves as educators, and mothers tend to resent this occupational assumption.[8,55] In recent years, the medical profession too has discussed a direct health education role for doctors;[14,50] health education sessions are now being promoted at surgeries. Whilst the liberal consensus is that doctors should tell people what they think, and that people should take such thoughts seriously, it is a large and problematic step from there to the doctor as health educator.[56] People who ask for help have not agreed to become pupils, and may be made resistant to behaviour change if a top-down education model presses heavily on them. On the other hand, partnership between health staff and patients may be improved if health education takes the form of egalitarian discussion of factors leading to good health, and of a range of measures, behavioural and social, to achieve it.

So, an important means of developing a constructive partnership between parents and health staff is through the demedicalizing of encounters. The difficulties both staff and parents may have in giving a voice to parental and child perspectives may be tackled through, for instance, group work, the harnessing the skills of a range of staff; community projects and self-help groups.[16] Such less formal meetings may provide a forum where children themselves may make themselves heard.[13] This may be particularly appropriate in school settings, and where children with chronic conditions are assuming responsibility for daily management. Staff with the highest status have a responsibility to think out carefully their role in such meeting grounds, so that they do not dominate discussions.[57]

Gender issues

The aim of providing responsive and appropriate services requires, as one condition, that staff be aware of gender issues. In their dealings with mothers, staff should stay alert to societal assumptions that we can take for granted both mothers' child-care work and the conditions – social, economic and psychological – in which mothers do this work. In a society which is increasingly reliant on the unpaid work of women to do the caring, it should be a part of the work of health staff to give recognition to that unpaid work, and to try to improve mothers' access to services which release them from some of the tasks, some of the time.

As regards fathers, health staff might plan for father-friendly services. These could comprise a dual-pronged approach, both responding to fathers' interest in their children and supporting the further assumption of labour and responsibility where fathers seem willing.

If, as one may hope, local research on people's wishes for health services is increasingly an important part of policy development within the health service, such research should aim to provide data on what fathers, mothers and children see as appropriate services.

Children

It is important for good health care that both parents and health staff remain alert to and respond to children's perspectives: the part children wish to play in their own health care, and in discussions about it.

I have suggested above the de-medicalization of meetings as a means of giving children a more user-friendly service. As regards school health services, whatever arrangements may be made in districts, it seems appropriate to consider children's active participation in health care discussions, as regards both their own health problems and health care strategies more generally conceived.[58] Health education in schools is an area where health staff and health education staff may work together with the children.

Assigning divisions of health care responsibilities between parents and children is a matter for continuous negotiation between children, parents and staff.[59,60] Research on consultations in hospital clinics has suggested that mothers tend to be judged as over-protective if they answer for the child, and as irresponsible if they suggest that the child is or should be responsible for their own health care.[13] However, we probably need to know more about children's perspectives on health care, as regards healthy, acutely ill and handicapped children.

Finally, we perhaps need a re-think of the character of services for teenagers or adolescents. A survey of paediatric text books in the British Medical Association and London University libraries indicates that, as compared to the USA, British paediatricians have given less thought to the provision of suitable services. Relevant here are young people's perceptions of their health problems. Community studies have indicated concern about acne, being overweight, menstruation, sex, and psychosocial problems (living with parents, coping with school); young people may not relish bothering the doctor with them.[61,62] It is also clear that some teenagers rate individual health behaviour low, since they perceive themselves to live in unhealthy environments; for them, coping with family, housing, employment and traffic problems rates more highly than giving up smoking.[63]

Evidence such as this suggests that conventional medical consultations and health education methods may be inappropriate. Local authorities and voluntary sector services have led the way here, with their drop-in services which offer informal settings for young people to discuss their problems. Health services might well follow their lead, and indeed the provision of services in places where teenagers gather – clubs, shopping streets, employment agencies, schools – may make for more approachable and successful meeting places between young people and health staff. We could also develop on the lines of well-woman clinics, well-teenager clinics. Finally, it may be productive to involve young people in the planning and management of primary health services, and in provision too, for instance as discussants and counsellors.[64]

This chapter has raised some issues for the consideration of community paediatric staff, necessarily general in the space allowed. I look forward to seeing detailed implementation.

References

1 Zola, I.K. Medicine as an institution of social control. *Sociol Rev* 1972; **20**: 487–509.

2 Foucault, M. *The Birth of the Clinic*. London: Tavistock, 1976.

3 Donzelot, J. *The Policing of Families*. London: Hutchinson, 1980.

4 Graham, H., Oakley, A. Competing ideologies of reproduction: medical and maternal perspectives on pregnancy. In: Currer, C., Stacey, M., eds. *Concepts of Health, Illness and Disease*. Leamington Spa: Berg, 1986.

5 Denzin, N.K. *Childhood Socialisation*. San Francisco: Jossey-Bass, 1977.

6 Skolnick, A. The limits of childhood: conceptions of child development and social context. *Law Contemp Problems* 1975; **39**: 38–77.

7 Hallden, G. Parental belief systems and time: parents' reflections on development and child-rearing. Stockholm: Institute of Education, Stockholm University, 1988. (Research Bulletin 13).

8 Mayall, B., Foster, M.-C. *Child Health Care: Living with Children, Working for Children*. Oxford: Heinemann, 1989.

9 Buswell, C. Social acceptability: how mothers perceive normal growth and development in their first child. Paper given at Medical Sociology Conference, York University, September 1983.

10 Alanen, L. Growing up in the modern family: re-thinking socialisation, the family and childhood. In: *Proceedings of a Conference: Growing into a Modern World*, (Vol 2). Trondheim, June 1987.

11 Illingworth, R.S. *The Normal Child: Some Problems of the Early Years and their Treatment*, 5th edn. London: Churchill Livingstone, 1972.

12 Aronsson, K., Rundstrom, B. Child discourse and parental control in paediatric consultations. *Text* 1988; **8**: 159–189.

13 Silverman, D. *Communication and Medical Practice: Social Relations in the Clinic*. London: Sage, 1987.

14 Royal College of General Practitioners. *Healthier Children: Thinking Prevention*. London: RCGP, 1982.

15 Inner London Education Authority. Improving secondary schools. *Report of the Committee on the Curriculum and Organisation of Secondary Schools* (Hargreaves Report). London: ILEA, 1984.

16 Elfer, P., Gatiss, S. *Charting Child Health Services*. London: National Children's Bureau, 1986.

17 Cohen, B. Caring for children: services and policies for childcare and equal opportunities in the United Kingdom. *Report for the European Commission's Childcare Network*. London: Commission of the European Communities, 1988.

18 Glendinning, C. Impoverishing women. In: Walker, A., Walker, C., eds. *The Growing Divide: a Social Audit 1979–87*. London: Child Poverty Action Group, 1987.

19 Baldwin, S., Glendinning, C. Employment, women and their disabled children. In: Finch, J., Groves, D.A., eds. *Labour of Love: Women, Work and Caring*. London: Routledge, Kegan Paul, 1983.

20 Hearn, G. The need to study men and masculinity. *Soc Sci Teacher* 1989; **18**: 7–9.

21 Mayall, B. The division of labour in early child care: mothers and others. *J Soc Policy* 1990; **19**: 299–330.

22 Lewis, C., O'Brien, M., eds. *Reassessing Fatherhood*. London: Sage, 1987.

23 Segal, L. *Slow Motion: Changing Masculinities, Changing Men*. London: Virago, 1990.

24 Preschool Play Association. *Parents and Playgroups*. London: Allen and Unwin, 1981.

25 Mayall, B. *Parents in Secondary Education*. London: Calouste Gulbenkian Foundation, 1990.

26 Brooke, E., Davis, A., eds. *Women, the Family and Social Work*. London: Tavistock, 1985.

27 Marsh, P. Social work and fathers: an exclusive practice. In: Lewis, C., O'Brien, M., eds. *Reassessing Fatherhood*. London: Sage, 1987.

28 Russell, G. *The Changing Role of Fathers*. Milton Keynes: Open University Press, 1983.

29 Lewis, C. *Becoming a Father*. Milton Keynes: Open University Press, 1986.

30 Urwin, C. Constructing motherhood: the persuasion of normal development. In: Steedman, C., Urwin, C., Walkerdine, V. *Language, Gender and Childhood*. London: Routledge, Kegan Paul, 1985.

31 Meerabeau, L. Images of fatherhood in ante-natal literature. *Health Visitor J* 1987; **60**: 116–117.

32 Hernes, H.M. Women and the welfare state: the transition from private to public dependence. In: Sassoon, A.S., ed. *Women and the State: the Shifting Boundaries of Public and Private*. London: Hutchinson, 1987.

33 Lewis, J. *The Politics of Motherhood: Child and Maternal Welfare in England 1900–39*. London: Croom Helm, 1980.

34 Lewis, J., ed. The working class wife and mother and state intervention 1870–1918. In: *Labour and Love: Women's Experience of Home and Family 1850–1940*. Oxford: Basil Blackwell, 1986.

35 Robson, P. The development of health visiting in North East England: A case study in social policy. In: While, A., ed. *Research in Preventive Community Nursing Care: 15 Studies in Health Visiting*. Chichester: John Wiley, 1986.

36 Davies, C. The health visitor as mother's friend: a woman's place in public health 1900–1914. *Soc History Med* 1988; **1**: 39–59.

37 Committee on Child Health Services. *Fit for the Future*. (Court Report). London: HMSO, 1976. (Cmnd 6684).

38 Townsend, P., Davidson, N. *Inequalities in Health: the Black Report*. Harmondsworth: Penguin, 1982.

39 Blaxter, M. *The Health of the Children*. London: Heinemann Educational Books, 1981.

40 Walker, A., Walker, C., eds. *The Growing Divide: a Social Audit 1979–87*. London: Child Poverty Action Group, 1987.

41 Whitehead, M. *The Health Divide: Inequalities in Health in the 1980s*. London: Health Education Council, 1987.

42 Graham, H. *Caring for the Family*. London: Health Education Council, 1985. (Research Report, no. 5).

43 Burghes, L. *Living from Hand to Mouth: a Study of 65 Families Living on Supplementary Benefit*. London: Family Service Units and Child Poverty Action Group, 1980. (Poverty Pamphlet no. 50).

44 Mayall, B. *Keeping Children Healthy*. London: Allen and Unwin, 1986.

45 Stacey, M., Graham, H. Socio-economic factors related to Child Health. In: McFarlane, A., ed. *Progress in Child Health*. Edinburgh: Churchill Livingstone, 1984.

46 Charles, N., Kerr, M. *Women, Food and Families*. Manchester: Manchester University Press, 1988.

47 Tizard, B., Hughes, M. *Young Children Learning*. London: Fontana, 1984.

48 David, M. Motherhood and social policy: a matter of education? *Crit Soc Policy* 1985; **12**: 28–43.

49 Policy and Practice Review Group. *Investing in the Future: Child Health Ten Years after the Court Report*. London: National Children's Bureau, 1987.

50 Royal College of General Practitioners. *Health and Prevention in Primary Care*. London: RCGP, 1981. (Report from General Practice 18).

51 Hall, D.M.B. *Health for All Children*. Oxford: Oxford Medical Publishers, 1989.

52 Woodruffe, C., Kurtz, Z. *Working for Children? Children's Services and the NHS Review*. London: National Children's Bureau, 1989.

53 Hogg, C. *The NAWCH Quality Review: Setting Standards for Children in Health Care*. London: National Association for the Welfare of Children in Hospital, 1989.

54 Tuckett, D., Boulton, M., Olson, C., Williams, A. *Meetings Between Experts: an Approach to Sharing Ideas in Medical Consultations*. London: Tavistock, 1985.

55 McIntosh, J. *A Consumer Perspective on the Health Visiting Service*. Glasgow: Social Paediatric and Obstetric Research Unit, University of Glasgow, 1987.

56 Calnan, M., Boulton, M., Williams, A. Health education and GPs: a critical appraisal. In: Rodmell, S., Watt, A., eds. *The Politics of Health Education*. London: Routledge, Kegan Paul, 1986.

57 Perkins, E., Spencer, N. Experimental group work – a lost opportunity. In: While, A., ed. *Research in Preventive Community Nursing Care*. London: John Wiley, 1986.

58 Whiting, K. Towards a school health service for adolescents: the teacher–health worker team. *Child Soc* 1990; **4**: 225–234.

59 Alderson, P. *Choosing for Children: Parents' Consent to Surgery*. Oxford: Oxford University Press, 1990.

60 Alderson, P. *Children's Consent to Surgery*. Milton Keynes: Open University Press, 1993.

61 Epstein, K., Rice, P., Wallace, P. Teenagers' health concerns: implications for primary health care professionals. *J Roy Coll Gen Practit* 1989; **39**: 247–249.

62 Bewley, B.R., Higgs, R.H., Jones, A. Adolescent patients at an inner London GP: their attitudes to illness and health care. *J Roy Coll Gen Practit* 1984; **34**: 543–546.

63 Harding, G. Adolescence and health: a literature review. In: Smith, M., Harding, G., eds. *Health Education and Young People*. London: Thomas Coram Research Unit, 1989. (TCRU Occasional Paper no. 9)

64 World Health Organization *Young People's Health: a Challenge for Society*. Geneva: WHO, 1986. (Technical Report Series 731).

Chapter 22

Support services for families with children with disabilities and special needs

Philippa Russell

The background to living with disability – family dynamics and special needs

It has been estimated that there are about 360 000 children with disabilities living in the UK.[1] The vast majority (355 000) live with natural or foster parents in their local community. The same survey tells us that many families are unaware of the sources of help available to them; 38% of families had never belonged to a voluntary organization (and did not know they existed). Only 27% of parents knew that respite care existed; and only 4% actually used it. The most common professionals cited by parents as being 'most often seen' were general practitioners (GPs), hospital doctors and consultants, followed by teachers and health visitors. Despite the significance of the Children Act 1989 and the community care arrangements, only 12% of parents of children living at home saw a social worker regularly. One-third of those children who were living in communal (i.e. residential) establishments were there because parents or foster families found their health or behaviour problems too difficult to cope with and, presumably, because inadequate support at home was available. The families had generally lower incomes than their equivalents in the community and single parents were likely to rely wholly on state benefits. Although the Office of Population and Census Surveys (OPCS) figures make gloomy reading, they also indicate the importance of information and of communication with parents. Practical parenting means receiving financial allowances, knowing about voluntary organizations and using respite care. It also means taking power and acting confidently in asking for help. This chapter considers a number of crucial needs for families and how parents may be best encouraged to use available services.

The birth of *any* child can be a traumatic as well as a happy event for the parents concerned. Parenthood brings alarming new responsibilities, as well as pleasures. When a new baby has a disability, the initial diagnosis may be devastating for the parents. Recent research by Cunningham and Davis[2,3] and others clearly shows us how important it is to recognize the impact of disability on parental expectations and self-image. But, as Hewett[4] noted in 1970, 'the general tendency to characterise parents of handicapped children as guilt-ridden, anxiety-laden ... over-protective and rejecting beings' is unfair. They are, rather, vulnerable families faced with a major challenge for which they require support as well as counselling, and respect rather than any global assumptions about 'pathological abnormality'. Many disabled children require high levels of practical support in their day-to-day lives. A study by Glendinning[5] found that 50.1% of the 361 severely disabled children in her survey could not be left alone and unsupervised for more than 10 minutes at a time in any one day. Wilkin[6] and Baldwin[7] have emphasized the burdens placed upon mothers with little support from neighbours or other relatives.

Cooke and Bradshaw[8] found that disabled children in a study of families using the Family Fund were more likely than other children to experience at least one spell in a one-parent family. These spells were longer than for families with non-disabled children and those families with the more severely disabled children were less likely to be reconstituted into new marriages or relationships. It is obvious that physical restrictions of care will limit families' social networks. But the Cooke and Bradshaw research indicates the importance of looking at the family networks and structures and individual needs when there is a disabled child, and at the implications for care and support within that family. Wolkind[9] and others have shown the high incidence of depression and low self-esteem among all young parents in disadvantaged inner-city areas. The social context of disability is therefore of crucial importance in determining whether positive approaches to parent support will be effective for both family and child. Supporting disabled children and their families will require a range of services.[10,11] However, ensuring that services are effective, fully used and sensitive to consumer needs requires constant review and assimilation by professionals, carers and managers. The significance of recent research for the development of good quality community services is often not appreciated or considered in setting priorities for the future. Such priorities for support should include access to services in statutory and voluntary agencies, respite day care and financial advice to reduce the additional costs of disability in the family.

Respite or short-term care – getting a break

The large majority of disabled children live at home. However, the development of respite care over the past decade (with some three hundred schemes now in operation) has shown the importance that parents place upon having a break and the value for children of opportunities to sample another family's lifestyle and leisure activities. Historically respite care developed as an emergency service, usually providing short-term care within a long-stay hospital or other institution in order to meet a family crisis. Such respite care was often offered in block bookings for summer holidays or other periods and was often distant from families and friends. However, there has been increasing effort to develop flexible and local family support services which include respite care as one of a range of options for individual families and children.[12] This shift in thinking sees respite care as part of an integrated service and not a special one-off intervention. In Maureen Oswin's words,[13,14] 'short term care should be regarded as a very specialist service needing clearly defined aims based on principles of child care practice and requiring continuous monitoring of standards with an emphasis on how it might be affecting individual children.' Taking a child away may not solve the problems in a family where there are other factors (such as not coping with difficult behaviour) which await the child on his or her return home. A number of studies on respite care have suggested that there are certain key principles to be followed when offering this care to a family:

1 That it should be a local service, where children can continue to attend school as if living at home.
2 That the service offers good quality child care. Although 10 000 individual respite care placements took place in mental handicap hospitals in 1988/9, hospitals are not good places for giving families breaks and every effort should be made to find community support.
3 It should be available on demand. Many parents want very short periods of respite care often on a baby-sitting rather than residential basis. But they need it to be available at short notice. A number of schemes operating respite on demand (such as the Somerset and Leeds respite family schemes) have proved that families do not abuse the service and welcome the ordinariness of being able to leave their children as if he or she did not have a disability.[15]

Under-use of some respite care arrangement usually indicates parental doubts about quality or lack of knowledge of what is available. A range of options (including additional help in the home, substitute families, residential homes or holiday schemes) should be offered. Although a number of children still receive respite care in NHS provision such as small units or paediatric wards because of lack of alternative provision, every effort should be made to avoid hospital admissions for so-called community relief. Voluntary organizations as well as social services run a number of respite programmes, but paediatricians may need to remind their social services departments of the need to pay for such provision and the long-term benefits of substitute families contributing in their local communities.

Evidence about the ability of short-term respite care to alleviate family stress is inevitably subjective. The Avon evaluation[16] emphasizes the fallacy of assuming that respite care is a universal panacea for all family problems. This study found that 'many of the user families had unmet needs as did many of the non-user families'. The Honeylands evaluation[17] suggests that many families may in fact need relief, but will still only use respite services on an incremental basis. Hence family relief may not be instantaneous and, indeed, measurements of stress levels in families in the Honeylands studies suggested that some families were actually *more* stressed at the start of using a service than before they did so.

The stresses associated with letting a child go to another family or unit for the first time are frequently underestimated. The DH Inspectorate Report in Oxfordshire made a similar point, noting the stages through which parents needed to go in becoming positive utilizers of respite services.[18] This study identified three hurdles for potential users to overcome, namely using the service chosen for the first time; leaving the child overnight and placing the child for a longer period. Although there has been no comparative research into parental satisfaction with different models of respite care, it seems that parents are more likely to be satisfied if a service is clearly linked to a voluntary organization, school or a wider service like Honeylands in order to put the service in context and to ensure that respite care is a rewarding experience for the child.

The evaluation of Honeylands and of Preston Skreens[17,19] found that parents of children with the most difficult behaviour problems were often the least likely to use respite care, although they needed it for a break. Other parents felt that no one would want to care for their child because of the behaviour problems and were frightened of being rebuffed if they wanted help. Parents themselves may have strong preferences about where respite care is given (in the family home, in a substitute family or in a residential unit). It is important, therefore, that paediatricians have information on the full range of local services and that they understand the different referral routes. Social services departments have new duties under the Children Act 1989 to provide and disseminate information on local services for parents of children in need. Paediatric services will need to liaise closely to ensure that they have access to this information and also to make certain that the registers of disabled children required by the Children Act accurately reflect the needs of the local population.

Supporting substitute families: developments in foster care and adoption

When children cannot live with their natural parents, there have been encouraging developments in substitute family care. Indeed foster families now form a significant group of carers with whom paediatricians will be sharing the care of children with a disability. Many local authorities now run foster schemes for disabled children, some using the specialist fostering schemes of Barnardo's, the British Adoption and Fostering Agencies or Parents for Children. The past 5 years have seen major advances in successful fostering for even the most severely disabled children, with enhanced allowances and a range of support services ranging from loan of equipment to home helps and respite care.

Foster parents with disabled children also have a special role in maintaining links and helping natural parents and siblings to keep in touch. However, many parents of disabled children still feel ambivalent about the use of foster placements (which are often seen as indicating an incompetent parent). Advocates of foster placements should emphasize the positive contribution of shared care for the child concerned and create time and space for natural and substitute families to get to know each other. If children are moving out of residential care (particularly residential care in a hospital or NHS setting), there may be major anxieties not only about the quality of care but the security of the placement being offered. Parents whose children live in NHS provision are not required to contribute to the residential costs. Local authorities may (and many do) waive charges, but they may legally require parents to contribute on a means-tested scale to their child's placement costs. Some parents have been particularly indignant when they had not accepted the need for the move, and have not realized the financial consequences. Shared care is likely to increase for disabled children and will necessitate constant professional support.

The decision to agree that a child with a disability should be adopted can also be very problematic and, wherever possible, parents should be helped to come to a voluntary agreement. Foster and adoptive parents are of course eligible for disability living allowance and other Department of Social Security allowances relating to disability.

Sources of financial help

The 1989 OPCS report on the prevalence of disability and the financial and other circumstances of people with disability and their families clearly indicated the serious consequences of any disability on the family budget. The fifth report[20] on the financial circumstances of children found that there was a lower rate of earned income among all men with disabled children and two parent families had a lower equivalent income than their counterparts in the general population. Three-quarters of the single parents with disabled children were wholly dependent on state benefits for their main source of income, often because of the impossibility of finding adequate day care for children. Families regularly spent an extra £6.54 a week because of disability and this sum excluded money spent on major purchases such as cars, household equipment or wheelchairs. It showed that such families spent more money on transport and at chemists than their equivalents in the wider community. Helping families to obtain allowances and benefits to which they are entitled should therefore be a priority for all professionals. Many families will not know where or how to apply and others imagine that their need is not as great as others'. The following section looks at the main financial benefits and allowances available to families and how to be successful in applying for them.

The disability living allowance

In April 1992, two new benefits were introduced – the disability living allowance (DLA) and the disability working allowance. The DLA replaced the attendance allowance and the mobility allowance which become the care component and the mobility component of the new allowance. Each component has a new lower level so there are now three different levels at which the allowance can be paid.

Children or adults who were already receiving the attendance or mobility allowances were automatically eligible for the new disability living allowance. Others may find that they can now claim either the care or the mobility components for the first time because of the new lower level. Four new disability tests are added to the long-term tests for assessing eligibility for attendance or mobility allowance. These are:

1 The applicant needs part-time help during the day.
2 The applicant is over 16 years and cannot prepare a cooked main meal unaided.
3 The applicant has severe mental impairment and has behaviour so difficult and disruptive that significant help is required (and already receives the higher rate of care component). The applicant may be automatically eligible for the higher rate of the mobility component of the allowance even though able to walk.
4 The applicant needs help or watching over in order to walk safely out of doors, and may be eligible for the newer lower rate of the mobility component.

The above four tests mean that there should be greater flexibility in awarding the allowances and that, for the mobility component in particular, there is recognition that many people with a mental handicap or learning disability can walk, but are unsafe to do so without constant supervision and help.

The DLA is tax free, not means tested and does not require any national insurance contributions. Providing that the individual has satisfied the criteria for the allowance, it can be paid over and above any other income. It is a benefit for the disabled person, not for the carer or parent. Those claiming the DLA should have experienced the same difficulties for 3 months before application, but application can be made from birth if a child is regarded as being terminally ill for the care component. The mobility component cannot be claimed until the child is 4 years and 9 months old.

The system for applying for the DLA is different to that for the old-style attendance or mobility allowance. Applicants should use the DSS Benefits Enquiry Line (0800 88 22 00 – Freecall) and ask for a copy of the DLA 1 Claimpack. If an application is successful it can be back-dated to the date of this first call, so it is important that parents make the call and ensure that their names are registered. The pack contains a self-assessment questionnaire for applicants. Thus, for the first time, initial decisions about eligibility for the allowance will be made by lay adjudication officers not doctors. The intention is to follow the approach used in many EC countries where simple questionnaires are used which are designed to be user friendly and collect the necessary information as quickly as possible. Many parents will need help in completing a lengthy and quite detailed questionnaire, which is designed to elicit the necessary information, and should help to avoid cases which go to appeal because families have not provided the necessary evidence to back their applications. The adjudicators will call upon doctors and any other relevant professionals for confirmation of diagnosis or to give evidence as required. Applicants will be expected to agree to medical examinations if requested. Medical advice may be sought from the applicant's own medical adviser or from the Benefits Agency Medical Services or the Disability Living Allowance Advisory Board.

Proving eligibility for the DLA

a The care component

To qualify, the need for care must arise from physical or mental disability. The applicant must require care, supervision or watching over from another person because of the disability. Thus the applicant must demonstrate the following needs:

DURING THE DAY

1 Frequent attention throughout the day in connection with bodily functions.
2 Continual supervision throughout the day in order to avoid substantial danger (to the applicant or to others).

AT NIGHT

3 Prolonged or repeated attention in connection with bodily functions.
4 In order to avoid substantial danger to the applicant or others, another person (is required) to be awake for a prolonged period or at frequent intervals.

PART-TIME DAY CARE (a new third level)

5 Help with bodily functions for a significant portion of the day (whether during a single period or a number of periods).
6 The applicant cannot prepare a cooked main meal unaided.

All three levels of need carry different rates. In addition to the above, there is an additional test for children. A child must be shown to have needs which are 'substantially in excess of the normal requirements of persons of his or her age' or if the child has 'substantial' care or supervision needs 'which younger persons in normal physical or mental health may also have but which persons of (his or her age) and in normal physical or mental health would not have'. Parents are likely to need advice from their own medical advisers in responding to these questions, and providing relevant evidence if necessary.

The so-called cooking test mentioned in number 6 above applies to young people of 16 years and over. The onus is on applicants to demonstrate that they can not only cook but prepare a meal. The Disability Rights Handbook 1993 points out that the questions asked in the self-assessment form included in the DLA claim pack clearly mean that this should be a 'traditional, labour intensive and by implication edible main meal, freshly cooked on a traditional cooker', that is to say not a frozen pizza or instant meal removed from freezer to microwave! The same handbook points out that being able to prepare and cook means being able to carry out all of the stages appropriately. If for example the applicant could not lift a hot pan off the cooker; manage to drain cooked vegetables safely from the pan or sequence the cooking process with suitable timings, then he or she should not pass the test. As with the old attendance allowance, it may be helpful to keep a detailed diary over a week to show what difficulties the applicant has and when he or she requires help.

b The mobility component

As with the mobility allowance, to qualify for the higher rate, the applicant must prove that he or she is 'unable to walk' or 'virtually unable to walk'. The applicant must also have a physical disability (although mental handicap or learning disabilities may qualify if there is a physical cause). However there are now new qualifications which should extend eligibility. These new conditions include:

- The fact that exertion in walking would constitute a possible danger to life or would be likely to lead to serious deterioration in health.
- If the applicant has no legs or feet (from birth or amputation). In these circumstances the fact that the applicant can walk with artificial limbs etc. is disregarded.
- If the applicant receives the higher rate care component of DLA and is severely mentally impaired with very disruptive and potentially dangerous behaviour problems.
- If the applicant is deaf and blind. In this case it must be shown that the person concerned 'because of the effects of these conditions in combination with each other (is unable) without the assistance of another person to walk to any intended or required destination while out of doors.'

Importantly these new criteria mean that application is not barred to those who can physically walk, but who could not do so without considerable support from another person. The new lower rate extends this provision by disregarding whether or not the applicant can walk and stating that the individual must be 'so severely disabled physically or mentally that disregarding any ability (he or she) may have to use routes which are familiar ... on their own, (they) cannot take advantage of the faculty out of doors without guidance or supervision from another person for most of the time.'

There is also an extra test for children under 16 years. Children must show that they require substantially more guidance or supervision from another person than would be expected for a child of a similar chronological age. The guidance stresses that applicants must demonstrate that they need extra help whereas other children of the same age 'in normal physical or mental health would not require such guidance or supervision.'

As noted above, the new self-assessment form and the provision of a comprehensive pack (as opposed to a simple leaflet) should enable more families to make successful applications. The introduction of a third tier of financial assistance is also helpful. However many parents will be unclear about how best to present their case and help with the self-assessment forms will be crucial for many potential applicants.

If a child or young person is eligible for the higher rate of the mobility component of DLA, they will probably be eligible for other help as well. *Door to Door* is a useful free guide on all mobility matters and is available from the Department of Transport. Motability is a voluntary organization set up by the government and designed to help people use the higher rate mobility component to purchase or hire a car. There are two schemes available, for either hiring or hire purchase. Under the hire purchase scheme it is possible to obtain an electric wheelchair or a good used car as well as a new vehicle. Further information is available from Motability. It is important to remind parents that they can make an application on behalf of their children.

Recipients of the higher rate of the mobility component have other opportunities to achieve greater mobility and reduce the costs. The Orange Badge scheme allows a car to be parked, without charge or time limit, on parking meters or in streets where waiting would be otherwise limited. Local authorities issue orange badges and may make a small charge. Families going on holiday abroad should remember that orange badge holders have similar advantages in certain countries which make similar parking concessions to their own disabled citizens. Before using an orange badge abroad it is important to get information from either the main motoring organizations or the Department of Transport.

If a car is used 'solely or only for the purpose of the disabled person', and the disabled person receives the higher rate of the mobility component, it should be eligible for exemption from vehicle excise duty. There is currently no precise legal definition of what 'solely or only for the purpose of the disabled person' means. The disabled person does not have to be in the car if it is used to do shopping or perform other errands. However, the use of an exempt car for purposes unrelated to the disabled person is illegal. No one has been prosecuted for infringing this requirement but theoretically prosecution is possible if, for example, a non-disabled person used the car to go to and from work.

It is important to advise parents that they can also claim exemption from vehicle excise duty under the disabled passengers scheme. Applicants must receive the DLA and be under 5 or over 65 years; be unable or virtually unable to walk and need to be driven (i.e. be unable to drive themselves) and be in need of attendance for which they receive the middle or higher rate of the DLA (care component), and have a car registered in their name. A car can easily be registered in a child's name if the exemption is claimed on his or her behalf.

Invalid care allowance

Invalid care allowance (ICA) is a benefit for people of working age who cannot work because they have to care for a severely disabled person. The allowance is not means-tested and does not depend upon payment of national insurance contributions. It is taxable and is therefore affected by any other income which a family receives.

To qualify for ICA, the carer must spend at least 35 hours a week caring for a person who receives the care component of the DLA at the middle or higher rate. Until 1987 married women were excluded unless they were sole supporters of their families. However, this ruling was overturned by the International Court at Strasbourg and men and women are now equally eligible. An added advantage of receiving ICA is that the recipient is credited with a weekly class 1 national insurance contribution credit. Fifty-two credits in a year constitute a 'qualifying year' for retirement pensions (an important consideration now that state pensions are contributory and not automatically available on reaching retirement age). ICA is payable during school holidays (for example when a child comes home from a residential school). Respite care is not usually affected, but parents may need to be reminded that eligibility is based upon a notional 35 hours a week care with permitted time off for holidays and other short periods but not for long periods in any circumstances.

The family fund

The family fund was established by the government, under the administration of the Joseph Rowntree Memorial Trust, to provide financial support for the special needs of families with disabled children under the age of 16 years. The fund aims to bridge the gaps between statutory services and in the provision of equipment which is urgently needed by families.

Parents can approach the fund directly, requesting an application form and stating their needs. They will be visited by one of the family fund social workers (who are appointed on a regional basis), who will be responsible for assessing their need and the degree of disability of the child. Normally receipt of the disability living allowance will be regarded as proof of severe disability, but the fund can be flexible. The range of provision offered is very varied, including washing machines and driers; holidays; furniture and carpets; special clothing; driving lessons and play activities. The fund will not normally finance equipment or services which should be provided by a statutory service. In the light of recent changes in the social security system, it is particularly useful to note that the family fund can provide financial support for visiting a child in hospital.

The family fund is not means tested, but works within guidelines laid down by central government. General social and economic circumstances are therefore sympathetically considered. The fund is increasingly giving support literally from birth, although its original brief was to provide support from the age of 2 years onwards.

Changes in the social security system

The Social Security Act 1986 made major changes to the way in which disabled people and their families can get help with day-to-day living expenses. Supplementary benefit has disappeared and has been replaced with income support. *Income support* is a new means-tested benefit, which is intended to provide a more streamlined approach to helping families who need financial support. People receiving income support will automatically have a passport to other benefits such as housing benefit, free prescriptions and dental treatment, vouchers for spectacles and fares to hospital. However, the much valued Single Payments (which often provided extra help with heating, essential household equipment and clothing and dietary requirements) have disappeared.

Income support is based upon the idea of applicable amounts for each applicant. The applicable amount means the income necessary for an individual or family to live on. The applicable amount is made up of:

1 A personal allowance: the basic scale for a single person or couple.
2 A dependant's allowance: the basic scale rate for each dependent child within a family eligible for income support.
3 Certain housing costs (to be met through housing benefit).

Families with dependent children will receive both a family and a dependent child premium. If the child is disabled, a double premium (to include the disabled child premium) is payable. There is an additional weekly payment for a single parent family. The disability premium is payable for disabled people aged between 16 and 60 years. Receipt of the disability living allowance or severe disablement allowance will be regarded as providing eligibility subject to other conditions for income support being met. A severe disablement premium may be awarded on top of the disability premium.

Family credit is a new social security benefit for working people who are employed or self-employed and have at least one child. It is intended to boost family income in low income families. But early evidence suggests that the application process is so complicated that many families are reluctant to apply. A major government publicity campaign was launched in the spring of 1989 to persuade parents to apply.

One of the most controversial changes has been the introduction of the *social fund*. This fund is intended to replace the old system of grants and exceptional needs payments with, in most cases, a system of interest free loans. The grants are divided into three main categories. *Budgeting loans* are intended to cover essential bedding, furniture, repairs, bottled fuel and removal expenses and similar needs. Money will no longer be available for school uniforms, fuel costs (for example with gas or electricity bills), school meals or tools.

Crisis loans are, as they suggest, for unexpected sudden time of expenditure, in particular for preventing serious risks to the health and safety of the applicant that could occur without the extra help. Loans will normally be expected to be repaid within 18 months, though this can be extended. Repayment rates are usually 15% of the weekly benefit, although in exceptional circumstances the DHSS can lower the repayment to 5%.

Community care grants are not loans to be repaid, and are made either to help keep people in their own homes rather than in hospital, to help them move out of hospital or for families in stress which include those which have broken up so that two homes need to be equipped. To be eligible for a community care grant, the applicant must either receive income support or be within 6 weeks of discharge from a residential setting and be likely to qualify for income support. Community care grants will be important for people with disabilities because they are non-repayable grants. But there is already concern that different DSS offices will interpret eligibility in different ways and that the grant is essentially one off and does not take account of subsequent wear and tear on furnishings and equipment. Additionally it focuses upon people moving into the community and takes no account of the considerable needs of disabled people and carers already living in their own homes.

Because of growing anxiety about disabled people and the loss of the additional payments under the former supplementary benefit system, the Government introduced an independent living fund. This fund, administered by the Disablement Income Group together with the DSS, could make payments for personal and domestic help in order to enable severely disabled people to remain at home. The creation of the independent living fund caused some disagreement in the disability world, with many people seeing it as a very poor substitute for proper income support for disabled people. Others, however, accepted the fund as a concession to the needs of disabled people and as a prelude to a future review of disability allowances, following the publication of the Office of Population and Census Surveys' reports on disability (OPCS, 1989). It was one of the few sources of financial support for additional care costs, apart from charities and was particularly important as disabled people increasingly demanded to be allowed to live in the community with appropriate support and not to spend unnecessary time in institutional care. In 1993, the Government established two new funds to replace the independent living fund. One fund provides support for existing independent living fund users. The other is designed to help a specific group of severely disabled people whose costs for home care will exceed those of residential or nursing care. These funds, like the independent fund, provide for *adult* disabled people, but paediatrician and child health services are likely to find themselves increasingly involved in community care assessments for adult life and will find it useful to be aware of them. The *Disability Rights Handbook* (Disability Alliance, 1994) provides annually updated advice on all disability benefits for children and adults.

Planning for transition to adult life has always been challenging and community child health services will wish to make good use of the new requirement under Part III of the Education Act 1993 to create a *Transition Plan* for young people at their fourteen-plus annual review. Although the LEA takes the lead in convening this annual review (and annual reviews in each of the subsequent years until the young person leaves school), it *must* involve health and social services in assessment and planning and it is hoped that the new requirement will enable more effective and better integrated planning as young people with disabilities move towards adult life. Few local authorities' community care arrangements have yet developed clear and accessible arrangements for *young* adults with disabilities or special health care needs and the 1993 Education Act (with an associated statutory Code of Practice which lays duties on health as well as education and social services) provides an important opportunity for joint assessment and for care planning.

Housing benefit is a means-tested benefit paid by local councils to help people who need help to pay their rent. Housing benefit may also be claimed to cover the costs of hostel, guest-house, hotel or similar accommodation and can help with mortgage interest repayments provided that the applicant also gets income support. The level of housing benefit is calculated on any earnings, any unearned income and savings, but the calculation also takes into account a personal allowance, a dependant's allowance (if the claimant has a child or other person living with him or her) and certain premiums for special needs (for example for disability, caring for children or old age). Housing benefit is awarded for limited periods which are set by the council. These are known as benefit periods. A fresh claim has to be made at the end of each benefit period. Students should note that special rules apply to their applications. Housing benefit (subject to all the conditions being met) can cover *all* of the rent and council tax, but all tenants have to pay rates for water and other benefits. As noted above, housing benefit may also cover interest repayments on mortgages (although there are now limits on the levels of repayment which will be accepted). But it should be noted that mortgage interest repayments will only be paid if the claimant is receiving income support. Further information is provided in DSS leaflet RR1, *Housing Benefit – Help with Your Rent* or Leaflet FB 28, *Sick or Disabled? A Guide to Benefits if You're Sick or Disabled for a Few Days or More.* Both leaflets are available from DSS offices, citizens advice bureaux or the local council.

Charges for residential care

Residential care in a hospital or NHS nursing home is free of charge (although certain benefits and allowances may be discontinued if the person concerned is in hospital for a period of time). Residential schools are usually fully covered by the local education authority (LEA), although in some instances social services may pay for the care element. If a child is in a residential home paid for by the social services department, parents may be asked to make a contribution on a means-tested basis. Charging policies vary according to the local authority in question and many local authorities do not ask for parental contributions when a child is disabled. Young adults living away from home in a residential setting formerly received an allowance from social security which was usually 'topped up' by the local authority of the young person's place of origin to cover the total costs. Since the implementation of the NHS and Community Care Act only those with 'residual protection' (i.e. who were receiving a social security allowance for residential care prior to implementation) continue to receive the social security allowance. Local authorities now receive what is intended to be the equivalent of the social security monies for residential and other forms of community care and must make community care plans and individual assessment and care manage-

ment arrangements for those needing community care. Young people and their advisers must therefore now look to the local authority rather than the social security system for support. There may be wide local variations as to what a local authority can or will pay for young people living away from home. However, if a local authority social services department assesses an individual as needing a particular service under the community care arrangements, the authority *must* provide the service and cannot claim expense as a reason for not meeting the specified need. It is therefore extremely important that young people with disabilities have assessments for their community care needs and that these clearly state what is needed and what will be provided. Local authorities may expect a disabled person to contribute to the costs of a service if he or she has sufficient resources. Community care guidance notes that parents or relatives may choose a more expensive home or service than is specified in a community care assessment and may 'top up' fees to enable a relative to live in particular provision.

Self-help: the changing role of parent organizations

The voluntary sector has always been a rich and creative resource for consumer groups in the UK. The major national voluntary organizations like Mencap and the Spastics Society have always played an important advisory role for parents of children with special needs. An emerging trend in the 1980s has been that of coalition groups (for instance Parents in Partnership, KIDS, Contact a Family and Action 81) which are non-denominational in terms of specific disabilities and which work with parents of all children with a range of special needs.

There are probably over 1000 local and national voluntary organizations in the UK concerned with disability. A list of the major *national* organizations is given at the end of this chapter. Most have local groups and increasingly collaborate with other organizations in the wider voluntary sector. Apart from providing personal support for parents, they offer a range of practical services ranging from loans of equipment and holiday playschemes to residential or education services. All provide information and most counselling and advice.

In practice, changes in official policy and legislation have been insufficiently utilized to promote partnership with parents through the use of parent groups. Part III of the 1993 Education Act requires health authorities to notify parents of any voluntary organizations likely to be able to help them. In practice, as a survey from the National Deaf Children's Society found in 1987,[21] few make such referrals. Although health authorities and social services departments have used joint finance money (often with voluntary organizations) to support parent-led activities, there has been too little participation by education authorities. However, there have been some notable exceptions. The three South Wales education departments have collaborated with the Spastics Society, Mencap in Wales and the Wales Council for the Disabled to establish SNAP (the Special Needs Advisory Project) which has clearly demonstrated the effectiveness of recruiting, training and supporting parents and other volunteers as parent advisers and advocates during assessment. The Elfrida Rathbone Parent Advisory Project in Camden similarly showed the need for many parents to have independent advice and counselling during assessment.[22]

One important asset in any parent organization is the ability to listen. An evaluation of a parent-adviser scheme at the London Hospital[3] has shown that many of the most vulnerable parents benefit from sensitive counselling and listening, even without explicit professional advice. In effect empowerment and partnership, however defined, are unlikely to be effective without time, continuity and an awareness of the multifaceted nature of family life, where special needs may be only one of a cluster of problems affecting parents at any one time. It is important to remember the great variety of parent organizations. Small neighbourhood groups offer local friendships and support. Major national voluntary organizations have local groups, but they also offer a range of services and information on current policy and practice. Some parents may wish to use three or four in different ways at the same time. For example a parent of a child with Down syndrome may use a local pre-school playgroup run by the Pre-school Playgroups Association, borrow toys from a local toy library, belong to the Down's Children's Association and Mencap to keep in touch with national developments and advice, and also regularly attend a Contact a Family local group. Each organization offers special support and will augment statutory services in a number of ways.

The OPCS Report[1] showed that only 38% of parents interviewed had ever heard of a voluntary organization. As only 12% of parents regularly saw a social worker, the number is perhaps not surprising. But referral to parent organizations right from the start will be a major step towards making sure that families know of all available services. Sixty-three per cent of the OPCS families had never heard of respite care. A mere 4% used it. It is hard to believe that wider family needs would not have been better met if the families concerned had been introduced to local and national voluntary agencies from the first diagnosis.

An evaluation of Contact a Family's parent groups in Wandsworth[23] clearly found that participants were more confident and optimistic. They were more likely to make good use of all available services and they felt able to negotiate on their own behalf with professionals. Many parent groups will offer practical advice as well as ongoing support. They all offer solidarity and friendship when families feel at their most vulnerable.

An individualized family service plan?

One way of ensuring that parents do know all about relevant sources of help, and are given appropriate advice about which of the often confusing melange of support systems to use, is the US concept of the individualized family service plan (IFSP). The IFSP was introduced as Public Law 99-457 to replace the individual education programme (IEP) for children between birth and 3 years of age. As the plan's name indicates, it addresses both the needs for the child and the needs of the family. The concept of a family plan is based on an acknowledgement, sadly often lacking in special needs services, that a balance needs to be struck between the best interests of the child, parents, siblings and the ability and desirability of parents to play a role as educators, care-takers or indeed their right to be ordinary parents.

The concept of a family plan also makes it easier to acknowledge cultural and other differences in child-rearing practices and to ensure that practical problems like money, housing and equipment can be resolved quickly and efficiently. Hopefully family plans will also avoid families being offered excessive numbers of professional advisers often with apparently conflicting advice. They should also (a) avoid inappropriate pathological perceptions of families with a special needs child as handicapped families, and (b) promote the recognition that all families are different in composition, needs, cultural heritage, past experiences and life stages. The philosophy behind such a family plan, which may gain legal recognition through the redefinition of children in need in the Children Act, is encapsulated in Peter Mittler's[24] citation of key factors for achieving the elusive and much-pursued partnership with parents; namely that:

1 Growth and learning can only be understood in children in relation to the various environments within which the children are living.
2 Parents and professionals concerned about a child with special needs share a number of common goals.
3 Parents and the extended family are the most accessible adults when helping a child.
4 Parents and professionals each have essential information which needs to be shared among all who are concerned with the child's development.

Looking to the 1990s, we have many of the successful ingredients for such partnership, but parity of esteem between parents, their professional advisers and the voluntary sector will only be achieved by continuous vigilance. In both the USA and the UK we have education legislation which has begun to bridge the gap between child, educators, family and community. No one group is subordinate to another and all of us must accept the challenge of being equal partners with differing strengths, addressing the shared task of education and growth of children and support for their families. In effect family life and a child's individual needs will best be strengthened if we remember that 'the most important thing that happens when a child with disabilities or special needs arrives in a family is that a child is born. The most important thing that happens when a couple become parents of a child with disabilities or special needs is that the couple have become parents.'[25,26] Hence even the most specialist services need to become ordinary and the ordinary special. They will also need to be appropriate to the major social and demographic changes and to recognize that shared information is a major first step to helping families.

List of useful organizations

Action for Sick Children
Argyle House
29–31 Euston Road
London NW1 2SD
Tel: 0171 833 2041

Action Research for the Crippled Child
Vincent House, North Parade
Horsham
West Sussex RH12 2DA
Tel: 01403 64101

Advisory Centre for Education
18 Aberdeen Studios
22 Highbury Grove
London N5 2EA
Tel: 0171 354 8318

Arthritis Care
18 Stephenson Way
London NW1 2HD
Tel: 0171 916 1500

AFASIC
347 Central Markets
Smithfield
London EC1A 9NH
Tel: 0171 236 3632/6487

Association for the Education and Welfare of the Visually Handicapped
24 Vicarage Road
Harborne
Birmingham B17 0SP
Tel: 0121 426 6815

Association for Spina Bifida and Hydrocephalus
Ashbah House
42 Park Road
Peterborough PE1 2UQ
Tel: 01733 555988

Association of Parents of Vaccine Damaged Children
2 Church Street
Shipston-on-Stour
Warwickshire CV46 4AP
Tel: 016086 61595

Association to Combat Huntingdon's Disease
108 Battersea High Street
London SW11 3HP
Tel: 0171 223 7000

Bobath Centre for Physically Handicapped Children
5 Netherhall Gardens
London NW3 5RN
Tel: 0171 794 6084

British Diabetic Association
10 Queen Anne Street
London W1M 0BD
Tel: 0171 323 1531

British Dyslexia Association
98 London Road
Reading
Berkshire RG1 5AU
Tel: 01734 688271

British Epilepsy Association
Anstey House
40 Hanover Square
Leeds LS3 1BE
Tel: 01132 439393

British Heart Foundation
14 Fitzhardinge Street
London W1H 4DH
Tel: 0171 935 0185

British Institute of Learning Disabilities
Wolverhampton Road
Kidderminster
Worcestershire DY10 3PP
Tel: 01562 850251

British Kidney Patient Association
Bordon
Hants GU35 9JZ
Tel: 01420 472021

British Polio Fellowship
Bell Close
West End Road
Ruislip
Middlesex HA4 6PL
Tel: 01895 675515

British Red Cross Society
9 Grosvenor Crescent
London SW1X 7EJ
Tel: 0171 235 5454

British Sports Association for the Disabled
Haward House
Barnard Crescent
Aylesbury
Bucks HP21 8PP
Tel: 01296 27889

British Bone Society
Ward 8
Strathmartine Hospital
Strathmartine,
Dundee DD3 0PG
Tel: 01382 817771

Centre on Environment for the Handicapped
Nutmeg House
60 Gainsford Street
London SE1 2NY
Tel: 0171 357 8182

Chest, Heart and Stroke Association
CHSA House
123-127 Whitecross Street
London EC1Y 8JJ
Tel: 0171 490 7999

Child Poverty Action Group
1 Bath Street
London EC1V 9PY
Tel: 0171 253 3406

Children's Legal Centre
20 Compton Terrace
London N1 2UN
Tel: 0171 359 0302

College of Speech Therapists
7 Bath Place
Rivington Street
London EC2A 3DR
Tel: 0171 613 3855

Colostomy Welfare Group
15 Station Road
Reading RG1 1LG
Tel: 01734 391537

Compassionate Friends
53 North Street
Bristol BS3 1EN
Tel: 01179 539639

Contact a Family
170 Tottenham Court Road
London W1P 0HA
Tel: 0171 383 3555

Council for Disabled Children
8 Wakley Street
London EC1 7QE
Tel: 0171 843 6061

Cystic Fibrosis Research Trust
5 Blyth Road
Bromley
Kent BR1 3RS
Tel: 0181 464 7211

Department of Transport
2 Marsham Street
London SW1

Disability Alliance
1st Floor East
Universal House
88-94 Wentworth Street
London E1 7SA
Tel: 0171 247 8763

Disabled Drivers Association
Ashwelthorpe Hall
Ashwelthorpe
Norwich
Tel: 0150841 449

Disablement Income Group
Unit 5
Archway Business Centre
19-23 Wedmore Street
London N19 4RZ
Tel: 0171 790 2424

Disabled Living Foundation
380–384 Harrow Road
London W9 2HU
Tel: 0181 289 6111

Down's Syndrome Association
155 Mitcham Road
London SW17 9PG
Tel: 0181 682 4001

ENABLE
6th Floor
7 Buchanan Street
Glasgow G1 3HL
Tel: 0141 226 4541

Family Fund Beverley House
PO Box 50
York YO3 2ZX
Tel: 01904 621115

Friedreich's Ataxia Group
Cranleigh Works
The Common
Cranleigh
Surrey GU6 8SB
Tel: 01483 272741

Greater London Association for the Disabled
336 Brixton Road
London SW9
Tel: 0171 274 0107

Haemophilia Society
123 Westminster Bridge Road
London SE1 7HR
Tel: 0171 928 2020

Handicapped Adventure Playground Association
Fulham Palace Playground
Bishops Avenue
London SW6 6AE
Tel: 0171 736 4443

Hyperactive Children's Support Group
71 Whyke Lane
Chichester
West Sussex
PO19 2LD
Tel: 01903 725182

Ileostomy Association of Great Britain and N. Ireland
Amblehurst House
Black Scotch Lane
Mansfield
Notts NG18 4PF
Tel: 01623 28099

Invalid Children's Aid Association
10 Bowling Green Lane
London EC1R 0BD
Tel: 0171 253 9111

John Groom's Association for the Disabled
10 Gloucester Drive
London N4 2LP
Tel: 0181 802 7272

Joint Committee on Mobility for the Disabled
Woodcliff House
51A Cliff Road
Weston-Super-Mare
Avon BS22 9SE
Tel: 01934 642313

KIDS
80 Waynflete Square
London W10 6UD
Tel: 0181 969 2817

Kith and Kids
404 Camden Road
Islington
London N7 05J
Tel: 0171 700 2755

Lady Hoare Trust for Physically Disabled Children
4th Floor
Mitre House
44-46 Fleet Street
London EC4Y 1BN
Tel: 0171 583 1951

Leukaemia Care Society
PO Box 82
Exeter
Devon EX2 5DP
Tel: 01392 218514

Medic Alert Foundation
12 Bridge Wharf
156 Caledonian Road
London N1 9UU
Tel: 0171 833 3034

MENCAP
117-123 Golden Lane
London EC1Y 0RT
Tel: 0171 454 0454

MIND
(National Association for Mental Health)
22 Harley Street
London W1N 2ED
Tel: 0171 637 0741

Motability
The Gate House
West Gate, The High
Harlow
Essex CM10 1HR
Tel: 01279 635666

Multiple Sclerosis Society
25 Effie Road
London SW6 1EE
Tel: 0171 736 6267

Muscular Dystrophy Group of Great Britain
7-11 Prescott Place
London SW4 6BS
Tel: 0171 720 8055

National Association for Deaf/Blind and Rubella
Handicapped (SENSE)
11-13 Clifton Terrace
Finsbury Park
London N4 3SR
Tel: 0171 272 7774

National Association of Swimming Clubs for the
Handicapped
The Willows
Mayles Lane
Wickham
Hants PO17 5ND
Tel: 01329 833689

National Autistic Society
276 Willesden Lane
London NW2 5RB
Tel: 0181 451 1114

National Children's Bureau
8 Wakley Street
London EC1V 7QE
Tel: 0171 843 6000

National Council for Voluntary Organizations
Regents Wharf
8 All Saints Street
London N1 9RL
Tel: 0171 713 6161

National Deaf Children's Society
45 Hereford Road
London W2 5AH
Tel: 0171 229 1891

National Eczema Society
6 Tavistock Place
London WC1H 9RA
Tel: 0171 388 9433

National Federation of Gateway Clubs
117 Golden Lane
London EC1Y 0RT
Tel: 0171 253 9433

National Listening Library
12 Lant Street
London SE1
Tel: 0171 407 9417

National Playing Fields Association
25 Ovington Square
London SW3 1LQ
Tel: 0171 584 6445

Partially Sighted Society
Queens Road
Doncaster
S. Yorks DN1 2NX
Tel: 01302 323132

Physically Handicapped and Able Bodied
(PHAB)
14 London Road
Croydon CR0 2TA
Tel: 0181 667 9443

Pre-School Playgroups Association
61–63 Kings Cross Road
London WX1X 9LL
Tel: 0171 833 0991

Queen Elizabeth's Foundation for the Disabled
Leatherhead Court
Leatherhead
Surrey KT22 0BN
Tel: 0137284 2204

Riding for the Disabled Association
Avenue R
National Agricultural Centre
Kenilworth
Warwickshire CV8 2LY
Tel: 01203 696510

Royal Association for Disability and Rehabilitation
12 City Forum
250 City Road
London EC1V 8AF
Tel: 0171 250 3222

Royal National Institute for the Blind
224 Great Portland Street
London W1N 6AA
Tel: 0171 388 1266

Royal National Institute for the Deaf
105 Gower Street
London WC1E 6AH
Tel: 0171 387 8033

Royal Society for the Prevention of Accidents
Canon House
Priory Queensway
Birmingham B4 6BS
Tel: 0121 200 2461

Scope
12 Park Crescent
London W1N 4EQ
Tel: 0171 636 5020

Scottish Council for Spastics
Wallace Court
191 Main Road
Elderslie
Paisley PA5 9ES
Tel: 01505 331804

Scottish Council on Disability Information Department
Princes House
5 Shadwick Place
Edinburgh EH2 4RG
Tel: 0131 229 8632

Scottish Society for the Mentally Handicapped
13 Elmbank Street
Glasgow G2 4PB
Tel: 0141 226 4541

Scottish Spina Bifida Association
190 Queensferry Road
Edinburgh EH4 2BW
Tel: 0131 332 0743

SEQUAL
(Special Equipment and Aids for Living)
Ddol Hir
Glyn Seirog
Llangollen LL20 7NP
Tel: 01691 72331

Shaftesbury Society
18-20 Kingston Road
London SW19 1JZ
Tel: 0181 956 6634

SKILL
(National Bureau for Handicapped Students)
336 Brixton Road
London SW9 7AA
Tel: 0171 274 0565

Spinal Injuries Association
Newpoint House
76 St James Lane
London N10 3DF
Tel: 0181 444 2121

References

1 Office of Population Censuses and Surveys. *Report 6, Disabled Children: Services, Transport and Education.* London: HMSO, 1989.
2 Cunningham, C., Davis, H. Early parent counselling. In: Craft, M., Bicknell, J., Hollins, S., eds. *Mental Handicap a Multidisciplinary Approach.* London: Bailliere Tindall, 1985.
3 Cunningham, C., Davis, H. *Working with Parents; Frameworks for Collaboration.* Milton Keynes: Open University Press, 1985.
4 Hewett, S. *Handicapped Children and their Families, a Survey.* Nottingham University Child Development Research Unit; 1970.
5 Glendinning, C. *Unshared Care – Parents and their Disabled Children.* London: Routledge & Kegan Paul, 1983.
6 Wilkin, D. *Caring for the Mentally Handicapped Child.* London: Croom Helm, 1979.
7 Baldwin, S. *The Costs of Caring.* London: Routledge & Kegan Paul, 1985.
8 Cooke, K., Bradshaw, J. Child disablement, family dissolution and reconstitution. *Dev Med Child Neurol* 1986; **28**: 610–616.
9 Wolkind, S. Depression in mothers of young children. *Arch Dis Child* 1981; **56**: 1–3.
10 Russell, P. *The Wheelchair Child.* London: Souvenir Press, 1989.
11 Russell, P., Griffiths, M. *Working Together with Handicapped Children.* London: Souvenir Press, 1985.
12 DHSS Social Services Inspectorate (NW Division). *Care for a Change?* London: HMSO, 1988.
13 Oswin, M. *They Keep Going Away.* Oxford: Blackwells/King's Fund Centre, 1983.
14 Oswin, M. *The Empty House.* London: Penguin, 1971.
15 Factsheet of family based respite care. London: NCB, 1991.
16 Robinson, C. *Avon Short Term Respite Care Scheme: Evaluation Study.* Department of Mental Health, University of Bristol, 1986.
17 Brimblecombe, F., Russell, P. *Honeylands: Developing a Service for Families with Handicapped Children.* London: National Children's Bureau, 1987.
18 Banks, S., Grizzell, R. *A Study of Family Placement Schemes for the Shared Care of Handicapped Children in Norfolk and Oxfordshire.* DHSS Social Services Inspectorate. London: HMSO, 1984.
19 Pahl, J., Quine, E. *Families with Mentally Handicapped Children: a Study of Stress and a Service Response.* Health Services Research Unit, University of Kent, 1984.
20 Office of Population Censuses and Surveys. *Report 5, The Financial Circumstances of Families with Disabled Children Living in Private Households.* London: HMSO, 1989.
21 Implementation of Section 10 of the 1981 Education Act: a survey. London: National Deaf Children's Society, 1987.
22 Nelson, J., Mair, S. *The Maze: Parents Experience of the Assessment Procedure Established by the 1981 Education Act.* London: Elfrida Rathbone, 1990.
23 Hatch, S., Hinton, T. *Self Help in Practice: a Study of Contact a Family in Wandsworth.* London: Community Care/Social Work Monographs, 1987.
24 Mittler, P. Family supports in England. In: Lipsky, D., ed. *Family Supports with Disabled Member.* New York: World Rehabilitation Fund, 1987.
25 Lipsky, D., Gartner, A. *Beyond Separate Education: Quality Education for All.* Baltimore: Brookes Publishing Co, 1989.
26 Ferguson, P., Asch, A. Lessons from life: personal and parental perspectives on schooling, childhood and disabilities. In: Ferguson, D., ed. *School and Disability.* Chicago: National Society For Education, 1989.

Appendix

UK immunization schedule

Vaccine		Age	Notes
D/T/P and polio Hib	1st dose 2nd dose 3rd dose	2 months ⎫ 3 months ⎬ [1] 4 months ⎭	Primary Course
Measles/mumps/ rubella (MMR)		12-18 months	Can be given at any age over 12 months
Booster D/T and polio, MMR (if not previously given)		4-5 years	
Rubella		10-14 years	GIRLS ONLY
BCG		10-14 years or infancy	Interval of 3 weeks between BCG and rubella
*Booster tetanus and polio		15-18 years	

*From October 1994 combined tetanus toxoid and low dose diphtheria toxoid (Td)
will replace the booster dose of tetanus toxoid.

Index